Dietary Reference Intakes: Recommended levels for individual intake[a]

Life-Stage Group	Calcium (mg/d)	Phosphorus (mg/d)	Magnesium (mg/d)	Vitamin D[b,c] (μg/d)	Fluoride (mg/d)	Thiamin (mg/d)	Riboflavin (mg/d)	Niacin[d] (mg/d)	Vitamin B-6 (mg/d)	Folate[e] (μg/d)	Vitamin B-12 (μg/d)	Pantothenic Acid (mg/d)	Biotin (μg/d)	Choline[f] (mg/d)
Infants														
0–6 mo	210*	100*	30*	5*	0.01*	0.2*	0.3*	2*	0.1*	65*	0.4*	1.7*	5*	125*
7–12 mo	270*	275*	75*	5*	0.5*	0.3*	0.4*	4*	0.3*	80*	0.5*	1.8*	6*	150*
Children														
1–3 y	500*	**460**	**80**	5*	0.7*	**0.5**	**0.5**	**6**	**0.5**	**150**	**0.9**	2*	8*	200*
4–8 y	800*	**500**	**130**	5*	1.1	**0.6**	**0.6**	**8**	**0.6**	**200**	**1.2**	3*	12*	250*
Males														
9–13 y	1,300*	**1,250**	**240**	5*	2.0	**0.9**	**0.9**	**12**	**1.0**	**300**	**1.8**	4*	20*	375*
14–18 y	1,300*	**1,250**	**410**	5*	3.2	**1.2**	**1.3**	**16**	**1.3**	**400**	**2.4**	5*	25*	550*
19–30 y	1,000*	**700**	**400**	5*	3.8	**1.2**	**1.3**	**16**	**1.3**	**400**	**2.4**	5*	30*	550*
31–50 y	1,000*	**700**	**420**	5*	3.8	**1.2**	**1.3**	**16**	**1.3**	**400**	**2.4**	5*	30*	550*
51–70 y	1,200*	**700**	**420**	10*	3.8	**1.2**	**1.3**	**16**	**1.7**	**400**	**2.4**[g]	5*	30*	550*
> 70 y	1,200*	**700**	**420**	15*	3.8	**1.2**	**1.3**	**16**	**1.7**	**400**	**2.4**[g]	5*	30*	550*
Females														
9–13 y	1,300*	**1,250**	**240**	5*	2.0	**0.9**	**0.9**	**12**	**1.0**	**300**	**1.8**	4*	20*	375*
14–18 y	1,300*	**1,250**	**360**	5*	2.9	**1.0**	**1.0**	**14**	**1.2**	**400**[h]	**2.4**	5*	25*	400*
19–30 y	1,000*	**700**	**310**	5*	3.1	**1.1**	**1.1**	**14**	**1.3**	**400**[h]	**2.4**	5*	30*	425*
31–50 y	1,000*	**700**	**320**	5*	3.1	**1.1**	**1.1**	**14**	**1.3**	**400**[h]	**2.4**	5*	30*	425*
51–70 y	1,200*	**700**	**320**	10*	3.1	**1.1**	**1.1**	**14**	**1.5**	**400**	**2.4**[g]	5*	30*	425*
> 70 y	1,200*	**700**	**320**	15*	3.1	**1.1**	**1.1**	**14**	**1.5**	**400**	**2.4**[g]	5*	30*	425*
Pregnancy														
≤ 18 y	1,300*	**1,250**	**400**	5*	2.9	**1.4**	**1.4**	**18**	**1.9**	**600**[i]	**2.6**	6*	30*	450*
19–30 y	1,000*	**700**	**350**	5*	3.1	**1.4**	**1.4**	**18**	**1.9**	**600**[i]	**2.6**	6*	30*	450*
31–50 y	1,000*	**700**	**360**	5*	3.1	**1.4**	**1.4**	**18**	**1.9**	**600**[i]	**2.6**	6*	30*	450*
Lactation														
≤18 y	1,300*	**1,250**	**360**	5*	2.9	**1.5**	**1.6**	**17**	**2.0**	**500**	**2.8**	7*	35*	550*
19–30 y	1,000*	**700**	**310**	5*	3.1	**1.5**	**1.6**	**17**	**2.0**	**500**	**2.8**	7*	35*	550*
31–50 y	1,000*	**700**	**320**	5*	3.1	**1.5**	**1.6**	**17**	**2.0**	**500**	**2.8**	7*	35*	550*

[a] Recommended Dietary Allowances (RDAs) are presented in bold type and Adequate Intakes (AIs) in ordinary type followed by an asterisk (*). RDAs and AIs may both be used as goals for individual intake. RDAs are set to meet the needs of almost all (97% to 98%) individuals in a group. For healthy breast-fed infants, the AI is the mean intake. The AI for other life-stage and gender groups is believed to cover needs of all individuals in the group, but lack of data or uncertainty in the data prevents being able to specify with confidence the percentage of persons covered by this intake. *Source:* The National Academy of Sciences. © 1998.

[b] As cholecalciferol, 1 μg cholecalciferol = 40 IU vitamin D.

[c] In the absence of adequate exposure to sunlight.

[d] As niacin equivalents (NE). 1 mg niacin = 60 mg tryptophan; 0 to 6 mo = preformed niacin (not NE).

[e] As dietary folate equivalent (DFE). 1 DFE = 1 μg food folate = 0.6 μg folic acid (from fortified food or supplement) consumed with food = 0.5 μg synthetic (supplemental) folic acid taken on an empty stomach.

[f] Although AIs have been set for choline, there are few data to assess whether a dietary supply of choline is needed at all stages of the life cycle, and it may be that the choline requirement can be met by endogenous synthesis at some of these stages.

[g] Because 10% to 30% of older people may malabsorb food-bound vitamin B-12, it is advisable for those older than 50 years to meet their RDA mainly by consuming foods fortified with vitamin B-12 or a supplement containing vitamin B-12.

[h] In view of evidence linking folate intake with neural tube defects in the fetus, it is recommended that all women capable of becoming pregnant consume 400 μg synthetic folic acid from fortified foods and/or supplements in addition to intake of food folate from a varied diet.

[i] It is assumed that women will continue consuming 400 μg folic acid until their pregnancy is confirmed and they enter prenatal care, which ordinarily occurs after the end of the periconceptional period—the critical time for formation of the neural tube.

Source: Yates, A. A., Schlicker, S. A., and Suitor, C. Dietary Reference Intakes: The new basis for recommendations for calcium and related nutrients, B-vitamins, and choline. J. Am. Diet. Assoc. 98:699–706, 1998.

Recommended Dietary Allowances,[a] Revised 1989

Designed for the maintenance of good nutrition of practically all healthy people in the United States[b]

Category	Age (years) or Condition	Protein (g)	Vitamin A (μg RE)	Vitamin E (mg α-TE)	Vitamin K (μg)	Vitamin C (mg)	Iron (mg)	Zinc (mg)	Iodine (μg)	Selenium (μg)
Infants	0.0–0.5	13	375	3	5	30	6	5	40	10
	0.5–1.0	14	375	4	10	35	10	5	50	15
Children	1–3	16	400	6	15	40	10	10	70	20
	4–6	24	500	7	20	45	10	10	90	20
	7–10	28	700	7	30	45	10	10	120	30
Males	11–14	45	1,000	10	45	50	12	15	150	40
	15–18	59	1,000	10	65	60	12	15	150	50
	19–24	58	1,000	10	70	60	10	15	150	70
	25–50	63	1,000	10	80	60	10	15	150	70
	51+	63	1,000	10	80	60	10	15	150	70
Females	11–14	46	800	8	45	50	15	12	150	45
	15–18	44	800	8	55	60	15	12	150	50
	19–24	46	800	8	60	60	15	12	150	55
	25–50	50	800	8	65	60	15	12	150	55
	51+	50	800	8	65	60	10	12	150	55
Pregnant		60	800	10	65	70	30	15	175	65
Lactating	1st 6 months	65	1,300	12	65	95	15	19	200	75
	2nd 6 months	62	1,200	11	65	90	15	16	200	75

[a]The allowances, expressed as average daily intakes over time, are intended to provide for individual variations among most normal persons as they live in the United States under usual environmental stresses. Diets should be based on a variety of common foods in order to provide other nutrients for which human requirements have been less well defined.

[b]Weights and heights of Reference Adults are actual medians for the U.S. population of the designated age, as reported by NHANES II. The median weights and heights of those under 19 years of age were taken from Hamill et al. (1979). The use of these figures does not imply that the height-to-weight ratios are ideal.

Median Heights and Weights and Recommended Energy Intake From the RDA

Category	Age (years) or Condition	Weight (kg)	Weight (lb)	Height (cm)	Height (in)	REE[a] (kcal/day)	Average Energy Allowance (kcal)[b]: Multiples of REE	Per kg	Per day[c]
Infants	0.0–0.5	6	13	60	24	320		108	650
	0.5–1.0	9	20	71	28	500		98	850
Children	1–3	13	29	90	35	740		102	1,300
	4–6	20	44	112	44	950		90	1,800
	7–10	28	62	132	52	1,130		70	2,000
Males	11–14	45	99	157	62	1,440	1.70	55	2,500
	15–18	66	145	176	69	1,760	1.67	45	3,000
	19–24	72	160	177	70	1,780	1.67	40	2,900
	25–50	79	174	176	70	1,800	1.60	37	2,900
	51+	77	170	173	68	1,530	1.50	30	2,300
Females	11–14	46	101	157	62	1,310	1.67	47	2,200
	15–18	55	120	163	64	1,370	1.60	40	2,200
	19–24	58	128	164	65	1,350	1.60	38	2,200
	25–50	63	138	163	64	1,380	1.55	36	2,200
	51+	65	143	160	63	1,280	1.50	30	1,900
Pregnant	1st trimester								+0
	2nd trimester								+300
	3rd trimester								+300
Lactating	1st 6 months								+500
	2nd 6 months								+500

[a]Calculation based on FAO equations, then rounded.

[b]In the range of light to moderate activity the coefficient of variations is ±20%.

[c]Figure is rounded.

Tolerable Upper Intake Levels[a] (ULs) for Certain Nutrients

Life-Stage Group	Calcium (g/d)	Phosphorus (g/d)	Magnesium[b] (mg/d)	Vitamin D (μg/d)	Fluoride (mg/d)	Niacin[c] (mg/d)	Vitamin B-6 (mg/d)	Synthetic Folic Acid[c] (μg/d)	Choline (g/d)
0–6 mo	ND[d]	ND	ND	25	0.7	ND	ND	ND	ND
7–12 mo	ND	ND	ND	25	0.9	ND	ND	ND	ND
1–3 y	2.5	3	65	50	1.3	10	30	300	1.0
4–8 y	2.5	3	110	50	2.2	15	40	400	1.0
9–13 y	2.5	4	350	50	10	20	60	600	2.0
14–18 y	2.5	4	350	50	10	30	80	800	3.0
19–70 y	2.5	4	350	50	10	35	100	1,000	3.5
>70 y	2.5	3	350	50	10	35	100	1,000	3.5
Pregnancy									
≤18 y	2.5	3.5	350	50	10	30	80	800	3.0
19–50 y	2.5	3.5	350	50	10	35	100	1,000	3.5
Lactation									
≤18 y	2.5	4	350	50	10	30	80	800	3.0
19–50 y	2.5	4	350	50	10	35	100	1,000	3.5

[a] UL = the maximum level of daily nutrient intake that is likely to pose no risk of adverse effects. Unless otherwise specified, the UL represents total intake from food, water, and supplements. Due to lack of suitable data, ULs could not be established for thiamin, riboflavin, vitamin B-12, pantothenic acid, or biotin. In the absence of ULs, extra caution may be warranted in consuming levels above recommended intakes.
[b] The UL for magnesium represents intake from a pharmacological agent only and does not include intake from food and water.
[c] The ULs for niacin and synthetic folic acid apply to forms obtained from supplements, fortified foods, or a combination of the two.
[d] ND: Not determinable due to lack of data of adverse effects in this age group and concern with regard to lack of ability to handle excess amounts. Source of intake should be from food only to prevent high levels of intake.

Source: Yates A. A., Schlicker, S. A., and Suitor, C. W. Dietary Reference Intakes: The new basis for recommendations for calcium and related nutrients, B vitamins, and choline. J. Am. Diet. Assoc. 98:699–706, 1998.

Cover Photo Credit:Charles D. Winters
Frontispiece: © Linda Burgess/Tony Stone Images
Part Opening Photo Credits:
Part Opener I: © Christel Rosenfeld/Tony Stone Images
Part Opener II: © Vadim Sokolov/Picture Perfect
Part Opener III: © John Gajda/FPG International
Part Opener IV: © Guy Marche/FPG International
Part Opener V: © Charles Sleicher/Tony Stone Images

Nutrition: Science and Applications, Third Edition
ISBN: 0-470-002034
Library of Congress Catalog Card Number: 99-62661

Printed in the United States of America

10 9 8 7 6 5

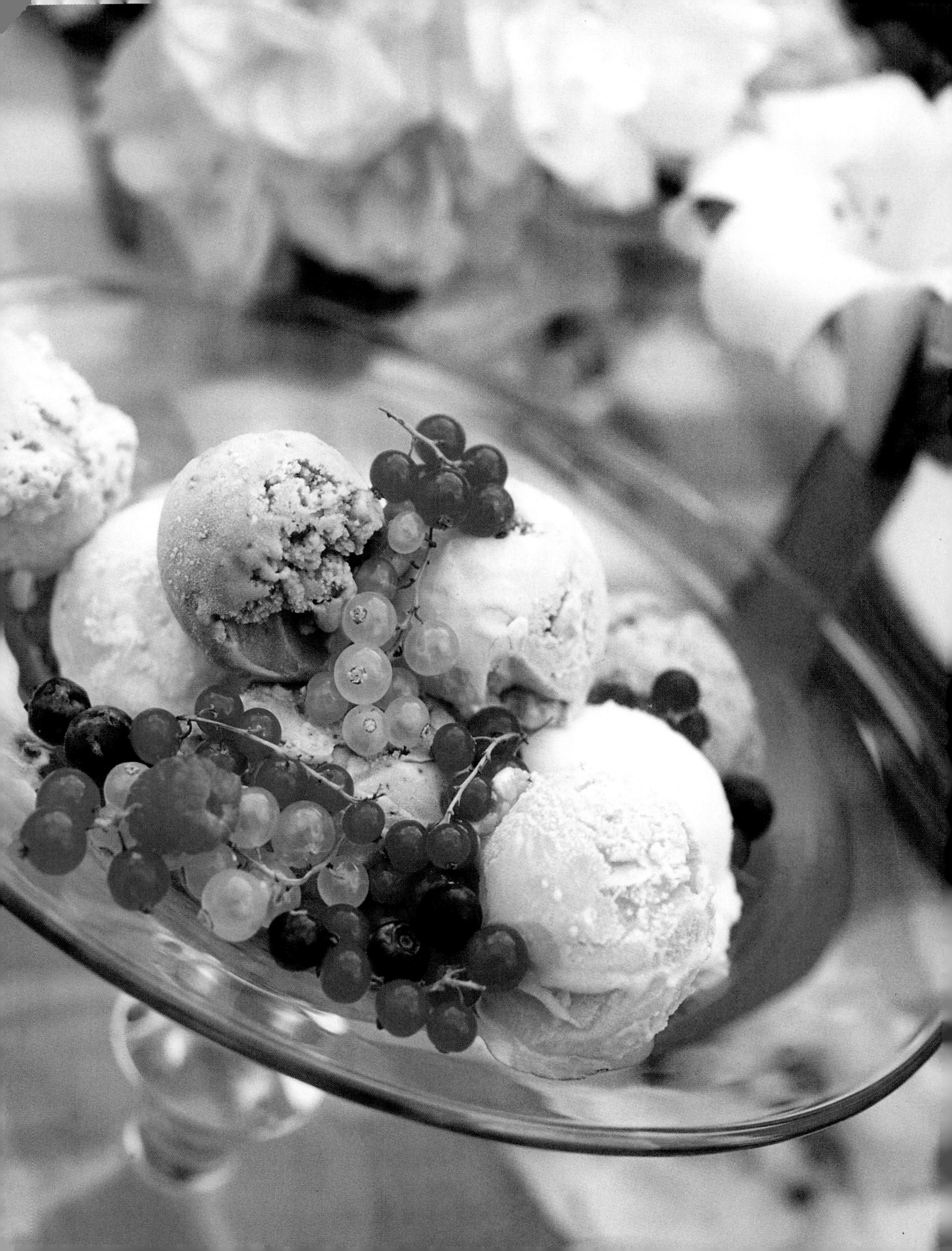

Nutrition

SCIENCE & APPLICATIONS

third edition

Lori A. Smolin, Ph.D.
University of Connecticut

Mary B. Grosvenor, M.S., R.D.

John Wiley & Sons, Inc.

To our sons, Zachary and Max and David and John.
Their view of the world helps us to keep life in perspective.

To our husbands, David Knecht and Peter Ambrose,
who have given their support, patience, and understanding
over the years as well as their expertise as
computer and literary consultants.

About the Authors

Lori A. Smolin, Ph.D. Lori Smolin received her B.S. degree from Cornell University, where she studied human nutrition and food science. She received her doctorate from the University of Wisconsin at Madison. Her doctoral research focused on B vitamins, homocysteine accumulation, and genetic defects in homocysteine metabolism. She completed postdoctoral training both at the Harbor–UCLA Medical Center, where she studied human obesity, and at the University of California at San Diego, where she studied genetic defects in amino acid metabolism. She has published in these areas in peer-reviewed journals. Dr. Smolin is currently at the University of Connecticut, where she has been involved in teaching, course development, and writing. She teaches both in the Department of Nutritional Science and in the Department of Molecular and Cell Biology. Courses she has taught include introductory nutrition, lifecycle nutrition, food preparation, nutritional biochemistry, general biochemistry, and biology.

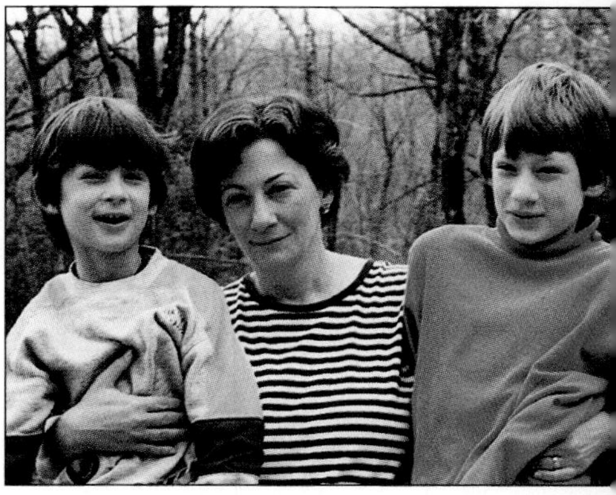

Mary B. Grosvenor, M.S., R.D. Mary Grosvenor received her B.A. degree in English from Georgetown University and her M.S. in Nutrition Sciences from the University of California at Davis. She is a registered dietitian who worked for many years managing nutrition research studies at the General Clinical Research Center at Harbor–UCLA Medical Center. She has published in peer-reviewed journals in the areas of nutrition and cancer and methods of assessing dietary intake. She has taught introductory nutrition at the community college level and currently lives with her family in a small town in Colorado. She is continuing her teaching and writing career and is still involved in nutrition research via the electronic superhighway.

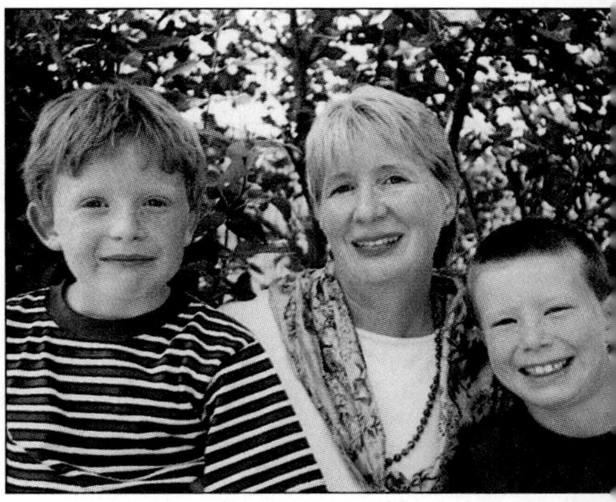

Preface

Life is full of choices. Whether you choose plain vanilla ice cream, raspberry sorbet, or fresh raspberries depends on many factors, including nutrition. How this choice affects your nutritional health depends on the other choices you make. This text conveys to students that each dietary choice makes up only one component of the overall diet. So, no one choice is a bad one as long as the sum of food choices over a period of days or weeks makes up a healthy overall diet. Knowing how to make wise choices is the key to applying nutritional principles. The third edition of *Nutrition: Science and Applications* continues with and expands upon the theme of choice that was used in the second edition.

The goal of the authors is to provide a text that teaches students both the basic principles of nutrition science and how to apply them to choices about the foods they eat and the information they encounter. Students frequently ask: Is this food good for me or bad for me? Should I be eating a lowfat diet? Should I take a protein supplement to improve my athletic performance? How can I lose 10 pounds? The answers to all these questions involve choices. And it is these personal concerns that trigger student interest in nutrition. When introductory nutrition classes and textbooks present the basics—What is carbohydrate? Protein? Fat?—but fail to prepare students to make choices about foods and popular nutrition issues, students cannot apply what they have learned. *Nutrition: Science and Applications* presents a complete introduction to the science of nutrition and can be used to teach students how to use a scientific approach in making decisions about the nutrition issues they face every day.

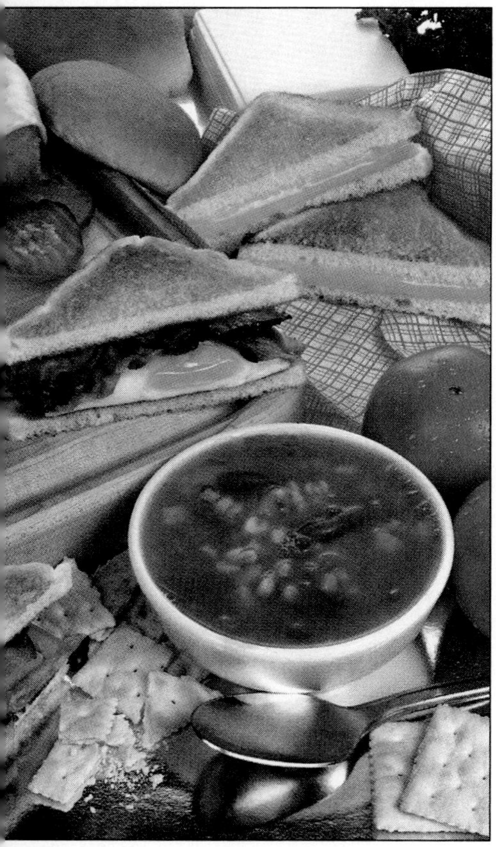

Approach

A scientific approach is employed throughout the text. Our goal is to teach students how to apply the logic of science to their own nutrition concerns. We present the process of scientific inquiry and demonstrate how it is used to evaluate the role of nutrition in health. The text contains all of the information students need to analyze and modify their own diets to promote health and reduce the risk of deficiencies and chronic diseases related to nutrition. *Critical Thinking* exercises in each chapter demonstrate to students how to logically evaluate diets, dietary supplements, and other aspects of nutrition science.

The third edition continues the integrated approach that was so successful in the first two editions. Health and disease, metabolism, cultural diversity, and life-stage topics are incorporated into each chapter. For example, the relationship of dietary fat intake, lipid metabolism and transport, and heart disease is discussed in the lipids chapter. In addition, how this information applies to young children, pregnant women, and older adults is also presented. This integration engages students early on because it presents the topics of greatest interest to them, such as the role of nutrition in health and disease, and the use of dietary supplements, along with basic nutrition principles. Students are then more motivated to learn the basics and are prepared to make decisions about their personal health and nutrition.

The writing style is concise, consistent, engaging, and easy to read. The organization from chapter to chapter is uniform, each chapter starting with a "friendly" or familiar topic to capture students' interest. The food composition information given throughout the chapters is consistent with that in the appendices and the food composition database. Throughout the book, similar illustration designs—such as those depicting the metabolism of carbohydrate, fat, and protein; the macronutrient content of foods; and the nutrients provided by the recommendations in the Food Guide Pyramid and the Dietary Guidelines—help students identify analogous information and reinforce and build upon knowledge acquired in previous sections. Colors are also used consistently to represent carbohydrate, fat, and protein and to identify certain steps in metabolism.

Features of the Third Edition

As the field of nutrition moves into the new millennium, attention has focused on the importance of both the total dietary pattern as well as individual nutrients in health and disease. Nutrition scientists and policy makers are developing a new set of dietary recommendations called the Dietary Reference Intakes and have broadened their view of nutrition recommendations to include the role of nutrients in prevention of chronic disease as well as deficiency disease. Advances in genetics have expanded our understanding of how nutrients and nutritional status affect gene expression and how genetic traits interact with our environment and lifestyle choices to determine our risk of chronic disease. The third edition of *Nutrition: Science and Applications* has kept abreast of nutrition science and policy with expanded coverage and new and enhanced features, including:

The Dietary Reference Intakes (DRIs) The DRIs are a set of dietary recommendations that are new to the field of nutrition. They are currently being developed to replace the Recommended Dietary Allowance (RDA) concept that has been used since the 1940s. The DRIs are explained in Chapter 2 and information is given throughout the text on all nutrients for which DRIs have thus far been developed. Because the field of nutrition is expanding so rapidly, it is impossible to publish a text that has all the latest information even six months after publication. Therefore, we have developed **Nutrition Update**, a supplement that will be available twice during the life of this edition, to update students and instructors on the DRIs, changes in the Dietary Guidelines, and other advances in the field of nutrition. In addition, the diet analysis software Total Diet Assessment will be updated annually to reflect the latest nutritional values.

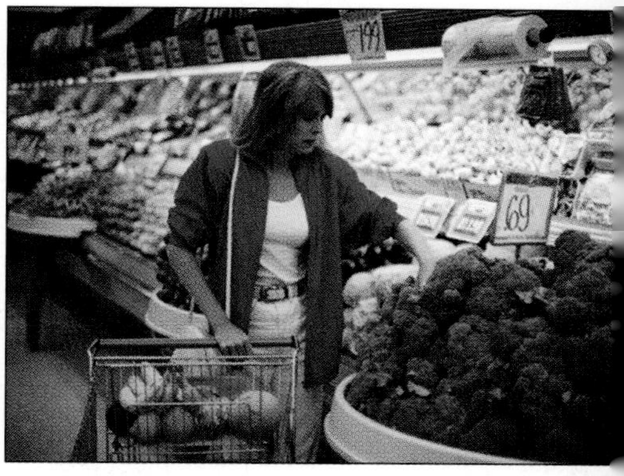

Nutrition and Gene Expression Our knowledge of nutrient function and the impact of nutrition on chronic disease risk is expanding in part due to our increasing understanding of genes. The third edition has expanded coverage of the role of nutrition in gene expression. In Chapter 1, the relationship between nutrition, genetic background, lifestyle, health, and disease is emphasized. Chapter 6 has expanded coverage of how genes make proteins, and in Chapter 9, the mechanism of how vitamins A and D function through gene expression is explained. Throughout the text the importance of nutrition in modulating one's genetic predisposition for chronic disease is addressed.

Regulation of Body Weight The text has been updated to include advances in our understanding of how body weight is regulated. For example, how can an abnormal gene result in too much body fat? Expanded coverage of the role genetics plays in obesity helps students understand the interplay between genetics and lifestyle choices and how they are related to energy balance and the potential for treatment of obesity. The area of obesity has also been updated to include new guidelines for assessing body weight and composition and recommendations for ranges of body weight and composition that do not increase the risk of chronic disease.

The Total Diet Scientists are placing more emphasis on the importance of dietary patterns rather than a single food or nutrient in health. This concept has been further strengthened in this edition by including sections that address the role of a nutrient as one part of the total diet. These sections stress the importance of a diet based on grains, fruits, and vegetables and the importance of meeting nutrient needs with a variety of foods. Foods contain phytochemicals and other nonnutrient substances that are important to health. These substances are provided by plant foods and are lacking when people rely on vitamin and mineral supplements, rather than foods, to meet their nutrient needs. Several of the *Critical Thinking* exercises help illustrate that each dietary change affects more than one nutrient in the diet. This focus on the importance of the diet as a whole rather than on single foods or nutrients helps students understand that one choice does not make or break a diet.

Dietary Supplements As the popularity of dietary supplements has increased, so too has the challenge of providing students with up-to-date information on the risks and benefits of a host of supplements, including those containing substances not classified as nutrients. The Dietary Supplements Health and Education Act of 1994 helped define what a dietary supplement is and how it should be labeled, but this does not help students assess the risks and benefits of these products. This topic has been expanded in the third edition so that students have a place to go for reliable information on supplements. Coverage includes sections that discuss supplements related to each nutrient as well as other sections such as ones related to herbal supplements in Chapter 9 and popular ergogenic aids in Chapter 12.

Easy-to-Understand Metabolism Information Metabolism is one of the most challenging topics for students. To prevent students from being overwhelmed, this text integrates coverage of metabolism with discussions of the macronutrients rather than concentrating it into one long chapter. This approach allows information on metabolism to build on and reinforce what was learned in the previous chapter. For example, the information on fat metabolism in Chapter 5 builds on that presented about carbohydrates in Chapter 4. Chapter 7 integrates all of the information on energy production. Chapters 8 through 11 discuss the role of micronutrients in metabolism, and Chapter 12 provides an overview and review by applying this knowledge to the discussion of fitness and the exercising body.

Environmental Issues Discussions of environmental issues are included because they can have an impact on the nutrient composition of foods as well as on food choices. For example, the amounts of certain nutrients in a food, such as iodine and selenium, depend on the environmental conditions where that food is produced. In addition, the foods we choose are often affected by our concern for the environment. For instance, as discussed in Chapter 6, the perception that meatless diets have less impact on the environment is responsible for some of the recent increase in vegetarianism.

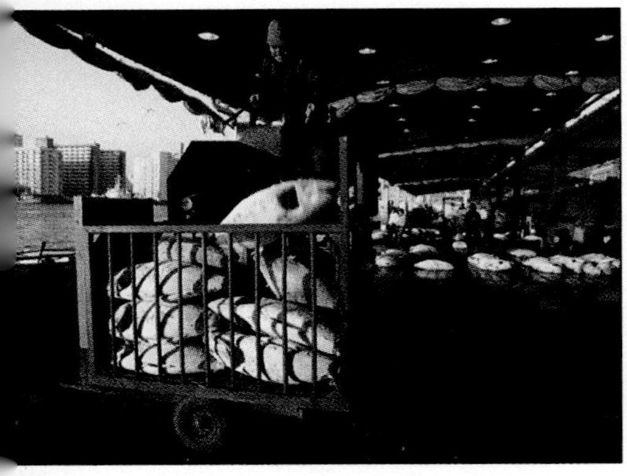

Ethnic Diversity This text uses statistics and examples reflecting the broad cultural base of a diverse student population. Incorporating ethnic foods in text examples and in *Critical Thinking* exercises throughout make the book more applicable to this audience. In addition, these examples expose students to the foods and eating patterns of other cultures. For example, in Chapter 5, Asian and Mediterranean diets are discussed in relation to the risk of heart disease.

Learning Aids in the Third Edition

Just a Taste These questions provide a simple self-test that targets common nutrition misconceptions to pique the student's interest before starting the chapter.

Chapter Outline This outline of the chapter's content provides students and teachers with an overview of all material presented in the chapter.

Chapter Concepts Each chapter opens with a list of the concepts to be explored. These aid students in understanding up front how the material will be covered and serve as a study guide once the chapter is completed.

***Off the Shelf* Boxes** *Off the Shelf* features discuss issues that relate to items that can be obtained off the shelves of stores, such as foods, books, and supplements. They focus on consumer issues and choices and on evaluating nutrition information. These discussions are a unique aspect of this text, briefly highlighting topics of special interest that deserve more explanation than the scope of a one-semester course allows. These can be read separately or in conjunction with the body of the text. In the third edition, 11 such features have been updated or are entirely new.

***Off the Label* Boxes** *Off the Label* features present in-depth information on food labels as they apply to specific nutrients or issues. The most up-to-date information is included. In the third edition, nine are new or updated.

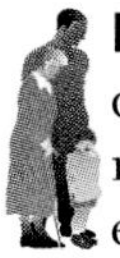

Life Stage Icon In each chapter, life stage icons highlight issues and recommendations that apply to specific stages and circumstances of life. The diversity of the material contained in each chapter is thereby increased, offering information relevant to students in all phases of life. This information also helps students understand how nutrient requirements are affected by one's life stage even if there is not time in a one-semester course to cover the separate chapters that provide complete information about this topic.

Margin Definitions Bold-faced type is used throughout the text to identify important terms and concepts. All bold-faced terms are defined in the margin as an easy reference glossary and a study aid. These terms and many others are also included in the main glossary at the back of the book.

***Critical Thinking* Exercises** The *Critical Thinking* exercises used in the first two editions have been updated and new ones added to reflect new issues that affect students. For example, the *Critical Thinking* exercise in Chapter 8, *Four Hundred of Fortified Folate,* addresses how to meet the new recommendations for folate intake, and in Chapter 10, *A Diet for Health* illustrates how dietary patterns can reduce the risk of more than one chronic disease. These exercises use case histories to guide students through the logical thought processes involved in solving nutrition problems. Some questions are answered to provide a model for students, and others require students to think through the answers themselves (solutions are included in the Appendices). These exercises also provide a guide for students to use when answering Applications at the end of the chapter.

Applications These exercises give students an opportunity to apply the critical thinking skills developed in *Critical Thinking* exercises and the knowledge gained throughout the chapter to their own diets and lifestyles.

Art and Photography Much of the existing line art has been revised to improve clarity and to match the level of the text. The illustrations were developed by the authors to better correspond to material in the text and to avoid using terminology that has not been explained. Many of these are reproduced as overhead transparencies to accompany the text. The photographs were carefully chosen to enhance the student's understanding of and interest in the material and to continue the sophisticated visual appeal of the previous editions.

Nutrition Web Links This new section has been added to guide students and instructors to a wealth of additional nutrition information available through the *Nutrition Science and Applications* Web site and the Internet in general. The Nutrition Web Links section highlights the different types of sites that can be accessed through the text Web site. Actual URLs have not been given, to allow the Web page the flexibility of adding new links and updating old ones as the Web evolves.

Chapter Summary A summary at the end of each chapter parallels but provides more detail about the concepts used to introduce each chapter. This summary of important information can be used by students to review the chapter topics.

Review Questions These brief questions direct students to the most important concepts covered in the chapter. They are designed to review in a simple manner the key points of each chapter and to serve as a study guide.

Updated References and Resources Nutrition knowledge is expanding rapidly. In response, we have included the most recent findings and research articles in this edition. The updating process has continued throughout the production of the text, providing the most up-to-date information and interpretations available. The majority of references are from 1995 or later. The authors would be happy to provide references for information that is not referenced in the text.

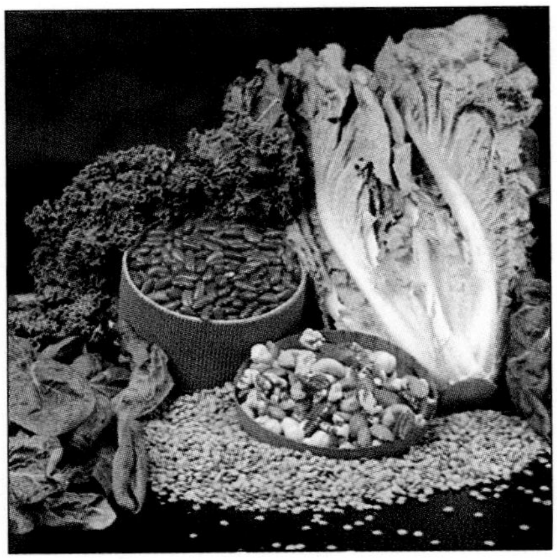

Inside the Covers Inside the front and back covers you will find information that is needed frequently during your study. This easily accessible information includes current recommended nutrient intakes: DRI values when available and 1989 RDAs and ESADDI values for other nutrients. The Food Guide Pyramid, a sample food label, and a metric conversion table are also included.

Appendices Thorough appendices can be found at the end of the text. These include a comprehensive food composition table containing information on energy and 25 nutrients in about 4000 foods, including fast foods and convenience foods. Other appendices include standards for nutritional indices, such as height and weight charts and tables for infants through the elderly; normal blood values; a list of reliable sources of nutrition information; dietary recommendations from the United States, Canada, and other countries; recommendations for risk reduction from various special interest groups, such as the American Heart Association; the objectives of Healthy People 2010; the Exchange Lists; ethnic and life-stage versions of the Food Guide Pyramid; an extensive review of food labeling guidelines; energy expenditure values; and answers to *Critical Thinking* exercises.

Glossary An extensive glossary of terms is included at the end of the text to provide a quick reference for terminology with which students may be unfamiliar or for which they require review.

Index The text is well indexed to allow students to easily cross-reference material of interest.

The Third Edition, Chapter-by-Chapter

The text is divided into five parts. Part I, "Nutrition: Sorting Fact From Fantasy," introduces the reader to the basic concepts of nutrition, the scientific method, and the principles of digestion and absorption necessary to understand issues presented throughout the book. Part II, "Energy-Containing Nutrients," includes chapters on carbohydrates, lipids, and proteins, as well as a chapter that covers energy balance, weight control, and eating disorders. Part III, "Water and the Micronutrients," examines the non-energy-containing nutrients: water, vitamins, and minerals. Part IV, "Applying Nutrition to Life," applies the basics of nutrition to different lifestyles and stages of development. Exercise is presented in this section as a lifestyle factor that affects nutritional status and nutritional needs. The final part, "Nutrition in Today's World," addresses food safety and discusses issues related to malnutrition in North America and the world. The material is presented in a consistent and logical order that will capture the student's interest, but the chapters and sections can be taught in any order.

Chapter 1, "Nutrition: Everyday Choices," provides an overview of the nutrients and their roles in the body, and introduces the scientific method. Chapter 1 teaches students how to identify accurate nutrition information. A mock ad featuring a protein supplement for athletes is used to help students learn how to interpret nutrition information from many sources.

Chapter 2, "Applying the Science of Nutrition," shows how the results of scientific studies are used to develop dietary standards and guidelines. The Dietary

Reference Intakes (DRIs) are introduced here. Guidelines for health promotion and disease prevention, such as Dietary Guidelines for Americans, are discussed, and tools for diet planning, including the Food Guide Pyramid, Exchange Lists, and food labels, are presented so that students can begin applying them to their own diets. The final section of this chapter discusses how these and other tools can be used to assess the health of populations and individuals. Information from the most up-to-date surveys (CSFII) and programs (Healthy People 2010) is provided here and throughout the text. The *Critical Thinking* exercise in this chapter demonstrates how to plan diets using the Food Guide Pyramid. A new figure shows students how to interpret information from computer diet analyses.

Chapter 3, "The Human Body: From Meals to Molecules," presents digestion and absorption by showing how a particular meal is digested, its nutrients absorbed into the body and transported to the cells where metabolism occurs, and finally how wastes are removed.

Chapters 4, 5, and 6 discuss carbohydrates, lipids, and proteins. Each begins with information on the types of foods that contain these nutrients, followed by a discussion of the basic chemistry of these nutrients. Key points about the digestion and absorption of these nutrients are followed by a section addressing the nutrient's role in the body. In each chapter, energy production is summarized using a figure that illustrates how the metabolism of each nutrient interfaces with that of others. A separate section on health and disease is followed by a section that discusses the role of each nutrient as one part of the total diet. Nutrient requirements and how they vary through life, as well as how to make dietary choices to help meet recommendations, are presented. To teach students how to select a healthy diet, the recommendations of the Dietary Guidelines are integrated with the information provided by food labels and the Food Guide Pyramid.

Chapter 4 has been expanded to include a discussion of what cancer is and how it can be affected by nutrition. This chapter also includes information on the role of fiber in gastrointestinal health. Chapter 5 includes an updated section on the role of diet in the development of heart disease. A new *Off the Shelf* feature discussing supplements that are claimed to lower cholesterol has been added. Improvements and additions to the art program help students to better understand lipid structure, digestion, absorption, and metabolism. In Chapter 6, the discussion of protein synthesis has been strengthened and the concept of gene expression is introduced. Protein deficiency and excess as well as the risks and benefits of vegetarian diets are discussed in this chapter. The vegetarian Food Guide Pyramid has been updated and a new *Off the Shelf* feature has been added to address the potential health benefits of soy protein.

Chapter 7, "Energy Balance and Weight Management," presents the concept of energy balance and applies it to weight management. This chapter reflects the newer view of obesity as a disease that can be treated in an individualized fashion with diet, exercise, behavior modification, and, when appropriate, medication. The genetic determinants of body weight are discussed from the standpoint of body weight management and the potential for improved treatment. A new *Off the Shelf* feature discusses the pros and cons of weight-loss drugs, and a new figure illustrates how leptin helps regulate body weight. The health risks of too much or too little body fat as well as of eating disorders are addressed in this chapter.

Chapter 8, "A Vitamin Primer and the Water-Soluble Vitamins," begins with a general overview of vitamins—where they are found in the diet, factors affecting bioavailability, and how they function. The B vitamins and vitamin C are discussed individually, but the B vitamins are grouped according to common roles as coenzymes in energy production, amino acid metabolism, and cell division. Discussions of each of the water-soluble vitamins include sources in the diet, functions in the body, impact on health, recommended intakes, supplement use, and potential for toxicity. This chapter presents the DRIs for the B vitamins and choline, a substance that is not currently classified as a vitamin but one for which DRIs have been established. The new recommendations on folate intake for women of childbearing age are included along with a discussion of the regulations for and impact of the folic acid fortification of foods. In addition, new recommendations for vitamin B_{12} intake in older adults are explained. Improved line art helps point out functional relationships between the B vitamins. The section on vitamin C includes an expanded discussion of oxidative stress and the role of antioxidants in protecting the body from damage.

Chapter 9, "Fat-Soluble Vitamins and Meeting Vitamin Needs," presents each of the fat-soluble vitamins and discusses sources in the diet, functions in the body, impact on health, recommended intakes, supplement use, and potential for toxicity. Improved coverage (including new line art) of how vitamins A and D act by affecting gene expression is presented in this chapter. The chapter closes with a discussion of the advantages and disadvantages of meeting vitamin needs with foods versus supplements. It emphasizes that food sources of vitamins provide nonnutrient substances, such as phytochemicals, that may promote health. An expanded section on dietary supplements uses a risk-benefit approach to help students evaluate all products defined as dietary supplements. An *Off the Shelf* feature on the risks and benefits of herbal supplements has been added. (Discussions of dietary supplements are also integrated throughout the book, with applicable topics.)

Chapter 10, "The Internal Sea: Water and the Major Minerals," presents information on where these nutrients are found and discusses their function in the body, their relationship to health and disease, and recommended intakes. The electrolytes sodium, potassium, and chloride are discussed together, as are calcium, phosphorus, and magnesium—the minerals involved in bone formation. DRI values are included for calcium, phosphorus, and magnesium. Health and disease topics addressed here include hypertension and osteoporosis. Advances in our understanding of the impact of total dietary patterns on hypertension are stressed by an expanded discussion of the DASH diet, a dietary pattern that has been shown to lower blood pressure. A *Critical Thinking* exercise that focuses on the DASH diet in relation to health maintenance has been added.

Chapter 11, "The Trace Minerals: Our Elemental Needs," discusses the trace elements in a format similar to that used for other micronutrients. Rather than using a typical laundry list approach, the book presents the minerals in an order that emphasizes similarities in function and the interactions that exist among them. Discussions of the health issues related to these nutrients help create interest, as do discussions of the pros and cons of mineral supplements. For example, the discussion of iron has been expanded to place emphasis on the problems of iron overload as well as iron deficiency, and a new *Off the Shelf* feature on the effectiveness of zinc lozenges for treating cold symptoms has been included.

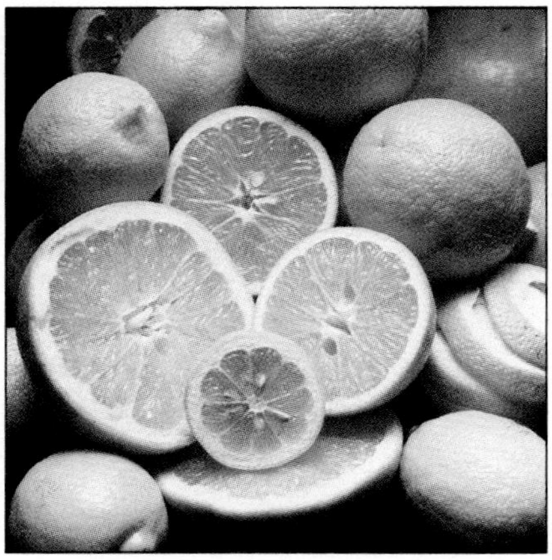

Chapter 12, "Fueling Fitness: Nutrition and Exercise," is designed to emphasize the importance of fitness to nutritional health as well as to provide information on nutrition and athletic performance. A number of new recommendations for exercise have been added, and the Activity Pyramid is included to illustrate these. This chapter serves as a review of metabolism, which was introduced in Part II, in relation to energy production. By this point in the text students have studied all the essential nutrients, so a complete discussion of the macronutrient and micronutrient needs for energy production can be included. There is an expanded discussion of ergogenic aids for more competitive athletes that directs students to use a risk-benefit analysis of these products before deciding whether or not to use them. A new *Off the Shelf* feature discusses anabolic steroids, androstenedione, and creatine.

Chapter 13, "In the Beginning: Nutrition for Mothers and Infants," addresses the role of nutrition in development by discussing the nutritional needs of the mother during pregnancy and lactation and the nutritional needs of the infant. Current recommendations and practical information about breast and formula feeding of infants are given. The new DRI recommendations for pregnancy and lactation are included. New line art illustrates the formation of the neural tube. Material on introducing solid food to the infant diet is now included in Chapter 14.

Chapter 14, "The Growing Years: Infancy to Adolescence," begins by discussing the importance of learning healthy eating habits early in life. The chapter discusses nutrient needs from the first solid foods offered to infants to the independent choices of adolescents. Exercise recommendations for children and an activity pyramid for kids have been added. A new *Off the Shelf* feature on peanut allergies helps students understand this issue. A discussion of nutrition and alcohol consumption is included in this chapter because whether or not to use alcohol is an important choice often made by adolescents.

Chapter 15, "Nutrition and Aging: The Adult Years," addresses how nutrition affects aging and how aging affects nutrition. It includes updated information on the interrelationships between aging and nutritional status. Nutrient-drug interactions are discussed, and nutrition programs such as the Older Americans Act and the Nutrition Screening Initiative are presented. The chapter includes a new *Off the Shelf* feature on dietary supplements marketed to alleviate arthritis as well as one that addresses the risks and benefits of alcohol consumption.

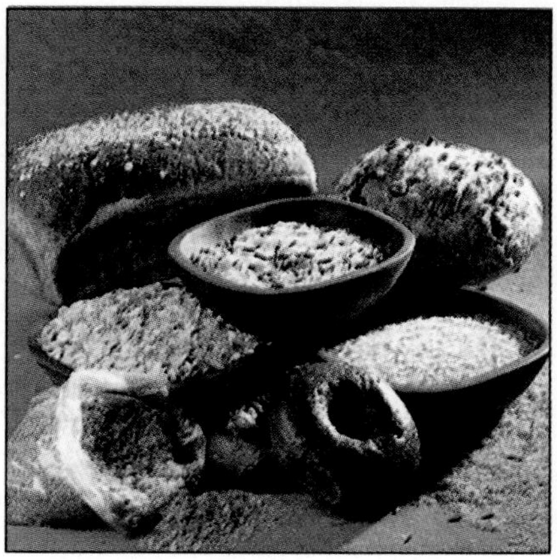

Chapter 16, "How Safe Is Our Food Supply?" discusses the risks and benefits of the U.S. food supply and includes information on the impact of microbial hazards, chemical toxins, food additives, irradiation, and genetically engineered foods. The directives of the Food Safety Initiative are addressed, including the use of a system called HACCP (Hazard Analysis Critical Control Point) to ensure safe food and advances in technology that help identify the sources of food-borne illness.

Chapter 17, "The Global View: Feeding the World," deals with the problems of hunger and malnutrition both at home and globally. It discusses the issue of providing enough of the right kinds of food and distributing it equitably. The causes of world hunger are examined, along with potential solutions. The World Food Conference is discussed and updated information on the status of world hunger and micronutrient deficiencies is presented. Finally, the health impact of the "Westernization" of the diet in many developing countries is discussed.

Ancillaries

This third edition of *Nutrition: Science and Applications* is accompanied by a complete set of supplementary teaching and learning materials. The materials available for students are as follows:

Nutrition Update This newsletter will be published twice during the life of this edition to inform students and instructors of the progress in updating the DRIs, the Healthy People 2010 initiatives, changes in the Dietary Guidelines, and other advances in nutrition science. The *Nutrition Update* newsletter will be free and included with all new copies of the book.

Diet Analysis Software The diet analysis software package that accompanies this book was used by the authors when developing examples and *Critical Thinking* exercises. It has been expanded to include values for energy and 25 nutrients and about 4000 foods. It includes a feature that allows users to add 30 foods to the database to keep pace with the ever-growing market of available products. The database has been designed to incorporate the foods mentioned throughout the text, including foods from a variety of cultures. The database includes updated folate values for all non-brand-name foods and for many brand-name items. The software in the third edition has been updated to include an analysis of the diet based on the number of servings recommended by the Food Guide Pyramid.

Clinical Cases Supplement This supplement, written by the authors, will expand on the *Critical Thinking* approach by including clinically oriented critical thinking problems that focus on health and disease, as well as some exercises that relate to institutional food production.

Study Guide This guide, written by Melanie Burns of Eastern Illinois University, includes chapter outlines, multiple-choice questions, matching exercises, short-answer review questions, and a variety of learning activities designed for use by individual students and by groups in the classroom.

The teaching materials available to instructors include the following:

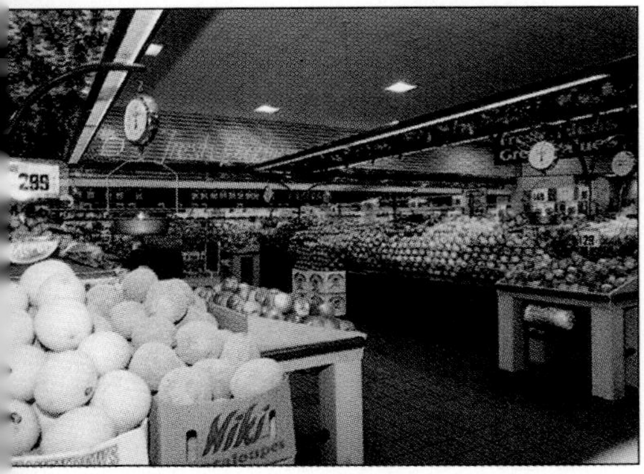

Instructor's Manual with Test Bank The Instructor's Manual, written by the authors, includes key concepts, complete chapter outlines, new *Critical Thinking* exercises, diet assessment forms, key terms, student self-assessment forms, and sources of other materials, including useful Web sites. The Test Bank, written by Kathy Beerman and Lois Jensen, both of Washington State University, includes multiple-choice and short-answer questions as well as short case studies with attendant questions that encourage students to apply what they have learned. There is also a selection of masters that supplement the images available in the basic overhead transparency package (see below).

ExaMaster+ This is a computerized version of the printed Test Bank that makes preparing clear, concise tests quick and easy. It is available for both Macintosh and PC computers.

Overhead Transparencies This set of 100 full-color overheads helps instructors illustrate the book's more complicated concepts in the classroom. The set can be supplemented by using the image bank from the Instructor's Resource CD-ROM for Nutrition (see below) or the transparency masters available in the Instructor's Manual.

Instructor's Resource CD-ROM for Nutrition This dual-platform presentation CD-ROM (for Macintosh and Windows) features all of the illustrations and approximately 100 photographs from the text. A PowerPoint slide presentation, prepared by Wendy White of Iowa State University, is loaded onto the CD-ROM. It can also be used with Persuasion images.

Please contact your Wiley sales representative for more information. Don't know who your Wiley representative is? Go to: www.wiley.com/college/rep.

Acknowledgments

The authors wish to thank the many professors and students who helped in the development of this text. Their endless hours of careful reading and their many thorough suggestions from many diverse viewpoints have helped to make this text the best available on today's market. The reviewers, who offered comments and suggestions on both the presentation and the accuracy of this information, include the following: Janet B. Anderson, Utah State University; Sarah Long Anderson, Southern Illinois University—Carbondale; Garry Auld, Colorado State University; L. Rao Ayyagari, Lindenwood University; Joye M. Bond, Mankato State University; Patsy Brannon, University of Maryland; N. Shane Broughton, University of Wyoming; Melanie Burns, Eastern Illinois University; John Capeheart, University of Houston—Downtown; Linda Drake, University of Connecticut—Storrs; Roberta Durschlag, Boston University; Anne Fortini, Mt. San Antonio College; Nancy P. Garnett-Thomas, East Greenwich, Rhode Island; Leonard Gerber, University of Rhode Island; William Helferich, University of Illinois—Urbana-Champaign; Robert Jackson, University of Maryland; Judy Kaufman, Monroe Community College; Chen Hey Kim Lee, Northern Arizona University; Khosla Pramod, Wayne State University; Elaine M. Long, Boise State University; Teresa Marcus, Chattanooga State Technical Community College; Marilyn Mook, Michigan State University; Barbara North, North Dakota State University; Thaddeus Osmolski, University of Massachusetts—Lowell; Erwina Peterson, Yakima Valley Community College; Michelle Pierce, University of Connecticut—Storrs; Roseann Poole, Tallahassee Community College; Joanne Slavin, University of Minnesota—St. Paul; Samuel Smith, University of New Hampshire; Joanne Spaide, University of Northern Iowa; Leslie Spencer, Rowan University; Diane

Stadler, University of Utah; Georgeanne P. Syler, Southeast Missouri University; Suzanne Vieira, Johnson and Wales University; Wendy S. White, Iowa State University; Anne Wilcox, Eastern Illinois University; Fred Wolfe, University of Arizona; Jean Zancanella, University of Utah.

We are grateful to the editorial and production staff at Saunders College Publishing for their help and support. We thank our Acquisitions Editors Edith Beard Brady and Nedah Rose for their support, our Developmental Editor Lee Marcott for hours of expert advice and moral support, and our Marketing Strategist, Erik Fahlgren, for coordinating the advertising, marketing, and sales efforts for the book and its supplements. We also thank our Photo Editor Walter Neary for ensuring the outstanding quality of the photos in this text, our Art Director Caroline McGowan for delivering an attractively designed text with high-quality artwork, our studio, Rolin Graphics, for translating our sketches into effective figures, and our Project Editors, Anne Gibby and Bonnie Boehme, for their patience in guiding this project through production.

To the Student

Most nutrition texts choose to put a photo of fruits, vegetables, or grain products on the cover. This is because these foods make up the basis of a healthy diet. We put ice cream and fruit on our cover to emphasize the concept of choice. Fresh raspberries may provide more nutrients with fewer kcalories than ice cream, but ice cream can be part of a healthy diet if your total diet is based on grains, vegetables, and fruits. Good nutrition does not mean giving up all the foods you like; it means making wise choices to select an overall diet that promotes health, protects you from disease, and provides enjoyment. Each food and lifestyle choice you make depends on other choices you have made or intend to make. To help you with these nutrition choices we have provided a text that bridges the gap between popular nutrition and nutrition science. Our goal is not to tell you, for instance, that you should or should not eat potato chips. Instead, we have provided you with the information you need to make informed decisions for yourself. This text takes nutrition science out of the classroom and allows you to apply it to the choices you make about foods, nutritional supplements, and other lifestyle factors important to your health. We have included the latest tools for selecting a healthy diet, such as the Food Guide Pyramid, the Dietary Guidelines, and information on food labels. We hope that the knowledge you gain from this book will help you choose a healthy diet while allowing you to enjoy the diversity of flavors, textures, and tastes that are available in today's food supply.

Lori Smolin
Storrs, Connecticut

Mary Grosvenor
Delta, Colorado

July 1999

Contents Overview

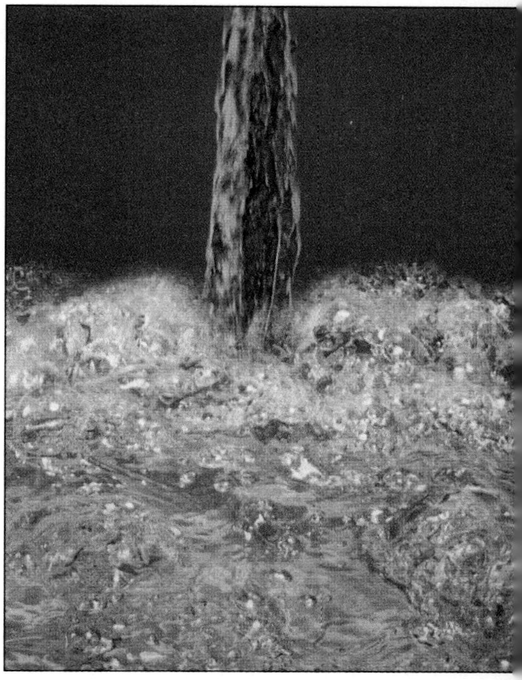

Contents

I

Nutrition: Sorting Fact From Fantasy

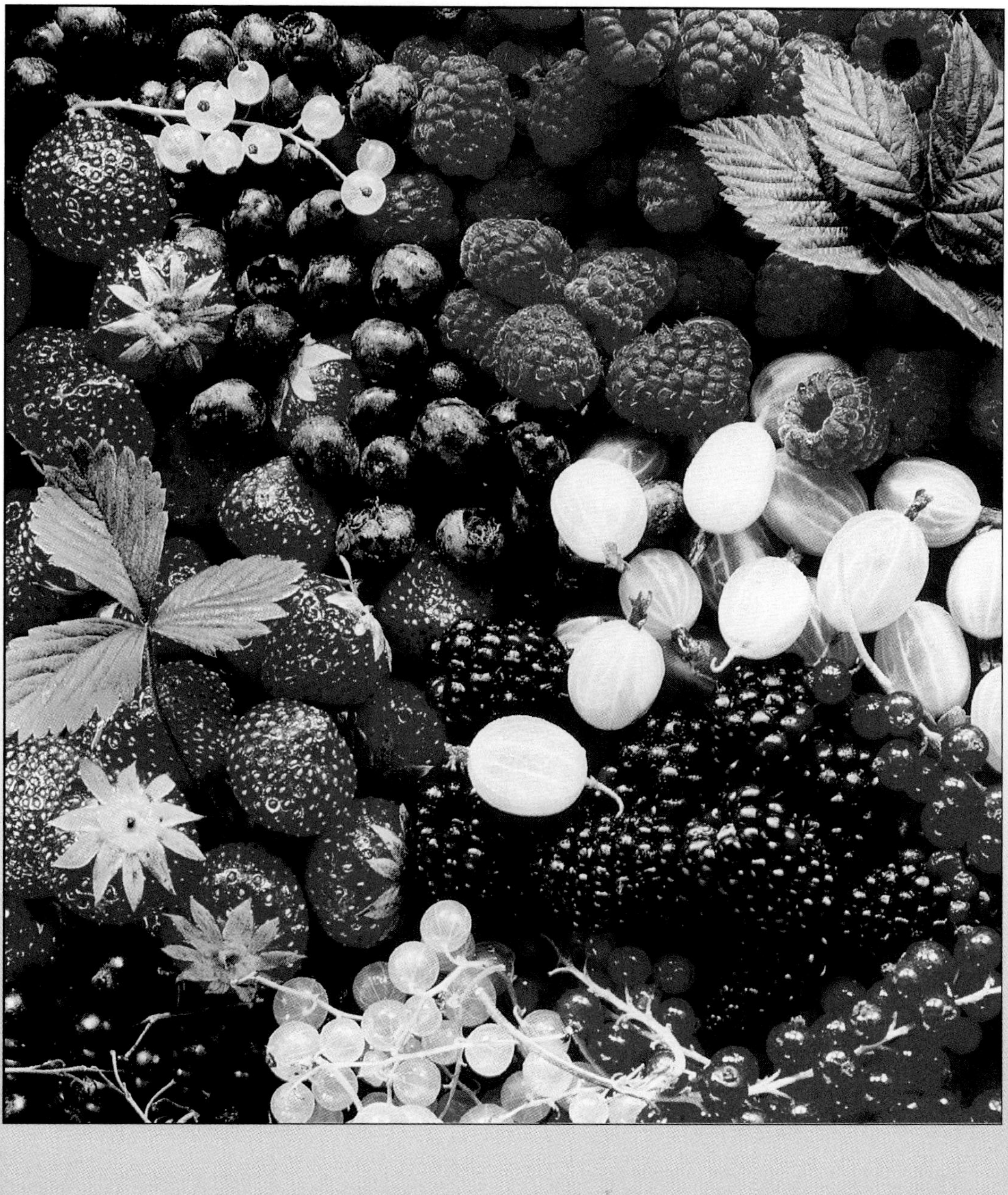

Chapter 1

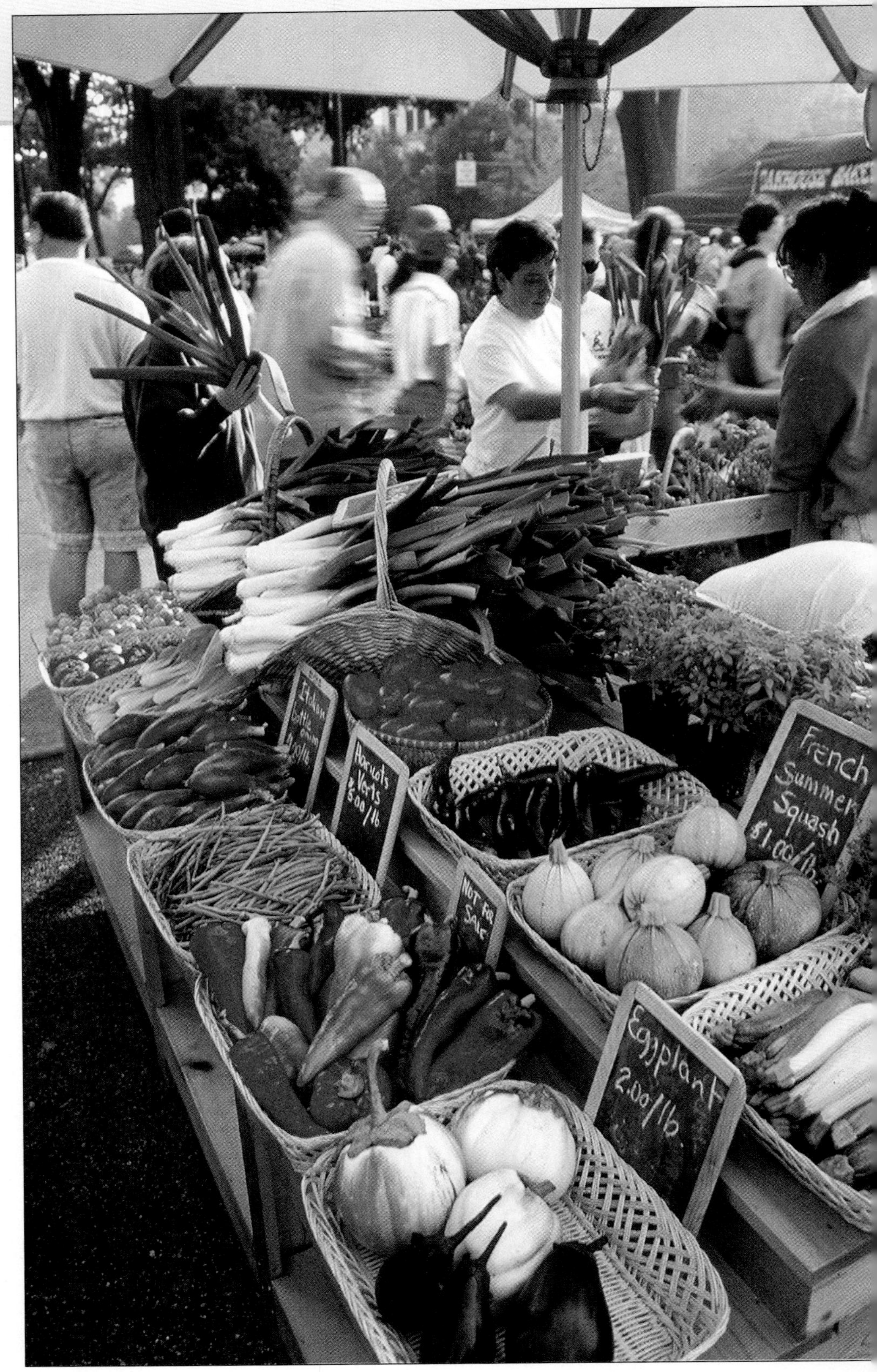

(© Zane Williams/Tony Stone Images)

Chapter Outline

What Is Nutrition?

What Are Nutrients?

What Do Nutrients Do?

How Much of Each Nutrient Do We Need?

Effects of Poor Nutrient Intake

What Are We Choosing?

How Healthy Is the American Diet?

How Do We Make Food Choices?

What Is Reliable Nutrition Information?

Understanding the Process of Science: The Scientific Method

How Scientists Study Nutrition

Judging Nutrition Information

Nutrition: Everyday Choices

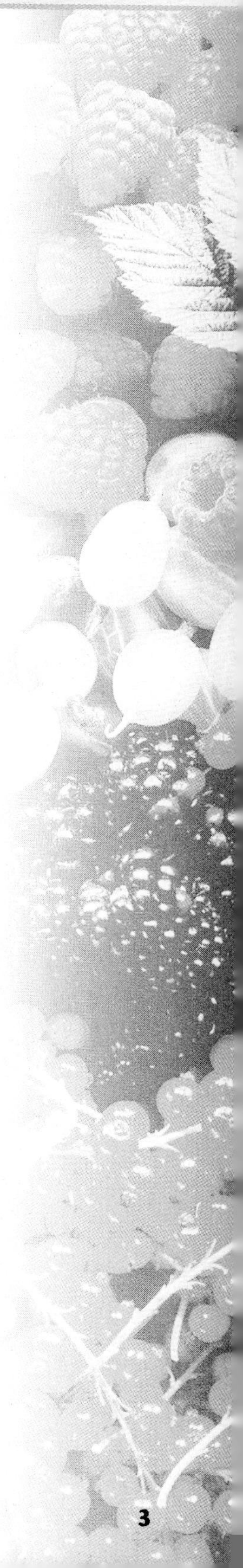

Chapter Concepts

1. Nutrition involves all of the interactions of living organisms with food.
2. Nutrients are substances found in food that provide energy, structure, and regulation for the body processes of maintenance and repair, growth, and reproduction.
3. Nutrients must be consumed in the proper amounts and proportions to meet nutritional needs and maintain health.
4. Any food can be part of a healthy diet as long as it is balanced with other food choices, but your overall pattern of food choices should be consistent with recommendations for a healthy diet.
5. Our food choices are based on what is available, what we like and are culturally conditioned to eat, as well as what we think we should be eating.
6. Advances in our understanding of nutrition are made by using the scientific method. This involves making observations, formulating hypotheses, testing hypotheses by experimentation, and developing theories from the results.
7. Well-conducted experiments must use objective measurements, proper experimental controls, and the right experimental population. Results must be carefully interpreted.
8. Many types of research are used to study relationships among diet, health, and disease. Epidemiological observations can be used to formulate hypotheses. Intervention and laboratory studies are conducted to test hypotheses, explore nutrient functions, and develop theories.
9. Choosing reliable nutrition information can be difficult. Consumers must be skeptical and analyze how the information was developed, who developed it, and who stands to benefit from it.

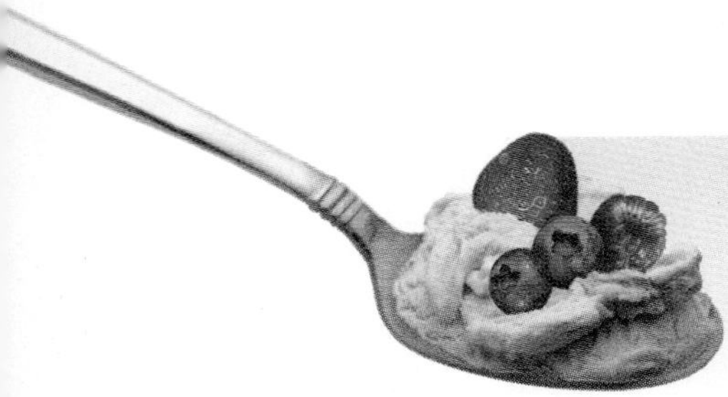

Just a Taste

Can ice cream be part of a healthy diet?

Can your food choices today affect your future health?

Which nutrition headlines should you believe?

Ice cream—cold, creamy, delicious—but is it nutritious? Should it be a part of your diet? The answer depends on the choices you make. Ice cream and other frozen desserts come in many colors, flavors, and varieties: Neapolitan, rainbow sherbet, heavenly hash, fudge swirl, frozen yogurt, sorbet, fat-free, sugar-free. . . . Each tastes different, looks different, and makes a different contribution to your total diet. None of these choices is bad, nor is the decision to include ice cream in your diet, as long as it constitutes one part of an overall healthy diet.

Whether you are deciding to have a bowl of ice cream or wondering if you should believe a news headline—the choices you make depend on who you are, what your individual goals are, and what your genetic and cultural background is. Are you an athlete? Are you planning a pregnancy, breast feeding an infant, or trying to prevent the physical decline that occurs with aging? Did your mother die of a heart attack? Does cancer run in your family? Are you trying to keep kosher, lose weight, or eat a vegetarian diet? Is your heritage Asian, African, European, Central or South American? In order to choose foods that satisfy your personal and cultural preferences but also contribute to a healthy diet and prevent chronic diseases, you must have information about what nutrients you require, what role they play in health and disease, and what foods contain them. Do you wonder if you should be taking antioxidants, eating fat-free foods, or taking calcium supplements? Should you believe the story you saw on the news about vitamin E and heart disease? Filtering out the worthless and understanding the worthwhile can be a mind-boggling task. It requires an understanding of the principles of nutrition; the nutrient content of foods; the interactions of nutrition, health, and disease; and how scientists study nutrition.

The purpose of this text is to provide an understanding of the basics of nutrition in a way that will allow you to make informed choices about the foods you consume and the information you encounter.

What Is Nutrition?

Nutrition A science that studies the interactions that occur between living organisms and food.

Nutrition is a science that studies all the interactions that occur between living organisms and food. It studies the psychological, social, cultural, economic, and technological factors that influence which foods we choose to eat. The science of nutrition also studies the biological processes by which we consume food and utilize the nutrients it contains.

What Are Nutrients?

Nutrients are substances contained in food that are necessary to maintain life and allow growth and reproduction. Nutrients provide energy, contribute to structure, and regulate biological processes. To date, approximately 45 nutrients are considered essential to human life. **Essential nutrients** are those substances necessary to support life that must be supplied in the diet because they either cannot be made by the body or cannot be made in large enough quantities to meet needs. Protein, for example, is an essential nutrient needed for the growth and maintenance of body tissues and the synthesis of regulatory molecules. Food also contains substances classified as nonessential. Some are not essential to sustain life but have health-promoting properties. For example, a **phytochemical** found in broccoli, called sulforaphane, is not essential but may reduce the risk of cancer. Other substances are required by the body but can be produced in sufficient amounts to meet needs. For example, lecithin, which is needed for nerve function, is not an essential nutrient because it can be manufactured in the body.

Chemically, there are six classes of nutrients: carbohydrates, lipids, proteins, water, vitamins, and minerals. Carbohydrates, lipids, and proteins provide energy to the body and thus are referred to as energy-containing nutrients. Along with water, they constitute the major portion of most foods. They are referred to as **macronutrients** because they are required in relatively large amounts ("macro" means large). Their requirements are measured in kilograms (kg) or grams (g) (see Table 1.1 and the back cover for metric conversions). Alcohol also provides energy but is not considered a nutrient because it is not needed to support life.

Carbohydrates include sugars such as those in table sugar, fruit, and milk, and starches such as those in vegetables and grains. Sugars are the simplest form of carbohydrate, and starches are more complex carbohydrates made of many

Nutrients Chemical substances in foods that provide energy, structure, and regulation of body processes.

Essential nutrients Nutrients that must be provided in the diet because the body either cannot make them or cannot make them in sufficient quantities to satisfy its needs.

Phytochemical A substance found in plant foods that is not an essential nutrient but may have health-promoting properties.

Macronutrients Nutrients needed by the body in large amounts. These include water, and the energy-yielding nutrients carbohydrates, lipids, and proteins.

Table 1.1 *Measures Used in Nutrition*

Metric	English
Measures of weight	
1 kilogram (kg) = 1000 grams (g)	= 2.2 pounds (lb)
454 grams	= 1 pound = 16 ounces (oz)
28.4 grams	= 1 ounce
4 grams of sugar or salt	= about 1 teaspoon (tsp)
1 gram = 1000 milligrams (mg)	
1 milligram = 1000 micrograms (µg or mcg)	
Measures of volume	
1 liter = 1000 milliliters (ml)	= approximately 1 quart (qt) = 4 cups
240 milliliters	= 1 cup = 8 oz
5 milliliters	= 1 teaspoon
15 milliliters	= 1 tablespoon (Tbsp) = 3 teaspoons
30 milliliters	= approximately 1 fluid ounce
Measures of length	
1 meter (m) = 1000 centimeters (cm) = 1000 millimeters (mm)	= 39.4 inches (in.) = 1.09 yards (yd)
2.54 centimeters	= 1 inch

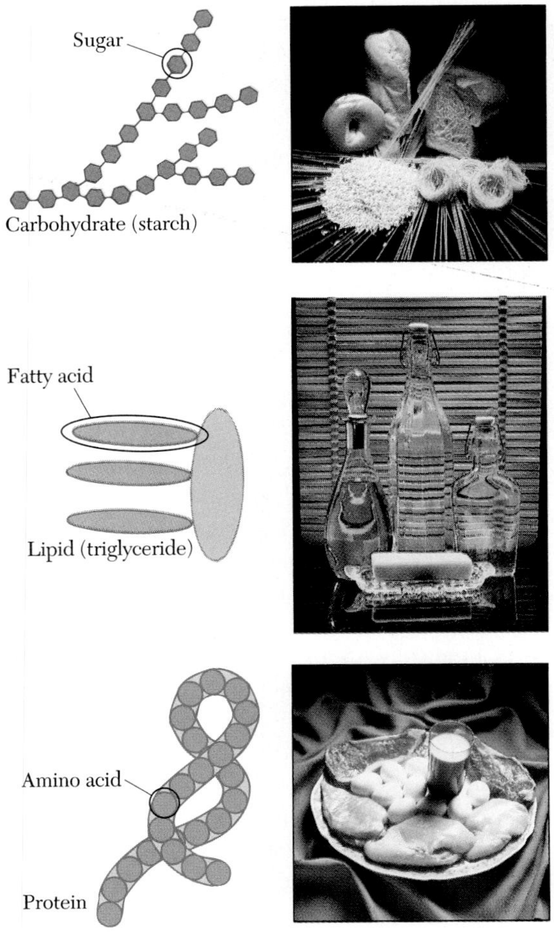

Figure 1.1
Starches are made of sugars linked together; most lipids such as the triglyceride shown here contain fatty acids; and proteins are made of amino acids linked together. (Photographs, Charles D. Winters)

sugars linked together (Figure 1.1). Carbohydrates provide a readily available source of energy to the body. Most fiber is also carbohydrate. It cannot be completely broken down by the body, so it provides little energy. However, it is important for gastrointestinal health. Fiber is found in vegetables, fruits, legumes, and whole grains.

Lipids, commonly referred to as fats and oils, provide a storage form of energy. Lipids in our diets come from foods that naturally contain fats, such as meat and whole milk, and from processed fats, such as vegetable oils and butter, that we add to food. Most lipids contain fatty acids, some of which are essential in the diet. The amount and type of lipid in the diet affects the risk of cardiovascular disease and certain types of cancer.

Protein, such as that in meat, fish, poultry, milk, grains, and legumes, is needed for growth and maintenance of body structures and regulation of body processes. Protein is made up of units called amino acids. Some amino acids can be made by the body, and others are essential in the diet. Dietary protein must meet the need for the essential amino acids.

Water is a nutrient in a class by itself. Water makes up about 60% of the human body and is required in kilogram amounts in the daily diet. It is a macronutrient that doesn't provide energy. Water serves many functions in the body, including acting as a lubricant, a transport fluid, and a regulator of body temperature.

Micronutrients Nutrients needed by the body in small amounts. These include vitamins and minerals.

Vitamins and minerals are classified as **micronutrients** because they are needed in small amounts in the diet ("micro" means small). The amounts required are expressed in milligrams (1 mg = 1/1000 g) or micrograms (1 μg =

1/1,000,000 g). They do not provide energy, but many help regulate the production of energy from carbohydrates, lipids, and proteins. They also have unique roles in processes such as bone growth, oxygen transport, and tissue growth and development. Vitamins and minerals are found in most of the foods we eat. Fresh foods are a good source of vitamins and minerals; however, losses may occur with storage. Although processing and cooking can cause micronutrient losses, frozen, canned, and otherwise processed foods are still good sources of vitamins and minerals. In some cases cooking releases nutrients making them more available to the body. Many micronutrients are added to food during processing. For example, breakfast cereals are a good source of iron because it is added during processing. Vitamin and mineral supplements are also a common source of micronutrients in today's diet.

What Do Nutrients Do?

Together, the macronutrients and micronutrients provide energy, structure, and regulation, which are needed for growth, maintenance and repair, and reproduction. Each nutrient provides one or more of these functions, but all nutrients together are needed to maintain health.

Carbohydrates, lipids, and proteins provide the fuel or energy that is required to maintain life. If less energy is consumed than is needed, the body will burn its own fat as well as carbohydrate and protein to meet its energy needs. If more energy is consumed than is needed, the extra is stored as body fat. The energy needed for all body processes and activities is measured in **kilocalories** (abbreviated as *kcalories* or *kcals*) or in **kilojoules** (abbreviated as *kjoules* or *kJs*). The more common term "calorie" is technically 1/1000 of a kilocalorie, but when spelled with a capital "C" it indicates kilocalories. For instance, the term "Calories" on food labels actually refers to kilocalories. One gram of carbohydrate or protein provides 4 kcalories. One gram of fat provides 9 kcalories. Alcohol contributes about 7 kcalories per gram (Table 1.2).

Kilocalorie A unit of heat that is used to express the amount of energy provided by foods.

Kilojoule A measure of work that can be used to express energy intake and energy output; 4.18 kjoules = 1 kcalorie.

Nutrients are also needed to form and maintain body structures. Water, proteins, lipids, and minerals are important structural nutrients. For example, muscle is made up primarily of protein and water, and bone is composed of a protein framework embedded with minerals. Nutrients also regulate biochemical reactions in the living body. Together all of the reactions that occur in the body are referred to as **metabolism.** Metabolic processes must be regulated to maintain a constant environment inside the body, referred to as **homeostasis.** Vitamins, minerals, water, and proteins are important regulatory nutrients. For example, water helps to regulate body temperature. When body temperature increases, water lost through sweat helps to cool the body. Protein, vitamins, and minerals help to speed up or slow down the reactions of metabolism as needed to maintain homeostasis.(See Table 1.3 for further examples.)

Metabolism The sum of all the chemical reactions that take place in a living organism.

Homeostasis A physiological state in which a stable internal body environment is maintained.

Table 1.2 ***Energy Content of Carbohydrate, Protein, Lipid, and Alcohol***

	Kcalories/gram	Kjoules/gram
Carbohydrate	4	16.7
Protein	4	16.7
Lipid	9	37.6
Alcohol	7	29.3

Table 1.3 *Examples of How Nutrients Function in the Body*

Function	Nutrient	Example
Energy	Carbohydrate	Blood glucose is a carbohydrate that fuels body cells.
	Lipid	Fat is the most plentiful source of stored fuel in the body.
	Protein	Protein consumed in excess of protein needs will be used for energy.
Structure	Lipid	The membranes that surround each cell are primarily lipid.
	Protein	Connective tissue protein holds bones together and holds muscles to bones.
	Minerals	The minerals calcium and phosphorus make teeth and bones hard.
Regulation	Lipid	Estrogen is a lipid hormone that helps regulate the reproductive cycle in women.
	Protein	Leptin is a protein that helps regulate body fat.
	Water	Water lost as sweat helps cool the body to regulate body temperature.
	Vitamins	B vitamins regulate the use of macronutrients for energy.
	Minerals	Sodium helps regulate blood volume.

How Much of Each Nutrient Do We Need?

In order to support life, an adequate amount of each essential nutrient must be consumed in the diet. The amount of a nutrient that is optimal is an amount that will avoid deficiencies and excesses and optimize short-term and long-term health. The exact amount that is optimal is different for each individual. It depends on genetic makeup and overall diet. A person with a genetic predisposition to heart disease needs to consume different amounts of certain nutrients to maintain long-term heart health than does a person with no genetic risk of heart disease. The amount of each nutrient required is also dependent on the other nutrients and non-nutrient substances present in the diet. For example, adequate fat is essential for the absorption of vitamin A. The amount of vitamin E that is optimal may be affected by the amount of selenium, vitamin C, and beta-carotene available; the amount of iron absorbed is affected by the presence of vitamin C and calcium. Therefore, it is difficult to make generalizations about how much is enough or too much without considering both individual needs and overall diet.

Effects of Poor Nutrient Intake

Malnutrition Any condition resulting from an energy or nutrient intake either above or below that which is optimal.

Undernutrition Any condition resulting from an energy or nutrient intake below that which meets nutritional needs.

Overnutrition Poor nutritional status resulting from a dietary intake in excess of that which is optimal for health.

Consuming either too much or too little of one or more nutrients or energy can cause **malnutrition** (Figure 1.2). We usually think of malnutrition as **undernutrition,** a deficiency of energy or nutrients. Undernutrition may occur due to a deficient intake of energy or nutrients, increased requirements, or an inability to absorb or use nutrients. Starvation, the most severe form of undernutrition, is a deficiency of energy that causes weight loss, poor growth, the inability to reproduce, and if severe enough, death. Iron deficiency is common in young children and adolescents because their rapid growth increases the need for iron. Older adults are at risk for vitamin B_{12} deficiency because changes in the stomach that often occur with age decrease vitamin B_{12} absorption. When undernutrition is caused by a specific nutrient deficiency the symptoms often reflect the body functions that rely on the deficient nutrient. For example, vitamin A is necessary for vision; a deficiency of vitamin A can result in blindness.

Overnutrition, an excess of nutrients, is also a form of malnutrition. When food is consumed in excess of energy need, the extra is stored as body fat. Some

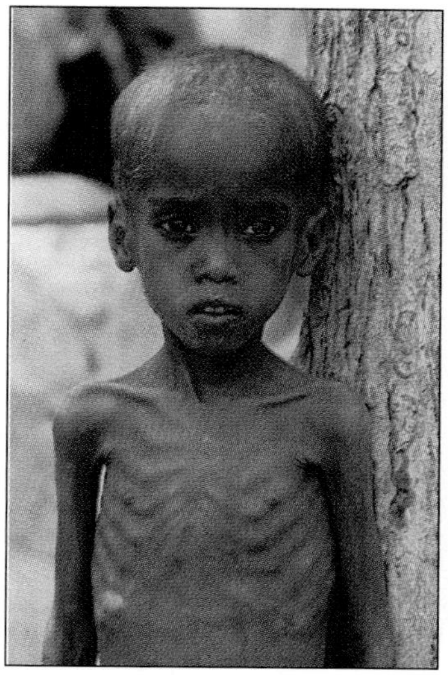
 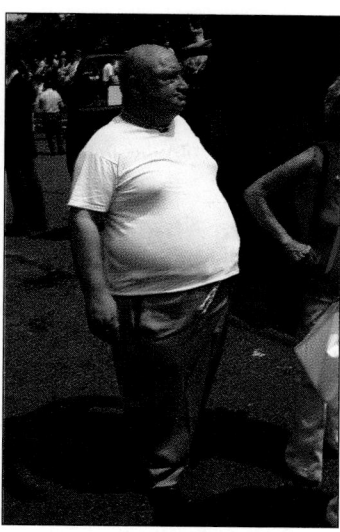

Figure 1.2
Malnutrition includes both undernutrition and overnutrition. (*Left,* Gamma Liaison/Camera Pix. *Right,* © Van Bucher/Photo Researchers, Inc.)

fat is necessary as insulation and an energy store, but an excess of body fat, called obesity, increases the risk for high blood pressure, heart disease, diabetes, and other chronic health problems. When excesses of specific nutrients are consumed, an adverse or **toxic** reaction may occur. Foods generally do not contain high enough concentrations of nutrients to cause a toxic reaction. A rare example of a food that has caused a nutrient toxicity is polar bear liver. It is extremely high in vitamin A. There are reported cases of illness and death among Arctic explorers who consumed it. Most nutrient toxicities result from the overconsumption of vitamin and mineral supplements.

Toxic The capacity to produce injury at some level of intake.

The symptoms of a nutritional deficiency or excess may appear rapidly or take a lifetime to develop. Both short-term and long-term nutritional effects have important health implications. For example, an athlete exercising in hot weather may become dehydrated in a matter of hours, developing symptoms such as headache and dizziness. Drinking water relieves the symptoms as rapidly as they appeared. Nutritional imbalances that take weeks or months to manifest themselves are no less important. For example, if excess energy is consumed, body fat is deposited, but it may take months before a significant amount of weight is gained. Likewise, as anyone who has tried to lose weight knows, it can take months of reduced energy consumption to use up the excess fat.

Risk factor A characteristic or circumstance that is associated with the occurrence of a particular disease.

Nutritional effects that occur over a much longer time are also an important health concern. An individual's nutrient intake today may affect the development of osteoporosis, cancer, or heart disease 20, 30, or 40 years from now. The effects of nutrition on the development of chronic disease are difficult to determine because other variables or **risk factors,** such as age, genetics, and gender, are also often involved. These risk factors cannot be changed, but nutrition is a lifestyle variable that is determined by individual choices.

What Are We Choosing?

We need nutrients to survive—but we eat food, not nutrients (Figure 1.3). There are hundreds of food choices to make and hundreds of reasons for making them. Each of these choices contributes to our total nutrient intake. Some foods are rich in protein and minerals, others in vitamins and phytochemicals. Choosing a healthy diet does not mean you have to give up favorite foods. None of the foods we choose are good or bad in and of themselves, but combined they make up a healthy or a not-so-healthy diet.

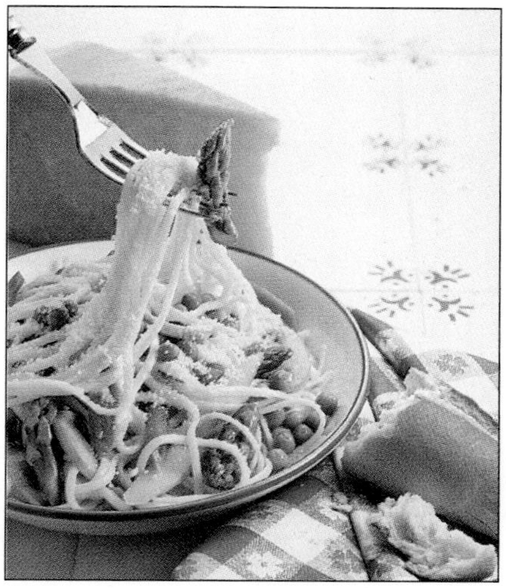

Figure 1.3
We don't eat nutrients, we eat foods that we choose for a variety of reasons including taste, color, and texture. (Charles Gold/The Stock Market)

The reasons for our choices are as varied as the foods we choose to eat: a food tastes good, it's good for us, it isn't bad for us, it costs less, it comes in an appealing package, it's consistent with personal religious practices, it's the kind you always buy, or even because the manufacturer is environmentally responsible and promotes minorities and women.

How Healthy Is the American Diet?

Recommendations for a healthy diet suggest that we should consume a diet that provides about 55 to 60% of energy from carbohydrate, 10 to 15% from protein, and 30% or less from fat. The typical diet in the United States comes close to these recommendations. As a nation we eat about 52% carbohydrate, 15% protein, and 33% fat (Figure 1.4).[1] The percentages of energy from macronutrients in the American diet have improved over the last 20 years. In 1980 we consumed 36% of our energy from fat.[2] Despite this, the American diet is not as healthy as it could be. The diet should be based on whole grains, vegetables, and fruits, with smaller amounts of dairy products and high protein foods and limited amounts of fats and sweets, as illustrated by the Food Guide Pyramid (see Chapter 2 and Figure 1.5a). As a population, we don't eat enough fruits, vegetables, and dairy products.[3] We eat too few whole grains, too little fiber, too much sugar, and we consume more energy than we expend (Figure 1.5). These dietary patterns increase the risk of developing chronic diseases, such as diabetes, obesity, heart disease, and cancer, which are the major causes of illness and death in our population. In the United States today, 16 million adults have diabetes,[4] 35 to 55% of adults are overweight depending on how overweight is defined,[5,6] and heart disease and cancer remain the leading causes of death.[7] Our dietary pattern along with a lack of physical activity are major contributors to these diseases. Recommendations for reducing disease risk focus on changes in the foods we choose. (See *Off the Shelf: What's a Healthy Choice? What's a Healthy Diet?*)

How Do We Make Food Choices?

Why do we choose the foods we do? Most Americans understand that nutrition is important to their health, yet only 39% believe they are doing everything they can to eat healthfully.[8] People don't want to give up their favorite foods and they don't want to eat foods they don't like. Our food choices and food intake are affected not only by nutrient needs but also by what is available to us, where we live, what is within our budget and compatible with our lifestyle, what we like, what is culturally acceptable, what mood we are in, and what we think we should eat.

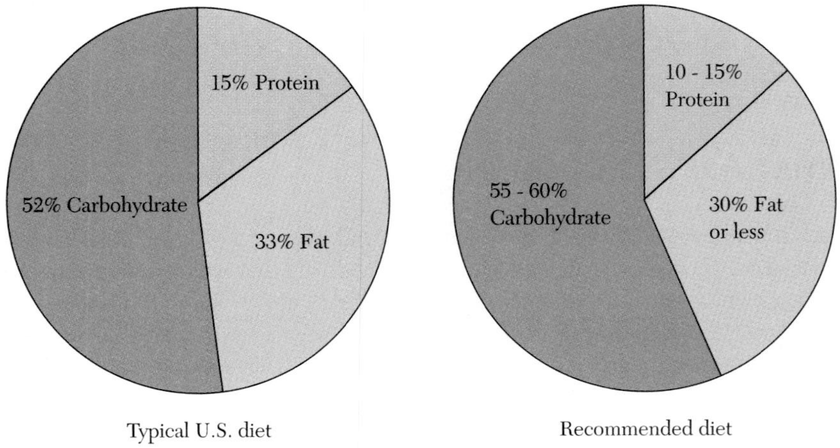

Figure 1.4
Americans are now eating a diet that contains amounts of carbohydrate, fat, and protein that are close to recommendations.

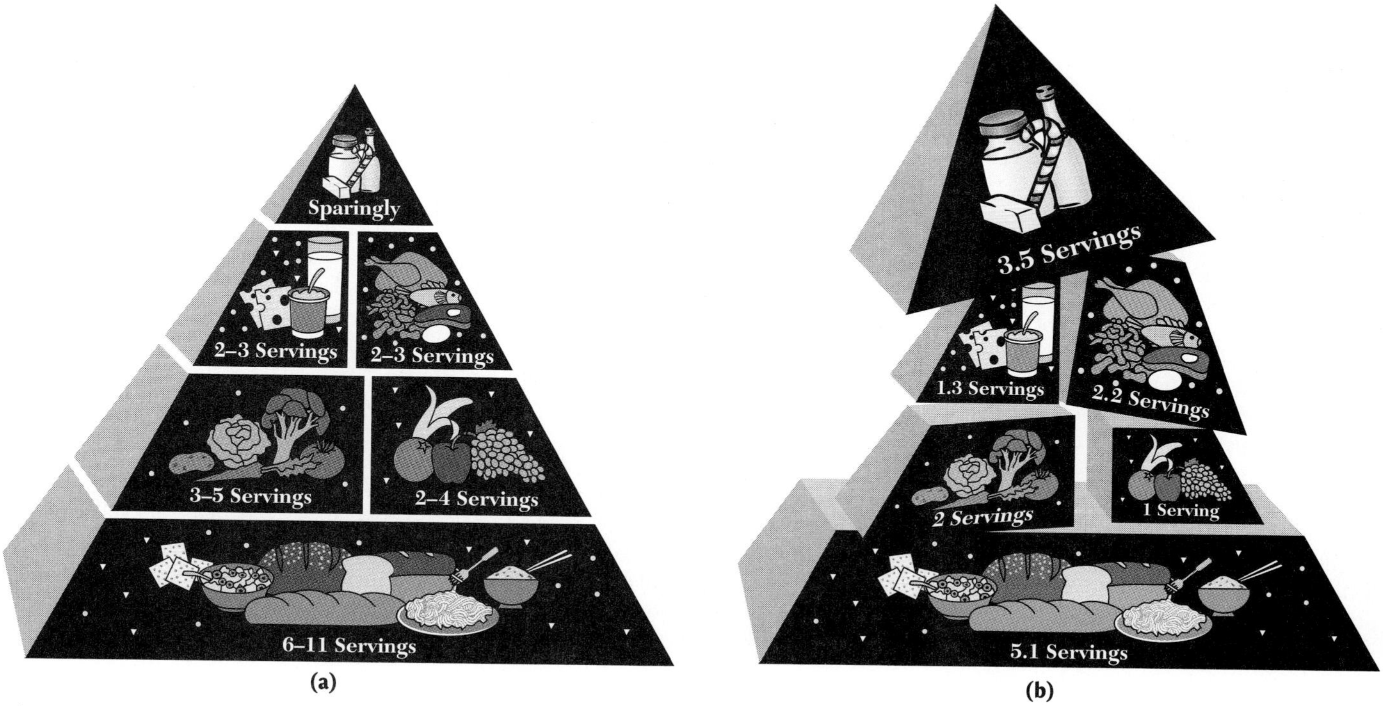

Figure 1.5
(a) The Food Guide Pyramid is a guide for planning diets that meet nutritional recommendations. (b) The typical American diet forms a top-heavy pyramid, with too many fats and sweets and too few fruits and vegetables and grains.

Availability The food available to an individual or a population is affected by geography, socioeconomics, and health status. In many parts of the world, food choices are limited to foods produced locally. Nutrients that are lacking in local foods will be lacking in the population's diet. In more developed parts of the world, the ability to store, transport, and process food allows year-round access to seasonal foods and foods grown and produced at distant locations. Grocery stores stock thousands of items from all over the world (Figure 1.6). Pasta from Italy and chocolates from Switzerland are processed and packaged for sale in North America. Mexican, Chinese, and Japanese foods can be found in Denver and Toronto. Pacific salmon is available in Iowa, and Chilean grapes are sold in Wyoming grocery stores.

Even if foods are available in the store, it doesn't mean that they are available to all individuals. Socioeconomic factors such as income level, living conditions, and lifestyle as well as education affect the types and amounts of foods that are available. Individuals with limited incomes can choose only the types and amounts of foods that they can afford. Individuals who don't own cars can only purchase what they can carry home on the bus or subway. Lack of food storage and cooking facilities affects what foods can be prepared at home. Knowledge of cooking and menu planning can also affect what foods are available. For example, if you don't know how to plan or cook a meal, you are limited to prepared meals and restaurants. Busy lifestyles and full schedules also affect what foods are available. For example, individuals who travel for a living are often forced to eat in restaurants several times a day. Individuals with jobs and families and little time to cook must select foods that can be prepared quickly and simply.

Health status also affects the availability of food. People who cannot carry heavy packages are limited in what they can purchase. People with food allergies,

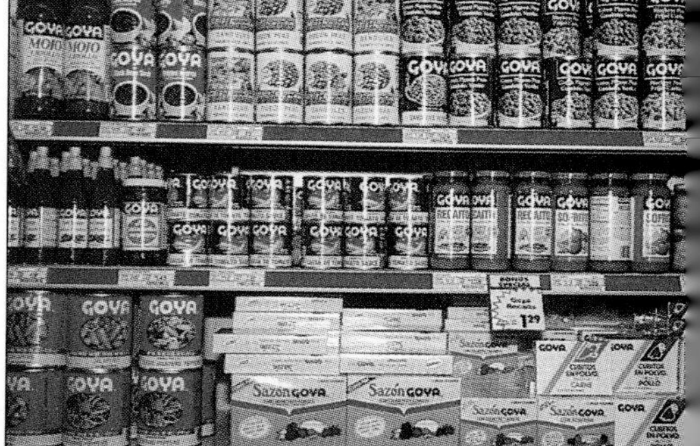

Figure 1.6
Modern processing and transportation make foods from around the world available in local grocery stores. (George Semple)

Off the Shelf

What's a Healthy Choice? What's a Healthy Diet?

Collard greens are rich in vitamin A. Potato chips are high in fat. Does that mean you should eat collard greens every day and swear off potato chips? What if the collard greens are swimming in pork fat? What if the potato chips are fat free? Are they healthy choices then? Can they be part of a healthy diet?

The first step toward making healthy choices is understanding that there is no such thing as a good food or a bad food—any food can be part of a healthy diet. A healthy diet does not need to exclude the foods you love. Whether your cravings are for ice cream or potato chips, you can fit favorite foods into your diet. High-fat foods must be balanced with lower fat choices and sweet treats offset by foods naturally low in sugar. Choosing special foods like fat-free chips, sugar-free soda, or lowfat cookies doesn't guarantee a healthy diet. These foods are lower in fat and/or sugar, but they still add kcalories to the diet and contribute few other nutrients.

A healthy diet is based on grains, fruits, vegetables, milk, and meats or meat substitutes. It includes a wide variety of foods we enjoy. But selecting a diet based on these is not necessarily easy. The multitude of choices that modern food production and processing provides makes choosing difficult. Chicken, rice, and vegetables sounds like a healthy meal. But even purchasing the foods for such a simple meal involves hundreds of decisions that can impact on the overall healthiness and appeal of the diet. Is it lower in fat if you purchase a whole raw chicken, boneless, skinless chicken breasts, or frozen breaded nuggets of chicken? Is brown rice healthier than white because it adds more fiber to the diet? Instant rice is convenient, but is it as nutritious and does it taste good? Is the packaged rice with added flavorings too high in fat and salt? The healthiness of the diet is also a concern when choosing produce. You need to decide not only which vegetable to eat, but whether you want it grown organically and whether to buy it fresh, frozen, or in a can. And variety is important too. Carrots every day is not bad, but a variety of vegetables is even better. Foods like cherimoya, chayote, and bok choy can add variety to your vegetable choices. But how do you prepare them?

A healthy choice can be any choice that is part of an overall healthy diet. For example, fat-free ice cream does not make a diet healthy if the diet's overall fat content is too high and it is low in whole grains, fruits, and vegetables; but a diet rich in whole grains, fruits, and vegetables can still be healthy even if you have regular ice cream for dessert. Subsequent chapters and *Off the Shelf* boxes throughout this text provide information that will help you understand what makes a healthy diet and how to make wise decisions about individual foods and supplements you buy off the shelf.

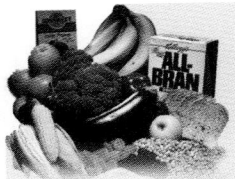

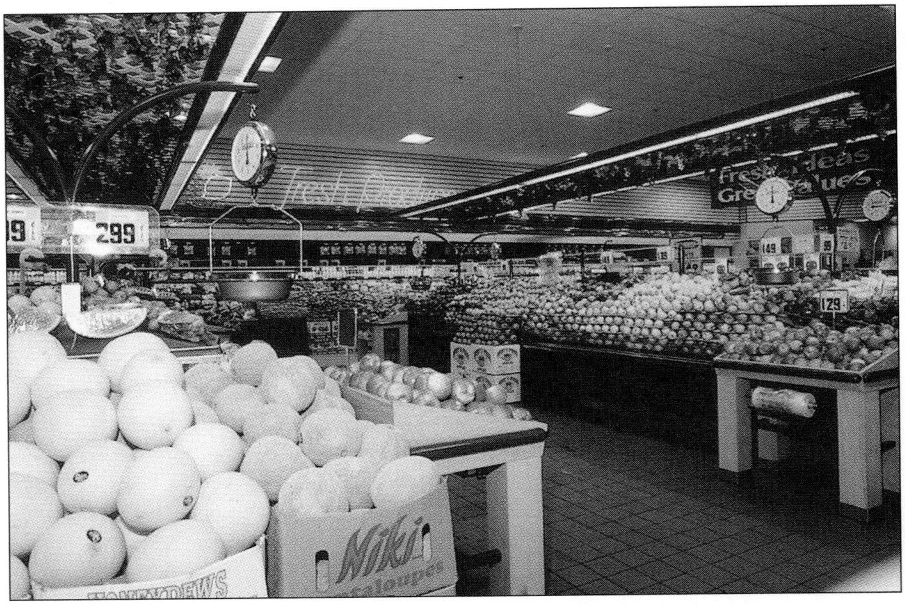

(George Semple)

digestive problems, and dental disease are limited in the foods they can consider for consumption. People consuming special diets for disease conditions are limited to foods that meet their dietary prescriptions.

Personal and Cultural Preferences. Availability affects the foods we have to choose from; but individual palates and convictions determine what we actually consume, and tradition and social values may dictate what foods we consider appropriate. Personal preferences for taste, smell, appearance, and texture affect which foods we select. Presentation and packaging can also affect food choices. If a food doesn't appeal to us, we won't eat it, and if we like it, it is difficult to eliminate from the diet. This is demonstrated by the fact that not wanting to give up the foods they like is the number one reason people give for not choosing a healthier diet.[8]

Food preferences and eating habits are learned as part of each individual's family, cultural, national, and social background. They are among the oldest and most entrenched features of every culture.[9] An individual of Asian descent may consider rice the focus of the meal, whereas Italians may include pasta with every meal. The foods we are exposed to as children influence what foods we buy and cook as adults. If your mother never served artichokes or Swiss chard you may not consider eating them as an adult. If you grow up eating turkey on Thanksgiving and tamales at Christmastime you will likely continue these traditions. Religious background also affects food intake: Seventh-Day Adventists are vegetarians; Jews and Muslims do not eat pork. Even for those who choose not to observe religious dietary rules, habit may dictate many mealtime decisions. Jewish kosher laws prohibit the consumption of meat and milk in the same meal. Even Jews who do not follow kosher law may choose not to serve milk at dinner because they never had it as children.

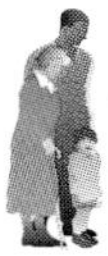

Food is a focus for social interaction and may be a determinant of social acceptance. Peer pressure exerts a tremendous influence on what foods we choose. For an adolescent, stopping for a cheeseburger or taco after school can be the basis for acceptance by one's peers. If all of your peers are choosing fish and chicken, you may not select the 16-ounce steak that you really want. These pressures change as society's values change and can influence food choices.

Food is also an expression and a moderator of mood and emotional states. Some of us eat more when we are upset, while others eat less. Food and certain specific foods are associated with comfort, love, and security.

What We Think We Should Eat Our attitudes about what foods we think are good for us also affect what we choose. We think that low fat is healthy for our hearts, high fiber protects us from cancer, eating less helps us live longer, antioxidants keep us young. . . . The health and nutrition information that shapes our attitudes about what we should and should not eat comes to us in a variety of ways.

Some nutrition information comes from individual contact with physicians and dietitians; some is printed on food labels and in educational pamphlets; but much of it reaches us through television, radio, newspapers, and magazines (Figure 1.7). Mass media are very powerful tools in promoting health and nutrition messages. Information that would take individual health-care workers years to disseminate can reach millions of individuals in a matter of hours or days. Although dietitians and physicians are viewed as the most valuable source of nutrition information, Americans today get most of their food and nutrition information from television, magazines, and newspapers.[8] Much of this information is reliable, but the nutrition messages promoted by the mass media can be misleading. The motivation for news stories is often to sell subscriptions or improve ratings, not to promote the nutritional health of the population. Some nutrition and health information originates from food manufacturers. It is usually in the form of marketing and advertising designed to sell existing products or target new ones. This promotional information can be confusing to the consumer, who may not know how to interpret it. For instance, the scientific evidence that reducing dietary fat intake can protect you from heart disease and help maintain a healthy weight has created a vast market for products low in fat. Food manufacturers responded by creating fat-free, lowfat, and reduced-fat products at an astonishing rate. Weight- and health-conscious consumers responded by increasing their consumption of fat-free foods, but the girth of American waists continued to increase. The message that reducing fat intake promotes health was received, but consumers did not understand that fat-free foods are not kcalorie free and simply adding lowfat foods to the diet was not a prescription for good health. Knowing what information to believe and how to use this information to choose a diet can be difficult. (See *Off the Label: Read the Whole Label to Know What You Are Choosing.*)

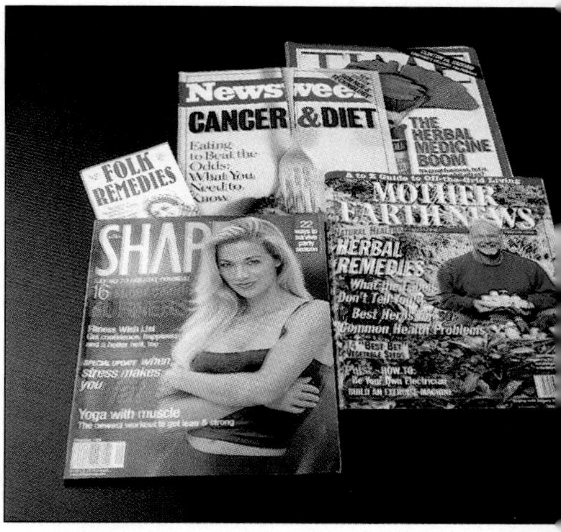

Figure 1.7
Nutrition information often makes the headlines but does not always provide an accurate presentation of new discoveries. (George Semple)

Off the Label

Read the Whole Label to Know What You Are Choosing

Healthy! Fresh! Light! The first thing that may catch your eye when shopping is a large-print banner describing some nutritious feature of a product. Food labels with eye-catching banners and names sell better. Although food labels must conform to federal guidelines and use standard definitions for most terms, they can still be misleading. Understanding what these terms mean on food labels will help you know what you are choosing and how it fits into your diet.

Many of these descriptors highlight individual nutrients, and just as no single food determines the healthiness of a diet, no single nutrient makes a food good or bad for you. Look beyond the banner and see what other contribution the food makes to your diet. For example, chocolate cookies labeled "fat free" may not be your best choice if you are trying to reduce your sugar intake or increase the amount of fiber in your diet. A food labeled "fresh" may sound appealing. Any raw food that has not been frozen, heat processed, or otherwise preserved can be labeled fresh. The term "fresh" however, doesn't provide any information about the nutrient content of the product or how long it took for this food to travel from the farm to the grocery store shelf. "Healthy" is another attractive byline that applies to more than a single nutrient. It implies that the product is wholesome and nutritious. In fact, to use the term "healthy" a food must be low in fat and saturated fat, contain no more than 360 mg of sodium and 60 mg of cholesterol per serving, and be a good source of one or more important nutrients. Since vegetables, fruits, and grain products are an important part of a healthy diet, fresh fruits and vegetables and some canned and frozen ones as well as enriched grain products may be labeled healthy even if they are not a good source of one or more of the specified nutrients.[1] While all of the qualities specified by the term "healthy" are part of a healthy diet, foods that fit this definition are not necessarily the basis for a healthy diet. For instance, some fat-free brownies fit the labeling definition of healthy. They are low in fat, saturated fat, cholesterol, and sodium, and supply 10% of the recommended intake for iron. But they are only a good choice in limited quantities because they are high in sugar and contain few other nutrients. Likewise, a food that doesn't meet the labeling definition of healthy is not necessarily a poor choice. Vegetable soup, for example, contains more sodium than the definition of healthy will allow, but if the rest of the diet is not high in sodium, the soup can be a healthy choice.

Enticing product names can also be misleading. However, unless you have memorized the U.S. Department of Agriculture (USDA) and Food and Drug Administration (FDA) labeling regulations you can't tell exactly what you are buying. These standards determine how much beef is in a beef enchilada, how much chicken is in chicken soup, and how much fruit is in a Fruit Roll-Up. Product names must comply with legal definitions, but they don't have to make sense to consumers. For example, "lasagna with meat sauce" must be 6% meat, but "lasagna with meat and sauce" must be 12% meat.

To get the whole picture, you need to look beyond the healthy sounding banner and the name of the product. Since the nutrient content of foods must be listed, as well as information on how a food fits into the diet as a whole, reading the label thoroughly will provide you with the information you need to make wise choices. Chapter 2 and *Off the Label* boxes throughout this book provide more information on how to read food labels.

[1]More foods can carry 'healthy' label. FDA Consumer 32:2, July–Aug. 1998.

WHAT IS RELIABLE NUTRITION INFORMATION?

We are bombarded with nutrition information. Some of what we hear is accurate and some of it is incorrect or exaggerated to sell products or make news headlines more enticing: oat bran lowers cholesterol, beta-carotene prevents cancer, obesity is genetic, vitamin C cures the common cold, vitamin E slows aging. Sifting through this information and distinguishing the useful from the useless may seem overwhelming. An understanding of the process of science and how it is used to study the relationship between nutrition and health will allow you to develop the nutrition sense needed to judge the validity of nutrition headlines.

Understanding the Process of Science: The Scientific Method

Scientific method The general approach of science that is used to explain observations about the world around us.

Advances in nutrition are made using the **scientific method.** The scientific method offers a systematic, unbiased approach to evaluating the relationships between food and health. The first step of the scientific method is to make an observation and ask questions about the observation. The next step is to propose an

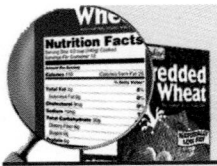

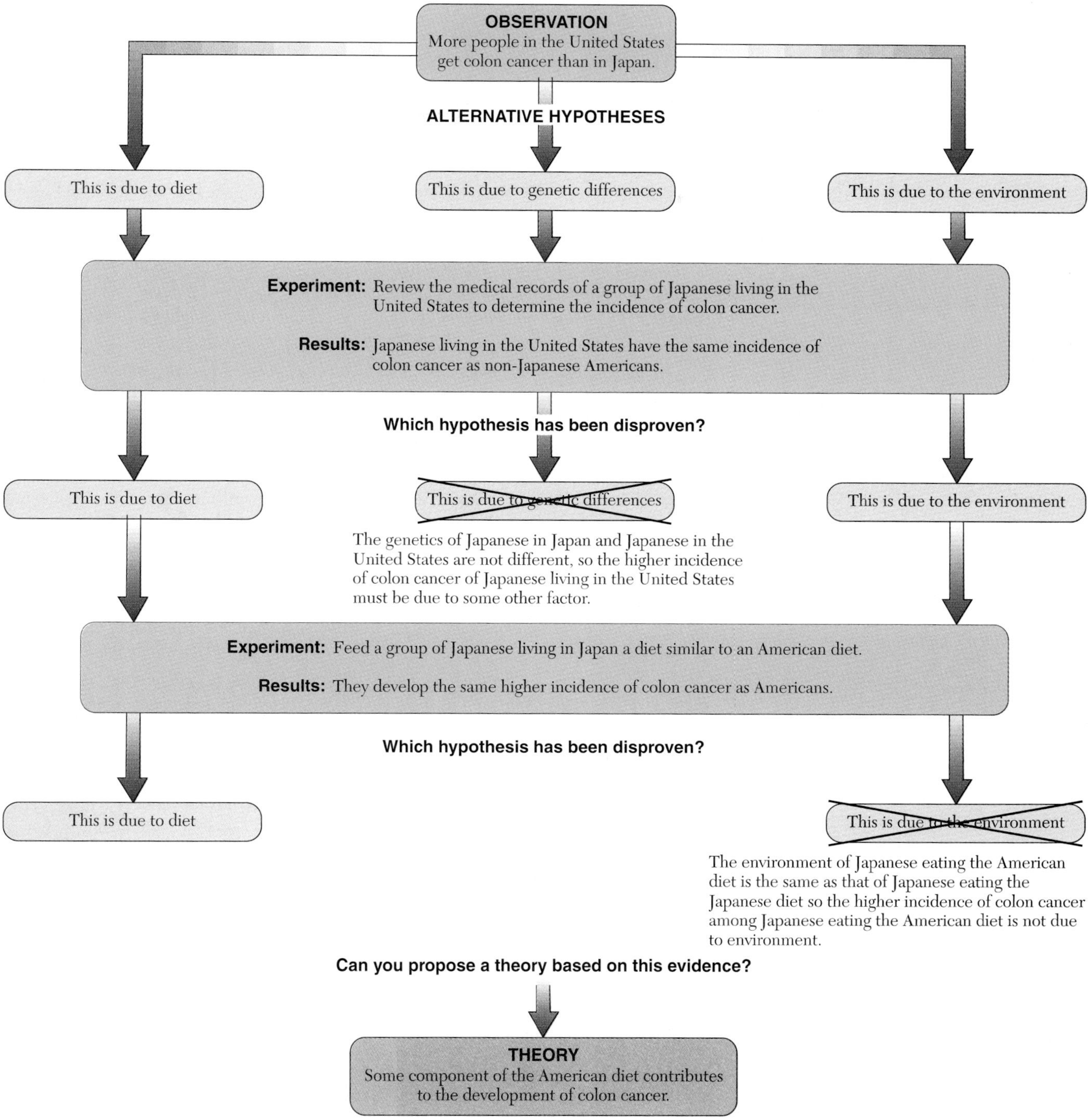
OBSERVATION
More people in the United States get colon cancer than in Japan.
ALTERNATIVE HYPOTHESES
This is due to diet
This is due to genetic differences
This is due to the environment
Experiment: Review the medical records of a group of Japanese living in the United States to determine the incidence of colon cancer.
Results: Japanese living in the United States have the same incidence of colon cancer as non-Japanese Americans.
Which hypothesis has been disproven?
This is due to diet
This is due to genetic differences
This is due to the environment
The genetics of Japanese in Japan and Japanese in the United States are not different, so the higher incidence of colon cancer of Japanese living in the United States must be due to some other factor.
Experiment: Feed a group of Japanese living in Japan a diet similar to an American diet.
Results: They develop the same higher incidence of colon cancer as Americans.
Which hypothesis has been disproven?
This is due to diet
This is due to the environment
The environment of Japanese eating the American diet is the same as that of Japanese eating the Japanese diet so the higher incidence of colon cancer among Japanese eating the American diet is not due to environment.
Can you propose a theory based on this evidence?
THEORY
Some component of the American diet contributes to the development of colon cancer.

Figure 1.8
This example illustrates how the scientific method can be used to formulate hypotheses based on observations, design experiments to test these hypotheses, and interpret the results to support or disprove the hypotheses, helping establish a theory.

explanation for the observation. This explanation is called a **hypothesis.** Once a hypothesis has been proposed, experiments can be designed to test it. The experiments must provide objective results that can be measured and repeated. If the experimental results do not prove the hypothesis to be wrong, a **theory,** or a scientific explanation based on experimentation, can be established (Figure 1.8). Scientific theories are accepted only as long as they cannot be disproved and continue to be supported by all new evidence that accumulates. Even a theory that has been accepted by the scientific community for years can be proved wrong.

Hypothesis An educated guess made to explain an observation or to answer a question.

Theory An explanation based on scientific study and reasoning.

This flux allows the body of knowledge to increase, but it can be confusing as old theories give way to new ones.

The discovery of the relationship between nutrition and pellagra, a disease now known to be caused by a deficiency of the vitamin niacin, is an example of how the scientific method has been used in nutrition research. The events leading to this discovery began with the observation that prisoners suffered from pellagra, but their jailers did not. If pellagra was an infectious disease, both populations would be equally affected. The hypothesis proposed was that pellagra was due to a deficiency in the prisoners' diets. To test this hypothesis, nutritious foods such as fresh meats and vegetables were added to the diet of prisoners. The symptoms of pellagra disappeared, supporting the hypothesis that pellagra is due to a deficiency of something in the diet. This experiment and others led to the theory that pellagra is caused by a dietary deficiency. This theory, further developed by the discovery of the vitamin niacin, still holds today.

For the scientific method to generate reliable theories, the experiments done to test hypotheses must generate reliable results and be interpreted accurately. The public hears about nutrition-related experiments in the news, and reads about them in magazines or in advertisements and promotional material for nutritional products. For example, the advertisement for Power Boost illustrated in Figure 1.9 discusses one study which supports its claim to increase muscle mass and decrease body fat. Was this experiment conducted properly? Do the results mean that Power Boost will increase your muscle mass?

What Makes a Good Experiment? A well-conducted experiment must use objective measurements, proper experimental controls, and the right experimental population.

Objective Measurements Scientific experiments are designed to provide measurable data that can be quantified and repeated. For instance, how much people weigh and how high their blood pressure is are parameters that can be measured reliably. Feelings are more difficult to assess. They can be quantified with standardized tests, but people's statements about how they feel are considered subjective, rather than objective. Subjective claims that come from individual testimonies or opinions, referred to as **anecdotal,** have not been measured objectively. In the Power Boost ad, the quotes from users who report increased muscle strength and pumped-up motivation are anecdotal and are not objective measures. The increase in muscle mass and loss of fat determined by underwater weighing are objective measurements that can be quantified and repeated.

Anecdotal Information based on a story of personal experience.

Proper Controls **Experimental controls** ensure that each factor or **variable** studied can be compared with a known situation. A **control group** acts as a standard of comparison for the treatment being tested. A control group is treated in the same way as the **experimental groups** except no experimental treatment is implemented. For example, in the experiment described in the Power Boost ad the experimental group consists of athletes consuming the Power Boost drink for four weeks. An appropriate control group would consist of athletes of similar age, gender, and ability eating similar diets and following similar workout regimens, but not consuming Power Boost. Both groups would have their body fat measured before and after the four-week period.

In order to make the control and experimental groups indistinguishable, a **placebo** is sometimes used. A placebo is a treatment that is identical in appearance to the actual treatment but has no therapeutic value. In the Power Boost example (Figure 1.9), the experimental group is consuming a protein drink. An appropriate placebo for the control group would be a drink that looks and tastes just like Power Boost but doesn't contribute any nutrients. By using a placebo, participants in the experiment would not know if they are receiving the actual supplement. When the subjects do not know which treatment they are receiving,

Experimental controls Factors included in an experimental design that limit the number of variables, allowing an investigator to examine the effect of only the parameters of interest.

Variable A factor or condition that is changed in an experimental setting.

Control groups Groups of participants in an experiment that are identical to the experimental group except that no experimental treatment is used. They are used as a basis of comparison.

Experimental groups Groups of participants in an experiment who are subjected to an experimental treatment.

Placebo A fake medicine or supplement that is indistinguishable in appearance from the real thing. It is used to disguise the control and experimental groups in an experiment.

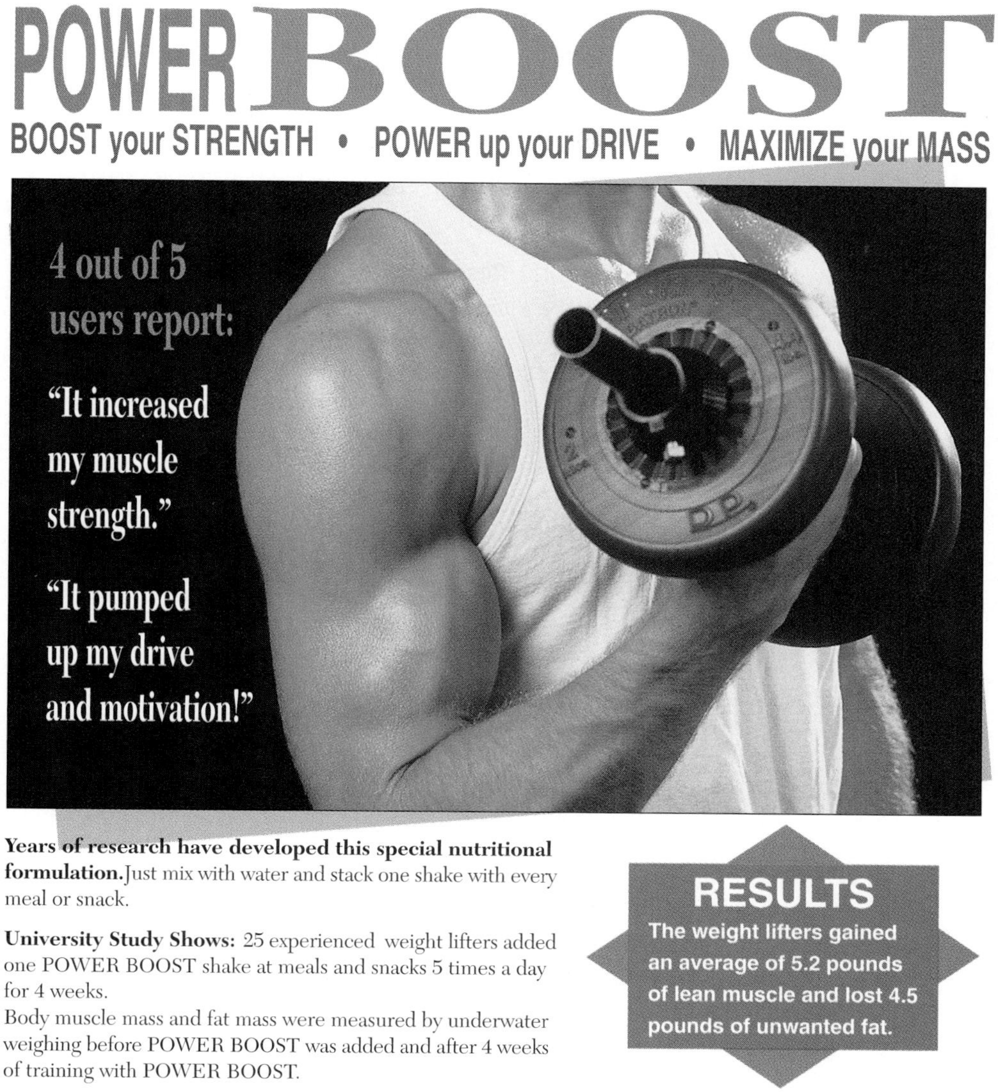
POWER BOOST
BOOST your STRENGTH • POWER up your DRIVE • MAXIMIZE your MASS
4 out of 5 users report:
"It increased my muscle strength."
"It pumped up my drive and motivation!"
Years of research have developed this special nutritional formulation. Just mix with water and stack one shake with every meal or snack.
University Study Shows: 25 experienced weight lifters added one POWER BOOST shake at meals and snacks 5 times a day for 4 weeks.
Body muscle mass and fat mass were measured by underwater weighing before POWER BOOST was added and after 4 weeks of training with POWER BOOST.
RESULTS
The weight lifters gained an average of 5.2 pounds of lean muscle and lost 4.5 pounds of unwanted fat.

Figure 1.9 This hypothetical advertisement illustrates the types of nutrition claims that consumers must be prepared to evaluate. (Lawrence Migdale/Photo Researchers, Inc.)

the study is called a **single-blind study.** Using a placebo in a single-blind study helps to prevent the expectations of subjects from biasing the results. For example, if the athletes think they are taking Power Boost, they may be convinced that they are getting stronger and as a result work harder in their training, and develop bigger muscles even without the supplement. Errors can also occur if investigators allow their own desire for a specific result to affect the interpretation of the data. This type of error can be avoided by designing a **double-blind study,** in which neither the subjects nor the investigators know who is in which group until after the results have been analyzed.

Single-blind study An experiment in which either the study participants or the researchers are unaware of who is in a control or an experimental group.

Double-blind study An experiment in which neither the study participants nor the researchers know who is in a control or an experimental group.

The Appropriate Experimental Population In order for an experiment to produce reliable results, it must be conducted in the right population. Therefore, if Power Boost claims to improve performance in trained athletes, it should be tested on trained athletes.

The number of subjects included in a study is also important. To be successful, an experiment must show that the treatment being tested causes a result to occur more frequently than it would occur by chance. Fewer subjects are needed to demonstrate an effect that rarely occurs by chance. For example, if only one person in a million can increase muscle mass by weight training for four weeks, then the experiment to see if Power Boost increases muscle mass in athletes weight training for four weeks would require only a few subjects to demonstrate an effect. If one in four athletes can improve his muscle mass by weight training for four weeks, then many more subjects are needed. Statistical methods should be applied before a study is conducted to determine how many subjects are needed to show the effect of the experimental treatment. The number of subjects will depend on the type of study and the effect being tested. The fewer variables included in a study, the fewer experimental subjects needed to demonstrate an effect.

Interpretation of Experimental Results In science, the interpretation of results is as important as the way studies are done. If Power Boost is tested in experienced weight lifters, the product cannot claim that it will help novices in the gym. One way to ensure that experiments are correctly interpreted is to use a **peer-review** system. Most scientific journals require that reports of studies be reviewed by two or three experts in the field who did not take part in the research that is being evaluated. Before an article can be published in the journal, these scientists must agree that the experiments were well conducted and that the results were interpreted fairly. Nutrition articles can be found in peer-reviewed journals such as *The American Journal of Clinical Nutrition, The Journal of Nutrition, Journal of the American Dietetic Association, The New England Journal of Medicine,* and *International Journal of Sport Nutrition.*

Peer review Review of the design and validity of a research experiment by experts in the field of study who did not participate in the research.

How Scientists Study Nutrition

Nutrition research studies are done to determine nutrient requirements, to learn more about the metabolism of nutrients, and to understand the role of nutrition in health and disease. Perfect tools do not exist for addressing all these questions. However, many types of research can be useful, including epidemiological observations, human intervention studies, and a variety of types of laboratory studies.

Epidemiological Observations **Epidemiology** is the study of patterns that occur within populations. In nutrition, epidemiological studies are used to suggest relationships between diet and health. For instance, epidemiology can be used to estimate nutrient needs by examining the typical intake of a nutrient in a healthy population. **Cross-sectional data** can be collected from a cross section of the population at one point in time, or **longitudinal data** can be collected from the same group of individuals over a period of time.

Epidemiology does not determine cause and effect relationships—it just identifies patterns. For instance, epidemiology was used to identify the association, or **correlation,** between high-fat diets and heart disease. This was done by looking at the incidence of heart disease in different countries and then finding dietary factors that follow the same pattern (Figure 1.10). From the observation that populations with high dietary fat intakes also have high incidences of heart disease, one possible hypothesis is that a high intake of fat in the diet predisposes to cardiovascular disease. This hypothesis must then be tested by controlled intervention and laboratory studies.

Epidemiology The study of the interrelationships between health and disease and other factors in the environment or lifestyle of different populations.

Cross-sectional data Information obtained by a single broad sampling of many different individuals in a population.

Longitudinal data Information obtained by repeatedly sampling the same individuals in a population over time.

Correlation Two or more factors occurring together.

Human Intervention Studies The observations and hypotheses that come from epidemiology can be tested in human **intervention studies.** This type of experiment actively intervenes in the lives of individuals in a population and examines the effect of this intervention. Nutrition intervention studies generally explore the effects of altering people's diets. For example, if it is determined by epidemiology that populations who eat a lowfat diet have a lower incidence of heart disease, an intervention trial may be designed with an experimental group that consumes a diet lower in fat than is typical in the population and a control group that consumes the typical higher fat diet. The groups can be monitored to see if the dietary intervention affects the incidence of heart disease over the long term.

Intervention study A study of a population in which there is an experimental manipulation of some members of the population; observations and measurements are made to determine the effects of this manipulation.

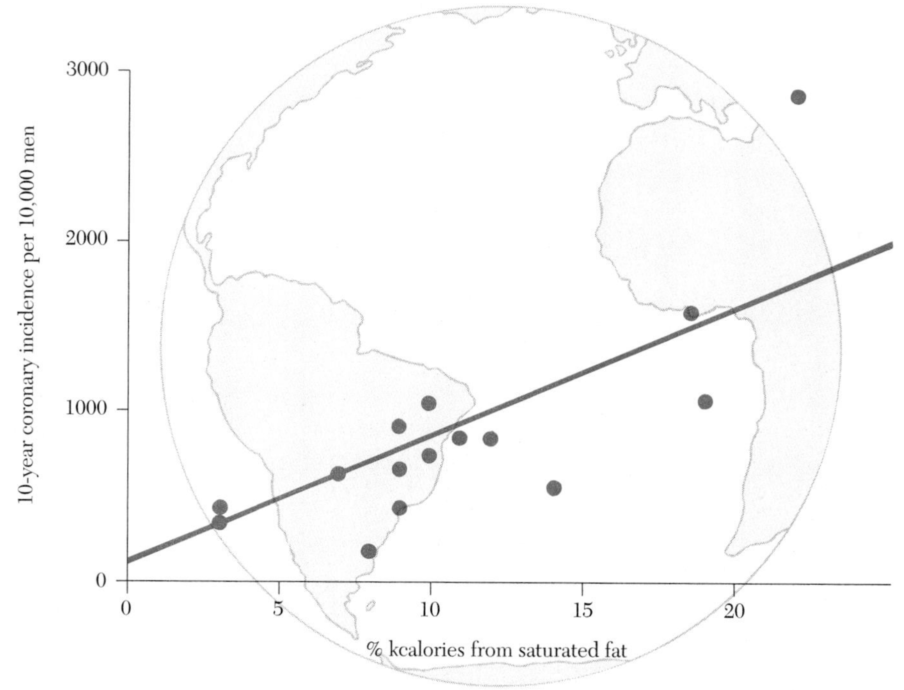

Figure 1.10
This graph shows the incidence of coronary heart disease versus the amount of saturated fat in the diet of different populations. As the amount of saturated fat in the diet increases, so does the incidence of coronary heart disease. (Keys, A. *Seven Countries: A Multivariate Analysis of Deaths and Coronary Heart Disease.* Cambridge, MA: Harvard University Press, 1980)

Laboratory Studies Laboratory studies are used to test hypotheses; to learn more about how nutrients function; and to evaluate the relationships among nutrient intake, levels of nutrients in the body, and health. They may study nutrient requirements and functions in whole organisms, or they may focus on nutrient functions at the cellular level. Some studies of human nutrition use animals to model what may happen in people.

Studies Using Whole Organisms Many nutrition studies are done by feeding a specific diet to a person or animal and monitoring the physiological effects of that diet. **Depletion-repletion studies** are a classic method for studying the functions of nutrients and estimating the requirement of a particular nutrient. They involve depleting a nutrient by feeding a subject a diet devoid of that nutrient. After a period of time, if the nutrient is essential, symptoms of a deficiency will develop. The symptoms provide information on how the nutrient is functioning in the body. The nutrient is then added back to the diet, or repleted, until the symptoms are reversed. The requirement for that nutrient is the amount needed to reverse the deficiency symptoms. For example, depletion of magnesium from the diet causes a lack of muscle coordination. This tells scientists that magnesium is needed for muscle contraction. When enough magnesium is again added to the diet, muscle control returns; the requirement for magnesium is determined to be the amount of magnesium needed to return muscle control to normal.

Depletion-repletion study A study that feeds a diet devoid of a nutrient until signs of deficiency appear, and then adds the nutrient back to the diet to a level at which symptoms disappear.

Another method for determining nutrient functions and requirements is to compare the intake of a nutrient with its excretion. This type of study is known as a **balance study.** If more of a nutrient is consumed than is excreted, it is assumed that the nutrient is being used or stored by the body. If more of the nutrient is excreted than is consumed, some is being lost from body stores. When the amount consumed equals the amount lost, the body is neither gaining nor losing that nutrient and is said to be in balance (Figure 1.11). By varying the amount of a nutrient consumed and then measuring the amount excreted, it is possible to determine the minimum amount of that nutrient needed to replace the body losses. This minimum amount is set as the requirement.

Balance study A study that compares the total amount of a nutrient that enters the body with the total amount that leaves the body.

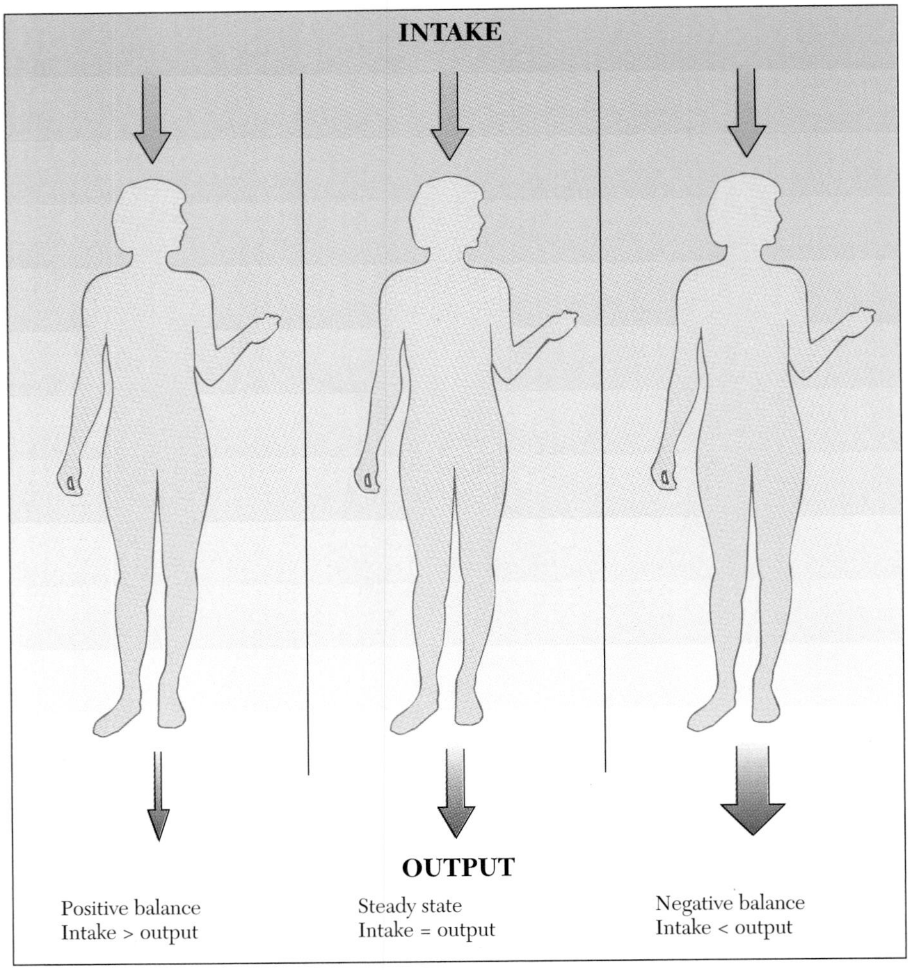

Figure 1.11
The concept of nutrient balance is illustrated here. If more of a nutrient is consumed than excreted, balance is positive; if the same amount is consumed and excreted, balance or a steady state exists; and if less is consumed than excreted, balance is negative.

Molecular biology The study of cellular function at the molecular level.

DNA (deoxyribonucleic acid) The genetic material that codes for the synthesis of proteins.

Gene A length of DNA that provides instructions for heritable traits.

Studies Using Cells More information about what nutrients do at the cellular level can be obtained using biochemical and molecular biological techniques to study cells either extracted from humans or animals or grown in the laboratory (Figure 1.12). Biochemistry studies how nutrients are used for energy and how they regulate chemical reactions in cells. **Molecular biology** studies how **DNA (deoxyribonucleic acid),** the genetic material in cells, dictates and regulates the functions of body cells. The types and amounts of nutrients available to cells can affect the action of DNA. Certain nutrients, such as vitamin A, can directly activate or inactivate segments of DNA called **genes.** Using molecular biology to study nutrition helps to explain nutrient function and identify processes that can be influenced by inadequate or excessive nutrient supplies. For example, molecular biology can be used to explore how vitamin A deficiency affects vision by studying genes related to the eye that are altered by a vitamin A-deficient diet.

Knowledge gained from studying molecules and genes can be used to study nutrition-related conditions that affect the entire organism. For example, molecular biology helps us understand the hereditary basis of diseases like heart disease, cancer, and obesity. These advances are enhancing our understanding of diet-disease relationships and enable us to identify individuals who are susceptible to specific diseases so that intervention can begin early. For example, it may someday be possible to identify individuals at high risk of developing heart disease by analyzing their DNA. These individuals could then modify their diet and lifestyle to delay or prevent disease onset.

Why Use Animals to Study Human Nutrition? Ideally, studies of human nutrition should be done in humans. A well-controlled human balance study involves measuring all the nutrients that subjects consume and collecting and analyzing all sources of nutrient losses, including urine, feces, sweat, sloughed skin and hair, and other body secretions. Study subjects must be housed under carefully controlled conditions for lengthy periods. Because studying humans is costly, time consuming, inconvenient for subjects, and in some cases impossible for ethical reasons, many studies are done in animals.

An ideal animal model is one with metabolic and digestive processes similar to those in humans. For example, cows are rarely used in human nutrition research because they digest their food in four stomach-like chambers as opposed to a single stomach. Pigs, on the other hand, are a good model because they digest food in a manner similar to that of humans. However, in addition to digestion and metabolism, factors such as cost and time must be considered. Pigs and other large animals are expensive to use, and they take a long time to develop nutrient deficiencies. Smaller laboratory animals, such as rats and mice, are therefore the most common experimental animals. They are inexpensive, have short life spans, reproduce quickly, and the effects of nutritional changes develop rapidly. Their food intake can be easily controlled and their excretions measured accurately using special cages. Even when using small animals, the species of animal must be carefully chosen. For example, rats are more resistant to heart disease than are humans, so they are not a good model for studying the effect of diet on heart disease. Rabbits, on the other hand, do develop heart disease and can be used to study diet–heart disease relationships. Both rabbits and rats, however, are poor choices for a study of vitamin C requirements because they can synthesize this vitamin. Guinea pigs would be a better choice because the guinea pig is one of the few animals, other than humans, that cannot make vitamin C in its body (Figure 1.13). Even the best animal model is not the same as a human, and care must be taken when extrapolating the results to the human population. For example, a study that uses rats to show that a calcium supplement increases bone density can hypothesize, but not conclude, that the supplement will have the same effect in humans.

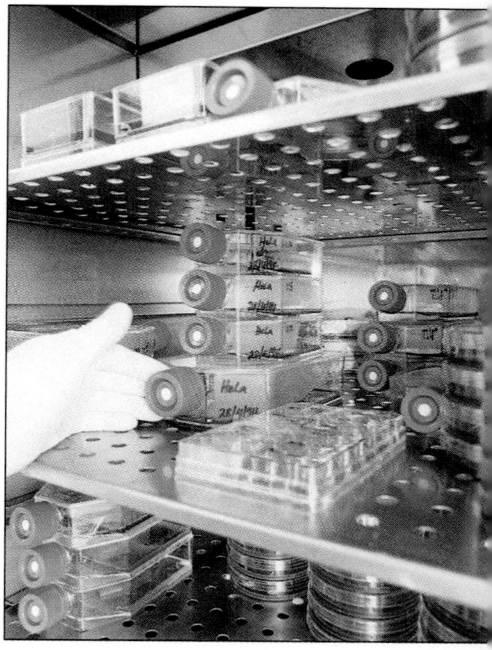

Figure 1.12
With technological advances, more and more research is being done using cells grown in the laboratory. *(James King-Holmes/Science Photo Library/Photo Researchers, Inc.)*

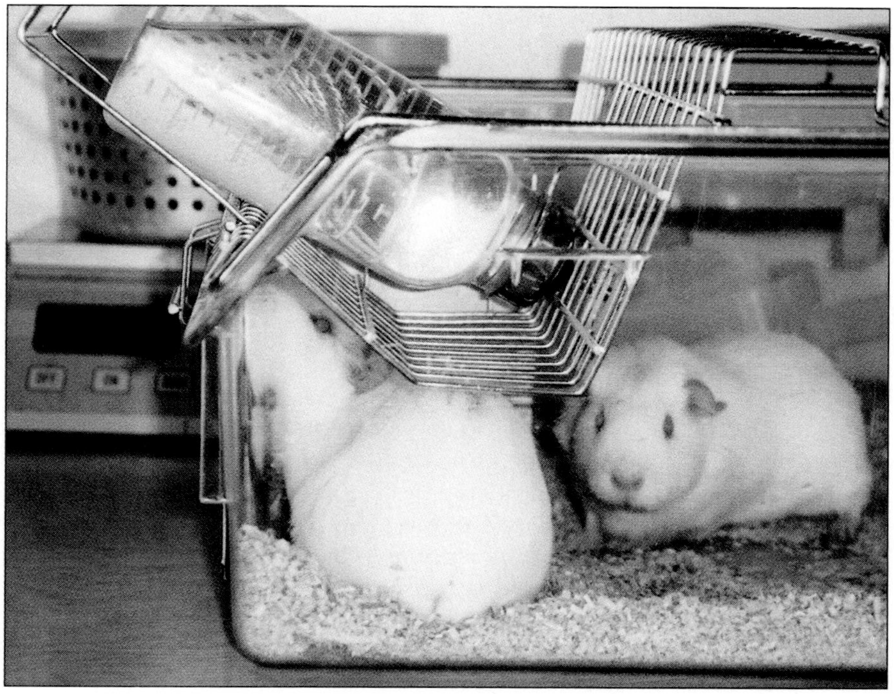

Figure 1.13
Laboratory animals, such as these guinea pigs, are used to study human nutrition. (Lori Smolin)

Ethical Concerns In order to better understand human nutrition scientists keep people in research facilities for months at a time; dissect rats; extract human cells and grow them in the laboratory; and alter human, animal, and plant genes. The ethics of all of these methods has been questioned. To avoid these issues, researchers use alternatives to humans or animals whenever possible. For example, some types of research now use computer models to predict how changes in nutrient intake affect body processes. Such alternatives cannot always be used—therefore, human and animal experimentation is still necessary to answer many questions. To protect the rights of humans and animals used in experimental research, government guidelines have been developed.

To conduct an experiment using human subjects, the study must first be reviewed by a human-use committee of scientists and nonscientists. The committee is responsible for ensuring that the rights of the subjects are respected and that the risk of physical, social, and psychological injury is balanced against the potential benefit of the research. This was not always the case. Much of what we know today about the effects of starvation in humans was determined during World War II by conducting depletion-repletion studies using conscientious objectors as experimental subjects. These subjects were monitored physically and psychologically while they were starved and then refed. Because starvation causes physical discomfort, these individuals experienced some level of suffering during the trials and risked longer lasting physical and psychological harm.

As with experiments involving humans, the federal government mandates that panels of scientists review experiments that propose to use animals. These panels consider whether the need for animals is justified and whether all precautions will be taken to avoid pain and suffering. Animal housing and handling is strictly regulated and a violation of these guidelines can close a research facility.

When studies are conducted using animal or human cells grown in the laboratory, individual people and animals are rarely harmed, but ethical issues still arise regarding the manipulation of genes. One concern relates more to the environment than to the consumer. Because the chemical makeup of DNA is similar in all living things, molecular biology can transfer genes from one species to another, creating characteristics in an organism that are unlikely to have arisen in nature. There is concern that organisms with these characteristics could find their way into the environment and affect the ecology of the planet. For example, if fish on a fish farm that are engineered to grow faster and produce more young escape into the wild, they might have an adaptive advantage over their wild relatives and ultimately eliminate other fish in their environment. Another concern is the ethics of cloning animals—producing exact copies. This has been done in sheep and mice and is theoretically possible in humans. This would allow the mass production of individuals with selected desirable characteristics—a scenario that has thus far only been the topic of science fiction. Although the benefits of genetic manipulation are huge, ranging from identifying genetic risks to curing genetic diseases, the ethics of manipulating genes is constantly being discussed to ensure the development of effective guidelines regarding the genetic manipulation of plant, animal, and human cells.

Judging Nutrition Information

Nutrition, like all science, continues to develop as new discoveries provide clues to the right combination of nutrients needed for optimal health. As knowledge and technology advance, new nutrition principles are developed. Sometimes, established beliefs and concepts must give way to new ideas. Yesterday's truths can be difficult to unlearn. Some of the nutrition principles we follow today would have seemed ridiculous to our great-grandparents and someday may be a source of humor to our great-grandchildren. One hundred and fifty years ago, fresh fruits and vegetables were thought to cause cholera; today, their use is promoted to reduce the risk of disease. As knowledge advances, recommendations change. Consumers may find this frustrating because the experts seem to change their minds so often. One day you are told margarine is better for you than butter; the next day a report says that it is just as bad. Which should you believe? Who are the experts?

Just as scientists use the scientific method to expand their understanding of the world around us, each of us can use an understanding of how science is done to evaluate nutrition claims. For example, the advertisement for Power Boost illustrated in Figure 1.9 states that this product contains protein essential for maximum weight-lifting performance. It claims to increase your muscle mass, decrease body fat, improve strength, and increase your drive. These claims are certainly appealing, but must be evaluated before they can be accepted.

Does the Information Make Sense? The first question to ask yourself when evaluating a nutrition claim is, Does the information make sense? (See Table 1.4.) Some claims are too outrageous to be true. If, for example, Power Boost had claimed to increase muscle mass and decrease body fat in only one week with no exercise or change in diet, common sense should tell you it is too good to be true. The claim that it will increase muscle mass over a four-week period with a strict training regimen is not so outrageous.

Where Did the Information Come From? If the claim seems reasonable, look to see where it came from. Was it a government recommendation or advice from a health professional? Was it the result of a research study, or one person's opinion? Is it in a news story or an advertising promotion?

Government recommendations regarding healthy dietary practices are developed by committees of scientists who interpret the latest well-conducted research studies and use their conclusions to develop recommendations for the population as a whole. The government provides information about food safety and recommendations on food choices and the amounts of specific nutrients needed to avoid nutrient deficiencies and excesses and to prevent chronic diseases. These recommendations are used to develop food-labeling regulations and are the basis for public health policies and programs. They are published in pamphlets and brochures designed for consumers.

Table 1.4 *Questions to Ask When Judging Nutrition Claims*

1. Does the information make sense?
    - Is it too outrageous to believe?
    - Is it based on a cultural or religious belief?
2. Where did the information come from?
    - Is it based on a government recommendation?
    - Is it based on a study in a peer-reviewed journal?
    - Is it based on the opinions of qualified individuals?
    - Is it based on personal experience?
3. Were the experiments well designed?
    - Were proper controls used?
    - Were enough study subjects used to get reliable results?
    - Were the experimental results interpreted correctly?
    - Was the importance of the study exaggerated?
4. Can the information be applied to humans?
    - Was the study done in animals?
    - Was the level of food or nutrient used compatible with amounts in a human diet?
    - Could the result be extrapolated to human health?
5. Who is making the recommendation and who stands to benefit?
    - Is it helping to sell a product?
    - Is it making a magazine cover or newspaper headline more appealing?
    - Is it designed to improve public health?

Research studies published in peer-reviewed journals are well scrutinized. But results presented at conferences or published in popular magazines, although they may be legitimate, have not been scrutinized by the scientific community to determine their quality and validity. Anecdotal claims that come from individual testimonies have not been tested by objective experimentation. The Power Boost ad states that the study was a university research study. They do not indicate if it was published, and if so, if it was published in a peer-reviewed journal. The claim that Power Boost increases muscle strength and improves drive and motivation is based on the experience of supplement users and is therefore anecdotal.

Was the Study Well Designed and Accurately Interpreted? If the source of the information seems reliable, ask if the study was well designed and if the results were interpreted accurately. Even well-designed, carefully executed, peer-reviewed experiments can be a source of misinformation if the experimental results are interpreted incorrectly or if the implications of the results are exaggerated. For example, a study that shows that rats fed a diet high in vitamin E live longer than those consuming less vitamin E could be the basis of the headline, "Vitamin E Supplements Increase Longevity." The fact that a diet high in vitamin E increased longevity does not mean that supplements will have the same effect. In addition, this study was done in rats. Can the result be extrapolated to human health? Just because rats consuming diets high in vitamin E live longer does not mean that the same is true for humans.

Some sources provide the details of how a study was done. For others it is not possible to evaluate how studies were done. For example, the Power Boost ad (Figure 1.9) gives some information on how the study was done. We know that 25 experienced weight lifters were studied and that underwater weighing was used to assess muscle mass and body fat at the beginning and end of the study. However, we don't know if there was a control group not taking Power Boost, or whether there was any control over what the subjects ate or how much they worked out. There is no mention of a placebo that would have made control and experimental groups indistinguishable. Without a placebo to eliminate bias, the athletes taking a supplement they believed would increase strength and muscle mass could have been motivated to eat better and work out more strenuously. We know that athletes taking Power Boost gained an average of 5.2 pounds of lean tissue, but we don't know if controls not taking Power Boost would have gained more, less, or the same amount of lean tissue.

Who Stands to Benefit? The final question in judging nutrition claims is, Who is presenting the information or who stands to benefit from the information? Is the claim making a magazine cover or newspaper headline more appealing? If a claim is part of a news headline, it may be true but exaggerated to sell newspapers and magazines. Is it helping to sell a product? The claims for Power Boost are part of an advertisement to increase sales. The company stands to profit from your believing the claim.

Is the individual making the claim going to benefit from the information? Most public health bulletins do not directly sell products. They are designed to improve the health of the population and, if followed, may reduce health-care costs to taxpayers. Care must be taken even when obtaining information from nutritionists. Although "nutritionists" and "nutrition counselors" may provide accurate information, it is important to determine the credentials of these individuals. The term nutritionist is not legally defined and is used by a wide range of individuals from college professors with doctoral degrees from reputable universities to sales clerks in health food stores. One reliable source of nutrition information is registered dietitians. Registered dietitians (RDs) are nutrition professionals who have completed a four-year college degree in a nutrition-related field and who have met established criteria to certify them in providing nutrition counseling (see *Critical Thinking: What Is Wrong With This Experiment?*)

Critical Thinking

What Is Wrong With This Experiment?

After seeing the advertisement for Power Boost in Figure 1.9, Jake wrote the company and asked about the "years of research" that was done to develop this product. He received the company's newsletter, which discussed these three experiments.

Experiment 1

Eight healthy male college students who regularly weight train were studied in two groups. They were asked to follow their regular weight-training regimens, but one group took Power Boost at every meal while the other group received a placebo. The study was double blind. After three weeks, the subjects were asked how energetic and motivated they felt during workouts. The individuals in the experimental group reported higher energy and motivation levels than those in the control group.

Was the study well controlled?

The study used a placebo control and was double blind; however, individuals were not asked to evaluate their motivation and energy level before the study started, so it cannot be concluded that the Power Boost improved their energy or motivation. The experimental group may have been more energetic and motivated even without taking Power Boost. In addition, the study did not control for differences in diet or training level among the subjects. A better controlled study would have evaluated the subjects both before and after Power Boost and would have standardized dietary intake and workout regimens.

Was the proper number of experimental subjects used?

No mention was made of a statistical analysis. It is unlikely that the small number of people in the experimental group could have conclusively demonstrated the advertised benefits of Power Boost.

Were the experimental data objective?

No. The data collected were all subjective, consisting of the opinions of the study subjects regarding their motivation or energy level. A measure of the amount of weight that a subject could lift before and after taking Power Boost would have provided more objective information.

Is the conclusion valid?

No. Because no data were collected prior to giving Power Boost or the placebo, it cannot be concluded that the effect seen was due to Power Boost.

Experiment 2

Five groups of rats were used to test the absorption and muscle-building properties of the nutrients contained in Power Boost. Each group of four rats was fed rat chow plus a different formulation of nutrients. Rat feces were collected and analyzed to see which nutrients were absorbed and which were excreted. To measure muscle mass, body composition was determined by carcass analysis at the end of the study. The average amount of muscle mass in one group was 1.2 grams greater than any other group. This same group of rats excreted smaller amounts of the supplemental nutrients in their feces. It was concluded that the formulation given to this group of rats was best absorbed and resulted in an increase in muscle mass.

Was the study well controlled?

No. There was no control group. All groups were taking some formulation of the supplement. No measurements of nutrient excretion or muscle mass were made at the beginning of the study before the supplement was given. Therefore, the change in nutrient excretion and muscle mass caused by adding these supplement formulations cannot be determined, only the differences between groups receiving the various formulations. There was also no control of activity, a variable that affects muscle development.

Was the proper number of experimental subjects used?

The use of four rats per group may have been sufficient, but no statistical analysis was reported to verify that one group was truly different from the others. An increase in average muscle mass of 1.2 grams may simply be due to one large rat in that group and may not reflect an increase in the muscle mass of all rats in the group.

Were the experimental data objective?

Yes. Measures of muscle mass and nutrients in the feces are both objective.

Given that this study was done in an experimental animal, is the conclusion valid?

Rats may have been an adequate experimental model for nutrient absorption, but showing that rats absorb the supplement does not necessarily mean that humans will. Further, a study that demonstrates increased muscle mass in rats cannot conclude that the same supplement will improve muscle mass in humans.

Experiment 3

Two groups of 25 nutrition majors were studied over a four-week period. At the beginning of the study, leg and arm muscle strength were measured in all participants. One group then added the Power Boost supplement at every meal and snack. The other group received no supplement. Both groups were instructed to consume their typical diet. After four weeks, arm and leg muscle strength were again measured. The group taking Power Boost increased leg muscle strength by 5 pounds. There was no difference in leg strength in the group not taking Power Boost or in arm strength in any group. It was concluded that Power Boost helps improve muscle strength.

Was the experiment subjected to the peer-review process?

No. This study, like the other two, was done and published by the company that makes the formula. There was no mention of a peer-review process by scientists who did not participate in the study.

Was the study well controlled? Was the proper number of experimental subjects used? Were the experimental data objective? Is the conclusion valid?

Answer:

APPLICATIONS

These exercises are designed to help you apply your critical thinking skills to your own nutrition choices.

1. List four food items you ate today or yesterday.
   a. For each, indicate the factor or factors that influenced your selection of that particular food. For example, if you ate a candy bar before your noon class, did you choose it because the machine was available outside the lecture hall, because you didn't have enough money for anything else, because you just like candy bars, because you were depressed, because all of your friends were eating them, because it is good for you or for some other reason?
   b. For each food, indicate what information you used in making the selection. For example, did you read the label on the product, or consider something you read or heard recently in the news media?
   c. List three factors that commonly influence your food choices.
   d. List three types of information you regularly use to make your food choices.
2. Examine a nutritional supplement ad provided by your instructor or select one from a health or fitness-related magazine.
   a. Is the claim made about this product believable?
   b. Does the ad refer to any research studies? If so, do they seem well controlled? Were the results based on objective measurements? Were the conclusions consistent with the results obtained? Were they published in peer-reviewed journals?
   c. Were claims based on anecdotal reports of individual users?
   d. Who stands to benefit if you spend money on this product?
   e. Based on this ad, would you choose to take this supplement?
3. Use an Internet search program to explore the types of nutrition information available over the Web. Search for the word nutrition. Make a list of four kinds of organizations that are listed under this heading. Why do these organizations have Web sites? For example, one might be listed to sell products directly to the consumer, whereas another might provide public health messages.

Summary

1. Nutrition is a science that encompasses all the interactions that occur between living organisms and food. These include the physiological processes by which an organism ingests and uses food; the biological actions and interactions of food with the body and their consequences for health and disease; and the psychological and sociocultural factors that influence what foods we eat.
2. Food contains nutrients that are needed by the body for growth, maintenance and repair, and reproduction. Nutrients are grouped into six classes: carbohydrates, lipids, proteins, water, vitamins, and minerals.
3. Nutrients provide energy, which is measured in kcalories or kjoules. They provide structure to the body and regulate the biochemical reactions of metabolism to maintain homeostasis. When energy or one or more nutrients are deficient or excessive in the diet, malnutrition may result.
4. Malnutrition includes both undernutrition and overnutrition. Its effects can occur in the short term or over the course of many weeks, months, or even years.
5. Consumers make many food choices every day. No one food choice is good or bad and no one choice can make a diet healthy or unhealthy—each choice contributes to the diet as a whole. The typical diet in North America does not meet the recommendations for a healthy diet and contributes to the incidence of chronic diseases such as diabetes, obesity, and heart disease.
6. Our food choices are affected by food availability, personal tastes, sociocultural influences, and what we think we should eat. What we think we should eat is affected by information received via media reports and advertising.
7. The science of nutrition uses the scientific method to determine the relationships between food and the nutrient needs of the body. The scientific method involves making observations of natural events, formulating hypotheses to explain these events, designing and performing experiments to test the hypotheses, and developing theories that explain the observed phenomenon based on the experimental results.
8. To be valid, a nutrition experiment must use objective measurements, appropriate controls, the right type and number of experimental subjects, and a careful interpretation of experimental results.
9. The science of nutrition uses many different types of experimental approaches to determine nutrient functions and requirements. Epidemiological observations identify relationships in populations. Intervention trials can test hypotheses developed from epidemiology. Laboratory studies, including those that study the whole organism such as depletion-repletion and balance studies, and those that study cells such as biochemical and molecular biological studies, are used to evaluate the relationships among nutrient intake, levels of nutrients in the body, and other parameters of metabolism or health.
10. When judging nutrition claims you need to consider whether the information makes sense, whether it came from a reliable source, whether the study was well done and accurately interpreted, and who stands to benefit from making the claim.

Review Questions

1. What is nutrition?
2. What is an essential nutrient?
3. List the energy-containing nutrients.
4. List three functions provided by nutrients.
5. What is malnutrition?
6. What is a toxicity?
7. How does the typical North American diet compare to recommendations for a healthy diet?
8. List three factors other than biological need that influence what we eat.
9. List the steps of the scientific method.
10. What is a control group?
11. What is a placebo?
12. What is a double-blind study?
13. What type of information can be obtained using epidemiology?
14. Why are animal studies used to determine human nutrient requirements?
15. What factors should be considered when judging nutrition claims?

Nutrition Web Links

To further explore areas related to the material in this chapter, go to the *Nutrition: Science and Applications* Web site at ***www.Wiley.com/college/Smolin*** and *click on* **Student Companion Site** for chapter-by-chapter links. Some Web sites related to the information in Chapter 1 include:

Organizations that provide consumer information, such as the U.S. Department of Agriculture, the U.S. Department of Health and Human Services, and Health Canada; American Dietetic Association; the American Cancer Society; and the American Heart Association.

Organizations that help identify what is valuable and what is misinformation, such as the American Dietetic Association and Stephen Barrett's Quackwatch.

Locations that allow you to search for additional scientific information, such as The National Library of Medicine's MEDLINE. This site provides access to almost 4000 scientific journals.

References

1. USDA, Agricultural Service, 1997. Results from USDA's 1994–1996 Continuing Survey of Food Intakes by Individuals and 1994–1996 Health Knowledge Survey. ARS Food Surveys Research Group. Online at http://www.barc.usda.gov/bhnrc/foodsurvey/home.htm
2. Healthy People 2000 Progress Report for Nutrition, July 5, 1994. Online at http://odphp.osophs.dhhs.gov/pubs/hp2000
3. Bowman, S. A., Lino, M., Gerrior, S. A., and Bastiotis, P. P. The Healthy Eating Index: 1994–96. U.S. Department of Agriculture, Center for Nutrition Policy and Promotion, 1998. CNPP-5. Online at http://www2.hqnet.usda.gov/cnpp/hei94-96.PDF
4. Leontos, C., Wong, F., and Gallivan, J., for National Diabetes Education Program Planning Committee. National Diabetes Education Program: opportunies and challenges. J. Am. Diet. Assoc. 98:73–75, 1998.
5. National Institutes of Health, National Heart, Lung, and Blood Institute, Clinical Guidelines on the Identification, Evaluation, and Treatment of Overweight and Obesity in Adults. Executive Summary, June 1998. Online at http://www.nhlbi.nih.gov/nhlbi/cardio/obes/prof/guidelines/ob_xsum.htm
6. Update: prevalence of overweight among children, adolescents, and adults—United States, 1988–1994. MMWR Morb. Mortal. Wkly. Rep., 46:198–202, 1998.
7. U.S. Department of Health and Human Services, Report from HHS Working Group on Sentinel Objectives, Leading Indicators for Healthy People 2010. U.S. DHHS Office of Disease Prevention and Health Promotion. Online at http://web.health.gov/healthypeople/
8. *American Dietetic Association 1997 Nutrition Trends Survey*, Executive Summary. Chicago: American Dietetic Association, 1997.
9. Pratt, E. L. Historical perspectives: food, feeding, and fancies. J. Am. Coll. Nutr. 3:115–121, 1984.

Chapter 2

Chapter Outline

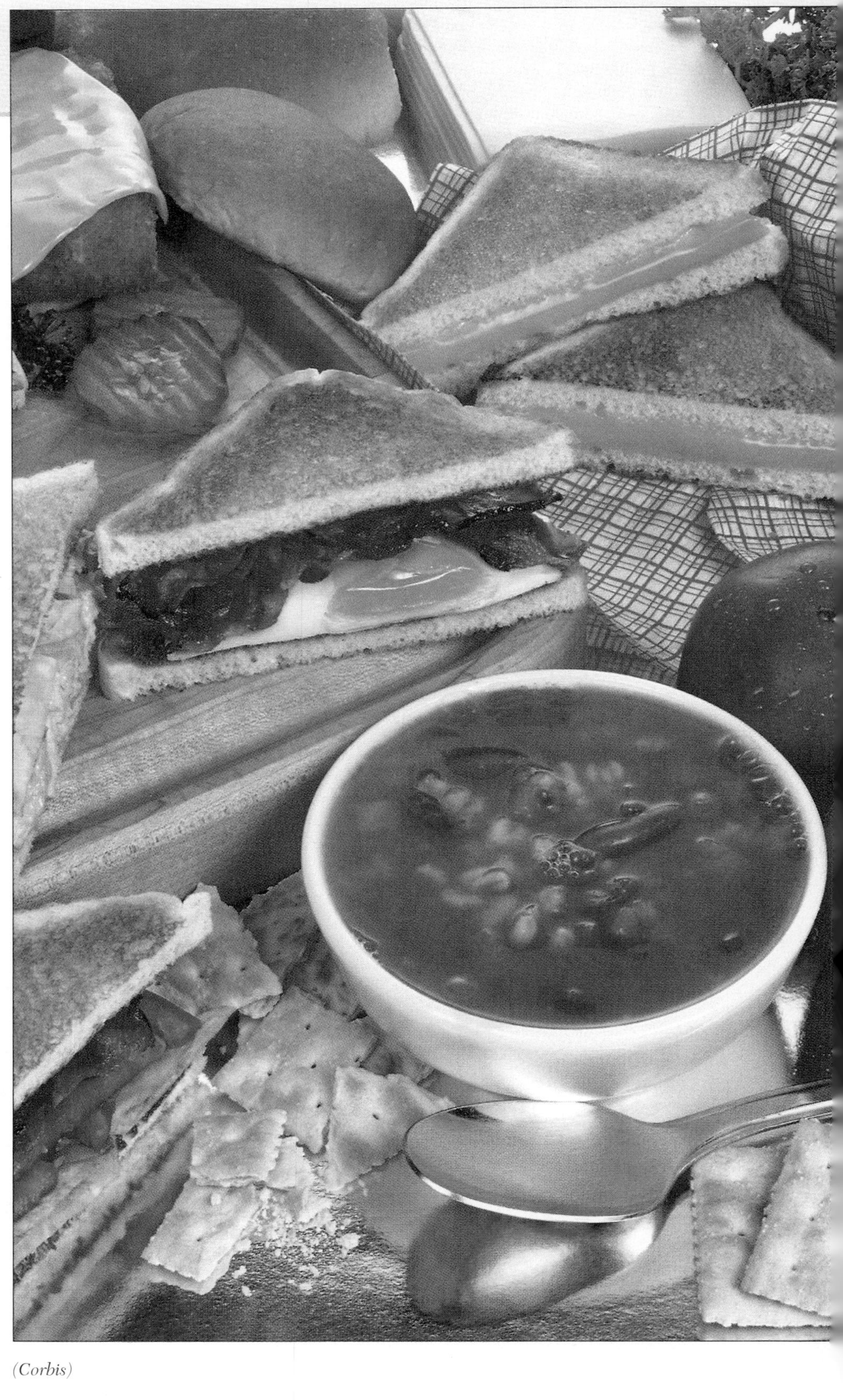

(Corbis)

Applying the Science of Nutrition

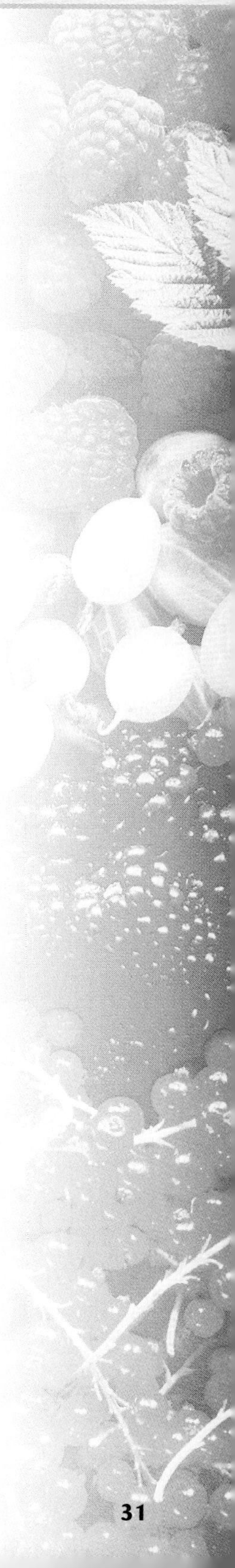

Chapter Concepts

1. Knowledge gained from nutrition research is used to establish dietary standards and guidelines for dietary intake by individuals and populations.
2. The Dietary Reference Intakes are a set of reference values for the amounts of nutrients and food components needed in the diets of healthy individuals. They can be used for planning and assessing the diets of healthy people in the United States and Canada.
3. The Dietary Guidelines for Americans are a set of nutrition recommendations that help consumers select healthful diets that may reduce the risks of chronic disease.
4. The Food Guide Pyramid is a tool that can be used by individual consumers to plan diets that meet nutrition recommendations.
5. The Exchange Lists are a system for grouping foods that was developed for use in planning diabetic diets. Exchange Lists can also be used for planning diets in general.
6. Food labels provide information about the nutrient content of individual foods and help consumers determine how specific food products fit into their total diet.
7. The nutritional status of the population is monitored by surveys that collect information about food consumption and health status and compare it to nutritional recommendations and health standards. Surveys can identify patterns and associations that occur among nutrient intake, health, and disease in the population.
8. An individual's nutritional status can be assessed by evaluating nutrient intake along with medical history and anthropometric and laboratory measures.

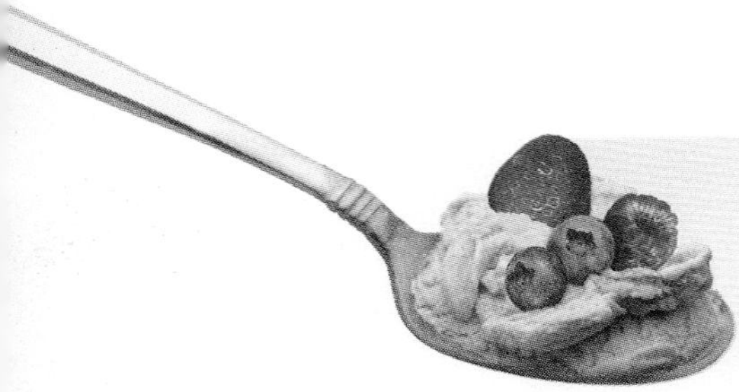

Just a Taste

How do you know if you are eating a healthy diet?

If your diet does not meet the RDAs, will you develop a nutrient deficiency?

Does what you eat for lunch affect what you should have for dinner?

People need to eat to survive, but health-conscious individuals want to do more than survive. They want to choose diets that will optimize their health. How do we know what an optimal diet is? We know it should contain just the right amount of each nutrient. But what is the right amount? Is it the amount needed to prevent a deficiency, the amount needed to maintain a certain nutrient level in the blood, the amount that minimizes cancer risk, maximizes immune function, or extends life span? For each nutrient, the optimal amount may vary depending on what parameter is being measured. The optimum is also different for each individual and depends on the amounts of other nutrients in the diet. Men have different needs from women, growing children have different needs from adults, athletes have different needs from sedentary individuals, and each of us has a unique genetic makeup that affects our nutrient requirements.

The science of nutrition has determined which nutrients are necessary for the survival of the species and how these needs change at different stages of life, such as pregnancy or infancy. But, it is not currently possible to determine the optimal amount of each nutrient that should be included in the diet of each individual. Instead, the methods of science have been used to establish general recommendations for the types and amounts of nutrients that will maintain the health of individuals and populations. To be useful to health-conscious consumers, these amounts have been translated into recommendations about food choices. These recommendations are also used as a standard of comparison to assess whether populations and individuals are consuming diets that promote health.

Guidelines for Health Promotion and Disease Prevention

Health is important to all of us—as individuals and as a population. Maintaining and improving a population's health increases its productivity and decreases health-care costs. In the interest of maintaining the public health, government agencies ask scientists to evaluate research data and make recommendations on healthy levels of nutrient intake. These levels are used by consumers and health professionals as dietary standards.

Dietary Standards

Some of the earliest dietary standards were developed in England in the 1860s. The Industrial Revolution had led to the rise of urban populations with large numbers of homeless and hungry people. To resolve this problem, the government wanted to know the least expensive way to keep these people alive and maintain the work force. As a result, a daily recommendation was established based on what the average working person ate in a typical day. This method of estimating nutrient needs was used until World War I, when the British Royal Society made specific recommendations about foods that not only would sustain life but also would be protective of health. They recommended that fruits and green vegetables be included in a healthy diet and that milk be included in the diets of all children. The United States government began considering recommendations for nutrient needs when food shipments were sent to its allies in Europe during World War I. But it was not until the early 1940s, when World War II created widespread food limitations at home, that the United States began considering nutrition or dietary standards for its own population (Figure 2.1).

Since World War II, the governments of many countries have established their own sets of dietary standards based on the nutritional problems and dietary patterns specific to their populations and the interpretations of their scientists. Most of the differences between guidelines from country to country are small. The World Health Organization and the Food and Agriculture Organization of the United Nations, organizations concerned with international health, publish a set of dietary standards to apply worldwide[1] (see Appendix F). The dietary standards developed in the United States were the Recommended Dietary Allowances (RDAs). The most recent revision of these values was published in 1989[2] and more recently they have been expanded into the **Dietary Reference Intakes (DRIs)**. In Canada, Health Canada set dietary standards called Recommended Nutrient Intakes (RNIs) (see Appendix E).[3] Because the United States and Canada are collaborating to develop the DRIs, the RNIs are also being replaced with these standards. This joint U.S.–Canadian effort (with input expected from Mexico) will help to harmonize recommendations for North America.

Dietary References Intakes (DRIs) A set of four reference values for the intake of nutrients and food components that can be used for planning and assessing the diets of healthy people in the United States and Canada.

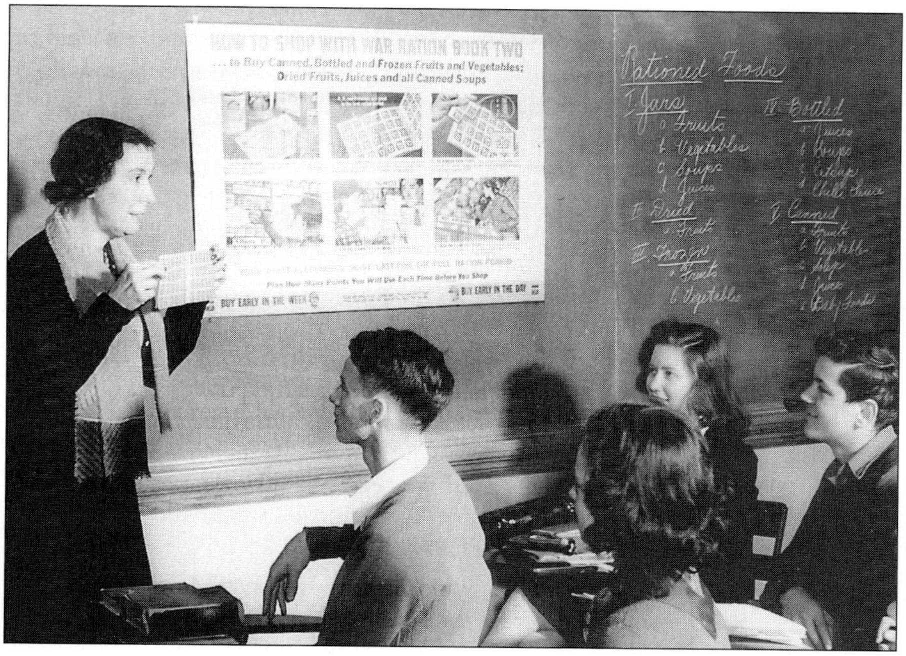
HOW TO SHOP WITH WAR RATION BOOK TWO
... to Buy Canned, Bottled and Frozen Fruits and Vegetables; Dried Fruits, Juices and all Canned Soups
BUY EARLY IN THE WEEK
BUY EARLY IN THE DAY
Rationed Foods

Figure 2.1
Food shortages during World War II prompted the U.S. government to establish dietary standards. (Office of War Information)

Dietary Reference Intakes

The Dietary Reference Intakes are a set of standards for the intake of nutrients and food components that can be used for planning and assessing the diets of healthy people in the United States and Canada. They provide recommendations for average daily intakes—not requirements that must be consumed each day.

How Do DRIs Differ From the Original RDAs? When the original RDAs were published in 1943, nutrient deficiency diseases were a public health concern. The Food and Nutrition Board of the National Research Council set the RDA values at levels that would prevent nutrient deficiencies. Recommendations were made for energy and nutrients at risk for deficiency—protein, vitamins, and minerals.

Today, as the DRIs are being developed, nutrient deficiencies are rare in the United States and chronic diseases such as heart disease and cancer are a major public health focus. Because of this, the DRIs are being developed to consider health promotion and a reduction of chronic disease as well as the prevention of deficiencies. Values are being set not only for energy, protein, and micronutrients but also for fat, carbohydrate, and food components, such as phytochemicals, which are not classified as nutrients.

Another difference between the original RDAs and the DRIs is the types of values. The original RDAs provided only a single set of values. The DRIs include four types of reference values so that appropriate standards are available for specific purposes. Each type of reference value includes recommendations that apply to different genders and life-stages based on age, and when appropriate, pregnancy and lactation. The life-stage groups are divided differently from those used in the original RDAs and in some cases are expanded to include additional categories.

The DRI Values The DRIs include Estimated Average Requirements, Recommended Dietary Allowances, Adequate Intakes, and Tolerable Upper Intake Levels.[4] The **Estimated Average Requirement (EAR)** is the amount of a nutrient that is estimated to meet the needs of 50% of people in the same gender and life-stage group. The new **Recommended Dietary Allowances (RDAs)** are recommendations calculated to meet the needs of nearly all healthy individuals in each gender and life-stage group. The RDAs are determined by starting with the EAR value and using the variability in the requirements among individuals to increase it to an amount that meets the needs of 97 to 98% of healthy individuals. **Adequate Intakes (AIs)** are estimates used when there is insufficient scientific evidence to set an EAR and calculate an RDA. The AIs are based on observed or experimentally determined approximations of the average nutrient intake by a healthy population. An AI value indicates that sufficient information on requirements is lacking and thus targets the need for more research on the requirement of that nutrient. The fourth set of values, the **Tolerable Upper Intake Levels (ULs)**, are the maximum level of daily intake of a nutrient that is unlikely to pose risks of adverse health effects to almost all individuals in the specified group. It is a level of intake that can probably be tolerated; it is not a recommended level. There is no established benefit of intakes above the RDA or AI for healthy individuals.

The DRIs are being developed for seven nutrient groups: calcium, phosphorus, magnesium, vitamin D, and fluoride; B vitamins and choline; antioxidants (e.g., vitamins C, vitamin E, selenium); macronutrients (e.g., protein, fat, carbohydrate); trace elements (e.g., iron, zinc, copper); electrolytes and water; and other food components (e.g., fiber, phytochemicals). Values for some groups have been established, others are in the process of being finalized, and others are still tentative and may be modified. An example of DRI values for calcium and phosphorus is shown in Table 2.1 and all values available at the time this text was published are given inside the front cover.

Estimated Average Requirements (EARs) Intakes that meet the estimated nutrient needs (as defined by a specific indicator of adequacy) of 50% of individuals in a gender and life-stage group.

Recommended Dietary Allowances (RDAs) Intakes that are sufficient to meet the nutrient needs of almost all healthy people in a specific life-stage and gender group.

Adequate Intakes (AIs) Intakes that should be used as a goal when no RDA exists. These values are an approximation of the average nutrient intake that appears to sustain a desired indicator of health.

Tolerable Upper Intake Level (UL) The maximum daily intake by an individual that is unlikely to pose risks of adverse health effects to almost all individuals in the specified life-stage and gender group.

Table 2.1 *Dietary Reference Intake Values for Calcium and Phosphorus*

	Calcium		Phosphorus			
Life-Stage Group*	AI (mg/day)	UL (mg/day)	EAR (mg/day)	RDA (mg/day)	AI (mg/day)	UL (mg/day)
0–6 months	210	ND†	—	—	100	ND
6–12 months	270	ND	—	—	275	ND
1–3 years	500	2500	380	460	—	3000
4–8 years	800	2500	405	500	—	3000
9–13 years	1300	2500	1055	1250	—	4000
14–18 years	1300	2500	1055	1250	—	4000
19–30 years	1000	2500	580	700	—	4000
31–50 years	1000	2500	580	700	—	4000
51–70 years	1200	2500	580	700	—	4000
>70 years	1200	2500	580	700	—	3000
Pregnancy						
≤18 years	1300	2500	1055	1250	—	3500
19–50 years	1000	2500	580	700	—	3500
Lactation						
≤18 years	1300	2500	1055	1250	—	4000
19–50 years	1000	2500	580	700	—	4000

*All groups except Pregnancy and Lactation contain both males and females.
† ND means Not Determined.

Determining Dietary Reference Intakes Designing standards to reduce the risk of chronic disease, developmental disorders, and other health problems—as well as prevent deficiency diseases—is challenging. In order to meet this goal, appropriate criteria of adequate intake must be established for each life-stage and gender group for each nutrient. A criterion of adequacy is an indicator that can be evaluated to determine the biological effect of a level of nutrient intake. One criterion may be best to determine the risk of deficiency, whereas another may help to assess the risk of chronic disease. For example, should the recommended amount of vitamin C be that which maintains blood concentrations at a level that prevents scurvy, or should it be the amount that reduces the risk of chronic disease, or should both criteria be considered?

For each nutrient, an EAR and RDA, or an AI is established to meet specific criteria for adequacy. The criteria may not be the same for different life-stage groups (Figure 2.2). For example, the AI for calcium for infants is based on the amount consumed in human milk. For children the AI is based on the amount needed to support maximal calcium accumulation to support bone growth. For older adults the AI is set to support maximal calcium retention, which may decrease the risk of bone fractures. One or more criterion may be used to establish each EAR or AI. For all DRI values, the recommendations consider how much of a nutrient in food is available to the body for use.

To establish Tolerable Upper Intake Levels, a specific adverse effect or indicator of excess is used. The lowest level of intake that causes the adverse effect is determined and the UL is set far enough below this level that even the most sensitive people in the population are unlikely to be affected. If adverse effects have been associated only with intake from supplements, the UL is based on this source only. Therefore, for some nutrients these values represent intake from supplements alone, for some, intake from supplements and fortified foods, and for others, total intake from food, fortified food, water, nonfood sources, and supplements. For many nutrients, data are insufficient to establish a UL value.

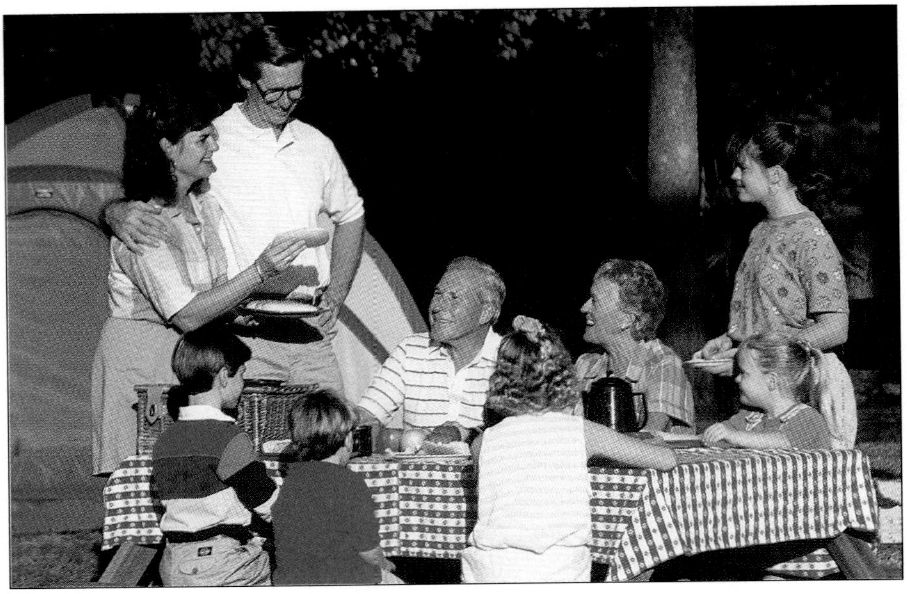

Figure 2.2
The criteria used to determine the DRI values for a particular nutrient may be different for different life-stage groups. (La Foto/H. Armstrong Roberts)

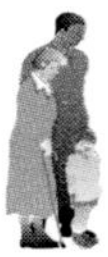

Life-Stage Groups The DRIs include values that apply to different life-stage groups. These have been modified from the categories used in the original RDAs. One difference is that the puberty/adolescence category begins at an earlier age because current information indicates that the physiological changes that mark the beginning of adolescence may occur earlier. The DRIs have expanded the adult age groups to include young adulthood, ages 19 through 30 years; middle ages, 31 through 50 years; adulthood, ages 51 through 70; and older adults, those over 70 years of age. The revised age categories recognize the possible higher nutrient intake needs of younger adults and the decline with age in the need for energy and nutrients related to energy metabolism. The addition of categories for older adults recognizes that most people today remain active until age 70, and after this, variability in health status and nutritional needs increases. Age categories have also been added to the pregnancy and lactation life stages to distinguish any unique nutritional needs of pregnancy and lactation in teenagers and older mothers.

Applications for Dietary Standards Dietary standards have many uses. They provide a set of standards that can be used to plan diets, to assess the adequacy of diets, and to make judgments about excessive intakes for individuals and populations.[4] The standards can be used to define food and nutrition regulations, plan and develop nutrition education programs, and evaluate the adequacy of the food supply.[2] They can serve as a standard for meals prepared for schools, hospitals and other health-care facilities, and for government feeding programs for the elderly and even meals for space-shuttle astronauts. Dietary standards can be used to determine standards for food labeling and to develop practical tools for diet planning, such as the Food Guide Pyramid.[5] They can also be used to interpret information gathered about the food consumed by a population to help identify potential nutritional inadequacies that may be of public health concern. They can serve as guidelines for recommending modifications to the diet or food supply. The original RDAs provide only a single standard, but while the DRI values are being developed, the 1989 RDA values are still being used for many purposes. DRIs give a more complete set of values, each with specific uses.

The Estimated Average Requirement is a value that is useful for evaluating the adequacy of nutrient intakes of population groups and planning for the nutrient intakes of groups. The prevalence of inadequate nutrient intakes can be estimated by looking at the proportion of the population with intakes below the EAR.

The RDA is the value that can be used by individuals as a guide to achieve adequate nutrient intake. The RDA is set at a value that should be adequate for 97 to 98% of all healthy individuals in a particular gender and life-stage group. The RDA is a target, and an intake less than the RDA does not necessarily indicate that the criterion of adequacy has not been met by the specific individual.[6] Since individual nutrient requirements are never known with certainty, the risk of a deficiency is low if intake meets the RDA and increases as an individual's average intake falls further below the RDA.

The Adequate Intake values, like the RDAs, can be used as a goal for individual intake. Even though they are derived from mean intakes of groups, not individuals, it is assumed that if healthy individuals have an intake that is at or above the AI there is a low risk that this intake is not adequate to maintain nutritional health.

Tolerable Upper Intake Levels are used as a guide for individuals to limit intake when planning diets and to evaluate the possibility of overconsumption. The exact level of intake that will cause an adverse effect cannot be known with certainty for each individual, but if an individual's intake is below the UL, there is good assurance that an adverse effect will not occur.

Despite their many uses, dietary standards cannot be used to identify with certainty whether a specific person has a nutritional deficiency or excess. To ascertain this, an evaluation of an individual's nutritional status using dietary, clinical, biochemical, and body-size measurements is needed.

Other Guidelines and Goals for Health Promotion and Disease Prevention

In the last 25 years, many different guidelines for health promotion and disease prevention have been developed by public health agencies. The first recommendation for health promotion—rather than just deficiency prevention—was the Dietary Goals for the United States, established in 1977 by the Senate Select Committee on Human Needs.[7] Since then, the dietary goals have been modified and are currently published as the **Dietary Guidelines for Americans,** 1995.[8] (Figure 2.3 and Appendix G). In addition to recommendations for a healthy diet, guidelines for reducing the risk of specific diseases have been published by special interest groups. Nutrition-related concerns have been incorporated into programs designed to improve the health of the population and the quality and availability of health care.

Dietary Guidelines for Americans A set of nutrition recommendations designed to promote population-wide dietary changes to reduce the incidence of nutrition-related chronic disease.

The Dietary Guidelines for Americans

The 1989 RDAs and the DRIs offer recommendations for the intake of specific amounts of about 40 nutrients. However, in planning our diets, we choose foods, not nutrients. To translate the recommendations for nutrients into food choices, the Dietary Guidelines for Americans make consumer-friendly recommendations on food choices that will reduce chronic disease risk. For instance, a diet high in plant foods is high in fiber and is associated with a reduced risk of a number of chronic diseases including certain forms of cancer. Therefore, the Dietary Guidelines recommend a diet that includes plenty of grains, vegetables, and fruits. The Dietary Guidelines are designed to promote health, support active lives, and reduce chronic disease risks in the general population. They are not meant to replace individual dietary prescriptions for disease conditions, or to recommend food choices that meet nutrient requirements. In Canada the issue of improving the nation's diet is addressed in *Canada's Guidelines for Healthy Eating* (see Appendix E).[9] Internationally, goals for nutrient intake are set by the World Health Organization (see Appendix F).

The Healthy People Initiative

The U.S. Public Health Service along with 300 private and public organizations have also developed a set of public health objectives called **Healthy People.** The first set, Healthy People 2000, developed in

Healthy People A set of national health promotion and disease prevention objectives for the U.S. population.

Figure 2.3
The Dietary Guidelines for Americans promote healthy diets. (USDA, DHHS, 1995)

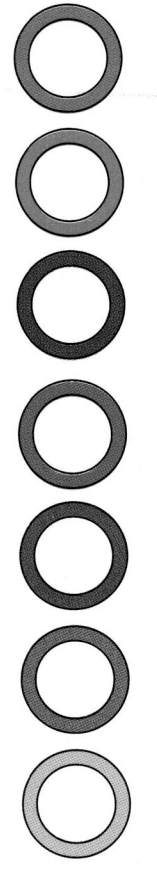

Nutrition and Your Health:

Dietary Guidelines for Americans

Eat a variety of foods. Foods contain combinations of nutrients and other healthful substances. No single food can supply all nutrients in the amounts you need. Choose the recommended number of daily servings from each of the five food groups of the Food Guide Pyramid.

Balance the food you eat with physical activity; maintain or improve your weight. Being overweight and gaining weight as an adult are linked to high blood pressure, heart disease, stroke, diabetes, certain types of cancer, and other illnesses. Most adults should not gain weight and if you are overweight you should try to lose weight.

Choose a diet with plenty of grain products, vegetables, and fruits. These foods provide vitamins, minerals, complex carbohydrates, and other substances that are important for good health. They are low in fat and are associated with a lower risk of many chronic diseases including certain types of cancer.

Choose a diet low in fat, saturated fat, and cholesterol. Fat supplies energy and essential fatty acids, and promotes the absorption of fat-soluble vitamins. However, high levels of saturated fat and cholesterol in the diet are linked to increased blood cholesterol and a greater risk of heart disease. Choose a diet that provides no more than 30% of total kcalories from fat.

Choose a diet moderate in sugars. Sugars occur naturally in many foods, including milk, fruits, and vegetables, that also supply other nutrients. Sugars added to food during processing add energy but no other essential nutrients. Both sugars and starch can promote tooth decay. Avoid excessive snacking and brush and floss teeth regularly.

Choose a diet moderate in salt and sodium. Salt and sodium are found mainly in processed and prepared foods. A high sodium intake is associated with high blood pressure. To reduce dietary sodium decrease the amount added in cooking and at the table and use the Nutrition Facts label to choose foods lower in sodium.

If you drink alcoholic beverages, do so in moderation. Alcoholic beverages supply kcalories but few or no nutrients. Alcohol alters judgment and can lead to dependency and other serious health problems including liver disease and birth defects.

1990, was directed toward the year 2000.[10] A new set of objectives, Healthy People 2010, targets the next decade. The goals for the Healthy People initiative include increasing the span of healthy life for Americans and eliminating health disparities among Americans. These goals are to be met through the broad approaches of promoting healthy behaviors, protecting health, assuring access to quality health care, and strengthening community prevention.[11] Many of these objectives are directed toward improving the nutritional status of the population (see Appendix H). For instance, Healthy People is working toward reducing the number of cancer and heart disease deaths and the prevalence of obesity in adults by promoting active lifestyles and diets low in fat and sodium and high in complex carbohydrate. It promotes a reduction in growth retardation in children by encouraging healthy feeding practices, including breast feeding for infants. Other nutrition-related objectives were designed to improve the delivery of nutrition information and services.[12]

Recommendations for Reducing Risks for Specific Diseases In addition to guidelines for a healthy diet for the general population, recommendations to populations at risk for certain diseases have been published by groups such as the American Heart Association and the American Institute for Cancer Research (see Appendix G). These groups base their recommendations on sound scientific literature, but because of their special interest in preventing a specific disease, their recommendations may differ slightly from one another in emphasis and focus. For example, to reduce the risk of heart disease, the guidelines developed by the

American Heart Association include a recommendation to restrict dietary cholesterol to less than 300 mg per day, whereas the recommendations of the American Institute for Cancer Research, which are designed to reduce the incidence of cancer, do not comment on cholesterol intake, since a correlation has not been established between cholesterol intake and cancer incidence. On the other hand, the American Institute for Cancer Research recommends a reduction in the consumption of cured and smoked meats because of a correlation with cancer, but these foods are not mentioned in the American Heart Association guidelines.

Tools for Diet Planning

How do you meet your need for a specific nutrient? The DRIs help you determine how much you should consume. The Dietary Guidelines tell you to eat a variety of foods. But, how much of which foods should you choose to ensure you consume the right amount of each nutrient? To help individuals follow the recommendations for a healthy diet, a number of systems have been developed to translate the recommendations for nutrient intake into food choices. The most commonly used tools are food groups. These divide foods into groups based on the nutrients they supply most abundantly and then recommend the number of servings from each group needed to provide a healthy diet. The most recent version of a food group system used in the United States is the Food Guide Pyramid (Figure 2.4). In Canada, the Food Guide to Healthy Eating is used (Figure 2.5 and Appendix E). The Exchange Lists are another type of food group system that can be used for planning diets. Food labels also provide information about the nutrient content of individual foods and how the amounts in a serving of the food compare to recommendations for health promotion and disease prevention.

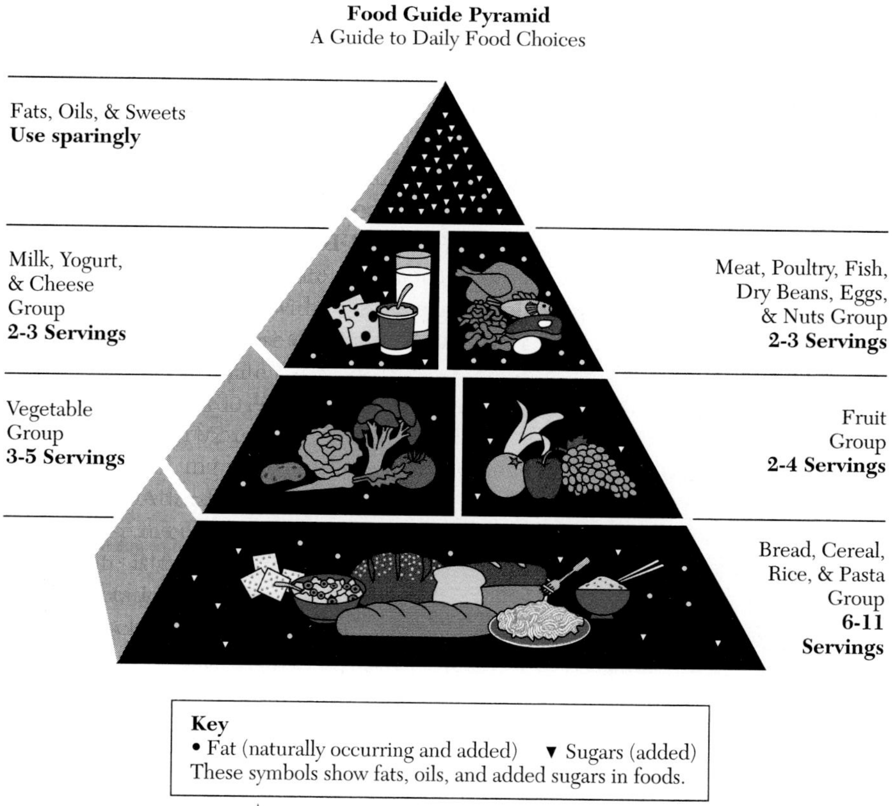

Figure 2.4
The Food Guide Pyramid. (USDA, 1992)

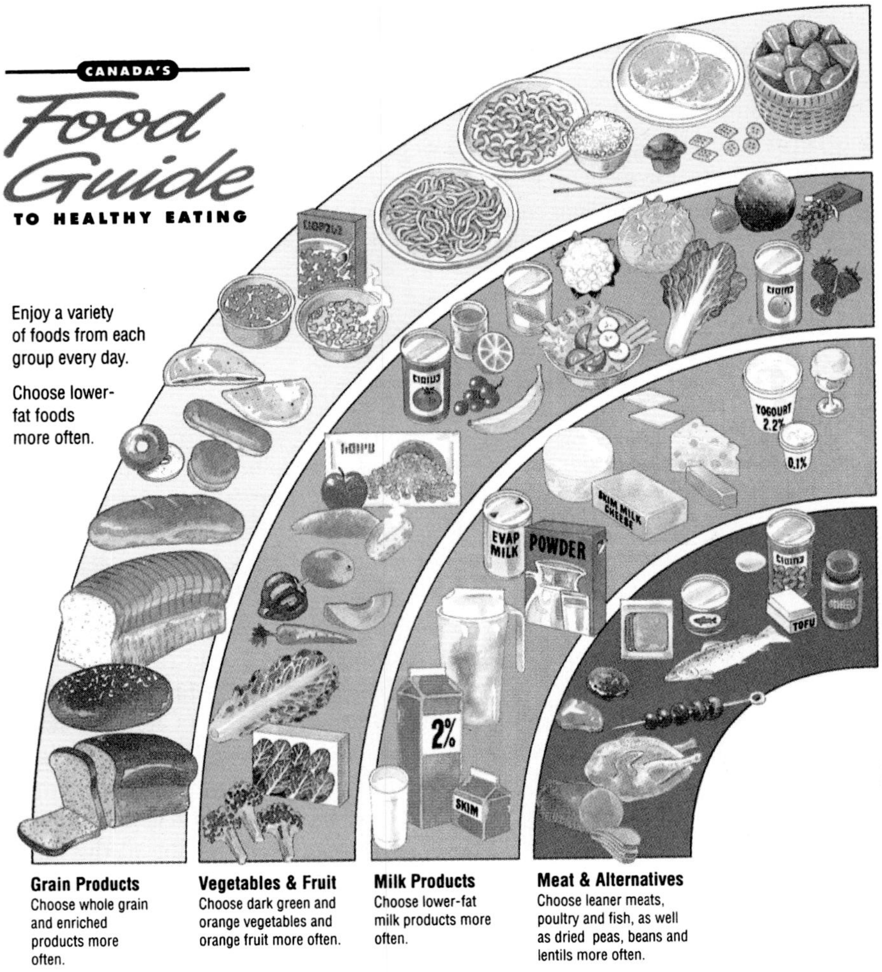
CANADA'S
Food Guide
TO HEALTHY EATING
Enjoy a variety of foods from each group every day.
Choose lower-fat foods more often.
EVAP MILK
POWDER
2%
SKIM
YOGOURT 2.2%
0.1%
TOFU
Grain Products
Choose whole grain and enriched products more often.
Vegetables & Fruit
Choose dark green and orange vegetables and orange fruit more often.
Milk Products
Choose lower-fat milk products more often.
Meat & Alternatives
Choose leaner meats, poultry and fish, as well as dried peas, beans and lentils more often.

Figure 2.5
Canada's Food Guide to Healthy Eating. (Health and Welfare Canada, 1992)

The Food Guide Pyramid

The Food Guide Pyramid is a guide for planning diets that meet nutrient requirements and the recommendations for health promotion and disease prevention. It proposes a diet plan based on servings from five food groups: Bread, Cereal, Rice, & Pasta; Vegetable; Fruit; Milk, Yogurt, & Cheese; and Meat, Poultry, Fish, Dry Beans, Eggs, & Nuts. The Pyramid also includes a recommendation to use Fats, Oils, & Sweets sparingly in the diet. The serving sizes within each group of the Pyramid are fairly constant. For instance, 1 serving from the grain group is 1 slice of bread; 1 ounce of dry cereal; or ½ cup of cooked cereal, rice, or pasta (see Table 2.2). Foods within each food group supply similar nutrients. For example, foods in the Milk, Yogurt, & Cheese Group are good sources of protein, calcium, and riboflavin.

Why Use a Pyramid Shape? The shape of the Pyramid helps emphasize the relative contribution each food group should make to the diet. The large base of the Pyramid is made up of foods that come from grains: bread, cereal, rice, and pasta. These high-carbohydrate foods are the foundation of a healthy diet; between 6 and 11 servings per day are recommended. In the next level of the Pyramid are two groups of plant foods: the Vegetable Group, of which 3 to 5 servings per day are recommended, and the Fruit Group, of which 2 to 4 servings per day are recommended. The next level, where the decreasing size of the Pyramid boxes reflects the smaller number of recommended servings, comprises 2 groups of foods that come primarily from animals: the Milk, Yogurt, & Cheese Group, of which 2 to 3 servings are recommended, and the Meat, Poultry, Fish, Dry Beans, Eggs, & Nuts Group, of which 2 to 3 servings a day are recommended. At the narrow tip of the Pyramid are Fats, Oils, & Sweets. These should be used sparingly after other nutrient needs have been met.

Table 2.2 *Servings and Selections From the Food Guide Pyramid*

Food Group/Serving Size	Nutrients Provided	Selection Tips
Bread, Cereal, Rice, & Pasta (6 to 11 servings)		
½ cup cooked cereal, rice, or pasta 1 ounce dry cereal 1 slice bread, 1 tortilla 2 cookies ½ medium doughnut	B vitamins, fiber, iron, magnesium, zinc, complex carbohydrates	Choose whole grain breads, cereals, and grains such as whole wheat or rye, oatmeal, and brown rice. Use high-fat, high-sugar baked goods such as cakes, cookies, and pastries in moderation. Limit fats and sugars added as spreads, sauces, or toppings.
Vegetable (3 to 5 servings)		
½ cup cooked or raw chopped vegetables 1 cup raw leafy vegetables ¾ cup vegetable juice 10 french fries	Vitamin A, vitamin C, folate, magnesium, iron, fiber	Eat a variety of vegetables, including dark-green leafy vegetables like spinach and broccoli, deep-yellow vegetables like carrots and sweet potatoes, starchy vegetables such as potatoes and corn, and other vegetables such as green beans and tomatoes. Cook by steaming or baking. Avoid frying, and limit high-fat spreads or dressings.
Fruit (2 to 4 servings)		
1 medium apple, banana, or orange ½ cup chopped, cooked, or canned fruit ¾ cup fruit juice ¼ cup dried fruit	Vitamin A, vitamin C, potassium, fiber	Choose fresh fruit, frozen without sugar, dried, or fruit canned in water or juice. If canned in heavy syrup, rinse with water before eating. Eat whole fruits more often than juices; they are higher in fiber. Regularly eat citrus fruits, melons, or berries rich in vitamin C. Only 100% fruit juice should be counted as fruit.
Milk, Yogurt, & Cheese (2 to 3 servings)		
1 cup milk or yogurt 1½ ounces natural cheese 2 ounces process cheese 2 cups cottage cheese 1½ cups ice cream 1 cup frozen yogurt	Protein, calcium, riboflavin	Use lowfat or skim milk for healthy people over 2 years of age. Choose lowfat and nonfat yogurt, "part skim" and lowfat cheeses, and lower-fat frozen desserts like ice milk and frozen yogurt. Limit high-fat cheeses and ice cream.
Meat, Poultry, Fish, Dry Beans, Eggs, & Nuts (2 to 3 servings)		
2–3 ounces cooked lean meat, fish, or poultry 2–3 eggs 4–6 tablespoons peanut butter 1 to 1½ cups cooked dry beans ⅔ to 1 cup nuts	Protein, niacin, vitamin B_6, vitamin B_{12}, other B vitamins, iron, zinc	Select lean meat, poultry without skin, and dry beans often. Trim fat, and cook by broiling, roasting, grilling, or boiling rather than frying. Limit egg yolks, which are high in cholesterol, and nuts and seeds, which are high in fat. Be aware of serving size; 3 ounces of meat is the size of an average hamburger.
Fats, Oils, & Sweets (use sparingly)		
Butter, mayonnaise, salad dressing, cream cheese, sour cream, jam, jelly		These are high in energy and low in micronutrients. Substitute lowfat dressings and spreads.

Human Nutrition Information Service. *The Food Guide Pyramid.* Home and Garden Bulletin No. 252. Hyattsville, Md: U.S. Department of Agriculture, 1992, 1996, revised.

In addition to recommended serving sizes and numbers of servings, the Food Guide Pyramid makes recommendations for food choices from within each group. Many of these suggestions are based on the nutrient density of the foods within groups. **Nutrient density** refers to the amounts of essential nutrients in a food relative to the energy provided. For example, both skim milk and ice cream are in the Milk, Yogurt, & Cheese Group. However, a 1-cup serving of skim milk provides 300 mg of calcium in 90 kcalories, whereas a cup of ice cream provides 168 mg of calcium in 265 kcalories. The skim milk is considered to have a higher nutrient density because it provides more nutrients per kcalorie than the ice cream. Selection tips for choosing high-nutrient-density foods from the Food Guide Pyramid are listed in Table 2.2.

Nutrient density A measure of the nutrients provided by a food relative to the energy it contains.

Table 2.3 *Number of Food Guide Pyramid Servings for 3 Daily Energy Levels**

	1600 kcalories (sedentary women and some older adults)	2200 kcalories (children, teenage girls, active women, and many sedentary men)	2800 kcalories (teenage boys, many active men, and some very active women)
Bread, Cereal, Rice, & Pasta Group	6	9	11
Vegetable Group	3	4	5
Fruit Group	2	3	4
Milk, Yogurt, & Cheese Group	2–3†	2–3†	2–3†
Meat, Poultry, Fish, Dry Beans, Eggs, & Nuts Group	2 (5 oz total)	2 (6 oz total)	3 (7 oz total)

*Assumes that food choices are mostly lowfat and low kcalorie.
†Women who are pregnant or breast feeding, teenagers, and young adults to age 24 need 3 servings.
Source: U.S. Department of Agriculture. *The Food Guide Pyramid*, Home and Garden Bulletin 252, 1992, slightly revised 1996.

Planning Diets Using the Food Guide Pyramid The Food Guide Pyramid is designed to be flexible enough to suit the needs and preferences of people from a variety of cultures and lifestyles. The Pyramid can be used by people with different energy requirements (see Appendix I). People who need 1600 kcalories per day could meet their needs by using the low end of the range of servings, for instance, 6 bread servings per day. People who need 2800 kcalories per day should choose from the high end of the range for each food group, for instance, 11 breads, 5 vegetables, 4 fruits, and so on. (See Table 2.3 for serving recommendations for various kcalorie levels.)

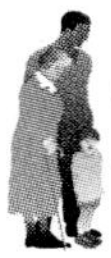

The Pyramid can also be modified for groups with special needs. Pregnant and lactating women, children, adolescents, and adults under 25 years of age should consume 3 servings from the milk group. Small children can follow the Pyramid guidelines by using smaller serving sizes (see Chapter 14). Vegetarians can use the Food Guide Pyramid by choosing meat alternatives such as legumes and nuts from the meat group (see Chapter 6).

To plan a diet that satisfies the recommendations of the Pyramid, several servings of breads and grains and fruits or vegetables should be included at each meal. From this base, servings from the milk and meat groups can be added. Mixed dishes can be planned with the Pyramid by considering the component parts. For example, a chicken taco consists of tortillas (a bread), chicken (a meat), and lettuce and tomatoes (vegetables). A beef with broccoli stir-fry consists of beef (a meat) and broccoli (a vegetable), served over rice (a grain) (see *Critical Thinking: Using the Food Guide Pyramid*).

CRITICAL THINKING

Using the Food Guide Pyramid

A few months ago, Naomi moved out of her parents' home and into her own apartment. For the first time in her life, all her food decisions are her own. She has gained a few pounds and is beginning to realize that she needs to pay more attention to the kinds of foods she eats. To evaluate her nutrient intake, Naomi records everything she consumes for one day and compares it with the number of servings recommended by the Food Guide Pyramid.

Food	Serving Size	Number of Servings	Food Group
Breakfast			
Cornflakes	¾ cup	1	Grain
Whole milk	½ cup	½	Milk
Orange juice	¾ cup	1	Fruit
Coffee	1 cup		
with cream	1 Tbsp		Fats and sweets
and sugar	1 tsp		Fats and sweets
Snack			
Doughnut	1	2	Grain
Lunch			
Tuna salad sandwich			
bread	2 slices	2	Grain
tuna	2 oz	1	Meat
celery	1 Tbsp	⅛	Vegetable
onions	1 Tbsp	⅛	Vegetable
mayonnaise	1 Tbsp		Fats and sweets
Pretzels	1 oz	1	Grain
Whole milk	1 cup	1	Milk
Snack			
French fries	10 pieces	1	Vegetable
Soda	1 can		Fats and sweets
Dinner			
Frozen lasagna			
noodles	½ cup	1	Grain
tomato sauce	¼ cup	½	Vegetable
ground beef	2 oz	1	Meat
cheese	1 oz	⅔	Milk
Soda	1 can		Fats and sweets
Ice cream	½ cup	⅓	Milk

Does Naomi's diet meet the minimum number of servings recommended by the Food Guide Pyramid?

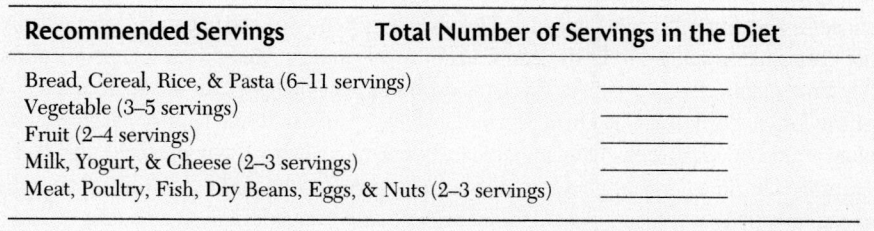

Recommended Servings	Total Number of Servings in the Diet
Bread, Cereal, Rice, & Pasta (6–11 servings)	________
Vegetable (3–5 servings)	________
Fruit (2–4 servings)	________
Milk, Yogurt, & Cheese (2–3 servings)	________
Meat, Poultry, Fish, Dry Beans, Eggs, & Nuts (2–3 servings)	________

To improve her diet, Naomi should increase her intake of vegetables and fruits. Although she likes vegetables, they take time to prepare. She decides she has time to cook some to add to her dinner and she can easily include a piece of fruit with lunch.

How many foods did she have during the day that contribute primarily sugar and/or fat?

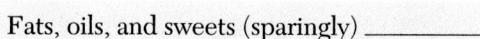

Fats, oils, and sweets (sparingly) ________

Many of Naomi's choices are of low nutrient density. How would different choices affect the energy content of her diet?

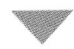

She used whole milk and chose to have a doughnut and french fries for snacks. By switching to lowfat milk she would reduce the energy and fat content of her diet.

What snacks could she substitute for doughnuts and french fries that would contribute less fat and sugar?

Answer:

Exchange Lists

Exchange Lists are another food group system. They were first developed in 1950 by the American Dietetic Association and the American Diabetes Association as a meal-planning tool for individuals with diabetes. Since then, their use has been expanded to planning weight-loss diets and diets in general. The latest revision of the Exchange Lists divides foods into three main groups based on their macronutrient content: the carbohydrate group, the meat and meat-substitute group, and the fat group. The carbohydrate group includes exchange lists for starches, fruits, milk, and vegetables. It also defines a list of other high-carbohydrate foods and indicates how to fit these foods into a diet based on exchanges. The meat and meat-substitute group includes an exchange list with four subgroups: very lean, lean, medium-fat, and high-fat meat. The fat group includes an exchange list with subgroups of monounsaturated, polyunsaturated, and saturated fats (Figure 2.6)[13] (see Appendix I). The serving sizes for foods within each exchange list are different from those in the Food Guide Pyramid. The exchanges are set so that each food within a list contains approximately the same amount of energy, carbohydrate, protein, and fat. For instance, each fruit in the fruit exchange list provides about 60 kcalories, 15 grams of carbohydrate, no protein, and no fat, whereas foods in the starch list provide about 80 kcalories, 15 grams of carbohydrate, 3 grams of protein, and 0 to 1 gram of fat. The Exchange Lists differ from the Food Guide Pyramid groups because the lists are designed to meet energy and macronutrient criteria, whereas the Pyramid groups are designed to be good sources of certain nutrients regardless of their energy content. For example, a potato is included in the starch exchange list because it contains about the same amount of energy, carbohydrate, protein, and fat as breads and grains, but in the Food Guide Pyramid a potato is in the Vegetable Group because it is a good source of vitamins, minerals, and fiber.

The exchange system can be used to design diets to meet individual tastes and preferences at specific energy levels. Calculating a diet using the Exchange Lists requires a thorough knowledge of the system as well as food composition; these diets are usually calculated by a registered dietitian or other health professional. Once the calculations have been completed, the consumer is instructed to select a specific number of foods from each exchange list. For example, a 1500-kcalorie diet providing 75 grams of protein and less than 30% fat could be designed and then the consumer would be instructed to choose 6 starch exchanges, 2 milk exchanges, 3 vegetable exchanges, and so on. Exchange Lists have also been developed to include the traditional foods of different ethnic groups (see Appendix J).

Carbohydrate Group

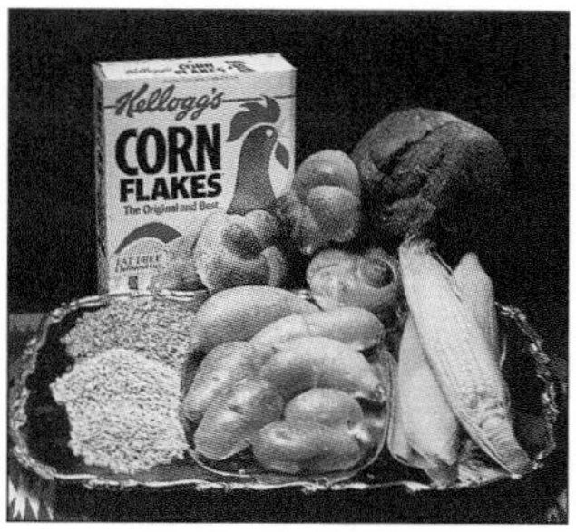

Starch List
1/2 cup cereal, grain, or starchy vegetable
1 slice bread
1 oz of most snack foods

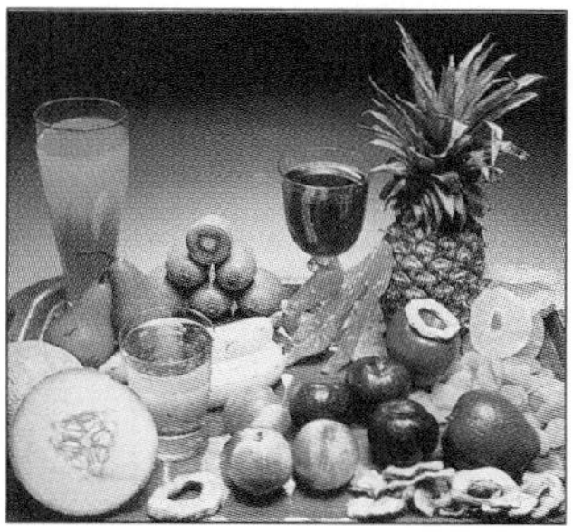

Fruit List
1 small to medium fresh fruit
1/2 cup canned or fresh fruit
1/2 cup fruit juice
1/4 cup dried fruit

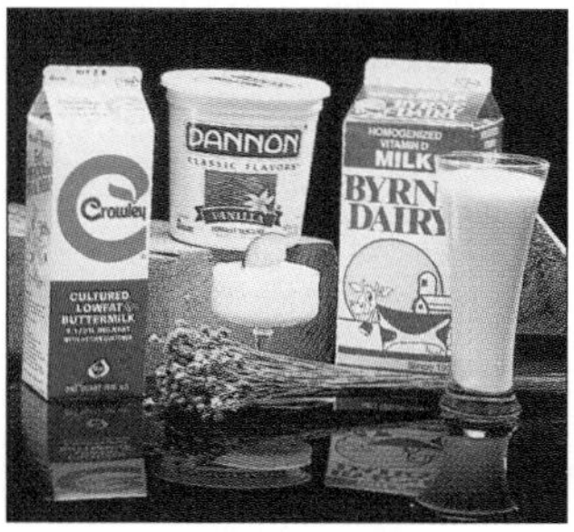

Milk List
1 cup milk
1 cup buttermilk
3/4 cup yogurt

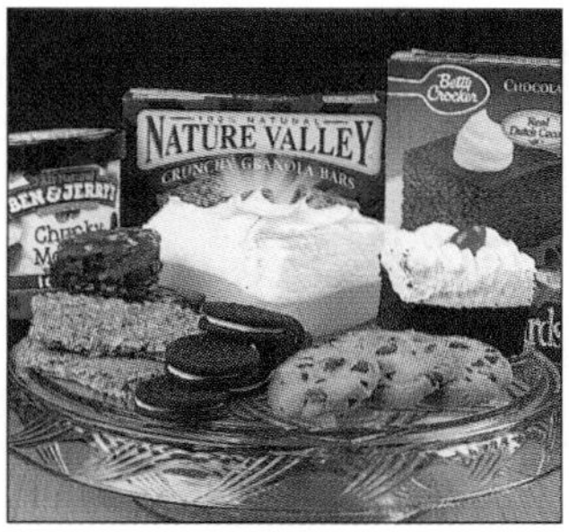

Other Carbohydrates List
2 inch square of cake
1 Tbsp jam or fruit spread
1/2 cup ice cream
2 small cookies

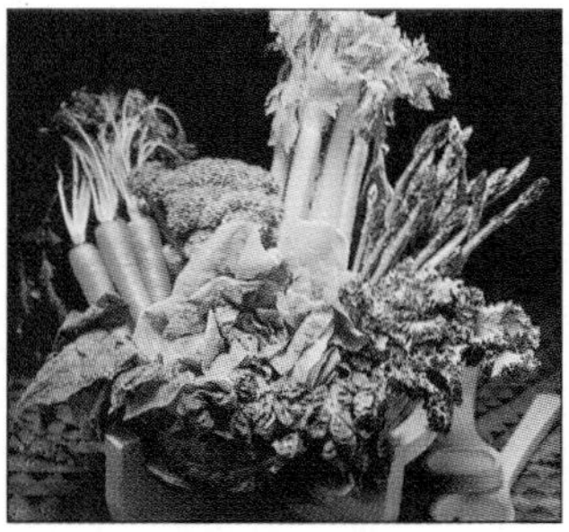

Vegetable List
1/2 cup cooked vegetables
1/2 cup vegetable juice
1 cup raw vegetables

Meat and Meat Substitutes Group

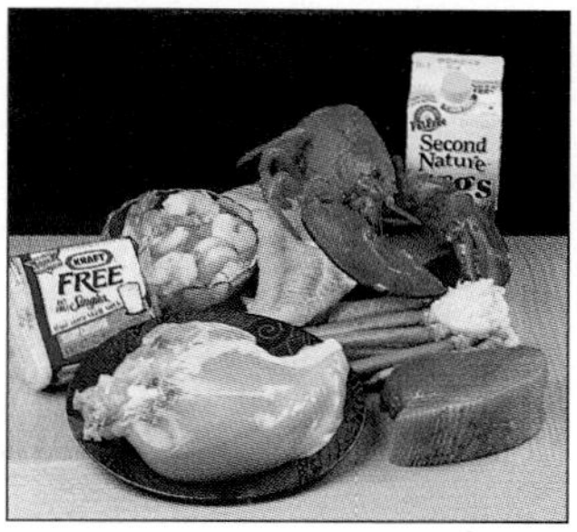

Very Lean Meat and Substitutes List
1 oz poultry, fish, or shellfish
1 oz fat-free cheese
1/2 cup dried beans

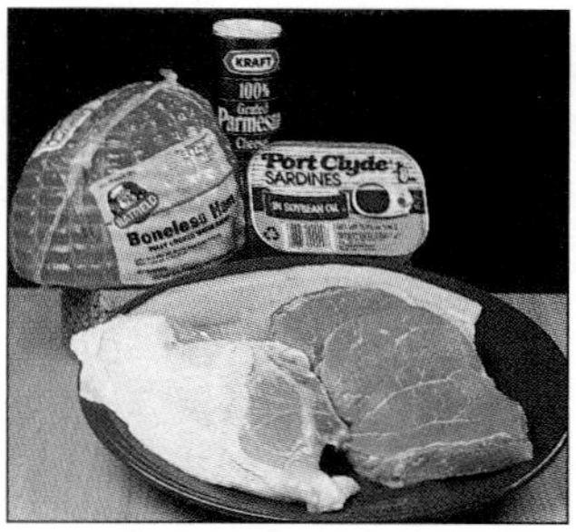

Lean Meat and Substitutes List
1 oz flank steak, lean pork, or catfish
1 oz lowfat cheese

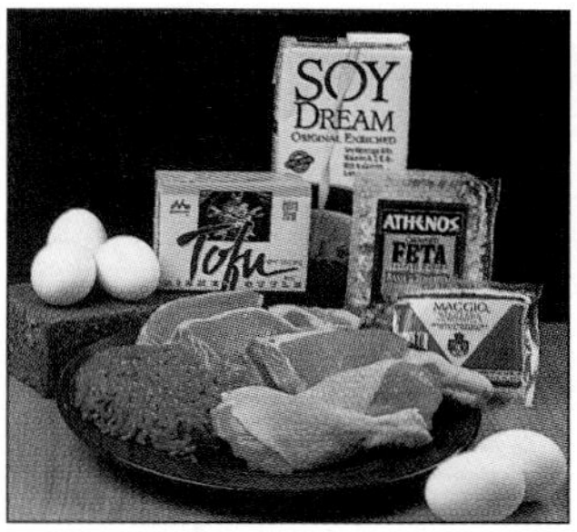

Medium-Fat Meat and Substitutes List
1 oz ground beef, pork chop, or fried fish
1 oz feta or mozzarella cheese
1 egg
1/2 cup tofu

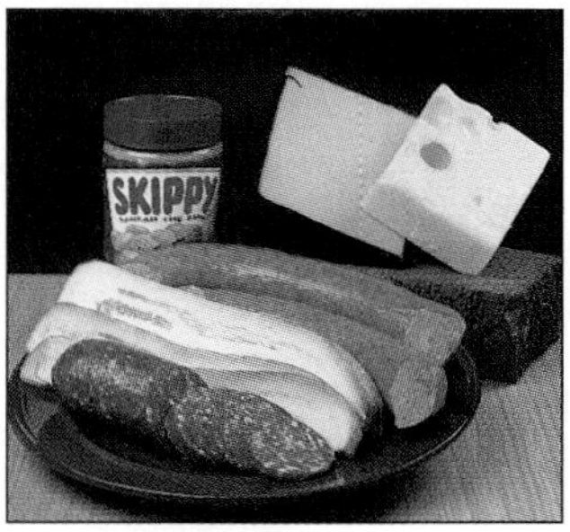

High-Fat Meat and Substitutes List
1 oz sausage or ground pork
1 oz American, cheddar, or Swiss cheese
2 Tbsp peanut butter

Fat Group

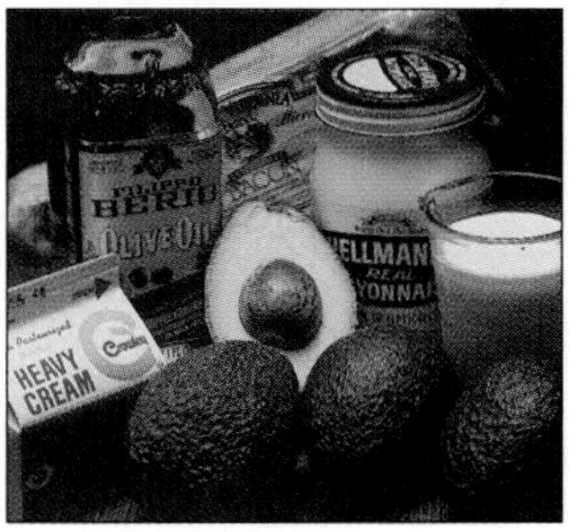

Fat List
1 tsp margarine, butter, or oil
1 Tbsp salad dressing
1 Tbsp sesame or sunflower seeds

Figure 2.6
These are examples of foods included in different Exchange Lists. Starches, milk, vegetables, and fruits are in the carbohydrate group. Meat, fish, eggs, and tofu are in the meat and meat-substitute group. Fats and oils are in the fat group. (*left 1, 2, 3, 5,* and *right 3, 5,* Charles D. Winters; *left 4* and *right 1, 2, 4,* George Semple)

Food Labels

Food labels are another tool that can be used in diet planning. They are designed to help consumers make food choices by providing information about the nutrient composition of foods and about how a food fits into the overall diet. To make this information uniform and easy to use, food labeling standards are specified by the Nutrition Labeling and Education Act of 1990.[14] Serving sizes and the format of food labels have been standardized to allow comparisons between products. For example, comparing the energy content of different types of crackers is simplified because all packages list values for a standard serving size of about 30 grams, the number of crackers per serving, and the kcalories per serving. On food labels, the term "Calorie" is used to refer to kcalories.

What Must Be Labeled Food labeling laws regulate about 75% of all food consumed in the United States.[15] The Food and Drug Administration (FDA) regulates the labeling of all foods except meat and poultry products, which are regulated by the U.S. Department of Agriculture (USDA). All packaged foods except those produced by small businesses and those in packages too small to fit the labeling information must be labeled. Some restaurant food and ready-to-eat food, such as that served in bakeries and delicatessens, is also exempt, but if a claim about a food's nutritional content or health benefits such as "lowfat" or "heart healthy" is included on a menu, the eating establishment must provide nutritional information about this food when requested.[16] (See *Off the Shelf: Choosing Off the Menu.*) Raw fruits, vegetables, fish, meat, and poultry are not required to carry individual labels. The FDA has asked grocery stores to voluntarily provide nutrition information for the raw fruits, vegetables, and fish most frequently eaten in the United States, and the USDA encourages voluntary nutrition labeling of raw meat and poultry. About 75% of stores comply with the request to provide nutrient information for raw produce and fish.[17] The information can appear on large placards or in consumer pamphlets or brochures (Figure 2.7). In Canada, nutrition labeling is voluntary but standardized and provides information similar to that on labels in the United States.[18]

What Must Be Listed All labels contain basic product information such as the name of the product; the net contents or weight; the date by which the product

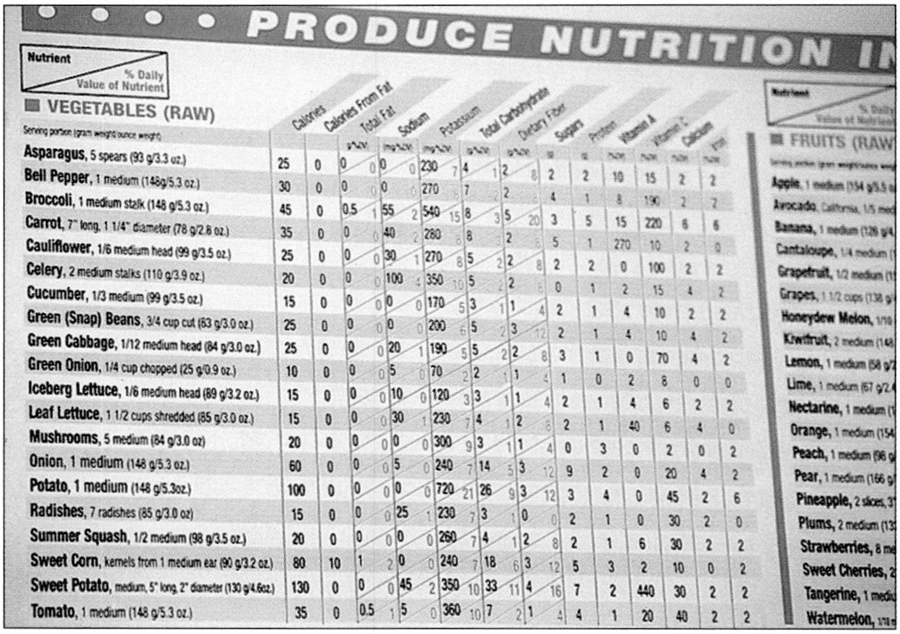

Figure 2.7
Fresh produce is not required to carry individual labels, but the information is usually displayed in the produce section of the store. (George Semple)

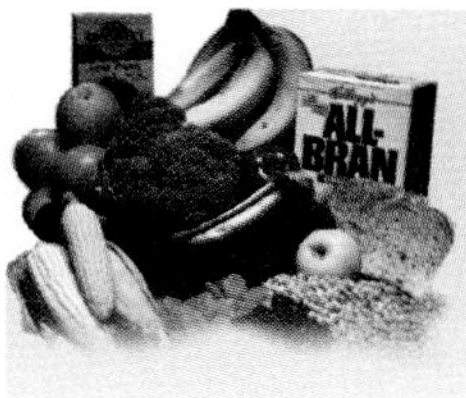

Off the Shelf

Choosing Off the Menu

Treating yourself to an occasional dinner out has little long-term impact on your total diet, but for many Americans eating out is more than an occasional treat. Today, more Americans than ever are eating away from home, and the restaurant meals they consume are usually higher in fat and cholesterol than meals eaten at home.[1] The change in our lifestyle to include more restaurant and fast-food meals has made choosing healthy foods from restaurant menus an important skill—but it can be a challenge.

Some healthy choices are easy, even at restaurants. If you are looking for a lowfat meal, skip the fried fish and have it broiled instead. Minimize sauces and spreads (like the honey butter on your corn bread) that add fat, sugar, and kcalories. Use less salad dressing by asking that it be served on the side. Be conscious of portion sizes. Those served in restaurants are often much larger than what we prepare at home. You don't have to finish everything—take it home for tomorrow's lunch.

Other restaurant choices are more difficult to make. Items that sound like part of a healthy diet are not always what they seem. What's in that house special turkey tetrazzini, beef lo mein, or a fajita wrap? Without the chef's recipe it is impossible to know. The amounts of specific nutrients are usually not given on menus and the ingredients can be a mystery. Even when you know what ingredients are usually in a dish like eggplant parmesan, you can never be sure how much oil or salt was used. Even an order of plain old green beans might come floating in butter.

Many restaurants and fast-food establishments have responded to consumer concern about healthy diets with healthier choices. Menus often highlight healthy items by making claims about nutrient content, such as lowfat tostados, low-salt lo mein, or reduced kcalorie lasagna. The food labeling laws that regulate packaged foods also apply to menus so the definition of these terms must match those used on food labels. For example, if you order lowfat tostados, the term "lowfat" should mean the same as it does on labeled packaged foods—that it contains 3 grams or less of fat per serving.

Menus may also include statements that give general dietary guidance or make specific claims about the relationship between a nutrient and a disease or health condition. For example, the salad section may start with the statement that "eating five fruits and vegetables a day is an important part of a healthy diet."[2] A dish that is low in fat, saturated fat, and cholesterol might carry a claim that diets low in saturated fat and cholesterol may reduce the risk of heart disease. To carry a health claim, menu items must contain a significant amount of at least one of six key nutrients (vitamin A, vitamin C, iron, calcium, protein, or fiber) and cannot contain a food substance at a level that increases the risk of a disease or health condition.

Nutrient content claims and health claims about items on the menu must be backed up with appropriate nutrition information when requested. This information can be on the menu or in accompanying nutrition information available upon request. It can be presented in any format, such as printed in a notebook or recited by the staff, and only needs to provide information about the nutrient or nutrients to which the claim is referring. Restaurants do not have to provide nutrition information about items that do not carry nutrient content or health claims or that are referred to in general dietary messages.

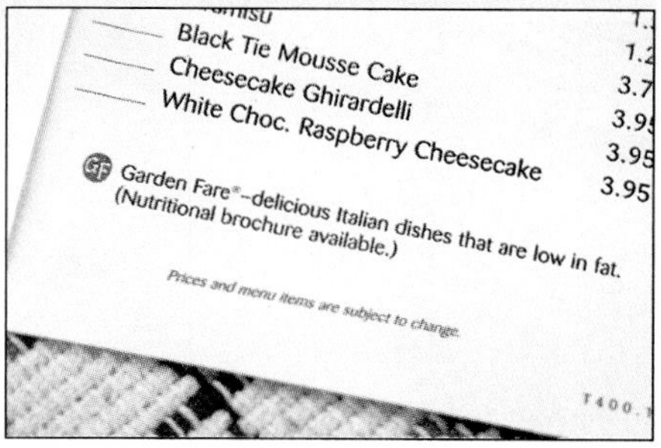

(George Semple)

When choosing from a menu, look for items that fit into an overall healthy diet—and are also things you enjoy. Choose foods you like and remember that a high-fat or high-kcalorie meal now and then doesn't make your overall diet unhealthy. But, if you eat out frequently, these meals make up a greater part of your overall diet and should be chosen carefully. Use nutrient content claims and health claims to choose items that meet your dietary needs.

[1]USDA, Agricultural Service, 1997, Results from USDA's 1994–1996 Continuing Survey of Food Intakes by Individuals and 1994–1996 Health Knowledge Survey. ARS Food Surveys Research Group. Online at http://www.barc.usda.gov/bhnrc/foodsurvey/home/htm

[2]Kurtzweil, P. Today's special nutrition information. FDA Consumer 31:21–25, May–June, 1997.

should be sold; and the name and place of business of the manufacturer, packager, or distributor. In addition, most food labels contain a list of the food's ingredients and information about the nutrient content of the product and its contribution to a healthy diet.

List of Ingredients The ingredients section of the label lists the contents of the product in order of their prominence by weight. An ingredient list is required on all products containing more than one ingredient. Food additives, including food colors and flavorings, must be listed among the ingredients.

Figure 2.8

The Nutrition Labeling Act of 1990 required standardization of the information on food labels. (FDA Consumer 27:23, May 1993)

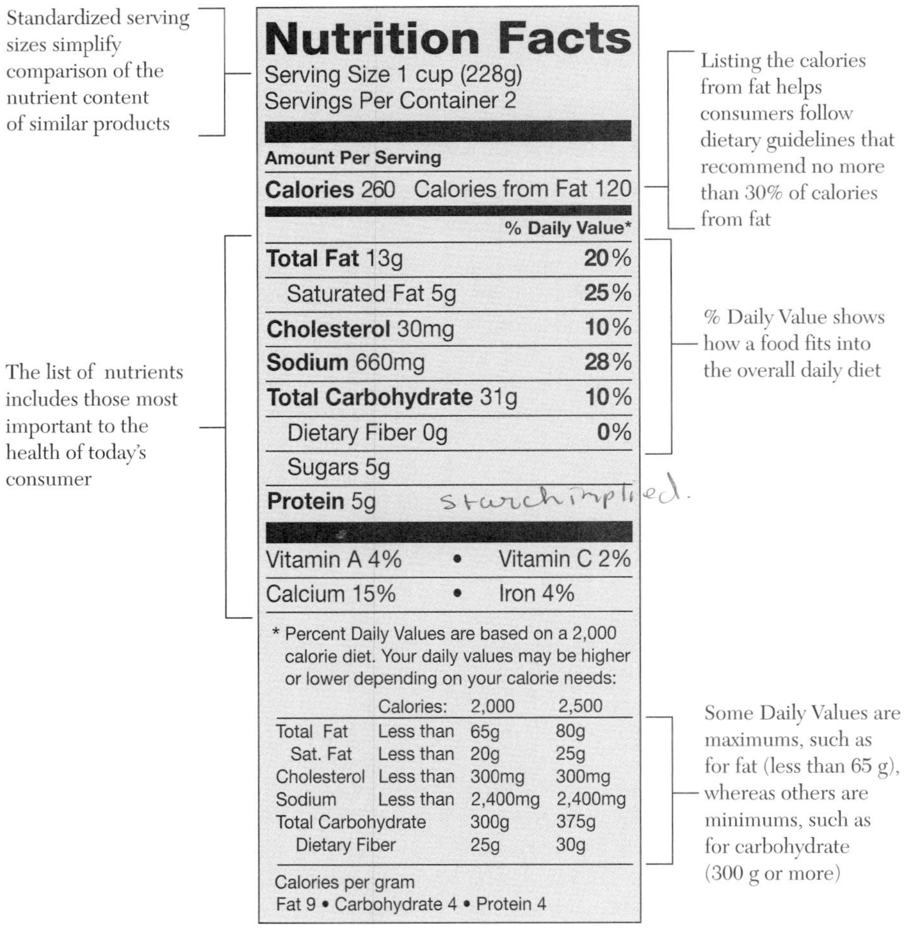

Nutrition Facts The nutrition information section of the label is entitled "Nutrition Facts" (Figure 2.8). In this section, the serving size is listed in common household and metric measures, and is based on a standard list of serving sizes designed to be representative of the serving sizes people choose. These serving sizes are not the same as the serving sizes in the Food Guide Pyramid. The serving size is followed by the number of servings per container. The label must then list the total kcalories, kcalories from fat, total fat, saturated fat, cholesterol, sodium, total carbohydrate, dietary fiber, sugars, and protein. The amounts of these nutrients are given per serving and most are also listed as a percentage of a standard called the **Daily Value.** Daily Values help consumers determine how a food fits into their overall diet. The percent Daily Value is the amount of a nutrient in a food as a percentage of the recommendation for a 2000-kcalorie diet. For example, if a food provides 10% of the Daily Value for dietary fiber, then the food provides 10% of the recommended daily intake for dietary fiber in a 2000-kcalorie diet. Daily Values are based on two sets of standards, the **Reference Daily Intakes (RDIs)** and the **Daily Reference Values (DRVs)**. To avoid confusion, only the term "Daily Value" appears on food labels.

Daily Values Nutrient reference values used on food labels to help consumers see how foods fit into their overall diets.

Reference Daily Intakes (RDIs) Reference values established for vitamins and minerals that are based on the highest amount of each nutrient recommended for any adult age group by the 1968 RDAs.

Daily Reference Values (DRVs) Reference values established for protein and seven nutrients for which no RDA has been established. The values are based on dietary recommendations for reducing the risk of chronic disease.

The Reference Daily Intakes (Table 2.4) are used to determine Daily Values for vitamins and minerals for which original RDAs were established. Although the name has changed, most of the current RDI values are the same as the old U.S. RDAs (U.S. Recommended Daily Allowances). They are based on the highest amount of each nutrient recommended for any adult age group by the 1968 RDAs. These may overestimate the amount of a nutrient needed for some groups, but they do not underestimate the requirement for any group (except pregnant and lactating women). Label regulations require that percent Daily Val-

Table 2.4 *Reference Daily Intakes**

Nutrient	Amount	Nutrient	Amount	Nutrient	Amount
Vitamin A	5000 IU (1000 μg)†	Vitamin E	30 IU (10 mg)	Biotin	300 μg
Vitamin C	60 mg	Vitamin B_6	2.0 mg	Pantothenic acid	10 mg
Thiamin	1.5 mg	Folic acid	400 μg	Vitamin K	80 μg
Riboflavin	1.7 mg	Vitamin B_{12}	6 μg	Chromium	120 μg
Niacin	20 mg	Phosphorus	1000 mg	Selenium	70 μg
Calcium	1000 mg	Iodine	150 μg	Molybdenum	75 μg
Iron	18 mg	Magnesium	400 mg	Manganese	2 mg
Vitamin D	400 IU (10 μg)	Zinc	15 mg	Chloride	3400 mg
		Copper	2 mg		

*Based on National Academy of Sciences' 1968 Recommended Dietary Allowances.
†The RDIs for some fat-soluble vitamins are expressed in International Units (IU). The RDAs use a newer system of measurement. Values that are approximately equivalent are given in parentheses.

ues, based on RDIs, be listed for vitamin A, vitamin C, calcium, and iron. In addition to these mandatory listings, a manufacturer may voluntarily include information about other nutrients.

Daily Reference Values are designed as standards to help consumers follow recommendations for health promotion and disease prevention. They have been established for fat, saturated fat, carbohydrate, fiber, cholesterol, sodium, potassium, and protein (Table 2.5). The DRV for fat, for example, is based on the recommendation that dietary fat should account for less than 30% of energy, or less than 65 grams for a 2000-kcalorie diet. The DRVs are used on food labels to calculate the percent Daily Values for nutrients based on a diet containing 2000 kcalories. To illustrate that the recommended intake of some nutrients depends on energy needs, Daily Values based on DRVs are listed on food labels for both a 2000- and a 2500-kcalorie diet.

Labeling Terminology and Health Claims In addition to the required nutrition information, food labels often highlight specific characteristics of a product that might be of interest to the consumer, such as "low in Calories" or "high in fiber." Definitions for nutrient content descriptors such as "free," "low," and "light" have been established by the FDA and are based on how these terms relate to nutrient content. In selecting a product labeled with a descriptor such as

Table 2.5 *Daily Reference Values*

Food Component	Daily Reference Value (2000 kcal)
Total fat	Less than 65 g (30% of energy)
Saturated fat	Less than 20 g (10% of energy)
Cholesterol	Less than 300 mg
Total carbohydrate	300 g (60% of energy)
Dietary fiber	25 g (11.5 g/1000 kcal)
Sodium	Less than 2400 mg
Potassium	3500 mg
Protein	50 g (10% of energy)

Table 2.6 *Nutrient Content Descriptors Commonly Used on Food Labels*

Free	Means that a product contains no amount of, or a trivial amount of, fat, saturated fat, cholesterol, sodium, sugars, or kcalories. For example, "sugar free" and "fat free" both mean less than 0.5 g per serving. Synonyms for "free" include "without," "no," and "zero."
Low	Used for foods that can be eaten frequently without exceeding the Daily Value for fat, saturated fat, cholesterol, sodium, or kcalories. Specific definitions have been established for each of these nutrients. For example, "lowfat" means that the food contains 3 g or less per serving, and "low cholesterol" means that the food contains less than 20 mg of cholesterol per serving. Synonyms for "low" include "little," "few," and "low source of."
Lean and extra lean	Used to describe the fat content of meat, poultry, seafood, and game meats. "Lean" means that the food contains less than 10 g fat, less than 4.5 g saturated fat, and less than 95 mg of cholesterol per serving and per 100 g. "Extra lean" means that the food contains less than 5 g fat, less than 2 g saturated fat, and less than 95 mg of cholesterol per serving and per 100 g.
High	Can be used if a food contains 20% or more of the Daily Value for a particular nutrient. Synonyms for "high" include "rich in" and "excellent source of."
Good source	Means that a food contains 10 to 19% of the Daily Value for a particular nutrient per serving.
Reduced	Means that a nutritionally altered product contains 25% less of a nutrient or of energy than the regular or reference product.
Less	Means that a food, whether altered or not, contains 25% less of a nutrient or of energy than the reference food. For example, pretzels may claim to have "less fat" than potato chips. "Fewer" may be used as a synonym for "less."
Light	May be used in different ways. First, it can be used on a nutritionally altered product that contains one third fewer kcalories or half the fat of a reference food. Second, it can be used when the sodium content of a low-calorie, lowfat food has been reduced by 50%. The term "light" can be used to describe properties such as texture and color as long as the label explains the intent, for example, "light and fluffy."
More	Means that a serving of food, whether altered or not, contains a nutrient that is at least 10% of the Daily Value more than the reference food. This definition also applies to foods using the terms "fortified," "enriched," or "added."
Healthy	May be used to describe foods that are low in fat and saturated fat and contain no more than 360 mg of sodium and no more than 60 mg of cholesterol per serving and provide at least 10% of the Daily Value for vitamins A or C, or iron, calcium, protein, or fiber.
Fresh	May be used on foods that are raw and have never been frozen or heated and contain no preservatives.

Federal Register 58, 1993, Jan. 6. U.S. Government Printing Office, Superintendent of Documents, Washington, D.C.

"fat free," consumers can be assured that the food meets the defined criteria, in this case that the product contains less than 0.5 gram of fat per serving. The specific definition of each of these descriptors is given in Table 2.6 and their use in relation to specific nutrients is discussed in *Off the Label* features throughout this text.

Food labels are also permitted to include a number of health claims if they are relevant to the product. Health claims refer to a relationship between a nutrient or a food and the risk of a disease or health-related condition. These

Table 2.7 Health Claims Allowed on Food Labels*

Calcium and osteoporosis	Adequate calcium intake throughout life helps maintain bone health and reduce the risk of osteoporosis.
Sodium and hypertension (high blood pressure)	Diets high in sodium may increase the risk of high blood pressure in some people.
Dietary fat and cancer	Diets high in fat increase the risk of some types of cancer.
Saturated fat and cholesterol and risk of coronary heart disease	Diets high in saturated fat and cholesterol increase blood cholesterol and, thus, the risk of heart disease.
Foods high in fiber and cancer	Diets low in fat and rich in fiber-containing grain products, fruits, and vegetables may reduce the risk of some types of cancer.
Foods high in fiber and risk of coronary heart disease	Diets low in saturated fat and cholesterol and rich in fruits, vegetables, and grain products that contain fiber, particularly soluble fiber, may reduce the risk of coronary heart disease.
Fruits and vegetables and cancer	Diets low in fat and rich in fruits and vegetables may reduce the risk of some types of cancer.
Folic acid and neural tube defect–affected pregnancy	Adequate folic acid intake by the mother reduces the risk of birth defects of the brain or spinal cord in her baby.
Foods high in soluble fiber from whole oats or psyllium husk and heart disease	Diets low in saturated fat and cholesterol that include soluble fiber from whole oats or psyllium husks may reduce the risk of heart disease.
Dietary sugar alcohol and dental caries	Sugar-free foods that are sweetened with sugar alcohols do not promote tooth decay and may reduce the risk of dental caries.

*A food carrying a health claim must be a naturally good source (10% or more of the Daily Value) for 1 of 6 nutrients (vitamin A, vitamin C, protein, calcium, iron, or fiber) and must not contain more than 20% of the Daily Value for fat, saturated fat, cholesterol, or sodium.

can help consumers choose products that will meet their dietary needs or health goals. For example, lowfat milk, a good source of calcium, might include on the label a statement indicating that a diet high in calcium will reduce the risk of developing osteoporosis. Only the claims listed in Table 2.7 are currently allowed.[19]

Despite the wealth of information available on food labels, today's consumer must be educated about the benefits and pitfalls of foods that are not labeled and about food and nutrition issues that are not addressed by food labels. Such issues include the advantages and disadvantages of fresh, frozen, and canned produce, and the safe selection, storage, and preparation of food. Food labels cannot tell you what you should eat, or how you should prepare it, but they are an important source of information about what you are eating. (See *Off the Label: Using Food Labels to Choose a Diet That Meets Recommendations.*)

Assessing Nutritional Health

To be healthy, populations and individuals need to consume nutrients from the right combination of foods in appropriate amounts. Scientists have developed standards for the amounts we need and tools for planning diets to meet these needs. But how do we know if the nutritional needs of a population or an individual are being met? Evaluating the **nutritional status** of populations and individuals can identify nutritional needs and be used to plan diets to meet these needs.

Nutritional status State of health as it is influenced by the intake and utilization of nutrients.

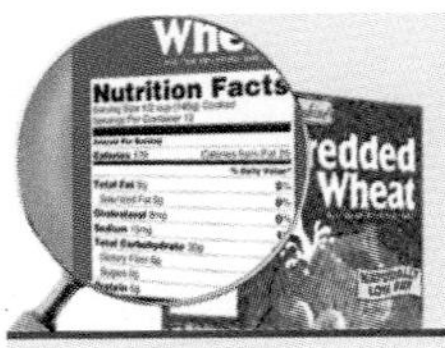

Off the Label

Using Food Labels to Choose a Diet That Meets Recommendations

Food labels can't help you include 3 to 5 servings of vegetables and 2 to 4 servings of fruit in your diet each day, or ensure that you select a diet with great variety, but they can help you choose packaged foods that meet the recommendations of the Dietary Guidelines and the Food Guide Pyramid.

Food labels are a readily available source of nutrition information. Yet 36% of Americans say they pay only slight or no attention to these valuable tools.[1] Reviewing labels while in the grocery store can have a big impact on your nutrient intake for the day. For example, if you are selecting foods for breakfast, your choice could be granola with whole milk or oatmeal made with skim milk. The labels on the milk and the cereal boxes can help you choose which fits best into a diet that is low in fat, moderate in sugar, and high in nutrient density. Whole milk provides 150 kcalories and 8 grams of fat in a cup. This 8 grams of fat represents 12% of the Daily Value—that is, 12% of the total amount of fat recommended per day for a 2000-kcalorie diet. The fat-free milk contains no fat and only 90 kcalories per cup. Both are sources of calcium and vitamins A and D, and both count as a serving from the milk group of the Food Guide Pyramid. In terms of meeting the the Dietary Guideline to choose a diet low in fat, saturated fat, and cholesterol, fat-free milk

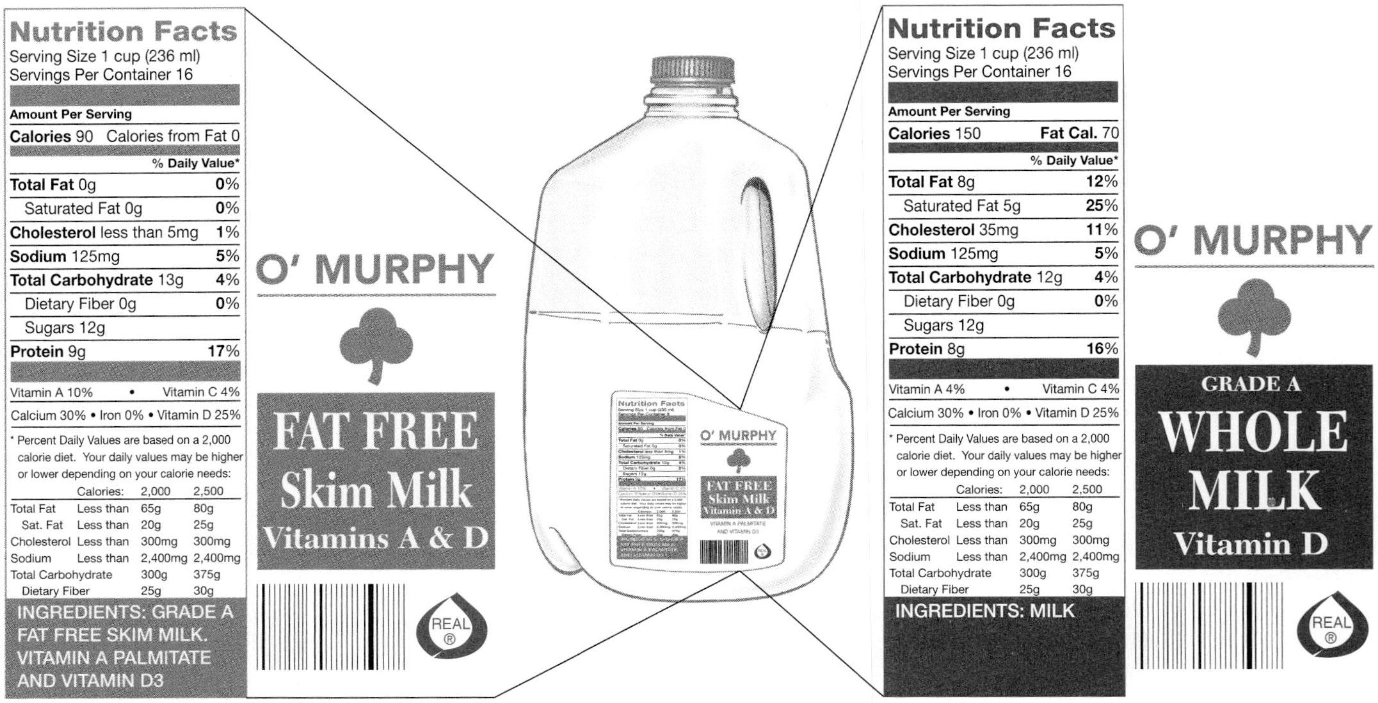

The Nutritional Health of the Population

We know that there is enough food available in the United States to meet the needs of the population. We also know that poor nutritional choices from this food supply result in diets high in some nutrients and low in others. This kind of information is obtained by monitoring what foods are available and what is consumed. In the United States, the National Nutrition Monitoring and Related Research Program is responsible for providing an ongoing description of nutrition conditions in the population by collecting information about food availability and consumption; food composition; and the eating behaviors, health, and nutritional status of the population.[20] These epidemiological data are used for the purpose of planning nutrition-related policies and programs and predicting future trends of public health importance.

The granola and the oatmeal both provide a serving from the grain group, but the amounts of fat and sugars differ. According to the labels, a serving of granola provides 230 kcalories and 9 grams of fat, whereas oatmeal provides only 150 kcalories and 3 grams of fat. A review of the ingredient list reveals that oatmeal contains only rolled oats, resulting in a food that is lower in both fat and refined sugars and is higher in nutrient density.

Knowing how to interpret the information on food labels can help you choose a diet that meets the recommendations of the Dietary Guidelines and follows the selection tips of the Food Guide Pyramid. This doesn't mean you can never choose the granola. This choice can be part of a healthy diet as long as it is balanced with healthy lowfat choices throughout the day. Remember, it is your total diet—not each choice—that counts.

[1]American Dietetic Association 1997 Nutrition Trends Survey, Executive Summary. Chicago: American Dietetic Association, 1997.

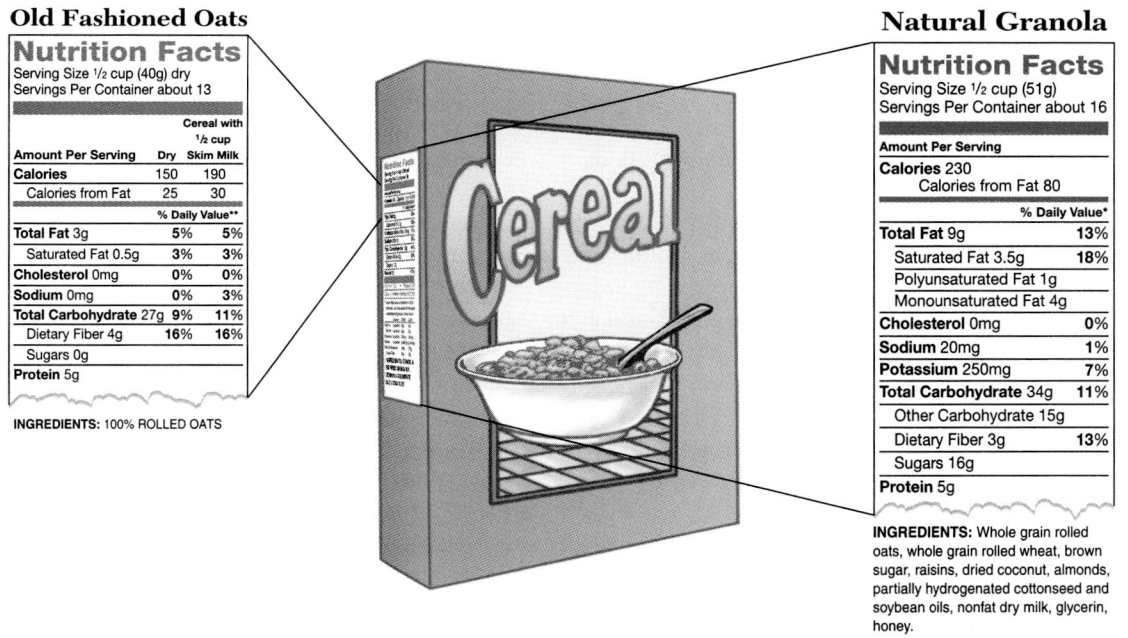

Old Fashioned Oats

Nutrition Facts
Serving Size 1/2 cup (40g) dry
Servings Per Container about 13

Amount Per Serving	Dry	Cereal with 1/2 cup Skim Milk
Calories	150	190
Calories from Fat	25	30
	% Daily Value**	
Total Fat 3g	5%	5%
Saturated Fat 0.5g	3%	3%
Cholesterol 0mg	0%	0%
Sodium 0mg	0%	3%
Total Carbohydrate 27g	9%	11%
Dietary Fiber 4g	16%	16%
Sugars 0g		
Protein 5g		

INGREDIENTS: 100% ROLLED OATS

Natural Granola

Nutrition Facts
Serving Size 1/2 cup (51g)
Servings Per Container about 16

Amount Per Serving	
Calories 230	
Calories from Fat 80	
	% Daily Value*
Total Fat 9g	13%
Saturated Fat 3.5g	18%
Polyunsaturated Fat 1g	
Monounsaturated Fat 4g	
Cholesterol 0mg	0%
Sodium 20mg	1%
Potassium 250mg	7%
Total Carbohydrate 34g	11%
Other Carbohydrate 15g	
Dietary Fiber 3g	13%
Sugars 16g	
Protein 5g	

INGREDIENTS: Whole grain rolled oats, whole grain rolled wheat, brown sugar, raisins, dried coconut, almonds, partially hydrogenated cottonseed and soybean oils, nonfat dry milk, glycerin, honey.

Monitoring the Food Supply The food available to a population is estimated using food disappearance surveys. The food supply includes all that is grown, manufactured, or imported for sale in the country. Food use or "disappearance" is estimated by measuring what food is sold. These types of surveys are used to estimate what is available to the population, provide year-to-year comparisons, and identify trends in the diet; but they tend to overestimate actual intake because they do not consider losses that occur during processing, marketing, and home use. Also, the surveys do not assess the distribution of food throughout the population. For example, Figure 2.9 illustrates the food disappearance data on milk consumption over the past 25 years. It shows that the consumption of whole milk, which is high in fat, has declined and the consumption of lower fat milks has increased since 1970. From this it can be concluded that fat intake from milk has declined. But the graph also indicates that total milk consumption has gone down

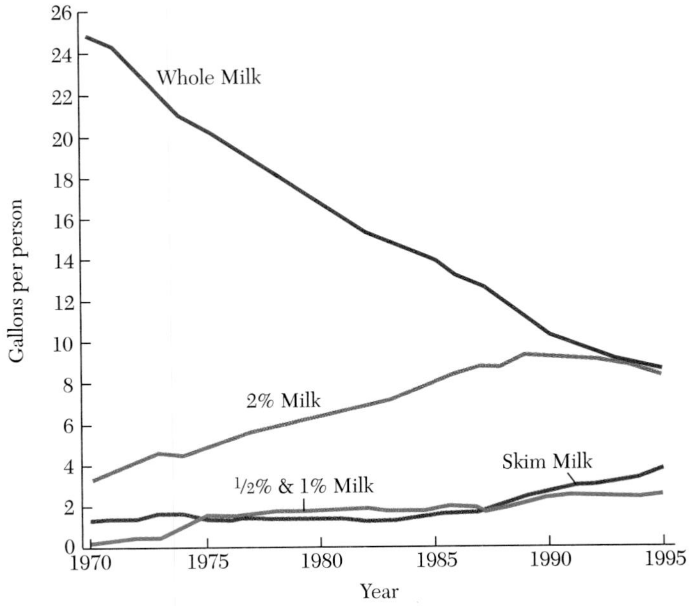

Figure 2.9
Food disappearance data can identify population trends in food intake such as the increase in the consumption of 2% milk and the decrease in whole milk consumption that occurred from 1970 to 1995.

over the last 25 years. This may alert the government that calcium intake from milk has decreased and calcium may therefore be at risk for deficiency in the population. The numbers in this graph do not give any information about how much milk each person is drinking or who is at risk of inadequate calcium intake.

Monitoring Nutritional Status The nutritional status of the population is monitored by examining and comparing trends in food intake and health. This is done by interviewing individuals within the population to determine what food is actually consumed, and collecting information on health and nutritional status. One series of surveys conducted by the U.S. Department of Agriculture is the Nationwide Food Consumption Surveys (NFCS), which collect information on the use of foods by households. The USDA also conducts the Continuing Survey of Food Intakes by Individuals (CSFII), which collects data on intakes of individuals within households. Together, these monitor the adequacy of food and nutrient intake by the population. The Department of Health and Human Services conducts the National Health and Nutrition Examination Survey (NHANES), which combines information on food consumption with medical histories, physical examinations, and laboratory measurements to monitor both nutritional and health information. These data on food and nutrient intake can be assessed by comparing population intakes with reference values such as the DRIs or with other guidelines such as the recommendations of the Dietary Guidelines or the Food Guide Pyramid. For example, we know that only 22% of people eat the 5 or more servings of fruits and vegetables per day recommended by the Food Guide Pyramid, that there has been a slight drop in dietary fat intake, and that the number of people who are overweight has increased in all adult age groups in the past decade.

A system that has been developed to evaluate the adequacy of the diet of Americans is the Healthy Eating Index.[21] This uses data from the USDA's CSFII and provides a measure that summarizes overall diet quality by scoring 10 components of the diet, each representing different aspects of a healthy diet. Five of these components measure how well a person's diet complies with the serving recommendations for the five food groups of the Food Guide Pyramid. The other five components score the diet based on how well it complies with the recommendations of the Dietary Guidelines regarding total fat, saturated fat, cholesterol, sodium, and variety. Each component has a maximum score of 10, so an individual who follows all of these guidelines would have a Healthy

Eating Index score of 100. Since the index was first computerized in 1989, the typical American diet has improved slightly from a score of 61.5 in 1989 to 63.8 in 1996.[21]

Individual Nutritional Health

What about your own nutritional status? Are you losing weight? Gaining weight? Do you have a history of heart disease in your family? Are you at risk for a nutrient deficiency because you can't get to the store, can't afford to buy healthy foods, or you don't know what to eat or how to cook? An individual **nutritional assessment** requires a review of past and present dietary intake, assessment of body size, medical history, and laboratory measurements. Even with all these tools, diagnosing a nutritional deficiency or excess is not trivial. Estimates of dietary intake are not always accurate and symptoms may be indistinguishable from other medical conditions.

Nutritional assessment The process of determining the nutritional status of individuals or groups for the purpose of identifying nutritional needs and planning personal health-care or community programs to meet these needs.

Estimating Dietary Intake A good place to start when evaluating people's nutritional status is to determine what they typically eat. Since this information relies on the memory and reliability of the individual, it is not always accurate. For instance, overweight persons tend to report smaller portions than they actually eat, and underweight individuals tend to overreport portions.[22] Despite this problem, the commonly used methods described below are the best tools available for evaluating dietary intake to predict nutrient deficiencies or excesses.

24-Hour Recall The most common method of assessing dietary intake is a 24-hour recall in which a trained interviewer asks people to recall exactly what they ate during the preceding 24-hour period. A detailed description of all food and drink, including descriptions of cooking methods and brand names of products, is recorded. Since food intake varies from day to day, repeated 24-hour recalls on the same individuals provide a more accurate estimate of typical intake.

Food Diary or Food Intake Record Food intake information can also be gathered by having people keep a daily record of all the food and drink they consume for a set period of time. Typically, this is done for two to seven days including at least one weekend day, since most people eat differently on weekends than during the school or work week. Foods may be weighed or portion sizes just estimated (Figure 2.10). The record should be as complete as possible, including all beverages,

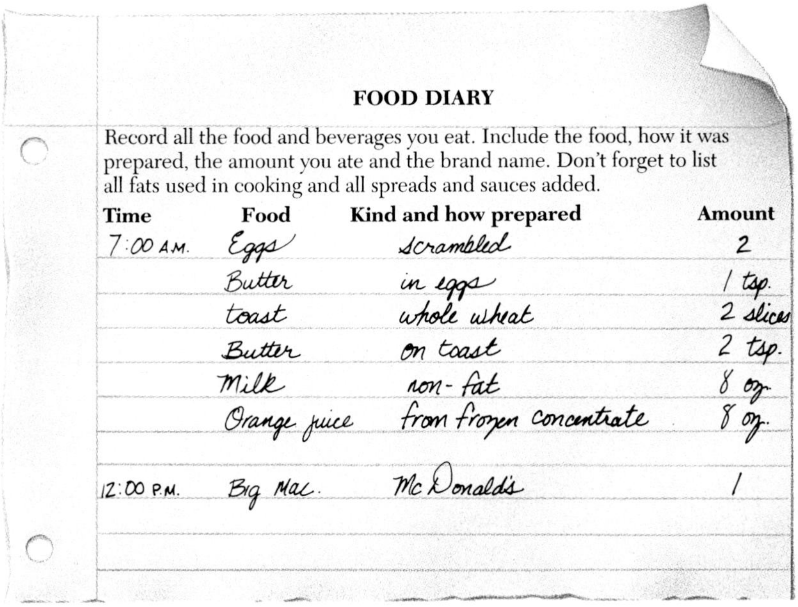
FOOD DIARY

Record all the food and beverages you eat. Include the food, how it was prepared, the amount you ate and the brand name. Don't forget to list all fats used in cooking and all spreads and sauces added.

Time	Food	Kind and how prepared	Amount
7:00 A.M.	Eggs	scrambled	2
	Butter	in eggs	1 tsp.
	toast	whole wheat	2 slices
	Butter	on toast	2 tsp.
	Milk	non-fat	8 oz.
	Orange juice	from frozen concentrate	8 oz.
12:00 P.M.	Big Mac.	McDonald's	1

Figure 2.10
Accurate food diaries require the recording of all food and drink consumed.

Figure 2.11
This section of a sample food frequency questionnaire obtains information about dairy product consumption patterns.

Food Frequency Questionnaire

On the following pages, please check the appropriate column indicating how often you consume each food.

	Once a day	Twice or more a day	Once a week	Twice or more a week	Once a month	Twice or more a month
Milk						
Whole						
Reduced fat						✓
Nonfat	✓					
Yogurt						
Whole						
Reduced fat			✓			
Nonfat						
Cheese						
Hard					✓	
Soft						✓
Reduced fat						
Ice cream						
Regular						
Reduced fat	✓					

condiments, and the brand names and preparation methods. The tedious nature of this type of record can be a disadvantage because in some cases it may cause the individual to change intake rather than record certain items.

Food Frequency To complete a food frequency questionnaire, individuals must respond to a series of questions about their patterns of intake. For example, "How often do you drink milk?" or "How many times a week do you eat red meat?" This doesn't itemize a specific day's intake, but it gives a general picture of patterns of food intake (Figure 2.11).

Diet History A diet history is a general term for information about dietary habits and patterns. It may include a history of eating habits: Do you cook your own meals? Do you skip lunch? Did you drink milk as an adolescent? It may also include a combination of other methods such as a 24-hour recall along with a food frequency questionnaire. The combination of two or more methods often provides more complete information than one method alone. For instance, if an individual's 24-hour recall does not include milk, but a food frequency questionnaire suggests that the individual usually drinks milk once a day, the two can be combined to provide a more accurate picture of this individual's typical intake.

Analyzing Nutrient Intake Once information on food intake has been obtained, the nutrient content of the diet can be compared to recommended intakes. This can be done in a number of ways. To get a general picture of dietary intake, an individual's food record can be compared with a guide for diet planning such as the Food Guide Pyramid. For example, does the individual consume the recommended number of servings of milk per day? If an evaluation of the energy and macronutrient content of the diet is needed, it can be estimated using the Exchange Lists. A more precise and extensive analysis of dietary intake can be done by totaling the nutrient content of each food item.

Nutrient composition information is available on food labels, in published food composition tables, and in computer databases. Information on food labels can be used to calculate the intake of some nutrients but since they are only included on packaged foods, food composition tables generated by government and industry laboratories are available (see Appendix A for an abbreviated list). The major source

3 Day Average September 8, 1998

Serving Size: 1585.31 g (55.92 oz-wt.)
Serves: 1.00

Nutrient	Value	Goal%
Basic Components		
Calories	1811.41	97%
Protein	95.48 g	219%
Carbohydrates	241.89 g	90%
Dietary Fiber	26.42 g	142%
Fat-Total	54.70 g	88%
Saturated Fat	22.70 g	122%
Mono Fat	16.63 g	73%
Poly Fat	8.10 g	39%
Cholesterol	195.20 mg	65%
Water	1174.44 g	
Vitamins		
Vitamin A RE	1780.71 RE	223%
Vitamin C	110.32 mg	184%
Thiamin-B1	1.78 mg	191%
Riboflavin-B2	2.33 mg	208%
Niacin-B3	26.03 mg	212%
Vitamin-B6	2.28 mg	142%
Folate	513.92 mcg	286%
Vitamin-B12	4.56 mcg	228%
Minerals		
Calcium	1069.14 mg	134%
Phosphorus	1712.86 mg	214%
Sodium	1851.02 mg	77%
Potassium	3462.69 mg	92%
Zinc	13.13 mg	109%
Iron	16.49 mg	110%
Magnesium	397.52 mg	142%

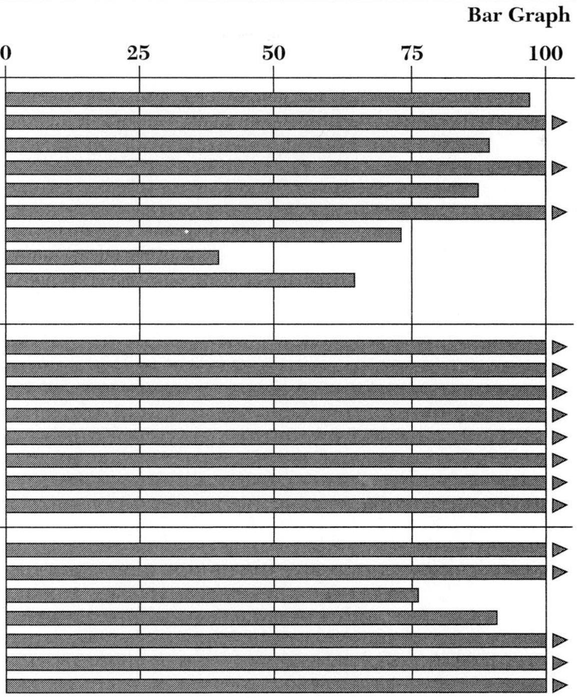

Figure 2.12

To be meaningful, the information on computer printouts from diet analysis must be accurately interpreted. This printout shows the average intake over three days. The "Value" column gives the average total amount of a nutrient consumed over three days and the "Goal %" column tells us how this amount compares to dietary standards. For example, the average calcium intake is 134% of the goal for this individual. For some nutrients such as fat, the recommended goal is a maximum recommended amount, so an intake below this is not a disadvantage.

of food composition data in the United States is USDA Nutrient Database for Standard Reference, which is available online.[23] Computer programs with food composition databases are now readily available for professionals and for home use.

To analyze nutrient intake using a computer program, each food and an exact portion consumed must be entered into the program. If a food is not found in the computer database, an appropriate substitute can be used or the food can be broken down into its individual ingredients. For example, homemade vegetable soup could be entered as generic vegetable soup, or as vegetable broth, carrots, green beans, rice, etc. If a new product has come on the market, the information from the food label can be added to the database. The advantage of computer diet analysis is that it is fast and accurate. A program can calculate the nutrients for each day or average them over several days. It can also compare nutrient intake to recommended amounts. However, the information generated by computer diet analysis is only useful if it is entered and interpreted correctly. Figure 2.12 shows a typical printout for a computerized diet analysis.

Height, Weight, and Body Size Evaluating nutritional health also involves an assessment of an individual's **anthropometric measurements,** that is, height, weight, and body size. These measurements can be compared with population standards (see Appendix B) or used to monitor changes in an individual over time (Figure 2.13). If an individual's measurements differ significantly from standards, he may have a nutritional deficiency or excess; however, this information should be evaluated only within the context of that person's personal and family history. For example, a child who is small for his age may have a nutritional deficiency or may simply have inherited his small body size. An individual whose weight is less than the standard may be adequately nourished if she has never weighed more than her current weight and is otherwise healthy.

Anthropometric measurements External measurements of the body, such as height, weight, limb circumference, and skinfold thickness.

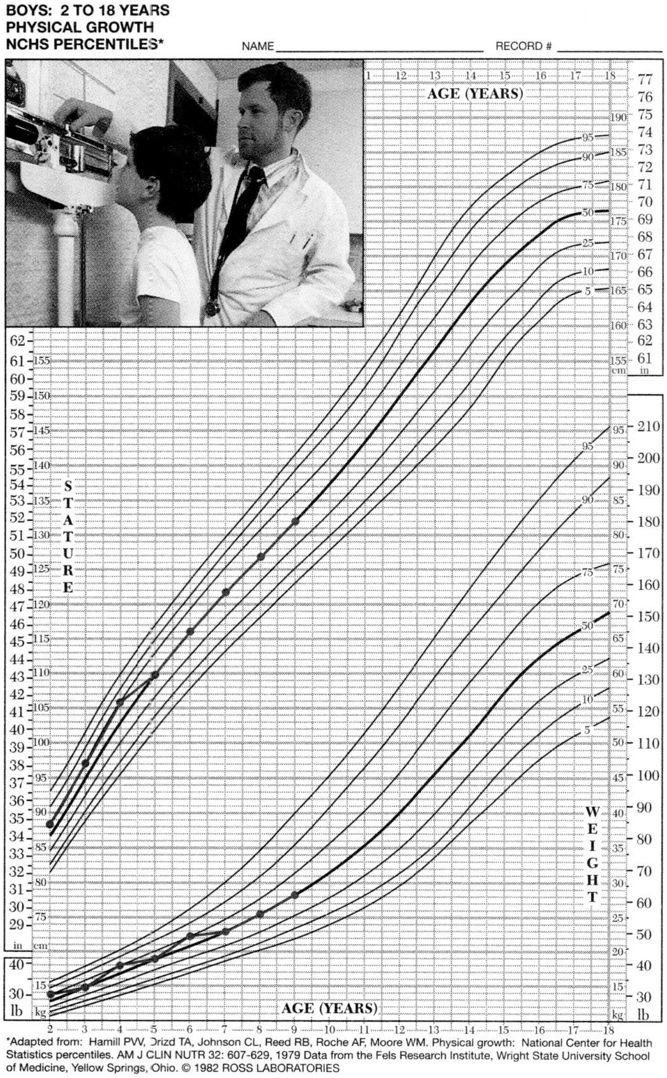

Figure 2.13
Changes in body weight can be indicators of nutritional status. (Photo, © Andy Levin/Photo Researchers, Inc.)

Medical History A medical history can also be used to assess symptoms of, or risk factors for, nutrition-related diseases. For instance, a medical history could reveal that an individual's mother died of a heart attack at age 50. This individual has a higher than average risk of developing heart disease and therefore would want to select a diet that reduces her risk of developing this disease (see Chapter 5). An individual who has a family history of diabetes has an increased risk of developing this disease especially if he carries excess body fat.

Other symptoms, such as dry skin, cracked lips, or lethargy, that may accompany nutrient deficiencies are noted in a clinical assessment. However, most of these are nonspecific and may or may not be due to nutritional status. Laboratory measurements may be used to determine whether a clinical symptom is due to malnutrition or another disease process.

Laboratory Measurements Measures of nutrients or their by-products in the blood, urine, or body compartments can be used to detect nutrient deficiencies and excesses. For instance, measuring the volume of red blood cells can be helpful in diagnosing iron deficiency anemia because red blood cells require iron for proper formation (see Chapter 11 and *Critical Thinking: Nutritional Assessment*). Because blood carries newly absorbed nutrients to the cells of the body, the amounts of some nutrients in the blood may reflect the amount in the current diet rather than the total body status of the nutrient. For some nutrients, it may be better to analyze the cells in the blood or other tissue samples (see Appendix C). If the measure does not reflect body status, then it is not useful in nutritional assessment. For instance, hair analysis has been suggested as a means of assessing body mineral levels. However, because many factors, including exposure to environmental contaminants, shampoos, and hair treatments, affect the mineral content of hair, this analysis may not provide much useful information about mineral status in the body.

Laboratory data can also be used to evaluate risk of nutrition-related chronic diseases. For instance, heart disease risk can be assessed by measuring levels of cholesterol in the blood. Measuring the amount of glucose in the blood can be used to diagnose diabetes. More sophisticated medical tests can be used to obtain additional information about the risk and progression of nutrition-related diseases. For example, procedures are available to determine the extent of coronary artery blockage in an individual with heart disease or to assess bone density in someone at risk for osteoporosis.

CRITICAL THINKING

Nutritional Assessment

Callie is 25 years old and has just started college. Recently she has been feeling tired and has had difficulty concentrating in class. She goes to the health clinic where she is weighed and measured. She is examined by the physician, who asks about her medical history. Blood and urine samples are taken for laboratory analysis and she is referred to a dietitian to assess her dietary intake. What do these assessment tools tell us?

Clinical assessment

The physician notes that she appears thin and pale. Anthropometric measurements of height and weight tell us that she is 5′4″ and weighs 114 pounds. She recalls that a year ago she weighed 120 pounds and hasn't been trying to lose weight.

Compare these values with the Standard Height–Weight Tables in Appendix B. Is her body weight in the normal range?

Although her body weight is in the normal range, her unintentional weight loss is a concern.

Dietary assessment

Callie tells the dietitian that she stopped eating red meat last year. Using information from a 24-hour recall, the dietitian enters her diet into a computer program. A portion of the analysis is shown below.

Nutrient	Value	Goal %
Kcalories	1500	68%
Protein	50 g	100%
Vitamin C	110 mg	183%
Vitamin A	1028 μg RE	128%
Iron	6 mg	40%
Calcium	1300 mg	130%

Use the values given on this computer printout to identify nutrients that do not meet recommendations.

She consumes adequate protein and more than the recommended amounts of vitamin A, vitamin C, and calcium. Her energy intake is less than the recommended amount and, since she is losing weight, is not enough to maintain her body weight. Her iron intake is well below the recommendation for young women.

Laboratory assessment

The results of her blood test indicate that blood hemoglobin level is 11.2 g per 100 ml of blood and her hematocrit, which measures the total volume of blood cells, is 35 ml per 100 ml of blood.

Look up the normal values for hemoglobin and hematocrit in Appendix C. Are her values in the normal range?

Her values for both hemoglobin and hematocrit are below normal. This along with her diet history suggests that she hasn't been consuming enough iron to produce adequate hemoglobin, the oxygen-carrying protein in red blood cells. This reduces her ability to deliver oxygen to her cells, which could be the cause of her tiredness and difficulty in concentrating. The dietitian recommends that she take an iron supplement for a few months and improve her diet to include vegetable sources of iron such as leafy green vegetables.

Should she be concerned about the nutrients she is consuming in excess of her goal? Use the DRI Tables to determine if her 1300 mg of calcium is likely to pose a risk.

Answer:

APPLICATIONS

These exercises are designed to help you apply your critical thinking skills to your own nutrition choices.

1. Make a form similar to the sample on page 61 or use one provided by your instructor to keep a food diary of everything you eat for three days. Since you may eat differently on weekends, record for two weekdays and one weekend day. To make sure you don't forget anything, carry your record with you and record food as it is consumed. This record will be used in Applications throughout this book to focus on particular nutrients. Make the record as complete as possible by using the following tips:

a. Include all food and drink, and be as specific as possible. For example, did you eat a chicken breast or thigh?
b. Estimate as carefully as possible the portion size that you ate; for example, ½ cup of rice, 10 potato chips, 2 ounces of tofu, and 6 ounces of milk.
c. Record the preparation or cooking method. For example, was your potato peeled? Was your chicken skinless? Was it baked or fried?
d. Include anything added to your food, for instance, butter, ketchup, or salad dressing.
e. Don't forget snacks, beverages, and desserts.
f. If the food is from a fast-food chain, list the name.
g. You may have to break down mixed dishes into their ingredients. For example, a tuna sandwich can be listed as 2 slices of whole wheat bread, 1 tablespoon of mayonnaise, and 3 ounces of tuna packed in water.

Food Record

Food or Beverage	How Prepared	Amount
Chicken salad sandwich:		
wheat bread		2 slices
chicken	skinless breast	½ cup
mayonnaise	lowfat	1 tablespoon
Diet cola		1 can

2. Make a form like the example shown here or use one provided by your instructor to list the foods from one day of your food record. Next to each food, list the Food Guide Pyramid food group to which it belongs. In the next column list the number of Food Guide Pyramid servings or fractions of servings it provides. For mixed foods, list all ingredients separately and identify the food groups and serving sizes that apply.

Food	Amount	Pyramid Group	Number of Servings
2 Egg rolls:			
wrappers	2	Grain	1
carrots	½ cup	Vegetable	1
pork	1 oz	Meat	½
peanut oil	1 Tbsp	Fats and sweets	
Rice	½ cup	Grain	1

a. How many servings from each food group did you consume?
b. Does your diet meet the guidelines of the Food Guide Pyramid? If not, what types of food(s) do you need to add to or eliminate from your diet?
c. Are your food choices consistent with the selection tips described in Table 2.2? How might you modify your food choices to more closely follow these suggestions?

3. From your kitchen cupboard or the grocery store, select three packaged foods with food labels.
a. What is the percent of kcalories from fat in each of these foods?
b. How much carbohydrate, fat, and fiber is in a serving of each?
c. How does each of these foods fit into your overall daily diet with regard to total carbohydrate? Total fat? Dietary fiber?
d. If you consumed a serving of each of these three foods, how much more fat could you consume without exceeding the recommendations? How much more total carbohydrate and fiber should you consume that day to meet recommendations for a 2000-kcalorie diet?

Summary

1. Nutrition recommendations made to the public for health promotion and disease prevention are based on available scientific knowledge. Dietary standards such as the Dietary Reference Intakes (DRIs) provide recommendations for intakes of nutrients and other food components that can be used to plan and assess the diets of individuals and populations. Intakes at these levels will avoid deficiencies and excesses and prevent chronic diseases in the majority of healthy persons.
2. The DRIs include four sets of standards. The Estimated Average Requirement (EAR) is the amount of a nutrient that is estimated to meet the needs of half of the people in a particular gender and life-stage group. The EARs can be used to evaluate and plan nutrient intakes for population groups and are the basis for the Recommended Dietary Allowances (RDAs). The RDAs are recommendations calculated to meet the needs of nearly all healthy individuals (97 to 98%) in a specific group and can be used by individuals as a guide to achieve an adequate intake. Adequate Intakes (AIs) serve the same purpose as the RDAs but are estimated from average intakes by healthy populations when there is insufficient scientific evidence to calculate an EAR and RDA. Tolerable Upper Intake Levels (ULs) provide a guide for a safe upper limit of intake.
3. The 1995 Dietary Guidelines for Americans, and Canada's Guidelines for Healthy Eating describe dietary patterns that promote good health and reduce the incidence of chronic diseases that are common in developed countries today.
4. A variety of tools have been developed for planning individual diets. The Food Guide Pyramid emphasizes variety and recommends servings from each of five major food groups to plan diets that meet recommendations.
5. The Exchange Lists are used to plan individual diets that provide specific amounts of energy, carbohydrate, protein, and fat.
6. Food labels assist food choices by providing information on the nutrient content of foods. The percent Daily Values show how foods fit into the recommendations for a healthy diet.
7. The nutritional status of populations is monitored by measuring what foods are available, what foods are consumed, and how nutrient intake is related to overall health.
8. Individual nutritional status is assessed by evaluating dietary intake, examining clinical parameters within the context of a medical history, and interpreting laboratory measurements.

Review Questions

1. What is the purpose of dietary standards?
2. Describe the four types of standards that make up the DRIs.
3. How can the DRIs be used for individuals? For population groups?
4. How does the type of recommendation made by the Dietary Guidelines differ from that made by the DRIs?
5. What is the basis for the shape of the Food Guide Pyramid?
6. List the food groups of the Food Guide Pyramid.
7. What is meant by nutrient density? Give an example.
8. How are the Exchange Lists used in planning diets?
9. What determines the order in which food ingredients are listed on a label?
10. How do the Daily Values help consumers determine how foods fit into their overall diets?
11. What is nutritional status?
12. List the components of individual nutritional assessment.

Nutrition Web Links

To further explore areas related to the material in this chapter go to the *Nutrition: Science and Applications* Web site at ***www.Wiley.com/college/Smolin*** and *click on* **Student Companion Site** for chapter-by-chapter links. Some Web sites related to the information in Chapter 2 include:

Government agency sites that provide additional information on tools for diet planning such as the USDA, which provides updated information about the Dietary Guidelines for Americans and the Food Guide Pyramid, the FDA, which gives additional information about food labels, and the National Academy of Sciences, which provides updates on the Dietary Reference Intakes.

Public health sites that provide information on health promotion and disease prevention programs such as Healthy People 2010.

Organizations that provide information on diet planning for disease control and prevention such as the American Dietetic and American Diabetes Associations.

Other locations that allow you to examine nutrition monitoring data for the U.S. population and those where you can search for the nutrient composition of foods, such as the USDA and the Standard Reference Database.

References

1. FAO/WHO/UNU. *Energy and Protein Requirements.* WHO Technical Report Series No. 724. Geneva: World Health Organization, 1985.
2. National Research Council, Food and Nutrition Board. *Recommended Dietary Allowances*, 10th ed. Washington, D.C.: National Academy Press, 1989.
3. Health and Welfare Canada. Nutrition Recommendations. *Report of the Scientific Review Committee*. Ottawa: Minister of Supply and Services Canada, 1990.
4. Institute of Medicine, Food and Nutrition Board. *Dietary Reference Intakes for Calcium, Phosphorus, Magnesium, Vitamin D, and Fluoride.* Washington, D.C.: National Academy Press, 1997.
5. U.S. Department of Agriculture. *The Food Guide Pyramid.* Home and Garden Bulletin No. 252. Hyattsville, Md: Human Nutrition Information Service, 1992, slightly revised, 1996.
6. Institute of Medicine, Food and Nutrition Board. *Dietary Reference Intakes for Thiamin, Riboflavin, Niacin, Vitamin B-6, Folate, Vitamin B-12, Pantothenic Acid, Biotin, and Choline.* Washington, D.C.: National Academy Press, 1998.
7. Report of the Select Committee on Nutrition and Human Needs, U.S. Senate. *Eating in America: Dietary Goals for the United States.* Cambridge, Mass.: MIT Press, 1977.
8. U.S. Department of Agriculture, U.S. Department of Health and Human Services. *Nutrition and Your Health: Dietary Guidelines for Americans*, 4th ed. Home and Garden Bulletin No. 232. Hyattsville, Md: U.S. Government Printing Office, 1995.
9. Health and Welfare Canada. Report of the Communications/Implementations Committee. Ottawa: Minister of Supply and Services Canada, 1992.
10. *Healthy People 2000: National Health Promotion and Disease Prevention Objectives.* Washington, D.C.: U.S. Department of Health and Human Services, 1990.
11. Maiese, D. R., and Fox, C. E. Laying the Foundation for Healthy People 2010—The First Year of Consultation. Online at http://www.health.gov/healthypeople
12. Healthy People 2000 Progress Report for Nutrition, July 5, 1994. Online at http://www.health.gov/healthypeople
13. The American Diabetes Association, Inc., and the American Dietetic Association. Exchange Lists for Meal Planning, 1995.
14. Federal Register 58, 1993, Jan. 6. Washington, D.C.: U.S. Government Printing Office, Superintendent of Documents.
15. United States Nutrition Labeling and Education Act of 1990. Nutr. Rev. 49:273–276, 1991.
16. Kurtzweil, P. Today's special nutrition information. FDA Consumer. 31:21–25, May–June, 1997.
17. Pennington, J. A. T., and Wilkening, V. L. Final regulations for the nutrition labeling of raw fruits, vegetables, and fish. J. Am. Diet. Assoc. 97:1299–1305, 1997.

18. Health and Welfare Canada. *Nutrition Labels—The Inside Story.* Ottawa: Minister of Supply and Services Canada, 1989.
19. Food and Drug Administration, Center for Food Safety and Applied Nutrition. A Food Labeling Guide. Appendix C, Health Claims, August 12, 1997. Online at http://vm.cfsan.fda.gov
20. Kuczmarski, M. F., Moshfegh, A., and Briefel, R. Update on nutrition monitoring activities in the United States. J. Am. Diet. Assoc. 94:753–760, 1994.
21. Bowman, S. A., Lino, M., Gerrior, S. A., and Bastiotis, P. P. The Healthy Eating Index: 1994–96. U.S. Department of Agriculture, Center for Nutrition Policy and Promotion, 1998. CNPP-5. Online at http://www2.hqnet.usda.gov/cnpp/hei94-96.PDF
22. Johansson, L., Solvoll, K., Bjørneboe, G-E. A., and Drevon, C. A. Under- and overreporting of energy intake related to weight status and lifestyle in a nationwide sample. Am. J. Clin. Nutr. 68:266–274, 1998.
23. USDA, USDA Nurientdatabase for Standard Reference. Online at http://www.nal.usda.gov/fnic/foodcomp/Data/SR12

Chapter 3

Chapter Outline

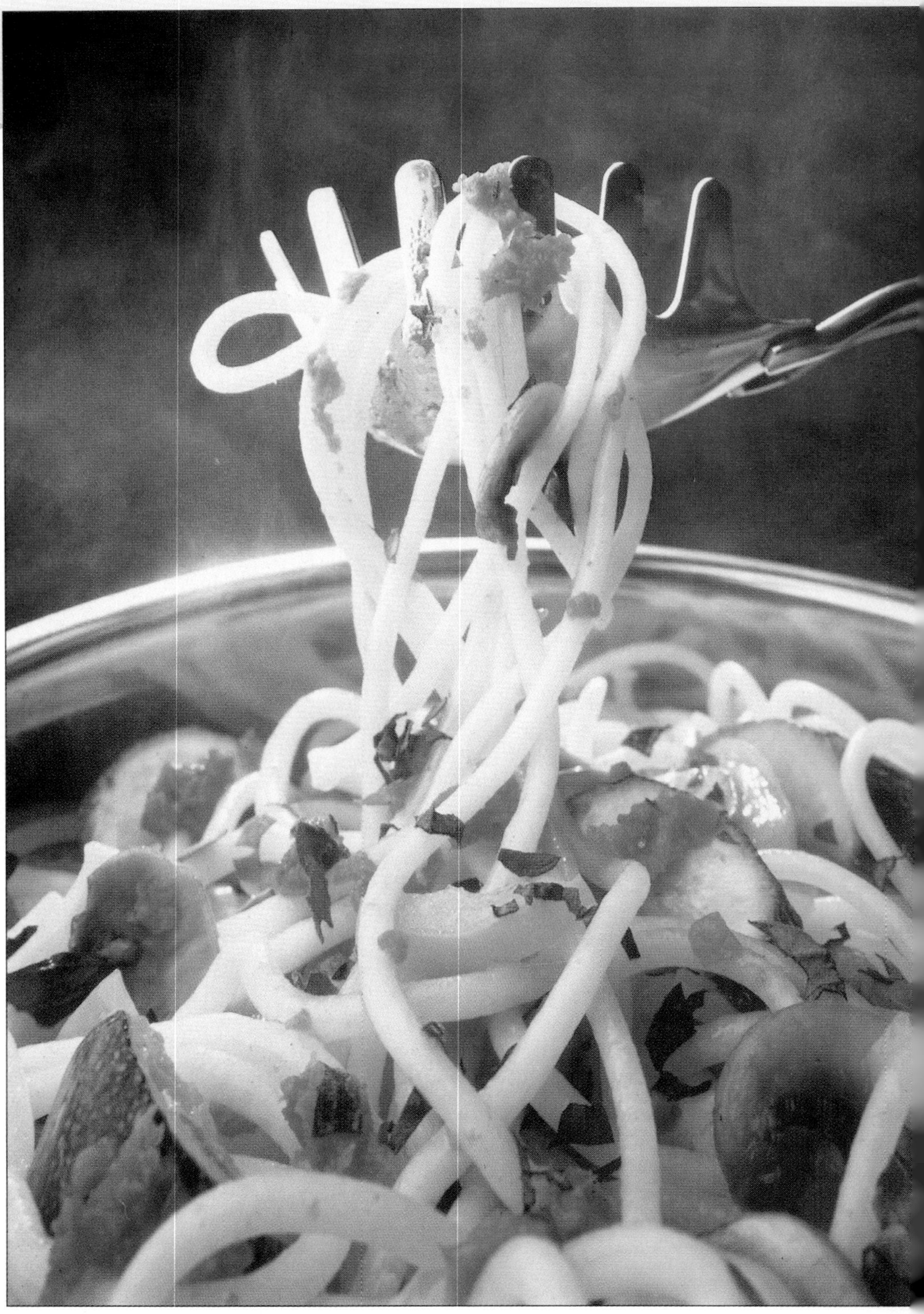

(© Ian O'Leary/Tony Stone Images)

The Human Body: From Meals to Molecules

Chapter Concepts

1. All plant and animal life is made up of atoms bound together to form molecules that are organized into cells. Cells form tissues that compose the organs and organ systems of a living organism.
2. The food we eat is digested in the gastrointestinal tract and nutrients are absorbed into the body. Food in the lumen of the digestive tract is technically outside the body until it is absorbed.
3. Hormones released into the blood and enzymes released into the gastrointestinal tract facilitate the digestion of food and the absorption of nutrients.
4. The small intestine is the primary site of digestion and absorption.
5. Water-soluble materials are absorbed into the blood. Most fat-soluble materials are absorbed into the lymph.
6. Nutrients delivered to the cells can be used to produce energy in the form of ATP, to synthesize molecules needed for immediate use, or to synthesize molecules for storage.
7. Materials that are consumed but not absorbed are excreted in feces. The waste products generated inside the body by metabolism are eliminated via the lungs, skin, and kidneys.

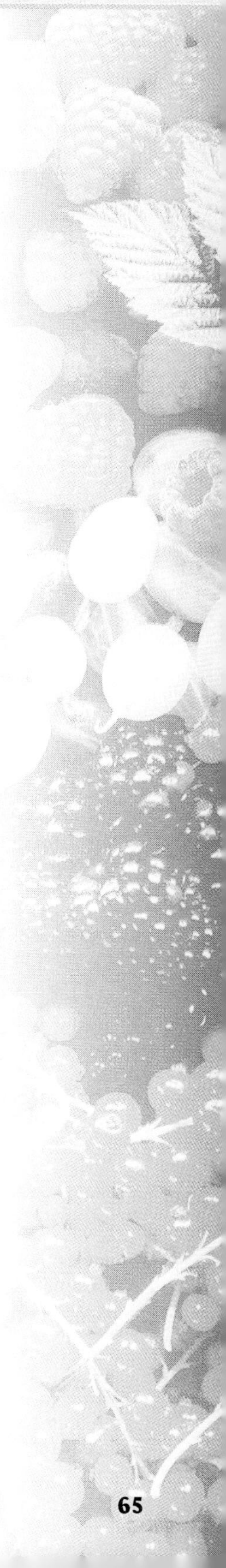

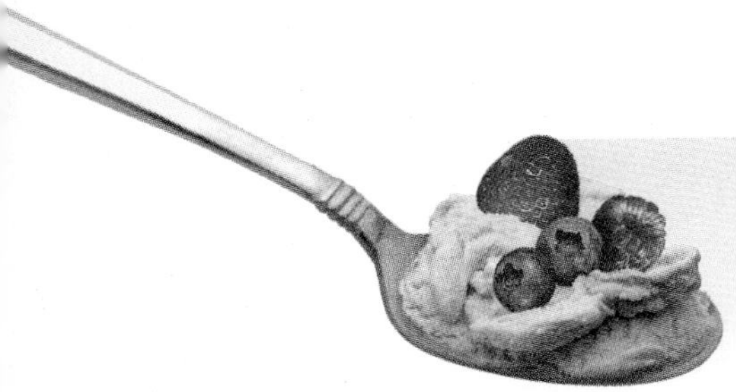

Just a Taste

Do carbohydrate, fat, and protein from the same meal interfere with each other's digestion?

Why are you hungry very soon after eating some meals while others stick with you longer?

Is it healthy to have bacteria living in your gastrointestinal tract?

No matter what food choices you make, the processes by which your body uses the nutrients in food are the same. After being consumed, food must be broken into smaller components, absorbed into the body, and then converted into forms that the body can use. Converting the meals we eat to energy or into molecules that are a part of our body involves the integration of a number of processes and interaction among almost all the systems of the body. Digestion breaks food into its component parts; absorption brings these components into the body; and metabolism uses the nutrients for energy production, building new tissues, maintaining and repairing existing tissues, and regulating these processes. Whether you choose to eat a burrito, a mango, and arroz con leche (rice with milk), or a turkey sandwich, an apple, and a glass of milk—if the food cannot be properly digested, absorbed, and metabolized by the body, it will be of little benefit.

An understanding of nutrition requires comprehending the processes by which food provides fuel and function to the human body. The unique features of the digestion, absorption, and metabolism of specific nutrients will be more thoroughly discussed in subsequent chapters.

Atoms The smallest units of an element that still retain the properties of that element.

Elements Substances that cannot be broken down into products with different properties.

Chemical bonds Forces that hold atoms together.

Molecules Units of two or more atoms of the same or different elements bonded together.

Organic molecules Molecules that contain carbon atoms.

Inorganic Substances that contain no carbon atoms.

Cells The basic structural and functional units of plant and animal life.

Organ A discrete structure composed of more than one tissue that performs a specialized function.

The Chemistry of Life

The organization of life, as of all matter, begins with **atoms.** Atoms are units of matter that cannot be further broken down by chemical means. Atoms of different **elements** have different characteristics. Carbon, hydrogen, oxygen, and nitrogen are the most abundant elements in our bodies and in the foods we eat. These atoms can be linked by forces called **chemical bonds** to form **molecules.** The chemistry of all life on earth is based on **organic molecules,** which are those that contain carbon. Carbohydrates, lipids, proteins, and vitamins are nutrient classes that are made up of organic molecules. Substances that do not contain carbon, such as water and minerals, are referred to as **inorganic.**

In any living system, whether a broccoli plant, a cow, or a human being, molecules are organized into structures that form cells, the smallest unit of life (Figure 3.1). **Cells** of similar structure and function are organized into tissues. The human body contains four types of tissues: muscle, nerve, epithelial, and connective. These tissues are organized in varying combinations into **organs,** which are discrete structures that perform specialized functions in the body (Figure 3.2). The stomach, for example, is an organ that contains all four types of tissue.

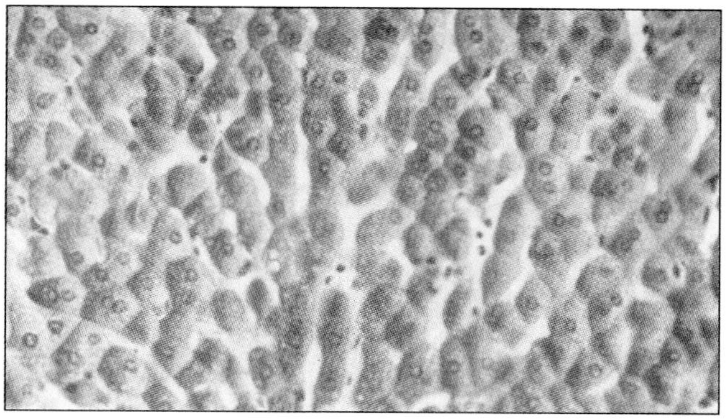

Figure 3.1
Living things are made up of cells such as these human liver cells. (Dr. Roger Wagner)

Most organs do not function alone but are part of a group of cooperative organs called an organ system. The organ systems in humans include the nervous system, respiratory system (lungs), urinary system (kidneys and bladder), reproductive system, cardiovascular system (heart and blood vessels), lymphatic system, muscular system, skeletal system, endocrine system (hormones), integumentary system (skin and body linings), and digestive system (Table 3.1). An organ may be part of more than one organ system. For example, the pancreas is part of the endocrine system as well as the digestive system.

The digestive system is the organ system primarily responsible for the movement of nutrients into the body; however, several other organ systems are also important in the process of using these nutrients. The endocrine system secretes chemical messengers that help regulate food intake and absorption. The nervous system aids in digestion by sending nerve signals that help control the passage of food through the digestive tract. Once absorbed, nutrients are transported to individual cells by the cardiovascular system. The body's urinary, respiratory, and integumentary systems allow for the elimination of metabolic waste products.

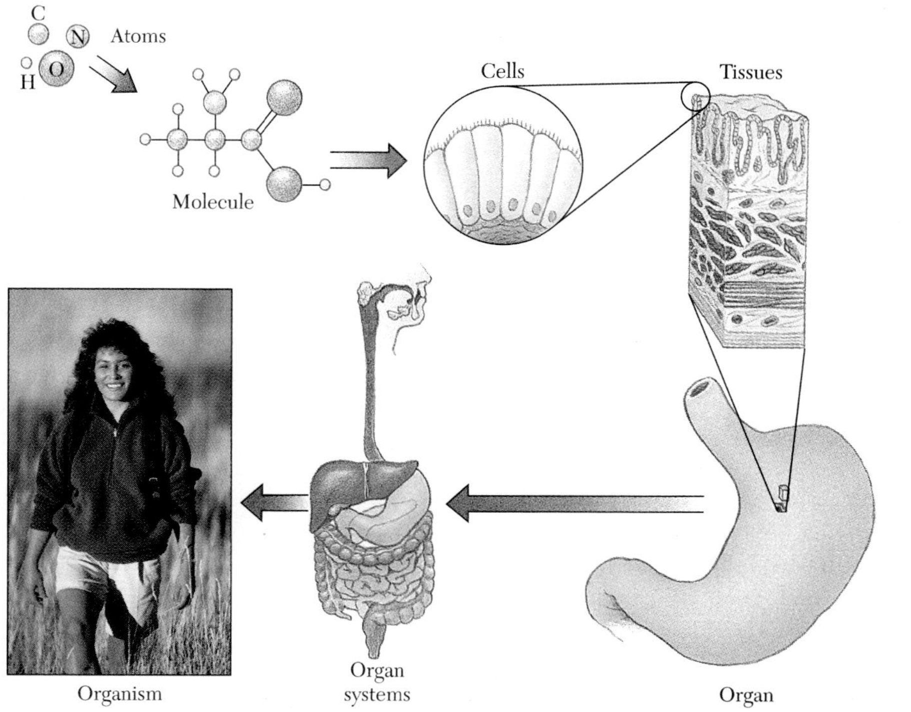

Figure 3.2
The organization of life begins with atoms that form molecules, which are then organized into cells to form tissues, organs, and organisms. (Photo, © Brian Bailey/Tony Stone Images)

Table 3.1 *The Role of Body Organ Systems*

Organ System	Components	Functions
Nervous	Nerves, sense organs, brain, and spinal cord	Responds to stimuli from the external and internal environment; conducts impulses to activate muscles and glands; integrates activities of other systems.
Respiratory	Lungs, trachea, and air passageways	Keeps blood supplied with oxygen and removes carbon dioxide.
Urinary	Kidney and bladder	Eliminates wastes and regulates water, electrolyte, and acid-base balance of the blood.
Reproductive	Testes, ovaries, and associated structures	Produces offspring.
Cardiovascular	Heart and blood vessels	Transports blood, which carries oxygen, nutrients, and wastes.
Lymphatic	Lymph and lymph structures	Defends against foreign invaders; picks up fluid leaked from blood vessels; and transports fat-soluble nutrients.
Muscular	Skeletal muscles	Provides movement and structure.
Skeletal	Bones and joints	Protects and supports the body and provides a framework for the muscles to use for movement.
Endocrine	Pituitary, adrenals, thyroid, and other ductless glands	Secretes hormones that regulate processes such as growth, reproduction, and nutrient use.
Integumentary	Skin, hair, nails, and sweat glands	Covers and protects the body; helps control body temperature.
Digestive	Mouth, esophagus, stomach, intestines, pancreas, liver, and gallbladder	Ingests and digests food; absorbs nutrients into the blood; and eliminates nonabsorbed food residues.

Marieb, E. N. *Human Anatomy and Physiology*, 4th ed. Redwood City, Calif.: Benjamin/Cummings Publishing Co., 1998.

THE DIGESTIVE SYSTEM: AN OVERVIEW

The digestive system provides two major functions: **digestion** and **absorption.** Carbohydrate, fat, and protein are digested and absorbed as sugars, fatty acids, and amino acids respectively. Some substances, such as water, can be absorbed without digestion, and others, such as dietary fiber, cannot be digested by humans and therefore cannot be absorbed. These unabsorbed substances pass through the digestive tract and are excreted in the **feces.**

The main part of the digestive system is the **gastrointestinal tract.** It is also referred to as the GI tract, gut, digestive tract, intestinal tract, or alimentary canal. It can be thought of as a hollow tube that runs from the mouth to the anus. The organs of the gastrointestinal tract include the mouth, pharynx, esophagus, stomach, small intestine, large intestine, and anus (Figure 3.3). The inside of the tube that these organs form is called the **lumen.** Food within the lumen of the gastrointestinal tract has not been absorbed and is therefore technically still outside the body. Only after food is transferred into the cells of the intestine by the process of absorption is it actually "inside" the body.

The amount of time it takes for food to pass from mouth to anus is referred to as **transit time.** In a healthy adult, transit time is about 24 to 72 hours. It is affected by the composition of the diet, physical activity, emotions, medications, and illnesses. To measure transit time, researchers add a nonabsorbable dye to a meal and measure the time between consumption of the dye and its appearance

Digestion The process of breaking food into components small enough to be absorbed into the body.

Absorption The process of taking substances into the interior of the body.

Feces Body waste, including unabsorbed food residue, bacteria, mucus, and dead cells, which is excreted from the gastrointestinal tract by passing through the anus.

Gastrointestinal tract A hollow tube consisting of the mouth, pharynx, esophagus, stomach, small intestine, large intestine, and anus, in which digestion and absorption of nutrients occurs.

Lumen The inside cavity of a tube, such as the gastrointestinal tract.

Transit time The time between the ingestion of food and the elimination of the solid waste from that food.

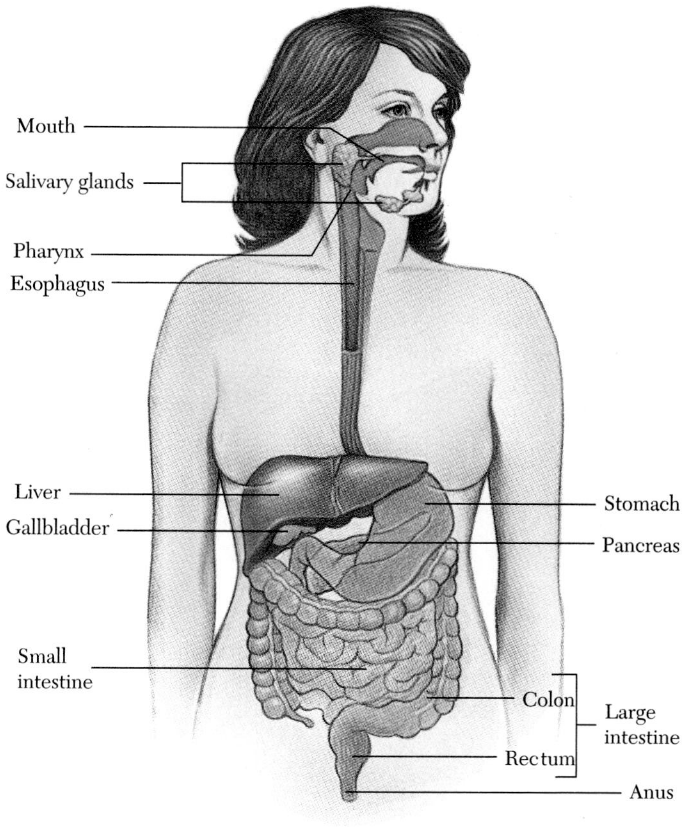

Figure 3.3
The digestive system consists of the organs of the gastrointestinal tract: the mouth, pharynx, esophagus, stomach, small intestine, large intestine, and anus, as well as a number of accessory organs: the salivary glands, liver, gallbladder, and pancreas.

in the feces. The shorter the transit time, the more rapid the passage through the digestive tract.

The digestive process is aided by substances that are secreted into the digestive tract both by cells lining the digestive tract and by a number of accessory organs. One of these substances is **mucus,** a viscous material produced by mucosal cells that line the gut. Mucus moistens, lubricates, and protects the digestive tract. **Enzymes,** protein molecules that speed up chemical reactions without themselves being consumed or changed by the reactions, are another component of digestive system secretions (Figure 3.4). In digestion, enzymes accelerate the

Mucus A thick fluid secreted by glands in the gastrointestinal tract and other parts of the body. It acts to lubricate, moisten, and protect cells from harsh environments.

Enzymes Protein molecules that accelerate the rate of specific chemical reactions without being changed themselves.

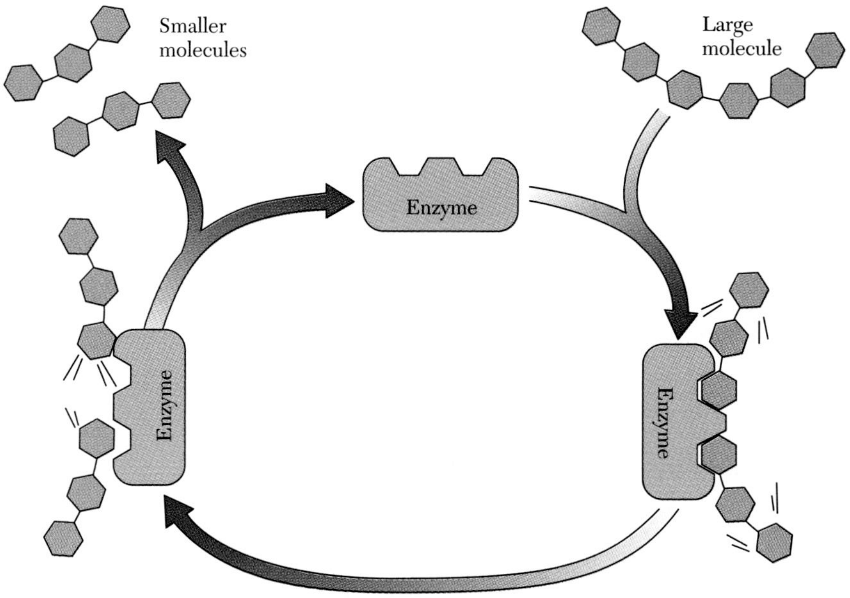

Figure 3.4
Enzymes speed up chemical reactions without themselves being altered by the reaction. In this example, an enzyme breaks a large molecule into two smaller ones.

Figure 3.5
This cross section through the wall of the small intestine shows the four tissue layers: mucosa, connective tissue, smooth muscle layers, and outer connective tissue layer. (Adapted from E. P. Solomon, R. R. Schmidt, and P. J. Adragna, *Human Anatomy and Physiology*, 2nd ed. Philadelphia: Saunders College Publishing, 1990.)

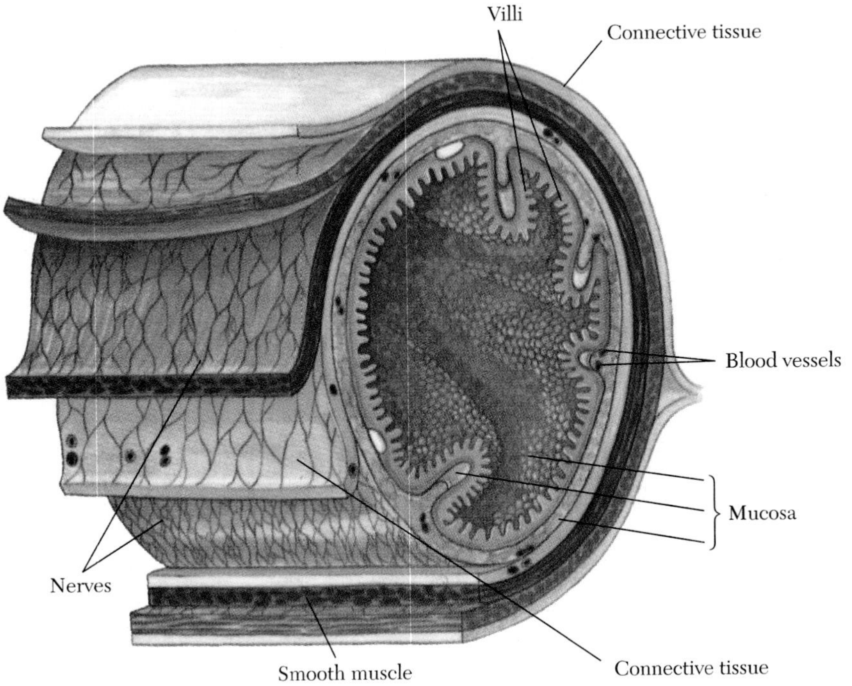

breakdown of food. Different enzymes are needed for the breakdown of different food components. For example, an enzyme that digests carbohydrate would have no effect on fat, and one that digests fat would have no effect on carbohydrate.

In addition to secreting substances into the lumen of the digestive tract, the digestive system secretes hormones into the bloodstream. **Hormones** are chemical messengers that are released into the blood by one organ to regulate body functions elsewhere. In the gastrointestinal tract, hormones send signals that help prepare different parts of the gut for the arrival of food and thus regulate the rate that food moves through the system.

Hormones Chemical messengers that are produced in one location, released into the blood, and that elicit responses at other locations in the body.

The wall of the gastrointestinal tract contains four layers of tissue (Figure 3.5). Lining the lumen is the **mucosa,** a layer of mucosal cells that secrete mucus into the lumen. The cells of the mucosa are in direct contact with churning food and harsh digestive secretions. Therefore, these cells have a short life span—only about two to five days. When these cells die, they are sloughed off into the lumen, where some components are digested and absorbed and the remainder are excreted in the feces. Because mucosal cells reproduce rapidly, the mucosa has high nutrient requirements and is therefore one of the first parts of the body to be affected by nutrient deficiencies. Surrounding the mucosa is a layer of connective tissue containing nerves and blood vessels. This layer provides support, delivers nutrients to the mucosa, and provides the nerve signals that control secretions and muscle contractions. Layers of smooth muscle—the type over which we do not have voluntary control—surround the connective tissue. The contraction of smooth muscles mixes food, breaks it into smaller particles, and propels it through the digestive tract. The final, external layer is also made up of connective tissue and provides support and protection.

Mucosa The layer of tissue lining the gastrointestinal tract and other body cavities.

DIGESTION AND ABSORPTION

To be used by the body, food must be eaten and digested, and the nutrients must be absorbed and transported to the cells of the body. The following sections of this chapter will trace a meal through all these processes, from the body's anticipation of the meal to its elimination of the waste products.

Imagine slices of oven-roasted turkey served on fresh baked bread accompanied by an apple and a glass of lowfat milk (Figure 3.6).

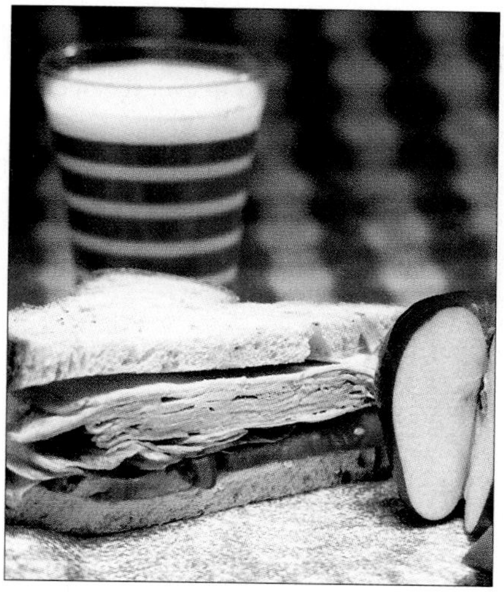

Figure 3.6
The sight, smell, and sounds of food preparation can initiate activity in the digestive tract. (Charles D. Winters)

Sights, Sounds, and Smells

Activity in the digestive tract begins before food even enters the mouth. As the meal is being prepared, sensory input such as the sight of a turkey being lifted out of the oven, the clatter of the table being set, and the smell of freshly baked bread may make your mouth become moist and your stomach begin to secrete digestive substances. This response occurs when the nervous system signals the digestive system to ready itself for a meal. This cephalic (pertaining to the head) response occurs as a result of external cues, such as sight and smell, even when the body is not in need of food.

The Mouth

The mouth is the entry point for food into the digestive tract. In the mouth, the taste of food continues the processes begun by the smells, sights, and sounds of food preparation. The presence of food in the mouth stimulates the flow of **saliva** from the salivary glands located internally at the sides of the face and immediately below and in front of the ears (see Figure 3.3). Saliva contains the enzyme **salivary amylase,** which begins the digestion of carbohydrate. Salivary amylase can break the long sugar chains of starch in the bread of the turkey sandwich into shorter chains of sugars. Saliva also lubricates the upper gastrointestinal tract and moistens the food so that it can easily be tasted and swallowed.

Saliva A watery fluid produced and secreted into the mouth by the salivary glands. It contains lubricants, enzymes, and other substances.

Salivary amylase An enzyme secreted by the salivary glands that breaks down starch.

Digestive enzymes can act only on the surface of food particles; therefore, chewing is important because it breaks food into small pieces, increasing the surface area in contact with digestive enzymes. Chewing also breaks apart fiber that traps nutrients in some foods. If the fiber is not broken, some nutrients cannot be absorbed. For example, the peel of the apple in the sample meal is a source of vitamins and minerals; however, these nutrients cannot be absorbed without first being released from the fiber in the peel. Adult humans have 32 teeth, specialized for biting, tearing, grinding, and crushing foods; thus, missing or decayed teeth can interfere with the proper digestion of food. Tooth decay, or caries, commonly called cavities, is caused by acid produced when bacteria break down carbohydrates (see Chapter 4).

The Pharynx

The meal that entered the mouth as a turkey sandwich, apple, and milk has now been formed into a bolus, a ball of chewed food mixed with saliva. From the mouth, the bolus moves into the **pharynx,** the part of the gastrointestinal tract responsible for swallowing. The pharynx is shared by the digestive tract and the respiratory tract: Food passes through the pharynx on its way to the stomach, and air passes here on its way to and from the lungs. During swallowing, the air passages are blocked by a valvelike flap of tissue called the epiglottis, so food passes to the stomach, not the lungs. Sometimes food can pass into an upper air passageway. It is usually dislodged with a cough, but if it becomes stuck it can block the flow of air and cause choking. A quick response is required to save the life of a person whose airway is completely blocked. The Heimlich maneuver, which forces air out of the lungs by using a sudden application of pressure to the upper abdomen, can blow an object out of the blocked air passage (Figure 3.7).

Pharynx A funnel-shaped opening that connects the nasal passages and mouth to the respiratory passages and esophagus. It is a common passageway for food and air and is responsible for swallowing.

The Esophagus

The **esophagus** passes through the diaphragm, a muscular wall separating the abdomen from the cavity where the lungs are located, to connect the pharynx and stomach. The bolus of food is moved along by rhythmic contractions of the

Esophagus A portion of the gastrointestinal tract that extends from the pharynx to the stomach.

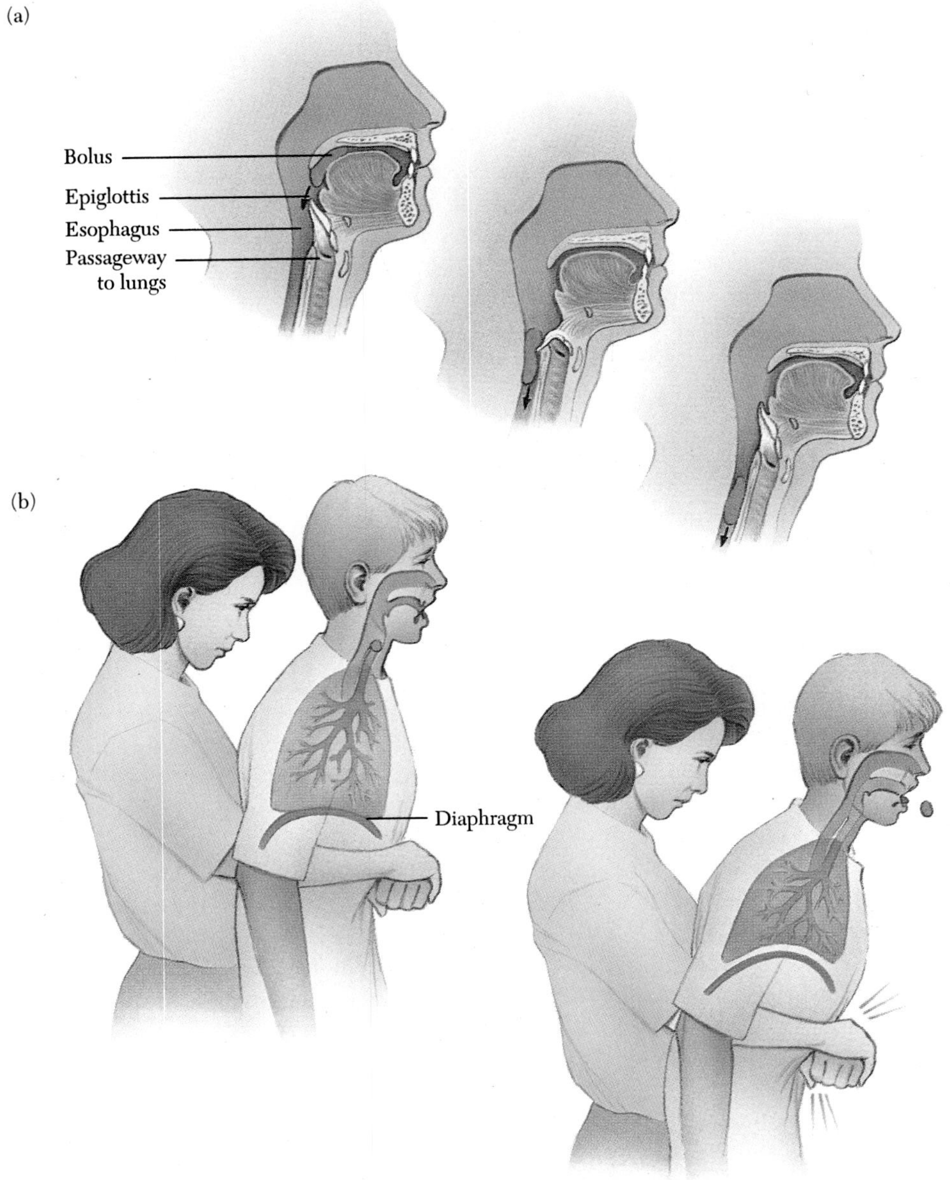

Figure 3.7
(a) When a bolus of food is swallowed, it pushes the epiglottis down over the opening to the air passageways. (b) If food does become lodged in the air passageways, it can be dislodged by the Heimlich maneuver, illustrated here.

Peristalsis Coordinated muscular contractions that move food through the gastrointestinal tract.

smooth muscles, a process called **peristalsis.** This contractile movement, which is controlled automatically by the nervous system, occurs throughout the gastrointestinal tract, pushing the food bolus along from the pharynx through the large intestine (Figure 3.8).

The Stomach

Sphincter A muscular valve that helps control the flow of materials in the gastrointestinal tract.

To move from the esophagus into the stomach, food must pass through a **sphincter,** a muscle that encircles the tube of the digestive tract and acts as a valve (see Figure 3.8). When the muscle contracts, the valve is closed. The gastroesophageal sphincter, located between the esophagus and the stomach, normally prevents foods from moving back out of the stomach. Occasionally, materials do pass out of the stomach through this valve. Heartburn occurs when some of the acidic stomach contents leak up and out of the stomach into the esophagus, causing a burning sensation. Vomiting is the result of a reverse peristaltic wave that causes the sphincter to relax and allow the food to pass upward out of the stomach toward the mouth.

The stomach is an expanded portion of the gastrointestinal tract that serves as a temporary storage place for food. While held in the stomach, the bolus is mixed with highly acidic stomach secretions to form a semiliquid food mass called **chyme.** The mixing of food in the stomach is aided by an extra layer of smooth muscle in the stomach wall. While most of the gastrointestinal tract is surrounded by two layers of muscle, the stomach contains a third layer, allowing for powerful contractions that thoroughly churn and mix the stomach contents. Some digestion takes place in the stomach, but, with the exception of some water, alcohol, and a few drugs such as aspirin and acetaminophen (Tylenol), very little absorption occurs here.

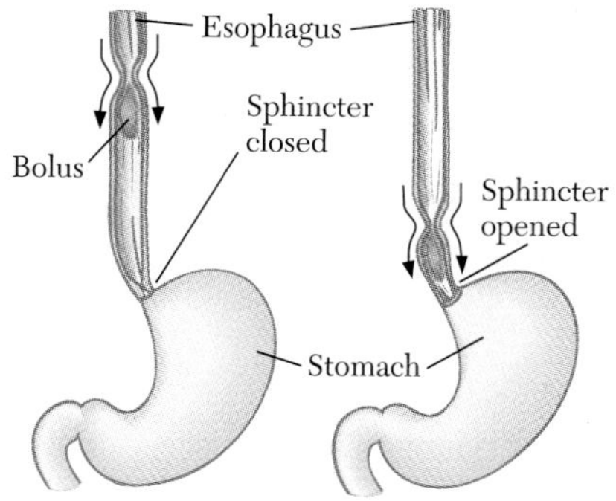

Figure 3.8
The rhythmic contractions of peristalsis propel food down the esophagus, through the open sphincter, and into the stomach.

Regulation of Gastric Secretion Gastric or stomach secretions are regulated by both nervous and hormonal mechanisms. Signals from three different sites—the brain, stomach, and small intestine—stimulate or inhibit gastric secretion. The three phases of gastric secretion are therefore called cephalic, gastric, and intestinal. The **cephalic phase** occurs before food enters the stomach. During this phase, the thought, smell, sight, or taste of food causes the brain to send nerve signals that increase gastric secretion. This prepares the stomach to receive food (Figure 3.9).

The second phase, referred to as the **gastric phase,** begins when food enters the stomach. The presence of food in the stomach causes gastric secretion by stretching local nerves, by signaling the brain, and by stimulating the secretion of the hormone **gastrin** from the upper portion of the stomach. Gastrin triggers the release of gastric juice, which is produced by digestive glands, called gastric glands, in the lining of the stomach. One of the components of gastric juice is hydrochloric acid. Hydrochloric acid stops the carbohydrate-digesting activity of salivary amylase and helps to begin the digestion of protein. It also serves to kill most bacteria present in food. Another component of gastric juice is pepsinogen. When pepsinogen is exposed to the acidity of the stomach, it is converted into the protein-digesting enzyme **pepsin,** which breaks proteins into shorter chains of amino acids called polypeptides. Pepsin is produced in an inactive form and activated in the stomach; otherwise, its active form would digest the glands that

Chyme A mixture of partially digested food and stomach secretions.

Cephalic phase The phase of gastric secretion that is stimulated by the sight, smell, and taste of food.

Gastric phase The phase of gastric secretion triggered by the entry of food into the stomach.

Gastrin A hormone secreted by the mucosa of the stomach that stimulates the secretion of enzymes and acid in the stomach.

Pepsin A protein-digesting enzyme produced by the stomach. It is secreted in the gastric juice in an inactive form and activated by acid in the stomach.

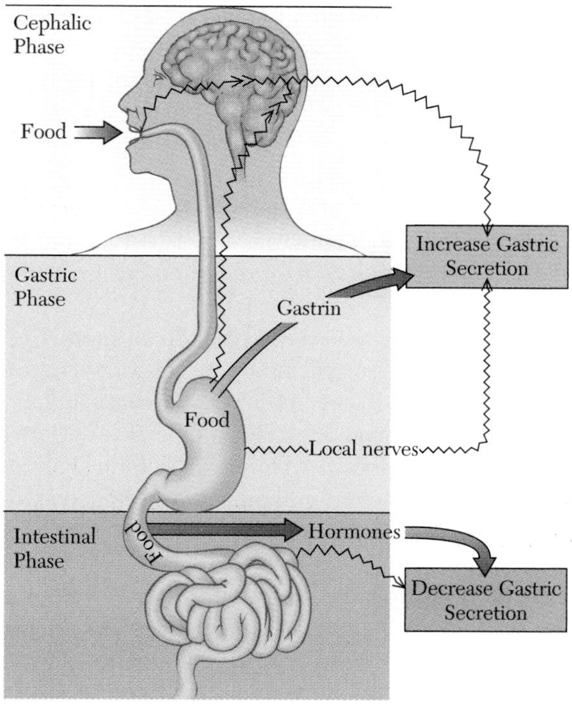

Figure 3.9
In the cephalic phase, the sight, smell, and taste of food cause the brain to signal an increase in gastric secretions. In the gastric phase, food entering the stomach stimulates gastric secretions by stretching local nerves, signaling the brain, and causing gastrin release. In the intestinal phase, food entering the small intestine inhibits gastric secretions by triggering nervous and hormonal signals.

produce it. Although salivary amylase function is stopped by the acidity of the stomach, pepsin functions best in acid. Therefore, digestion of starch from our sample meal stops in the stomach, and digestion of the protein from the turkey, milk, and bread begins. The protein of the stomach wall is protected from the acid and pepsin by a thick layer of mucus. If the mucus layer is penetrated, pepsin and acid can damage the underlying tissues and cause **peptic ulcers,** erosions of the stomach wall or some other region of the gastrointestinal tract. The leading cause of ulcers is acid-resistant bacteria that infect the lining of the stomach, causing damage to the gastrointestinal tract wall and destroying the protective mucosal layer.[1]

Peptic ulcer An open sore in the lining of the stomach, esophagus, or small intestine.

The third phase of gastric secretion, the **intestinal phase,** is begun by the passage of chyme into the small intestine. This triggers events that decrease stomach motility and secretions, and slow the release of food into the intestine. This ensures that the amount of chyme entering the small intestine does not exceed the ability of the intestine to process it.

Intestinal phase The phase of gastric secretion that is begun by the entry of food into the small intestine.

Control of Stomach Emptying Chyme normally leaves the stomach in 2 to 6 hours. The rate of stomach emptying is determined by the size and composition of the meal and controlled by signals from the small intestine. Chyme moving out of the stomach must pass through the pyloric sphincter. This sphincter helps regulate the rate at which food enters the intestine. The small intestine stretches as it fills with food. This distension inhibits stomach emptying. A large meal will take longer to leave the stomach than a small meal, and a solid meal will leave the stomach more slowly than a liquid meal. The nutritional composition of a meal also affects how long it stays in the stomach. The meal we have been following is of mixed composition. Together, the sandwich, apple, and milk contain about 25% of energy as protein, 45% as carbohydrate, and 30% as fat. The meal is partly solid and partly liquid, and so will be in the stomach for an average amount of time (about 4 hours). A high-fat meal will stay in the stomach the longest because fat entering the small intestine slows stomach emptying. A meal that is primarily protein will leave more quickly, and a meal of mostly carbohydrate will leave the fastest. The reason you are often ready to eat again soon after a meal of vegetables and rice is that this high-carbohydrate, lowfat meal leaves the stomach rapidly. Thus, what you choose for breakfast can affect when you become hungry for lunch. Toast and coffee will leave your stomach far more quickly than a larger meal with more protein and some fat, such as a bowl of cereal with lowfat milk, toast with peanut butter, and a glass of juice. Factors besides food composition also can affect gastric emptying. For example, sadness and fear tend to slow emptying, while aggression tends to increase gastric motility and speed emptying.

The Small Intestine

The small intestine is a narrow tube about 20 feet in length. It is divided into three segments. The first 12 inches are the duodenum, the next 8 feet are the jejunum, and the last 11 feet are the ileum. About 95% of digestion occurs in the small intestine.

Digestion in the small intestine is aided by secretions from the intestine itself and from the **gallbladder** and **pancreas.** The gallbladder stores and secretes **bile,** a substance produced in the liver that is necessary for fat digestion and absorption. The pancreas secretes pancreatic juice, containing digestive enzymes and bicarbonate ions. The bicarbonate neutralizes the hydrochloric acid in chyme. This reduction in acidity allows enzymes from the pancreas and small intestine to continue the digestion of carbohydrate, fat, and protein.

Gallbladder An organ of the digestive system that stores bile, which is produced by the liver.

Pancreas An organ that secretes digestive enzymes and bicarbonate ions into the small intestine during digestion.

Bile A substance made in the liver and stored in the gallbladder. It is released into the small intestine to aid in fat digestion and absorption.

Digestion of the Total Diet Most foods we consume are mixtures of carbohydrate, fat, and protein, and the physiology of the digestive tract is carefully designed to allow the digestion of all these components without competition among them. For example, as seen earlier, the digestion of carbohydrate from the bread in our sample meal begins in the mouth but stops in the acid environment of the stomach. However, the digestion of protein from the turkey, milk, and bread is begun by the acid and pepsin in the stomach. Once the food reaches the neutral environment of the small intestine, the enzyme pancreatic amylase continues the job of breaking starch into sugars that was started by salivary amylase. Protein-digesting enzymes such as trypsin and chymotrypsin, designed to work in the environment of the small intestine, continue to break protein into shorter and shorter chains of amino acids. Digestive enzymes found attached to or inside the cells lining the small intestine are involved in both the digestion of sugars into single sugar units and the digestion of small polypeptides into amino acids. Most of the digestion of fat, from the milk, mayonnaise, and turkey, occurs when the chyme reaches the small intestine. Here fat is mixed with bile, which emulsifies it, or breaks it into small droplets. These small droplets both allow pancreatic enzymes, called **lipases,** to more efficiently access the fat and digest it, and facilitate fat absorption.

Lipases Fat-digesting enzymes.

Several popular diet books have stated that foods must be eaten in the proper combinations to be digested and absorbed. These books claim that if a high-protein food such as turkey is consumed with a high-carbohydrate food such as bread, the gastrointestinal tract cannot digest both foods at once. This is not correct. The changing environments of the gastrointestinal tract are designed to allow the digestion of all the different food components in the same meal. Even a meal of only turkey or only bread contains more than one nutrient. Turkey contains protein and fat, and bread contains carbohydrate, protein, and a small amount of fat. A digestive system that could not break down all the nutrients present together in foods would not have allowed humans to thrive.

Hormonal Control of Secretions The release of bile and pancreatic enzymes into the small intestine is controlled by two hormones secreted by the mucosal lining of the duodenum. **Secretin** signals the pancreas to secrete bicarbonate ions and stimulates the liver to secrete bile into the gallbladder. **Cholecystokinin (CCK)** signals the pancreas to secrete digestive enzymes and causes the gallbladder to contract and release bile into the duodenum (Figure 3.10).

Secretin A hormone released by the duodenum that signals the pancreas to secrete bicarbonate ions and stimulates the liver to secrete bile into the gallbladder.

Cholecystokinin (CCK) A hormone released by the duodenum that signals the pancreas to secrete digestive enzymes and causes the gallbladder to contract and release bile into the duodenum.

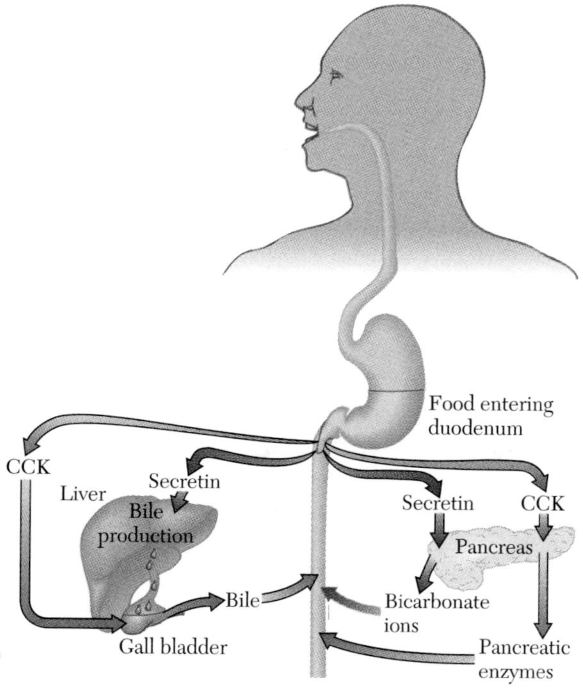

Figure 3.10
Food entering the duodenum triggers the release of the hormones secretin and cholecystokinin (CCK). Secretin increases the output of bile by the liver and the secretion of bicarbonate ions from the pancreas. CCK signals the release of bile by the gallbladder and the secretion of digestive enzymes from the pancreas.

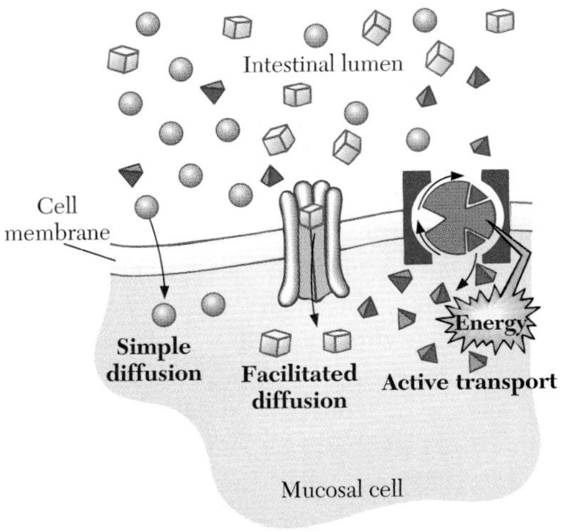

Figure 3.11
Nutrients are absorbed from the lumen across the cell membrane into the cell by simple diffusion, shown here by the purple balls that move from an area of higher concentration to an area of lower concentration; by facilitated diffusion, shown here by the yellow cubes that move from an area of higher concentration to an area of lower concentration with the help of a carrier; and by active transport, which requires energy and a carrier and is shown here by the red pyramids that move from an area of lower concentration to an area of higher concentration.

Absorption The small intestine is the primary site of absorption for water, vitamins, minerals, and the products of carbohydrate, fat, and protein digestion. Several different mechanisms are involved (Figure 3.11). Some molecules are absorbed by diffusion—the process by which a substance moves from an area of higher concentration to an area of lower concentration. Substances that move from higher to lower concentrations are said to move down their concentration gradient. When a concentration gradient exists and the nutrient can pass freely from the lumen of the GI tract across the cell membrane into the mucosal cell, the process is called **simple diffusion.** This process requires no energy. The water, small lipid molecules, and fat-soluble vitamins from the milk in our meal are absorbed by simple diffusion. Many nutrients, however, cannot pass freely across cell membranes; they must be carried by other molecules in a process called **facilitated diffusion.** Even though these nutrients are carried across the cell membrane by other molecules, they still move down a concentration gradient from an area of higher concentration to one of lower concentration without requiring energy; the sugar fructose found in the apple is absorbed by facilitated diffusion. Substances unable to be absorbed by diffusion must enter the body by **active transport,** a process that requires both a carrier molecule and energy. This use of energy allows substances to be transported against their concentration gradient from an area of lower concentration to an area of higher concentration. The sugar glucose, which makes up the starch of the bread, is absorbed by active transport. This allows glucose to be absorbed even when it is present in high concentrations inside the mucosal cells. More specific information about the absorption of the products of carbohydrate, fat, and protein digestion will be discussed in Chapters 4, 5, and 6 respectively.

Simple diffusion The movement of substances from an area of higher concentration to an area of lower concentration. No energy is required.

Facilitated diffusion The movement of substances across a cell membrane from an area of higher concentration to an area of lower concentration with the aid of a carrier molecule. No energy is required.

Active transport The transport of substances across a cell membrane with the aid of a carrier molecule and the expenditure of energy. This may occur against a concentration gradient.

Structure to Maximize Absorption The structure of the small intestine is specialized to allow maximal absorption of the nutrients. In addition to its length, the small intestine has three other features that increase the area of its absorptive surface (Figure 3.12). First, the intestinal walls are arranged in circular or spiral folds which increase the surface area in contact with nutrients. Second, its entire inner surface is covered with fingerlike projections called **villi** (singular, villus). And finally, each of these villi is covered with tiny **microvilli,** often referred to as the brush border. Together these features provide a surface area that is about the size of a tennis court (300 m^2 or 3229 ft^2). Each villus contains a blood vessel and a **lymph vessel** or **lacteal,** which are located only one cell layer away from the nutrients in the intestinal lumen. Nutrients must cross the mucosal cell layer to reach the bloodstream or lymphatic system for delivery to the tissues of the body.

Villi (villus) Fingerlike protrusions of the lining of the small intestine that participate in the digestion and absorption of foodstuffs.

Microvilli Minute brushlike projections on the mucosal cell membrane that increase the absorptive surface area in the small intestine.

Lymph vessel or **lacteal** A tubular component of the lymphatic system that carries fluid away from body tissues. Lymph vessels in the intestine are known as lacteals and can transport large particles such as the products of fat digestion.

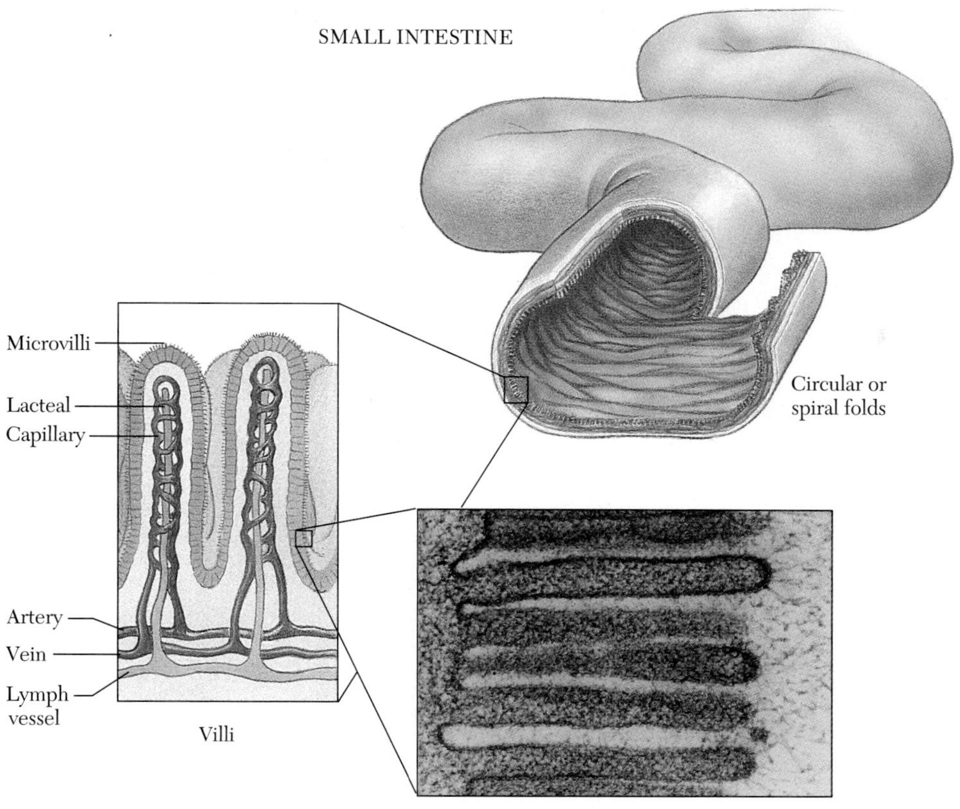

Figure 3.12
The small intestine contains folds, villi, and microvilli, which increase the absorptive surface area. (Photo, © S. Ito, D. W. Fawcett/Visuals Unlimited)

The Large Intestine

Components of chyme that are not absorbed in the small intestine pass through the ileocecal valve to the large intestine, which includes the **colon** and **rectum.** Although most absorption occurs in the small intestine, water and some vitamins and minerals are also absorbed in the colon. Peristalsis here is slower than in the small intestine. Water, nutrients, and fecal matter may spend 24 hours in the large intestine, in contrast to the 3 to 5 hours it takes for chyme to move through the small intestine. This slow movement favors the growth of bacteria, referred to as **intestinal microflora.** These bacteria are permanent beneficial residents of this part of the gastrointestinal tract (see *Off the Shelf: Feeding Your Flora*). The microflora act on unabsorbed portions of food, such as the fiber contained in the apple and whole grain bread, producing nutrients that they can use or, in some cases, that can be absorbed into the body.[2] The microflora also synthesize small amounts of some B vitamins and vitamin K, some of which can be absorbed. One additional by-product of bacterial metabolism is gas, which causes flatulence.

Colon The largest portion of the large intestine.

Rectum The portion of the large intestine that connects the colon and anus.

Intestinal microflora Microorganisms that inhabit the large intestine.

Materials not absorbed are excreted as waste products in the feces. The amount of water in the feces is affected by fiber and fluid intake. Fiber retains water, so when adequate fiber and fluid are consumed, feces have a high water content and are easily passed. When inadequate fiber or fluid is consumed, feces are hard and dry, and constipation can result.

The end of the colon is connected to the rectum, where feces are stored prior to defecation. The rectum is connected to the **anus,** the external opening of the digestive tract. The rectum and anus work with the colon to prepare the feces for elimination. Defecation is regulated by a sphincter that is under voluntary control. It allows the feces to be eliminated at convenient and appropriate times. The digestion and absorption of carbohydrate, fat, and protein are summarized in Figure 3.13.

Anus The outlet of the rectum through which feces are expelled.

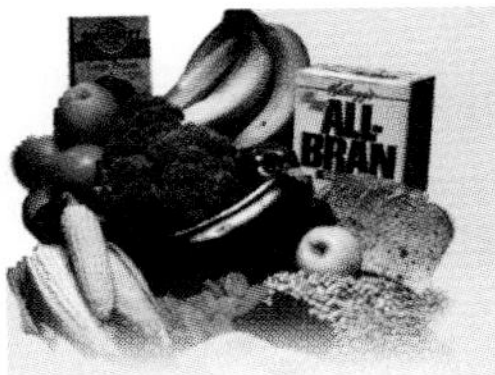

Off the Shelf

Feeding Your Flora

Bacteria growing in your gut? Sounds bad, but the large intestine of a healthy adult is home to several hundred species of bacteria. Some of these are beneficial and some are harmful.[1] Most of the time the microflora in our gastrointestinal tract have beneficial effects, but when the wrong bacteria take over, the result could be diarrhea, infections, and perhaps cancer. Should we be supplementing our diet with beneficial bacteria or eating certain foods to promote their growth?

The type and amount of bacteria in the gastrointestinal tract are affected by the diet and health of the host. In turn, the type and amount of bacteria affect the health of the host. The beneficial bacteria improve the digestion and absorption of essential nutrients; synthesize vitamins, some of which can be absorbed; and can metabolize harmful substances, such as ammonia, thus reducing levels in the blood. These bacteria are important for intestinal immune function, proper growth of cells in the colon, and optimal intestinal motility and transit time.[2] A strong population of healthful bacteria can also inhibit the growth of harmful bacteria.[3]

Obviously, it would be beneficial if we could encourage the growth of the good bacteria and not the bad. One way to increase the population of healthful bacteria is to eat the bacteria themselves. Two types of bacteria that are believed to have health-promoting properties are *Bifidobacterium* and *Lactobacillus*. These bacteria are contained in yogurt with live cultures and acidophilus milk. They can also be purchased in bottled suspensions or tablets. When eaten alive, some of these organisms survive passage through the upper GI tract and live temporarily in the colon before they are excreted in the feces.[4] The consumption of live beneficial bacteria, referred to as probiotics, has been hypothesized to reduce blood cholesterol, stimulate immune function, prevent cancer, and improve the integrity of the gastrointestinal mucosa. Research has supported some of these claims. The appropriate probiotic can stimulate immune function in the intestine[5] and prevent the formation and growth of cancerous cells in rats.[6] Probiotics may be useful in treating disorders in which the gut barrier is compromised, such as diarrhea, food allergies, and colitis,[7,8] as well as helping with constipation, flatulence, and gastric acidity. One problem with a probiotic is that when it is no longer consumed, the added bacteria are rapidly washed out of the colon.

Another approach to altering the intestinal microflora is to consume foods or other substances that encourage the growth of particular types of bacteria. These foods for bacteria, called prebiotics, are nondigestible food components that pass into the colon where they are used as a food source by the bacteria. A given type of prebiotic can selectively stimulate the growth of certain types of bacteria. For example, nondigestible carbohydrates extracted from chicory roots are a prebiotic that stimulates the growth of *Bifidobacteria*.[9]

Our understanding of how probiotics and prebiotics can be used to treat disease and promote health is still expanding. Today, healthy adults can eat yogurt or drink milk containing active cultures to get a dose of beneficial bacteria in a food. But soon we may be able to take probiotics, instead of antibiotics, to kill hazardous bacteria in the gut. And, we may be paying attention to what we are feeding our microflora—as well as ourselves.

[1]Gibson, G. R., and Roberfroid, M. B. Dietary modulation of the human colonic microbiota: introducing the concept of prebiotics. J. Nutr. 125:1401–1412, 1995.

[2]Roberfroid, M. B., Bornet, F., Bouley, C., and Cummings, J. H. Colonic microflora: nutrition and health. Summary and conclusions of an International Life Sciences Institute (ILSI) [Europe] workshop held in Barcelona, Spain. Nutr. Rev. 53:127–130, 1995.

[3]Drago, L., Gismondo, M. R., Lombardi, A., et al. Inhibition of *in vitro* growth of enteropathogens by new *Lactobacillus* isolates of human intestinal origin. FEMS Microbiol. Lett. 153:455–463, 1997.

[4]Marteau, P., Pochart, P., Bouhnik, Y., and Rambaud, J. C. The fate and effects of transiting nonpathogenic microorganisms in the human intestine. World Rev. Nutr. Diet 74:1–21, 1993.

[5]Majamaa, H., and Isolauri, E. Probiotics: a novel approach in the management of food allergy. J. Allergy Clin. Immunol. 99:179–185, 1997.

[6]Singh, J., Rivenson, A., Tomita, M., et al. *Bifidobacterium longum*, a lactic acid-producing intestinal bacterium inhibits colon cancer and modulates the intermediate biomarkers of colon carcinogenesis. Carcinogenesis 18:833–841, 1997.

[7]Guarino, A., Canani, R. B., Spagnuolo, M. I., et al. Oral bacterial therapy reduces the duration of symptoms and of viral excretion in children with mild diarrhea. J. Pediatr. Gastroenterol. Nutr. 25:516–519, 1997.

[8]Salminen, S., Isolauri, E., and Salminen, E. Clinical uses of probiotics for stabilizing the gut mucosal barrier: successful strains and future challenges. Antonie Van Leeuwenhoek 70: 347–358, 1996.

[9]Roberfroid, M. B. Functional effects of food components and the gastrointestinal system: chicory fructooligosaccharides. Nutr. Rev. 54(part II):S38–S42, 1996.

Digestive Problems and Solutions

Each of the organs and processes of the digestive system is necessary for the proper digestion and absorption of food. Problems at any step along the way can inhibit the ability to obtain nutrients from food and influence nutritional status. For example, the inability to chew food due to dental caries or loss of teeth can limit the types of food consumed or prevent digestive enzymes from coming in contact with the nutrients in food. A reduction in saliva that might be caused by

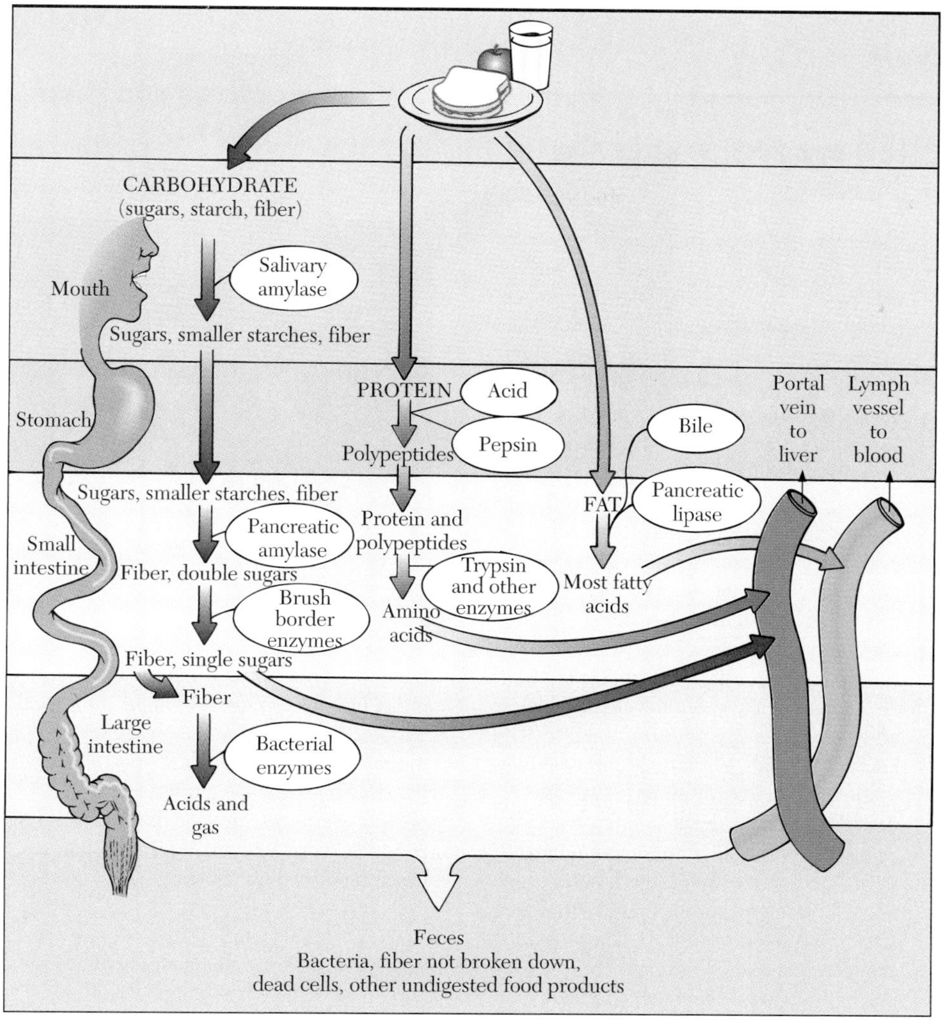

Figure 3.13
An overview of the digestion and absorption of a meal.

disease or medication can reduce the ability to taste foods and make swallowing difficult. A problem in the closure of the gastroesophageal sphincter can result in heartburn. Reduced acid production by the stomach can interfere with the absorption of vitamin B_{12}. Pancreatic problems can limit the availability of enzymes needed to digest protein. Gallbladder problems can interfere with fat absorption. Abnormalities in the small intestine can reduce nutrient absorption. A reduction in muscle tone in the large intestine can slow transit time and cause constipation. Some of these problems require adaptations in the way we obtain nutrients, whereas others are minor and can be treated with over-the-counter medications (see *Off the Shelf: Antacids: Risks, Benefits, and Nutritional Impact*).

For individuals who are unable to consume food or digest and absorb the nutrients needed to meet their requirements, several alternative feeding methods have been developed. People who are unable to swallow can be fed a liquid diet through a tube inserted into the stomach or intestine. Tube feeding with commercially prepared formula can provide a balanced diet containing all the essential nutrients. Tube feeding can be used in patients who are unconscious or have suffered an injury to the upper gastrointestinal tract. For individuals whose gastrointestinal tract is not functional, nutrients can be provided directly into the bloodstream. This is referred to as total parenteral nutrition (TPN). Carefully planned TPN can provide all the nutrients essential to life. When all nutrients are not provided in a TPN solution, nutrient deficiencies develop quickly. Inadvertently feeding patients incomplete TPN solutions has helped demonstrate the essentiality of several trace minerals.

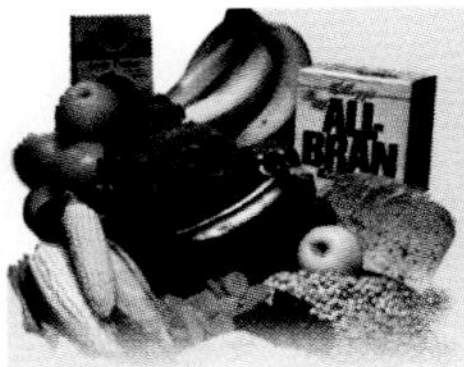

Off the Shelf

Antacids: Benefits, Risks, and Nutritional Impact

Heartburn remedies are among the most popular over-the-counter drugs. Although many of these medications are effective, they are not risk free and some have a nutritional impact. Since drugs are labeled differently from foods, it can be difficult to tell what you are getting.

Heartburn is caused by stomach acid leaking into the esophagus. Stomach acid is necessary for digestion; it enhances the absorption of certain nutrients and minimizes bacterial growth. But stomach acid can also cause pain and discomfort. It contributes to heartburn and ulcer formation and can irritate existing ulcers. Heartburn usually results from overeating and tends to occur about an hour after a large meal. Anxiety and stress may also cause heartburn by stimulating stomach acid production. The most common medications used to manage heartburn are antacids and drugs that block acid secretion.

Antacids work by making the gastric contents less acidic. In general, these over-the-counter products have been found to be safe and effective.[1] Most antacids contain the minerals calcium, sodium, aluminum, or magnesium and therefore have a nutritional impact. Calcium, as calcium carbonate, is found in antacids such as Tums. Calcium carbonate works rapidly and acts for a fairly long time.[2] These products are a good source of well-absorbed calcium.[3] For example, two extra-strength Tums contain 600 mg of calcium, which is 60% of the Daily Value. The active ingredient in sodium-containing antacids, such as Alka-Seltzer, is sodium bicarbonate. These also act rapidly and are especially good for relief after overeating. A problem with of this type of antacid is the high amount of sodium they contain—each tablet of Alka-Seltzer contains 567 mg of sodium, about 24% of the Daily Value. Sodium-containing antacids would not be recommended for someone on a sodium-restricted diet. Aluminum is also found in a number of antacids. Aluminum binds to phosphate in the gut and limits phosphorus absorption, and may cause constipation. Magnesium-containing products may cause diarrhea. In fact, when taken in higher doses, magnesium antacids such as Milk of Magnesia can be used as a laxative. In addition to minerals, many antacids contain sugar, which is added to make them more palatable. The amount is small, but individuals who have diabetes or are consuming low-kcalorie diets should consider it in diet planning.

A second type of medication used to treat heartburn reduces the amount of gastric acid released rather than neutralizing it after it has been produced. These agents are effective and easy to use.[4] Studies comparing these acid blockers to antacids found them to be equal in efficacy. Common over-the-counter acid blockers include Pepcid AC (famotidine), Tagamet (cimetidine), and Zantac (ranitidine). These drugs are effective longer than antacids (about 5 hours).

If you are looking for an over-the-counter medication to treat occasional heartburn, both antacids and acid blockers are effective. Acid blockers do not contribute minerals or kcalories to the diet, but sometimes this contribution is welcome. For example, someone who wants to boost her calcium intake might want a calcium carbonate antacid. In general, self-medication with antacids to treat heartburn should be limited because repeated use may stimulate the stomach to produce more acid and aggravate some gastrointestinal problems.

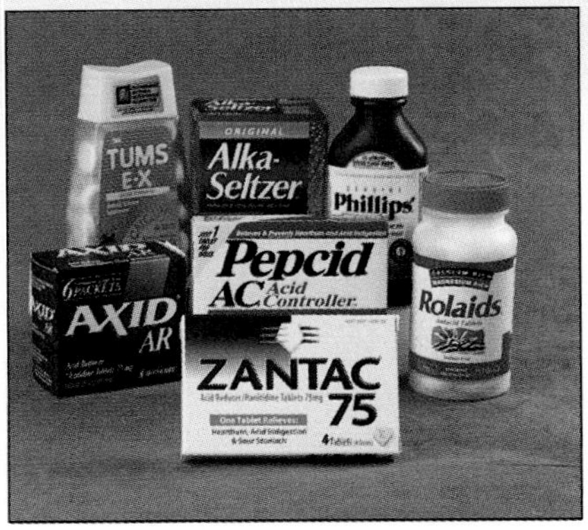

(George Semple)

[1]Brucker, M. C., and Faucher, M. A. Pharmacologic management of common gastrointestinal health problems in women. J. Nurse-Midwifery 42:145–162, 1997.

[2]Feldma, M. Comparison of the effects of over-the-counter famotidine and calcium carbonate antacid on postprandial gastric acid. J.A.M.A. 275:1438–1441, 1996.

[3]Mortensen, L., and Charles, P. Bioavailability of calcium supplements and the effect of vitamin D: comparisons between milk, calcium carbonate, and calcium carbonate plus vitamin D. Am. J. Clin. Nutr. 63:354–357, 1996.

[4]Shindelbeck, N. E., Klauser, A. G., Voderholzer, W. A., and Muller-Lissner, S. A. Empiric therapy for gastrointestinal reflux disease. Arch. Intern Med. 155:1808–1812, 1995.

Differences in the Digestive System Throughout Life

At different stages of life the digestive system may require special diets to maximize nutrient intake and absorption and minimize discomfort. Most of the unique aspects of digestion that occur during pregnancy, infancy, and advanced age do not affect nutritional status when the diet is properly managed.

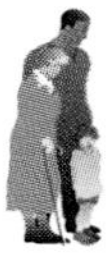

Pregnancy Physiological changes that occur during pregnancy may cause gastrointestinal problems. During the first three months, many women experience nausea, referred to as morning sickness. This term is a misnomer, because it can occur at any time of the day. Morning sickness is believed to be due to pregnancy-related hormonal changes. In most cases, it can be dealt with by eating frequent small meals and avoiding foods and smells that cause nausea. Eating dry crackers or cereal may also help. In severe cases where uncontrollable vomiting occurs, TPN may be needed to obtain adequate nutrition.

Later in pregnancy, the enlarged uterus puts pressure on the stomach and intestines, which can make it difficult to consume large meals. In addition, the placenta produces the hormone progesterone, which causes the smooth muscles of the digestive tract to relax. The muscle-relaxing effects of progesterone may relax the gastroesophageal sphincter enough to allow stomach contents to move back into the esophagus, causing heartburn. Symptoms of heartburn can be reduced by avoiding spicy foods; avoiding fatty foods, which slow the rate of stomach emptying; and remaining upright after eating. In the large intestine, relaxed muscles and the pressure of the uterus cause less efficient peristaltic movements and may result in constipation. Increasing water intake, eating a diet high in fiber, and exercising regularly can help relieve constipation.

Infancy The digestive system is one of the last to fully mature in developing humans. At birth, the digestive tract is functional, but a newborn is not ready to consume an adult diet. The most obvious difference between the infant and adult digestive tracts is that newborns are not able to chew and swallow solid food. They are born with a suckling reflex that allows them to consume liquids from a nipple placed toward the back of the mouth. A protrusion reflex causes anything placed in the front of the mouth to be pushed out by the tongue. As head control increases, this reflex disappears, making spoon feeding possible.

Digestion and absorption also differ between infants and adults. In infants, the digestion of milk protein is aided by rennin, an enzyme produced in the infant stomach that is not found in adults.[3] The stomachs of newborns also produce the enzyme gastric lipase, which begins the digestion of the fats in human milk. Low levels of pancreatic enzymes in infants limit starch digestion; however, enzymes at the brush border of the small intestine allow the milk sugar lactose to be digested and absorbed. The absorption of fat from the infant's small intestine is inefficient. However, the ability to absorb intact proteins is greater than in adults. The absorption of whole proteins can cause food allergies (see Chapter 14), but it also allows infants to absorb immune factors from their mother's milk. These proteins provide temporary immunity to certain diseases. The bacteria in the large intestine of infants are also different from those in adults because of the all-milk diet infants consume. This is the reason that the feces of breast-fed babies are almost odorless. Another feature of the infant digestive tract is the lack of voluntary control of elimination. Between the ages of two and three, this ability develops, and toilet training is possible.

Advanced Age Although there are few dramatic changes in the nutrient requirements of humans as they age, changes in the digestive tract and other systems may affect the palatability of food and the ability to obtain proper nutrition. The senses of smell and taste are often diminished or even lost with age, reducing the appeal of food. A reduction in the amount of saliva may make swallowing difficult, decrease the taste of food, and also promote tooth decay. Loss of teeth and improperly fitting dentures may limit food choices to soft and liquid foods or cause solid foods to be poorly chewed. Intestinal secretions may also be reduced, but this rarely impairs absorption because the levels secreted in healthy elderly are still sufficient to break down food into forms that can be absorbed. A condition that causes a reduction in the secretion of stomach acid is also common in the elderly. This may decrease the absorption of several vitamins and minerals and may allow bacterial growth to increase (see Chapter 15). Constipation in the elderly is caused by decreased motility and elasticity in the colon, weakened abdominal and pelvic muscles, and a decrease in sensory perception. Although constipation occurs in about the same frequency in all age groups,[4] it is estimated that 20 to 30% of individuals over 65 are dependent on laxatives[5] (see *Critical Thinking: Gastrointestinal Problems Can Affect Digestion and Absorption*).

CRITICAL THINKING

Gastrointestinal Problems Can Affect Digestion and Absorption

This chapter has followed the path of a turkey sandwich, an apple, and a glass of milk through the processes of digestion and absorption. During the journey from mouth to anus, many factors affect how well these processes work. For each situation described below, think about how digestion and absorption might be altered.

Mouth

An individual is taking medication that reduces the amount of saliva produced.

What effect would this have on nutrition?

When there is not enough saliva, the food is not tasted as well and it is difficult to swallow. Both of these factors are likely to decrease the appeal and therefore consumption of food. Since saliva helps protect teeth from decay, insufficient saliva also increases the likelihood of tooth decay and gum disease.

What nutrients might not be absorbed from the apple if an individual has just had some dental work done?

If the food is not well chewed, digestive enzymes cannot come in contact with all components of the food. If the fiber in the apple skin is not chewed, the vitamins and minerals it contains may not be available for absorption.

Stomach

After consuming the turkey sandwich, apple, and glass of milk, a large slice of high-fat cheesecake is added for dessert.

How would this affect transit time?

Transit time would increase because the cheesecake is high in fat, which slows stomach emptying. The meal would take more time to pass from mouth to anus.

Pancreas

An individual has a disease of the pancreas that causes a deficiency of pancreatic enzymes.

What effect would this have on the digestion and absorption of the sample meal?

Pancreatic enzymes are needed to digest carbohydrate, fat, and protein. If these enzymes are lacking, digestion will be incomplete, and nutrient absorption will be compromised. Carbohydrate-digesting enzymes in the mouth and intestinal brush border, as well as protein-digesting enzymes in the stomach and mucosal cells, can partially compensate for a reduction in pancreatic enzymes.

Small intestine

An individual has been malnourished. The malnutrition causes the intestinal villi to become flattened.

If the sample meal was consumed, how would nutrient absorption be affected?

The absorption of all nutrients depends on the health of the small intestine. If the villi are flattened, the absorptive area will be decreased, so fewer nutrients will be absorbed.

Large intestine

An individual eats the turkey sandwich and apple but chooses not to drink the milk or consume any other fluid.

How might this affect the feces?

A diet low in fluid and high in fiber could result in hard feces and constipation.

Gallbladder

An individual has gallstones, which cause pain when the gallbladder contracts.

What type of foods should be avoided?

Answer:

THE PATHS OF ABSORBED NUTRIENTS

Absorbed materials are delivered to body cells by the cardiovascular system, which consists of the heart and blood vessels. The path by which nutrients enter the bloodstream varies with the nutrient. Amino acids from protein, simple sugars from carbohydrate, and the water-soluble products of fat digestion are absorbed directly into the bloodstream. The products of fat digestion that are not water soluble are taken into the lymphatic system before entering the blood.

The Cardiovascular System

The cardiovascular system is a closed network of tubules through which blood is pumped. Blood carries nutrients and oxygen to the cells of all the organs and tissues of the body and removes waste products from these same cells. Blood also carries other substances, such as hormones, from one part of the body to another (Figure 3.14).

The heart is the workhorse of the cardiovascular system. It is a muscular pump with two circulatory loops—one that delivers blood to the lungs and one that delivers blood to the rest of the body. The blood vessels that transport blood and dissolved substances toward the heart are called **veins,** and those that transport blood and dissolved substances away from the heart are called **arteries.** As arteries carry blood away from the heart, they branch many times to form smaller and smaller blood vessels. The smallest arteries are called arterioles. Arterioles then branch to form **capillaries.** Capillaries are thin-walled vessels that are just large enough to allow one red blood cell to pass at a time. From the capillaries, oxygen and nutrients carried by the blood pass into the cells, and waste products pass from the cells into the capillaries. In the capillaries of the lungs, blood releases carbon dioxide to be exhaled and picks up oxygen to be delivered to the cells. In the capillaries of the GI tract, blood picks up water-soluble nutrients absorbed from the diet. Blood from capillaries then flows into the smallest veins, the

Veins Vessels that carry blood toward the heart.

Arteries Vessels that carry blood away from the heart.

Capillaries Small, thin-walled blood vessels where the exchange of gases and nutrients between blood and cells occurs.

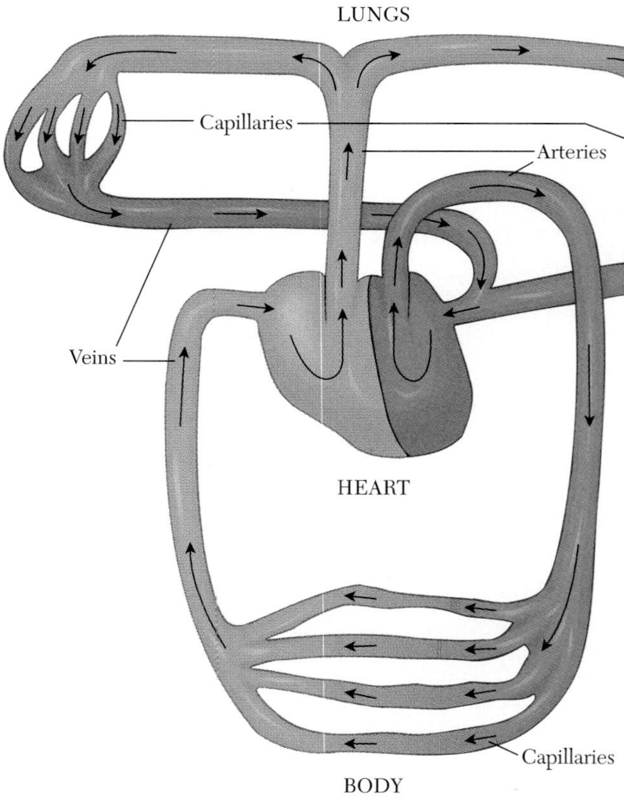

Figure 3.14
Blood is pumped from the heart through the arteries to the capillaries of the lungs, where it picks up oxygen. It then returns to the heart via the veins and is pumped out again into the arteries that lead to the rest of the body. In the capillaries of the body, blood delivers oxygen and nutrients and picks up wastes before returning to the heart via the veins. In this figure, red indicates blood that is rich in oxygen, and blue represents blood that is oxygen-poor and carrying more carbon dioxide.

venules, which converge to form larger and larger veins for return to the heart. Therefore, blood starting in the heart is pumped through the arteries to the capillaries of the lungs where it picks up oxygen. It then returns to the heart via the veins and is pumped out again into the arteries that lead to the rest of the body. In the capillaries of the body, blood delivers oxygen and nutrients and removes wastes before returning to the heart via the veins.

The volume of blood flow, and hence the amounts of nutrients and oxygen that are delivered to an organ or tissue, depends on the need. When a person is resting, about 24% of the blood goes to the digestive system, 21% to the skeletal muscles, and the rest to the heart, kidneys, brain, skin, and other organs.[6] After a large meal, a greater proportion will go to the intestines to support digestion and absorption and to transport nutrients. When a person engages in strenuous exercise, about 85% of blood flow will be directed to the skeletal muscles to deliver nutrients and oxygen and remove carbon dioxide and waste products. Attempting to exercise after a large meal creates a conflict. The body cannot direct blood to the intestines and the muscles at the same time. The muscles win, and food remains in the intestines, often resulting in cramps.

Hepatic Portal and Lymphatic Circulation

Nutrients enter the blood circulation by either the **hepatic portal circulation** or the the **lymphatic system.** The villi of the intestine contain both capillaries, which are part of the portal circulation, and lacteals, which are small vessels of the lymphatic system.

Hepatic portal circulation The system of blood vessels that collects nutrient-laden blood from the digestive organs and delivers it to the liver.

Lymphatic system The system of vessels, organs, and tissues that drains excess fluid from the spaces between cells and contributes to immune function.

The Hepatic Portal Circulation In the small intestine, water-soluble molecules, including amino acids, sugars, water-soluble vitamins, and water-soluble products of fat digestion, cross the mucosal cells of the villi and enter capillaries. These capillaries merge to form venules at the base of the villi. The venules then merge to form larger and larger veins, which eventually form the **hepatic portal vein.** The hepatic portal vein transports blood directly to the liver, where absorbed nutrients are processed before they enter the general circulation (Figure 3.15).

Hepatic portal vein The vein that transports blood from the gastrointestinal tract to the liver.

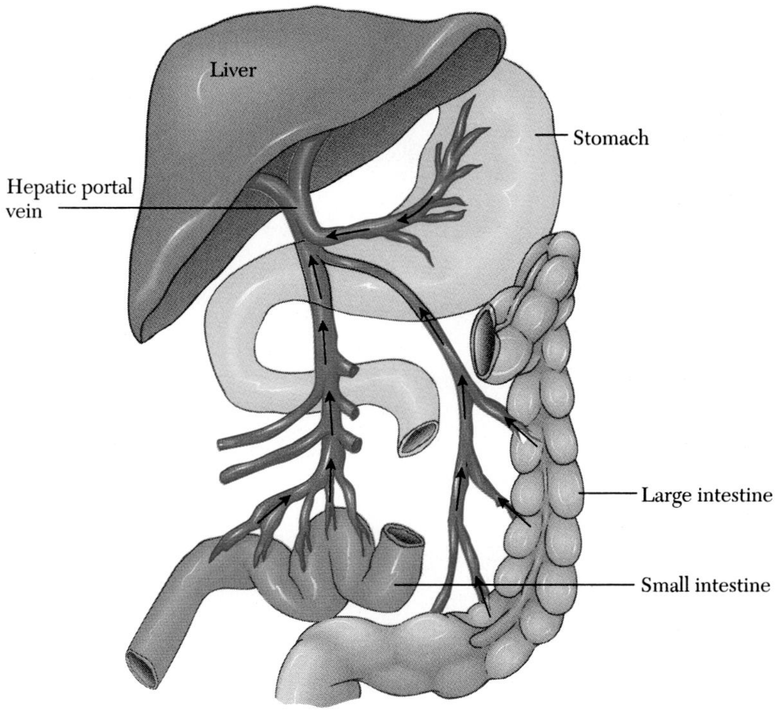

Figure 3.15
The hepatic portal circulation carries blood from the stomach and intestines to the hepatic portal vein and then to the liver.

The liver acts as a gatekeeper between substances absorbed from the intestine and the rest of the body. Some nutrients are stored in the liver, some are changed into different forms, and others are allowed to pass through unchanged. Based on the immediate needs of the body, the liver decides whether individual nutrients will be stored or delivered directly to the cells. For example, the liver, with the help of hormones from the pancreas, keeps the concentration of sugar in the blood constant. The liver modulates blood glucose by removing absorbed glucose from the blood and storing it, by sending absorbed glucose on to the tissues of the body, or by releasing liver glucose (from stores or synthesis) into the blood. The liver is also important for the synthesis and breakdown of amino acids, proteins, and fats. It modifies the products of protein breakdown to form molecules that can be safely transported to the kidney for excretion. The liver also contains enzyme systems that protect the body from toxins that are absorbed by the gastrointestinal tract.

The Lymphatic System The lymphatic system consists of a network of vessels that drain excess tissue fluid from the space between cells, called interstitial space, and return it to the bloodstream. Unlike the blood vessels, which carry substances to and from tissues, the lymphatic system only carries fluid away from the tissues. Fluid that is pushed out of capillaries by the force of the blood moves into the interstitial space and is then collected by the lymph vessels. The lymphatic system prevents fluid from accumulating and causing the tissues to swell. Fat-soluble substances—such as triglycerides, cholesterol, and fat-soluble vitamins—and other absorbed materials too large to enter the intestinal capillaries are transported from the villi by the lymphatic system (see Chapter 5). Lymph vessels from the intestine and most other organs of the body drain into the thoracic duct, which empties into the bloodstream near the neck. Therefore, substances that are absorbed into the lymph do not pass through the liver before entering the blood circulation.

In addition to its role in nutrient absorption and fluid balance, the lymphatic system is an extremely important part of the immune system. The role of nutrition in immune function is discussed with specific nutrients in later chapters.

Cell membrane The membrane that surrounds the cell contents.

Selectively permeable Describes a membrane or barrier that will allow some substances to pass freely but will restrict the passage of others.

Destination: The Cell

For nutrients to enter a cell, they must first cross the **cell membrane.** The cell membrane maintains homeostasis in the cell by controlling what enters and what exits. It is **selectively permeable** because some substances, such as water, can

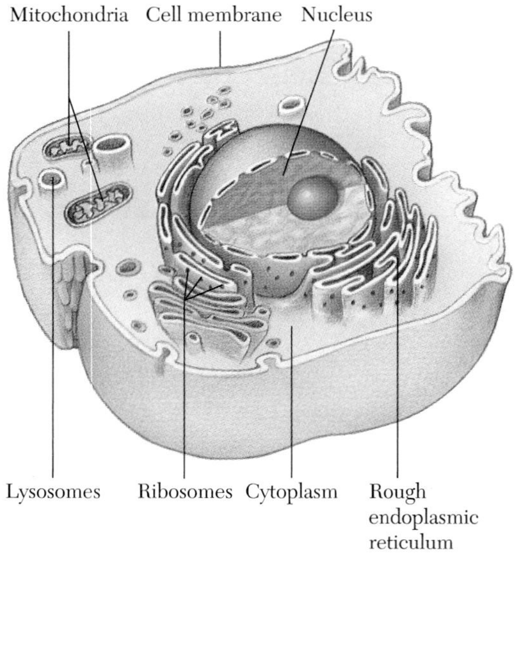

Figure 3.16
Structure of a general animal cell. Almost all human cells contain the organelles illustrated here.

pass freely back and forth, whereas the passage of others is regulated. Nutrients and other substances from the bloodstream are transported into cells by simple and facilitated diffusion and active transport. Once the nutrients have crossed the cell membrane and entered the cell, they can be broken down and used for energy, or they can be used to build the types of carbohydrates, lipids, and proteins that are needed by the human body. Inside the cell membrane is the **cytoplasm,** or cell fluid that contains the cell **organelles** that perform functions necessary for cell survival. Organelles are also surrounded by membranes. The largest organelle is the nucleus, which contains the cell's genetic material (Figure 3.16).

Cytoplasm The cellular material outside the nucleus that is contained by the cell membrane.

Organelles Cellular organs that carry out specific metabolic functions.

Metabolism: Making and Breaking Molecules

To stay healthy our bodies use nutrients to produce energy and to manufacture structural and regulatory molecules. The sum of the chemical reactions that occur inside body cells is collectively referred to as metabolism. If the proper amounts and types of nutrients are not delivered to cells, the reactions of metabolism cannot proceed optimally, resulting in poor health. Each nutrient plays a unique role in metabolism. The following discussion provides only a brief overview. Details about the metabolism of each nutrient will be discussed in later chapters.

Many of the reactions of metabolism occur in series known as metabolic pathways. Molecules that enter these pathways are modified at each step of the pathway with the help of enzymes. Some of the pathways are **anabolic,** using energy to build body structures, whereas others are **catabolic,** breaking large molecules into smaller ones and releasing energy. If a nutrient needed for these pathways to proceed is missing, the production of important body structures, chemical compounds, or energy may be impaired. The consequences may be as severe as a life-threatening deficiency disease or as mild as impaired athletic performance.

Anabolic and catabolic processes occur in different cellular organelles. An example of an anabolic organelle is the endoplasmic reticulum, which is a maze of internal membranes. One type of endoplasmic reticulum specializes in the synthesis of lipid-based compounds such as the sex hormones estrogen and testosterone. Another type of endoplasmic reticulum is covered with organelles called ribosomes, which are the site of protein synthesis. Proteins such as digestive enzymes are made here. Lysosomes are catabolic organelles that act as a kind of digestive system for the cell. Lysosomes contain enzymes capable of breaking down carbohydrates, fats, proteins, and other types of molecules that originate both inside and outside the cell.

The **mitochondrion** is a catabolic organelle that obtains energy from carbohydrates (Chapter 4), fats (Chapter 5), and proteins (Chapter 6) by **cellular respiration.** This process completely metabolizes these macronutrients in the presence of oxygen to produce carbon dioxide, water, and a form of energy that can be used by cells called **ATP (adenosine triphosphate).** The chemical bonds of ATP are very high in energy, and when they break, the energy is released. The energy contained in ATP can be used to do work such as pump blood or contract muscles—or it can be used to synthesize new molecules needed to maintain and repair body tissue.

The meal consumed at the beginning of this chapter has now been delivered to the cells. The carbohydrate in the bread has been broken down into glucose. The cells can use glucose to produce ATP or to synthesize other molecules for immediate use or storage. The protein in the turkey, milk, and bread has been broken down into amino acids that can be used by cells to synthesize needed protein, make glucose if it is in short supply, or produce ATP (Figure 3.17). The fat in the milk, turkey, and mayonnaise has been broken down into fatty acids. These can be used to make ATP or to produce lipids needed for body function, or they can be stored as body fat for later use.

Anabolic Energy-requiring processes in which simpler molecules are combined to form more complex substances.

Catabolic The processes by which substances are broken down into simpler molecules releasing energy.

Mitochondrion The cellular organelle responsible for generating energy in the form of ATP for cellular activities.

Cellular respiration The reactions that break down carbohydrates, fats, and proteins in the presence of oxygen to produce energy in the form of ATP.

ATP (adenosine triphosphate) The high-energy molecule used by the body to perform energy-requiring activities.

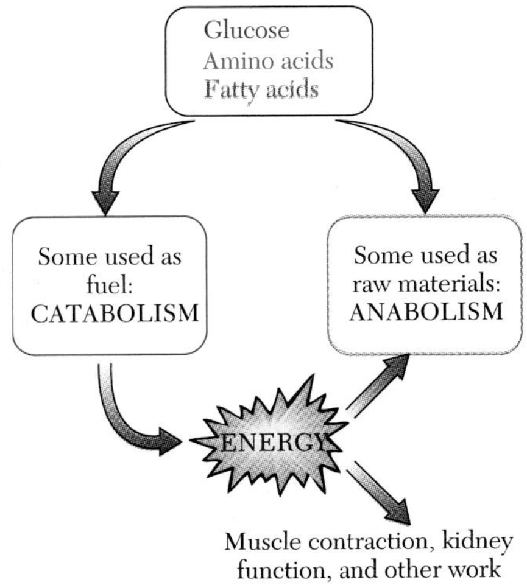

Figure 3.17
Nutrients delivered to cells can be used either to produce energy or as raw materials for the synthesis of carbohydrates, fats, and proteins in the body.

Elimination of Wastes

The waste products left over from the digestion and metabolism of the meal must be removed from the body. Substances such as fiber that are not absorbed from the intestine are eliminated from the gastrointestinal tract in the feces. The waste products of cellular metabolism are eliminated by the lungs, the skin, and the kidneys. Carbon dioxide produced by cellular respiration leaves the cells and is transported to the lungs by red blood cells. At the lungs, red blood cells release their load of carbon dioxide, which is then exhaled into the environment. In addition to carbon dioxide, the lungs lose a significant amount of water by evaporation. Water, along with protein breakdown products and minerals, is also lost through the skin in perspiration or sweat.

The kidney is the primary site for the excretion of water, nitrogen, and other dissolved metabolic waste products. These are excreted in the urine. The amounts of water and other substances excreted in the urine are regulated so that homeostasis is maintained (see Chapters 10 and 12).

Applications

These exercises are designed to help you apply your critical thinking skills to your own nutrition choices.

1. Imagine you wake up on a Sunday morning and join some friends for a large breakfast consisting of: a cheese omelet and sausage (foods high in fat and protein); a croissant with butter (which contains carbohydrate but is also very high in fat); and a small glass of orange juice. After the meal, you remember that you have plans to play basketball with a friend in just an hour.
   a. If you keep your plans and play basketball, what problems might you experience while exercising?
   b. Had you remembered your plans for strenuous exercise before you had breakfast, what type of meal might you have selected to ensure that your stomach would empty more quickly?
2. There are hundreds of products available to aid digestion. Go to the drug store, health food store, or search the Internet and select a product claiming to aid digestion.
   a. List the claims made for the product.
   b. Using the information in Chapter 1 on judging nutritional claims, analyze the information given.
   c. Does the product make any nutritional contributions to the diet?
   d. Does it carry any risk?
   e. Would you take it? Why or why not?

Summary

1. The organization of all matter begins with the same basic structure—the atom. Atoms are linked by chemical bonds to form molecules. The cell is the smallest unit of life. Cells of similar structure and function are organized into tissues, and tissues into organs and organ systems.
2. The digestive system is the organ system primarily responsible for the movement of nutrients into the body. The digestive system provides two major functions: digestion and absorption. Digestion is the process by which food is broken down into units that are small enough to be absorbed. Absorption is the process by which nutrients are transported into the body.
3. The gastrointestinal tract consists of a hollow tube that begins at the mouth and continues through the pharynx, esophagus, stomach, small intestine, large intestine, and anus. The passage, digestion, and absorption of food in the lumen of this tube are aided by the secretion of mucus, enzymes, and hormones.
4. The processes involved in digestion begin in response to the smell or sight of food and continue as food enters the digestive tract at the mouth, where it is broken into smaller pieces by the teeth and mixed with saliva. Carbohydrate digestion is begun in the mouth by salivary amylase. From the mouth, food passes through the pharynx and into the esophagus. The rhythmic contractions of peristalsis propel it down the esophagus to the stomach.
5. The stomach acts as a temporary storage site for food. The muscles of the stomach mix the food into a semiliquid mass called chyme, and gastric juice containing hydrochloric acid and pepsin begins protein digestion. Stomach emptying is regulated by the amount and composition of food consumed and by nervous and hormonal signals from the small intestine.
6. The small intestine is the primary site of nutrient digestion and absorption. In the small intestine, bicarbonate from the pancreas neutralizes stomach acid, and pancreatic and intestinal enzymes digest carbohydrate, fat, and protein. The diges-

tion of fat in the small intestine is aided by bile from the gallbladder. Bile helps break fat into small droplets accessible to fat-digesting enzymes. Secretions from the pancreas and liver are regulated by the hormones secretin and cholecystokinin, produced by the duodenum.

7. The absorption of food across the intestinal mucosa occurs by several different processes. Simple and facilitated diffusion do not require energy but depend on a concentration gradient. Active transport requires energy but can transport substances against a concentration gradient. The absorptive surface of the small intestine is increased by folds and fingerlike projections called villi, which are covered with tiny projections called microvilli.
8. Components of chyme that are not absorbed in the small intestine pass on to the large intestine, where some water and nutrients are absorbed. The large intestine is populated by bacteria that digest some of these unabsorbed materials, such as fiber, producing small amounts of nutrients and gas. The remaining unabsorbed materials are excreted in feces.
9. Absorbed nutrients are delivered to the cells of the body by the cardiovascular system. The heart pumps blood to the lungs to pick up oxygen and eliminate carbon dioxide. From the lungs, blood returns to the heart and is pumped to the rest of the body to deliver oxygen and nutrients and remove carbon dioxide and other wastes before returning to the heart. Blood is pumped away from the heart in arteries and returned to the heart in veins. Exchange of nutrients and gases occurs at the smallest blood vessels, the capillaries.
10. The products of carbohydrate and protein digestion and the water-soluble products of fat digestion enter capillaries in the intestinal villi and are transported to the liver via the hepatic portal circulation. The liver serves as a processing center, removing the absorbed substances for storage, converting them into other forms, or allowing them to pass unaltered. The liver also protects the body from toxic substances that may have been absorbed.
11. The fat-soluble products of digestion and other large materials enter lacteals in the intestinal villi. The nutrients absorbed via the lymphatic system enter the blood circulation without first passing through the liver.
12. Cells are the final destination of absorbed nutrients. To enter the cells, nutrients must be transported across cell membranes. Within the cells, some organelles are catabolic, specializing in the breakdown of nutrients to produce energy. Others are anabolic, specializing in the synthesis of molecules needed by the body. The sum of all the chemical reactions of the body is called metabolism. The reactions that completely break down macronutrients in the presence of oxygen to produce water, carbon dioxide, and energy are referred to as cellular respiration.
13. Unabsorbed materials are excreted in the feces. The waste products of metabolism are excreted by the lungs, skin, and kidneys.

Review Questions

1. What is an organic molecule?
2. What is the smallest unit of plant and animal life?
3. List three organ systems involved in the digestion and absorption of food.
4. How do teeth function in digestion?
5. What is peristalsis?
6. List two functions of the stomach.
7. List three mechanisms by which nutrients are absorbed.
8. Where does most digestion and absorption occur?
9. How does the structure of the small intestine aid absorption?
10. What products of digestion are transported by the lymphatic system?
11. What path does an amino acid follow from absorption to delivery to the cell? What path does a large fatty acid follow from absorption to delivery to the cell?
12. What is the form of energy used by cells?
13. List four ways that waste products are eliminated from the body.

Nutrition Web Links

To further explore areas related to the material in this chapter, go to the *Nutrition: Science and Applications* Web site at ***www.Wiley.com/college/Smolin*** and *click on* **Student Companion Site** for chapter-by-chapter links. Some Web sites related to the information in Chapter 3 include:

Sites that provide additional information about the structure and function of the cells and organs that make up the digestive tract.

Sites that provide additional information about cellular structure and metabolism in general.

Locations such as the National Institutes of Diabetes and Digestive and Kidney Diseases and the Digestive Diseases Information Center that provide information about heartburn, constipation, peptic ulcers, diverticular disease, and other digestive diseases.

References

1. Damianos, A. J., and McGarrity, T. J. Treatment strategies for *Helicobacter pylori* infection. Am. Fam. Physician 55:2765–2774, 1997.
2. Roberfroid, M. B., Bornet, F., Bouley, C., and Cummings, J. H. Colonic microflora: nutrition and health. Summary and conclusions of an International Life Sciences Institute (ILSI) [Europe] workshop held in Barcelona, Spain. Nutr. Rev. 53:127–130, 1995.
3. Marieb, E. N. *Human Anatomy and Physiology*, 4th ed. Redwood City, Calif.: Benjamin/Cummings Publishing Co., 1998.
4. Harari, D., Gurwitz, J. H., Avorn, J., et al. Bowel habit in relation to age and gender: findings from the National Health Interview Survey and clinical implications. Arch. Intern. Med. 156:315–320, 1996.
5. Brucker, M. C., and Faucher, M. A. Pharmacologic management of common gastrointestinal health problems in women. J. Nurse-Midwifery 42:145–162, 1997.
6. Rhoades, R., and Pflanzer, R. *Human Physiology*, 3rd ed. Philadelphia: Saunders College Publishing, 1996.

II

Energy-Containing Nutrients

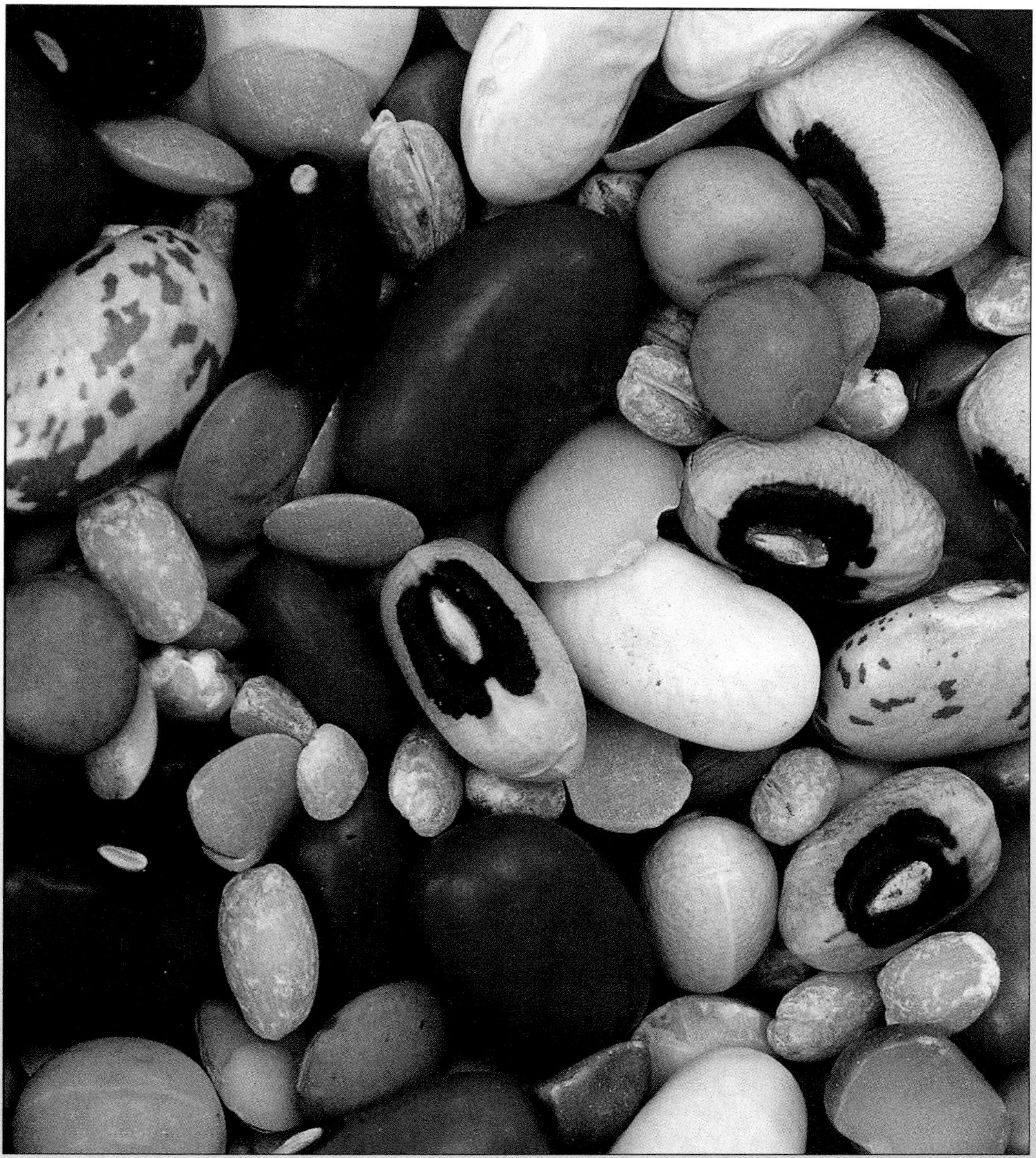

Chapter 4

Chapter Outline

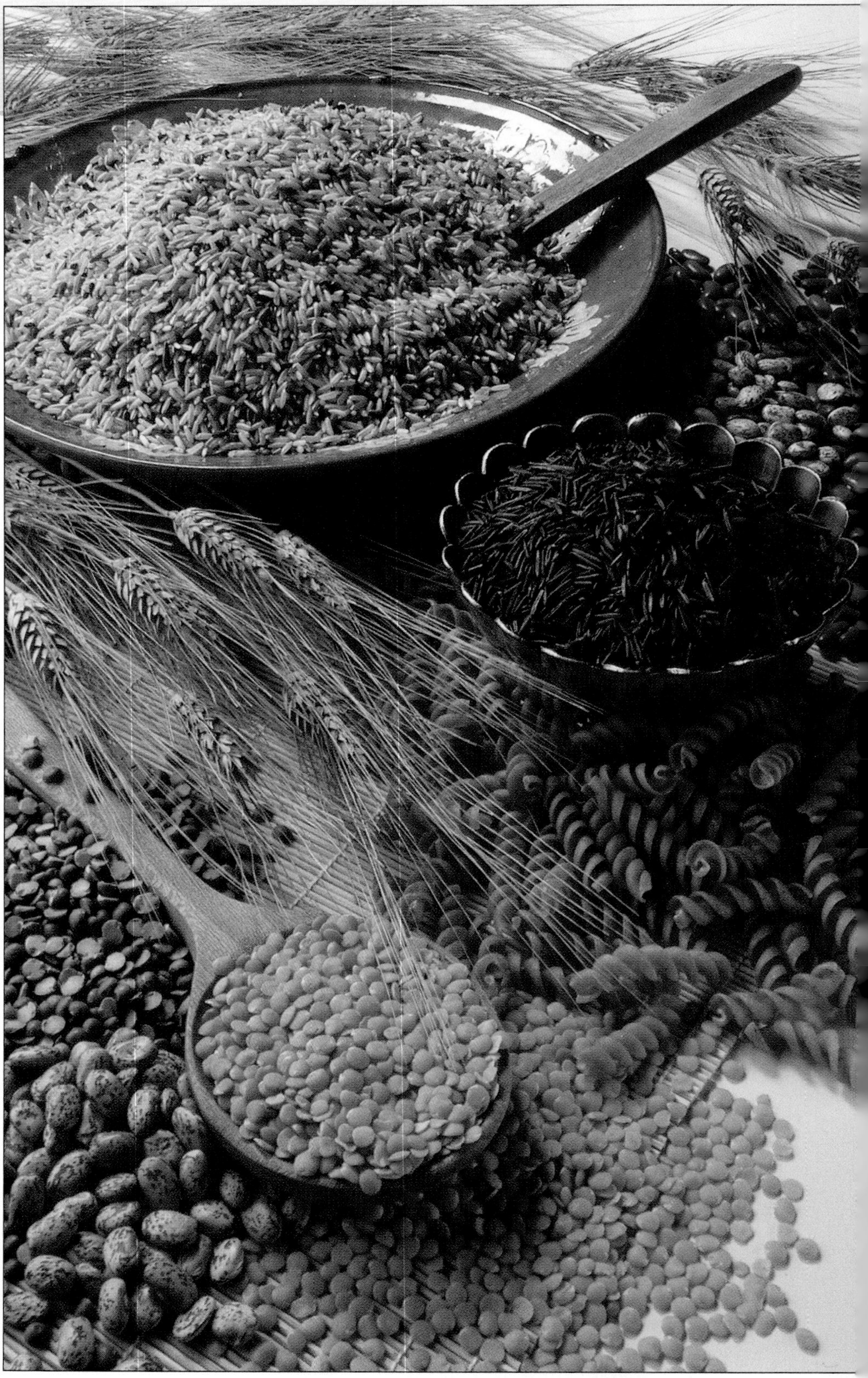

(© *Picture Perfect*)

Carbohydrates: Sugars, Starches, and Fiber

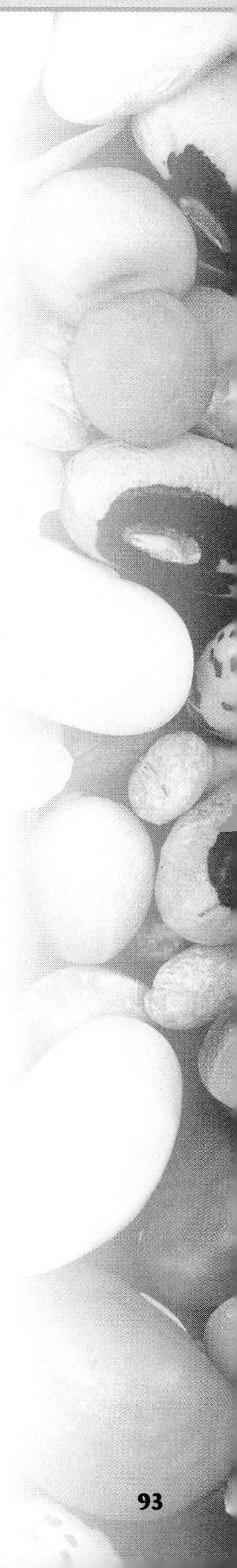

Chapter Concepts

1. Foods high in complex carbohydrates, such as rice, beans, and corn, are the basis of the diet for most of the world.
2. Carbohydrates include simple carbohydrates, such as those in table sugar and fruit, and complex carbohydrates, such as starch and fiber found in legumes and grains.
3. Fiber cannot be absorbed into the body because it cannot be digested by enzymes produced by the human gastrointestinal tract.
4. Carbohydrates provide a readily available source of energy and are central to energy production in the human body.
5. Diabetes is a disease of carbohydrate transport and metabolism that has serious complications. It is characterized by abnormally high levels of blood glucose.
6. Foods high in unrefined complex carbohydrates are rich sources of other nutrients and phytochemicals. Diets high in fiber may protect against bowel disorders, heart disease, and cancer.
7. Diets high in carbohydrates, particularly simple sugars, promote tooth decay. Foods high in refined sugar are low in nutrient density.
8. The typical intake of carbohydrates in the North American diet is below the recommended level of 55 to 60% of total energy.
9. Carbohydrates are added in processing to sweeten, preserve, stabilize, or thicken foods.
10. Artificial sweeteners, also called sugar substitutes, are used to reduce the sugar and energy content of foods.

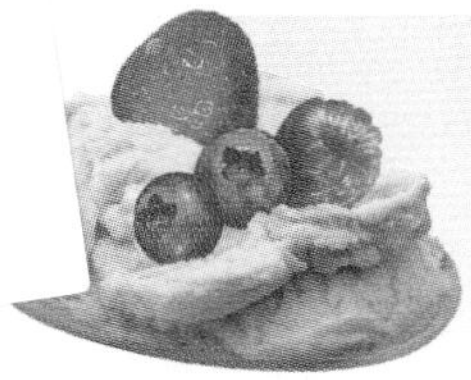

Just a Taste

Is sugar bad for you?

Are carbohydrates fattening?

Is whole wheat bread better for you than white bread?

Carbohydrate-rich foods provide the basis of the diet for most of the world. Rice is the dietary staple in much of Asia, corn in South America, and cassava, a starchy root vegetable, in parts of Africa. Although every culture eats carbohydrates, the amount and type consumed often depend on the wealth and prosperity of the society. As countries become more affluent, animal foods become more affordable, so the intake of carbohydrate from grains and vegetables typically decreases as the intake of fat and protein from animal foods increases. For example, in developing countries today, two thirds of the energy in the diet comes from carbohydrates, whereas in more economically developed countries, the typical intake of carbohydrate accounts for only about half of the energy intake.

The affluence of the society also influences the form of carbohydrate consumed. Throughout history peasants have eaten dark breads and brown rice while the aristocracy has consumed refined white flour, white sugar, and polished rice. Is the peasant diet the one we should be following? Recommendations for a healthy diet promote diets high in whole grains, vegetables, and fruits and limited in refined and added carbohydrates. Do we need to give up white bread, soft drinks, and sugared cereals to consume a healthier diet?

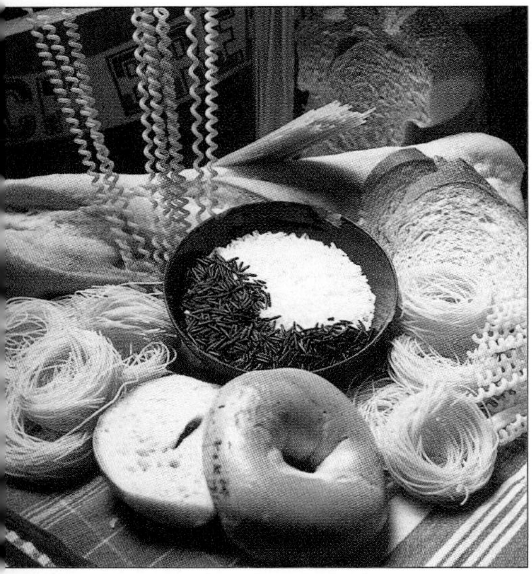

Figure 4.1
Grains, breads, and legumes are sources of dietary carbohydrate. (Charles D. Winters)

What Are Carbohydrates?

Carbohydrates Compounds containing carbon plus hydrogen and oxygen in the same proportions as in water. They include sugars, starches, and fibers.

Simple carbohydrates Carbohydrates known as sugars that include monosaccharides and disaccharides.

Refined Refers to the process whereby the coarse parts of foods are removed, leaving behind a product of more uniform composition.

Empty kcalories Refers to foods that contribute energy but few other nutrients.

Chemically, **carbohydrates** are compounds that contain carbon (*carbo*), as well as hydrogen and oxygen in the same proportion as in water (*hydrate*). They are found in grains, breads, legumes, fruits, vegetables, and milk, as well as in sweeteners such as honey and table sugar (Figure 4.1). Carbohydrates provide about 52% of the energy in the American diet.

Simple carbohydrates, or sugars, provide about 21% of the energy in the U.S. diet. Half of this is from sugars naturally present in whole foods such as milk or fresh fruit.[1] The rest is from **refined** sugars added to foods. Added refined sugars are not nutritionally or chemically different from sugars occurring naturally in foods. The only difference is that they have been separated from their plant sources, such as sugar cane and sugar beets. Refined sugars are considered **empty kcalories** because they are low in nutrient density, containing energy but few other nutrients. Whole foods, such as fruits, contain vitamins, minerals, fiber, and phytochemicals as well as energy. Therefore they have a higher nutrient density—that is, they contain more nutrients per kcalorie than refined sugars. For example, a tablespoon of sugar contains about 50 kcalories but almost no nutrients other than sugar. A small orange also has about 50

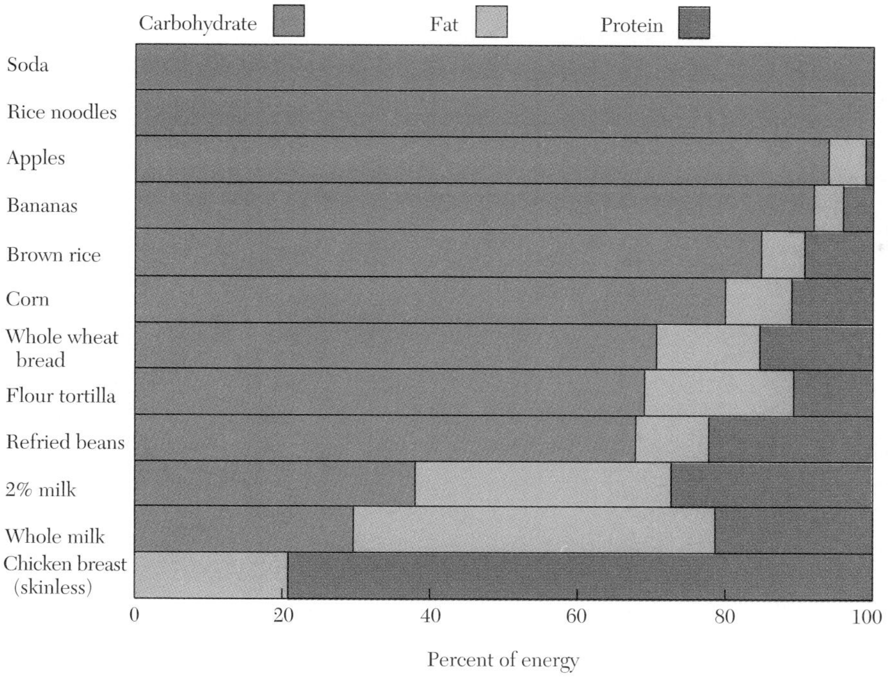

Figure 4.2
Most of these foods are sources of carbohydrate, and most also contain protein and fat.

kcalories but contributes vitamin C, folate, potassium, and some calcium as well as fiber.

Grains are the major source of **complex carbohydrates** in the North American diet. Grains provide a mixture of starch and fiber along with protein, lipids, vitamins, and minerals. Other plant foods such as vegetables and legumes are also sources of both fiber and starch as well as protein, vitamins, and minerals (Figure 4.2). The pulp of starchy vegetables such as potatoes provides starch, whereas the skins are a source of fiber. Dried legumes, such as pinto and kidney beans, are excellent sources of starch and fiber and are good sources of protein. Other vegetables such as green beans and broccoli are lower in starch and high in fiber and water. Whether starch or sugar, carbohydrates provide about 4 kcalories per gram. They are the primary source of energy used to fuel the body.

Complex carbohydrates Carbohydrates composed of sugar molecules linked together in straight or branching chains. They include starches and fibers.

Simple Carbohydrates

The basic unit of carbohydrate is a single sugar molecule, a **monosaccharide** (*mono* means one). When two sugar molecules combine, they form a **disaccharide** (*di* means two). Monosaccharides and disaccharides are known as simple sugars, or simple carbohydrates. The three most common monosaccharides in the diet are glucose, fructose, and galactose. Each contains 6 carbon, 12 hydrogen, and 6 oxygen atoms but differs in their arrangement (Figure 4.3). **Glucose,** commonly referred to as blood sugar, is the most important carbohydrate fuel for the body. It is produced in plants by the process of **photosynthesis,** which uses energy from the sun to combine carbon dioxide and water

Monosaccharide A single sugar molecule, such as glucose.

Disaccharide A sugar formed by linking two monosaccharides.

Glucose A monosaccharide that is the primary form of carbohydrate used to produce energy in the body. It is the sugar referred to as blood sugar.

Photosynthesis The metabolic process by which plants trap energy from the sun and use it to make sugars from carbon dioxide and water.

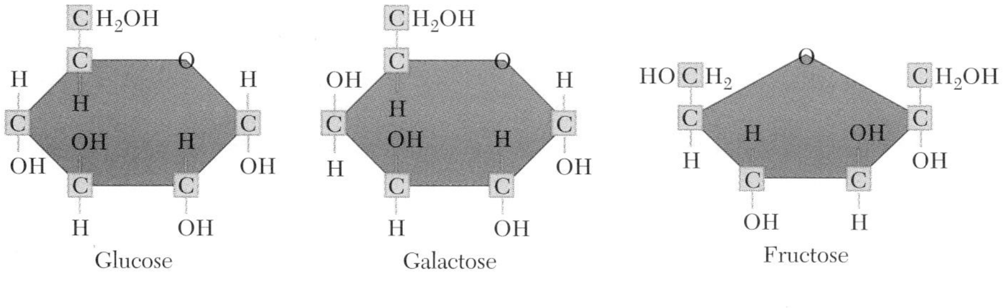

Figure 4.3
Common monosaccharides.

Figure 4.4
The process of photosynthesis uses energy from the sun to synthesize glucose from carbon dioxide and water. Glucose can then be stored as starch.

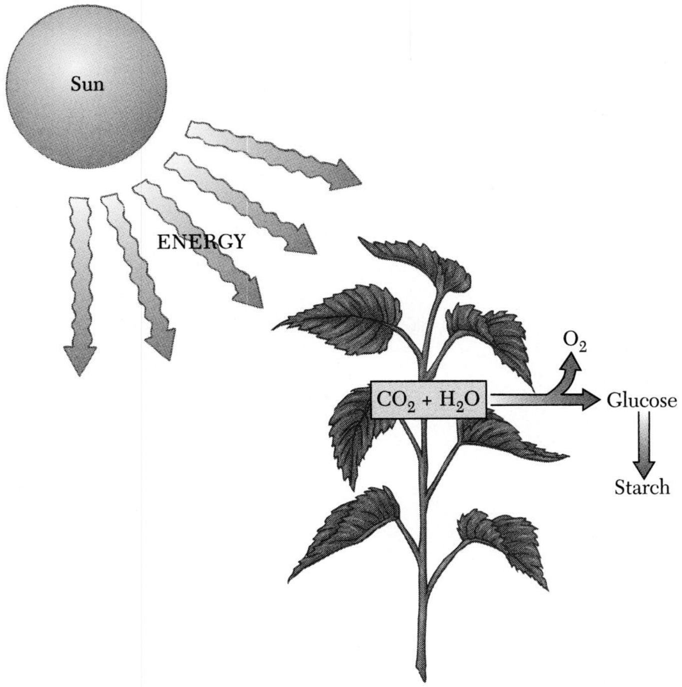

(Figure 4.4). Glucose rarely occurs as a monosaccharide in food. It is most often found as part of a disaccharide or starch. Fructose is a monosaccharide that tastes sweeter than glucose. It is found in fruits and vegetables and makes up more than half the sugar in honey. Galactose occurs most often as a part of lactose, the disaccharide in milk, and is rarely present as a monosaccharide in the food supply.

Disaccharides are simple carbohydrates made up of two monosaccharides linked together (Figure 4.5). Maltose is a disaccharide consisting of two molecules of glucose. This sugar is made whenever starch is broken down. For example, it is responsible for the slightly sweet taste experienced when bread is held in the mouth for a few minutes. As salivary amylase begins digesting the starch, some sweeter-tasting maltose is formed. Sucrose, or common white table sugar, is the disaccharide formed by linking glucose to fructose. It is found in sugar cane, sugar beets, honey, and maple syrup. Sucrose is the only sweetener that can be called "sugar" in the ingredient list on food labels in the United States. Lactose, or milk sugar, is glucose linked to galactose. Lactose is the only sugar found naturally in animal foods. It contributes about 30% of the energy in whole cow's milk and about 40% of the energy in human milk.

Complex Carbohydrates

Complex carbohydrates are made up of many monosaccharides linked together in chains. They are generally not sweet to the taste like simple carbohydrates. Short chains of three to ten monosaccharides are called **oligosaccharides** and longer chains are called **polysaccharides** (*poly* means many). The polysaccharides include glycogen in animals and starch and fiber in plants (Figure 4.6).

Oligosaccharides Short chain carbohydrates containing 3 to 10 sugar units.

Polysaccharides Carbohydrates containing many sugar units linked together.

Oligosaccharides Oligosaccharides such as raffinose and stachyose are found in beans and other legumes. These cannot be digested by enzymes in the human stomach and small intestine, so they pass undigested into the large intestine. Here bacteria digest them, producing gas and other by-products. This gas produced by the intestinal microflora can cause abdominal discomfort and flatulence. Over-the-counter enzyme tablets and solutions (such as Bean-O) can be consumed to break down oligosaccharides before they reach the intestinal bacteria, thereby reducing the amount of gas produced.

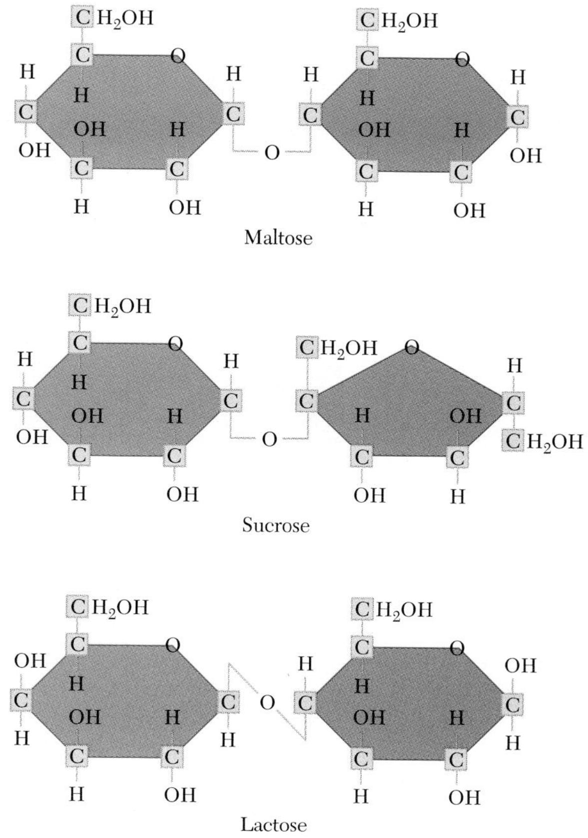

Figure 4.5
Common disaccharides.

Glycogen **Glycogen** is the storage form of carbohydrate in animals. It is made up of highly branched chains of glucose molecules. The branched structure allows it to be broken down quickly when glucose is needed. In humans, glycogen is stored in the muscles and in the liver. Muscle glycogen provides glucose to the muscle as a source of energy during activity; liver glycogen provides glucose to cells throughout the body via the bloodstream.

The amount of glycogen in the body is relatively small—about 200 to 500 grams.[2] The amount of glycogen stored in muscle can be temporarily increased by a diet and exercise regimen called **carbohydrate loading** or **glycogen supercompensation.** This regimen is often used by endurance athletes to build up glycogen stores before an event. Extra glycogen can mean the difference between running only 20 miles or finishing a 26-mile marathon before exhaustion takes over. Glycogen supercompensation is discussed in more detail in Chapter 12.

Glycogen A carbohydrate made of many glucose molecules linked together in a highly branched structure. It is the storage form of carbohydrate in animals.

Carbohydrate loading or **glycogen supercompensation** A regimen of diet and exercise that is designed to load muscle glycogen stores beyond their normal capacity.

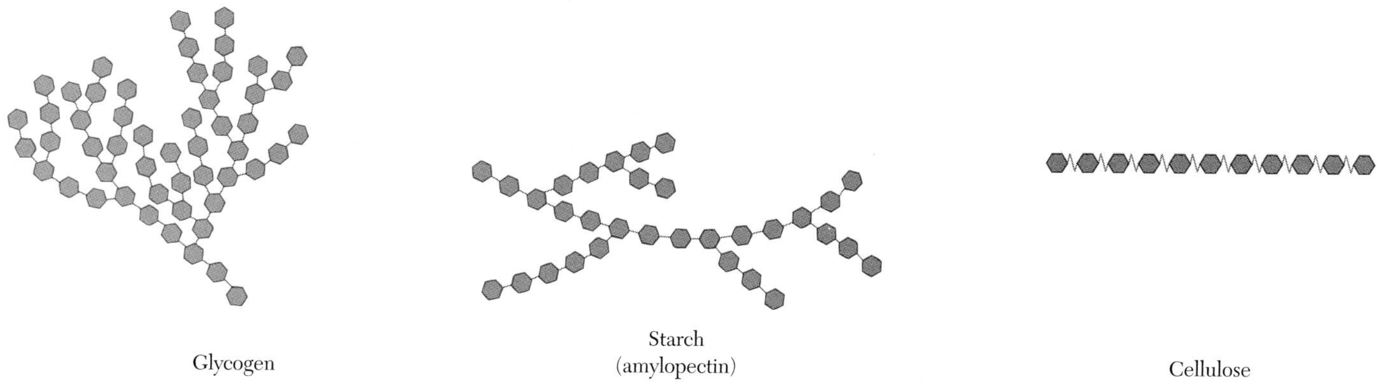

Figure 4.6
Complex carbohydrates are made up of straight or branching chains of monosaccharides.

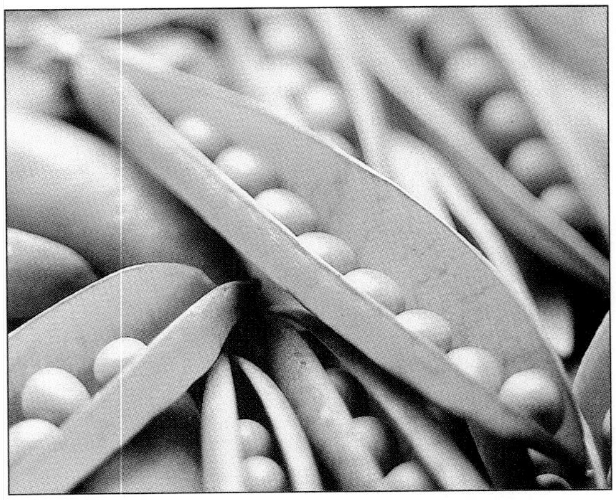

Figure 4.7
Legumes like these peas are seeds that grow in a pod. (© Chris Everard/Tony Stone Images, Inc.)

Starch A carbohydrate made of many glucose molecules linked in straight or branching chains. The bonds that hold the glucose molecules together can be broken by the human digestive enzymes.

Bran The protective outer layers of whole grains. It is a concentrated source of dietary fiber.

Germ The embryo or sprouting portion of a kernel of grain. It contains vegetable oil and vitamins.

Endosperm The largest portion of a kernel of grain. It is primarily starch and serves as a food supply for the sprouting seed.

Enrichment The addition of nutrients lost in processing to a level equal to or higher than that originally present.

Dietary fiber Nonstarch polysaccharides in plant foods that are not broken down by human digestive enzymes.

Insoluble fiber Fiber that, for the most part, does not dissolve in water. It includes cellulose, hemicelluloses, and lignin.

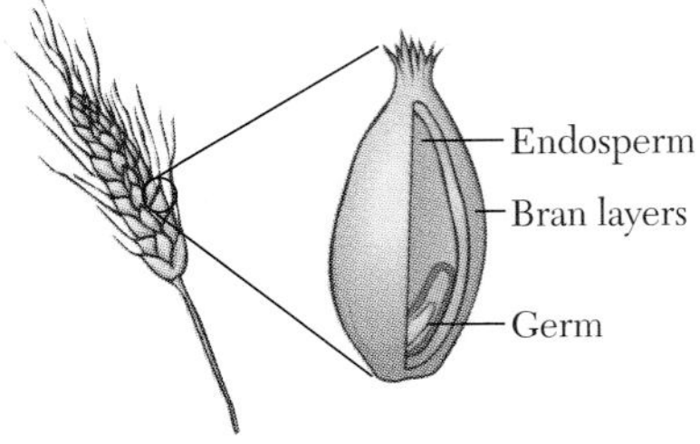

Figure 4.8
A grain of wheat contains outer layers of bran, the plant embryo or germ, and a carbohydrate-rich endosperm.

Starches **Starch** is the storage form of carbohydrate in plants. It is found in two forms: amylose, which consists of long straight chains of glucose molecules, and amylopectin, which consists of branched chains of glucose molecules. Starch accumulates in roots and tubers (the underground energy storage organ of some plants) where it provides energy for the growth and reproduction of the plant. It accumulates in seeds as an energy source for the developing plant embryo.

In our diet, we take advantage of these plant energy stores. When we eat potatoes or yams, we are eating tubers, and when we eat cassava, a food common in West Africa, a starchy root is being used as a food source. When we eat legumes such as lentils, soybeans, and kidney beans, we are eating a starchy seed from a plant that produces seeds in a pod (Figure 4.7). When we eat products made from corn, rice, wheat, or oats, we are also eating the starch from a seed.

If we eat the entire kernel or seed from a grain we are eating a whole grain product (Figure 4.8). The outermost part of a kernel of grain, the **bran,** contains most of the fiber and is a good source of B vitamins. The **germ,** which lies at the base of the kernel, is the plant embryo where sprouting occurs. It is the source of vegetable oils such as corn or safflower oil, and is rich in vitamin E. The remainder of the kernel is the **endosperm,** which is the starchy food supply for the sprouting embryo. The endosperm is primarily starch but also contains most of the protein and some vitamins and minerals. During the milling of grain into flour, the grinding detaches the germ and bran from the endosperm. Whole grain flours such as whole wheat flour include most of the bran, germ, and endosperm. When flours are refined, these components are separated; white flour is produced from just the endosperm. Fiber and some vitamins and minerals naturally found in the whole grain are lost. The process called **enrichment** adds back some, but not all, of the nutrients lost in processing. For example, vitamin E, magnesium, and vitamin B_6 are removed by milling and are not added back in the enrichment process (see Chapter 8).

Dietary Fiber **Dietary fiber** consists of substances that cannot be digested in the stomach and small intestine because humans lack the enzymes necessary to break the bonds that connect the monosaccharide units. Since fiber cannot be digested, it cannot be absorbed into the body and used for energy. Some fiber is digested by microflora in the large intestine, producing gas and short chain fatty acids, small quantities of which can be absorbed.

Fibers are categorized by their ability to dissolve in water. **Insoluble fibers** are primarily those that are derived from the structural parts of plants, such as the cell walls. These substances include cellulose and some hemicelluloses, which are carbohydrates, and lignins, which technically are not carbohydrates but are classified as insoluble fiber. Food sources of insoluble fiber include wheat bran and rye bran, which are mostly hemicellulose and cellulose, and vegetables such as broccoli, which contain woody fibers composed partly of

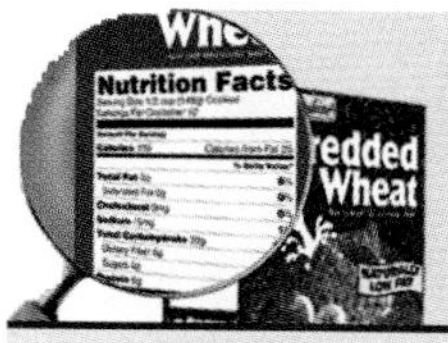

Off the Label

Finding Fiber

Consumers often choose brown breads and colored pasta in an effort to increase the fiber in their diet. The color of a product, however, often reveals little about the fiber content. Better places to look are the list of ingredients and the Nutrition Facts section of the food label.

On the ingredient list of breads, cereals, pastas, crackers, and other grain products, the term "whole" before the name of the grain indicates that the bran layer is still present in the food. Wheat flour, used to describe refined white flour made from wheat, is often confused with whole wheat flour. Only when whole wheat flour is the first ingredient, as it is in the label shown here from whole wheat bread, is the product made with mostly wheat flour containing the bran layer. The first ingredient on the "wheat bread" label shown in the figure is enriched wheat flour, rather than whole wheat flour. For products containing oats, the term "rolled" indicates that the whole oat grain has been used. Fiber added to processed foods can also be identified from the list of ingredients. Insoluble fibers, such as the wheat bran added to the wheat bread shown here, are usually added to decrease the energy content of a product or to meet consumer demands for a high-fiber product. The soluble fiber oat bran is also added for these reasons, but most added soluble fibers, such as pectins and gums, are used to thicken and stabilize foods and rarely contribute a significant amount of fiber.

The Nutrition Facts section of a food label provides information about how much dietary fiber is in a product and how it fits into the recommendations for an overall diet. It lists the total amount of dietary fiber contained in a serving of the product; the amounts of soluble and insoluble fiber are not mandatory, but some manufacturers choose to include them. The percent Daily Value, based on the Daily Value for fiber of 25 grams for a 2000-kcalorie diet, is also listed. For example, the whole wheat bread shown here contains 2 grams of fiber per serving, which is 8% of the recommended 25 grams. Foods that contain 20% or more of the Daily Value for fiber per serving can state on the label that they are "high in dietary fiber." Products containing 10 to 19% of the Daily Value can state that they are "a good source of dietary fiber."

Food labels may also carry health claims related to fiber and chronic disease risk. Fiber-containing grain products, fruits, and vegetables that contain at least 2.5 grams of fiber per serving and are low in fat may claim to reduce the risk of cancer. Fruits, vegetables, and grain products that are low in total fat, saturated fat, and cholesterol and that contain at least 0.6 gram of soluble fiber per serving, and foods that contain at least 0.75 gram of soluble fiber per serving from whole oats or psyllium husks, may claim to reduce the risk of heart disease.

Although whole grain breads are usually brown in color, the dark color may also be due to ingredients such as molasses that contribute no fiber. The green, orange, and red colors of some pasta products are due to the addition of such vegetable extracts as spinach, carrot, or tomato. These vegetables may add some micronutrients but the amounts are usually too small to make a significant contribution to fiber intake. So, when looking for fiber, look beyond the color of the products you choose, and read the label.

Whole Wheat Bread

Nutrition Facts
Serving Size 1 Slice (27g)
Servings Per Container 17
Calories 70
Calories from Fat 10

Amount/Serving	%DV*	Amount/Serving	%DV*
Total Fat 1g	2%	**Total Carb.** 12g	4%
Sat. Fat 0g	0%	Dietary Fiber 2g	8%
Cholesterol 0mg	0%	Sugars 2g	
Sodium 10mg	0%	**Protein** 2g	

Vitamin A 0% • Vitamin C 0% • Calcium 4% • Iron 4%
Thiamin 4% • Riboflavin 2% • Niacin 4%

*Percent Daily Values (DV) are based on a 2,000 calorie diet. Your daily values may be higher or lower depending on your calorie needs:

	Calories:	2,000	2,500
Total Fat	Less than	65g	80g
Sat Fat	Less than	20g	25g
Cholesterol	Less than	300mg	300mg
Sodium	Less than	2,400mg	2,400mg
Total Carbohydrate		300g	375g
Dietary Fiber		25g	30g

NOT A SODIUM FREE FOOD

INGREDIENTS: WHOLE WHEAT FLOUR, WATER, SWEETENERS (HIGH FRUCTOSE CORN SYRUP, MOLASSES), WHEAT GLUTEN, SOYBEAN OIL, CONTAINS 2% OR LESS OF THE FOLLOWING: YEAST, DOUGH CONDITIONERS (MONO & DIGLYCERIDES, ETHOXYLATED MONO & DI-GLYCERIDES, CALCIUM STEAROYL-2-LACTYLATE), YEAST NUTRIENTS (CALCIUM SULFATE, MONO- CALCIUM PHOSPHATE), CALCIUM PROPIONATE (A PRESERVATIVE).

Wheat Bread

Nutrition Facts
Serving Size 1 Slice (28g)
Servings Per Container 20
Calories 80
Calories from Fat 15

Amount/Serving	%DV*	Amount/Serving	%DV*
Total Fat 1g	2%	**Total Carb.** 13g	4%
Sat. Fat 0g	0%	Dietary Fiber 1g	4%
Cholesterol 0mg	0%	Sugars 2g	
Sodium 190mg	8%	**Protein** 2g	

Vitamin A 0% • Vitamin C 0% • Calcium 4% • Iron 4%
Thiamin 4% • Riboflavin 4% • Niacin 4%

*Percent Daily Values (DV) are based on a 2,000 calorie diet. Your daily values may be higher or lower depending on your calorie needs:

	Calories:	2,000	2,500
Total Fat	Less than	65g	80g
Sat Fat	Less than	20g	25g
Cholesterol	Less than	300mg	300mg
Sodium	Less than	2,400mg	2,400mg
Total Carbohydrate		300g	375g
Dietary Fiber		25g	30g

INGREDIENTS: ENRICHED WHEAT FLOUR, (WHEAT FLOUR, BARLEY MALT, NIACIN, IRON, THIAMIN MONONITRATE, RIBOFLAVIN), WATER, WHOLE WHEAT FLOUR, SWEETENERS, (HIGH FRUCTOSE CORN SYRUP, MOLASSES, HONEY), WHEAT BRAN, YEAST, SOYBEAN OIL, CONTAINS 2% OR LESS OF THE FOLLOWING: SALT, DOUGH CONDITIONERS (MONOGLYCERIDES, SODIUM STEAROYL LACTYLATE), YEAST NUTRIENTS (AMMONIUM SULFATE, CALCIUM SULFATE), CALCIUM PROPIONATE (A PRESERVATIVE).

Figure 4.9
These foods are good sources of dietary fiber. (Charles D. Winters)

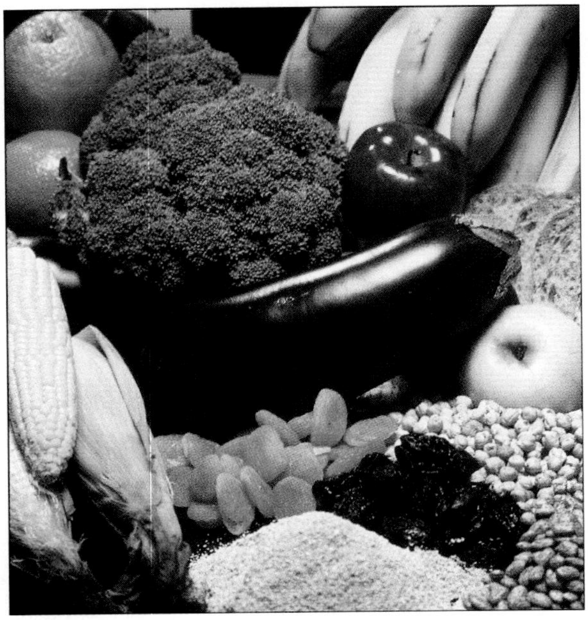

Soluble fiber Fiber that either dissolves when placed in water or absorbs water. It includes pectins, gums, and some hemicelluloses.

lignins. **Soluble fibers** are found around and inside plant cells. These carbohydrates either absorb water or dissolve in water. They include pectins, gums, and some hemicelluloses. Food sources of soluble fibers include oats, apples, beans, and seaweed. Pectins from fruit are used to gel jams and jellies. Gums found in seaweed are often added to processed foods as thickeners; for example, gums are used to thicken reduced-fat salad dressings and frozen desserts. Most foods of plant origin contain mixtures of soluble and insoluble fibers (Figure 4.9; see also *Off the Label: Finding Fiber*, p. 99).

CARBOHYDRATES IN THE DIGESTIVE TRACT

The majority of disaccharide and starch digestion occurs in the small intestine. Substances that are not completely digested in the small intestine pass into the large intestine. Here the enzymes of the intestinal microflora further break down these substances. When the sugar lactose is not digested, as is the case in many people, this bacterial degradation can cause abdominal discomfort. On the other hand, when fiber passes undigested into the large intestine, as occurs in everyone, the effects are beneficial to the health of the gastrointestinal tract.

Sugars and Starches

The digestion of starch begins in the mouth, where the enzyme salivary amylase starts breaking it into shorter polysaccharides (see Figure 4.10). In the small intestine, pancreatic amylases complete the job of breaking starch into maltose. The digestion of disaccharides is completed by enzymes attached to the brush border of the villi in the small intestine. Here maltose is broken down into two glucose molecules by maltase, sucrose is broken down by the enzyme sucrase to glucose and fructose, and lactose is broken down by lactase to form glucose and galactose. The resulting monosaccharides—glucose, galactose, and fructose—are then absorbed and transported to the liver via the hepatic portal circulation.

Lactose Intolerance

Lactase, needed for lactose digestion, is normally produced by all humans at birth. Lactase levels decrease with age and in many individuals decline so much

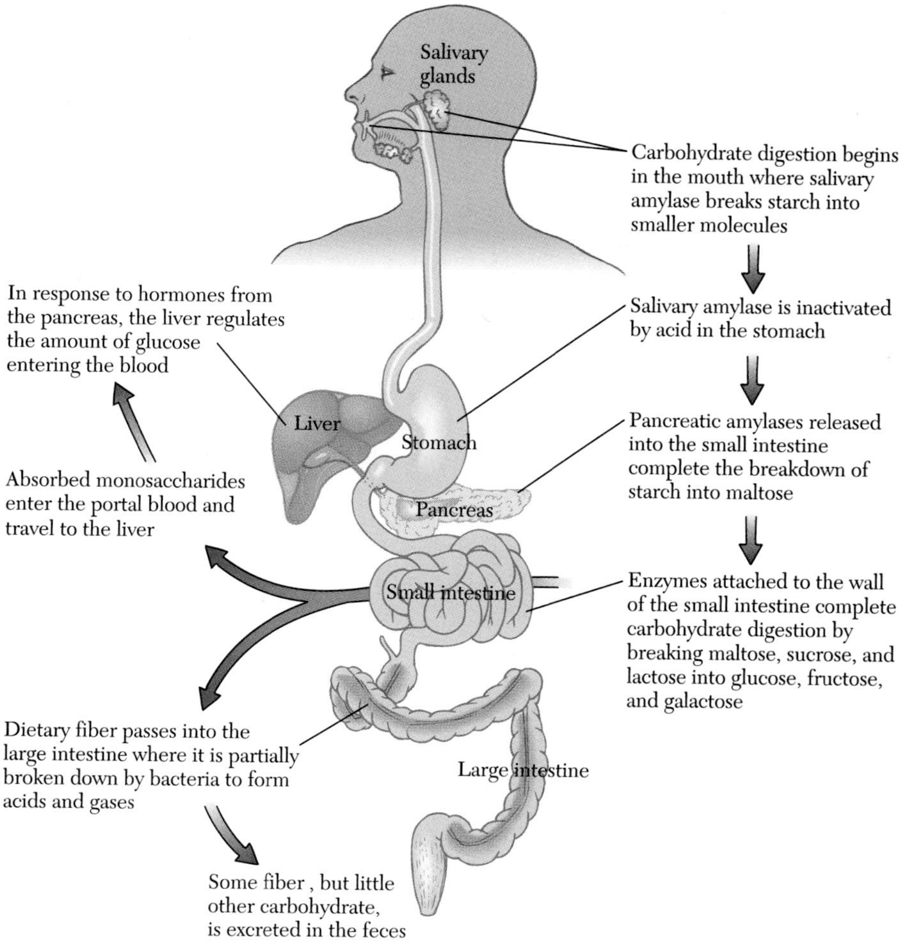
Salivary glands
Carbohydrate digestion begins in the mouth where salivary amylase breaks starch into smaller molecules
Salivary amylase is inactivated by acid in the stomach
Pancreatic amylases released into the small intestine complete the breakdown of starch into maltose
Enzymes attached to the wall of the small intestine complete carbohydrate digestion by breaking maltose, sucrose, and lactose into glucose, fructose, and galactose
In response to hormones from the pancreas, the liver regulates the amount of glucose entering the blood
Liver
Stomach
Pancreas
Absorbed monosaccharides enter the portal blood and travel to the liver
Small intestine
Dietary fiber passes into the large intestine where it is partially broken down by bacteria to form acids and gases
Large intestine
Some fiber , but little other carbohydrate, is excreted in the feces

Figure 4.10
An overview of carbohydrate digestion and absorption.

that lactose cannot be completely digested. In these individuals, lactose consumed in dairy products passes into the large intestine, where it is metabolized by bacteria. The undigested lactose and the acids and gas produced by the bacteria can draw water into the intestine and cause abdominal distension, flatulence, cramping, and diarrhea. This condition is called **lactose intolerance.**

Lactose intolerance The inability to digest lactose because of a deficiency of the enzyme lactase. It causes symptoms including intestinal gas and bloating after dairy products are consumed.

The percentage of adults with lactose intolerance ranges from a low of 5% or less in northwestern European populations to nearly 100% in Asian populations and parts of Africa.[3] In the United States, it is estimated that about 25% of the total adult population is lactose intolerant, but the incidence varies enormously depending on ethnic background. For instance, 80% of African Americans and 90% of Asian Americans experience symptoms after consuming lactose.[4] Lactose intolerance may also occur as a result of an intestinal infection or other disease. It is then referred to as secondary lactose intolerance and may disappear when the other condition is resolved.

The severity of lactose intolerance also varies. Some individuals cannot tolerate any lactose, whereas others can consume small amounts without symptoms. Because some of the lactose in yogurt and cheese is digested or lost in processing, many individuals with lactose intolerance can tolerate these products. Although individuals with lactose intolerance must determine their own threshold for consuming dairy products without experiencing symptoms, research has shown that most individuals can consume 1 to 2 servings of dairy products daily if they are spread out over the course of the day.[4]

Because dairy products are an important source of dietary calcium, individuals with lactose intolerance must consume other sources of calcium to meet their needs. In cultures where lactose intolerance is common, traditional diets provide sources of calcium other than milk. For example, in Asia, tofu and fish consumed with bones

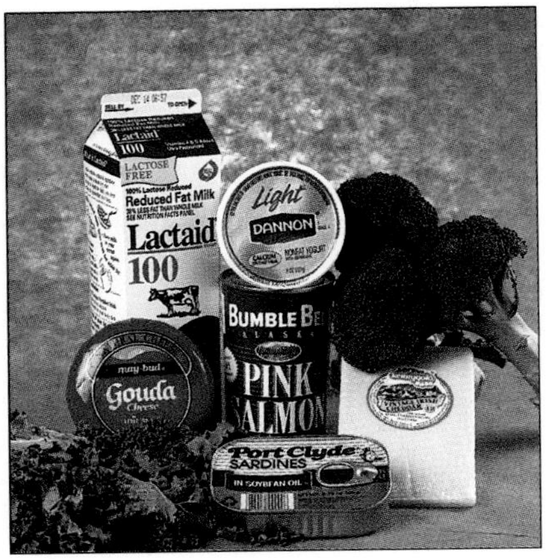

Figure 4.11
These foods are good sources of calcium and are also low in lactose. (George Semple)

supply calcium, and in the Near East, fermented cheese and yogurt provide much of the calcium. In the United States, milk is the most important source of calcium. The Food Guide Pyramid recommends 2 to 3 servings from the Milk, Yogurt, & Cheese Group each day. Those who can tolerate lactose in small doses can divide the 2 to 3 servings into many smaller portions. Those who cannot tolerate any lactose can meet their calcium needs with tofu, fish, calcium-rich vegetables, milk treated with the enzyme lactase, or calcium-fortified foods or supplements (Figure 4.11). Lactase tablets, which can be consumed with or before milk products, are also available. The enzymes in these tablets digest the lactose before it passes into the large intestine.

Fiber

Fiber cannot be digested by human digestive enzymes; however, fiber does have important properties that affect the digestive tract and maintain healthy bowel function. Soluble fibers, such as pectins and gums, absorb water. For example, the soluble fiber in a carrot can hold 20 to 30 times its weight in water. In the gastrointestinal tract, soluble fibers absorb water, forming viscous solutions that slow the rate at which nutrients are absorbed. Insoluble fibers, such as wheat bran, increase the amount of material in the intestine. Together, the increased bulk of insoluble fibers and the fluid drawn in by soluble fibers result in an increased volume of material in the intestine. This allows for easier evacuation of the stool. It also promotes healthy bowel function because it stimulates peristalsis, causing the muscles of the colon to work more, become stronger, and function better. The increase in peristalsis also reduces transit time—the time it takes food and fecal matter to move through the intestine. In African countries, where the diet contains 40 to 150 grams of fiber per day, the transit time is 36 hours or less. In the United States, where the usual fiber intake is 14 to 15 grams per day,[5] it is not uncommon for transit time to be as long as 96 hours.

CARBOHYDRATES IN THE BODY

The major function of carbohydrate in the body is to provide energy. The main source of this energy is glucose. In addition, carbohydrate has several other functions. The monosaccharide galactose is an important molecule in nervous tissue. It also combines with glucose to make lactose in women who are producing breast milk. Two other monosaccharides that are of great importance to the body are deoxyribose and ribose. These sugars are components of DNA and RNA (ribonucleic acid) respectively, which contain the genetic information for the synthesis of proteins. Deoxyribose and ribose can be synthesized by the body and are not found in significant amounts in the diet. Ribose is also a component of the vitamin riboflavin. Oligosaccharides are also important in our bodies. They are found attached to proteins or lipids on the surface of cells where they help to signal information about cells.

Carbohydrate Metabolism

Body cells receive a constant supply of glucose via the bloodstream. This supply is regulated by the liver and by hormones secreted from the pancreas. Once glucose reaches the cells, it is metabolized to produce energy.

Delivery of Glucose to Cells After a meal, monosaccharides are absorbed and travel via the hepatic portal vein to the liver where much of the fructose and galactose is converted into glucose. Glucose is then transported in the blood, reaching cells throughout the body. The amount of glucose in the blood is regulated at about 60 to 100 mg per 100 ml of blood (70 to 120 mg/100 ml serum). This ensures adequate glucose delivery to body cells, which is particularly important for brain and red blood cells, which rely almost exclusively on glucose as an energy source. If blood glucose levels rise too high or drop too low, hormones from the pancreas act to decrease or increase levels.

How quickly blood glucose levels rise after a meal, referred to as the **glycemic index,** or **glycemic response,** is affected by the composition of the food or meal. Fat and protein consumed with high-carbohydrate foods cause the stomach to empty more slowly and therefore delay the rate at which glucose enters the small intestine, where it is absorbed. This causes a slower rise in blood glucose. Fiber also slows the rise in blood glucose both because foods high in fiber take longer to leave the stomach and because fiber in the small intestine slows absorption. Consuming sugar alone—for example, drinking a sugar-sweetened soft drink on an empty stomach—will cause blood glucose to increase rapidly. After a mixed meal, such as chicken, rice, and green beans, which contains starch, fat, protein, and fiber, it will take 30 to 60 minutes before blood glucose begins to rise.

Glycemic index or **glycemic response** A measure of how quickly blood glucose levels increase after a food or a meal is consumed.

A rise in blood glucose triggers the pancreas to secrete the hormone **insulin,** which allows glucose to be taken into the cells of the body. In the liver, insulin promotes the storage of glucose as glycogen and, to a lesser extent, fat. In muscle, insulin stimulates the uptake of glucose for energy production and the synthesis of muscle glycogen for energy storage. In fat-storing cells, insulin increases glucose uptake from the blood and stimulates lipid synthesis. All of these actions remove glucose from the blood, decreasing levels to the normal range (Figure 4.12).

Insulin A hormone made in the pancreas that allows the uptake of glucose by body cells and has other metabolic effects such as stimulating the synthesis of glycogen in liver and muscle.

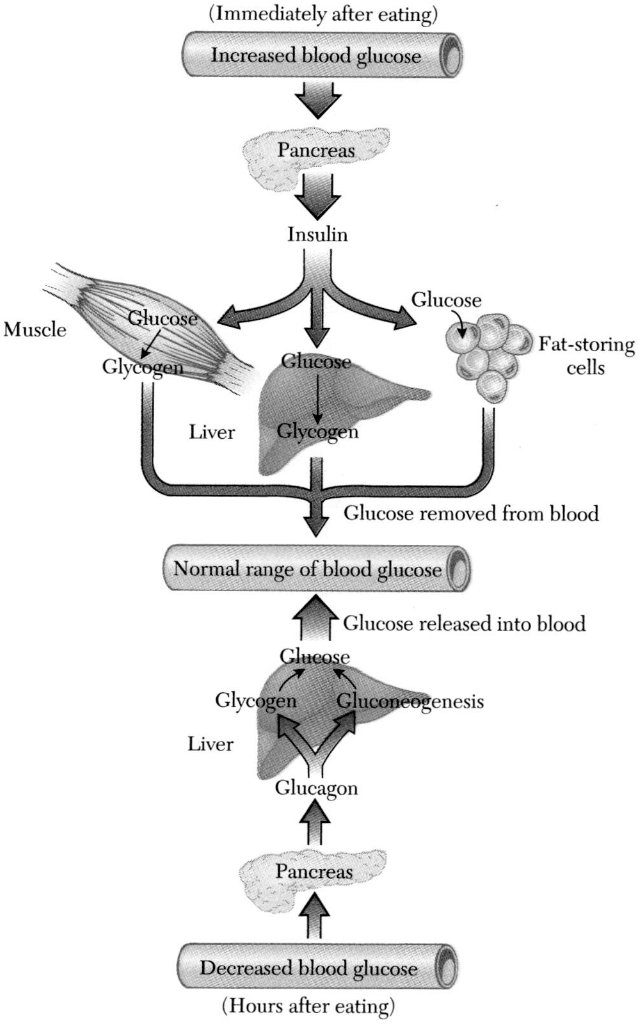

Figure 4.12

Blood glucose is regulated by hormones secreted by the pancreas. Immediately after a meal, when blood glucose increases, insulin is released and stimulates the uptake and storage of glucose. Several hours after a meal, when blood glucose levels begin to decrease, glucagon is released and stimulates the breakdown of glycogen into glucose and glucose production via gluconeogenesis.

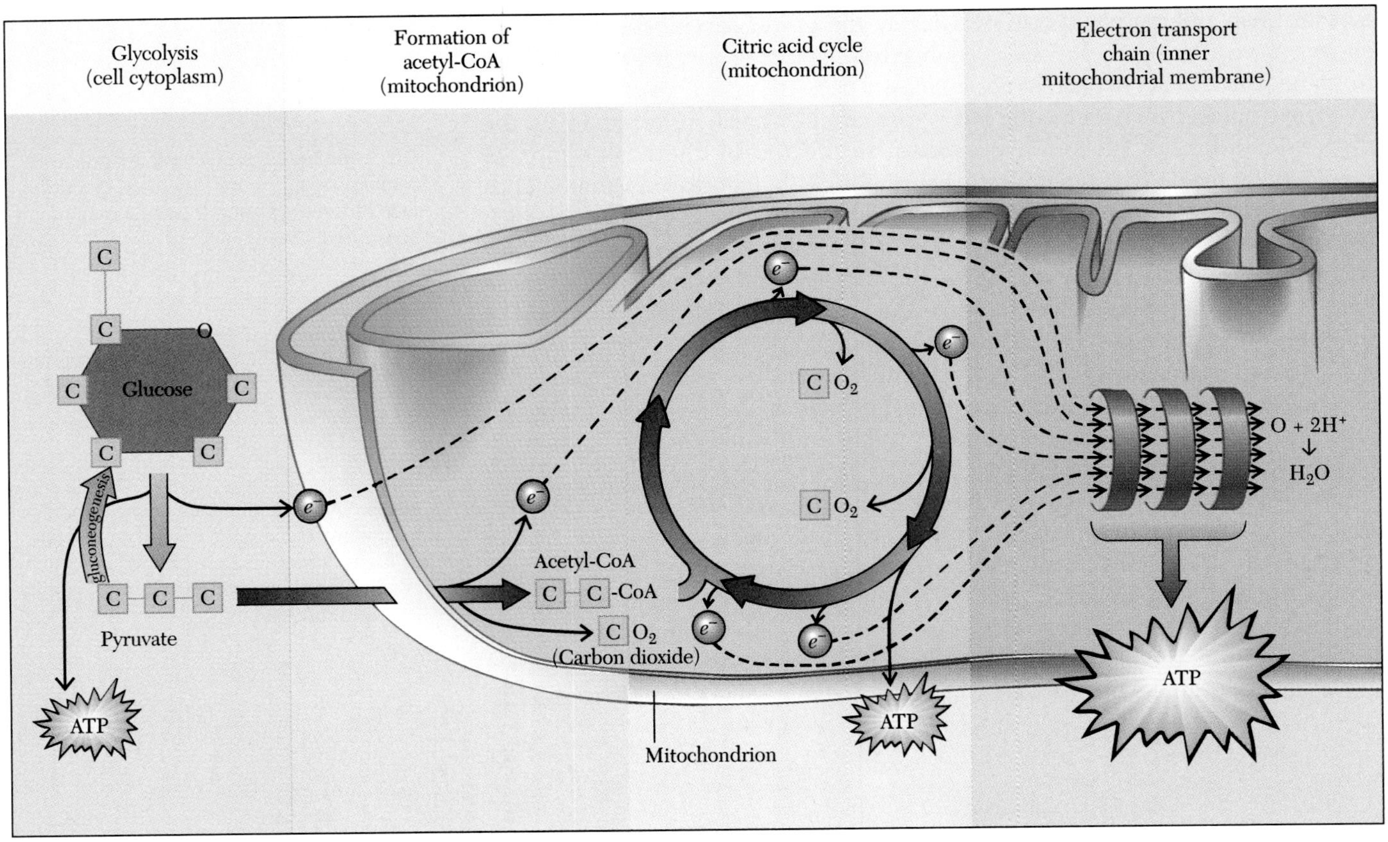

Figure 4.13
An overview of glucose metabolism. In the cytoplasm, glycolysis breaks glucose into two 3-carbon pyruvate molecules that enter the mitochondria, where they are converted into acetyl-CoA, which enters the citric acid cycle. High-energy electrons are released and transferred to the electron transport chain, where their energy is trapped to produce ATP.

Glucose Metabolism Once glucose has left the bloodstream and been taken up by a cell, it can be metabolized through cellular respiration to produce carbon dioxide, water, and energy in the form of ATP. Providing energy through cellular respiration involves four interconnected stages. The first takes place in the cytoplasm of the cell and is called **glycolysis** (meaning glucose breakdown). In glycolysis, the 6-carbon sugar glucose is broken into two 3-carbon pyruvate molecules and produces 2 molecules of ATP (Figure 4.13).

In the next stage, which occurs in the mitochondria, 1 carbon is removed from pyruvate, leaving 2 carbons that form acetyl-CoA. Acetyl-CoA then enters the third stage of breakdown, the **citric acid cycle.** To begin the cycle, acetyl-CoA combines with a 4-carbon molecule, oxaloacetate, derived from carbohydrate to form a 6-carbon molecule. The citric acid cycle then removes 1 carbon at a time, as carbon dioxide, from this molecule until the 4-carbon oxaloacetate is reformed. These chemical reactions produce 2 ATP molecules per glucose molecule but also remove **electrons,** which are passed to shuttling molecules for transport to the last stage of cellular respiration, the **electron transport chain.** The electron transport chain involves a series of molecules, most of which are proteins, associated with the inner membrane of the mitochondria. These molecules accept the electrons from the shuttling molecules and pass them from one to another down the chain until they are finally combined with oxygen to form water. As the electrons are passed along, their energy is trapped and used to make ATP. The reactions of cellular respiration are central to all energy-producing processes in the body.

Glycolysis A metabolic pathway in the cytoplasm of the cell that splits glucose into two 3-carbon pyruvate molecules. The energy released from 1 molecule of glucose is used to make 2 ATP molecules.

Citric acid cycle Also known as the Krebs cycle or the tricarboxylic acid cycle, this is the stage of respiration in which acetyl-CoA is broken down into 2 molecules of carbon dioxide.

Electrons Negatively charged high-energy particles that orbit the nucleus of an atom.

Electron transport chain The final stage of cellular respiration in which electrons are passed down a chain of molecules to oxygen to form water and produce ATP.

Using Protein to Make Glucose If no carbohydrate has been eaten for a few hours, the glucose level in the blood—and consequently glucose available to the cells—begins to decrease. This triggers the pancreas to secrete the hormone **glucagon** (see Figure 4.12). Glucagon signals liver cells to break down glycogen into glucose, which is released into the bloodstream. Glucagon also stimulates the synthesis of new glucose molecules, using a pathway called **gluconeogenesis** (meaning production of new glucose). Gluconeogenesis occurs in liver and kidney cells and requires energy in the form of ATP. This pathway makes glucose from 3-carbon molecules. Three-carbon molecules come primarily from amino acids because the reactions that break down fatty acids produce 2-carbon molecules (acetyl-CoA). Newly synthesized glucose is released into the blood to prevent blood glucose from dropping below the normal range. Gluconeogenesis can also be stimulated by the hormone epinephrine, also known as adrenaline. This hormone enables the body to respond to emergencies. For example, epinephrine is released in response to dangerous or stressful situations. It causes a rapid release of glucose into the blood to supply the energy needed for action.

Gluconeogenesis is essential for meeting the body's immediate need for glucose, particularly when carbohydrate intake is very low, but it uses protein that could be used for other essential functions such as growth and maintenance of muscle tissue. When carbohydrate is adequate in the diet, protein is not needed to synthesize glucose. Therefore, carbohydrate is said to spare protein.

Glucagon A hormone made in the pancreas that stimulates the breakdown of liver glycogen and the synthesis of glucose to increase blood sugar.

Gluconeogenesis The synthesis of glucose from simple noncarbohydrate molecules. Amino acids from protein are the primary source of carbons for glucose synthesis.

Carbohydrate Is Needed to Produce Energy From Fat To completely metabolize fat, a small amount of carbohydrate must be available. This is because fatty acids are broken into molecules of acetyl-CoA. Acetyl-CoA can be used to produce energy via the citric acid cycle only if it can combine with a 4-carbon oxaloacetate molecule derived from carbohydrate metabolism. When carbohydrate is in short supply, oxaloacetate is limited and acetyl-CoA cannot be metabolized to carbon dioxide and water. Instead, the liver converts it into compounds known as **ketones** or **ketone bodies** (Figure 4.14). The liver releases ketones into the blood that can be used for energy by tissues, such as those in the heart, muscle, and kidney. Ketone production is a normal response to starvation or a very low carbohydrate diet. Even the brain, which requires glucose, can adapt to obtain a portion of its energy from ketones. Excess ketones are excreted by the kidney in

Ketones or **ketone bodies** Molecules formed when there is not sufficient carbohydrate to completely metabolize the acetyl-CoA produced from fat breakdown.

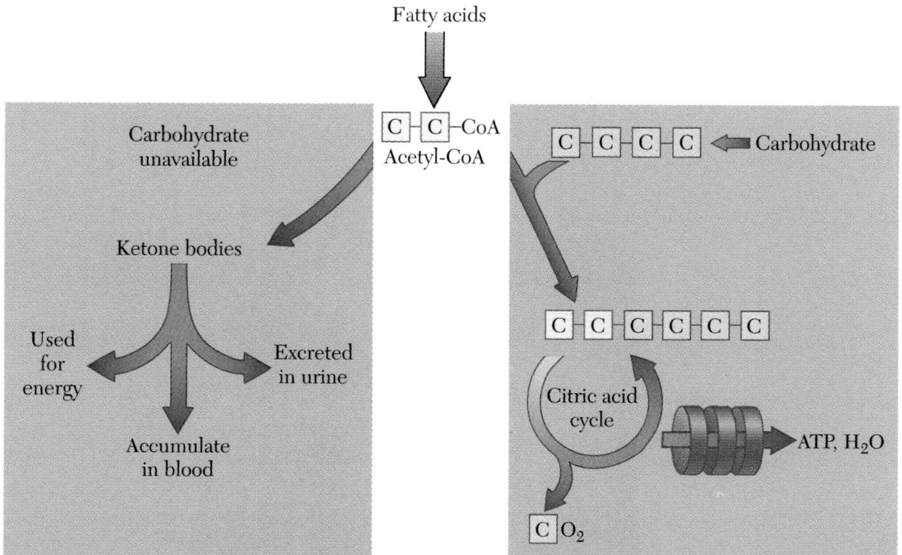

Occurs when carbohydrate is in short supply as in starvation, a low-carbohydrate diet, or diabetes

Occurs when cells have a plentiful supply of carbohydrate

Figure 4.14
If carbohydrate is in short supply, the acetyl-CoA from fatty acid breakdown is unable to enter the citric acid cycle and instead is used to make ketone bodies.

urine. However, if fluid intake is too low to produce enough urine to excrete ketones or if ketone production is high, ketones can build up in the blood, causing **ketosis.** Mild ketosis, which occurs with moderate kcalorie restriction such as that during a weight-loss diet, produces symptoms including headache, dry mouth, foul-smelling breath, and, in some cases, a reduction in appetite (see *Critical Thinking: What Happens If You Consume Too Little Carbohydrate?*). High ketone levels, such as those produced by starvation or untreated diabetes (discussion follows), increase the acidity of the blood and can result in coma and death.

Ketosis High levels of ketones in the blood.

Abnormal Glucose Regulation

Blood glucose levels are normally tightly controlled by insulin, glucagon, and other hormones. Abnormal blood glucose levels can result from either abnormal levels of the hormones that regulate blood glucose levels or abnormal responses to these hormones. When glucose homeostasis is not maintained and levels rise above the normal range, as occurs in diabetes, or drop below the normal range, as occurs in hypoglycemia, overall health can be affected.

Diabetes **Diabetes mellitus** is a major public health problem in the United States today, accounting for about $98 billion in direct medical costs and indirect costs due to disability, lost work, and premature death.[6] This disease is characterized by high blood glucose levels. The elevated glucose is believed to bind proteins, alter their functions, and damage body tissues (Figure 4.15). Diabetes is the leading cause of blindness in adults, and accounts for 40% of all new cases of kidney failure and over half of all lower-limb amputations.[7] Diabetes increases the risk of heart disease and stroke.[8]

Diabetes mellitus A disease caused by either insufficient insulin production or decreased sensitivity of cells to insulin. It results in elevated blood glucose levels.

To reduce disability and death associated with diabetes and its complications, the National Institutes of Health and the Centers for Disease Control and Prevention have established the National Diabetes Education Program. This program is designed to increase public awareness of the seriousness of diabetes, promote better management among individuals with diabetes, and improve the quality of and access to health care. There are three types of diabetes: type 1, type 2, and gestational diabetes, which occurs during pregnancy.

Type 1 Diabetes Type 1 diabetes is usually diagnosed before the age of 30. It occurs in only 5 to 10% of diagnosed cases.[10] What triggers the disease is unknown, but it is believed to be an **autoimmune disease** in which the immune system destroys the insulin-secreting cells of the pancreas. Because these cells have been damaged or destroyed, insulin production is reduced or absent. Blood levels of glucose rise, but since insulin is unavailable, the glucose cannot enter cells to be

Autoimmune disease A disease that results from immune reactions that destroy normal body cells.

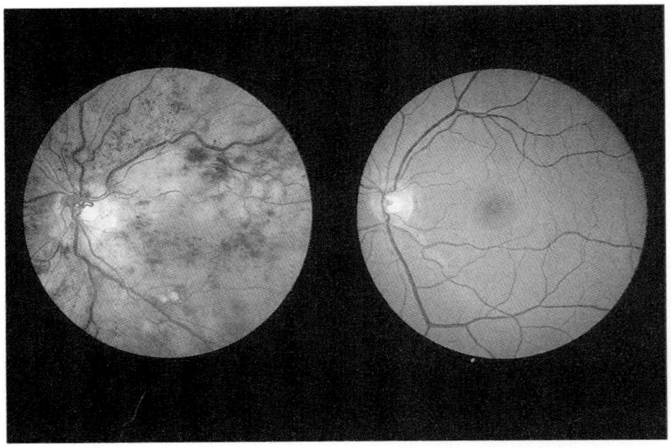

Figure 4.15
(*left*) Damaged blood vessels in the retina caused by diabetes. (*right*) Normal blood vessels in the retina of the eye. (© SBHA/Tony Stone Images, Inc.)

used or stored as an energy source. The body responds as it does in starvation, and fat is used for energy. Since glucose cannot enter cells, fat cannot be completely broken down and large quantities of ketones are produced, causing ketosis.

The goal in treating type 1 diabetes is to maintain blood glucose within the normal range to prevent tissue damage. This requires insulin injections, a modified diet, and adequate exercise. Insulin must be injected because it is a protein that would be broken down in the gastrointestinal tract if taken orally. Dietary intake should be modified, based on either the Exchange Lists or on a system of carbohydrate counting, to limit the amount of carbohydrate consumed at any given time.[11] Recommendations no longer restrict sugar intake but rather suggest that total carbohydrate consumption—whether sucrose, fructose (which causes a smaller rise in blood glucose than sucrose), or starch—be limited. Insulin injections and carbohydrate consumption must be coordinated so that glucose and insulin are available in the proper proportions at the same time to maintain normal blood glucose levels. The diet must be adequate in energy and micronutrients, and protein should provide 10 to 20% of energy. It should meet the Dietary Guidelines recommendation of no more than 30% of energy from fat, with 10% from saturated fat. Adherence to this type of treatment regimen along with monitoring of blood glucose levels throughout the day can reduce the incidence of elevated blood glucose levels and the complications it causes.

Exercise is also an important component of diabetes management. Exercise can reduce blood glucose levels, so individuals with diabetes are encouraged to maintain regular exercise patterns. Because exercise increases the sensitivity of body cells to insulin, an increase in the amount of exercise an individual gets may reduce the amount of insulin required.

Type 2 Diabetes Type 2 diabetes is the more common form.[10] It affects almost 16 million adults in the United States.[7] The incidence is higher among minority groups, particularly African Americans, Hispanic Americans, and Native Americans.[7] This form of diabetes usually appears in persons over the age of 40. Risk is increased in individuals who are overweight, in those who have a body type with more fat in the abdominal region, and in those with a family history of diabetes. In type 2 diabetes, insulin secretion may be normal but blood glucose rises because body cells are resistant to the effects of insulin (Figure 4.16).[10] Large amounts of insulin are therefore required for cells to take up enough glucose to meet their energy needs. Since some glucose does enter the cells, ketosis rarely occurs in this form of diabetes. Type 2 diabetes is believed to be due to a combination of genetic, dietary, and lifestyle factors. There is now evidence that diets

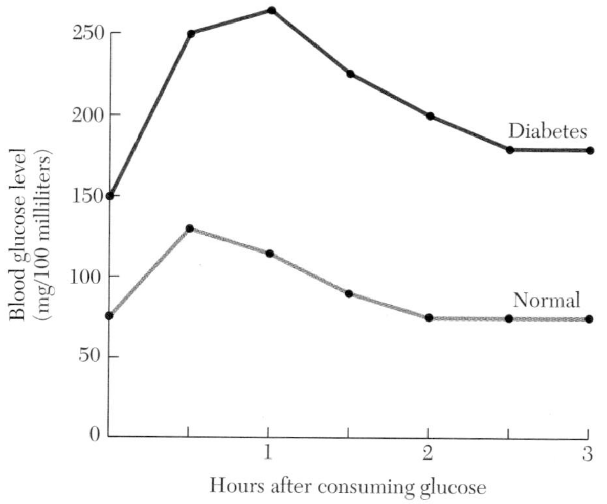

Figure 4.16

These glucose tolerance curves compare normal blood sugar patterns with those commonly seen in individuals with type 2 diabetes. The values are measured from blood drawn every 30 minutes for 3 hours after an individual consumes 75 grams of glucose.

high in refined carbohydrates and low in fiber may increase the risk of developing type 2 diabetes.[12,13]

Treatment for type 2 diabetes includes diet, exercise, and, in many cases, drug therapy. The primary goal of diet modification in type 2 diabetes is to normalize blood glucose as well as blood cholesterol and triglyceride levels (see Chapter 5). A diet and exercise program that limits the amount of carbohydrate consumed at each meal or snack, increases exercise, and, for overweight individuals, restricts energy, can be beneficial for maintaining blood glucose levels in the normal range.[11] When these treatments fail to normalize blood sugar, medications that increase pancreatic insulin production and, in about 40% of type 2 diabetes cases, insulin itself, are prescribed. As with type 1 diabetes, blood glucose should be monitored frequently to assure that treatment is keeping glucose levels within the normal range.

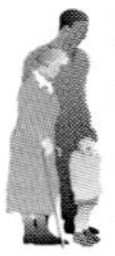

Gestational Diabetes A third form of diabetes, called gestational diabetes, sometimes occurs in women during pregnancy. This form of diabetes may be caused by the hormonal changes that occur during pregnancy. The high levels of glucose in the mother's blood increase the risk of complications for the unborn child (see Chapter 13). Gestational diabetes usually disappears once the pregnancy is complete and hormones return to nonpregnant levels. However, individuals who have had gestational diabetes have an increased risk for developing type 2 diabetes in the future.[14]

Hypoglycemia A low blood glucose level, usually below 40 to 50 mg of glucose per 100 ml of blood.

Hypoglycemia **Hypoglycemia,** or low blood glucose, results from an overproduction of insulin or other hormones involved in blood sugar regulation. The symptoms of hypoglycemia include irritability, nervousness, sweating, shakiness, anxiety, rapid heartbeat, headache, hunger, weakness, and sometimes seizure and coma. There are two forms of hypoglycemia. Reactive hypoglycemia occurs in response to the consumption of high-carbohydrate foods. The rise in blood glucose from the carbohydrate stimulates insulin release. However, too much insulin is secreted, resulting in a rapid fall in blood glucose to an abnormally low level. The treatment for reactive hypoglycemia is a diet that prevents rapid changes in blood glucose. Small, frequent meals low in simple carbohydrates and high in protein and fiber are recommended. The second form of hypoglycemia, fasting hypoglycemia, is not related to food intake. In this disorder, abnormal insulin secretion results in episodes of low blood glucose levels. This condition is often caused by pancreatic tumors.

CRITICAL THINKING

What Happens If You Consume Too Little Carbohydrate?

Bob weighs about 30 pounds more than he wants to weigh, so he decides to try to shed pounds quickly with a low-carbohydrate weight-loss diet. The diet allows an unlimited amount of beef, chicken, and fish as well as limited fruits and vegetables; breads, grains, and cereals are not allowed. Bob is overjoyed with his initial rapid weight loss, but after about a week his weight loss slows down and he begins to feel tired and light-headed. He is having headaches and notices a funny smell on his breath.

Nutritional assessment

A nutritional assessment suggests that Bob needs about 2500 kcalories a day to maintain his weight. His weight-loss diet provides about 1000 kcalories, 25 grams of carbohydrate, 125 grams of protein, and 44 grams of fat per day. He consumes only about 3 cups of fluid daily.

What's wrong with Bob's diet plan?

Bob's diet is very low in energy and carbohydrate. This low energy intake causes Bob to use stored fat to meet his energy needs. Because his diet does not contain enough carbohydrate to allow fat to be metabolized completely, ketones are produced and begin to accumulate in his blood. Some of the ketones are used by cells for energy; some are excreted in the urine. However, since Bob is not consuming much fluid, the rate of ketone production exceeds the ability of his kidneys to excrete them, and ketone levels in his blood increase. Also, it is unlikely that he will be able to meet his micronutrient needs on a 1000-kcalorie diet without taking a vitamin and mineral supplement.

Ketone accumulation causes Bob's symptoms

High blood ketone levels probably are causing the headaches and light-headedness Bob is experiencing. Some blood ketones are lost through the lungs, giving him funny-smelling breath.

What will happen if Bob increases the carbohydrate and fluid content of his diet but keeps the energy level the same?

A diet this low in energy will still result in some ketone production, but including at least 50 grams of carbohydrate will allow Bob's body to burn fat more completely so fewer ketones will be produced. Also, a high fluid intake will increase his urine production, allowing more ketone excretion and lowering his blood ketone level.

Why can type 1 diabetics develop ketosis even when consuming plenty of carbohydrate?

Answer:

Carbohydrates and Health

The consumption of carbohydrates has been blamed for a host of chronic health problems, from hyperactivity to obesity, and from diabetes to heart disease.[12,15,16] Meanwhile, guidelines for a healthy diet are recommending that Americans increase their carbohydrate intake. This dichotomy relates to the type of carbohydrates: Foods high in complex carbohydrates, particularly whole grains, are good

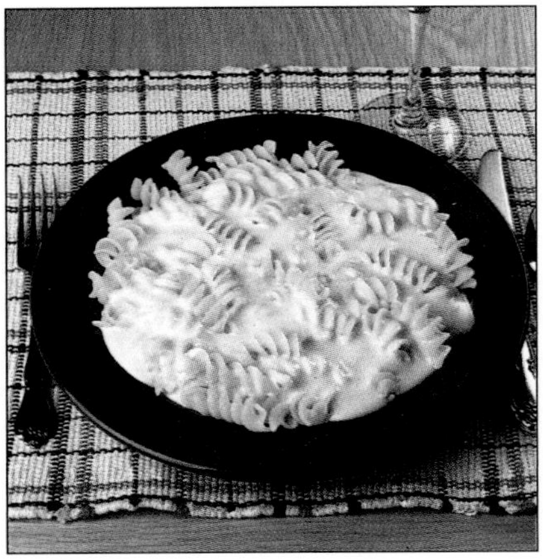

Figure 4.17
High-carbohydrate foods are not high in kcalories, but the toppings used on them often are. (George Semple)

sources of micronutrients, phytochemicals, and fiber, while foods high in sugar generally contribute little more than energy. This is reflected in nutrition messages from the Dietary Guidelines, food labels, and the Food Guide Pyramid, all of which recommend that we increase our intake of complex carbohydrates but limit our refined sugar intake.

What's So Good About Complex Carbohydrates?

Diets high in plant foods have been the staple of the world's diet for centuries. A diet based on whole grains, fruits, and vegetables is high in complex carbohydrates, including fiber, generally moderate in energy, low in fat, and a good source of other nutrients and phytochemicals. This dietary pattern has been associated with reduced risk of a variety of chronic diseases. Whole grain consumption has been found to reduce the risk of heart disease.[17] Diets high in cereal fiber and low in refined carbohydrates are also associated with a lower risk of developing diabetes.[12,13] Evidence is accumulating that perhaps greater emphasis should be placed on using whole grains as a source of complex carbohydrates.[18]

Carbohydrates are not "fattening." They provide 4 kcalories per gram compared with 9 kcalories per gram provided by fat. This is not to say that starch consumed in excess of energy needs will not add pounds. Any energy source consumed in excess of requirements can cause weight gain. But carbohydrate is no more fattening than any other energy source. In fact, excess carbohydrate in the diet is less efficient at producing body fat than excess fat in the diet (see Chapter 7). It is the fat that we add to our starches that increases the kcalorie tally. A medium baked potato provides about 110 kcalories, but the 2 tablespoons of sour cream you add brings the total to 175 kcalories. A plate of plain pasta has about 200 kcalories, but with a high-fat sauce, the kcalories rise to 300; add sausage and the meal is now 450 kcalories (Figure 4.17).

Dietary fiber is plentiful in plant foods that are low in fat and rich in nutrients and phytochemicals. Fiber itself also provides other health benefits. Epidemiological research comparing the incidence of certain chronic diseases in populations with different fiber intakes found high-fiber diets to be associated with a lower incidence of certain bowel disorders, heart disease, and colon cancer.[5]

Hemorrhoids Swollen veins in the anal or rectal area.

Diverticula Sacs or pouches that protrude from the wall of the large intestine in the disease diverticulosis. When these become inflamed, the condition is called diverticulitis.

Dietary Fiber and Chronic Bowel Disorders A diet high in fiber can relieve or prevent some chronic bowel disorders. Fiber adds bulk and absorbs water, making the feces larger and softer and reducing the amount of pressure needed for defecation. This helps to reduce the incidence of constipation and **hemorrhoids,** the swelling of veins in the rectal or anal area. Reducing the pressure in the lumen of the colon can also reduce the possibility of developing diverticulosis, a condition in which the intestinal wall forms outpouches called **diverticula** (Figure 4.18). In the United States, about 50% of elderly people have diverticulosis. Fecal matter may occasionally accumulate in these outpouchings, causing irritation, pain, inflammation, and infection. This condition is known as diverticulitis. Treatment of diverticulitis usually includes antibiotics to reduce bacterial growth and a temporary decrease in fiber intake to prevent irritation of the inflamed tissues. Once the inflammation is resolved, however, a high-fiber intake is recommended to increase fecal bulk, decrease transit time, ease stool elimination, and reduce future attacks.[5]

Dietary Fiber and the Risk of Heart Disease Blood cholesterol levels can be reduced by increasing the consumption of fiber-rich foods.[5] High blood cholesterol levels are a risk factor for the development of heart disease (see Chapter 5). By reducing blood cholesterol levels, the risk of heart disease is reduced. Not all dietary fiber, however, has a cholesterol-lowering effect. Studies in humans indicate that soluble fiber such as that in legumes, rice and oat bran, guar gum, pectin, and psyllium (a grain used in over-the-counter bulk-forming laxatives such as

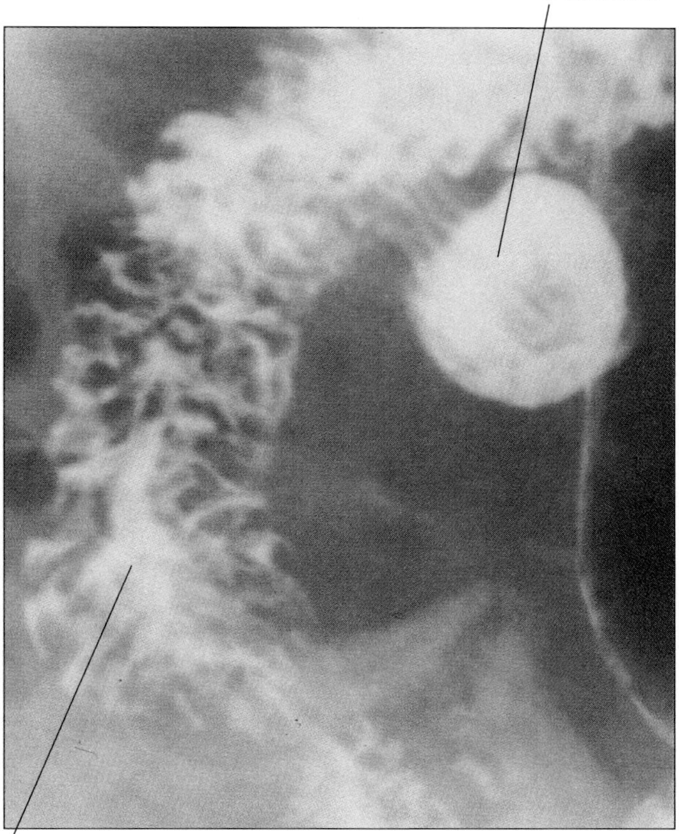

Figure 4.18
Diverticulum in the colon. (L. V. Bergman/The Bergman Collection)

Metamucil) are more effective at lowering blood cholesterol levels than insoluble fibers such as wheat bran or cellulose.[5] This may be due to the ability of soluble fibers to bind cholesterol and **bile acids,** which are made from cholesterol, in the digestive tract. Normally, bile acids secreted into the GI tract are absorbed and reused. When bound to fiber, cholesterol and bile acids are excreted in the feces rather than being absorbed. The liver must then use cholesterol from the blood to synthesize new bile acids. This provides a mechanism for eliminating cholesterol from the body and reducing blood cholesterol levels (Figure 4.19). Another theory as to how soluble fiber reduces blood cholesterol suggests that the short chain fatty acids produced by the microbial digestion of fiber enter the circulation and travel to the liver where they inhibit cholesterol synthesis.[19] Regardless of the mechanism, diets high in soluble fiber help to reduce blood cholesterol levels.

Bile acids Emulsifiers present in bile that are synthesized by the liver from cholesterol.

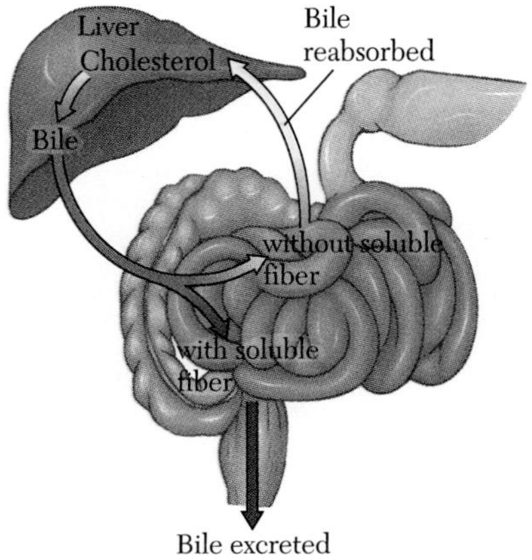

Figure 4.19
When the diet is low in soluble fiber, bile, which contains cholesterol and bile acids made from cholesterol, is absorbed and returned to the liver. When soluble fiber is present, it binds cholesterol and bile acids so they are excreted rather than absorbed.

Dietary Fiber and Colon Cancer Epidemiological studies have shown that the incidence of colon cancer is lower in populations consuming diets high in fiber.[5] In order to understand the role of fiber in cancer prevention or development, it is helpful to understand what cancer is.

What Is Cancer? Cancer is a disease that affects the way cells behave. Different cancers originate in different parts of the body and have different causes and effects. However, all cancer cells share two traits that distinguish them from other body cells. First, they reproduce without restraint. Normal body cells reproduce only to replace lost cells or to accommodate normal growth, but cancer cells divide continuously, forming enlarged cell masses known as tumors. Second, they invade and colonize areas reserved for other cells. A normal mucosal cell in the colon will stay in the colon, but a cancerous cell could travel to the liver, bone, or other tissue and begin dividing in the new location. Therefore, cancer cells eventually crowd out the normal cells, robbing them of nourishment and preventing them from functioning properly.

Mutations Changes in DNA caused by chemical or physical agents.

Cells become cancerous as a result of **mutations** in their genetic material. The type of cancer depends on the type of cell that is originally affected—for example, lung, breast, or colon—and on how the genetic material is altered by the mutations. Most mutations are thought to be caused by environmental factors, such as diet, tobacco use, or air pollution. In the case of the colon, mutations may be caused by substances consumed in the diet or produced in the gastrointestinal tract that come in contact with mucosal cells. Any substance that causes a cell to have cancerous potential is called a **tumor initiator.** Tumor initiators sow the seeds of cancer, but alone do not create cancerous cells. For the affected cell to begin growing and dividing as a cancer cell, it must be exposed to a **tumor promoter.** Although tumor promoters allow mutated cells to begin dividing, they do not cause mutations themselves.

Tumor initiator A substance that causes mutations and therefore may predispose a cell to becoming cancerous.

Tumor promoter A substance that stimulates a mutated cell to begin dividing.

The Role of Fiber The role of fiber in preventing the development of colon cancer may be related to its ability to decrease contact between the mucosal cells of the large intestine and the fecal contents, which may contain tumor initiators or tumor promoters. Fiber increases fecal bulk, dilutes the colon contents, and speeds transit, thereby decreasing contact time between the mucosal cells and potentially cancer-causing substances.

Problems With Excessive Fiber Intake Although a diet that meets the recommendation for fiber intake has many benefits, too much fiber or a rapid increase in the fiber content of the diet can decrease the energy density of the diet, reduce nutrient absorption, and, if the diet is not adequate in fluid, cause constipation.

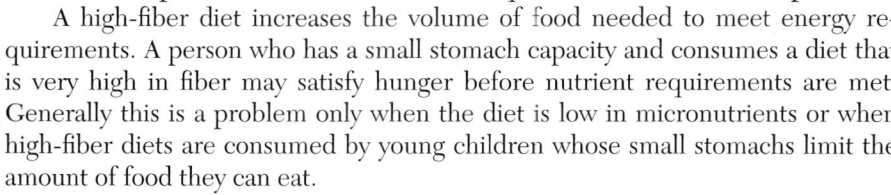

A high-fiber diet increases the volume of food needed to meet energy requirements. A person who has a small stomach capacity and consumes a diet that is very high in fiber may satisfy hunger before nutrient requirements are met. Generally this is a problem only when the diet is low in micronutrients or when high-fiber diets are consumed by young children whose small stomachs limit the amount of food they can eat.

A high-fiber diet may decrease nutrient absorption for two reasons. First, the increased volume of intestinal contents that occurs with a high-fiber diet may prevent enzymes from coming in contact with food. If a food cannot be broken down, nutrients may not be absorbed. Second, fiber may bind some micronutrients, preventing their absorption. For instance, wheat bran fiber binds the minerals zinc, calcium, magnesium, and iron, reducing their absorption. When mineral intake meets recommendations, a reasonable intake of high-fiber foods does not compromise mineral status.

A sudden increase in the fiber content of the diet can cause abdominal discomfort, gas, and diarrhea due to the bacterial breakdown of fiber. If fluid intake is too low, fiber can also cause constipation. The more fiber there is in the diet, the more water is needed to keep the stool soft. When too little fluid is consumed, the stool becomes hard and difficult to eliminate. In severe cases when fiber intake is excessive and fluid intake is low, intestinal blockage can occur.[20] To avoid these problems, the fiber and fluid content of the diet should be increased gradually.

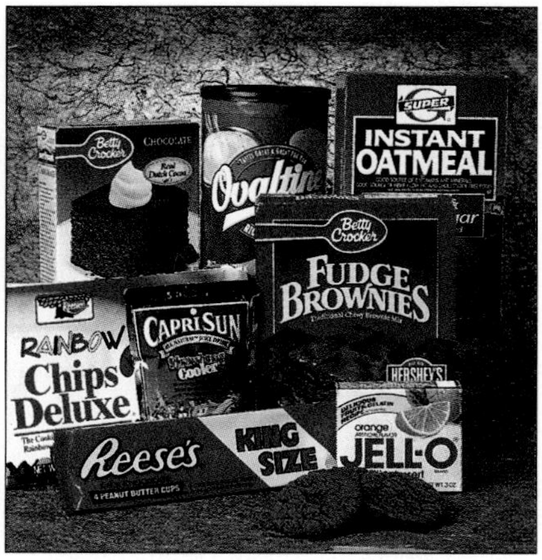

Figure 4.20
These foods are high in added refined sugar. (George Semple)

Is Sugar Really That Bad?

Despite the negative press that has hounded sugar, very few diseases are directly related to a high sugar intake. Then why the recommendations to consume it in moderation? The problem with sugar is that it is a source of empty kcalories, and when it replaces more nutrient-dense foods, it reduces the nutritional value of the diet as a whole. There is nothing wrong with an occasional sweet treat. However, nutritional deficiencies may result when a large percentage of the energy in the diet is from low-nutrient-density foods (Figure 4.20).

Sugar Intake and Disease Sugar has been accused of increasing the risk of heart disease and diabetes and causing obesity. There is some evidence that high sugar intake can affect the risk of heart disease but little data to indicate that it alone contributes to either diabetes or obesity. In the case of heart disease, risk is affected by blood cholesterol levels—and high levels of simple sugars can alter levels of some types of cholesterol in the blood.[21] Diabetes is characterized by high blood sugar levels, but the increase in blood glucose that occurs after a meal depends on the composition of the total meal, not just the amount of sugar.[22] Therefore, it is the effect of the total diet, not sugar intake specifically, that may affect the risk of diabetes. High intakes of sugar also do not cause obesity.[23] Obesity is caused by consuming more kcalories than are expended. Although many high-kcalorie foods are high in sugar, sugar itself does not cause obesity.

The most significant health problem associated with a diet high in simple carbohydrates is **dental caries,** or tooth cavities. Dental caries are formed when bacteria that live in the mouth metabolize sugar from the diet and produce acid. The acid can then dissolve the enamel and underlying structure of the teeth. Simple carbohydrate, particularly sucrose, is the most rapidly utilized food source for these microbes; however, any carbohydrate-containing foods that stick to the teeth can also cause cavities. The length of time that carbohydrate is in contact with the teeth determines the likelihood that a cavity will develop. Certain foods, such as sticky candies, cereals, crackers, and cookies, tend to remain on the teeth longer, providing a continuous supply of nutrients to decay-causing bacteria. Other foods, such as chocolate, ice cream, and bananas, are rapidly washed away from the teeth. Frequent snacking also increases contact time by providing a continuous food supply for the bacteria. Limiting sugar can help prevent dental caries, but since starch is also eventually metabolized into acid, proper dental hygiene is important even if the diet is low in sugar.[24]

Dental caries The decay and deterioration of teeth caused by acid produced when bacteria on the teeth metabolize carbohydrate.

Sugar and Behavior It has been hypothesized that carbohydrate can affect behavior. Controlled experiments have not supported a link between the consumption of sugary foods and either criminality or hyperactive behavior. But support for an effect of carbohydrate consumption on the brain and mood is strong. Carbohydrate craving is believed to play a role in disorders ranging from obesity to several types of depression.

Sugar and Criminal Behavior In 1978, Dan White blamed overconsumption of Hostess Twinkies for the mental state that led him to gun down the mayor and city supervisor of San Francisco. This became known as the "Twinkie Defense." In response to the idea that high sugar consumption leads to criminal behavior, some correctional facilities removed candy machines and reduced the sugar in their menus. However, controlled studies have not found a significant relationship between sugar intake and aggressive behavior.[16]

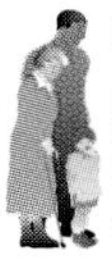

Sugar and Hyperactivity The consumption of sugary foods has also been suggested as a cause of hyperactivity in children (see Chapter 14). The increase in blood glucose after a meal high in simple carbohydrates is hypothesized to provide the energy for the excessive activities of a hyperactive child. However, research on sugar intake and behavior has failed to support the hypothesis that sugar contributes to behavioral changes.[25] Hyperactive behavior that is observed after sugar consumption is likely the result of other circumstances in that child's life. For example, the excitement of a birthday party rather than the cake is more likely the cause of hyperactive behavior. Other situations that might cause hyperactivity include lack of sleep, overstimulation, the desire for more attention, or lack of physical activity.

Carbohydrate Craving An abnormal craving for carbohydrate-rich foods has been identified in individuals with a variety of disorders including obesity, premenstrual syndrome, bulimia, depression, and seasonal affective disorder.[26,27] An

Neurotransmitter A chemical substance produced by a nerve cell that can stimulate or inhibit another cell.

abnormality in the regulation of brain levels of the **neurotransmitter** serotonin, which functions in the sleep center of the brain, is believed to be related to carbohydrate craving. In most people, a high-carbohydrate meal causes the amount of serotonin in the brain to increase, which results in sleepiness and the inability to concentrate. In carbohydrate-cravers, carbohydrate intake causes brain levels of serotonin to increase, but the effect is different: For carbohydrate-cravers, the rise in serotonin alleviates tension, anxiety, and mental fatigue, allowing them to feel calm and clearheaded after their carbohydrate "fix."

CARBOHYDRATE: ONE PART OF THE TOTAL DIET

The amount and source of carbohydrate in the diet impacts the healthiness of the diet as a whole. Diets that are high in complex carbohydrates from whole grains, legumes, and vegetables and in simple carbohydrates from whole foods such as fresh fruit are high in fiber, micronutrients, and phytochemicals, and low in fat. In this section we will discuss the recommendations for carbohydrate intake, how to determine the amount of carbohydrate and fiber in a diet, how to modify it to meet recommendations, and what carbohydrate choices contribute best to the overall healthiness of the diet (see *Critical Thinking: Carbohydrates in the Total Diet*).

Recommendations for Carbohydrate Intake

In a diet that meets energy needs, a minimum of about 50 to 100 grams of carbohydrate is needed to meet glucose needs and prevent ketosis. This amount of carbohydrate is easy to obtain in a normal diet. For example, two slices of toast and a cup (240 ml) of juice provide about 60 grams. If, however, only this small amount of carbohydrate was consumed, the total diet would be higher in fat and protein than is desirable.

In a typical North American diet, carbohydrate provides about 52% of the energy. Recommendations for a healthy diet suggest that the carbohydrate content be increased to 55 to 60% of the total energy intake and that refined sugar be limited (Figure 4.21). The Dietary Guidelines, Healthy People 2010, food labels, and the Food Guide Pyramid recommend that this be accomplished by increasing consumption of grains, vegetables, and fruits, and limiting bakery products, candy, and soft drinks. An increase in dietary fiber above the current average intake of 15 grams per day is also recommended. Expert panels in both Canada and the United States recommend 10 to 13 grams of fiber per 1000 kcalories, or about 20 to 35 grams of fiber per day for adults.

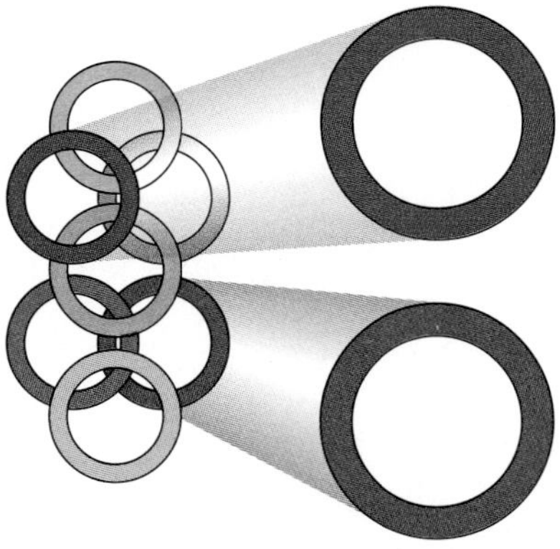

Choose a diet with plenty of grain products, vegetables, and fruits.

Choose a diet moderate in sugars.

Figure 4.21
The Dietary Guidelines for Americans recommend a diet high in complex carbohydrates with moderate amounts of refined sugars. (USDA, DHHS, 1995)

Determining Your Carbohydrate Intake

How does your diet compare to the recommendation of 55 to 60% carbohydrate? To calculate carbohydrate intake as a percent of energy, you need to know the grams of carbohydrate in the diet and the amount of energy consumed. For example, if you know a diet contains 2500 kcalories and 350 grams of carbohydrate, you can calculate the percent of energy as carbohydrate as follows:

$$350 \text{ g of carbohydrate} \times 4 \text{ kcal/g} = 1400 \text{ kcal of carbohydrate}$$

$$\frac{1400 \text{ kcal}}{2500 \text{ total kcal}} \times 100 = 56\% \text{ energy (kcal) as carbohydrate}$$

This same equation can be used to calculate the percent of energy as carbohydrate in individual foods. For example, a tortilla that contains 14 grams of carbohydrate and 70 kcalories contains 80% of its energy as carbohydrate ([(14 g ×

4 kcal/g)/70 kcal] × 100). The amount of carbohydrate in a diet can be calculated using values from food labels, food composition tables (see Appendix A), computer databases, or the Exchange Lists.

Food labels list the grams of total carbohydrate, fiber, and sugars. Total carbohydrate and fiber are also listed as a percent of the Daily Value. The Daily Value for total carbohydrate is calculated as 60% of the energy. For a 2000-kcalorie diet this represents 300 grams of carbohydrate ([2000 kcal × 0.6]/4 kcal/g of carbohydrate = 300 g). The Daily Value for fiber is based on a recommended intake of about 11.5 grams per 1000 kcalories, which is rounded to 25 grams in a 2000-kcalorie diet. No Daily Value has been established for sugars, but labels can help identify high-sugar products. The number of grams of sugars listed in the Nutrition Facts includes all monosaccharides and disaccharides but does not distinguish between refined and naturally occurring sugars. For example, the fructose found naturally in frozen strawberries, and that added as high-fructose corn syrup in soft drinks, are both listed as sugars. Nutrient claims provide some information about whether a food contains added refined sugar. The presence of a claim such as "no added sugar" or "without added sugar" indicates that no sugars have been added in processing. The list of ingredients also provides information about the types of sweeteners added to a food. Only added sugars are listed here and the only type of sweetener that can be called "sugar" is sucrose. Since sucrose may represent only one of many added sweeteners, consumers need to increase their carbohydrate vocabulary to recognize all the sweeteners on the label. High-fructose corn syrups, invert sugar, dextrose, lactose, honey, and mannitol are just a few (see *Off the Shelf: Are "Natural" Sugars Better?*).

The Exchange Lists can be used to give a quick estimate of the total amount of carbohydrate in a food or in the diet (Table 4.1). One serving of bread or fruit provides 15 grams of carbohydrate, 1 milk serving provides 12 grams, and 1 vegetable serving provides about 5 grams. Meats and fats provide no carbohydrate. The Exchange Lists cannot be used for calculating fiber intake, but Table 4.2 offers a method for estimating fiber in foods.

Table 4.1 *Using Exchange Lists to Calculate the Carbohydrate Content of a Diet*

Exchange Groups/Lists	Serving Size	Carbohydrates (g)
Carbohydrate Group		
Starch	1/2 cup rice, cereal, potatoes; 1 slice bread	15
Fruit	1 small apple, peach, pear; 1/2 banana; 1/2 cup canned juice-pack fruit	15
Milk	1 cup milk or yogurt	
Nonfat		12
Lowfat		12
Reduced fat		12
Whole		12
Other carbohydrates	Serving sizes vary	15
Vegetables	1/2 cup cooked vegetables, 1 cup raw	5
Meat/Meat Substitute Group	1 oz meat or cheese, 1/2 cup legumes	
Very lean		0
Lean		0
Medium fat		0
High fat		0
Fat Group	1 tsp butter, margarine, or oil, 1 Tbsp salad dressing	0

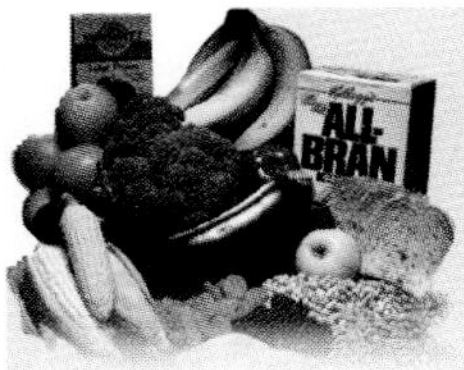

Off the Shelf

Are "Natural" Sugars Better?

Is honey healthy? Honey, blackstrap molasses, and other less-refined sugars have been promoted as healthier alternatives to table sugar, since they contain some nutrients that have been processed out of pure white table sugar. Candy and baked products made with these sweeteners are marketed as more nutritious. Although these sweeteners do have more micronutrients than table sugar, the amounts are too small to add much to the diet.

Honey is derived from the nectar of flowering plants, which contains sucrose. Bees collect the nectar and convert some of the sucrose into fructose and glucose. The color, flavor, and proportions of the sugars in honey vary with the source of the nectar. Honey supplies a concentrated source of energy but only traces of vitamins and minerals, so it cannot be considered a nutrient-dense food. Since sucrose from any source is broken into glucose and fructose before it is absorbed in the small intestine, the body cannot distinguish whether the glucose and fructose it absorbs come from honey or from refined white table sugar. The benefit of honey mixed with lemon juice as a home remedy for a cough is only anecdotal. Honey is somewhat sweeter than sucrose, so smaller amounts may be used for the same level of sweetness. Because honey may contain spores of the bacterium *Clostridium botulinum* (see Chapters 14 and 16), it should not be fed to infants.

Blackstrap molasses is a by-product of the refining of sucrose from sugar cane or sugar beets. It is a thick brown syrup that remains after the sucrose has crystallized. Refining of blackstrap molasses produces light and medium molasses. Curative properties for cancer and other disorders have been attributed to molasses, but there is no scientific support for these claims. Unlike any other concentrated nutritive sweetener, molasses does contain significant amounts of some minerals. For example, when it is made in old-fashioned iron vats with iron pipes, it is rich in iron.

Other sweeteners such as brown sugar, maple syrup, and fruit juices are also believed by some to be healthier than sucrose. In fact, most are not significantly different from sucrose. Most brown sugar is simply refined white sugar containing some molasses to color it brown. Maple syrup is formed by boiling down the sap of maple trees. It is composed primarily of sucrose, which has been browned by the heat involved in processing. Fruit juices are also used as sweeteners. These may add small amounts of micronutrients but contribute primarily the sugar fructose to the product.

Sweeteners promoted as "natural," such as honey, molasses, brown sugar, and maple syrup, are all processed in some way, either by humans or, in the case of honey, by bees. Though these sweeteners contribute distinctive flavors to the foods to which they are added, their nutritional contribution is not significantly different from that of refined white sugar.

Foods that are high in added refined sugars provide energy but few nutrients. So, guidelines for a healthy diet recommend that refined sugars be consumed in moderation. There are some easy ways to do this—use less sugar in coffee or on cereal and reduce sweetened soft drink consumption. But finding and eliminating other sources of refined sugar in the diet isn't always easy. Consumers need to understand the information provided on food labels before they can sort out their sugar intake.

Nutritional Value of Various Sweeteners
(nutrients per tablespoon of sweetener)

	Daily Value*	Light Molasses	Medium Molasses	Blackstrap Molasses	Honey	Brown Sugar	Table Sugar
Energy (kcal)	—	40	38	35	61	52	46
Protein (g)	50	0.4	0.4	0.4	0.1	0	0
Carbohydrate (g)	300	10	9	8	16.5	13.4	11.9
Calcium (mg)	1000	25	44	103	1	11	0.7
Phosphorus (mg)	1000	7	10	13	1	5	0
Sodium (mg)	<2400	2	6	14	1	3	0
Magnesium (mg)	400	31	31	31	1	9	0
Potassium (mg)	3500	138	159	439	10	32	0.7
Iron (mg)	18	0.6	0.9	2.4	0.1	0.4	0
Zinc (mg)	15	0.1	0.1	0.1	0.1	0.1	0

* Daily Value for a 2000-kcalorie diet.

Table 4.2 *A System for Estimating the Fiber Content of a Diet*

	High Fiber	Medium Fiber	Low Fiber
Bread, Cereal, Rice, & Pasta Group			
fiber per serving	*5 grams*	*2 grams*	*0.5 gram*
Breads (1 slice)	—	Whole wheat Rye	White bread Bagel (1/2) Tortilla Roll (1/2) English muffin (1/2) Graham cracker
Cereals (1/2 cup)	All Bran Bran Buds 100% Bran Flakes	40% Bran Shredded Wheat	Cheerios Rice Krispies
Rice and pasta (1/2 cup)	—	Whole wheat pasta Brown rice	Macaroni Pasta White rice
Fruit Group			
fiber per serving	*4 grams*	*2 grams*	*1 gram*
Fruits (1 medium or 1/2 cup)	Berries Prunes	Apple Apricot Banana Orange Raisins	Melon Canned fruit Juices
Vegetable Group			
fiber per serving	*4 grams*	*2 grams*	*1 gram*
Vegetables (1/2 cup)	Peas Broccoli Spinach Beans: pinto, red, kidney Blackeyed peas	Green beans Carrots Eggplant Cabbage Potatoes with skin Corn	Asparagus Cauliflower Celery Lettuce Tomatoes Zucchini Peppers Potatoes without skin Onions

Adapted from Bright-See, E., Benda, C., Vartouhi, J., et al. Development and testing of a dietary fibre exchange system. Can. Diet. Assoc. J. 47:199–205, 1986; and Marlett, J. A. Content and composition of dietary fiber in 117 frequently consumed foods. J. Am. Diet. Assoc. 92:175–186, 1992.

A Diet to Meet Recommendations: Choose More Grains, Fruits, and Vegetables

To meet the recommendations of 55 to 60% of energy from carbohydrate and a moderate intake of refined sugar, most people need to increase the total carbohydrate in their diets but limit their intake of sugar. To do this without increasing energy, complex carbohydrates should be substituted for foods high in refined sugar, fat, and protein. For example, choosing a stir-fry meal of a few ounces of beef and vegetables on rice or a meal of spaghetti and meat sauce can provide the same energy but more carbohydrate than a dinner of a 12-ounce steak and french fries. These carbohydrate-based meals are also lower in fat and cost less than meat-based meals. To limit refined sugars, soft drinks and candy bars should be rare treats, and fruits should be substituted for sugary desserts.

The recommendations of the Food Guide Pyramid can be used to plan a diet high in complex carbohydrates. Six to 11 servings should be selected from the Bread, Cereal, Rice, & Pasta Group, the base of the Pyramid. If whole grain products are selected, this group will also provide excellent sources of fiber. The next level of the Pyramid contains the Vegetable Group and Fruit Group, which are also good sources of complex carbohydrates, fiber, and naturally occurring

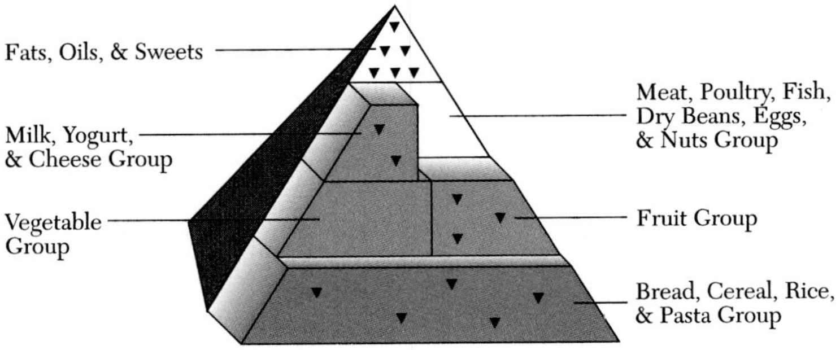

Figure 4.22

The Food Guide Pyramid groups that are sources of naturally occurring simple and complex carbohydrates are raised and colored red. The darker shades indicate groups with a greater proportion of high-carbohydrate foods. The ▼ symbol indicates sources of added sugars.

simple carbohydrates. It is recommended that 3 to 5 servings from the Vegetable Group and 2 to 4 servings from the Fruit Group be consumed each day. On the next level of the Pyramid, the Milk, Yogurt, & Cheese Group provides unrefined simple carbohydrate in the form of lactose. To emphasize moderation in the consumption of refined sugar, the Food Guide Pyramid recommends that added sweeteners be used sparingly. The relative amounts of added sugar in each of the food groups are indicated by an upside-down triangle symbol (▼). The food groups that contain a higher proportion of foods with added sugar have more of these symbols. For example, the tip of the Pyramid, which includes sweets along with fats and oils, has the highest concentration of these symbols; the grain group, which includes sweetened bakery products like cakes and cookies, has a moderate concentration of symbols; and the Vegetable Group, which includes almost no foods with added sugar, has no symbols (Figure 4.22).

A diet based on the Pyramid will meet the recommendations for carbohydrate and fiber intake if care is used in choosing from the food groups. For example, switching from a breakfast of ham and eggs to one of cereal and toast will increase carbohydrate but will not add much fiber unless whole grains are chosen. Breakfast cereals all fit into the grain group, yet choosing one over another can make a big difference in sugar and fiber intake. A serving of Frosted Flakes has about 120 kcalories with 1 gram of fiber and 13 grams of sugars. A serving of bran flakes has about 100 kcalories but 5 grams of fiber and only 6 grams of sugars.

Table 4.3 *How to Choose Carbohydrates Wisely*

1. Increase intake of whole grains, fruits, and vegetables.
2. Use whole grain products such as oatmeal, brown rice, and whole wheat bread.
3. Increase consumption of legumes such as kidney, black, and pinto beans.
4. If fresh fruits are not available, choose frozen or canned fruits without added sugar.
5. Choose packaged foods that contain 10% or more of the Daily Value for fiber.
6. When baking at home, substitute whole grain flour for one fourth to one half of the amount of flour specified in the recipe.
7. When cooking at home, use less sugar; try adding one-fourth less sugar than called for in the recipe.
8. Use less added sugar in beverages and on cereals and pancakes.
9. Eat fewer high-sugar prepared foods such as cookies and candies.
10. Read food labels to choose foods low in added sugars and high in fiber.

Using fresh instead of canned fruit can also help increase fiber and decrease refined sugars. For example, half a cup of pear halves canned in heavy syrup provides 90 kcalories, 1 gram of fiber, and almost 20 grams of sugar, most of which is added in the syrup. One large fresh pear would provide 90 kcalories, 4 grams of fiber, and no refined sugar (see Table 4.3). Choosing fresh fruit over juice also adds fiber. An apple provides about 80 to 90 kcalories and 2.7 grams of fiber, whereas a cup of apple juice provides the same amount of energy but almost no fiber (0.2 gram).

CRITICAL THINKING

Carbohydrates in the Total Diet

Mercedes knows that a healthy diet is important but is confused as to what makes a diet healthy. She tries to follow the recommendations of the Food Guide Pyramid but rarely consumes the number of servings of grains, vegetables, and fruits that are recommended. So she meets with a dietitian to evaluate her diet.

Nutritional assessment

Mercedes's nutritional assessment suggests that her diet contains about 2000 kcalories, 20% of which come from protein, 41% from fat, and 39% from carbohydrate, and she consumes 8 grams of fiber. Her diet is higher in fat and lower in carbohydrate than recommended.

How many more grams of carbohydrate would Mercedes need to meet the recommendation of 55 to 60% of energy from carbohydrate?

Her diet provides approximately 39% carbohydrate and 2000 kcal:

$$\frac{39 \times 2000 \text{ kcal}}{100} = 780 \text{ kcal from carbohydrate}$$

$$\frac{780 \text{ kcal from carbohydrate}}{4 \text{ kcal per gram}} = 195 \text{ grams of carbohydrate}$$

A 2000-kcalorie diet with 55% of energy from carbohydrate would provide:

$$\frac{55 \times 2000 \text{ kcal}}{100} = 1100 \text{ kcal from carbohydrate}$$

$$\frac{1100 \text{ kcal from carbohydrate}}{4 \text{ kcal per gram}} = 275 \text{ grams of carbohydrate}$$

Mercedes's diet therefore needs to provide at least 80 additional grams of carbohydrate (275 grams recommended − 195 grams consumed = 80 grams).

Does Mercedes's original diet meet the recommendations for 2–4 servings of fruits, 3–5 servings of vegetables, and 6–11 servings of grains?

Answer:

Original Diet			Modified Diet	
Food	**Carbohydrate (g)**	**Fiber (g)**	**Food**	**Carbohydrate (g)**
Breakfast				
Coffee	0	0	Coffee	0
White toast (2)	30	1	White toast (2)	30
Margarine	0	0	Margarine	0
Jelly	4	0	Jelly	4
Chorizo (sausage) (~~2 oz~~)	0	0	Chorizo (sausage) (1 oz)	0
Orange juice (1 cup)	30	1	Orange juice (1 cup)	30
Lunch				
Burritos:			Burritos:	
Tortilla (2)	30	1	Tortilla (2)	30
Beef (3 oz)	0	0	Beef (3 oz)	0
~~Cheese (1 oz)~~	0	0	Beans (1/2 cup)	15
Milk (1 cup)	12	0	Milk (1 cup)	12
Cookies (2)	15	0.5	Cookies (2)	15
			Canned pears (1 cup)	30
Snack				
Diet soda	0	0	Diet soda	0
Pretzels (1 oz)	15	0.5	Pretzels (1 oz)	15
Dinner				
Carne asada (beef) (~~4 oz~~)	0	0	Carne asada (beef) (2 oz)	0
Potatoes (1 cup)	30	4	Potatoes (1 cup)	30
			Green beans (1/2 cup)	5
			Salad (1/2 cup)	5
Milk (1 cup)	12	0	Milk (1 cup)	12
~~Ice cream (1/2 cup)~~	15	0	Nonfat frozen yogurt (1 cup)	19
			w/berries	15
Snack				
			Graham crackers (3 squares)	15
Total	**193**	**8**		**282**

To improve her total diet and increase her complex carbohydrate intake without increasing her total energy intake, the dietitian suggests some ways Mercedes could increase her intake of fruits, vegetables, legumes, and grains. The carbohydrate content of her original diet and a sample modified diet are estimated using the Exchange Lists (see Table 4.1). The modifications decrease her fat intake and increase her carbohydrate intake to the recommended level.

Are the carbohydrate sources in her modified diet from whole or refined sources?

Answer:

How does fiber factor into her diet?

Mercedes estimates the fiber content of her original diet using Table 4.2. The 8 grams of fiber in her diet falls short of the recommended fiber intake of 10 to 13 grams per 1000 kcalories.

How much fiber should Mercedes's diet provide?

$$\frac{2000 \text{ kcal}}{1000} = 2.0$$

$$2.0 \times 10\text{g fiber} = 20\text{g fiber} \quad \text{and} \quad 2.0 \times 13\text{g fiber} = 26\text{g fiber}$$

Therefore she needs to obtain 20 to 26 grams of fiber from her diet.

How many grams of fiber are in Mercedes's modified diet? Does it meet the recommendations?

Answer:

Carbohydrates and Food Technology

Many forms of carbohydrate are added in the manufacture of processed foods. Carbohydrates are added for sweetness, to change food texture or color, to thicken, and to preserve food. Some of these make only a small contribution to the overall carbohydrate content of the diet, whereas others may contribute significantly to the amounts and types of carbohydrates consumed.

Complex Carbohydrates as Additives

Starch is found as small granules in plants. When heated with water, these granules swell, and the solution becomes thicker. This property makes starches useful

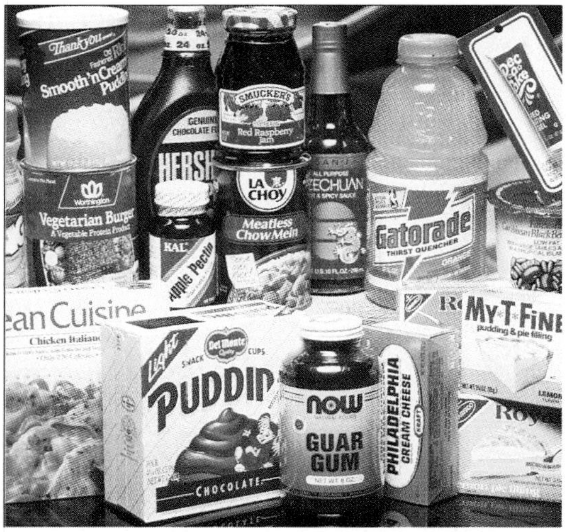

Figure 4.23
Modified food starch, pectin, and gums are used as stabilizers and thickeners in processed foods. (Charles D. Winters)

Modified starch or **modified food starch** Starch that has been treated to enhance its ability to thicken or form a gel.

as thickeners in foods such as sauces, puddings, and gravies. As a starch-thickened mixture cools, bonds form between the molecules, creating a gel. For example, cornstarch is frequently added to thicken or gel sauces and puddings. Food manufacturers also use a product called **modified starch,** or **modified food starch.** This is starch that has been treated to cause it to form a more stable gel.

The soluble fiber pectin, common in fruits and vegetables, is also used as a thickener. Pectin forms a gel when sugar and acid are added, such as in the preparation of jams and jellies. Commercial pectin, which is sold as a thickener for home-canned fruits and jellies, is refined from citrus peels and apples. Pectin is added to thicken tomato paste and to prevent the fine particles in orange juice from settling out. Carbohydrate gums are used as thickeners and stabilizers because they combine with water to keep solutions from separating. Gravies, pie fillings, jellies, and puddings are examples of products that contain such stabilizers and thickeners. Pectins and gums are also used in reduced-fat products to mimic the texture and viscosity of fat. Gums used in food processing include gum arabic, gum karaya, guar gum, locust bean gum, xanthan gum, and gum tragacanth. These gums are extracted from shrubs, trees, and seed pods. Agar, carrageenan, and alginates, which come from seaweeds, are also used as thickeners and stabilizers (Figure 4.23).

Simple Carbohydrates as Additives

Americans consume about 150 pounds of sweeteners per person per year.[28] The simple carbohydrates added to foods as sweeteners include not only sucrose but also fructose, high-fructose corn syrup, corn syrup, maltose, honey, molasses, and others. They can be added in dry form or dissolved in water to form syrups. Simple carbohydrates can also be used as a preservative, as in jams and jellies, since high concentrations of sugar hold water and prevent the growth of microorganisms. They are also used to color foods, since they darken or caramelize when heated. Caramelized sugar is responsible for the brown color of caramel candy and the dark color of maple syrup.

Fructose is a component of a number of sweeteners, including sucrose, honey, and high-fructose corn syrup. High-fructose corn syrup is produced by modifying starch extracted from corn to produce a syrup that is approximately half glucose and half fructose. Fructose dissolves more readily than sucrose, so it is preferred in soft drinks and canned fruits. It is also sweeter than sucrose. Fructose intake from sweeteners like high-fructose corn syrup, honey, and sucrose now makes up about 5% of the total energy intake in the United States.[1] Since fructose does not cause as great a rise in blood glucose, it is sometimes used as an alternative to sucrose in products for diabetics. Although current levels of fructose consumption are considered safe, fructose, like other simple sugars, can promote tooth decay and, in sensitive individuals, has been reported to cause an increase in insulin levels, blood lipids, and blood uric acid.[29] Fructose consumed in fruits or juices can also cause diarrhea in children.[30]

Artificial Sweeteners: Sugar Substitutes

America's love of sweets and the bad press surrounding sugar have driven the technological development of an increasing number of artificial and non-nutritive sweeteners. These sugar substitutes, which provide little or no energy, are added to a host of low-kcalorie and "light" foods such as yogurts, ice creams, and soft drinks. Although many sugar substitutes are technically not carbohydrates, they were developed to replace simple sugars in food products or as a replacement for table sugar at home. Their potential benefits include reducing the amount of energy consumed, not contributing to tooth decay, and not causing a rise in blood glucose. Although the use of artificial sweeteners has not affected the incidence of obesity in the American population, these products may facilitate weight loss and long-term weight maintenance when used by individuals as part of a weight-control program.[31]

The main competitors in the artificial sweetener market in the United States today are saccharin and aspartame. Acesulfame K (acesulfame potassium) and sucralose are also FDA-approved sugar substitutes. These are used alone or in combination to sweeten a variety of foods sold in the United States. Cyclamate, an artificial sweetener that was popular in the 1960s, was banned by the FDA in 1969. It is still sold in Canada and some 50 other countries. Sugar alcohols are also considered sugar substitutes even though they provide energy.

Saccharin Saccharin is a sweetener that is 200 to 700 times sweeter than sugar. In 1977, after large doses of saccharin were found to increase the incidence of bladder cancer in rats, the FDA proposed banning saccharin. However, the public and industry protested. In response to the outcry, Congress imposed a moratorium on the banning of saccharin. This moratorium has been extended every few years since. In the United States, all products containing saccharin must display a warning on the label informing the public that it may cause cancer (Figure 4.24). In Canada, the sale of products containing saccharin is banned in grocery stores, but saccharin with a warning label is available in pharmacies.

Intake of saccharin in the United States is estimated to be about 50 mg per person per day. The FDA has set an acceptable daily intake (ADI), which is an estimate of the amount an individual can safely consume every day over a lifetime without risk, of 5 mg per kg body weight per day. For a 145-pound (70 kg) individual, this would be 350 mg per day or 500 mg per day for a 220-pound (100 kg) individual.[32] A packet of sweentener contains 36 mg of saccharin.

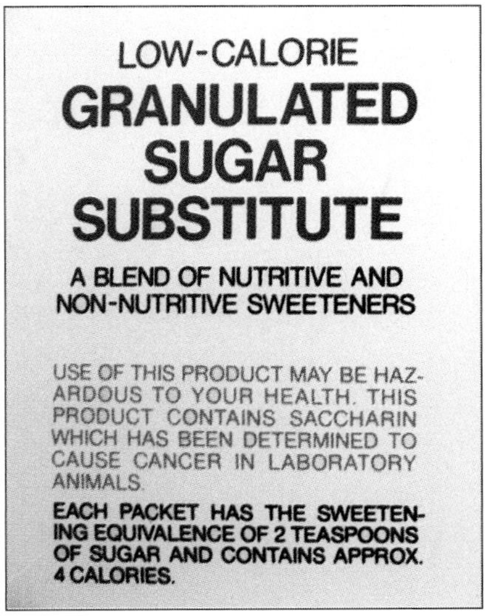

LOW-CALORIE
GRANULATED SUGAR SUBSTITUTE
A BLEND OF NUTRITIVE AND NON-NUTRITIVE SWEETENERS
USE OF THIS PRODUCT MAY BE HAZARDOUS TO YOUR HEALTH. THIS PRODUCT CONTAINS SACCHARIN WHICH HAS BEEN DETERMINED TO CAUSE CANCER IN LABORATORY ANIMALS.
EACH PACKET HAS THE SWEETENING EQUIVALENCE OF 2 TEASPOONS OF SUGAR AND CONTAINS APPROX. 4 CALORIES.

Figure 4.24
Products that contain saccharin must provide this warning. (Gregory Smolin)

Aspartame In 1965, James Schlatter, at the pharmaceutical company G. D. Searle, was working with a chemical made up of two amino acids when he spilled some of the chemical on his fingers. Shortly afterward, he licked his finger to pick up a piece of paper and discovered an intensely sweet taste. This accidental discovery led to the development of the artificial sweetener aspartame. Since aspartame is made of two amino acids, the building blocks of protein, it is not a carbohydrate. It was approved for some uses in 1981 and for use in soft drinks in 1983. Because aspartame breaks down when heated, it works best in products that are not cooked, such as chewing gum, breakfast cereals, fruit spreads, yogurt, and beverages. Common trade names for this sweetener include NutraSweet,

Equal, and NutriTaste. Each gram of aspartame contains 4 kcalories, but since it is about 200 times as sweet as sugar, only 1/200 as much of it needs to be used to achieve the same level of sweetness.

As with other artificial sweeteners, safety concerns have been raised about aspartame. It contains the amino acid phenylalanine and therefore can be dangerous to individuals with a genetic disorder called phenylketonuria (PKU). These individuals have an abnormality that affects the metabolism of phenylalanine. They must restrict their intake of this amino acid to prevent brain damage (see Chapter 6). There is also a concern that consuming aspartame might cause dangerously high blood phenylalanine levels in the general public. Phenylalanine occurs naturally in protein. A 4-ounce hamburger has 12 times more phenylalanine than a 12-ounce aspartame-sweetened soft drink. However, when phenylalanine is ingested without the other amino acids found in high-protein foods, blood or brain levels increase to a greater extent. There have been reports of headaches, dizziness, seizures, nausea, allergic reactions, and other side effects following ingestion of aspartame; however, double-blind placebo-controlled studies have not been able to reproduce these symptoms.[32] There has also been concern that the use of aspartame might be associated with an increased risk of brain cancer in children, but controlled studies found no evidence that aspartame is a carcinogen.[33] Overall, the consensus of the scientific community is that aspartame is safe for most people.

The FDA has set an ADI of 50 mg of aspartame per kg of body weight. A packet of sweetener contains about 37 mg of aspartame. A 12-ounce soft drink sweetened with aspartame contains about 225 mg. To exceed the ADI, a 70-kg adult would have to consume almost 16 aspartame-sweetened soft drinks a day, and a 35-kg child would have to consume almost 8 soft drinks.[32]

Acesulfame K Marketed as Sunette, acesulfame K is 200 times as sweet as sugar and provides no energy. It was approved for use in 1988 and is found in chewing gum, powdered drink mixes, gelatins, puddings, soft drinks, and nondairy creamers. It is heat stable, so it can be used in baking. The ADI has been set at 15 mg per kg body weight. A packet of sweetener contains about 50 mg of acesulfame K.

Sucralose Sucralose (trichlorogalactosucrose) has been used in Canada for many years and was approved for use in the United States in 1998. It is about 600 times sweeter than sucrose. It is sold as Splenda and can be used as a tabletop sweetener that is added directly to foods. Since it is heat stable it can be used in baked goods.[32] It is used in beverages, chewing gum, frozen desserts, puddings, jams and jellies, syrups, and many other products.

Sugar Alcohols Sugar alcohols such as sorbitol, mannitol, lactitol, and xylitol are chemical derivatives of sugar. They provide energy, but since they are not digested, absorbed, or metabolized to the same extent as monosaccharides and disaccharides, they generally provide less energy. For example, lactitol is a sugar alcohol that provides 2 kcalories per gram and is about 40% as sweet as sugar.[34]

The bacteria in the mouth cannot metabolize sugar alcohols as rapidly as sucrose. Therefore, sugar alcohols are less likely to promote tooth decay.[32] They are used in "sugar-free" gum and candies. Since sugar alcohols are not monosaccharides or disaccharides, they can be used in products labeled "sugar free." Sugar-free products sweetened with sugar alcohols may carry the health claim statement that they do not promote tooth decay. Consumption of large amounts of sugar alcohols (more than 50 grams of sorbitol or 20 grams of mannitol per day) can cause diarrhea.

APPLICATIONS

These exercises are designed to help you apply your critical thinking skills to your own nutrition choices. Many are best performed using a diet analysis software program. If you do not have access to a computer program, the exercises can be hand calculated using the information in this text and its appendices.

1. Calculate your average carbohydrate and energy intake from the three-day diet record you kept in Chapter 2.
   a. What is the percent of energy from carbohydrate in your diet?
   b. How does this compare with the recommended 55 to 60% of energy from carbohydrate?
   c. If your diet does not meet the recommendations, modify it to increase your carbohydrate intake without changing your energy intake.
   d. How does the fat content of your original diet compare with your modified diet?
   e. List some foods in your diet that are high in simple carbohydrates and some that are high in complex carbohydrates. Classify the simple carbohydrates as either whole or refined. Are the complex carbohydrates from refined or whole sources?
2. Calculate the grams of fiber in your modified diet from question 1 above using a computer software program or the exchanges in Table 4.2.
   a. How many grams of fiber does your diet provide?
   b. How many grams of fiber per 1000 kcalories does your diet provide?
   c. If your diet does not meet recommendations, modify it to meet them.

Summary

1. Carbohydrates from grains are the basis of the diet in most of the world. Dietary recommendations in the United States suggest that carbohydrate intake be increased to 55 to 60% of energy.
2. Carbohydrates are chemical compounds that contain carbon, hydrogen, and oxygen. In food, they include sugar, starch, and fiber. Simple carbohydrates include monosaccharides and disaccharides and are found in foods such as table sugar, honey, milk, and fruit. Complex carbohydrates are oligosaccharides and polysaccharides. Polysaccharides include glycogen in animals and starch and fiber in plants. Sources of starch and fiber in the diet include whole grains, legumes, vegetables, and fruits.
3. Fiber cannot be digested by enzymes in the human stomach or small intestine and therefore is not absorbed into the body. Fiber benefits gastrointestinal function by increasing the amount of water and bulk in the intestine, which increases the ease and rate at which material moves through the gastrointestinal tract.
4. In the body, carbohydrate, primarily as glucose, provides a source of energy. Glucose is metabolized through cellular respiration, involving glycolysis, which breaks glucose into pyruvate; the citric acid cycle, which produces carbon dioxide and electrons; and the electron transport chain, which produces water and ATP. Several tissues, including the brain and red blood cells, require glucose as an energy source.
5. The bloodstream delivers glucose to body cells. Blood glucose levels are maintained by the hormones insulin and glucagon. When blood glucose rises, insulin is released from the pancreas to allow body cells to take up the glucose. When blood glucose falls, glucagon is released to increase blood glucose.
6. Diabetes is a disease in which high blood glucose damages tissues and causes complications including heart disease, stroke, high blood pressure, kidney failure, blindness, and amputations. This occurs either because insufficient insulin is produced or because there is a decrease in the sensitivity of body cells to insulin. It is a major public health problem.
7. Hypoglycemia is a condition in which blood glucose falls to abnormally low levels, causing symptoms such as sweating, headaches, and rapid heartbeat.
8. Diets high in complex carbohydrates from whole grains, vegetables, fruits, and legumes are good sources of fiber, vitamins, minerals, and phytochemicals. Diets high in fiber reduce the risk of chronic bowel disorders, heart disease, and colon cancer.
9. Diets high in simple sugars are low in nutrient density and increase the risk of dental caries.
10. Guidelines for healthy diets recommend an increase in the intake of complex carbohydrate and a moderate sugar intake. Whole grains, legumes, fruits, and vegetables should be increased in the diet, and foods high in refined sugars should be consumed in moderation. Fiber intake should be increased to 10 to 13 grams per 1000 kcalories per day.
11. Carbohydrates are added to foods in processing as preservatives and to provide flavor, texture, and color. Complex carbohydrates are added as thickeners and stabilizers. Simple carbohydrates are most frequently added as sweeteners.
12. Artificial sweeteners or sugar substitutes are used to replace energy-containing sweeteners. They do not contribute to tooth decay.

Review Questions

1. What is the basic unit of carbohydrate?
2. List three common simple carbohydrates. In what foods are they found?
3. What is complex carbohydrate? What foods are good sources?
4. Why is refined sugar considered a source of empty kcalories?
5. How much energy is provided by a gram of carbohydrate?
6. Why do we say that fiber does not provide energy?
7. Why is carbohydrate said to spare protein?

8. What is the main function of glucose in the body?
9. What is diabetes? Why is ketosis a problem only in type 1 diabetes?
10. What health benefits are associated with a diet high in complex carbohydrates?
11. List some functions of carbohydrates added to processed foods.
12. How can you use the information on food labels to help you identify foods that are high in refined sugars?
13. What are the risks and benefits of artificial sweeteners?

Nutrition Web Links

To further explore areas related to the material in this chapter, go to the *Nutrition: Science and Applications* Web site at ***www.Wiley.com/college/Smolin*** and *click on* **Student Companion Site** for chapter-by-chapter links. Some Web sites related to the information in Chapter 4 include:

Organizations that provide information about carbohydrate intake and health, such as the National Institute of Dental and Craniofacial Research and the National Food Safety Database.

Organizations that provide information on diabetes management, such as the American Diabetes Association and the American Dietetic Association.

Locations that provide information on digestive problems associated with carbohydrates, including the International Food Information Council and the National Institutes of Diabetes and Digestive and Kidney Diseases.

References

1. Giboney, M., Sigman-Grant, M., Stanton, J. L., and Keast, D. R. Consumption of sugars. Am. J. Clin. Nutr. 62(suppl):178S–194S, 1995.
2. Flatt, J. P. Use and storage of carbohydrates. Am. J. Clin. Nutr. 61(suppl):952S–959S, 1995.
3. Lee, M.-F., and Krasinski, S. D. Human adult-onset lactase decline: an update. Nutr. Rev. 56:1–8, 1998.
4. McBean, L. D., and Miller, G. D. Allaying fears and fallacies about lactose intolerance. J. Am. Diet. Assoc. 98:671–676, 1998.
5. American Dietetic Association. Position of the American Dietetic Association: health implications of dietary fiber. J. Am. Diet. Assoc. 97:1157–1160, 1997.
6. American Diabetes Association. Economic consequence of diabetes mellitus in the United States in 1997. Diabetes Care 21:296–309, 1998.
7. National Institutes of Diabetes and Digestive and Kidney Diseases, National Institutes of Health, National Diabetes Information Clearinghouse. Fact Sheet on Diabetes Statistics, NIH Publication No. 98-3926, Nov. 1997, updated Feb. 1998. Online at http://www.niddk.nih.gov/health/diabetes/pubs/dmstats/dmstats.htm
8. Leontos, C., Wong, F., and Gallivan, J., for National Diabetes Education Program Planning Committee. National Diabetes Education Program: opportunities and challenges. J. Am. Diet. Assoc. 98:73–75, 1998.
9. National Institutes of Diabetes and Digestive and Kidney Diseases, National Institutes of Health. National Diabetes Education Program Fact Sheet. Available online at http://www.niddk.nih.gov/health/diabetes/ndep/ndep.htm
10. Report of the Expert Committee on the Diagnosis and Classification of Diabetes Mellitus. Diabetes Care 20:1183–1197, 1997.
11. Schafer, R. G., Bohannon, B., Franz, M., et al. Translation of the diabetes nutrition recommendations for health care institutions: technical review. J. Am. Diet. Assoc. 97:43–51, 1997.
12. Salmeron, J., Ascherio, A., Rimm, E.B., et al. Dietary fiber, glycemic load, and risk of NIDDM in men. Diabetes Care 20:545–550, 1997.
13. Salmeron, J., Manson, J. E., Stampfer, M. J., et al. Dietary fiber, glycemic load, and the risk of noninsulin-dependent diabetes mellitus in women. J.A.M.A. 277:472–477, 1997.
14. Pasei, K., and McFarland, K. F. Management of diabetes in pregnancy. Am. Fam. Physician 55:731–738, 1997.
15. Frayn, K. N., and Kingman, S. M. Dietary sugars and lipid metabolism. Am. J. Clin. Nutr. 95(suppl):250S–263S, 1995.
16. White, J. W., and Wolraich, M. Effect of sugar on behavior and mental performance. Am. J. Clin. Nutr. 62(suppl): 242S–249S, 1995.
17. Jacobs, D. R., Meyer, K. A., Kushi, L. H., and Folsom, A. R. Whole-grain intake may reduce the risk of ischemic heart disease death in postmenopausal women: the Iowa Women's Health Study. Am. J. Clin. Nutr. 68:248–257, 1998.
18. Willett, W. C. The dietary pyramid: does the foundation need repair? Am. J. Clin. Nutr. 68:218–219, 1998.
19. Marlett, J. A. Sites and mechanisms for the hypocholesterolemic actions of soluble dietary fiber sources. In Kritevsky, D., and Bonfield, C., eds. *Fiber in Human Health and Disease,* New York: Plenum Press, 1997, 109–121.
20. Miller, D. L., Miller, P. F., and Dekker, J. J. Small bowel obstruction from bran cereal. J.A.M.A. 263:813–815, 1990.
21. Starc, T. J., Shea, S., Cohn, L. C., et al. Greater dietary intake of simple carbohydrates is associated with lower concentrations of HDL cholesterol in hypercholesterolemic children. Am. J. Clin. Nutr. 67:1147–1154, 1998.
22. Wolever, T. M. S., and Miller, J. B. Sugars and blood glucose control. Am. J. Clin. Nutr. 62(suppl):212S–227S, 1995.
23. Hill, J. O., and Prentice, A. M. Sugar and body weight regulation. Am. J. Clin. Nutr. 62(suppl):264S–274S, 1995.
24. Konig, K. G., and Navia, J. M. Nutritional role of sugars in oral health. Am. J. Clin. Nutr. 62(suppl):275S–283S, 1995.

25. Wolraich, M. L., Wilson, D. B., and White, J. W. The effect of sugar on behavior or cognition in children: a meta analysis. J.A.M.A. 274:1617–1618, 1995.
26. Wurtman, R. J., and Wurtman, J. J. Brain serotonin, carbohydrate craving, obesity and depression. Obes. Res. 4:477S–480S, 1995.
27. Kurzer, M. S. Women, food, and mood. Nutrition Reviews 55:268–276, 1997.
28. USDA. Food Consumption, Prices, and Expenditures, 1997.
29. Glinsmann, W. H., and Bowman, B. A. The public health significance of dietary fructose. Am. J. Clin. Nutr. 58(suppl):820S–823S, 1993.
30. Dennison, B. A. Fruit juice consumption by infants and children: a review. J. Am. Coll. Nutr. 15:4S–11S, 1996.
31. Blackburn, G. L., Kanders, B. S., Lavin, P. T., et al. The effect of aspartame as part of a multidisciplinary weight-control program on short- and long-term control of body weight. Am J. Clin. Nutr. 65:409–418, 1997.
32. American Dietetic Association. Position of the American Dietetic Association: use of nutritive and non-nutritive sweeteners. J. Am. Diet. Assoc. 98:580–587, 1998.
33. Gurney, J. G., Pogoda, J. M., Holly, E. A., et al. Aspartame consumption in relation to childhood brain tumor risk: results from a case-control study. J. Nat. Cancer Inst. 89:1072–1074, 1997.
34. Blackers, I. Properties and applications of lactitol. Food Technol. 49:66–68, 1995.

Chapter

5

Chapter Outline

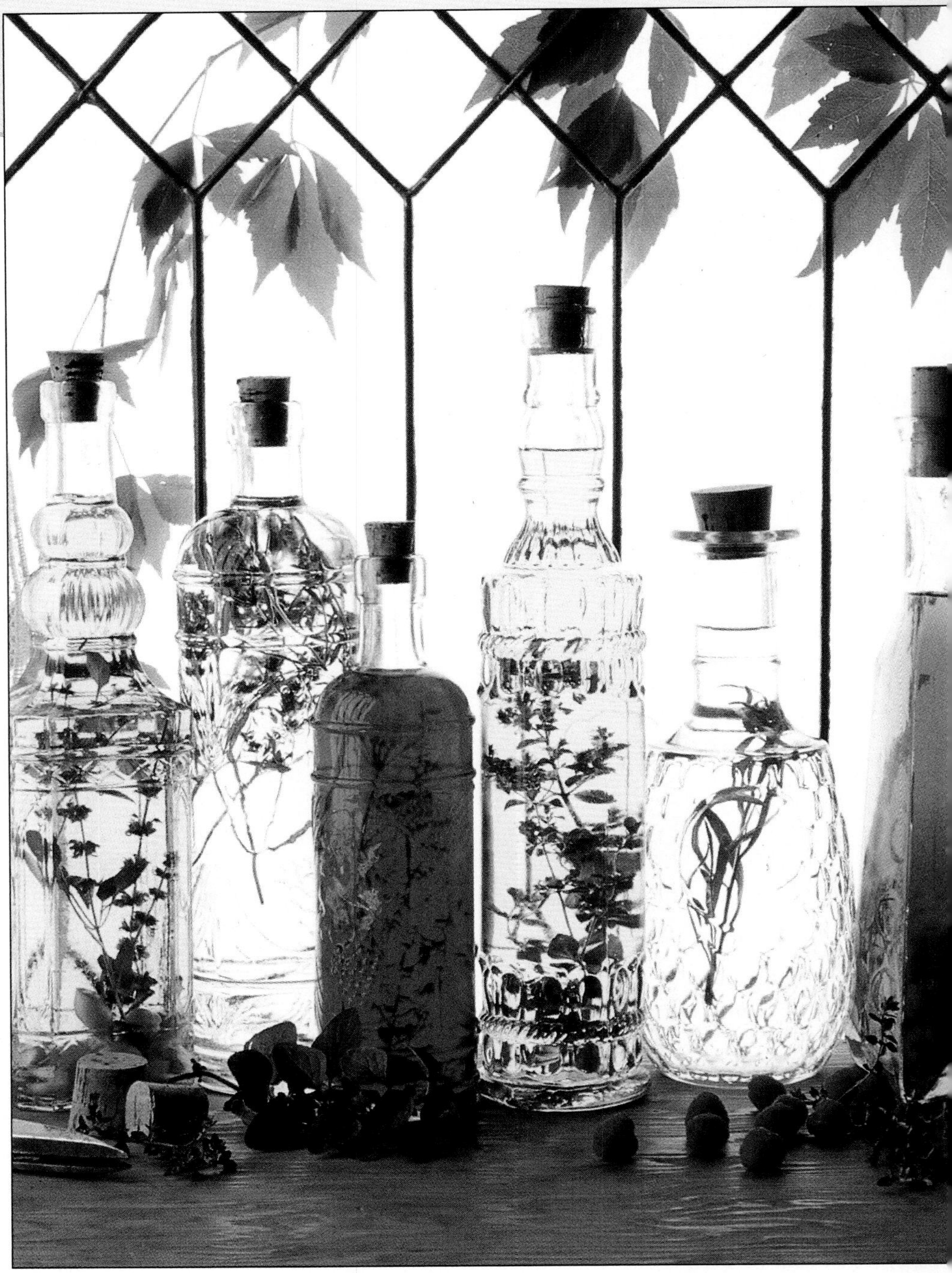

(Carol Guenzi Agents /Index Stock Photography)

Lipids: How Much of a Good Thing?

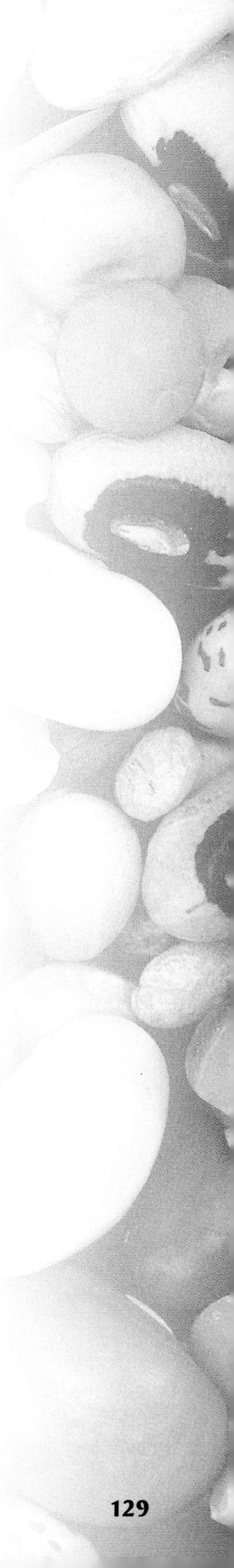

Chapter Concepts

1. Lipids, often referred to as fats, add flavor to food and provide a concentrated source of energy.
2. Most people in North America consume more fat and saturated fat than is recommended.
3. The major types of lipids in the body are fatty acids, glycerides, phospholipids, and sterols.
4. Fatty acids are made of chains of carbons. The length of the chain and the types and locations of the carbon-carbon bonds affect their characteristics in food and functions in the body.
5. Triglycerides (triacylglycerols) provide a concentrated source of energy in our food and in our bodies. They are composed of three fatty acids attached to a glycerol backbone.
6. Phosphoglycerides are important because they dissolve in both water and lipids; they are composed of two fatty acids and a phosphate group attached to a glycerol backbone.
7. Cholesterol is a sterol that is both made in the body and consumed in the diet.
8. For transport in the blood, lipids combine with protein to form lipoproteins.
9. Diets high in some types of fat are associated with an increased risk of heart disease and cancers of the breast, colon, and prostate.
10. Public health guidelines recommend a reduction in total fat, saturated fat, and cholesterol intake, and an increase in the consumption of grains, vegetables, and fruits, to reduce the risks of developing chronic disease.
11. During food processing, fats may be added to foods, and the fats in food may be modified, to change the stability or shelf life of the product.
12. A number of artificial fats have been developed that add texture and taste without increasing the fat in foods.

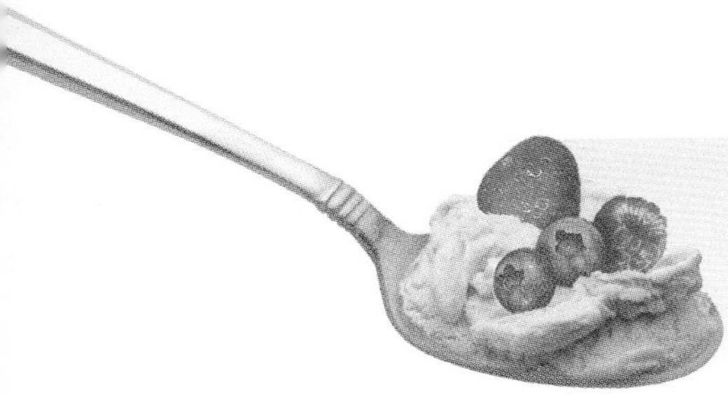

Just a Taste

Which is better for you: butter, margarine, or olive oil?

Is fat more fattening than other nutrients?

Will reducing your fat intake eliminate your risk of heart disease?

Should you put butter or margarine on your toast? Should you use canola or corn oil in cooking? There are hundreds of oils and butters and margarines from which to choose. Some are solid, some are liquid, some come from plants, some come from animals. Which are healthier for your heart? For reducing your risk of cancer? For your budget? Consumers need to know what foods to choose, which fats, if any, to avoid, and how to negotiate the obstacle course of advertising and product availability to make appropriate dietary choices.

The relationship between the amount and the type of dietary fat needed to optimize health is complicated. Epidemiological studies have shown that, in general, countries that have high intakes of fat and saturated fat tend to have higher incidences of heart disease and certain types of cancer. Yet not all countries follow this trend. Some Mediterranean countries have a high fat intake and yet the incidence of heart disease is extremely low.

How much fat and what type of fat should we be consuming? Fat is high in energy and promotes body fat storage, which is undesirable for weight management. Saturated fat and trans fat may increase the risk of heart disease. Polyunsaturated vegetable oils may reduce heart disease risk but promote certain types of cancers. Monounsaturates may reduce heart disease and breast cancer risk. So which fat should you choose? This chapter describes the types of fats, the risks and benefits associated with their intake, and the role of fat in the diet as a whole.

Lipid A group of organic molecules, most of which do not dissolve in water. They include fatty acids, glycerides, phospholipids, and sterols.

What Are Lipids?

Lipid is the chemical term for what is commonly known as fats or oils. They contribute to the texture, flavor, and aroma of our food. It is the high fat content of ice cream that gives it its smooth texture and rich taste. Olive oil imparts a unique taste to salads, and sesame oil gives Chinese food its distinctive aroma.

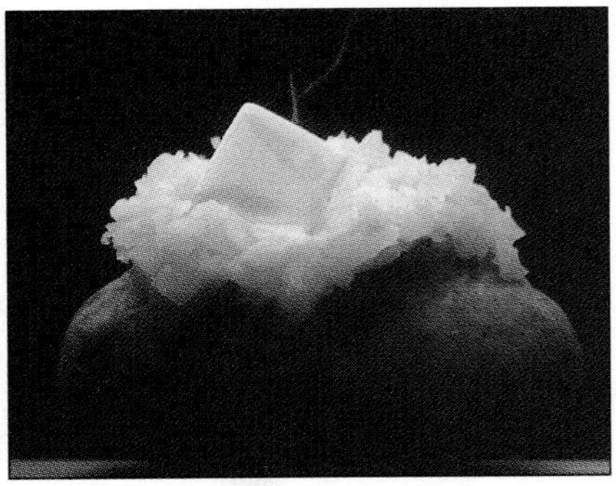

Figure 5.1
Butter on a hot baked potato is a visible source of dietary fat. (© Picture Perfect)

In our diets, some sources of fat are obvious, such as the fat on the outside of a cut of meat, or a pat of butter melting on a hot baked potato (Figure 5.1). Other fats are hidden. Baked goods such as cakes and cookies are usually high in fat, as are crackers, croissants, and some muffins. Even milk and cheese can be high in fat (Figure 5.2).

In the body, lipids have a number of essential roles in addition to providing a concentrated source of energy. Each gram of fat provides 9 kcalories, compared

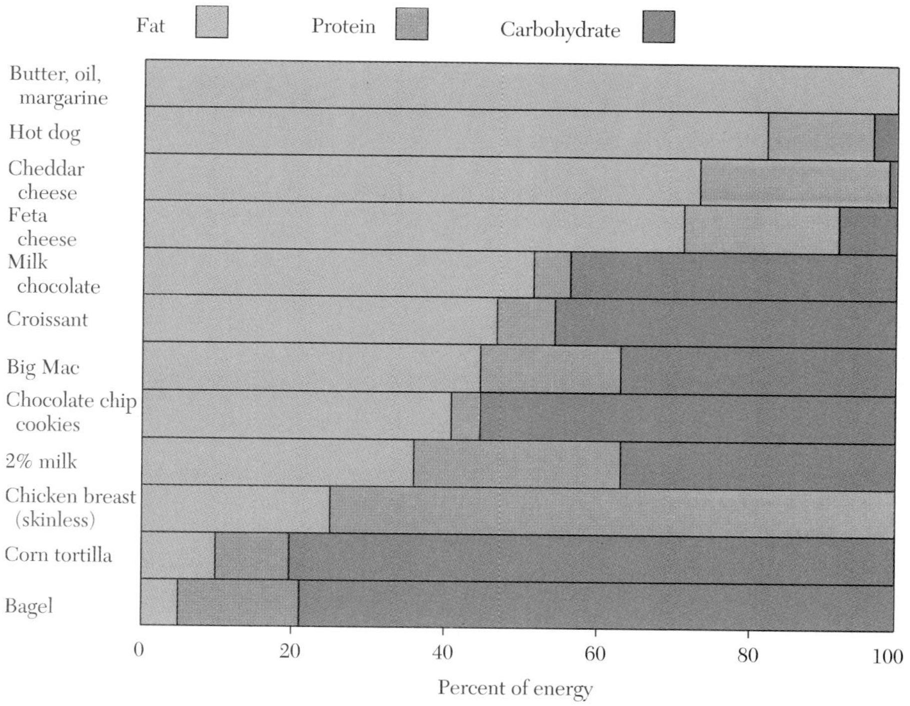

Figure 5.2
These foods all contain some fat, and most are also sources of protein or carbohydrate.

with only 4 kcalories per gram from carbohydrate or protein. Lipids found in the body and in the diet include fatty acids, glycerides, phospholipids, and sterols. Each has a different structure and function.

Fatty Acids

A **fatty acid** is a chain of carbon atoms linked together by chemical bonds. Fatty acids are typically found bound to other molecules. For example, most fatty acids in foods and in the body are bound to glycerol to form triglycerides.

Fatty acid An organic molecule made up of a chain of carbons linked to hydrogens with an acid group at one end.

The carbon chains of fatty acids vary in length from a few to 20 or more carbons. Each carbon atom forms four bonds to link it to four other atoms. If a carbon is not bound to four other atoms, double bonds are formed. At one end of the carbon chain, the omega or methyl end, the carbon atom is attached to another carbon and three hydrogens (CH_3); at the other end of the chain is an acid group formed by joining the carbon to an oxygen by a double bond and an OH group (COOH). Each of the carbons between is attached to two other carbons and up to two hydrogens (Figure 5.3).

Categories of Fatty Acids Fatty acids are categorized based on the number of carbons in their carbon chain as well as the types and locations of bonds between the carbons. These structural features affect their physical properties. One way to categorize fatty acids is by chain length. Short chain fatty acids range from four to seven carbons in length. They remain liquid at colder temperatures. For example, the short chain fatty acids in whole milk remain liquid even in the refrigerator. Medium chain fatty acids, such as those in coconut oil, range from 8 to 12 carbons. They solidify in the refrigerator but remain liquid at room temperature. Long chain fatty acids (greater than 12 carbons), such as those in beef fat, usually remain solid at room temperature. Most fatty acids in plants and animals, including humans, contain between 14 and 22 carbons.

Fatty acids are also categorized by the types of bonds between carbons in the chain. A fatty acid in which the chain is saturated with hydrogens so that each carbon has two hydrogens bound to it is called a **saturated fatty acid.** The most common saturated fatty acids are palmitic acid, which has 16 carbons, and stearic

Saturated fatty acid A fatty acid in which the carbon atoms are bound to as many hydrogens as possible and which therefore contains no carbon-carbon double bonds.

Figure 5.3
The structure of common saturated, monounsaturated, and polyunsaturated fatty acids.

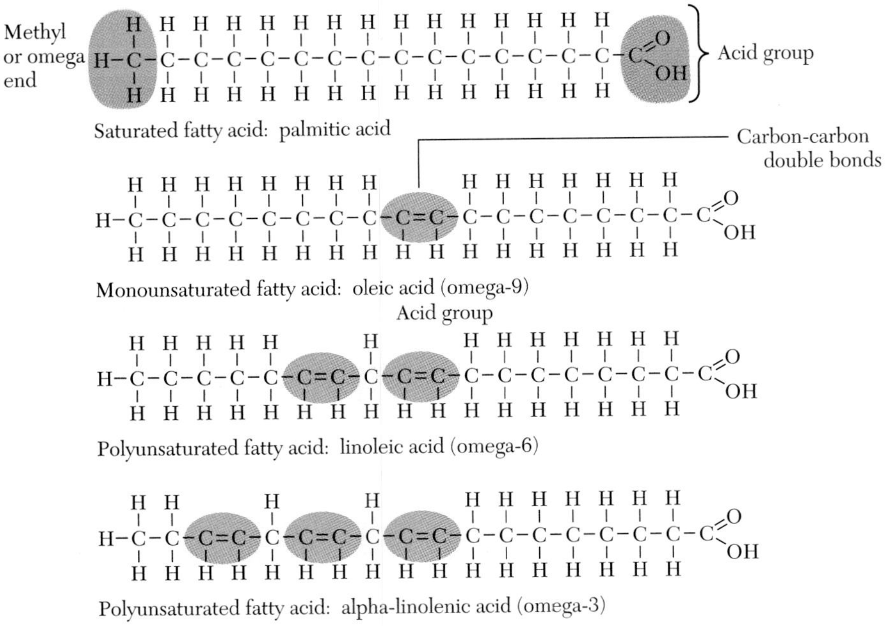

acid, which has 18 carbons. These are found most often in animal foods such as meat and dairy products. Vegetable sources of saturated fatty acids include palm oil, palm kernel oil, and coconut oil. These are often called **tropical oils** because they are found in plants common in tropical climates.

Tropical oils A term used in the popular press to refer to the saturated oils—coconut, palm, and palm kernel oil—that are derived from plants grown in tropical regions.

Unsaturated fatty acid A fatty acid that contains one or more carbon-carbon double bonds.

Monounsaturated fatty acid A fatty acid that contains one carbon-carbon double bond.

Polyunsaturated fatty acid A fatty acid that contains two or more carbon-carbon double bonds.

An **unsaturated fatty acid** contains some carbons that are not saturated with hydrogens. The carbons within the chain contain double bonds formed between carbons that are bound to only one hydrogen (see Figure 5.3). A fatty acid containing one double bond in its carbon chain is called a **monounsaturated fatty acid.** In our diets, the most common monounsaturated fatty acid is oleic acid, which is prevalent in olive and canola oils. A fatty acid with more than one double bond in its carbon chain is said to be a **polyunsaturated fatty acid.** The most common polyunsaturated fatty acid is linoleic acid, found in corn, safflower, and soybean oils. Unsaturated fatty acids melt at cooler temperatures than saturated fatty acids of the same chain length. Therefore, the more unsaturated bonds a fatty acid contains, the more likely it is to be liquid at room temperature. For example, margarine, which has more unsaturated bonds than butter, is more likely to melt at room temperature. Fats in our diets contain combinations of saturated, monounsaturated, and polyunsaturated fatty acids.

There are different categories of unsaturated fatty acids, depending on the location of the first double bond in the chain. If the first double bond occurs between the third and fourth carbons, counting from the omega (CH_3) end of the chain (see Figure 5.3), the fat is said to be an **omega-3 (ω-3) fatty acid.** Alpha-linolenic acid, found in vegetable oils, and eicosapentaenoic acid (EPA) and docosahexaenoic acid (DHA), found in fish oils, are omega-3 fatty acids. If the first double bond occurs between the sixth and seventh carbons (from the omega end), the fatty acid is called an **omega-6 (ω-6) fatty acid.** Linoleic acid, found in corn and safflower oils, is the major omega-6 fatty acid in the North American diet.

Omega-3 (ω-3) fatty acid A fatty acid containing a carbon-carbon double bond between the third and fourth carbons from the omega end.

Omega-6 (ω-6) fatty acid A fatty acid containing a carbon-carbon double bond between the sixth and seventh carbons from the omega end.

The position of the hydrogen atoms around a double bond is another way of classifying unsaturated fatty acids. Most unsaturated fatty acids found in nature have both hydrogen atoms on the same side of the double bond, called the *cis* configuration. When the hydrogens are on opposite sides of the double bond, called the *trans* configuration, the fatty acid is a **trans fatty acid** (Figure 5.4). A trans fatty acid has a higher melting point than the same fatty acid in the *cis* con-

Trans fatty acid An unsaturated fatty acid in which the hydrogens are on opposite sides of the double bond.

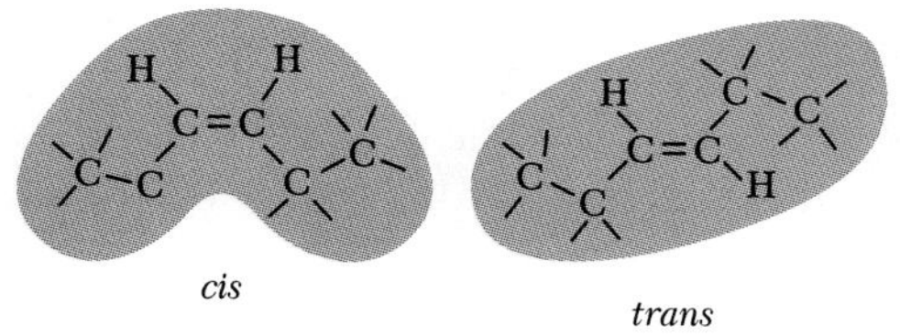

Figure 5.4
The orientation of hydrogens around the double bond distinguishes *cis* and *trans* fatty acids. In *cis* fatty acids, the hydrogens are on the same side of the double bond and cause a bend in the carbon chain. In *trans* fatty acids the hydrogens are on opposite sides of the double bond and the carbon chain is straighter.

figuration. Trans fatty acids are found in small amounts in nature and are formed during the **hydrogenation** of vegetable oils.[1] For instance, margarine containing **partially hydrogenated vegetable oil** is made by adding hydrogen atoms to some of the unsaturated bonds in vegetable oil. During the process, some of the remaining unsaturated bonds are converted from the *cis* to the *trans* configuration. The resulting product is semisolid at room temperature and contains more trans fatty acids than the original oil.

Hydrogenation The process whereby hydrogens are added to the carbon-carbon double bonds of unsaturated fatty acids, making them more saturated.

Partially hydrogenated vegetable oil Vegetable oil that has been modified by hydrogenation to decrease the number of unsaturated bonds, therefore raising the melting point and improving the storage characteristics.

Essential Fatty Acids The body is capable of synthesizing most of the fatty acids it needs from glucose or other sources of carbon, hydrogen, and oxygen. However, humans are not able to synthesize double bonds in the omega-6 and omega-3 positions. Therefore, the fatty acids, linoleic acid (omega-6), and alpha-linolenic acid (omega-3), are **essential fatty acids.** They must be consumed in the diet to make other omega-6 and omega-3 fatty acids. Omega-6 fatty acids are important for growth, skin integrity, fertility, and maintaining red blood cell structure. Omega-3 fatty acids are important for the structure and function of cell membranes, particularly in the retina of the eye and the central nervous system. If these are not consumed in adequate amounts, an **essential fatty acid deficiency** will result. Symptoms include scaly, dry skin, liver abnormalities, poor healing of wounds, growth failure in infants, and impaired vision and hearing. Essential fatty acid deficiency is rare because the requirement for essential fatty acids is well below the typical intake. Deficiencies have been seen in infants and young children fed lowfat diets, individuals who are unable to absorb lipids, and in adults consuming a weight-loss diet consisting of only skim milk.

Essential fatty acids Fatty acids that must be consumed in the diet because they cannot be made by the body or cannot be made in sufficient quantities to meet needs.

Essential fatty acid deficiency A condition characterized by dry scaly skin and poor growth that results when the diet does not supply sufficient amounts of the essential fatty acids.

There are some fatty acids needed in the body that are synthesized from the essential fatty acids. If the diet is low in linoleic acid or alpha-linolenic acid, the fatty acids synthesized from them become dietary essentials. Arachidonic acid is an omega-6 fatty acid synthesized from linoleic acid. Arachidonic acid is considered essential only when the diet is low in linoleic acid. It is found in both animal and vegetable fats. EPA and DHA are omega-3 fatty acids synthesized from alpha-linolenic acid. Arachidonic and DHA are necessary for normal brain development in infants and young children. The rate at which these are synthesized may not be sufficient to meet body needs, particularly in preterm infants.[2]

Glycerides

Most fatty acids in food and in the body are found attached to a backbone of the three-carbon molecule glycerol. When three fatty acids are attached, the molecule is called a **triacylglycerol,** commonly known as a **triglyceride** (Figure 5.5). When one fatty acid is attached, the molecule is called a **monoacylglycerol,** or **monoglyceride,** and when two fatty acids are attached, it is a **diacylglycerol,** or **diglyceride.** Triglycerides may contain any combination of fatty acids: long, medium, or short chain, saturated or unsaturated. Triglycerides make up most of the lipids in our food and in our bodies and are usually what are referred to when the term "fat" is used.

Triacylglycerol (triglyceride) The major form of lipid in food and in the body. It consists of three fatty acids attached to a glycerol molecule. When only one fatty acid is attached, it is a **monoacylglycerol** or **monoglyceride,** and when two are attached, it is a **diacylglycerol** or **diglyceride.**

The types of fatty acids in triglycerides determine their texture, taste, and physical characteristics. For example, the triglycerides in red meat contain predominantly long chain saturated fatty acids; thus the fat on a piece of steak is solid

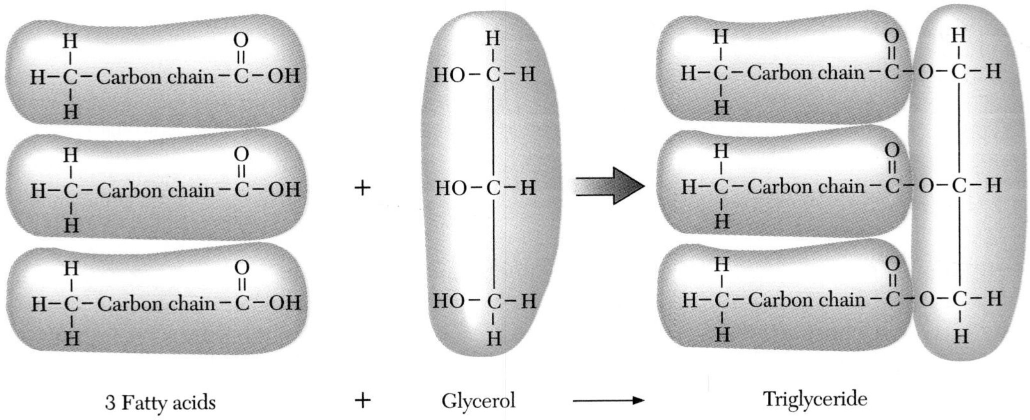

Figure 5.5
A triglyceride (triacylglycerol) is three fatty acids attached to a molecule of glycerol.

at room temperature. The amounts and types of fatty acids in chocolate allow it to remain brittle at room temperature, snap when bitten into, and then melt quickly and smoothly in the mouth (Figure 5.6).

Phosphoglycerides A type of phospholipid composed of a glycerol backbone with two fatty acids and a phosphate group attached.

Emulsifiers Substances that allow water and fat to mix.

Lipid bilayer Two layers of phosphoglyceride molecules oriented so that the fat-soluble fatty acid tails are sandwiched between the water-soluble phosphate-containing heads.

Lecithin A phosphoglyceride composed of a glycerol backbone, two fatty acids, a phosphate group, and a molecule of choline.

Cholesterol A lipid made only by animal cells that consists of multiple chemical rings.

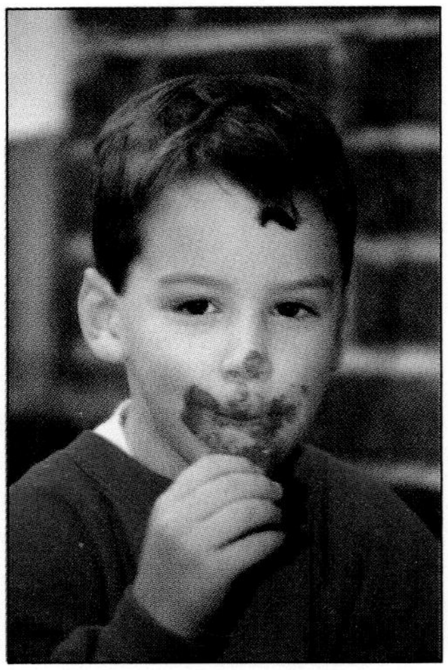

Figure 5.6
Because of its fatty acid content, chocolate is solid at cold temperatures but melts rapidly at body temperature. (George Semple)

Phospholipids

Phospholipids are lipids attached to a chemical group containing phosphorus called a phosphate group. The **phosphoglycerides** are the major class of phospholipids. Like triglycerides, they have a backbone of glycerol. However, they have only two fatty acids attached. In place of the third fatty acid is a phosphate group, which is then attached to a variety of other molecules. The fatty acid end of phosphoglycerides is soluble in fat, whereas the phosphate end is water soluble. This allows phosphoglycerides to mix in both water and fat—a property that makes them important for many functions in foods and in the body.

In foods, the ability of phospholipids to mix in water and fat allows them to act as **emulsifiers,** substances that allow water and fat to mix by breaking large fat globules into smaller ones. Egg yolk, which contains phospholipids, functions as an emulsifier in food; the egg yolk in cake batter allows the oil and water to mix. In the body, cell membranes contain phospholipids that form a **lipid bilayer,** allowing an aqueous (water) environment both inside and outside the cell with a lipid environment sandwiched between them (Figure 5.7).

The specific function of a phosphoglyceride depends on the molecule that is attached to the phosphate group. If a molecule of choline is attached, the phosphoglyceride is **lecithin.** In the body, lecithin is a major constituent of cell membranes and is required for their optimal function. It is also used to synthesize the neurotransmitter acetylcholine, which is important in the memory center of the brain. Based on these functions, lecithin is marketed to consumers as a supplement that improves memory and maintains proper cell function. However, lecithin is made in ample amounts by the body, and large doses in supplements have been shown to cause gastrointestinal upsets, sweating, and loss of appetite.[3] Eggs and soybeans are natural sources of lecithin. Lecithin is also used by the food industry as an additive to margarine, salad dressings, chocolate, frozen desserts, and baked goods to keep the oil from separating from the other ingredients.

Sterols

Structurally, sterols are composed of multiple rings, which makes them very different from triglycerides and phosphoglycerides. Like other lipids, they do not dissolve well in water. **Cholesterol** is probably the best-known sterol (Figure 5.8). In the diet, cholesterol is found only in foods from animal sources. Egg yolks

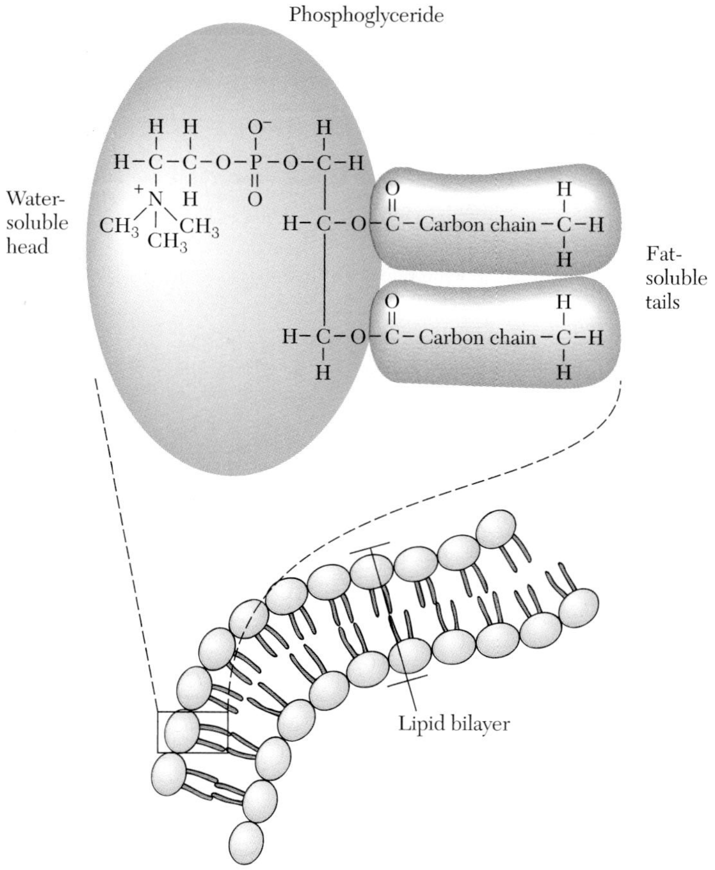

Figure 5.7
Phosphoglycerides, such as the lecithin molecule shown here, consist of a water-soluble head containing a phosphate group and a lipid-soluble tail of fatty acids. In cell membranes, phosphoglycerides form a lipid bilayer by orienting the water-soluble portion toward the water environment of the cell.

and organ meats such as liver and kidney are high in cholesterol. One egg yolk contains about 213 mg of cholesterol. Organ meats contain about 300 mg per 3-ounce (85 g) serving. Lean red meats and skinless chicken contain about 90 mg, whereas fish contains 50 mg in 3 ounces. Plant foods do not contain cholesterol unless animal products are combined with them in cooking or processing.

Cholesterol is necessary in the body, but because it is manufactured by the liver, it is not essential in the diet. More than 90% of the cholesterol in the body is found in cell membranes. It is also part of myelin, the coating on many nerve cells. Cholesterol is needed to synthesize vitamin D in the skin; cholic acid, a component of bile; and some hormones, such as testosterone and estrogen, which promote growth and the development of sex characteristics, and cortisol, which promotes glucose synthesis in the liver. The drugs known as **anabolic steroids,** which mimic the action of hormones that stimulate muscle growth, are also sterols. Their use has been popular in athletes trying to increase muscle strength and muscle mass; however, their use is illegal and can cause liver damage and other negative long-term health effects (see Chapter 12).

Anabolic steroids Synthetic fat-soluble hormones used by some athletes to increase muscle mass.

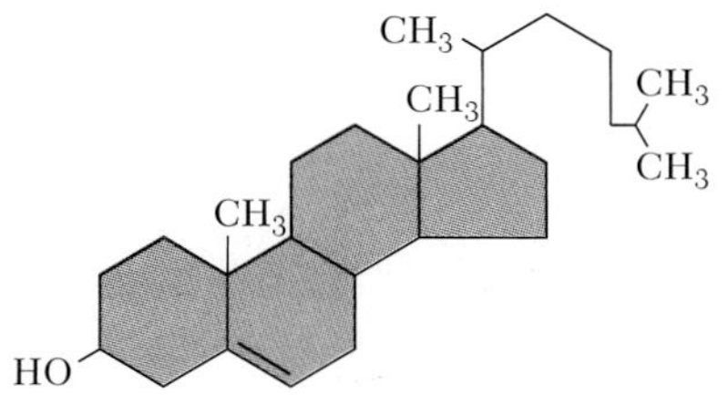

Figure 5.8
Cholesterol structure. The four colored rings indicate the backbone structure common to all sterols.

Lipids in the Digestive Tract

Some lipid digestion begins in the stomach due to the action of lipases produced in the mouth and stomach. These enzymes work best on triglycerides containing short and medium chain fatty acids such as those in milk, and so are particularly important in infants.[4] In healthy adults, most of the digestion of dietary fat takes place in the small intestine due to the action of lipases secreted by the pancreas

Figure 5.9
An overview of lipid digestion and absorption.

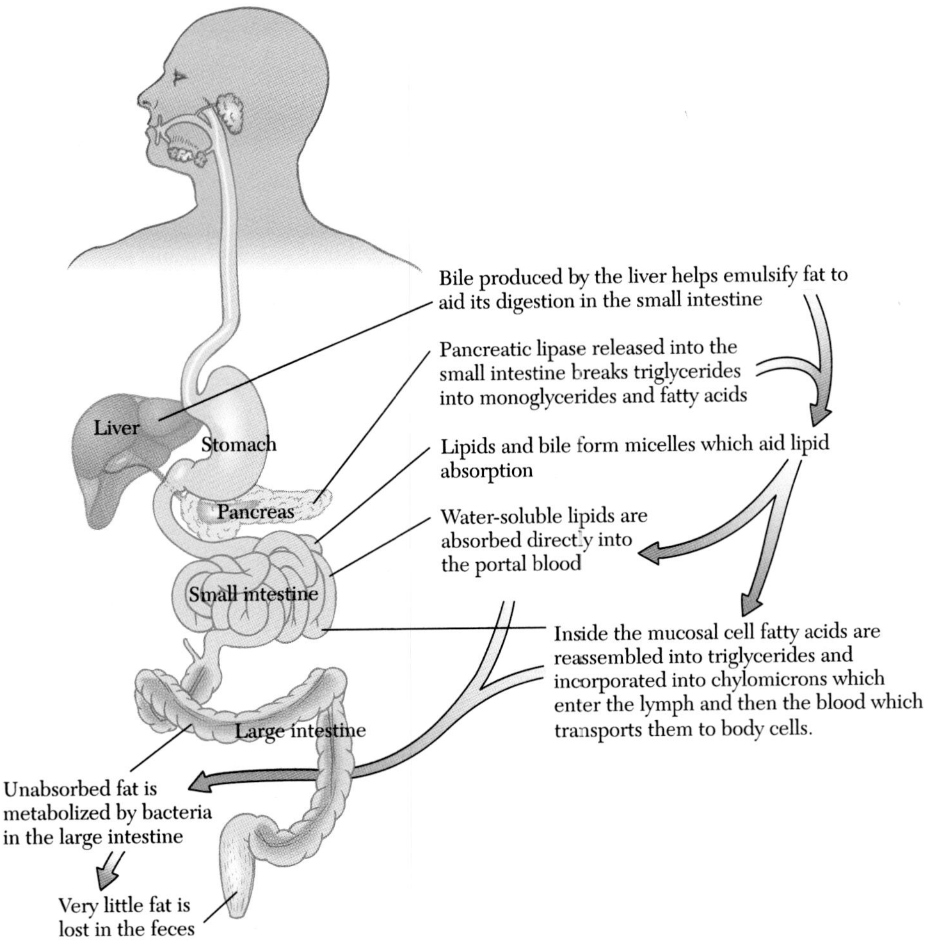
Liver
Stomach
Pancreas
Small intestine
Large intestine
Bile produced by the liver helps emulsify fat to aid its digestion in the small intestine
Pancreatic lipase released into the small intestine breaks triglycerides into monoglycerides and fatty acids
Lipids and bile form micelles which aid lipid absorption
Water-soluble lipids are absorbed directly into the portal blood
Inside the mucosal cell fatty acids are reassembled into triglycerides and incorporated into chylomicrons which enter the lymph and then the blood which transports them to body cells.
Unabsorbed fat is metabolized by bacteria in the large intestine
Very little fat is lost in the feces

Micelles Particles formed in the small intestine when droplets of lipid are surrounded by bile acids.

(Figure 5.9). Here, bile from the gallbladder emulsifies fat to form **micelles.** Micelles have a fat-soluble center surrounded by a coating of bile acids (Figure 5.10). Bile acids allow water-soluble enzymes access to triglycerides, and micelles facilitate the absorption of lipids into the mucosal cells. Triglycerides are digested primarily into monoglycerides and fatty acids that diffuse into the mucosal cell when the micelle comes in contact with the intestinal brush border. These processes, necessary for fat digestion and absorption, are also necessary for the absorption of the fat-soluble vitamins, as well as of other fat-soluble molecules present in foods, such as beta-carotene. These lipid-soluble molecules must be incorporated into micelles to be absorbed and therefore their absorption depends on the presence of dietary fat. Most of the bile acids in micelles are also absorbed and returned to the liver, where they can be reused.

LIPIDS IN THE BODY

Adipose tissue Tissue found under the skin and around body organs that is composed of fat-storing cells.

In the body, lipids can be used as an immediate source of energy or stored for future use. Most lipids in the body are triglycerides stored in **adipose tissue** that lies under the skin and around internal organs. Because triglycerides are a concentrated energy source (9 kcal/g), a large amount of energy can be stored without a great increase in body size or weight. Adipose tissue also insulates the body from changes in temperature, and provides a cushion to protect against shock.

Eicosanoids Regulatory molecules that can be synthesized from omega-3 and omega-6 fatty acids.

Lipids are an important structural component of cells, particularly in the brain and nervous system. As components of all cell membranes, lipids protect the internal environment of cells. Lipids also have a regulatory role. Both omega-3 and omega-6 fatty acids are precursors of compounds called **eicosanoids** that help regulate blood clotting, blood pressure, immune function, and other body

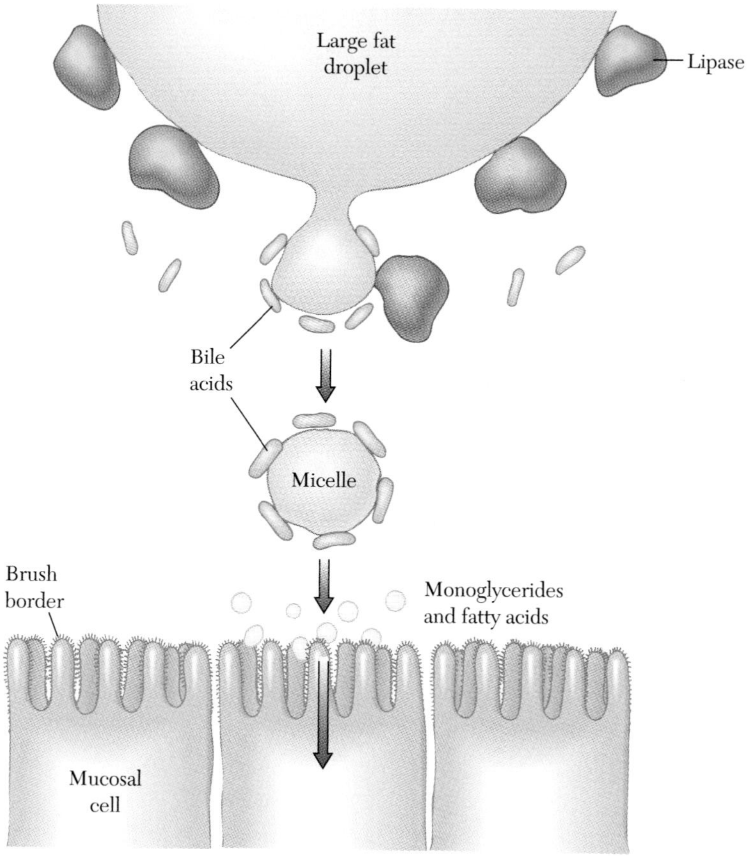

Figure 5.10
Bile acids help break fats into small droplets called micelles that facilitate the absorption of monoglycerides and fatty acids into the mucosal cells of the small intestine.

processes.[5] The effect of an eicosanoid depends on the fatty acid from which it is made. For example, when the omega-6 fatty acid arachidonic acid is the starting material, the eicosanoid synthesized increases blood clotting; when the eicosanoid is made from the omega-3 fatty acid EPA, it decreases blood clotting. The correct ratio of the two is necessary to allow appropriate blood clotting.

Transporting Lipids in the Body

Because most lipids are not soluble in water, they require unique handling to be transported through the aqueous bloodstream to reach the cells of the body. Some fat-soluble vitamins are transported along with dietary lipids while others utilize different methods of transport. Water-insoluble lipids are transported through the blood, coated in a water-soluble envelope created when the lipids combine with phospholipids and proteins to form transport particles called **lipoproteins.** Lipoproteins help transport both dietary lipids from the small intestine and stored or newly synthesized lipids from the liver.

Lipoproteins Particles containing a core of lipids surrounded by a shell of protein and phospholipid that transport lipids in blood and lymph.

Transport From the Small Intestine After absorption into the intestinal mucosal cells, lipids that are somewhat water soluble, such as short and medium chain fatty acids and phospholipids, can enter the blood. Lipids that are not soluble in water, such as long chain fatty acids and cholesterol, cannot enter the bloodstream directly. Absorbed monoglycerides and long chain fatty acids are first resynthesized into triglycerides by the mucosal cell. These triglycerides are then combined with cholesterol, phospholipids, and a small amount of protein to form lipoproteins called **chylomicrons.** Chylomicrons are absorbed into the lymphatic system and then enter the bloodstream without first passing through the liver.

Chylomicrons Lipoproteins that transport lipids from the mucosal cells of the intestine to other body cells.

As chylomicrons circulate in the blood, the enzyme **lipoprotein lipase,** present on the surface of the cells lining the blood vessels, breaks the triglycerides down into fatty acids and glycerol, which enter the surrounding cells. The fatty

Lipoprotein lipase An enzyme attached to cell membranes that breaks down triglycerides into fatty acids and glycerol.

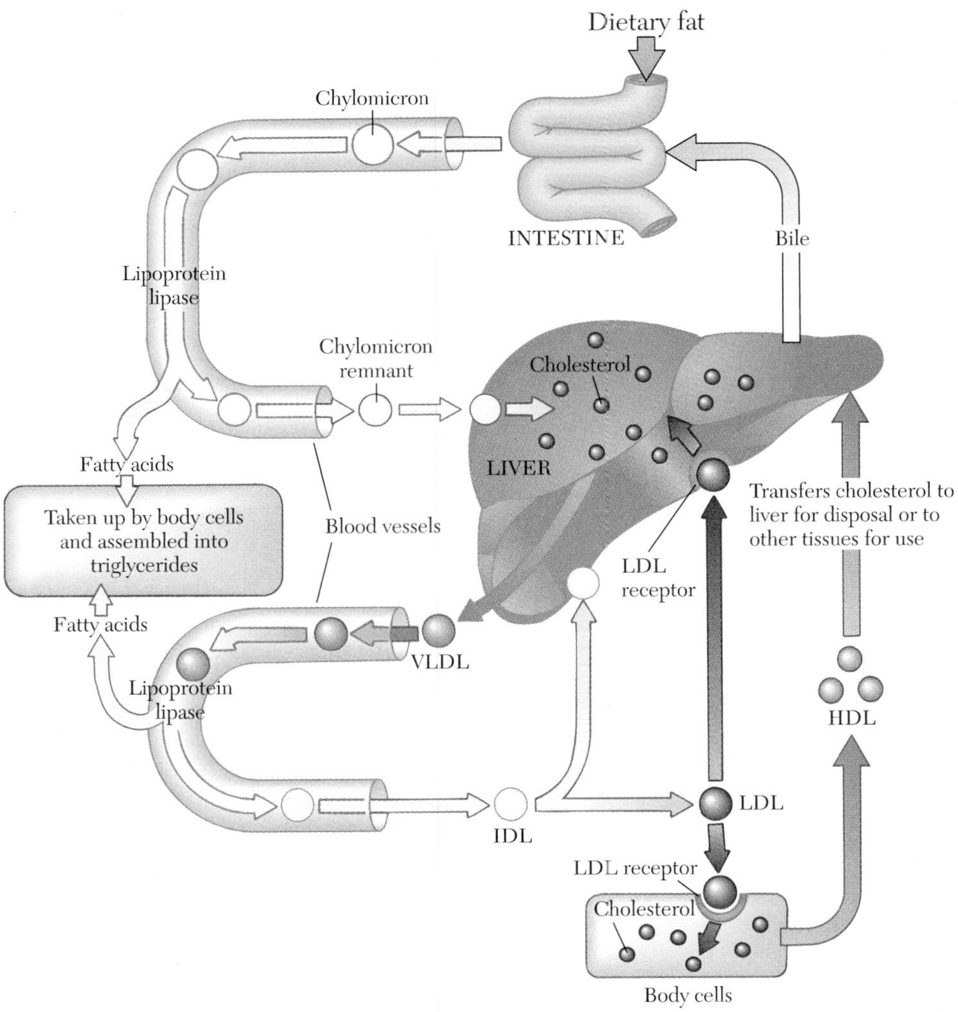

Figure 5.11
Chylomicrons carry lipids from the intestines and deliver triglycerides to body cells. VLDLs carry lipids from the liver and deliver triglycerides to body cells. LDLs are derived from IDLs and are the primary cholesterol delivery system for body cells. HDLs carry cholesterol away from cells to the liver.

acids can be either used as fuel or resynthesized into triglycerides for storage. What remains of the chylomicron is a chylomicron remnant composed mostly of cholesterol and protein. This goes to the liver and is disassembled (Figure 5.11).

Transport From the Liver The liver is the major lipid-producing organ in the body. Here excess protein, carbohydrate, or alcohol can be broken down and used to make triglycerides or cholesterol. Triglycerides made in the liver are incorporated into lipoprotein particles called **very-low-density lipoproteins (VLDLs).** Cholesterol synthesized in the liver or returned in chylomicron remnants can also be incorporated into VLDLs or can be used to make bile. VLDLs transport lipids out of the liver and deliver triglycerides to body cells. As with chylomicrons, the enzyme lipoprotein lipase breaks down the triglycerides in VLDLs so that the fatty acids can be taken up by surrounding cells. Once the triglycerides are removed from the VLDLs, a denser, smaller, intermediate-density lipoprotein (IDL) remains. About two thirds of the IDLs are returned to the liver, and the rest are transformed in the blood into **low-density lipoproteins (LDLs).** LDLs contain an even higher proportion of cholesterol than VLDLs and are the primary cholesterol delivery system for cells (Figure 5.12). High levels of LDLs in the blood have been associated with an increased risk for heart disease. For LDLs to be taken up by cells, a protein on the surface of the LDL particle must bind to a receptor protein on the cell membrane, called an **LDL receptor.** This binding allows LDLs to be removed from circulation and enter cells where their cholesterol and other components can be used (see Figure 5.11).

Very-low-density lipoproteins (VLDLs) Lipoproteins assembled by the liver that carry lipid from the liver and deliver triglycerides to body cells.

Low-density lipoproteins (LDLs) Lipoproteins that transport cholesterol to cells. Elevated LDL cholesterol increases the risk of cardiovascular disease.

LDL receptor A protein on the surface of cells that binds to LDL particles and allows their contents to be taken up for use by the cell.

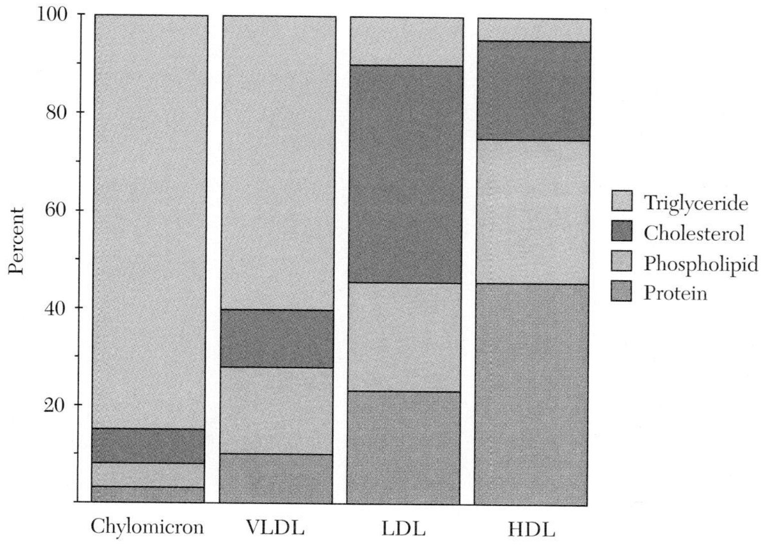

Figure 5.12

All lipoproteins consist of a shell of phospholipid, protein, and cholesterol and a center of triglycerides and cholesterol, but they vary in size and density. Particles with proportionately more triglyceride and less protein are larger and less dense. Chylomicrons are the largest, least-dense particles and contain the most triglyceride, whereas HDLs are the smallest, densest particles and have the greatest percentage of protein.

Since most body cells have no system for breaking down cholesterol, it must be returned to the liver to be eliminated from the body. This reverse cholesterol transport is accomplished by the densest of the lipoprotein particles, called **high-density lipoproteins (HDLs).** These particles originate from the intestinal tract and liver and circulate in the blood, picking up cholesterol from other lipoproteins and body cells. They function as a temporary storage site for lipid. Some of the cholesterol in HDLs is taken directly to the liver for disposal, and some is transferred to organs that have a high requirement for cholesterol, such as those involved in steroid hormone synthesis. High levels of HDL in the blood are associated with a reduction in heart disease risk.

High-density lipoproteins (HDLs) Lipoproteins that pick up cholesterol from cells and transport it to the liver so that it can be eliminated from the body. A low level of HDL increases the risk of cardiovascular disease.

Lipid Metabolism: Fat for Fuel and for Storage

Fatty acids can be used directly for energy or reassembled into triglycerides for storage. In muscle cells, fatty acids and glycerol from triglycerides are used primarily to produce ATP. The carbon chain of fatty acids is broken into two-carbon units that form acetyl-CoA. Acetyl-CoA can then enter the citric acid cycle which passes electrons to the electron transport chain to generate ATP (Figure 5.13). The glycerol can also be used to produce ATP.

In adipose tissue cells, fatty acids are usually reassembled into triglycerides for storage. Throughout the day, stored triglycerides are continuously broken down and reformed depending on the immediate energy needs of the body. For example, after a meal, some triglyceride will be immediately stored; then between meals, some of the stored triglyceride will be broken down to provide energy. When the energy in the diet equals the body's energy requirements, the net amount of stored triglyceride in the body does not change.

Feasting When energy is ingested in excess of needs, the excess can be converted into triglycerides and stored in adipose tissue. Excess dietary fat is transported directly to the adipose tissue in chylomicrons. Excess dietary carbohydrate and protein must first go to the liver, where they can be used, although inefficiently, to synthesize fatty acids; these fatty acids are then assembled into triglycerides, which are transported to the adipose tissue in VLDLs. Lipoprotein lipase at the membrane of cells lining the blood vessels breaks down the triglycerides from both chylomicrons and VLDLs so that the fatty acids can enter the cells, where they are reassembled into triglycerides for storage (Figure 5.14). The ability of the body to store fat is theoretically limitless. Fat cells can increase in weight by about 50 times, and new fat cells can be made when existing cells reach their maximum size (see Chapter 7).

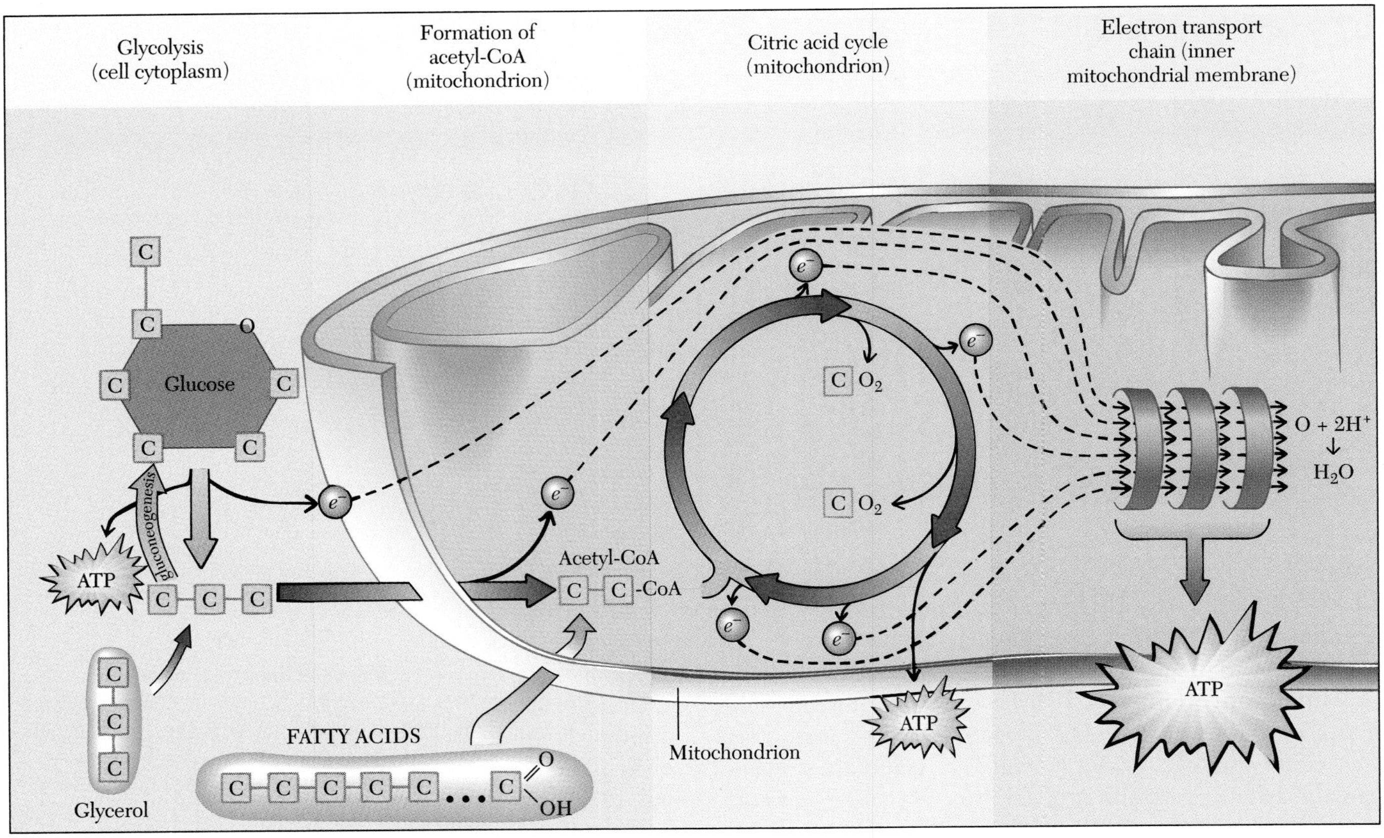

Figure 5.13
Triglycerides can be used to produce energy. Fatty acids break into two-carbon units and enter the citric acid cycle as acetyl-CoA. Glycerol is a three-carbon molecule that can be converted into pyruvate.

Hormone sensitive lipase An enzyme present in adipose cells that responds to chemical signals by breaking down triglycerides into fatty acids and glycerol for release into the bloodstream.

Fasting When less energy is consumed than is needed, the body obtains energy from fat stores. In this situation, the enzyme **hormone sensitive lipase** inside the fat cells receives a signal to break down stored triglycerides. The fatty acids and glycerol are released directly into the blood to be taken up by body cells to produce ATP. If there is not enough carbohydrate to allow acetyl-CoA from fat breakdown to enter the citric acid cycle, it will be used to make ketones (see Chapter 4). Some of these ketones can be used for fuel. For instance, the brain can adapt to use ketones to meet about half of its energy needs. For the other half, it must use glucose. Fatty acids cannot be used to make glucose, but a small amount of glucose can be made from glycerol.

LIPIDS AND HEALTH

Diets high in fat are associated with an increased risk for many chronic diseases. The development of cardiovascular disease has been linked to diets high in fat, especially saturated fat.[6] The risk of certain types of cancer, including that of the breast, colon, and prostate, has also been associated with fat intake.[7] Populations that have a high intake of total fat have a higher incidence of these cancers than populations that have a lower intake.[8] Obesity is also associated with diets high in fat because high-fat diets are usually high in energy and promote storage of body fat. Excess body fat in turn is associated with an increased risk of diabetes and high blood pressure.

In general, populations that consume high-fat diets have a higher incidence of heart disease,[9] but this does not always hold true. It is not only the amount of

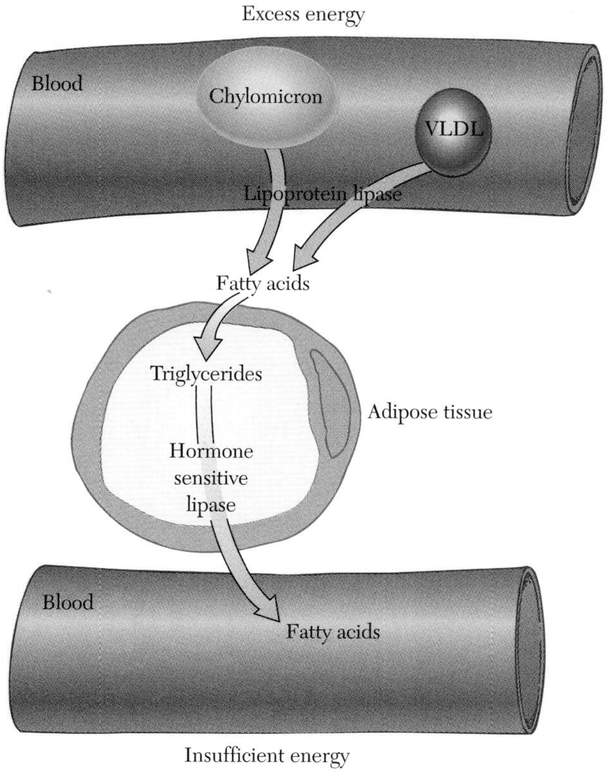

Figure 5.14
When excess dietary energy is available, lipoprotein lipase helps remove triglyceride from chylomicrons and VLDLs so it can be stored in adipose tissue. When dietary energy is insufficient, the enzyme hormone sensitive lipase helps break down stored triglycerides to make fatty acids available as an energy source.

fat that affects risk. The type of fat and other dietary and lifestyle factors are also important. Populations that consume a diet high in omega-3 fatty acids, such as the Inuits in Greenland, have a low incidence of heart disease.[10] In Mediterranean countries, where the diet is high in monounsaturated fat as well as grains and vegetables, deaths from both heart disease and cancer are low.[11,12] Thus, the type of fat consumed, in addition to the higher intake of grains and vegetables, and the active, low-stress lifestyles found in many Mediterranean populations may be as important as overall fat intake in reducing disease risk and maintaining health. Our understanding of how diet, and fat in particular, affects disease risk is still developing.

Dietary Fat and Heart Disease

Over 58 million people in the United States suffer from one or more forms of **cardiovascular disease,** which is any disease that affects the heart and blood vessels. There are many dietary and lifestyle factors associated with cardiovascular disease, including the intake of fat, saturated fat, fruits and vegetables, fiber, antioxidants, and phytochemicals, as well as smoking and activity level. The relationship between dietary fat, saturated fat, and heart disease risk is one that has been extensively studied.

Cardiovascular disease Any disease affecting the heart and blood vessels.

How Does Atherosclerosis Develop? **Atherosclerosis** is a type of cardiovascular disease in which lipids are deposited in the artery walls, reducing elasticity and eventually blocking the flow of blood. It was originally hypothesized that this was caused by dietary cholesterol transported into the bloodstream and deposited in the arteries.[13] Since this initial hypothesis, a great deal of research has been done to determine how cholesterol deposits form in arteries, how diet affects blood cholesterol levels, and whether changes in diet can decrease the risk of developing atherosclerosis.

Atherosclerosis A type of cardiovascular disease that involves the buildup of fatty material in the artery walls.

Our current understanding of how atherosclerosis develops is based on the work of Michael Brown and Joseph Goldstein, who were awarded the Nobel

Prize in 1985 for their discoveries. Their work identified LDL receptors on cells and demonstrated how they bind LDL particles in the blood, allowing them to be taken up by the cells. When LDL particles enter body cells, the amount of LDL cholesterol in the blood is reduced. If the amount of LDL cholesterol in the blood exceeds the amount that can be taken up by cells—due to either too much LDL cholesterol or too few LDL receptors—the result is a high level of LDL cholesterol.[14] Excess LDL cholesterol in the blood can lead to the deposition of cholesterol in the artery walls, causing atherosclerosis.

The exact events that cause the buildup of cholesterol in arterial walls are still not fully understood. One theory is that an injury to the arterial wall—possibly caused by high blood pressure, high cholesterol levels, microorganisms, chemicals, or some other factor—begins the process. Once the initial injury has occurred, LDL particles, white blood cells, and blood cell fragments involved in blood clotting (called platelets) enter the artery wall. Inside the artery wall, LDL

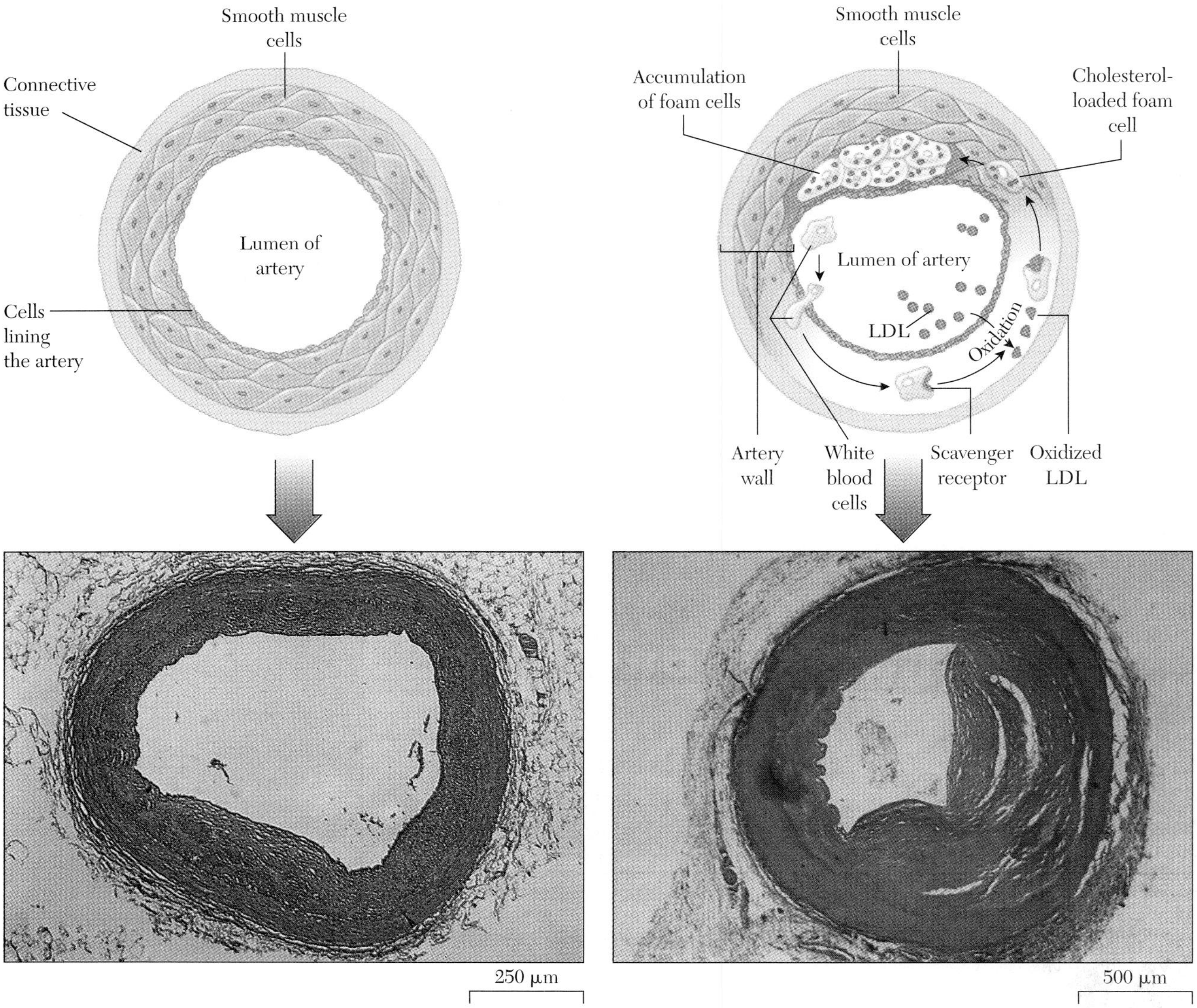

Figure 5.15

On the left are a drawing and photograph of a normal artery. On the right are a diagram showing the development of an atherosclerotic plaque and a photograph of a cross section of an artery blocked by atherosclerotic deposits. Plaque develops when white blood cells and LDL particles penetrate the artery wall. LDLs become oxidized and enter the white blood cells by binding to scavenger receptors. The cholesterol-filled white blood cells are transformed into foam cells that burst, depositing cholesterol in the artery wall. *(left,* © Cabisco/Visuals Unlimited; *right,* © Ober/Visuals Unlimited)

that comes in contact with highly reactive oxygen molecules is transformed into **oxidized LDL cholesterol.** Oxidized LDL cholesterol binds to scavenger receptors on the surface of white blood cells and is transported into these cells.[15] As white blood cells fill with more and more oxidized LDL cholesterol, the white blood cells are transformed into cholesterol-filled foam cells. Foam cells accumulate in the artery wall and then burst, depositing cholesterol to form a fatty streak. Platelets signal muscle cells to invade the fatty streak and secrete fibrous proteins. The result is a mass of cholesterol, muscle cells, and fibrous tissue called a **plaque** (Figure 5.15). Eventually, calcium collects in the plaque and causes it to harden. Blood clots form around the plaque and it continues to enlarge, causing the artery to narrow and lose its elasticity. The buildup of material can become so large that it completely blocks the artery, or a blood clot can break loose and block an artery elsewhere. When an artery is blocked, blood can no longer move through it to supply oxygen and nutrients to the cells, and they die quickly. If blood flow to the heart muscle is interrupted, heart cells die, resulting in a heart attack or myocardial infarction. If the blood flow to the brain is interrupted, a stroke results.

Oxidized LDL cholesterol A substance formed when the cholesterol in LDL particles is oxidized by reactive oxygen molecules. It is key in the development of atherosclerosis because it is taken up by scavenger receptors on white blood cells.

Plaque The cholesterol-rich material that is deposited in the blood vessels of individuals with atherosclerosis. It consists of cholesterol, smooth muscle cells, fibrous tissue, and calcium.

Risk Factors for Heart Disease High blood pressure, diabetes, obesity, and high blood cholesterol levels increase the risk of developing heart disease. Other factors that affect risk include age, gender, genetics, and lifestyle factors such as smoking, exercise, and diet. These may directly affect risk or act indirectly by altering blood cholesterol levels, blood pressure, body weight, or the risk of diabetes (see Table 5.1).

Table 5.1 *Factors That Affect Heart Disease Risk*

Age: Risk increases with increasing age.

Sex: Males have a higher risk until age 65, then risks do not differ between the sexes.

Disease factors:

Diabetes: fasting blood sugar greater than 180 mg/100 ml

High blood pressure: greater than 140/90

Obesity: body mass index greater than 27*

High blood lipid levels:

	Low Risk	Moderate Risk	High Risk
Total cholesterol (mg/100 ml)	<200	200–239	≥ 240
LDL cholesterol (mg/100 ml)	<130	130–159	≥ 160
HDL (mg/100 ml)	≥ 35	<35	<35

Lifestyle:

Cigarette smoking increases risk.

Regular exercise decreases risk.

Diet: Risk is increased by:

High total fat intake

High saturated fat intake

High cholesterol intake

Low intake of omega-3 fatty acids

High intake of trans fatty acids

Low fiber intake

Low intake of fruits and vegetables

Low intake of antioxidant nutrients such as vitamin E

*See Chapter 7 for information about body mass index and how it can be calculated.

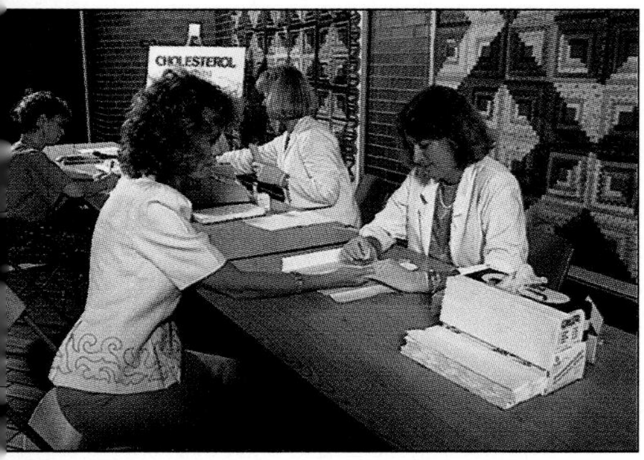

Figure 5.16
The National Cholesterol Education Program recommends that all adults have their blood cholesterol levels checked at least every five years. (© Blair Seitz/Photo Researchers, Inc.)

Diabetes, High Blood Pressure, Obesity, and Blood Cholesterol Levels The high levels of blood glucose that can occur in diabetes damage blood vessels, but even when blood glucose is under control, diabetes increases the risk of heart disease. Elevated blood pressure may damage blood vessels and make the heart work harder, causing it to enlarge and weaken over time. Obesity both increases the amount of work required by the heart and affects blood pressure, blood cholesterol levels, and the risk of diabetes. High blood cholesterol levels, and, in particular, high levels of LDL cholesterol, may also injure artery walls as well as promote plaque formation.

The desirable level for total blood cholesterol in adults is below 200 mg per 100 ml of blood. LDL levels should be below 130 mg per 100 ml. Since HDL cholesterol has a protective effect against heart disease, an HDL cholesterol level of 35 mg per 100 ml or greater is beneficial. Currently, 51% of American adults have blood cholesterol levels of 200 or more, and 20% have values of 240 mg per 100 ml or greater.[16] The National Cholesterol Education Program (NCEP), a nationwide program designed to evaluate and reduce the risks of heart disease, recommends that all adults have their blood lipids measured every five years (Figure 5.16).[17] Individuals with an LDL cholesterol level above 160 mg per 100 ml, and those with levels between 130 and 159 mg per 100 ml who also have heart disease or two other risk factors for heart disease, should begin a dietary program to reduce blood cholesterol levels.

Age, Gender, Genetics, and Lifestyle Factors The risk of heart disease increases with age; four out of five people who die of heart disease are 65 or older.[18] Men and women are both at risk, but men are generally affected a decade earlier than women.[19] This is due in part to the protective effect of the hormone estrogen in women. As women age, the effects of menopause—including the decline in estrogen level and gain in weight—increase heart disease risk. Although it is unclear why, the incidence of heart disease among men has been declining since the 1950s, whereas the incidence among women has increased.[20] Heart disease is currently the single largest killer of American women. Genetics, including ethnic background, also affect risk. Individuals with a male family member who exhibited heart disease before the age of 55 or a female family member who exhibited heart disease before the age of 65 are considered to be at greater risk. African Americans are at greater risk than other ethnic groups; the death rate from cardiovascular disease is 49% higher in African American men and 67% higher in African American women than among male and female Caucasians respectively.[16]

Age, gender, and genetics are risks that cannot be changed, but diet and lifestyle factors can be modified to reduce risk. The amount and type of fat consumed in the diet, as well as the intake of other nutrients, affect heart disease risk.[21] Some types of dietary lipids increase risk. Other lipids, as well as fiber, phytochemicals, and antioxidant vitamins and minerals, offer a protective effect. An inactive lifestyle increases the risk of heart disease, as do cigarette smoking and stress. On the other hand, regular exercise decreases risk by promoting the maintenance of a healthy body weight, reducing the risk of diabetes, increasing HDL cholesterol, and reducing blood pressure[22] (see *Critical Thinking: Dietary Fat and Heart Disease Risk*).

Dietary Factors That Promote Heart Disease Intakes of cholesterol, saturated fat, trans fatty acids, and excess energy tend to increase the risk of cardiovascular disease. Some or all of their effect is due to their influence on blood cholesterol levels.

Dietary Cholesterol The extent to which cholesterol intake affects blood levels depends on an individual's genes. Cholesterol in the blood comes from cholesterol both consumed in the diet and made by the liver. Generally, about three to four times more cholesterol is made by the body than is consumed in the diet. In some individuals, as dietary cholesterol increases, liver cholesterol synthesis decreases so that blood levels do not change.[23] In others, however, liver synthesis does not decrease in response to an increase in dietary cholesterol, so blood cholesterol levels rise.

Dietary Saturated Fat Diets high in some types of saturated fat increase LDL cholesterol in the blood. Increased LDL then increases the risk of atherosclerosis. It is hypothesized that when the diet is high in these saturated fatty acids, there are fewer LDL receptors in the liver, so that LDL cholesterol cannot be removed from the blood. When the diet is low in these saturated fats, the number of LDL receptors increases, allowing more cholesterol to be removed from the bloodstream.[24] There are some saturated fats, such as stearic acid found in chocolate and beef, that do not increase blood cholesterol levels.[25] However, these may contribute to heart disease by affecting blood platelets and blood clotting, both of which are involved in plaque formation.[26]

Trans Fatty Acids Both clinical and epidemiological studies provide evidence that trans fatty acid intake increases the risk of heart disease.[27] Epidemiological studies indicate that an increase in the amount of trans fatty acids in the diet increases the risk of heart disease even more than an equivalent increase in saturated fat.[21] Trans fatty acid intake increases blood cholesterol levels less than an equivalent amount of saturated fatty acids but more than the same amount of polyunsaturated fatty acids. Therefore when partially hydrogenated vegetable oils high in trans fatty acids replace unhydrogenated vegetable oils in the diet, the total and LDL cholesterol concentrations in the blood increase and HDL concentrations decrease.[27] When partially hydrogenated vegetable oils, such as those in stick margarine, replace fats rich in saturated fatty acids, such as those in butter, total as well as LDL and HDL cholesterol concentrations in the blood decrease.[28]

Excess Energy Excess energy intake increases the risk of heart disease because it increases body fat, which is a separate risk factor for elevated blood cholesterol levels, high blood pressure, diabetes, and heart disease in general. A reduction in body weight has been shown to reduce blood cholesterol levels, blood pressure, and heart disease risk, and to help control diabetes.[29]

Dietary Factors That Protect Against Heart Disease Both omega-6 and omega-3 polyunsaturated fats as well as monounsaturated fat, plant foods, and moderate alcohol consumption tend to decrease the risk of heart disease. Some reduce risk by reducing LDL cholesterol and increasing HDL cholesterol. Some protect against heart disease in other ways.

Dietary Polyunsaturated Fat: Omega-6 and Omega-3 When saturated fat in the diet is replaced by any type of polyunsaturated fat, there is a beneficial decrease in LDL cholesterol.[24] However, a high intake of omega-6 polyunsaturated fatty acids may also decrease HDL cholesterol, which is undesirable in terms of heart disease risk. Omega-3 fatty acids have a similar effect on LDL levels but do not lower HDL cholesterol.[30] Studies show that replacing some of the fat in the diet with omega-3 polyunsaturated fatty acids reduces the incidence of heart disease. In addition to these effects on blood lipids, omega-3 fatty acids may reduce heart disease risk by preventing the growth of atherosclerotic plaque and by affecting blood clotting, blood pressure, and immune function.[31,32] The beneficial effects are greater when the omega-3 fatty acids are consumed in fish, such as salmon and albacore tuna, rather than in supplements.[33]

Dietary Monounsaturated Fat Populations with diets high in monounsaturated fats, such as those in Mediterranean countries where olive oil is commonly used, have a mortality rate from heart disease that is half of that in the United States.

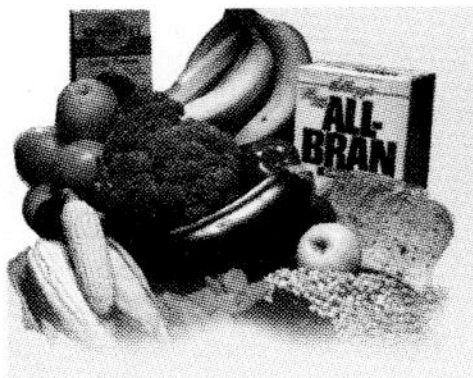

Off the Shelf

Are Supplements a Safe Way to Reduce Blood Cholesterol?

Is your blood cholesterol above 200 mg per 100 ml, or are you trying to keep it from getting there? A trip to the drugstore will reveal a whole host of over-the-counter cholesterol-lowering remedies. Could you benefit from one of these? Do they work? What are the risks?

These supplements include everything from fibers and vitamins to garlic and phytochemicals. The safest supplements for lowering cholesterol are probably soluble fibers such as psyllium, pectin, guar gum, or locust bean gum. Many studies have shown that fiber supplements lower total and LDL cholesterol in those with elevated levels. The effectiveness depends on how the fiber is processed and thus varies with the brand of fiber supplement. An alternative to fiber supplements for lowering your cholesterol is to increase your intake of high-fiber foods such as beans, whole oats, and fruit. These add not only soluble fiber to your diet but also the other nutrients and phytochemicals present in these foods.

A vitamin that can lower blood cholesterol is niacin. In doses of 2 to 3 grams per day, niacin has been shown to lower LDL cholesterol and raise HDL.[1,2] It is recommended by the National Cholesterol Education Program as a treatment for high blood cholesterol. But at doses this high, niacin is not really a vitamin, it is a drug. The amount used to treat high blood cholesterol is well above the Tolerable Upper Intake Level of 35 mg per day that has been set for adults.[3] High doses can cause liver damage, ulcers, impaired glucose tolerance, headaches, flushing, nausea, heartburn, and diarrhea. Although readily available over the counter, niacin should not be taken at these high doses without a doctor's supervision.

Garlic has been used medicinally for centuries. Many health-promoting phytochemicals have now been identified in garlic, and today one of the promises used to market garlic supplements is that they will lower blood cholesterol. Some reports have found that garlic supplements are effective at reducing blood cholesterol[4,5] whereas others have found no effect.[6,7] The doses used in these studies are equivalent to consuming one or more cloves of raw garlic daily. The primary side effect of this is a strong garlic body odor. You do not have to eat the raw garlic, however; garlic supplements are available as capsules containing garlic extract or garlic oil and as garlic powder or garlic powder tablets. If you don't want to smell like an Italian restaurant, some of these preparations are odorless.

Phytosterols are phytochemicals that are sold as a cholesterol-lowering supplement. Phytosterols resemble cholesterol chemically, making it difficult for the digestive tract to distinguish them from cholesterol. They are believed to lower blood cholesterol by inhibiting cholesterol absorption.[8] A Western diet provides about 200 to 400 mg of phytosterols a day from foods such as soybeans, wheat, and rice.[9] Intakes of 1.5 to 3 grams a day have been shown to reduce total and LDL cholesterol levels in the blood and to have no effect on HDL cholesterol. A tablet of the phytosterol supplement Cholestatin contains 380 mg, so it would take 4 to 8 tablets a day to supply the amounts that have been shown to reduce cholesterol in these studies. Phytosterols have been found to lower blood cholesterol when consumed in margarines into which phytosterols have been incorporated.[10] No side effects have been reported with phytosterol consumption.[8]

Compounds called tocotrienols, which are related to vitamin E, have also been sold to lower cholesterol. They are found in rice, oat bran, and barley. They are believed to lower cholesterol by interfering with the liver's ability to make it. One study found that a dose of 200 mg a day for a month lowered LDL cholesterol by 13% in

---

This is true even when total fat intake provides 40% or more of energy intake.[34] Substituting monounsaturated fat for saturated fat reduces LDL cholesterol without decreasing HDL cholesterol and makes LDL cholesterol less susceptible to oxidation.[1,30] However, the type of fat in the diet is unlikely to be the only factor involved in the differences in the incidence of heart disease between the Mediterranean countries and the United States. As already mentioned, the Mediterranean diet is higher in fruits and vegetables, lower in animal products, includes more wine, and is consumed in countries where the lifestyle includes more day-to-day activity and has fewer of the stresses of modern life.

Plant Foods: Fiber and Antioxidants Epidemiology has shown that a diet high in plant foods is associated with a lower risk of heart disease. Plant foods such as fruits, vegetables, grains, and legumes are a good source of fiber, vitamins, minerals, and phytochemicals. Different types and amounts of dietary fiber can affect blood cholesterol levels. Soluble fibers, such as those in oat bran, legumes, psyl-

subjects with high cholesterol.[11] Tocotrienols have potential benefit, but to obtain these effects would require taking 4 to 8 times the dosage recommended on supplement packages.

To assess your risk of heart disease you should have your blood cholesterol measured. If it is higher than recommended you should be under a doctor's care. The best treatment can only be determined by following a physician's assessment of the levels of all types of lipid fractions in your blood. The use of over-the-counter supplements should be discussed with your doctor, since they may impact the effectiveness of other treatments. In addition, dietary supplements are not tested as extensively as drugs, so less is known about their safety and effectiveness. For example, Cholestin, a supplement made from Chinese red yeast rice, contains the chemical lovastatin. Lovastatin is the active ingredient in some prescription cholesterol-lowering medications. Unlike prescription lovastatin, the amount of this drug in each dose of Cholestin is not regulated and may vary. Lovastatin causes serious side effects and should not be used by people with infections or organ transplants and those who consume more than two alcoholic beverages a day.

Since most of the active ingredients contained in these supplements can be obtained from foods, eating a healthy diet may be just as effective at lowering cholesterol. Even when taking a drug or supplement to lower cholesterol, it should not take the place of adequate exercise and a diet low in total fat, saturated fat, and cholesterol and high in fiber, fruits, vegetables, and whole grains. This type of diet can benefit not only blood cholesterol levels but blood pressure, body weight, and cancer risk.

[1]O'Connor, P. J., Rush, W. A., and Trence, D. L. Relative effectiveness of niacin and lovastatin for treatment of dyslipidemias in a health maintenance organization. J. Fam. Pract. 44:462–467, 1997.

[2]McKenney, J. M., McCormick, L. S., Weiss, S., et al. A randomized trial of the effects of atorvastatin and niacin in patients with combined hyperlipidemia or isolated hypertriglyceridemia. Collaborative Atorvastin Study Group. Am. J. Med. 104:137–143, 1998.

[3]Institute of Medicine, Food and Nutrition Board. *Dietary Reference Intakes for Thiamin, Riboflavin, Niacin, Vitamin B-6, Folate, Vitamin B-12, Pantothenic Acid, Biotin, and Choline.* Washington, D.C.: National Academy Press, 1998.

[4]Adler, A. J., and Holub, B. J. Effect of garlic and fish oil supplementation on serum lipid and lipoprotein concentrations in hypercholesterolemic men. Am. J. Clin. Nutr. 65:445–450, 1997.

[5]Bordia, A., Verma, S. K., and Srivastava, K. C. Effect of garlic (Allium sativum) on blood lipids, blood sugar, fibrinogen and fibrinolytic activity in patients with coronary artery disease. Prostaglandins Leukot. Essent. Fatty Acids 58:257–263, 1998.

[6]Berthold, H. K., Sudhop, T., and von Bergmann, K. Effect of garlic oil preparation on serum lipoproteins and cholesterol metabolism: a randomized controlled trial. J.A.M.A. 279: 1900–1902, 1998.

[7]Isaacsohn, J. L., Moser, M., Stein, E.A., et al. Garlic powder and plasma lipids and lipoproteins: a multicenter, randomized, placebo-controlled trial. Arch. Intern. Med. 158:1189–1194, 1998.

[8]Ling, W. H., and Jones, P. J. Dietary phytosterols: a review of metabolism, benefits and side effects. Life Sci. 57:195–206, 1995.

[9]Jones, P. J., MacDougall, D. E., Ntanios, F., and Vanstone, C. A. Dietary phytosterols as cholesterol-lowering agents in humans. Can. J. Physiol. Pharmacol. 75:217–227, 1997.

[10]Weststrate, J. A., and Meijer, G. W. Plant sterol–enriched margarines and reduction of plasma total- and LDL-cholesterol concentrations in normocholesterolemic and mildly hypercholesterolemic subjects. Eur. J. Clin. Nutr. 52:334–343, 1998.

[11]Qureshi, A. A., Bradlow, B. A., Brace, L., et al. Response of hypercholesterolemic subjects to administration of tocotrienols. Lipids 30:1171–1177, 1995.

lium, pectin, and gums, have been shown to reduce blood cholesterol levels. These fibers are believed to bind cholesterol and bile acids in the small intestine and cause them to be excreted in the feces (see Figure 4.18). Many of the vitamins, minerals, and phytochemicals in plant foods have antioxidant functions. Antioxidants are postulated to protect against plaque formation by decreasing the formation of oxidized LDL cholesterol[1] (see *Off the Shelf: Are Supplements a Safe Way to Reduce Blood Cholesterol?*).

Moderate Alcohol Consumption Moderate alcohol consumption has been shown to reduce stress and to raise levels of HDL cholesterol. This has a protective effect against heart disease. Some of the protection may also be due to compounds in red wine known as phenols, which may act as antioxidants and protect against lipoprotein oxidation, thereby preventing the development of atherosclerotic plaques.[35] The Dietary Guidelines recognize the benefits of moderate alcohol consumption. An intake of one to two drinks per day has been shown to reduce cardiovascular disease risk and is not believed to increase the risk of other diseases. Greater intakes of alcohol increase the risk of accidental deaths as well as heart disease and should be avoided.

Dietary Fat and Cancer

Cancer is the second leading cause of death in the United States, and it is estimated that 30 to 40% of cancers are directly linked to dietary choices.[36] As with cardiovascular disease, there is a body of epidemiological evidence correlating diet and lifestyle with the incidence of cancer, particularly cancers of the esophagus, breast, prostate, and colon. Diets high in fat and low in fiber and plant foods are correlated with an increased risk of cancer.[8] The mechanism whereby a high intake of dietary fat increases the incidence of various cancers is less well understood than the relationship between dietary fat and cardiovascular disease; however, dietary fat has been suggested to be both a tumor promoter and tumor initiator.

Dietary Fat and Breast Cancer Breast cancer is the leading form of cancer in women worldwide. In the United States it affects 182,000 women annually. The incidence is similar among all ethnic groups, but the mortality is higher among minority women. Breast cancer is more common in postmenopausal women, in women who have had no children or who had children late in life, and in women with a family history of the disease. In populations where the diet is high in fat and low in fiber, the incidence of breast cancer is high. In populations where the typical fat intake is low, the incidence is lower and the survival rate is better in people with the disease. Currently, several major studies are under way to determine if reducing fat intake to less than 15% of energy will reduce breast cancer risk or mortality.

As is the case with heart disease, the type of fat is as important as the total amount of fat in determining risk. The incidence of breast cancer in Mediterranean women who rely on olive oil, which is high in monounsaturated fat, as a source of dietary fat is low despite a total fat intake similar to that in the United States.[37] Epidemiology also supports a protective effect from an increased intake of omega-3 fatty acids from fish, such as in the native Eskimos of Alaska and Greenland.[38] A higher intake of trans fatty acids found in foods such as stick margarines, however, may increase the risk of breast cancer.[39]

The mechanism by which diet affects breast cancer has been studied in laboratory animals. Since most laboratory animals do not get breast cancer tumors, studies are conducted by implanting breast tumors and examining how diet affects their growth. The tumors are more likely to grow in mice fed a high-fat diet than in those fed a lowfat diet. The type of fat also affects growth; diets high in linoleic acid, which is found in polyunsaturated vegetable oils, are stronger tumor promoters than diets high in saturated fatty acids or omega-3 fatty acids.[40] So, unlike heart disease, where polyunsaturated fats reduce risk, a high polyunsaturated fat intake may be detrimental in terms of cancer risk.

Diet and Colon Cancer Epidemiology has correlated the incidence of colon cancer with high-fat, low-fiber diets.[41] The correlation is stronger for diets high in animal fats, in particular those from red meats.[42] The connection between dietary fat and colon cancer may be related to the breakdown products of fat in the large intestine. Here, bacteria metabolize dietary fat and bile, producing substances that may cause mutations. These mutation-producing substances, or mutagens, may act as tumor initiators. A high intake of fiber tends to dilute these mutagens by increasing the volume of feces. High-fiber diets also decrease transit time. Both of these effects reduce the exposure of the intestinal mucosa to the hazardous substances (see Chapter 4).

CRITICAL THINKING

Dietary Fat and Heart Disease Risk

Rafael's mother died of a heart attack at age 60. Rafael is worried about his own heart disease risk, so he makes an appointment with his physician. He fills out a questionnaire about his medical history and lifestyle, meets with a dietitian to evaluate his diet, and has blood drawn for cholesterol analysis. The table below summarizes factors that may affect Rafael's risk of developing heart disease:

Sex	Male
Age	35
Family history	Mother had heart attack at age 60
Height/weight	68 inches/160 lb
Blood pressure	120/70
Stress level	Moderate
Smoker	Yes
Activity level	Sedentary
Blood values	
Total cholesterol	210 mg/100 ml
LDL cholesterol	160 mg/100 ml
HDL cholesterol	34 mg/100 ml
Typical daily intake from three-day food record:	
Percent energy from fat	39
Percent energy from saturated fat	17
Percent energy from polyunsaturated fat	7
Cholesterol	350 mg/day
Servings from groups of the Food Guide Pyramid:	
Bread, Cereals, Rice, & Pasta	11
Vegetable	2
Fruit	1
Milk, Yogurt, & Cheese	2
Meat, Poultry, Fish, Dry Beans, Eggs, & Nuts	4

What risk factors does Rafael have for developing cardiovascular disease?

He smokes cigarettes. He is inactive.
Other answers:

What dietary and lifestyle changes would you recommend to reduce his risks?

He could quit smoking.
Other answers:

If Rafael were to replace all of the added fat in his diet with olive oil, would he reduce his risk of cardiovascular disease to the level found in Mediterranean countries?

Answer:

LIPIDS: ONE PART OF THE TOTAL DIET

About 33% of the energy in the typical North American diet comes from lipids.[43] Guidelines for a healthy diet recommend a reduction in total and saturated fat intake and moderation in the use of other fats. In this section we will discuss how to determine the amount of fat in your diet, how to modify it to meet recommendations, and what dietary choices contribute best to the overall healthiness of the diet.

Recommendations for Fat Intake

Fat is an essential nutrient. Although there is no 1989 RDA for fatty acids, the recommendation for a minimally adequate adult intake is 1 to 2% of energy, or 3 to 6 grams per day, from the omega-6 fatty acid, linoleic acid. This is well below the approximately 7% of energy from linoleic acid in a typical adult diet in the United States. There is no 1989 RDA for omega-3 fatty acids, but DRIs are being considered. The Canadian RNIs recommend at least 3% of energy from omega-6 fatty acids and at least 0.5% of energy from omega-3 fatty acids, with the ratio of omega-6 to omega-3 in the range of 4:1 to 10:1.[44] The recommendations of the World Health Organization are similar, recommending a ratio of linoleic to alpha-linolenic acid in the diet between 5:1 and 10:1.[45]

The amounts of essential fatty acids needed are minuscule compared with the amount of fat most Americans consume. Of more concern than fatty acid deficiency is the chronic disease risk related to the typical American diet. Whether you are trying to consume a generally healthy diet or are concerned about your risk of heart disease or cancer, the recommendation is that most people should reduce their total fat intake while meeting their needs for essential fatty acids (Figure 5.17). Total dietary fat intake should be reduced to no more than 30% of energy, and the consumption of grains, vegetables, and fruits, which are high in fiber, micronutrients, and phytochemicals, should be increased. Total fat in the diet should be divided approximately equally between saturated fat, polyunsaturated fat, and monounsaturated fat. Cholesterol intake should be no more than 300 mg per day and trans fatty acid intake should not increase above the current level of intake—about 2 and 4% of energy.[46] These recommendations apply to the total diet as it is consumed over several days or a week; they are not meant as guidelines for a single meal or day. Differences in age, genetics, and disease risk may affect how these recommendations apply to an individual (see *Off the Label: Using Food Labels to Choose Your Fats*).

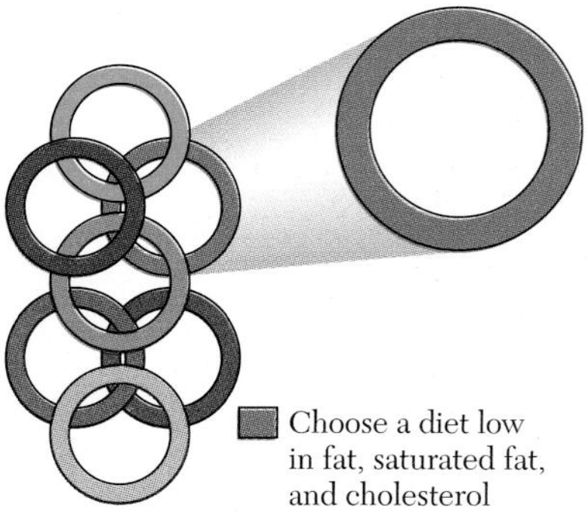
Choose a diet low in fat, saturated fat, and cholesterol

Figure 5.17
The Dietary Guidelines for Americans recommend a diet low in fat, saturated fat, and cholesterol. (USDA, DHHS, 1995)

Recommendations to Reduce Specific Risks Some dietary recommendations are made to target specific diseases. For example, the American Heart Association has developed recommendations to specifically reduce heart disease risk. They recommend that fish be included in the diet as a source of omega-3 fatty acids. They also stress that fiber intake should come from foods, not supplements (see Appendix G). The National Cholesterol Education Program (NCEP) recommends that individuals with elevated cholesterol reduce their total fat intake to no more than 30% of energy, their saturated fat intake to less than 10%, and their cholesterol intake to less than 300 mg per day. If, after six months of consuming this diet, blood cholesterol levels have not decreased, fat should be reduced to 20% and saturated fat to 7% of energy. The NCEP also recommends drug therapy in addition to diet therapy for individuals with extremely high cholesterol levels or those in whom diet therapy fails. Two types of drugs are used to lower blood cholesterol levels: One acts in the gastrointestinal tract by preventing cholesterol and bile absorption, and the other blocks cholesterol production in the liver.

To reduce cancer risk, the American Cancer Society recommends limiting your intake of high-fat foods, particularly those from animal sources; increasing consumption of foods from plants, such as fruits, vegetables, and grains; limiting alcohol consumption; and maintaining a physically active lifestyle (see Appendix G).[47]

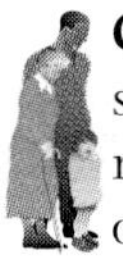

Guidelines for Special Groups The recommendations for fat intake are designed for all individuals over two years of age. None of the recommendations to restrict fat and cholesterol intake have been suggested for children under the age of two because of their high energy needs and because lipids are needed to support the rapid brain development that occurs in young children. After two years of age, fat intake should be gradually decreased until about age five when the diet should provide 30% or less of its energy as fat. Children between the ages of 2 and 19 with cholesterol levels of 170 mg per 100 ml or greater are at high risk for heart disease; they should reduce their fat intake and be monitored carefully by their physicians. The American Academy of Pediatrics specifies a lower limit of 20% of energy from total fat for children and adolescents.[48]

During pregnancy, there is an increase in blood cholesterol. This increase appears to be independent of diet, and levels return to normal about eight weeks after the baby is born. Reducing fat intake to 30% of energy intake has not been shown to be detrimental during pregnancy as long as energy, protein, and micronutrient needs are met.

In the elderly, the value of dietary fat reduction must be balanced with the risk of undernutrition. Reducing fat intake to 30% of energy causes little risk, though further reduction may increase the risk for protein or micronutrient malnutrition in this group.

Determining Your Fat Intake

How does your diet compare with the recommendation of less than 30% energy from fat? To calculate fat intake as a percent of energy, you need to know the number of grams of fat in the diet and how much energy is consumed. For example, if you know a diet contains 1800 kcalories and 68 grams of fat, you can calculate the fat intake as a percent of energy as follows:

$$68 \text{ g of fat} \times 9 \text{ kcal/g} = 612 \text{ kcal of fat}$$

$$\frac{612 \text{ kcal}}{1800 \text{ total kcal}} \times 100 = 34\% \text{ energy (kcal) as fat}$$

This same equation can be used to determine the percent of energy from fat in individual foods. For example, a glass of whole milk containing 8 grams of fat and 160 kcal provides 45% of its energy from fat ([8 g × 9 kcal/g]/160 kcal × 100).

Databases and food composition tables provide information on the number of grams of fat contained in a wide variety of foods. Food labels provide a more accessible source of information on packaged foods. The Nutrition Facts portion of food labels lists the amount in grams of total fat, saturated fat, and cholesterol

Off the Label

Using Food Labels to Choose Your Fats

The information about fat on food labels is designed to make it easier to identify the sources and types of fat in foods. Understanding how to use this information can help consumers make more informed choices about the fats they include in their diet.

Food labels provide a number of different types of information concerning the fat in a food. The ingredient list includes the source of fat, such as corn oil, soybean oil, or partially hydrogenated vegetable oil, and the Nutrition Facts section provides the number of kcalories from fat, the number of grams of fat and saturated fat, and the number of milligrams of cholesterol in a serving. These are also presented as a percent of the Daily Value. Daily Values are calculated for a diet containing 2000 kcalories and are based on the recommendation that the diet should contain no more than 30% of energy from fat (65 g), no more than 10% from saturated fat (20 g), and no more than 300 mg of cholesterol per day. The percent Daily Value allows consumers to tell at a glance how one food will fit into the recommendations for fat intake for the day. For example, if a serving provides 50% of the Daily Value for fat—that is, half the recommended maximum daily intake for a 2000-kcalorie diet—the rest of the day's intake will have to be carefully selected to not exceed the recommended maximum.

The amount of monounsaturated and polyunsaturated fat is voluntarily included on the labels of some products. For example, in addition to listing the 2 grams of saturated fat, the label on a bottle of olive oil may indicate that it contains 2 grams of polyunsaturated fat and 10 grams of monounsaturated fat per tablespoon. (There are no Daily Values for polyunsaturated and monounsaturated fat.) The amount of trans fat in a product is included in the total fat value but is not listed separately or as a component of the saturated, polyunsaturated, or monounsaturated values. Identifying foods low in trans fat is not easy. Some foods are labeled "trans free," and products likely to contain trans fats can be identified by looking at the ingredient list for partially hydrogenated vegetable oil. Many, but not all, partially hydrogenated oils are high in trans fat. At present, there is no way to determine exactly how much trans fat a product contains.

Food labels may also include terms such as "fat free," "low cholesterol," or "lean." These descriptors are added by manufacturers trying to capitalize on the public's interest in decreasing fat intake. To make these descriptors helpful to consumers as well as to manufacturers, food labeling regulations have developed standard definitions for these terms. For instance, a product labeled "lowfat" cannot contain more than 3 grams of fat in a serving (see the accompanying table). So reduced-fat (2%) milk, which contains 5 grams of fat per cup, cannot be labeled as lowfat, whereas 1% milk, with only 2.5 grams per cup, does fit the definition.[1] These terms can be used only in ways that do not confuse consumers. For instance, since saturated fat in the diet raises blood cholesterol, a food that is low in cholesterol but high in saturated fat, such as crackers containing coconut oil, cannot be labeled "low cholesterol," because it may actually raise blood cholesterol. Currently, the level of trans fat, a fat that increases the risk of heart disease, is considered when a food claims to be "saturated-fat free," but a product that is high in trans fat can claim to be "low cholesterol."

A component of food labels that may be confusing to consumers is the claim that a product is a certain percent fat free. This refers to percent by weight, not by energy. To avoid deception, labeling laws require that a product can claim to be a certain percent fat free only if it is also a

in the product, as well as the number of kcalories from fat in that food. Daily Values help determine how much fat, saturated fat, and cholesterol are in a food relative to the daily amount recommended for a 2000-kcalorie diet. The Daily Value for total fat is calculated as 30% of the energy required. For a 2000-kcalorie diet, this represents about 65 grams of fat (30% of 2000 kcal = 600 kcal from fat; 600 kcal ÷ 9 kcal/g = 67 g, which is rounded to 65 grams). For saturated fat, the Daily Value is based on 10% of energy, and the Daily Value for cholesterol is set at 300 mg per day regardless of the amount of energy in the diet. Unfortunately, food label information is not always available on fresh meats, which are one of the main contributors of fat in our diets.

The Exchange Lists can be used to give a quick estimate of the total amount of fat in a food or in the diet (Table 5.2; see also Appendix I). An exchange of fruits, vegetables, or breads contains 1 gram or less. The amount of fat in an exchange of dairy products depends on what items you choose to consume. A serving of nonfat milk provides less than a gram of fat, but a serving of whole milk

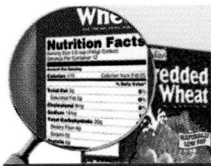

Descriptors Related to Fat and Cholesterol

Descriptor	Definition
Fat free	Contains less than 0.5 gram of fat per serving.
Lowfat	Contains 3 grams or less of fat per serving.
Percent fat free	May be used only to describe foods that meet the definition of fat free or lowfat.
Reduced or less fat	Contains at least 25% less fat per serving than the regular or reference product.
Saturated fat free	Contains less than 0.5 gram of saturated fat per serving and less than 0.5 gram trans fatty acids per serving.
Low saturated fat	Contains 1 gram or less of saturated fat and not more than 15% of kcalories from saturated fat per serving.
Reduced or less saturated fat	Contains at least 25% less saturated fat than the regular or reference product.
Cholesterol free	Contains less than 2 mg of cholesterol and 2 grams or less of saturated fat per serving.
Low cholesterol	Contains 20 mg or less of cholesterol and 2 grams or less of saturated fat per serving.
Reduced or less cholesterol	Contains at least 25% less cholesterol than the regular or reference product and 2 grams or less of saturated fat per serving.
Lean	Contains less than 10 grams of fat, 4.5 grams or less of saturated fat, and less than 95 mg of cholesterol per serving and per 100 grams.
Extra lean	Contains less than 5 grams of fat, less than 2 grams of saturated fat, and less than 95 mg of cholesterol per serving and per 100 grams.

fat-free or lowfat food. For example, lowfat hot dogs that are labeled 97% fat free contain 1.5 grams of fat per serving and therefore meet the definition of a lowfat food. Although packaged meats must be labeled, fresh raw meats such as steak, which are one of the greatest contributors of fat, are not required to carry standard labels. Labels on ground beef can be particularly misleading because they may mention a certain "% lean." In this case "% lean" refers to the weight of the meat that is lean. So when the label says it is 78% lean, it means that 22% of the weight of the meat is fat, or that there are 22 grams of fat in 100 g (3.5 ounces) of raw hamburger. This works out to about 55% of energy as fat. Only ground beef that is 90% lean or greater meets the government's definition of lean: less than 10 grams of fat per serving.

[1]Kurtzweil, P. Skimming the milk label. FDA Consumer 32:22–25, Jan./Feb., 1998.

contains 8 grams. Likewise, the amount of fat in a meat exchange depends on your choice; a very lean meat such as turkey breast contains 1 gram of fat or less, whereas a serving of bologna contains 8 grams. An exchange from the fat list contains 5 grams of fat (see *Critical Thinking: Fats in the Total Diet*).

A Diet to Meet Recommendations: Choose Fats Wisely

Choosing a diet that limits cholesterol and total fat; that divides fats equally among saturated, monounsaturated, and polyunsaturated; and that meets the recommendations for other nutrients sounds like an overwhelming task. In reality, meal planning does not need to be that difficult. Following the guidelines of the Food Guide Pyramid can provide a diet that meets all of these specifications.

The Food Guide Pyramid recommends a diet that is rich in grains, vegetables, and fruits, and that is low in fat. The concentration of high-fat choices in

Table 5.2 *Using Exchange Lists to Calculate the Fat Content of a Diet*

Exchange Groups/Lists	Serving Size	Fat (g)
Carbohydrate Group		
Starch	1/2 cup rice, cereal, potatoes; 1 slice bread	1 or less
Fruit	1 small apple, peach, pear; 1/2 banana; 1/2 cup canned juice-pack fruit	0
Milk	1 cup milk or yogurt	
Nonfat		0
Lowfat		2.5
Reduced fat		5
Whole		8
Other carbohydrates	Serving sizes vary	Varies
Vegetables	1/2 cup cooked vegetables, 1 cup raw	0
Meat/Meat Substitute Group	1 oz meat or cheese, 1/2 cup legumes	
Very lean		0–1
Lean		3
Medium fat		5
High fat		8
Fat Group	1 tsp butter, margarine, or oil; 1 Tbsp salad dressing	5

each of the Food Guide Pyramid groups is indicated by a circle (●) symbol (Figure 5.18). There are few of these at the base of the Pyramid. Grain products, vegetables, and fruits are naturally low in fat as long as fat is not added in preparation. The choices you make within these groups can significantly affect the fat content and nutrient density of your diet. For example, within the grain group, choosing high-fat baked goods such as doughnuts, cookies, and muffins adds more fat and energy and fewer nutrients than whole grain breads, rice, and pasta. Within the Fruit Group, fresh fruits are a nonfat choice while fruits that are baked into pies and tarts add fat and refined sugar. Most fresh vegetables have little or no fat, but fried vegetables such as french fries and fried onion rings are high in fat and energy (Table 5.3). High-fat snack foods such as potato chips and corn chips are a major contributor to the fat in the American diet.[49] To enjoy these snacks without adding excess fat and energy to the diet, about 75% of adult Americans and 93% of dieters consume reduced-fat snack products.[50] Using reduced-fat products has some advantages, but consumers should be aware that

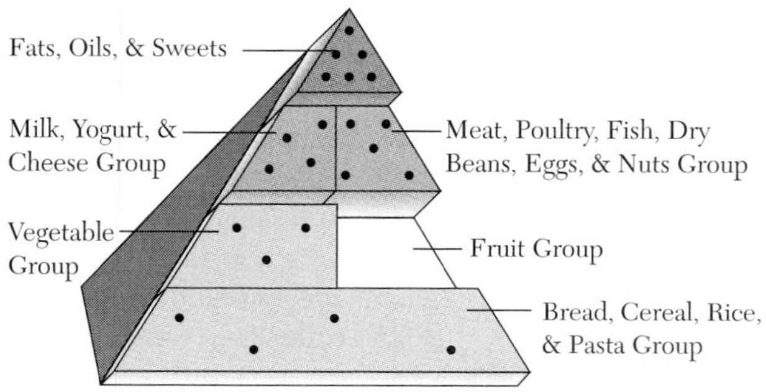

Figure 5.18

The groups that are sources of naturally occurring and added fat contain circles and are raised and colored orange. The darker the shade and the more circles, the more high-fat foods the group contains.

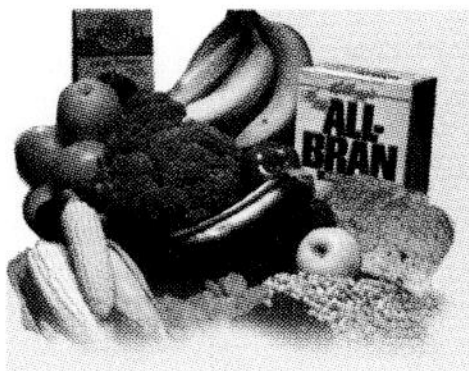

Off the Shelf

Can Lowfat Foods Improve Your Diet?

Fat-free and reduced-fat foods are everywhere. From chips and dip to cookies and ice cream, we have an abundant assortment of fat-free and lowfat foods to choose from. Since 1990, over a thousand reduced-fat foods have been introduced into the marketplace each year. Health-conscious consumers are using these products in their efforts to reduce fat and energy intake. In a recent survey, half of the respondents wanted even more of these types of products.[1] Can fat-modified foods help us lower our fat intake? Do they help with weight loss? Are these foods a healthy choice?

Lowfat products can help reduce fat intake when used in place of high-fat choices. For example, if a snack of salsa and regular tortilla chips is replaced with one of salsa and chips containing Olestra, fat intake will be reduced. However, just reducing fat intake does not make a diet healthy. If products containing fat substitutes replace whole grains, fruits, and vegetables, the result could be a diet low in fat but also low in fiber, vitamins, minerals, and phytochemicals.

Do fat-free foods help with weight loss? Studies show that switching from a high-fat to a lowfat diet does result in some weight loss—about 1 to 3 kg. And studies of products containing Olestra show that consumption of these foods is associated with lower fat and energy intakes.[2] Then why, with the multitude of fat-free foods available, are more Americans today overweight than ever before? One reason is that dieters do not always reduce energy intake when they reduce fat consumption. If lowfat foods are consumed liberally or added to a diet that is already high in energy, total energy intake will not be reduced and weight will not decrease. Even though the percent of energy from fat in our diets has decreased from about 40% of kcalories in the late 1950s and early 1960s to only 33% of kcalories today, the total amount of fat we eat has not really changed because we now consume more energy.[1]

Are fat-free foods a healthy choice? There is some concern that the use of fat-modified products will reduce the micronutrient content of the diet. This is a problem if they replace nutrient-dense choices, but as long as they are not consumed in large quantities, these foods do not have a great impact on the intake of nutrients other than fat. Because the majority of fat-modified foods we consume are sweets and snack foods—which are low in nutrient density to begin with—the impact of lowfat snack foods on the total micronutrient content of the diet is minimal. Foods that are lower in fat because fat has been removed or because less fat has been added may even have a higher nutrient density than the original product. For example, reduced-fat milk is higher in nutrient density than whole milk. This is also true of foods such as baked goods that have applesauce or other fruit puree added in place of oil. When nonabsorbable fats such as Olestra are used as fat replacers, the resulting product affects not only the nutrients that may be consumed, but also the availability of fat-soluble substances in the gastrointestinal tract. Olestra decreases the absorption of fat-soluble vitamins, cholesterol, beta-carotene, and other fat-soluble compounds. Although Olestra is fortified with vitamins A, D, E, and K, it does not contain beta-carotene or other fat-soluble phytochemicals, and it is not possible to ascertain the extent to which it impacts the absorption of these substances over the course of days or weeks.

Fat-free, lowfat, and reduced-fat foods do not make a diet healthy, but they can be part of a healthy diet.

[1]American Dietetic Association. Position of the American Dietetic Association: fat replacers. J. Am. Diet. Assoc. 98:463–468, 1998.

[2]Miller, D. L., Castellanos, V. H., Shide, D. J., et al. Effect of fat free potato chips with and without labels on fat and energy intakes. Am. J. Clin. Nutr. 68:282–290, 1998.

---

using these products does not transform a poor diet into a healthy one. This issue is discussed in more detail in the food technology section below and in *Off the Shelf: Can Lowfat Foods Improve Your Diet?*

The food groups closer to the top of the Food Guide Pyramid—the Milk, Yogurt, & Cheese Group and the Meat, Poultry, Fish, Dried Beans, Eggs, & Nuts Group—contain more high-fat choices. The animal foods in these groups contain saturated fat and are the only source of cholesterol in the diet. To reduce your saturated fat and cholesterol intake, choose lowfat or nonfat dairy products; choose lean meats, such as chicken, turkey, flank and round steak; and use vegetable sources of protein such as legumes.

The most concentrated sources of fat—oils, butter, margarine, and salad dressings—are separated into the narrow tip of the Pyramid. These should be added sparingly to the diet. To reduce your total fat consumption, limit the amount of fat added to food at the table and in cooking. Many lowfat and nonfat salad dressings and spreads are available that offer the taste and texture of the original products with much less fat. To reduce saturated fat intake, use vegetable oils such as canola and olive oil that are high in monounsaturated fat, and corn

Table 5.3 *Comparison of Lowfat and High-Fat Choices*

Food	Serving	Energy (kcal)	Fat (g)
Bagel	1 large	236	1.0
Doughnut, glazed	1 large	436	22.0
Egg noodles	1 cup	213	2.0
Ramen noodles	1 cup	180	7.0
Broiled chicken breast (no skin)	3 oz	140	3.0
Breaded chicken nuggets	3 oz	242	15.0
Fresh broccoli	1 cup	24	0.2
Frozen broccoli with cheese sauce	1 cup	220	15.0
Potato, no skin, boiled	1 medium	118	0.1
French fries	1 small order	202	10.0

and soybean oils that are high in polyunsaturated fat. To reduce your intake of trans fatty acids, consume soft margarine or liquid margarines and those that do not list partially hydrogenated fat as the first ingredient (see Table 5.4).

Following these recommendations will reduce your fat intake and increase your consumption of grains, vegetables, and fruits. This dietary pattern is more similar to the traditional diets of Asia and the Mediterranean, where the risk of heart disease and cancer is low. The Asian diet is based on rice and vegetables with small amounts of meats; the Mediterranean diet is also high in grains, vegetables, and fruit. Animal products such as cheese and yogurt, fish, poultry, eggs, and red meat represent a relatively small portion of the total diet (see Appendix J, the Asian and Mediterranean Food Guide Pyramids).

Table 5.4 *Suggestions for Reducing Fat Intake*

1. Instead of frying, bake, broil, or microwave.
2. Skip added fats like butter, margarine, mayonnaise, and salad dressing—or use lowfat or fat-free spreads and dressings.
3. Use egg whites or egg substitutes in baking.
4. Use cocoa instead of chocolate in baking.
5. Use reduced-fat milk instead of coffee creamer.
6. Use reduced-fat cheeses or limit the amounts consumed.
7. Reduce the emphasis on meat as the centerpiece of meals:
   - Base meals on whole grain products.
   - Reduce the portion size of meats served.
8. Trim visible fat from meats before cooking, and skin poultry before eating if not before cooking.
9. Choose meats with little marbling:
   - "Prime grade" contains an abundant amount of marbled fat.
   - "Choice grade" contains a modest amount of marbling.
   - "Select grade" contains a comparatively slight amount of marbling.

CRITICAL THINKING

Fats in the Total Diet

After reading about the relationship between dietary fat intake and chronic disease, Stella became concerned that her fat intake was too high. She understood the principles of a lowfat diet but wasn't sure she could change her own eating habits. She has a busy schedule—working full-time and going to school—and has little time to cook meals at home. She is lactose intolerant so can consume few dairy products. Currently, she relies on fast foods for breakfast and lunch and usually cooks a quick dinner when she gets home in the evening. To begin her new eating plan, she records everything that she eats for one day.

Original Diet			Modified Diet		
Food	Serving	Fat (g)	Food	Serving	Fat (g)
Breakfast					
~~Bran muffin~~	1	6	Bagel	1	1
~~Butter~~	1 tsp	5	Cream cheese	1 Tbsp	4.5
Coffee	1 cup	0	Coffee	1 cup	0
			Orange	1	0.2
Lunch					
~~Big Mac~~	1	25	Rice noodles	1 cup	0
~~French fries~~	20	16.6	Stir-fry vegetables	1 cup	2
			Chicken	2 oz	2.6
			in peanut oil	1 tsp	4.5
Soda	1 can	0	Soda	1 can	0
Apple	1	0	Apple	1	0
			Pretzels	5	2.1
Dinner					
~~Fish sticks~~	5	17	Tarpon fish	3 oz	1.7
~~Tater Tots~~	10	8	Rice	1 cup	0.5
			Long beans	1 cup	0.8
			Peanut oil	2 tsp	9
			Carrots	2	0.2
Cookies	2	4	Cookies	2	4
			Melon	1 cup	0.2
Tea	1 cup	0	Tea	1 cup	0
			Nonfat frozen yogurt	3/4 cup	1.5
Total		**81.6**			**34.8**

Does Stella's original diet meet the serving recommendations of the Food Guide Pyramid for grains, vegetables, and fruit? Do her choices from these groups follow the selection tips of the Food Guide Pyramid?

Answer:

A computer analysis shows that her total energy intake is 2100 kcalories. What is the percent of kcalories from fat in her original diet?

Answer:

What modifications could Stella make to decrease her fat intake?

A visit to her grandmother's house for dinner reminds her how much she enjoys traditional Filipino food, so she decides to incorporate these lowfat foods into her diet. For the Western foods she does not want to give up, she finds some lower-fat alternatives. Breakfast must be quick to prepare, but she can cut 5 grams of fat by eating a bagel rather than a bran muffin. For lunch, she begins taking rice noddles with vegetables and chicken to work that can be heated in the microwave. For dinner, she uses her grandmother's traditional recipes, which are low in fat. Since she doesn't need to lose weight, she'll make up the energy by increasing the servings of vegetables, adding pretzels for her snack, and enjoying some nonfat frozen yogurt at dinner. Her modified diet (shown on the right side of the table) provides comparable kcalories and less fat.

What is the percent of energy from fat in her modified diet, assuming it also contains 2100 kcalories? Does this diet meet the serving and selection recommendations of the Food Guide Pyramid for grains, vegetables, and fruit?

Answer:

Lipids and Food Technology

Fats may be added to foods during food processing, and the fats in food may be modified to change the stability or shelf life of the product. Which fats a product contains and how they are modified depends on the product and consumer demand (Figure 5.19).

Hydrogenated Vegetable Oils

The process of hydrogenation bubbles hydrogen gas into a liquid oil. This causes some of the double bonds in the oil to accept hydrogen atoms and become saturated. The resulting fat has more of the properties of a saturated fat, such as increased stability against rancidity and a higher melting point. Hydrogenated or partially hydrogenated vegetable oils are a primary ingredient in margarine and vegetable shortening because they raise the melting point of the products, making them more solid at room temperature. In breakfast cereals and other processed foods such as cookies, crackers, and potato chips, they are used to lengthen shelf life (Figure 5.20).

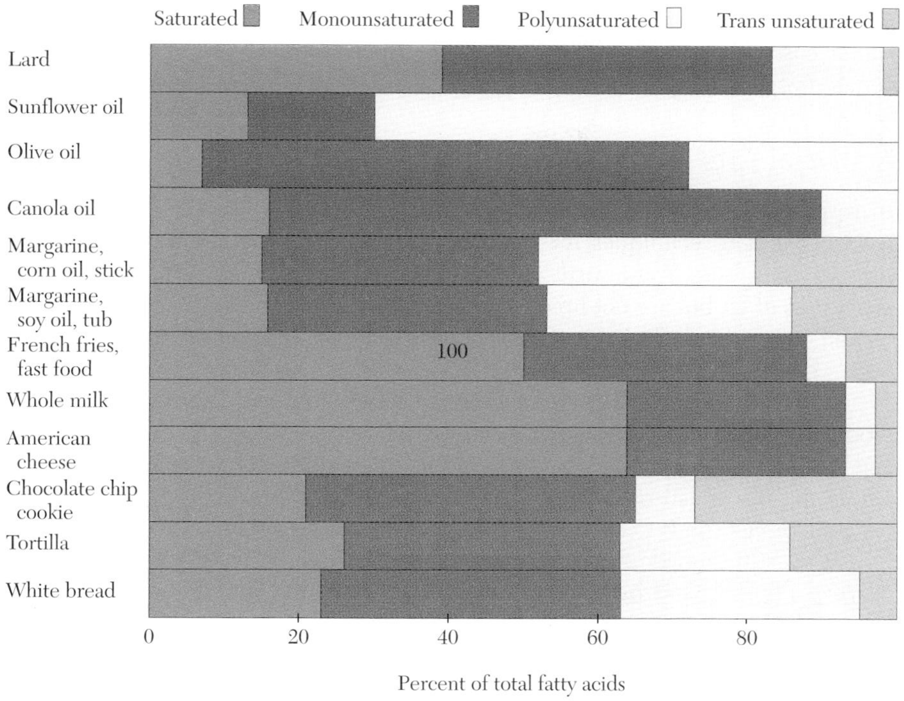

Figure 5.19
Foods have varying amounts of saturated, monounsaturated, polyunsaturated, and trans unsaturated fatty acids. This graph shows the amounts of these types of fatty acids as a percentage of the total amount of fat in the product. (From Fat and fatty acid content of selected foods containing trans fatty acids, USDA, ARS, Beltsville Human Nutrition Research Center, Special Purpose Table No. 1.)

Although good for food manufacturing, the use of hydrogenated vegetable oils has created some health concerns. As fatty acids lose their unsaturated bonds, they lose the health benefits associated with polyunsaturated fats. This is not as much of a problem as it may seem because partial hydrogenation generally changes fatty acids from polyunsaturated to monounsaturated, producing little saturated fat. For example, soybean oil is 17% saturated fat. When it is partially hydrogenated to make margarine, it becomes 20% saturated fat. Compared to butter, which is 66% saturated, margarine is still fairly low in saturated fat. But another health concern is that during hydrogenation, the percentage of trans fatty acids is increased. Trans fatty acid intake may increase the risk for both heart disease and cancer as discussed earlier. Trans fatty acids are present naturally in small amounts in animal fats, but can account for as much as 30 to 40% of the total fat in products such as margarine and shortening.[46] The amount of trans fatty acids in a food cannot be determined from the Nutrition Facts section of food labels, but foods that contain trans fats can be identified by the presence of hydrogenated or partially hydrogenated oils in the ingredient list.

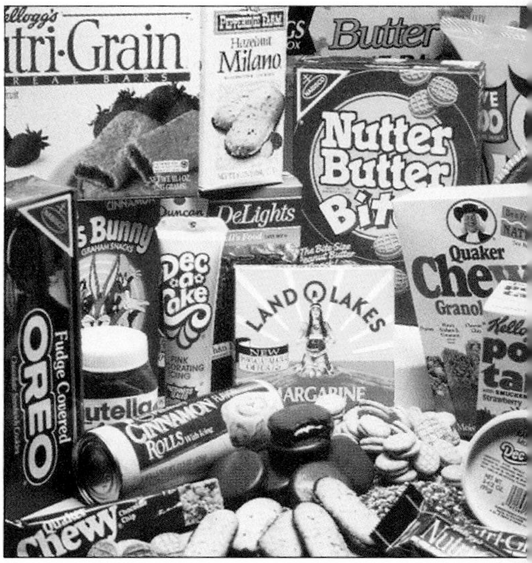

Figure 5.20
These products contain partially hydrogenated vegetable oil. (Charles D. Winters)

Tropical Oils: Saturated Vegetable Oils

Saturated vegetable oils such as the tropical oils—coconut, palm, and palm kernel oil—are rarely added to foods at home but are used by the food industry in cereals, crackers, salad dressings, and cookies. Products that contain these saturated fats are more resistant to rancidity and have longer shelf lives than those containing unsaturated fats.

Coconut, palm, and palm kernel oils provide only a small amount of the saturated fat in the American diet (3.8 g per day).[51] However, concern about the saturated fat content of the diet has led many of the large food manufacturers to reformulate some of their products to use unsaturated vegetable oils. This will reduce saturated fat intake but will not come without a cost to the consumer. Coconut oil, which comes primarily from the Philippines and Indonesia, and palm oil, which is imported from Malaysia, are usually cheaper than the soybean and corn oil produced in North America, so changing oils may increase the product

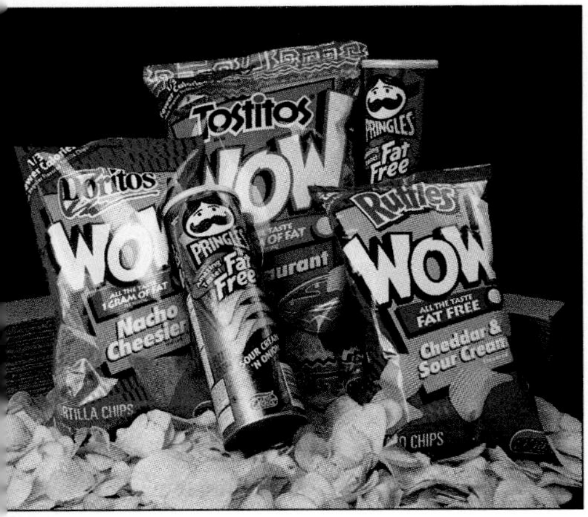

Figure 5.21
Products that contain Olestra (Olean), such as these snack chips, must carry the following health warning: This Product Contains Olestra. Olestra may cause abdominal cramping and loose stools. Olestra inhibits the absorption of some vitamins and other nutrients. Vitamins A, D, E, and K have been added. (George Semple)

price. Shorter shelf life and increased wastage of product will also increase consumer costs. To increase product shelf life, manufacturers can switch to hydrogenated vegetable oils or monounsaturated fats, or try new packaging techniques.

Artificial Fats

In response to consumer demand for lowfat, low-kcalorie foods, manufacturers have developed techniques for reducing the amount of fat contained in or absorbed from food. Some artificial fats replicate the taste, texture, and cooking properties of fat but are not lipids, and thus contribute less energy. Others reduce fat and energy intake because they are not well absorbed from the gastrointestinal tract.

Fat replacers have been engineered from carbohydrates and proteins, and by modifying fat itself.[52] Carbohydrate-based fat replacers such as various pectins and gums are often added to foods to mimic the texture that fat provides. For example, fat-free salad dressings contain gums. Protein-based fat replacers often use milk or egg solids to help emulsify and add a fatlike texture to food. Simplesse is a fat substitute made from egg white and milk proteins, which are modified by heating, filtering, and high-speed mixing. The resulting protein consists of millions of microscopic balls that slip and slide over each other to give it the creamy texture of fat. Because it is made from protein it contains energy, but because the protein is mixed with water, Simplesse contains only 1.3 kcalories per gram, which is much lower than the 9 kcalories per gram in fat. It is used in frozen desserts, cheese foods, and other products, but it cannot be used for cooking, because heat causes it to break down.[53]

Some fat substitutes are made from fats that have been modified to reduce their digestibility. Caprenin, for example, consists of a glycerol backbone with three poorly absorbed fatty acids attached. It is digested like fat, but the fatty acids are only partially absorbed, so it provides only 5 kcalories per gram.[53] The latest artificial fat approved by the FDA is Olestra, or sucrose polyester, which is made from sucrose with fatty acids attached. Olestra cannot be digested by either the human enzymes or the bacterial enzymes in the gastrointestinal tract. It is therefore excreted in the feces without being absorbed. One of the problems with Olestra is that it reduces the absorption of other fat-soluble substances, including the fat-soluble vitamins A, D, E, and K. To avoid depleting these vitamins, Olestra has been fortified with them. However, it is not fortified with beta-carotene and other fat-soluble substances that may be important for health. Another potential problem with Olestra is that it can cause gastrointestinal irritation, bloating, and diarrhea in some individuals because it passes into the colon without being digested.[53] Olestra has been approved by the FDA for use in snack foods such as chips and crackers. These products must carry a warning label about these potential problems (Figure 5.21).

Most lowfat and fat-free products contain a combination of ingredients that offer the texture of fat. In many products, fats are replaced with other energy-containing nutrients, so the energy content of fat-free foods may not be significantly reduced. For instance, a brownie contains about 6.5 grams of fat and 112 kcalories. A reduced-fat brownie contains 2 grams of fat and 89 kcalories, whereas a fat-free brownie contains no fat and 76 kcalories. As you can see, fat-free products can help reduce the amount of fat in the diet—but they cannot be eaten liberally without affecting energy intake.

APPLICATIONS

These exercises are designed to help you apply your critical thinking skills to your own nutrition choices. Many are best performed using a diet analysis software program. If you do not have access to a computer program, the exercises can be hand-calculated using the information in this text and its appendices.

1. Calculate your average fat, saturated fat, and cholesterol intake using the three-day food record you kept in Chapter 2.
   a. How many grams of fat and saturated fat do you consume?
   b. What percent of your energy intake is from fat? Saturated fat?
   c. How does your fat intake compare with the recommendation of no more than 30% of energy from total fat and no more than 10% from saturated fat?
   d. If your diet contains more than 30% of energy from fat, make food substitutions that would decrease your fat intake to 30% or less of energy without changing your energy intake. If your diet already contains less than 30% of energy from fat, list foods you typically consume that are high in fat and some lower-fat substitutes that you could try.
   e. If your diet contains more than 10% of energy from saturated fat, suggest food substitutions that would decrease the amount of saturated fat in your diet.
   f. How does your cholesterol intake compare with the suggested limit of 300 mg per day?
   g. Does your diet meet the recommendations of the Food Guide Pyramid?
2. Review all three days of the food record you kept in Chapter 2. Identify two foods from your diet that are sources of each of the following lipids. If your diet does not contain any foods that are sources of these, name foods that do contain them.
   a. Cholesterol
   b. Saturated fat
   c. Polyunsaturated fat
   d. Monounsaturated fat
   e. Omega-3 fatty acids
   f. Trans fatty acids
3. Using the example in *Critical Thinking: Dietary Fat and Heart Disease Risk*, assess your own risk of cardiovascular disease. Unless you have had a recent physical examination, you may not know your blood cholesterol values.
4. Using the Internet, locate the American Heart Association's Web page. Use their online health assessment, "What's your risk?" to determine your risk of cardiovascular disease.

Summary

1. Lipids are a diverse group of organic compounds, most of which do not dissolve in water. In the body, they provide a concentrated source of energy, insulate against shock and temperature changes, are a structural component of cell membranes, and are used to synthesize hormones and other molecules. In the diet, they provide energy and contribute to the texture and flavor of food.
2. Fatty acids consist of a carbon chain with an acid group at one end. The length of the carbon chain and the number and position of double bonds determine the characteristics of the fat. Linoleic acid (omega-6) and alpha-linolenic acid (omega-3) are considered essential fatty acids because they cannot be synthesized by the body. Other omega-6 and omega-3 fatty acids may become essential when they cannot be synthesized in adequate amounts for proper physiological function. In the body and in the diet, most fatty acids are found as part of triglycerides.
3. Triglycerides, commonly referred to as fat, are the storage form of fat. They consist of a backbone of glycerol with three fatty acids attached.
4. Phosphoglycerides consist of a backbone of glycerol, two fatty acids, and a phosphate group. Phosphoglycerides are an important part of cell membranes and lipoproteins because one end is water-soluble and one end is lipid-soluble.
5. Sterols, of which cholesterol is the best known, are made up of multiple chemical rings. Cholesterol is made by the body and consumed in animal foods in the diet. In the body, it is a component of cell membranes and is used to synthesize vitamin D, bile acids, and a number of hormones.
6. In the small intestine, fats from the diet form micelles with bile and are digested by pancreatic lipase. The products of fat digestion pass into the cells of the small intestine.
7. In body fluids, lipids are transported as lipoproteins. Lipids absorbed from the intestine are packaged with protein to form chylomicrons, which enter the lymphatic system before entering the blood. The triglycerides in chylomicrons are broken down by lipoprotein lipase on the surface of cells lining the blood vessels. Fatty acids are released and are taken up by surrounding cells. The chylomicron remnants that remain are returned to the liver.
8. Very-low-density lipoproteins (VLDLs) are lipoproteins synthesized by the liver. They deliver triglycerides to the tissues. Once the triglycerides have been removed, intermediate-density lipoproteins (IDLs) are transformed into low-density lipoproteins (LDLs). LDLs deliver cholesterol to tissues by binding to LDL receptors on the cell surface. High levels are associated with cardiovascular disease. High-density lipoproteins (HDLs) are made by the liver and small intestine. They help remove cholesterol from cells for disposal and protect against cardiovascular disease.
9. After eating, chylomicrons and VLDLs deliver triglycerides to cells for energy or storage. During fasting, triglycerides stored in adipose cells are broken down by hormone sensitive lipase and the fatty acids and glycerol are released into the blood.
10. The risk of heart disease is increased by diabetes, high blood pressure, obesity, and high blood cholesterol levels. High blood levels of total and LDL cholesterol are a risk factor for heart disease. High blood HDL cholesterol protects against heart disease.
11. The risk of heart disease is affected by age, gender, genetics, and lifestyle factors such as diet. Diets high in total fat, saturated fat, trans fatty acids, and cholesterol increase the risk of heart disease primarily by increasing blood cholesterol levels. Diets high in omega-6 or omega-3 polyunsaturated fatty acids, monounsaturated fatty acids, and plant foods containing fiber, antioxidants, and phytochemicals reduce the risk of

heart disease by affecting cholesterol levels and other risk factors.

12. Diets high in fat correlate with an increased incidence of certain types of cancer. In general, diets very low in fat are associated with a lower risk of breast cancer, and high intakes of linoleic acid may promote tumor growth. Diets high in fat and low in fiber increase colon cancer risk. As with heart disease, the overall diet is probably more important in cancer prevention than fat intake alone.
13. A minimum of 3 to 6 grams of linoleic acid is recommended. To reduce chronic disease risk, it is recommended that total fat in the diet be divided equally between saturated fat, polyunsaturated fat, and monounsaturated fat; that it account for no more than 30% of energy; and that dietary cholesterol be no more than 300 mg per day.
14. Reducing fat intake requires decreasing intake of obvious sources of fat such as butter and oils, as well as baked goods, fast foods, and processed convenience foods that contain hidden fats. To reduce health risks, the total diet, including consumption of grains, fruits, and vegetables, is as important as a low fat intake.
15. The types of fats used in processing depend on the desired characteristic. Partially hydrogenated vegetable oils and tropical oils are used to improve shelf life and increase the melting point. The trans and saturated fatty acids in these products may increase health risks.
16. Artificial fats are used to create reduced-fat products with taste and texture similar to the original. Some lowfat products are made by using mixtures of carbohydrates or proteins to simulate the properties of fat, and some use modified lipids that are not well absorbed.

Review Questions

1. What is a lipid?
2. Name four types of lipids found in the body.
3. What distinguishes a saturated fat from a monounsaturated fat? From a polyunsaturated fat?
4. Name two functions of fat in foods.
5. List three functions of fat in the body.
6. In the body, what is the advantage of storing energy as fat rather than as carbohydrate?
7. What is the function of bile in fat digestion?
8. How do chylomicrons and VLDLs differ?
9. How do HDLs differ from LDLs?
10. How are blood levels of LDLs and HDLs related to the risk of cardiovascular disease?
11. What types of foods contain cholesterol?
12. What are the recommendations for dietary fat intake?
13. What is hydrogenation and how is it related to trans fatty acids?
14. Is essential fatty acid deficiency common in developed countries? Why or why not?

Nutrition Web Links

To further explore areas related to the material in this chapter go to the *Nutrition: Science and Applications* Web site at ***www.Wiley.com/college/Smolin*** and *click on* **Student Companion Site** for chapter-by-chapter links. Some Web sites related to the information in Chapter 5 include:

Sites from government programs that provide recommendations on fat intake and disease prevention such as Healthy People 2010 and the National Cholesterol Education Program.

Sites from health promotion agencies that make recommendations regarding fat intake such as the American Cancer Society and the American Heart Association.

Sites from food companies that manufacture fat replacers and fat-modified foods such as Procter and Gamble and Nabisco.

References

1. Kwiterovich, P. O. The effect of dietary fat, antioxidants and pro-oxidants on blood lipids, lipoproteins and atherosclerosis. J. Am. Diet. Assoc. 97(suppl): S231–S241, 1997.
2. Crawford, M. A., Costeloe, K., Ghebremeskel, K., et al. Are deficits of arachidonic and docosahexaenoic acids responsible for the neural and vascular complications of preterm babies? Am. J. Clin. Nutr. 66(suppl): 1032S–1041S, 1997.
3. Wood, J. L., and Allison, R. G. Effects of consumption of choline and lecithin on neurological and cardiovascular systems. Fed. Proc. 41: 3015, 1982.
4. Hamosh, M., Iverson, S. J., Kirk, C. L., and Hamosh, P. Milk lipids and neonatal fat digestion: relationship between fatty acid composition, endogenous and exogenous digestive enzymes and digestion of milk fat. World Rev. Nutr. Diet. 75:86–91, 1994.
5. Gerster, H. The use of n-3 PUFAs (fish oil) in enteral nutrition. Int. J. Vitam. Nutr. Res. 65:3–20, 1995.
6. Krauss, R. M., Deckelbaum, R. J., Ernst, N., et al. Dietary guidelines for healthy American adults: a statement for health professionals from the Nutrition Committee, American Heart Association. Circulation 94:1795–1800, 1996.
7. Lichtenstein, A. H., Kennedy, E., Barrier, P., et al. Dietary fat consumption and health. Nutr. Rev. 56(II):S3–S28, 1998.
8. Kuller, L. H. Dietary fat and chronic diseases: epidemiologic overview. J. Am. Diet. Assoc. 97(suppl):S9–S15, 1997.
9. Keys, A. *Seven Countries: A Multivariate Analysis of Diet and Coronary Heart Disease.* Cambridge, Mass.: Harvard University Press, 1980.
10. Ascherio, A., Rimm, E. B., Stampfer, M. J., et al. Marine n-3 fatty acids, fish intake, and the risk of coronary disease among men. N. Engl. J. Med. 332:977–982, 1995.
11. Nestle, M. Mediterranean diets: historical and research overview. Am. J. Clin. Nutr. 61(suppl):1313S–1320S, 1995.
12. Keys, A. Mediterranean diet and public health: personal reflections. Am. J. Clin. Nutr. 61(suppl):1321S–1323S, 1995.
13. Gordon, T. The diet-heart idea. Am. J. Epidemiol. 127:220–223, 1988.

14. Brown, M. S., and Goldstein, J. L. How LDL receptors influence cholesterol and atherosclerosis. Sci. Am. 251:58–66, 1984.
15. Brown, M. S., and Goldstein, J. L. Scavenging for receptors. Nature 343:508–509, 1990.
16. American Heart Association, Cardiovascular Disease Statistics. Online at http://www.amhrt.org/Heart_and_Stroke_A_Z_Guide/cvds.html
17. Summary of the Second Report of the National Cholesterol Education Program. Expert Panel on detection, evaluation and treatment of high blood cholesterol in adults. J.A.M.A. 269:3015–3023, 1993.
18. Schaefer, E. J., Lichtenstein, A. H., Lamon-Fava, S., et al. Lipoproteins, nutrition, aging, and atherosclerosis. Am. J. Clin. Nutr. 61(suppl):726S–740S, 1995.
19. American and Canadian Dietetics Association. Position paper of the American Dietetic Association and the Canadian Dietetic Association on women's health and nutrition. J. Am. Diet. Assoc. 95:362–366, 1995.
20. Geil, P. B., Anderson, J. W., and Gustafson, N. J. Women and men with hypercholesterolemia respond similarly to an American Heart Association Step 1 Diet. J. Am. Diet. Assoc. 95:436–441, 1995.
21. Hu, F. B., Stampfer, M. J., Manson, J. E., et al. Dietary fat intake and the risk of coronary heart disease in women, N. Engl. J. Med. 337:1491–1499, 1997.
22. Sagiv, M., and Goldbourt, U. Influence of physical work on high density lipoprotein cholesterol: implications for the risk of coronary heart disease. Int. J. Sports Med. 15:261–266, 1994.
23. Denke, M. A. Review of human studies evaluating individual dietary responsiveness in patients with hypercholesterolemia. Am. J. Clin. Nutr. 62(suppl):471S–477S, 1995.
24. Dietschy, J. M. Dietary fatty acids and the regulation of plasma low density lipoprotein cholesterol concentrations. J. Nutr. 128:444S–448S, 1998.
25. Aro, A., Jauhiainen, M., Partanen, R., et al. Stearic acid, trans fatty acids and dairy fat: effects on serum and lipoprotein lipids, apolipoproteins, lipoprotein (a) and lipid transfer proteins in healthy subjects. Am. J. Clin. Nutr. 65:1419–1426, 1997.
26. Watts, G. F., Jackson, P., Burke, V., and Lewis, B. Dietary fatty acids and progression of coronary artery disease in men. Am. J. Clin. Nutr. 64:202–209, 1996.
27. Ascherio, A., and Willett, W. C. Health effects of trans fatty acids. Am. J. Clin. Nutr. 66(suppl):1006S–1010S, 1997.
28. Zock, P. L., and Katan, M.B. Butter, margarine and serum lipoproteins. Atherosclerosis 131:7–16, 1997.
29. Eckel, R. H., and Krauss, R. M. American Heart Association call to action: obesity is a major risk factor for coronary heart disease. AHA Nutrition Committee. Circulation 97:2099–2100, 1998.
30. Katan, M. B., Zock, P. L., and Mensink, R. P. Dietary oils, serum lipoproteins, and coronary heart disease. Am. J. Clin. Nutr. 61(suppl): 1368S–1373S, 1995.
31. Stone, N. J. Fish consumption, fish oil, lipids, and coronary heart disease. Am. J. Clin. Nutr. 65:1083–1086, 1997.
32. Connor, S. L., and Connor, W. E. Are fish oils beneficial in the prevention and treatment of coronary artery disease? Am. J. Clin. Nutr. 66(suppl):1020S–1031S, 1997.
33. Schoene, N. W., and Fitzgerald, G. A. Thrombogenic potential of dietary long-chain polyunsaturated fatty acids: session summary. Am. J. Clin. Nutr. 56(suppl):825S–826S, 1992.
34. Willett, W. C., Sacks, F., Trichopouluo, A., et al. Mediterranean diet pyramid: a cultural model for healthy eating. Am. J. Clin. Nutr. 61(suppl):1402S–1406S, 1995.
35. Waterhouse, A. L., German, B. L., Walzem, R. L., et al. Is it time for a wine trial? Am. J. Clin. Nutr. 68:220–221, 1998.
36. American Institute for Cancer Research, World Cancer Research Fund. Food, Nutrition and the Prevention of Cancer: A Global Perspective. Presented at the American Institute of Cancer Research Research Conference, Oct. 8–10, 1997.
37. Trichopoulou, A., Katsouyanni, K., Stuver, S., et al. Consumption of olive oil and specific food groups in relation to breast cancer risk in Greece. J. Natl. Cancer Inst. 87:110–116, 1995.
38. Rose, D. P. Dietary fatty acids and cancer. Am. J. Clin. Nutr. 66(suppl):998S–1003S, 1997.
39. Greenwald, P., Sherwood, K., and McDonald, S. Fat, caloric intake and obesity: lifestyle risk factors for breast cancer. J. Am. Diet. Assoc. (suppl):S24–S30, 1997.
40. Noguchi, M., Rose, D. P., Earashi, M., and Miyazaki, I. The role of fatty acids and eicosanoid synthesis inhibitors in breast carcinoma. Oncology 52:265–271, 1995.
41. Reddy, B. S. Nutritional factors and colon cancer. Crit. Rev. Food Sci. Nutr. 35:175–190, 1995.
42. LeMarchand, L., Wilkens, L. P., Hankin, J. H., et al. A case control study of diet and colorectal cancer in a multiethnic population in Hawaii: lipids and foods of animal origin. Cancer Causes Control 8:637–648, 1997.
43. USDA, Agricultural Service. Results from USDA's 1994–1996 Continuing Survey of Food Intakes by Individuals and 1994–1996 Health Knowledge Survey. ARS Food Surveys Research Group, 1997. Online at http://www.barc.usda.gov/bhnrc/foodsurvey/home/htm
44. Health and Welfare Canada. Nutrition Recommendations: The Report of the Scientific Review Committee. Ottawa: Minister of Supply and Services Canada, 1990.
45. WHO and FAO Joint Consultation. Fats and oils in human nutrition. Nutr. Rev. 53:202–205, 1995.
46. Emken, E. A. Trans fatty acids and coronary heart disease risk: physiochemical properties, intake and metabolism. Am. J. Clin. Nutr. 62(suppl):659S–669S, 1995.
47. American Cancer Society. 1996 Guidelines on Diet, Nutrition and Cancer Prevention. Online at http://www.cancer.org/frames.html
48. American Academy of Pediatrics Committee on Nutrition. Statement on cholesterol. Pediatrics 101:141–147, 1998.
49. Miller, D. L., Castellanos, V. H., Shide, D. J., et al. Effect of fat-free potato chips with and without nutrition labels on fat and energy intake. Am. J. Clin. Nutr. 68:282–290,1998.
50. Calorie Control Council. Light foods and beverages soar to new levels of popularity. Calorie Control Commentary 18:1–3, 1996.
51. Elson, C. E. Tropical oils: nutritional and scientific issues. Crit. Rev. Food Sci. Nutr. 31:79–102, 1992.
52. Sigmna-Grant, M. Can you have your low-fat cake and eat it too? The role of fat-modified products. J. Am. Diet. Assoc. 97(suppl):S76–S81, 1997.
53. American Dietetic Association. Position of the American Dietetic Association: fat replacers. J. Am. Diet. Assoc. 98:463–468, 1998.

Chapter 6

Chapter Outline

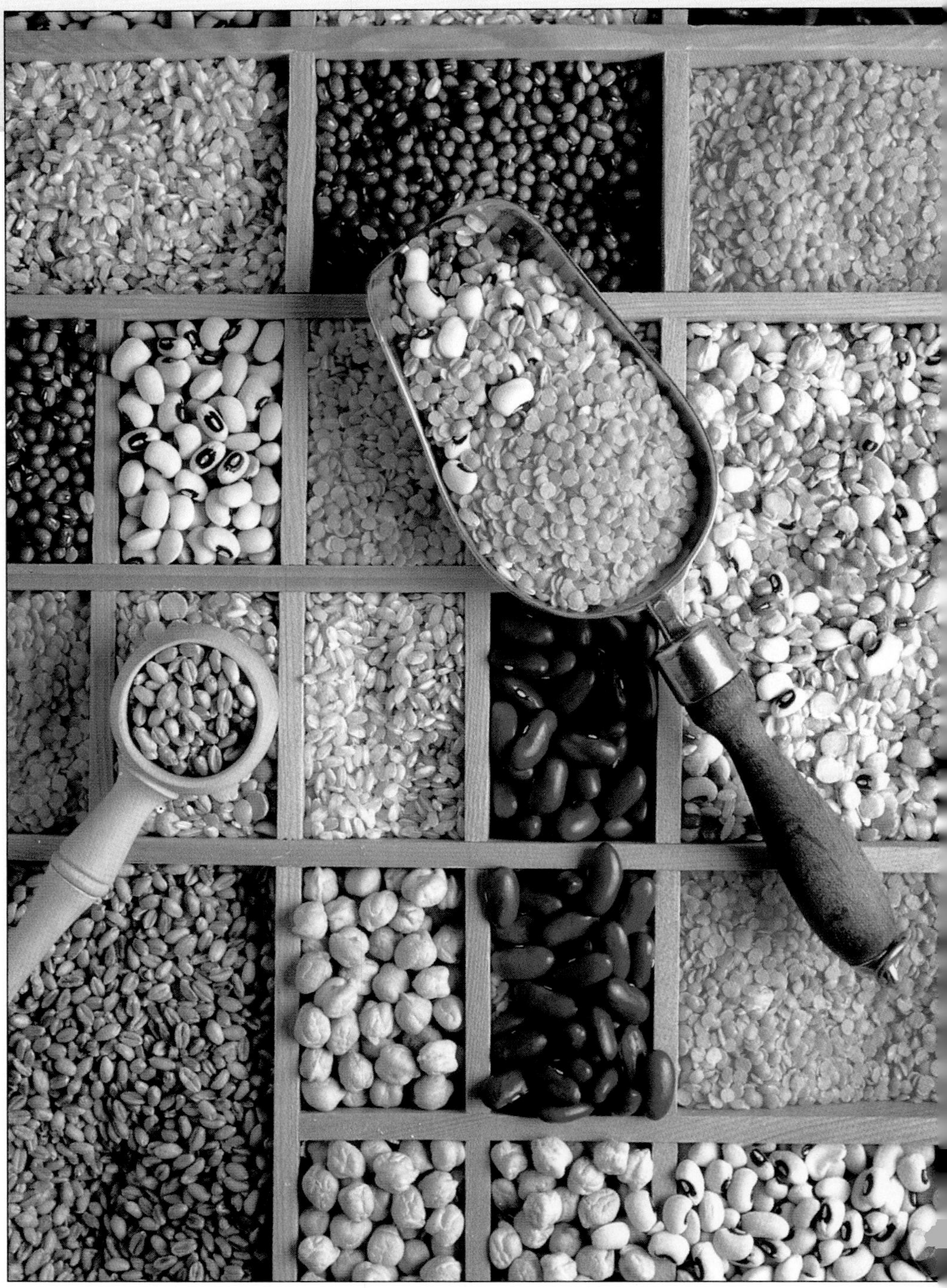

(© *Tony Craddock/Science Photo Library/Photo Researchers, Inc.*)

Protein: The Privileged Nutrient

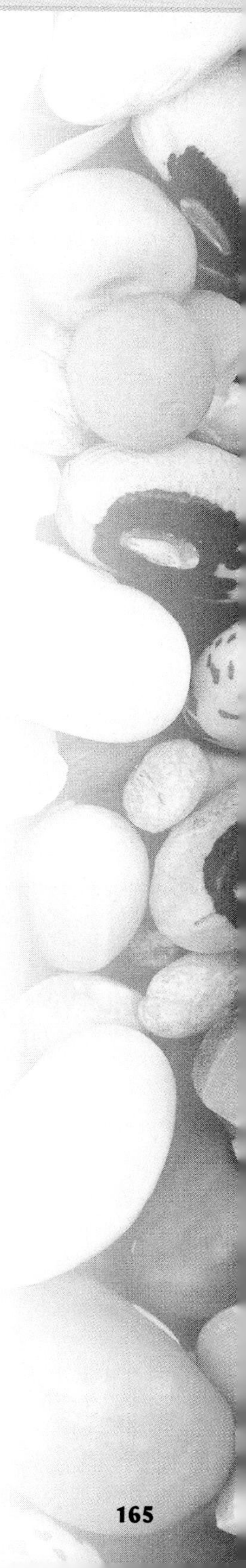

Chapter Concepts

1. Most people in economically developed countries eat more than enough protein.
2. Protein is found in both animal and plant foods.
3. Proteins are made up of chains of amino acids folded into three-dimensional shapes.
4. Amino acids that cannot be made by the body in amounts sufficient to meet needs are essential in the diet.
5. Amino acids can be used to synthesize body proteins, to synthesize nonprotein molecules, and to provide energy.
6. Protein is necessary to allow for growth as well as to maintain structure and regulate functions in the body.
7. The amino acid composition of a protein affects how efficiently it can be used to make body proteins. This is referred to as protein quality.
8. Animal sources of protein are generally of higher quality than plant sources.
9. Vegetarian diets rely on plant protein from varied sources to meet body needs.
10. Proteins and amino acids are added to alter the texture, flavor, and nutritional characteristics of food products.

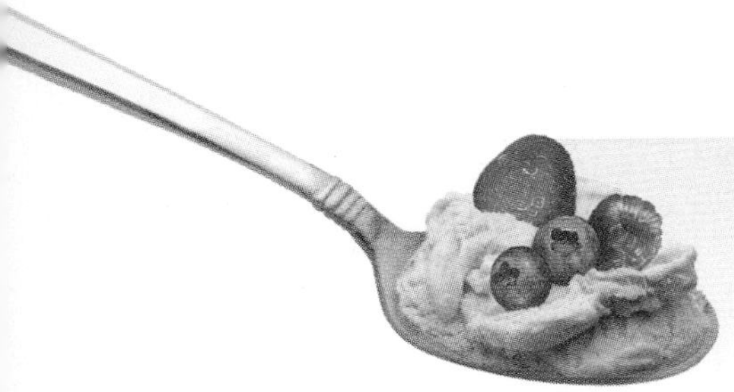

Just a Taste

Do you eat enough protein?

Does eating a high-protein diet make your muscles bigger?

Can you stay healthy eating a vegetarian diet?

Protein is a nutrient that conjures up images of vitality and strength. Unlike carbohydrate and fat, protein has had the privilege of being associated with positive effects. It has not been accused of being fattening, causing tooth decay, or increasing the risk of heart disease. It is associated with strong muscles and good health. As a result, protein is a "big seller." Protein drinks, pills, and powders fill the shelves of health food stores. Consumers often choose high-protein foods and supplements because of protein's association with good health. Is protein worthy of its lofty reputation? Do we need to worry about eating too much protein or which protein sources we choose?

Most of the world relies on plant foods such as grains and vegetables to meet their protein needs. There is growing evidence that this may be a healthier dietary pattern than one that relies heavily on animal foods. Although the Dietary Guidelines do not specifically address protein intake, following these recommendations will affect the amount and sources of protein in the overall diet. For example, the typical meat and potatoes diet of North America provides too few fruits and vegetables and too much fat. The Dietary Guidelines recommend a diet that contains plenty of grain products, vegetables, and fruits and is low in fat, saturated fat and cholesterol. Following these guidelines will decrease the amount of animal protein, and most likely total protein, in the diet. Is this a healthy dietary pattern? Does it reduce the risk of chronic disease? Or does it increase the possibility of protein and other nutrient deficiencies?

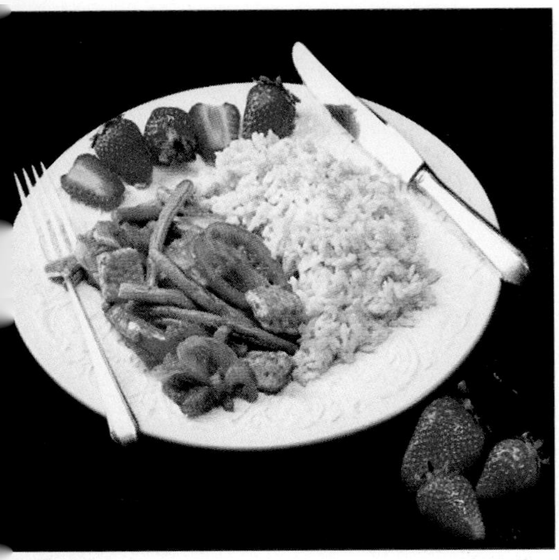

Figure 6.1
Foods of plant origin can supply plenty of protein. (ASAP/Photo Researchers, Inc.)

WHAT IS PROTEIN?

In a typical day, most Americans consume about 100 grams of protein—about twice their requirement. Most of this comes from animal sources such as meat, milk, and eggs—the most concentrated sources of protein. One egg or an ounce of meat contains about 7 grams of protein, and a cup of milk contains 8 grams. But plants also provide good sources of protein (Figure 6.1). Legumes, such as lentils, soybeans, peanuts, black-eyed peas, chickpeas, red beans, pinto beans, kidney beans, and black beans, provide 6 to 10 grams of protein per half-cup serving. Nuts and seeds are also good sources of protein, providing about 5 to 10 grams per quarter cup. A half-cup serving of vegetables or grains, such as rice or

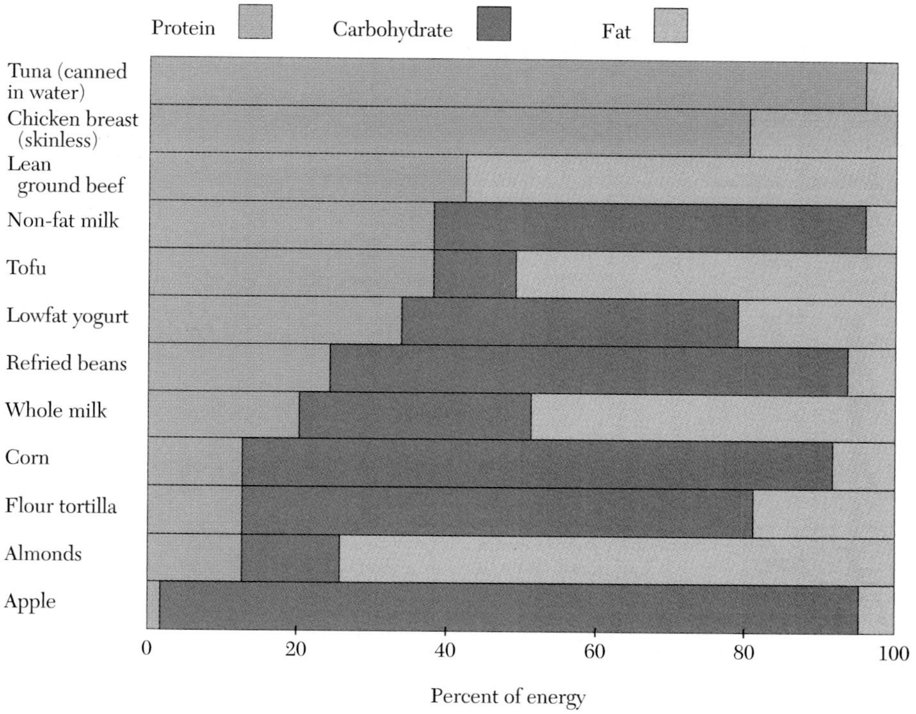

Figure 6.2
These foods provide varying amounts of dietary protein and also contain carbohydrate and fat.

pasta, provides 2 to 3 grams (Figure 6.2). Although plant proteins are not used as efficiently as animal sources to make body proteins, a diet including plant proteins from a variety of sources can easily meet most people's needs.

One way that protein is distinguished from carbohydrate and lipid is by the fact that it contains the element nitrogen. Protein in the diet provides the raw material to make all the various types of proteins that the body needs. These body proteins provide important structural and regulatory functions. In some circumstances protein can be used for energy, providing 4 kcalories per gram.

Amino acids The building blocks of proteins. Each contains a carbon atom bound to a hydrogen atom, an amino group, an acid group, and a side chain.

Essential or **indispensable amino acids** Amino acids that cannot be synthesized by the human body in sufficient amounts to meet needs and therefore must be included in the diet.

Nonessential or **dispensable amino acids** Amino acids that can be synthesized by the human body in sufficient amounts to meet needs.

Proteins Are Made of Amino Acids

A protein molecule, whether found in a steak, a kidney bean, or a part of the human body, is constructed of one or more folded, chainlike strands of **amino acids.** Each different protein contains a specific number of amino acids in specific proportions that are bound together in a specific order. Variations in the number, proportion, and order of amino acids allow for an infinite number of different protein structures.

There are approximately 20 amino acids commonly found in proteins. Each amino acid consists of a carbon atom bound to four chemical groups: a hydrogen atom; an amino group, which contains nitrogen; an acid group; and a fourth group called a side chain that varies in length and structure (Figure 6.3). Different side chains give specific properties to individual amino acids.

Of the 20 amino acids commonly found in protein, 9 cannot be made by the adult human body. These amino acids, called **essential** or **indispensable amino acids,** must be consumed in the diet (Table 6.1). If the diet is deficient in one or more of these amino acids, new proteins containing them cannot be made without breaking down other body proteins to provide them. The 11 **nonessential** or **dispensable amino acids** can be made by the human body and are not required in the diet. When a nonessential amino acid needed for protein synthesis is not available from the diet, it can be made in the body. Most of the nonessential

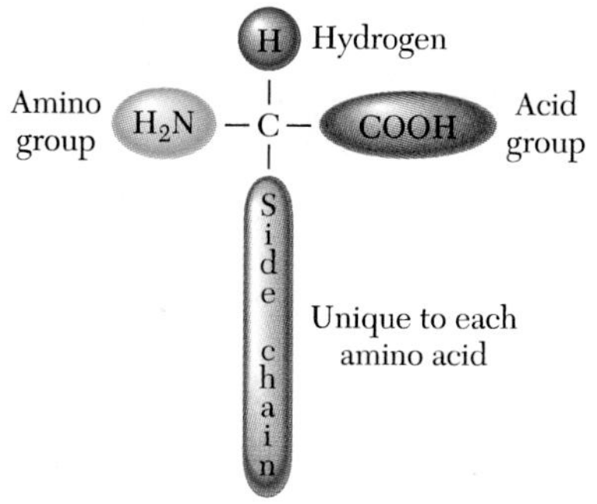

Figure 6.3
All amino acids have a similar structure, but each has a different side chain.

Table 6.1 *Classification of Amino Acids for Adult Humans*

Essential Amino Acids	Nonessential Amino Acids
Histidine	Alanine
Isoleucine	Arginine
Leucine	Asparagine
Lysine	Aspartic acid (aspartate)
Methionine	Cysteine (cystine)°
Phenylalanine	Tyrosine°
Threonine	Glutamic acid (glutamate)
Tryptophan	Glutamine
Valine	Glycine
	Proline
	Serine

°These amino acids are also classified as semiessential. If not enough is supplied in the diet, they must be made from essential amino acids. If those essential amino acids are in short supply, the semiessential amino acids can become essential.

Transamination The process by which an amino group from one amino acid is transferred to a carbon compound to form a new amino acid.

Semiessential or **conditionally essential amino acids** Amino acids that are essential in the diet only under certain conditions or at certain times of life.

amino acids can be made by the process of **transamination,** in which an amino group from one amino acid is transferred to a carbon-containing molecule to form a different amino acid (Figure 6.4).

Some amino acids are **semiessential** or **conditionally essential.** These are essential only under certain conditions. For example, the conditionally essential amino acid tyrosine can be made in the body from the essential amino acid phenylalanine. If phenylalanine is in short supply, tyrosine cannot be made and becomes essential in the diet. Likewise, the amino acid cysteine is only essential when the essential amino acid methionine is in short supply. Other amino acids may be essential under certain conditions, such as premature infancy.

Protein Structure

Amino acids are linked together to form proteins by a unique type of chemical bond called a peptide bond. This bond is formed between the acid group of one amino acid and the nitrogen atom of the next amino acid (Figure 6.5). When two

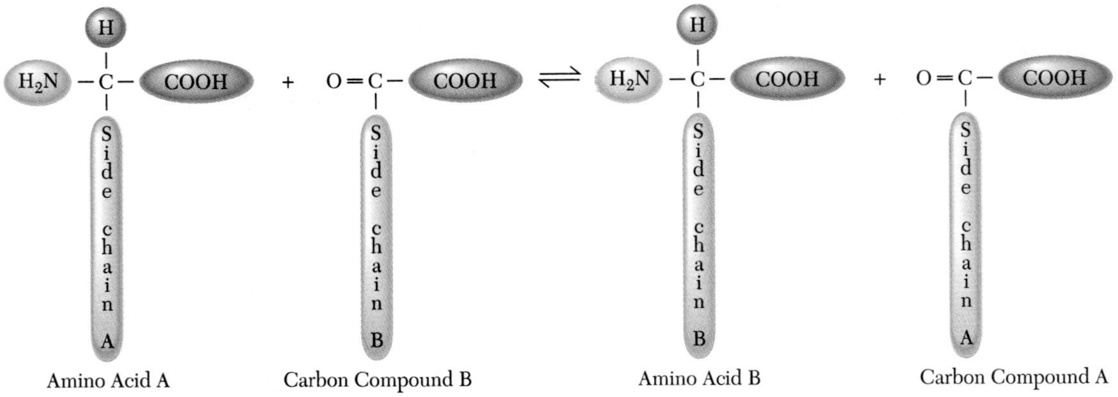

Figure 6.4
By the process of transamination, a carbon compound, shown as B in this figure, is combined with the amino group from a nonessential amino acid, shown as A in this figure, to form amino acid B and carbon compound A.

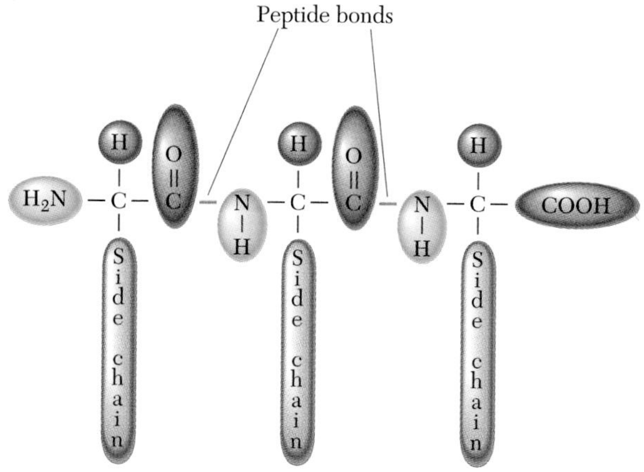

Figure 6.5
Amino acids in proteins are linked by peptide bonds.

amino acids are linked with a peptide bond, they are called a **dipeptide;** when three amino acids are linked, they form a **tripeptide.** Many amino acids bonded together constitute a **polypeptide.** A protein is made of one or more polypeptide chains folded into a complex three-dimensional shape. The three-dimensional shape of the protein is determined by the order of the amino acids, and it is the shape of a protein that determines its function.

Dipeptide Two amino acids linked by a peptide bond. A **tripeptide** is three amino acids linked by peptide bonds, and a **polypeptide** is a chain of three or more amino acids linked by peptide bonds.

If the shape of the protein changes, its function is altered. For example, the genetic disease sickle-cell anemia results from a change in only one of the amino acids in hemoglobin, the protein that carries oxygen in the blood. The altered amino acid chain causes the protein to change shape, which causes the characteristics of the hemoglobin molecule to change. Sickle-cell hemoglobin molecules bind together, forming long chains, whereas normal hemoglobin molecules do not bind together. A red blood cell containing normal hemoglobin is disc shaped, whereas a cell containing chains of sickle-cell hemoglobin is crescent or sickle shaped (Figure 6.6). These distorted red blood cells can block capillaries, causing inflammation and pain, and they rupture easily, leading to anemia from a shortage of red blood cells.

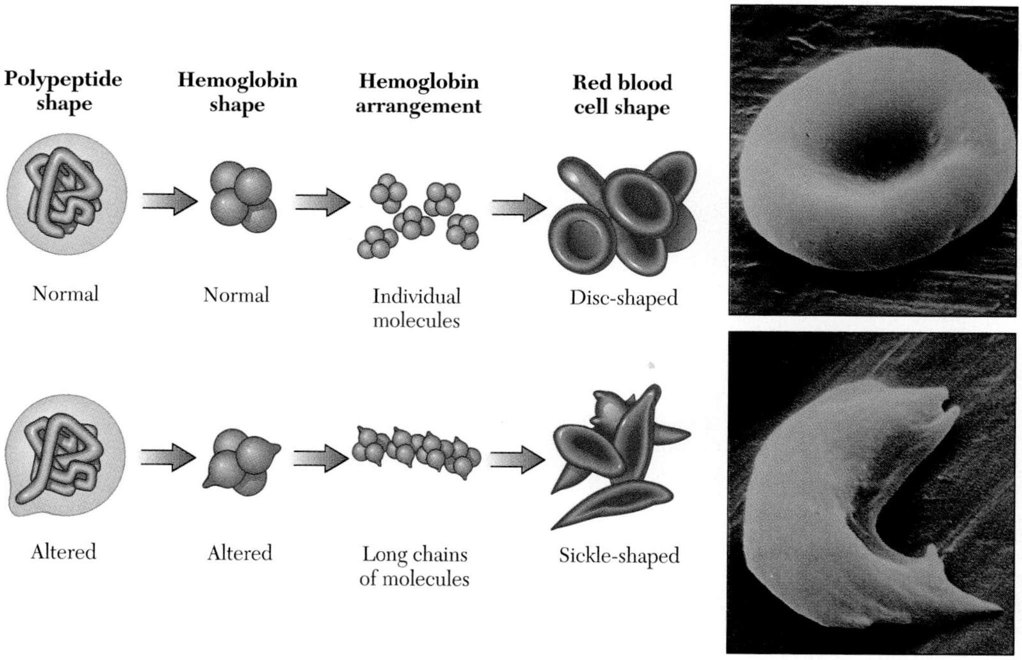

Figure 6.6
In sickle-cell anemia, a change in the sequence of amino acids in hemoglobin causes a change in the shape and function of the protein molecule. Sickle-cell hemoglobin forms long chains that distort the shape of red blood cells. (© Stan Flegler/ Visuals Unlimited)

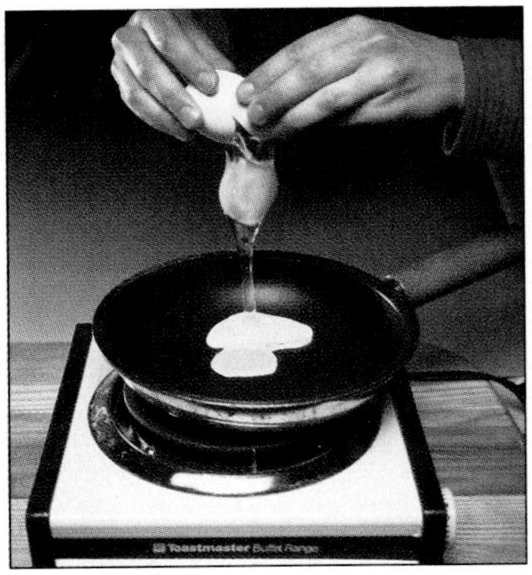

Figure 6.7
The protein in egg white is denatured by heat when the egg is cooked. (Charles D. Winters)

Denaturation The alteration of a protein's three-dimensional structure.

Changes in protein structure can also be caused by heat or acid. This change in structure is called **denaturation,** a change from the natural. In food, cooking denatures protein, thereby changing its shape and physical properties. For example, a raw egg white is clear and liquid, but once it has been denatured by cooking, it becomes white and firm (Figure 6.7).

PROTEIN IN THE DIGESTIVE TRACT

The digestion of protein begins in the stomach, where hydrochloric acid denatures proteins, opening up their folded structure to make them more accessible to enzyme attack. The acid also activates the protein-digesting enzyme pepsin, which breaks proteins into polypeptides and amino acids. When the polypeptides enter the small intestine, they are broken into smaller peptides by the enzymes trypsin and chymotrypsin, which are secreted by the pancreas. Small peptides are broken into single amino acids by protein-digesting enzymes from the small intestine. Single amino acids, dipeptides, and tripeptides can be absorbed by the mucosal cells of the small intestine. Once inside the mucosal cells, dipeptides and tripeptides are broken into single amino acids (Figure 6.8).

Amino acids cross the mucosal cell of the small intestine using one of several active transport systems. Amino acids with similar structures share the same transport system and therefore compete for absorption. If there is an excess of any one of the amino acids sharing a transport system, more of it will be absorbed, slowing the absorption of the other competing amino acids. This is generally not a

Figure 6.8
An overview of protein digestion and absorption.

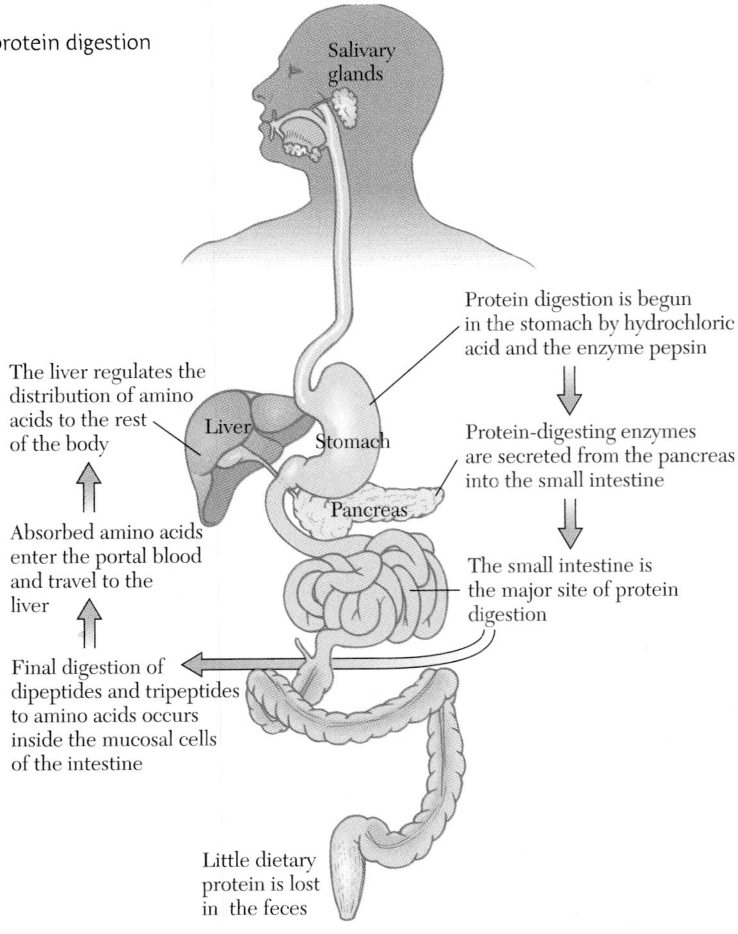
Salivary glands
Protein digestion is begun in the stomach by hydrochloric acid and the enzyme pepsin
The liver regulates the distribution of amino acids to the rest of the body
Liver
Stomach
Protein-digesting enzymes are secreted from the pancreas into the small intestine
Pancreas
Absorbed amino acids enter the portal blood and travel to the liver
The small intestine is the major site of protein digestion
Final digestion of dipeptides and tripeptides to amino acids occurs inside the mucosal cells of the intestine
Little dietary protein is lost in the feces

problem with foods because they contain a variety of amino acids. However, if one takes an amino acid supplement, the absorption of other amino acids that share the same transport system may be impaired (Figure 6.9). For example, weight lifters often supplement the amino acid arginine. Arginine shares the same transport system as lysine. If large doses of arginine are ingested, the absorption of lysine will be reduced.

If a protein from the diet is absorbed without being completely digested, an allergic reaction can occur (see Chapter 14). The absorbed protein is recognized as a foreign substance by the immune system, which mounts an attack. Symptoms of food allergies can include reactions of the respiratory tract (sneezing and asthma), skin (rashes or hives), nervous system (headache and dizziness), cardiovascular system (rapid heart rate), urinary tract (blood in the urine), or digestive system (vomiting and diarrhea). Allergies are most common both in people with gastrointestinal disease, because their damaged intestine allows the absorption of whole proteins, and in infants, because their immature gastrointestinal tracts are more likely to allow larger polypeptides to be absorbed. Once an infant's intestinal mucosa matures, absorption of whole proteins is less likely and food allergies usually disappear. The absorption of whole proteins by very young infants, however, can also be of benefit since antibody proteins absorbed from breast milk can provide temporary protection against certain diseases (see Chapter 13).

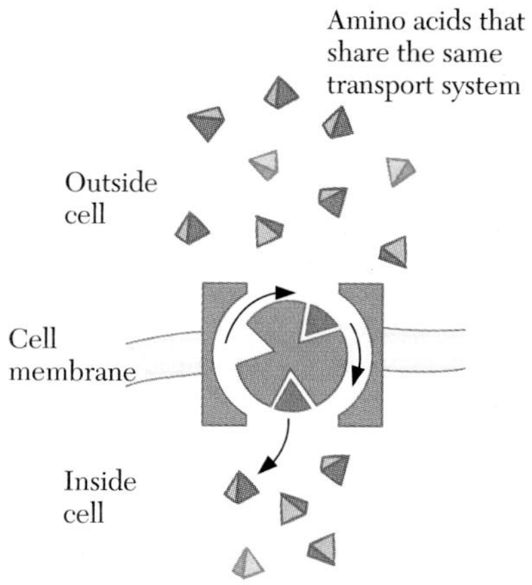

Figure 6.9
The amino acids in this figure share the same transport system, and since there are more of the purple ones than the green ones, more of the purple amino acids are able to cross the membrane into the cell.

PROTEINS IN THE BODY

Once dietary proteins have been digested and absorbed, their amino acids become available to synthesize proteins needed by the body, to synthesize nonprotein molecules, or to provide energy.

Protein Metabolism: Amino Acids for Synthesis and Energy

Once amino acids are absorbed, they enter the hepatic portal vein and travel to the liver. The liver plays an important role in determining how amino acids will be used by the rest of the body. The liver can use the amino acids to synthesize blood or liver proteins, release them into the general circulation for use by other tissues, or degrade them for energy. Some amino acids are also used by the liver and other tissues to form nonprotein molecules of biological importance such as neurotransmitters, which are chemical messengers that transmit nerve signals.

Recycling Amino Acids The amino acids present in body tissues and fluids are available for use and are referred to collectively as the body **amino acid pool.** Amino acids enter this so-called pool from protein in the diet as well as from the breakdown of body proteins. Of the approximately 300 grams of protein synthesized by the body each day, only about 100 grams are made of amino acids from the diet. The other 200 grams are made from amino acids recycled from protein broken down in the body. When dietary intake of protein and energy are adequate but not excessive, most amino acids in the amino acid pool are used to synthesize body proteins and other nitrogen-containing compounds (Figure 6.10). When the diet does not provide enough total energy and when protein is consumed in excess of need, amino acids are used for energy.

Amino acid pool All of the amino acids in body tissues and fluids that are available for protein synthesis.

Protein Synthesis Amino acids from the amino acid pool are used to make body proteins. Which proteins are made and when they are made are carefully regulated but both are dependent on the availability of amino acids. The blueprint for the synthesis of proteins is contained in the DNA in the nucleus of the cell. When a protein is needed, the process of protein synthesis is turned on; but if all the amino acids aren't available, the completed protein cannot be made.

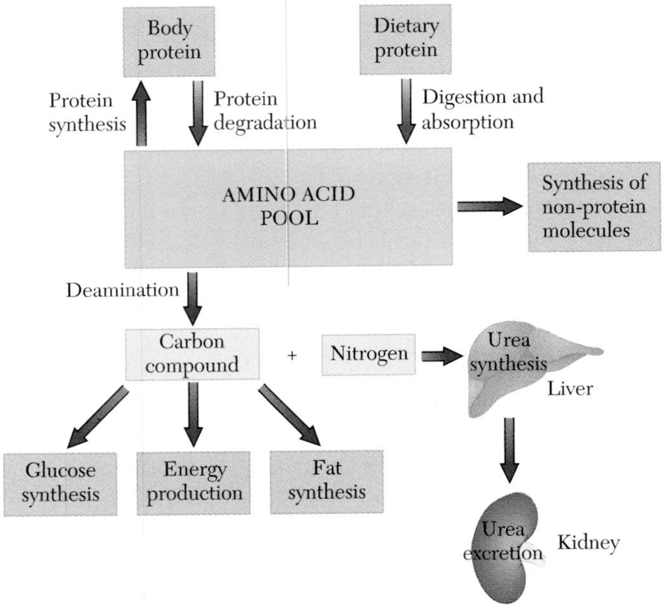

Figure 6.10
Amino acids enter the available pool from the diet and from the breakdown of body proteins. They are used to synthesize body proteins and nonprotein molecules and to provide energy.

Gene A section of DNA that codes for a protein.

Transcription The process of copying the information in DNA to a molecule of mRNA.

Translation The process of translating the RNA code into the amino acid sequence of a protein.

Gene expression Refers to the events of protein synthesis in which the information coded in a gene is used to synthesize a protein.

Gene Expression A **gene** is a stretch of DNA that provides the blueprint for the structure of a protein. For a protein to be made, the information in the gene must first be transferred or transcribed into a molecule of messenger RNA (mRNA). This process is called **transcription.** The mRNA takes this information from the nucleus to ribosomes in the cytoplasm of the cell where proteins are made. Here the information in mRNA is translated into a chain of amino acids in a process called **translation.** The mRNA message or code dictates which amino acids are used and in what order they will be bonded together (Figure 6.11). When the information in a gene is used to make a protein, **gene expression** is occurring. Not all genes are expressed in all cells or at all times. For example, the hormone insulin is a protein that is made in pancreatic cells. Insulin is not made by other body cells because the gene is not expressed in cells other than those in the pancreas. The expression of some genes changes depending on the need for the protein for which they code. For example, when iron intake is high, the expression of a gene that codes for ferritin, an iron-storage protein, is turned on. This allows more of this protein to be synthesized and the capacity to store iron is increased.[1]

Nutrients can affect how and when genes are expressed. As seen above, the amount of iron in the diet determines the amount of ferritin made. Vitamin A affects the expression of many genes involved in the maturation of cells, and vitamin D affects genes that code for calcium transport proteins (see Chapter 9). In

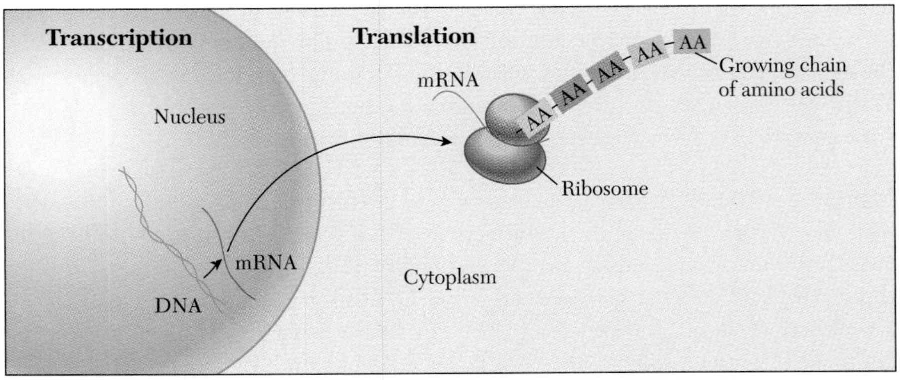

Figure 6.11
DNA in the nucleus of cells provides a blueprint for the sequence of amino acids in proteins. The information in DNA is transcribed into mRNA, which carries it to the ribosomes where it is translated into an amino acid sequence.

this way, levels of nutrients can determine which proteins are made and can therefore regulate body functions. Who we are and how healthy we are depend not only on which genes we have but which genes are expressed.

Limiting Amino Acids During the construction of a protein, a shortage of one needed amino acid can stop protein synthesis. Just as on an assembly line, if one part is missing, the line stops—a different part cannot be substituted. If the missing amino acid is a nonessential amino acid, it can be synthesized in the body and protein synthesis can continue. If the missing amino acid is an essential amino acid, the body can break down its own proteins to obtain this amino acid. If an amino acid cannot be supplied, protein synthesis will stop. The essential amino acid present in shortest supply relative to need is called the **limiting amino acid,** because lack of this amino acid limits the ability to make the protein. If all amino acids are present in adequate amounts at the time of synthesis, proteins will be completed and released for further processing by the cell.

Limiting amino acid The essential amino acid that is available in the lowest concentration in relation to the body's needs.

Synthesis of Nonprotein Molecules Some amino acids are also used to synthesize nonprotein molecules that contain nitrogen. These include a number of neurotransmitters. For example, the amino acid tryptophan is used to synthesize the neurotransmitter serotonin, which acts in the relaxation center of the brain. The units that make up DNA and RNA are another group of nitrogen-containing compounds that are derived in part from amino acids. Other molecules synthesized from amino acids include the skin pigment melanin, and histamine, which causes blood vessels to dilate.

Energy Production Although carbohydrate and fat are more efficient energy sources, protein can also be used for energy. This occurs both when the diet does not provide enough total energy to meet needs, as in starvation, and when protein is consumed in excess of needs.

When energy is deficient, proteins, such as enzymes and muscle proteins, are broken down into amino acids that can then be used as fuel. Before amino acids can be used for energy, the nitrogen-containing amino group must be removed in a process called **deamination.** The nitrogen is then converted by the liver into the waste product **urea,** which can be excreted by the kidneys. The carbon compounds remaining after nitrogen is removed from the amino acids can enter the citric acid cycle to produce ATP or be used to make glucose via gluconeogenesis (Figure 6.12). This provides energy in times of need, but it also robs the body of functional proteins.

Deamination The removal of the amino group from an amino acid.

Urea A nitrogen-containing waste product that is excreted in the urine.

Amino acids are also used for energy when protein intake exceeds protein needs. If the diet is adequate in energy and high in protein, the extra amino acids are used to produce ATP. If both energy and protein exceed needs, the extra amino acids are not stored as protein; rather, they are deaminated and converted into either glucose or fatty acids, depending on their structure.

Functions of Proteins in the Body

The number of different proteins made by the human body is vast. Each protein molecule has a specific function. Some provide structure and others help regulate body processes.

Structural Proteins Proteins provide structure to individual cells and to the body as a whole. In cells, proteins are an integral part of the cell membrane, the cytoplasm, and the organelles. Skin, hair, and muscle are composed largely of protein. Bones and teeth are made up of minerals embedded in a protein framework. When the diet is deficient in protein, these structures break down. The muscles become smaller, the skin loses its elasticity, and the hair becomes thin and can easily be pulled out by the roots. These outward signs of dietary protein

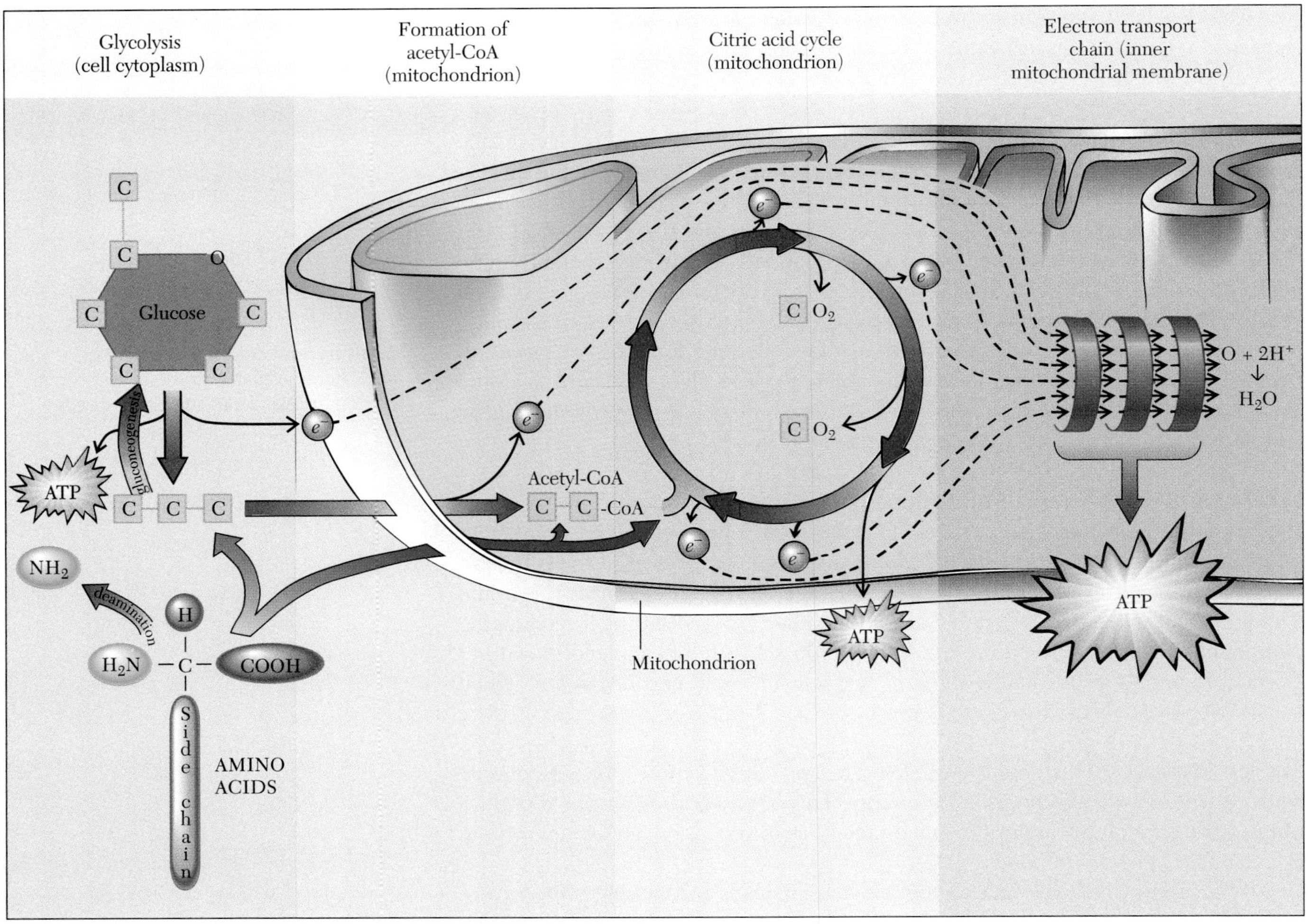

Figure 6.12

Amino acids must be deaminated to remove the nitrogen before they can be metabolized to produce energy or used to synthesize glucose.

deficiency have become marketing strategies for cosmetic companies. Shampoo and hand lotion manufacturers add protein to their products, suggesting that protein applied to the hair or skin will improve its structure. However, the proteins that make up hair and skin can only be made inside the body, so a healthy diet will do more for hair and skin quality than expensive protein shampoos or lotions.

Regulatory Proteins Proteins help regulate the body's many different processes to maintain homeostasis. Regulatory proteins include enzymes, transport proteins in the blood and in cells, immune system proteins, protein hormones, and proteins that aid in muscle contraction, fluid balance, and acid balance.

Enzymes Enzymes are protein molecules that speed up the metabolic reactions of the body but which are not used up or destroyed in these reactions. All the reactions involved in the production of energy and the synthesis and breakdown of carbohydrates, lipids, proteins, and other molecules are expedited by enzymes. Each reaction requires a specific enzyme with a specific structure. If the structure of the enzyme molecule is changed, it can no longer function in the reaction it is designed to accelerate.

Enzymes that function in the body are made by the body and therefore do not need to be consumed in the diet. Enzymes present in foods are denatured by the cooking process and are no longer functional when eaten. When raw foods are eaten, the enzymes present—such as papain in papaya—are broken down during digestion and are absorbed from the gastrointestinal tract as amino acids. Purified enzymes sold as dietary supplements are also broken down in the gut. These may provide some function in the gut; for example, lactase, taken by individuals with lactose intolerance, breaks down lactose that is consumed while the lactase is in the gut. Eventually, these enzymes are digested and absorbed as amino acids.

Transport Proteins Proteins transport substances throughout the body and into and out of individual cells. Transport proteins in the blood carry substances from one organ to another. For example, hemoglobin, the protein in red blood cells, picks up oxygen in the lungs and transports it to other organs of the body. The proteins in lipoproteins are needed to transport lipids from the intestines and liver to body cells. Some vitamins, such as vitamin A, must be bound to a specific protein to be transported in the blood. When protein is deficient, the nutrients that require protein for transport cannot travel to the cells. For this reason, a protein deficiency can cause a vitamin A deficiency; even if vitamin A is consumed in the diet it cannot be transported to the cells. At the cellular level, transport proteins present in cell membranes help move substances such as glucose and amino acids across the cell membrane. For example, transport proteins in the intestinal mucosa are necessary to absorb amino acids from the intestinal lumen into the mucosal cells.

Defense Proteins Proteins play an important role in protecting the body from injury and invasion by foreign substances. Skin, which is made up of protein, is the first barrier against infection and injury. Foreign particles such as dirt or bacteria that are on the skin cannot enter the body and can be washed away. If the skin is broken and blood vessels are injured, fibrinogen and thrombin, blood-clotting proteins, help prevent too much blood from being lost. If a foreign particle such as a virus or bacterium enters the body, the immune system fights it off by synthesizing proteins called **antibodies.** Each antibody has a unique structure that allows it to attach to a specific invader. When an antibody binds to an invading substance, the production of more antibodies is stimulated, and other parts of the immune system are signaled to help destroy the invader. The next time the same type of invading bacterium or virus enters the body, the immune system is already primed to produce specific antibodies to fight off the invader. This is also how immunizations against diseases, such as measles, work: A small amount of dead or inactivated virus is injected into the body; the injected material does not cause disease, but it does stimulate the immune system to produce antibodies to the virus, so the next time the body comes in contact with the virus, a large-scale immune attack is mounted and the infection is prevented. When the immune system malfunctions as a result of protein deficiency or other causes, such as HIV infection, the ability to protect the body from infection is compromised.

Antibodies Proteins produced by cells of the immune system that destroy or inactivate foreign substances in the body.

Contractile or Motile Proteins Some proteins give cells and organisms the ability to move, contract, and change shape. Actin and myosin function in the contraction of muscles. These two proteins slide past each other to shorten the muscle and cause contraction. For example, when you do a pull-up, the muscles in your arms shorten as the alternating actin and myosin proteins slide past one another (Figure 6.13). A similar process causes contraction in the heart muscle and in the muscles that cause constriction in the digestive tract, blood vessels, and body glands. Actin and myosin can also cause contraction in nonmuscle cells. This contraction may help individual cells, such as white blood cells, change shape and move. The energy for contraction comes from ATP, which is derived primarily from the metabolism of carbohydrate and fat.

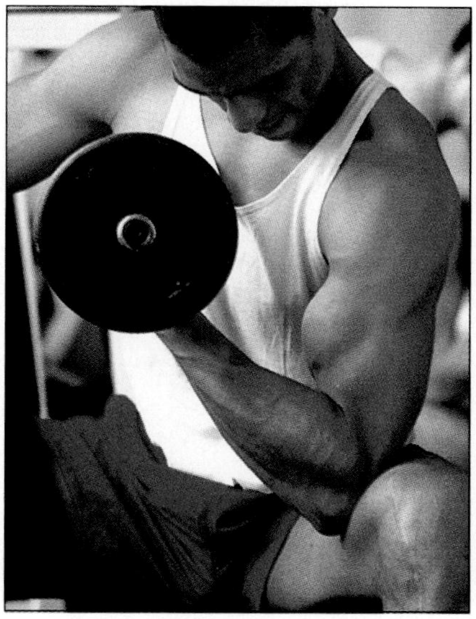

Figure 6.13
The proteins actin and myosin slide past each other to contract muscles. (© T. & D. McCarthy/The Stock Market)

Protein Hormones Hormones are chemical messengers that are secreted into the blood by one tissue or organ and act on target cells in other parts of the body.

Some hormones are made of lipid; others are made of amino acids and so are classified as peptide or protein hormones. For instance, insulin and glucagon are protein hormones.

Proteins in Fluid Balance The distribution of fluid in body cells, in the bloodstream, and in the interstitial space between cells is important for homeostasis. Fluid moves back and forth across membranes to maintain appropriate concentrations of particles and fluids inside and outside cells and tissues (see Chapter 10). Proteins help regulate this fluid balance in two ways. First, protein pumps located in cell membranes transport particles from one side of a membrane to another. Second, large protein molecules present in the blood keep fluid in the blood both by preventing it from being forced into tissues and by attracting fluid in tissues back into blood vessels. In cases of protein malnutrition, the concentration of these large proteins in the blood decreases, fluid is no longer held in the blood, and it accumulates in the tissues.

pH A measure of acidity.

Proteins in Acid Balance The chemical reactions of metabolism require a specific level of acidity, or **pH,** to function properly. In the gastrointestinal tract, acidity levels vary widely. The digestive enzyme pepsin works best in the acid environment of the stomach, whereas the pancreatic enzymes operate best in the more neutral environment of the small intestine. Inside the body, large fluctuations in pH can prevent metabolic reactions from proceeding. Proteins both within cells and in the blood help prevent large changes in acidity. For instance, the protein hemoglobin in red blood cells helps neutralize acid produced when carbon dioxide, a waste product of cellular respiration, reacts with water.

PROTEIN AND HEALTH

A diet adequate in protein is essential to health. Dietary protein is needed for growth and to replace protein that is broken down and lost each day. If too little protein is consumed, the consequences can be dramatic and devastating. Too much protein, particularly if it is derived primarily from animal sources, may also have negative health implications.

Protein-energy malnutrition (PEM) A condition characterized by wasting and an increased susceptibility to infection that results from the long-term consumption of insufficient energy and protein to meet needs.

Kwashiorkor A form of protein-energy malnutrition in which only protein is deficient. It is most common in young children who are unable to meet their high protein needs with the available diet.

Marasmus A form of protein-energy malnutrition in which a deficiency of energy in the diet causes severe body wasting.

Protein Deficiency

Because of the availability and variety of foods in developed countries, protein deficiency is uncommon. However, in developing nations, concerns about inadequate protein are very real. Diets deficient in protein are most often deficient in energy as well, but a pure protein deficiency can occur when food choices are extremely limited and the staple food of a population is very low in protein. The term **protein-energy malnutrition (PEM)** is used to refer to the continuum of conditions ranging from pure protein deficiency, called **kwashiorkor,** to energy deficiency, called **marasmus** (Figure 6.14).

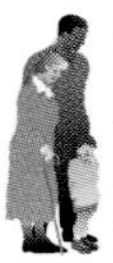

Kwashiorkor Kwashiorkor is typically a disease of children. The word "kwashiorkor" comes from the Ga tribe of the African Gold Coast. It means the disease that the first child gets when a second child is born.[2] When the new baby is born, the older child is no longer breast-fed. Rather than receiving protein-rich breast milk, the young child is fed a watered-down version of the diet eaten by the rest of the family. This diet is low in protein and is often high in fiber and difficult to digest. The child, even if able to get adequate energy, is not able to eat a large enough quantity to get adequate protein. Because children are growing, their pro-

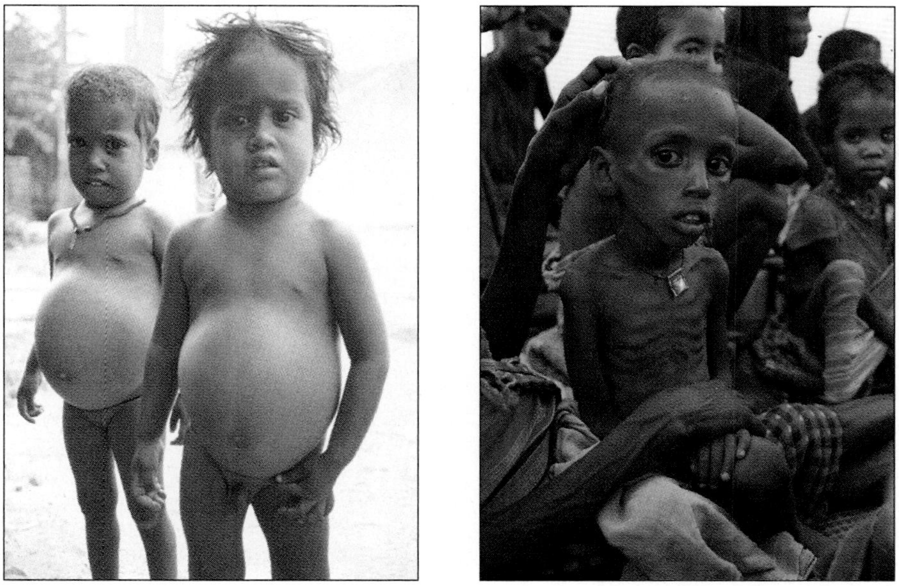

(a) (b)

Figure 6.14
Kwashiorkor (a) is characterized by a bloated belly, whereas marasmus (b) presents as severe wasting. Most protein-energy malnutrition is a combination of the two. (*a,* Food and Agriculture Organization of the United Nations; *b,* Scott Dani Peterson/Gamma Liaison, Inc.)

tein needs per unit of body weight are higher than those of adults, and the effects of a deficiency become evident much more quickly.

The symptoms of kwashiorkor can be predicted from the roles that proteins play in the body. Because protein is needed for the synthesis of new tissue, growth in height and weight is hampered. Because proteins are important in immune function, there is an increased susceptibility to infection. There are changes in hair color because the skin pigment melanin is not made; the skin flakes because structural proteins are not available to provide elasticity and support. Cells lining the digestive tract die and cannot be replaced, so nutrient absorption is impaired. The bloated belly typical of this condition is a result of both fat accumulating in the liver because there is not enough protein to transport it and fluid accumulating in the abdomen because there is not enough protein to keep fluid in the blood. Kwashiorkor occurs most commonly in Africa, South and Central America, the Near East, and the Far East. It has also been reported in poverty-stricken areas in the United States. Although kwashiorkor is often thought of as a disease of children, it is seen in hospitalized adults who have high-protein needs due to infection or trauma and a low-protein intake because they are unable to eat.

Marasmus At the other end of the continuum of protein-energy malnutrition is marasmus, meaning to waste away. Marasmus is due to a deficiency of energy, but protein and other nutrients are usually also insufficient to meet needs. Marasmus may have some of the same symptoms as kwashiorkor, but there are also differences. In kwashiorkor, some fat stores are retained, since energy intake is adequate. Marasmic individuals appear emaciated because their body fat stores have been used to provide energy. Since fat is a major energy source and carbohydrate is limited, ketosis may occur in marasmus. This is not so in kwashiorkor because carbohydrate intake is adequate—only protein is deficient.

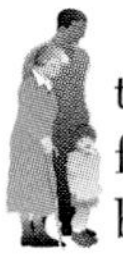

Marasmus occurs in individuals of all ages and is the form of malnutrition that occurs with eating disorders (see Chapter 7). It has devastating effects in infants and children because adequate energy is essential for growth. Because most brain growth takes place in the first year of life, malnutrition early in life causes a decrease in intelligence and learning ability that persists throughout life. Marasmus often occurs in children who are fed diluted infant formula prepared by caregivers trying to stretch limited supplies. Marasmus occurs less often in breast-fed infants.

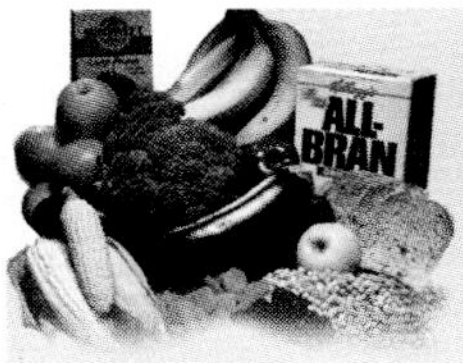

Off the Shelf

Is Soy the Perfect Protein?

Plant foods are the current rage, phytochemicals the current craze, and at the forefront of this trend is the soybean. The market for soy foods is huge. Soy food sales exceeded $1 billion in 1997—a jump from $300 million in 1980. Why has soy become so popular? Soy is a high-quality plant protein that is low in fat and high in phytochemicals. It has been suggested to reduce the risk of heart disease, cancer, and osteoporosis and lessen the symptoms of menopause. Can soy consumption really deliver on these promises? Is it the perfect protein source?

There is evidence that the consumption of soybeans and products made from soybeans may reduce the risk of heart disease. Compared to animal protein, soy is low in fat and saturated fat and contains no cholesterol. When soy protein is substituted for animal protein in the diet, it lowers blood levels of LDL cholesterol and either increases or causes no change in HDL levels.[1] Some of this effect on blood lipids is believed to be due to the phytochemicals in soy. One class of phytochemical, isoflavones, which are also known as plant estrogens or phytoestrogens, may also reduce the formation of plaque in artery walls and protect cholesterol from oxidation. The antioxidant effect of isoflavones, is similar in magnitude to that of vitamin E.[2] Taking supplements of isoflavones, however, does not have the same effect as consuming them in soy foods.[3] It is hypothesized that there is something else in soy protein that allows the phytoestrogens to act.

Soy may also be protective against cancer. Isoflavones are chemically similar to the hormone estrogen and may protect against hormone-related cancers, such as cancers of the breast, prostate, and endometrium.[4,5] The high intake of soy in traditional Asian diets has been hypothesized to be one reason that Asian women have a relatively low breast cancer incidence.[6] In cultured cells, soy protein preparations containing isoflavones prevent breast cancer cell growth. In animals, they reduce breast cancer initiation.

In addition to reducing the risks of heart disease and cancer, soy may reduce osteoporosis and alleviate some of the symptoms of menopause. Epidemiologic evidence suggests that populations who consume a large amount of soy have a lower incidence of osteoporosis.[7] Some soy products are a good source of calcium, but the effects on osteoporosis go beyond this. When compared to a soy-free diet, women consuming a soy-containing diet show an increase in bone mineral density. A synthetic isoflavone, called ipriflavone, is even used to treat women with osteoporosis.[8] Soy isoflavones may also be an alternative for hormone replacement therapy in postmenopausal women. In studies conducted in monkeys, phytoestrogens were as effective as standard hormone replacement therapy at limiting the buildup of plaque in the carotid artery.[9]

The health-promoting effects of soy are well documented—but how much do you need to eat to achieve these benefits? An analysis of the studies done on soy suggests that an intake of about 25 grams of soy protein per day is necessary to reduce cholesterol levels.[10] This is about half of a woman's daily protein requirement. How can you increase your intake of soy protein? Soy-based foods are available in many forms. Soybeans can be eaten boiled or roasted. Soybean sprouts can be added to salads. Tofu, also

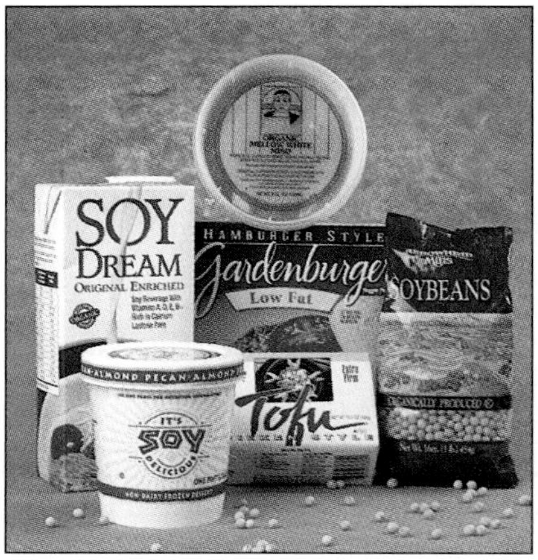

(George Semple)

Protein Excess

The body is very efficient at disposing of excess nitrogen; therefore, it is believed that protein intakes moderately above recommendations are safe. The National Research Council recommends that protein intakes not exceed twice the 1989 RDA.[3]

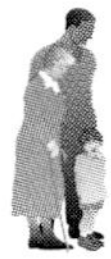

High-protein diets increase fluid needs. Protein requires about seven times more water for metabolism than does carbohydrate or fat. In addition, urea, which is produced from the breakdown of amino acids, requires large amounts of water for excretion in the urine. So unless sufficient fluid is consumed when protein intake is high, dehydration can result. Although not a problem for most people, this can be a problem if the kidneys are not able to concentrate urine, as is the case with the immature kidneys of newborns. Feeding an infant cow's milk, which is higher in protein than human milk, or formula that is too concentrated

Products Made From Soybeans

Food	Amount	Energy (kcal)	Protein (g)	Fat (g)
Soy milk, regular	1 cup	150	4	8
Soy milk, fat free	1 cup	89	4	0
Tofu, regular	1 oz	22	2.3	1.4
Tofu, lowfat	1 oz	10	1.7	0.3
Miso	1 Tbsp	35	2	1
Tempeh	1 Tbsp	21	2	1
Roasted soybeans	1/4 cup	203	15	11
Soybean sprouts	1 cup	85	9	4
Texturized soy protein (TSP)	1 oz	42	9	0.4
Veggie dogs	1 serving	112	10	6
Soy veggie burger	3 oz	120	15	5
Tofutti frozen dessert, regular	1/2 cup	120	2	2
Tofutti frozen dessert, lowfat	1/2 cup	87	2	0.2
Soy flour, regular	1 Tbsp	23	2	1
Soy flour, fat free	1 Tbsp	21	3	0

known as bean curd, is a soft cheese-like product made by curdling fresh hot soy milk. It can be consumed cooked or raw. Miso and tempeh are fermented soybean products that are used in soups and mixed dishes. Soy flour can be incorporated into baked goods. It is also used to make texturized soy protein (TSP). TSP is used to make vegetarian burgers and hot dogs. Although the evidence supporting the health-promoting effects of soy is strong, simply including soy-based foods, or any single food, in the diet is not the answer to good health. Replacing some of the animal sources of protein with soy protein may help protect your health, but other dietary and lifestyle factors also influence your overall risk.

[1]Potter, S. M. Soy protein and cardiovascular disease: the impact of bioactive components in soy. Nutr. Rev. 56:231–235, 1998.

[2]Tikkanen, M. J., Wahala, K., Ojala, S., et al. Effect of soybean phytoestrogen intake on low density lipoprotein oxidation resistance. Proc. Natl. Acad. Sci. USA 95:3106–3110, 1998.

[3]Nestel, P. J., Yamashita, T., Sasahara, T., et al. Soy isoflavones improve systemic arterial compliance but not plasma lipids in menopausal and perimenopausal women. Atheroscler. Thromb. Vasc. Biol. 17:3392–3398, 1997.

[4]Fair, W. R., Fleshner, N. E., and Heston, W. Cancer of the prostate: a nutritional disease? Urology 50:840–848, 1997.

[5]Goodman, M. T., Wilkens, L. R., Hankin, J. H., et al. Association of soy and fiber consumption with the risk of endometrial cancer. Am. J. Epidemiol. 146:294–306, 1997.

[6]Stoll, B. A. Eating to beat breast cancer: potential role for soy supplements. Ann. Oncol. 8:223–225, 1997.

[7]Adlercreutz, H., and Mazur, W. Phytoestrogens and Western diseases. Ann. Med. 29:95–120, 1997.

[8]Potter, S. M., Baum, J. M., Teng, H., et al. Soy protein and isoflavones: their effects on blood lipids and bone density in postmenopausal women. Am. J. Clin. Nutr. 68(suppl): 1375S–1379S.

[9]Clarkson, T. B., Anthony, M. S., Williams, J. K., et al. The potential of soybean phytoestrogens for postmenopausal hormone-replacement therapy. Proc. Soc. Exp. Biol. Med. 17:365–368, 1998.

[10]Anderson, J. W., Johnstone, B. M., and Cook-Newell, M. E. Meta-analysis of the effects of soy protein intake on serum lipids. N. Engl. J. Med. 333:276–282, 1995.

can increase fluid losses and lead to dehydration. It has been hypothesized, but not proven, that the long-term consumption of diets high in protein have a negative effect on kidney function.[4]

Diets that are high in protein are usually high in foods of animal origin. Diets high in animal products are generally high in fat and low in grains, vegetables, and fruits. Such diets are associated with a number of chronic diseases. Low intakes of grains, vegetables, and fruits have been associated with an increased incidence of cancer.[5,6] A diet high in animal protein may increase calcium losses, thereby increasing the risk of osteoporosis (see Chapter 10).[7] Diets high in animal protein are typically high in saturated fat and cholesterol and therefore increase the risk of heart disease (see Chapter 5). Diets high in animal protein are also usually high in energy and total fat, which may promote obesity (see Chapter 7). Reducing the amount of animal protein in the diet decreases the energy and fat content. For example, a quarter-pound hamburger patty contains 26 grams of protein along with

325 kcalories, 23 grams of fat, and 9 grams of saturated fat. Replacing half the protein with plant protein—for instance, having a cup of chili con carne with beans—would reduce the energy to 227 kcalories and the fat to 7 grams with 3 grams of saturated fat, and would increase the fiber and micronutrient content (see *Off the Shelf: Is Soy the Perfect Protein?*, p. 178).

Despite the high protein content of the American diet, protein and amino acid supplements remain popular. They promise to improve immune function, promote hair growth, and build muscle. Although protein is needed for all of these functions, a supplement will improve them only if the diet was deficient in protein in the first place. Increasing protein intake alone does not increase muscle growth; muscle growth is increased by exercising the muscle in the presence of adequate protein. Although protein supplements are not harmful for most people, they are an expensive and unnecessary way to increase protein intake. A typical protein drink provides 10 to 20 grams of protein per serving, or 20 to 40% of the Daily Value. It can add about 100 to 200 kcalories to the diet, and thus can contribute to weight gain. If consumed consistently, a high intake of protein from supplements or from foods may contribute to dehydration and promote calcium losses.

Amino acid supplements are also an unnecessary and expensive addition to a healthy diet. Many of these are marketed for specific reasons; for example, a metabolite of the amino acid tryptophan (5-hydroxy-L-tryptophan) is promoted to treat insomnia, and arginine is offered to increase lean body mass. Because amino acids share transport systems, a supplement of one may impair the absorption of another that shares the same transport system. In addition, because these are dietary supplements and not drugs, they are often not carefully tested for safety and purity. Supplements of L-tryptophan contained a contaminant that was associated with an outbreak of a rare blood disorder in 1989. L-tryptophan supplements can no longer be sold, but in 1998 similar impurities were found in 5-hydroxy-L-tryptophan.[8]

PROTEIN: ONE PART OF THE TOTAL DIET

In a typical North American diet, protein provides about 15% of the energy. While the recommendations do not suggest that we reduce our protein intake, there is a new emphasis on the source of protein—plant versus animal. The amount and source of dietary protein has an impact on the healthiness of the overall diet. In this section we will discuss the recommendation for protein intake, how to determine the amount of protein in your diet, and whether or not a vegetarian diet is the best choice for you.

Recommendations for Protein Intake

Historically, recommendations for protein intake were estimated from the amount of protein consumed by healthy working men in the general population. These protein levels were often as high as 150 grams per day. Current recommendations are generally lower than this and are based on balance studies used to measure the protein needs of the body (see below). Most people in developed countries such as the United States and Canada consume more than enough protein in their diets.

The 1989 RDA for dietary protein is 0.8 gram of protein per kilogram of body weight for adults. This value is calculated assuming that the diet contains both plant and animal sources of protein and is set to meet the needs of the majority of the population. For a person weighing 70 kg (154 lb), the recommended intake would be 56 grams of protein per day. The Canadian RNI for protein is similar: 0.86 gram per kilogram, or 60 grams for a 70-kg individual.

How Protein Requirements Are Determined Protein requirements are estimated using balance studies. Since protein is the only nutrient that contains nitrogen, the amount of protein used by the body can be calculated by comparing nitrogen intake with nitrogen loss. Nitrogen intake is calculated from dietary protein intake. Nitrogen loss or output is measured by totaling the amounts of nitrogen excreted in urine and feces and that lost from skin, sweat, hair, and nails. The majority of the nitrogen lost is excreted in the urine as urea. Comparing the amount of nitrogen consumed with the amount lost provides information about the amount of protein being synthesized and broken down within the body. An individual who is consuming enough protein to meet body needs is in protein or nitrogen balance. The amount of nitrogen or protein the individual consumes in the diet is enough to replace the amount that is lost from the body. If more nitrogen is lost than ingested, a negative nitrogen balance is said to exist. This indicates that more body protein is being broken down than is being consumed. This can occur when intake is too low or when the amount of protein breakdown has been increased by a stress such as injury, illness, or surgery. Positive nitrogen balance occurs when less nitrogen is lost than is ingested; this indicates that the body is using dietary protein for synthesis of new body proteins. This occurs when new tissue is synthesized, such as during growth, pregnancy, wound healing, or muscle building (Figure 6.15); see *Critical Thinking: What Does Nitrogen Balance Tell Us?*).

The protein requirement of a specific individual can be determined by doing a balance study for that individual. Because this procedure cannot be done for everyone, the protein needs of populations must be estimated from balance study data. Recommendations for protein intake for the general public are actually higher than the requirements determined by balance studies for individuals. This is to allow a margin of safety that will ensure the needs of the majority of the population are met.

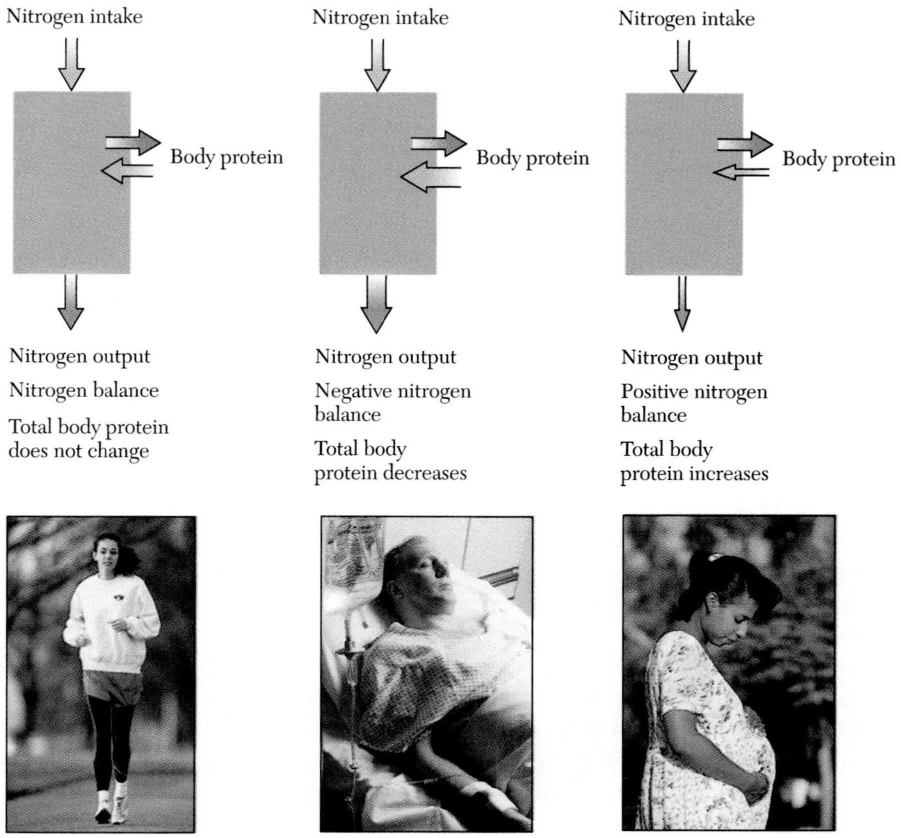

Figure 6.15
In nitrogen balance, nitrogen intake is equal to the nitrogen output; in negative balance, output exceeds intake because more body proteins are broken down than synthesized and the nitrogen is excreted; in positive balance, intake exceeds output because more protein is used to synthesize body proteins than is lost from protein breakdown. (Photos: *left,* Dennis Drenner; *center,* © Brian Yarvin/Photo Researchers, Inc.; *right,* © Myrleen Cate/Tony Stone Images, Inc.)

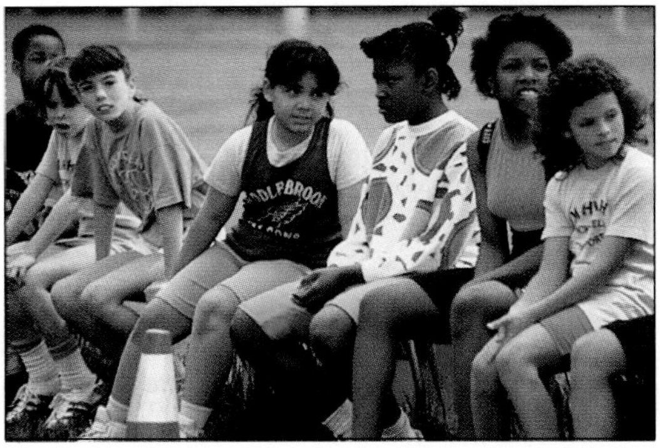

Figure 6.16
Protein needs are greater during periods of growth. (© Jeff Greenberg/Visuals Unlimited)

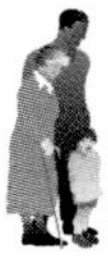

Recommendations for Special Groups Protein needs vary with life stage. Growth during childhood and pregnancy increases protein requirements. Lactation increases the body's protein demand, since milk is high in protein. Physical stress and exercise can also affect protein needs.

Growth During the first year of life, a large amount of protein is required to support the rapid growth rate. Thus, the 1989 RDA for the first six months of life is 2.2 grams per kilogram of body weight; for the second six months, 1.6 grams per kilogram is recommended. As the growth rate slows, requirements per unit of body weight decrease but continue to be greater than adult requirements until about 18 years of age (Figure 6.16).

Pregnancy Protein is needed in the pregnant woman's diet for the expansion of her blood volume, enlargement of her uterus and breasts, development of the placenta, and growth and development of the fetus. The 1989 RDA for pregnant women suggests an additional 10 grams per day above the nonpregnant recommendation. Most women in North America already consume this much protein in their typical diets.

Lactation The quantity of milk produced and the protein content of the milk determine the additional protein needs of lactation. The 1989 RDA recommends an additional 15 to 20 grams per day of dietary protein during lactation.

Physical Stress Extreme stresses on the body such as infections, fevers, burns, or surgery increase protein breakdown. These losses must be replaced by dietary protein. Requirements for these types of stresses must be assessed on an individual basis, depending on the extent of the losses. For example, a severe infection increases requirements by about one third. Burns can increase requirements to two to four times the normal level.

Exercise The marketing of protein powders and amino acid supplements to athletes might lead people to believe that protein is in short supply in the athlete's diet. In fact, athletes can obtain plenty of protein in their diets without supplements. Most athletes can meet their protein needs by consuming the 1989 RDA of 0.8 gram per kg of body weight. Those participating in endurance sports, in which protein is used for energy and to maintain blood glucose, may benefit from more protein—a total of 1.2 to 1.4 grams per kilogram per day. Strength athletes, such as weight lifters and body builders, may benefit from a total of 1.4 to 1.8 grams per kilogram per day.[9] Strength athletes require this extra protein to supply amino acids to build muscle protein; dietary protein in excess of this does not increase muscle growth. Muscle growth occurs in response to exercise, which is fueled primarily by glycogen stored in the muscles. Even endurance and strength athletes can meet their protein needs without supplements. For example, if a 200-pound (91-kg) man consumes 3600 kcal per day, 15% of which is from protein (approximately the amount contained in a typical North American diet), he will consume 135 grams of protein. This equals about 1.5 grams of protein per kilogram of body weight. The protein needs of athletes are also discussed in Chapter 12.

CRITICAL THINKING

What Does Nitrogen Balance Tell Us?

The Amecht Company wants to include nitrogen balance studies in the assays it performs in its clinical laboratory. To test their methodology, they analyze nitrogen balance (nitrogen intake − nitrogen output) in three subjects referred to as subjects A, B, and C. The technicians are given information about the daily nitrogen intake of these subjects and analyze samples of urine and feces to determine daily nitrogen losses.

$$\text{Nitrogen balance} = \text{Nitrogen In} - \text{Nitrogen Out}$$

Subject A consumed 6.4 grams of nitrogen. The laboratory determines that she lost 8.0 grams of nitrogen in her urine and feces. The nitrogen balance equation for subject A is

$$6.4\text{ g} - 8.0\text{ g} = -1.6\text{ g}$$

This result of a balance of −1.6 grams per day suggests that the individual is breaking down body protein to meet her needs.

Does this make sense metabolically?

Subject A is a 35-year-old woman who weighs 120 kg but is on a weight-loss diet. She is consuming only 500 kcalories and 30 grams of protein per day. To meet energy needs, her body is breaking down body protein, resulting in an increased excretion of nitrogen in the urine. A negative nitrogen balance would be expected for someone consuming such a low-energy, low-protein diet.

Subject B is a healthy 29-year-old male who weighs 82 kg and consumes an adequate diet of 2700 kcalories and 70 grams of protein a day. His nitrogen values are:

	Nitrogen In	Nitrogen Out
Subject B	11.2 g	11.2 g

What is his nitrogen balance?

Answer:

Does his nitrogen balance make sense metabolically?

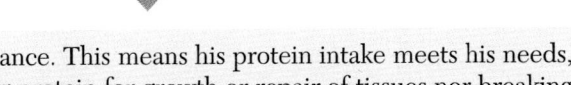

Yes. He is in nitrogen balance. This means his protein intake meets his needs, and he is neither retaining protein for growth or repair of tissues nor breaking down body protein for energy.

Subject C is a 31-year-old pregnant woman of average prepregnancy weight who is consuming 2500 kcalories and 80 grams of protein a day. Her nitrogen values are:

	Nitrogen In	Nitrogen Out
Subject C	12.8 g	10.4 g

What is her nitrogen balance?

Answer:

Does her nitrogen balance make sense metabolically?

Answer:

Determining Your Protein Intake

To determine if your protein intake meets recommendations, the protein content of your diet can be calculated using food composition tables or databases, the information on food labels, or Exchange Lists. Food composition tables and databases contain information on all types of foods and supplements. Food labels provide a more readily available source of information; however, since the labeling of raw meats and fish is voluntary, many of the greatest sources of protein in the diet do not carry food labels. Another way to estimate protein in the diet is to use the exchanges shown in Table 6.2. According to the Exchange Lists, a 1-ounce serving of meat (28 g) provides 7 grams of protein. One cup of milk provides 8 grams, and grains and vegetables provide 2 to 3 grams per serving. For diets based primarily on plant proteins, **protein quality** must also be considered.

Protein quality A measure of how efficiently a protein in the diet can be used to make body proteins.

Protein Quality The recommendations for protein intake assume that the diet contains proteins of various quality. Protein quality is a measure of how useful a protein in the diet is for building body protein. Animal proteins usually contain a pattern of amino acids closer to that needed by the body than do plant proteins. Therefore, they are said to be of higher quality. Plant proteins are limited in one or more amino acids and are therefore said to be of lower quality. Since foods

Table 6.2 ***Using Exchange Lists to Calculate the Protein Content of a Diet***

Exchange Groups/Lists	Serving Size	Protein (g)
Carbohydrate Group		
Starch	1/2 cup rice, cereal, potatoes; 1 slice bread	3
Fruit	1 small apple, peach, pear; 1/2 banana; 1/2 cup canned juice-pack fruit	0
Milk	1 cup milk or yogurt	
Nonfat		8
Lowfat		8
Reduced fat		8
Whole		8
Other carbohydrates	Serving sizes vary	Varies
Vegetables	1/2 cup cooked vegetables, 1 cup raw	2
Meat/Meat Substitute Group	1 oz meat or cheese, 1/2 cup legumes	
Very lean		7
Lean		7
Medium fat		7
High fat		7
Fat Group	1 tsp butter, margarine, or oil; 1 Tbsp salad dressing	0

with high-quality protein provide more of the essential amino acids in the proportions needed by the body than do foods with low-quality protein, less total protein is needed when the diet contains high-quality protein.

Measuring Protein Quality Protein quality is evaluated experimentally in a number of ways. One way is to compare the amino acid pattern of the food being evaluated with that found in a reference protein known to be of high quality, such as egg protein. A **chemical score** is calculated by comparing the amount of the limiting amino acid in the test protein with the amount of that amino acid in egg protein. In this analysis, proteins with the most desirable proportions of amino acids will have the highest scores. For example, if a test protein has a limiting amino acid that is present at 75% of the level found in egg, it will be assigned a chemical score of 75.

$$\text{Chemical score} = \frac{\text{mg of limiting amino acid per g of test protein}}{\text{mg of amino acid per g of egg protein}} \times 100$$

Chemical score is an easy way to estimate protein quality in theory, but it does not take into account how well the body can use the protein that is being evaluated. The simplest estimate of protein quality that takes into account usage by the body is the **protein efficiency ratio.** This is calculated by comparing the weight gain of growing animals fed a test protein with the weight gain of those fed a reference protein such as egg protein. Other methods use balance studies with humans or animals to measure not just weight gain but also how well a protein is used for growth and maintenance. **Net protein utilization** measures how much of the protein in the diet is retained for use by the body. Since not all the protein in the diet is absorbed, another measure, **biological value,** compares the amount of nitrogen retained in the body for maintenance and growth with the amount absorbed from the diet. The high-quality protein in egg has a biological value of 100, meaning that 100% of the egg protein that is absorbed is retained by the body.

Chemical score A measure of protein quality determined by comparing the amount of the limiting amino acid in a food with that in a reference protein.

Protein efficiency ratio A measure of protein quality determined by comparing the weight gain of a laboratory animal fed a test protein with the weight gain of an animal fed a reference protein.

Net protein utilization A measure of protein quality determined by comparing the amount of nitrogen retained in the body with the amount eaten in the diet.

Biological value A measure of protein quality determined by comparing the amount of nitrogen retained in the body with the amount absorbed from the diet.

The protein in corn has a biological value of only 60, meaning that only 60% of that which is absorbed is retained for use by the body.

$$\text{Net protein utilization} = \frac{\text{nitrogen retained}}{\text{nitrogen intake}} \times 100$$

$$\text{Biological value} = \frac{\text{nitrogen retained}}{\text{nitrogen absorbed}} \times 100$$

Each of these measures has scientific advantages and drawbacks. They are useful for determining the dietary protein quality available to populations. For example, the quality of protein in a dietary staple such as corn or cassava is extremely important in a country where both food and protein are scarce. In industrialized countries, where protein is usually not scarce, measuring protein quality is less crucial and is generally too cumbersome to be used for diet planning.

A more appropriate way of evaluating protein quality in an individual diet is to look at the sources of the protein. Foods of animal origin, because they supply essential amino acids in the proper proportions for human use, are sources of **complete dietary protein.** Plant foods, on the other hand, contain proteins that do not provide all the amino acids in the proper proportions required for protein synthesis in humans and are therefore said to be incomplete. If the protein in a diet comes from both complete and incomplete sources, it most likely contains adequate amounts of all the essential amino acids needed for protein synthesis. If the protein in a diet comes from incomplete sources, different types of incomplete protein must be combined so the amino acids provided complement each other to supply all the essential amino acids.

Complete dietary protein Protein that provides essential amino acids in the proportions needed to support protein synthesis.

A Diet to Meet Recommendations: Vegetarian or Not?

Populations around the world meet their protein requirements with different types and amounts of protein. In the United States and other affluent countries, the majority of dietary protein comes from animal sources—meat, poultry, fish, eggs, and dairy products—but in many cultures smaller amounts of animal proteins are used. To meet requirements, plant proteins are combined with small amounts of animal proteins or with other plant proteins containing different limiting amino acids. Plant protein–based or vegetarian diets have evolved mostly out of necessity because animal sources are unavailable physically or economically. In affluent societies, vegetarian diets are followed for a variety of reasons other than economics, such as health, religion, personal ethics, or environmental awareness (see *Off the Shelf: Are Vegetarian Diets Better for Our Environment?*).

Traditionally, **vegetarianism** is defined as abstinence from meat, fish, and fowl. The current interpretation of vegetarianism includes a wide variety of eating patterns depending on the degree of abstinence from animal products. Semivegetarians are those who avoid only certain types of red meat, fish, or poultry—for example, individuals who avoid all red meat but continue to consume poultry and fish. Lacto-ovo vegetarians are those who eat no animal flesh but do eat eggs and dairy products such as milk and cheese; lacto vegetarians are those who avoid animal flesh and eggs but do consume dairy products; and **vegans** are those who avoid all food of animal origin.

Vegetarianism A pattern of food intake that eliminates some or all animal products.

Vegan A pattern of food intake that eliminates all animal products.

Protein Complementation

Vegetarian diets meet protein needs by using **protein complementation,** a technique for combining foods containing different limiting amino acids in order to improve the protein quality of the diet as a whole. By eating plant proteins with complementary amino acid patterns, essential amino acid requirements can be met without consuming any animal proteins. The amino acids that are most often limited in plant proteins are lysine, methionine, cysteine, and tryptophan. As a general rule, legumes are deficient in methionine and cysteine but high in lysine. Grains and nuts and seeds are deficient in lysine but high in methionine and cysteine. Corn is deficient in lysine and tryptophan

Protein complementation Combining proteins from different sources so that they collectively provide the proportions of amino acids required to meet needs.

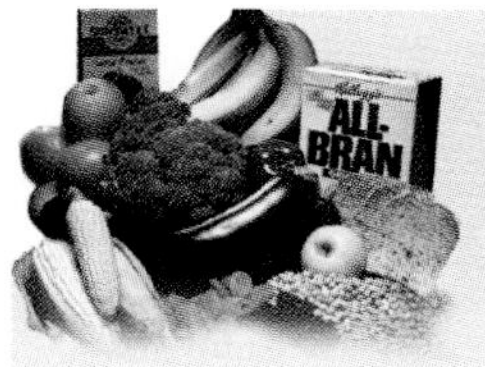

Off the Shelf

Are Vegetarian Diets Better for Our Environment?

Concern about the environment is one reason people choose to adopt vegetarian diets. Producing animal products consumes large amounts of energy, destroys forests and grazing lands, and pollutes the air and water. Should you become a vegetarian to save the planet from environmental destruction? To answer this question, you need to look at the role of animals in the ecosystem.

In developed nations, the drive to produce animals more efficiently and more profitably has moved them off the family farm and into large agribusinesses. This has had an impact on energy use, land and water use, and air quality. On a small farm, animals can consume crop wastes, kitchen scraps, and cellulose grasses that people cannot eat, and turn them into meat, milk, and eggs that make important contributions to the human diet. This is not true in large agribusinesses. Animals are fed grain rather than grasses and kitchen scraps. This is inefficient because humans who eat the animals get back only a fraction of the energy they could have gotten from eating the grain. For every 100 kcalories of plant material a cow eats, only 10 kcalories are stored in the cow and can be consumed by humans.[1] In the United States, 1 pound of pork provides 1000 to 2000 kcalories in the diet and costs 14,000 kcalories to produce. Worldwide, 38% of the total grain produced is fed to chickens, pigs, and cows. In the United States, as much as 70% of grain grown is fed to animals. Livestock production also uses water—430 gallons to produce 1 pound of pork in the United States. For the world to adopt the American diet would require "more grain than the world can grow and more energy, water, and land than the world can supply."[2]

In addition to feeding animals, we must also manage animal waste materials. On small farms, manure is used for fertilizer, but when thousands of animals are confined to a small area, as in agribusiness, manure runoff may pollute nearby rivers and lakes. This can cause algae overgrowth that kills other aquatic life and causes nitrate pollution of drinking water. Animal wastes also produce gases that are released into the atmosphere, contributing to acid rain and global warming.

The sheer number of domestic animals is also destructive to the environment. Pastures are overstocked and grazing lands are overgrazed, reducing the potential to continue to use these lands. Forests such as those in the Amazon are being cut down to create new grazing land for cattle. Forests serve to absorb carbon dioxide, therefore deforestation allows carbon dioxide to accumulate in the atmosphere and contributes to global warming. Whether domestic animals are confined or free, the natural resources of the earth are no longer able to sustain their increasing numbers without serious ecological consequences. Is the elimination of animal foods the answer to feeding the world and saving the planet?

Animal foods make important contributions to the human diet. In parts of the developing world, small amounts of meat and milk obtained from animals may mean the difference between survival and starvation. Animal products also make important economic contributions. Manure is a valuable fertilizer and a source of cooking fuel. When integrated into farming, animal products provide extra income during good times and insurance during bad times. In the United States, we rely on animal foods to provide vitamin B_{12}, much of our calcium, and highly absorbable sources of iron and zinc. Eliminating animals entirely would reduce both the variety of food and the nutrient content of the human diet.

The environmental problems caused by animal production occur both because of the way animals are raised and because there are too many of them, not because of their existence per se. If we are to both feed the world and preserve the environment, sustainable agricultural systems must be adopted. The aim of sustainable agriculture is to produce vegetable and animal foods while preserving the long-term fertility and productiveness of the planet. The natural ecosystems of the earth include both plants and animals, so it is not surprising that agricultural systems modeled after natural ecosystems would require both. For example, in a sustainable system, cattle and sheep would eat only from grazing lands unsuitable for growing crops, rather than being fed grains better consumed by humans. This agricultural method utilizes both unproductive and productive cropland in an ecologically sound manner. While this type of system uses fewer resources, it also produces many fewer animals than the present system. To absorb the decrease in production, demand for animal products would have to decrease in developed nations. Consuming a diet that is higher in grains, vegetables, and fruits and lower in animal products is therefore a goal that is compatible not only with the recommendations of the Dietary Guidelines but also with the ecology of the planet. Completely eliminating animal products is neither necessary nor beneficial. Both plants and animals are essential for a diversified ecosystem, and both plant and animal foods make valuable contributions to the diet.

[1]Raven, P. H., Berg, L. R., and Johnson, G. B. *Environment*, 2nd ed. Philadelphia: Saunders College Publishing, 1998.

[2]Durning, A. T. Fat of the land. World Watch 4:7–11, 1991.

but is a good source of methionine. Consuming a diet containing foods from various categories improves the amino acid composition of the diet as a whole. For example, when rice, which is limited in the amino acid lysine but high in methionine, is eaten with beans, which are high in lysine but limited in methionine, the combination will provide a much higher quality protein than if either is eaten alone.

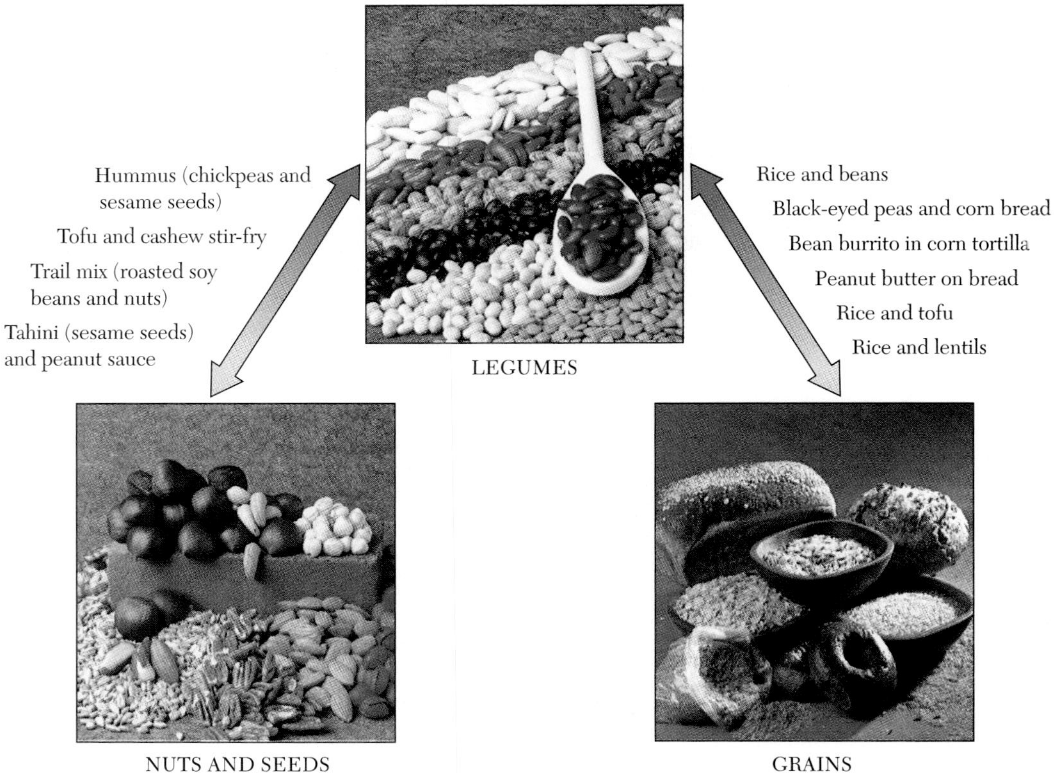

Figure 6.17
Combining complementary sources of incomplete plant proteins can provide a diet containing enough of all of the essential amino acids. (George Semple)

Common combinations of grains and legumes that have become cultural staples include beans and rice or beans and wheat or corn tortillas in Central and South America; rice and tofu in China and Japan; rice and lentils in India; rice and black-eyed peas in the southern United States; and peanut butter (peanuts are legumes) and bread throughout the United States (Figure 6.17). Plant proteins can also be complemented with animal protein in order to meet the need for essential amino acids. For example, in Asia rice is often flavored with a small amount of spiced beef, chicken, or fish. Although it is not necessary to consume complementary proteins at each meal, the entire day's diet should include proteins from complementary sources in order to satisfy the daily need for amino acids.[10]

Benefits and Pitfalls of Vegetarian Diets The health benefits of vegetarian diets have made them increasingly popular in affluent societies as people strive to adopt health-promoting lifestyles. Vegetarians have been shown to have lower risks for obesity, diabetes, cardiovascular disease, high blood pressure, and some types of cancer.[10,11] Studies of Seventh-Day Adventists, a religious group that espouses a diet containing no animal products as well as abstention from alcohol consumption and cigarette smoking, found that the incidence of heart disease is about half that of non–Seventh-Day Adventists living in the same area.[12] Even when lifestyle factors other than diet, such as abstinence from alcohol use and cigarette smoking, were kept constant by comparing Seventh-Day Adventists who do not consume vegetarian diets with their vegetarian counterparts, eating meat was associated with a higher incidence of heart disease.[13] Because vegetarian diets eliminate or limit the intake of animal foods, they are lower in saturated fat, cholesterol, and animal protein. The increased intakes of grains, legumes, vegetables, and fruits add fiber, vitamins (including antioxidant vitamins), minerals, and phytochemicals to the diet.[14,15] It is not known whether the reduction in chronic disease is due to the amount and type of fat in the diet, the source of the protein, or the increase in fiber, micronutrients, and phytochemicals. It is likely that the total dietary pattern rather than a single factor alone is responsible.

In addition to reducing disease risks, diets that rely more heavily on plant proteins are more economical. A meal based on rice, pasta, or beans with a small serving of meat costs less and can provide plenty of protein with less fat than a meal based on a large serving of meat. For example, a dinner of spaghetti with meat sauce costs about half as much as a meal of steak and potatoes. Yet both meals provide a significant portion of the day's protein requirement.

Despite the health and economic benefits, nutrient deficiencies can be a problem for people consuming unsupplemented vegetarian diets, particularly vegan diets. Most people can easily meet their protein needs with lacto and lacto-ovo vegetarian diets. These diets contain high-quality animal proteins from eggs or milk, which complement the limiting amino acids in the plant proteins. Protein deficiency is a potential risk when vegan diets are consumed by small children and adults with increased protein needs, such as pregnant women and those recovering from illness or injury. These individuals must consume carefully planned diets to meet their protein needs.

Deficiencies of some vitamins and minerals are a greater risk for vegetarians than protein deficiency.[10] Vitamin B_{12} is found almost exclusively in animal products; therefore, supplements or fortified foods must be used in vegan diets to meet needs. The major source of calcium in the North American diet is dairy products, so again, vegan diets must be carefully planned to meet calcium needs. Likewise, most dietary vitamin D comes from fortified dairy products, so vegans must get their vitamin D from sunshine (see Chapter 9) or consume other sources of this vitamin such as fortified soy milk. Iron and zinc may be deficient in vegetarian diets because the best sources of these minerals are red meats and these minerals are poorly absorbed from plant sources. Since iron and zinc are low in dairy products, lacto-ovo and lacto vegetarians as well as vegans are at risk for deficiencies. Vegetarian sources of these nutrients are listed in Table 6.3 and discussed in Chapters 8 to 11 (see *Critical Thinking: Choosing a Vegetarian Diet*).

Choosing a Diet to Meet Needs A simple way to ensure an adequate protein intake from a combination of plant and animal proteins is to follow the recommendations of the Food Guide Pyramid. The groups in the Food Guide Pyramid that are highest in protein are the Milk, Yogurt, & Cheese Group and the Meat, Poultry, Fish, Dry Beans, Eggs, & Nuts Group. These two food groups are in the upper sections of the Pyramid, indicating that these foods should make up a relatively small proportion of the day's intake. Two to three servings per day are

Table 6.3 ***Sources of Essential Nutrients in Vegan Diets***

Nutrient	Sources in Vegan Diets
Protein	Soy-based products, legumes, seeds, nuts, grains, and vegetables
Vitamin B_{12}	Supplements, fortified soy beverages and cereals
Calcium	Tofu processed with calcium, broccoli, kale, bok choy, legumes, and fortified soy beverages, cereals, and orange juice
Vitamin D	Fortified soy beverages, fortified margarine, sunshine
Iron	Legumes, tofu, green leafy vegetables, dried fruit, whole grains, iron-fortified cereals and breads
Zinc	Whole grains, legumes, nuts, and tofu

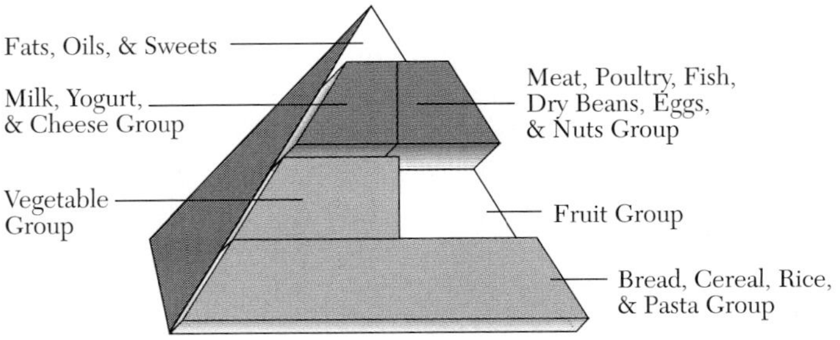

Figure 6.18
The Food Guide Pyramid groups that are raised and colored blue are good sources of protein. The groups shown in the darker shade contain a greater proportion of high-protein foods and are the only groups that include animal proteins.

recommended from each. Two 8-ounce glasses of milk and two 2-ounce servings of meat provide about 44 grams of protein. Consuming the minimum recommended servings from the Bread, Cereal, Rice, & Pasta Group and the Vegetable Group, 6 and 3 servings respectively, would bring the total to 71 grams of protein—more than enough to meet most people's needs (Figure 6.18).

Lacto vegetarians and vegans can meet their needs by following the recommendations of the modified Food Guide Pyramid shown in Figure 6.19. The food choices and recommended number of servings from the grains, vegetables, and fruits, found in the bottom two levels of this vegetarian pyramid, are the same as in the traditional Food Guide Pyramid. The groups in next level of the traditional Pyramid (meat and milk) include foods of animal origin. In the vegetarian pyramid, 2 to 3 servings from a group containing dry beans, nuts, seeds, eggs, and meat substitutes are recommended. Lacto vegetarians (those who consume dairy products) should also consume 2 to 3 servings from the milk group. Vegans (those who do not consume any animal foods) should consume milk substitutes fortified with calcium and vitamin D, or other foods high in these nutrients. To obtain adequate vitamin B_{12}, vegans must take B_{12} supplements or use products fortified with vitamin B_{12}.[10]

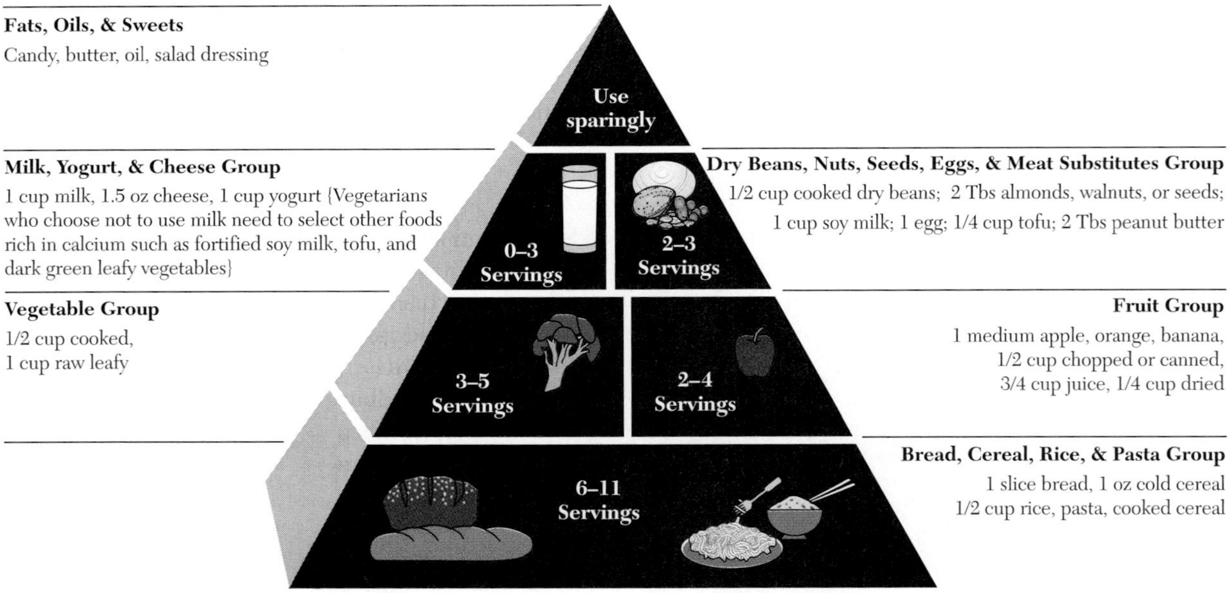

Figure 6.19
With a few modifications, the Food Guide Pyramid can be used to choose a balanced vegetarian diet. Instead of meats, servings of legumes, nuts and seeds, and eggs should be consumed each day. If dairy products are eliminated, other high-calcium foods such as fortified soy milk should be substituted. At least 2 servings of calcium-rich foods should be consumed daily. Vitamin B_{12} supplements or vitamin B_{12}–fortified foods are necessary to meet needs. (Modified from National Center for Nutrition and Dietetics, the American Dietetic Association; based on the USDA Food Guide Pyramid, © ADAF, 1997.)

CRITICAL THINKING

Choosing a Vegetarian Diet

A year ago Ajay decided to stop eating meat. While studying protein in his nutrition class, he became concerned that his diet did not correctly complement protein sources. Ajay is 26 years old and weighs 154 pounds. Does his diet meet his protein needs?

What is the 1989 RDA for protein for someone of his age and weight?

$$\frac{154 \text{ lb}}{2.2 \text{ lb/kg}} = 70 \text{ kg}$$

1989 RDA for adults = 0.8 g protein per kg body weight

$$70 \text{ kg} \times \frac{0.8 \text{ g}}{\text{kg}} = 56 \text{ g of protein}$$

He records his food intake for one day and then uses diet analysis software to calculate his protein intake.

Food	Amount	Protein (g)
Breakfast		
Grape Nuts	3 Tbsp	2.4
Milk, lowfat	1/2 cup	4
Orange juice	1/2 cup	0.8
Toast, wheat	2 slices	5
Peanut butter	1 Tbsp	4
Coffee	1 cup	0
Lunch		
Dahl (lentil soup)	1 cup	9
Rice	1 cup	6
Banana	1	1
Apple juice	1 cup	0
Dinner		
Green salad	1 cup	1
with dressing	1 Tbsp	0
Rice	1 cup	6
Curried potatoes	1/2 cup	1.5
and chickpeas	1/3 cup	5
Yogurt	1 cup	13
Poori (fried bread)	2 pieces	5
Ice cream	1/2 cup	2
Total		**65.7**

His diet provides 65.7 grams of protein, which exceeds his calculated 1989 RDA of 56 grams.

Do Ajay's food choices include complementary proteins?

At breakfast, he has milk, which is a high-quality protein, and bread and peanut butter, which contain proteins that complement each other (see Figure 6.17). At lunch, the protein in the dahl, which is made from lentils, complements the protein in the rice. At dinner, he has chickpeas, which complement both the rice and the wheat protein in the poori. He also has yogurt and ice cream, which provide high-quality proteins.

How much protein would this diet provide if he decided to eliminate dairy products?

Answer:

How would eliminating dairy products affect his calcium and vitamin D intake?

The major source of calcium in his diet is dairy products, so he would have to carefully plan his diet to include other calcium sources. Likewise, most of his dietary vitamin D comes from fortified dairy products, so he would need to be sure to get his vitamin D from sunshine or other fortified foods. Vegetarian sources of these nutrients are listed in Table 6.3 and discussed in Chapters 8 to 11.

Does his diet meet the serving recommendations of the vegetarian pyramid?

Answer:

PROTEINS, AMINO ACIDS, AND FOOD TECHNOLOGY

Protein in foods provides more than nutrients; it contributes to the texture, shape, and color of food. It is the protein in grains that provides the structure of breads and baked goods. Egg protein gives custard stability. The protein in cream allows it to be whipped into whipped cream; and myoglobin, the iron-carrying protein in muscle, gives meat its red color. These chemical and physical properties of proteins have made them important additives in processed foods.

Proteins in Processed Foods

Many proteins are added to foods in purified forms in order to contribute taste and texture. The milk protein casein (sodium caseinate) is used in coffee whiteners and frozen dessert toppings. The casein in these products helps simulate the taste and texture of cream. Gelatin, a protein derived from animal connective tissue, is used to gel yogurt; to whip foams such as cupcake fillings; to clear fruit juices, wines, and beer; to increase viscosity; and to prevent the growth of ice crystals in frozen desserts. Gelatin, although it is derived from an animal protein, is completely deficient in the essential amino acid tryptophan and low in other essential amino acids, so though a useful additive for the food industry, it is not a good source of high-quality dietary protein. **Protein hydrolysates** or **hydrolyzed proteins** are proteins that have been treated with acid or enzymes to break them down into amino acids and small peptides. They are used as flavorings, flavor enhancers, stabilizers, or thickening agents. Hydrolyzed proteins from plant sources are commonly added to packaged rice and potato products such as rice pilaf and potatoes au gratin.

Soy proteins are used in processed foods for many reasons. Soy protein concentrate is a derivative of soybeans that is used to aid in emulsification and provide texture in products such as canned gravies and candy bars. Soy protein isolates and texturized vegetable protein are types of soy protein that can be formed into chunks, woven or spun into fibers, or otherwise shaped and flavored to form meat substitutes. They are used to make imitation hot dogs, meatballs, chicken, and veal, or they can be added to animal protein as an extender or filler. Fish protein can also be restructured into new forms. A protein slurry can be made from minced fresh fish. This can then be washed, seasoned, flavored, and shaped to look and taste like lobster, crab, and other seafood (Figure 6.20).

An addition to the array of proteins used in processed foods is the fat substitute Simplesse. Simplesse is made from egg white and milk proteins that are modified by heating, filtering, and high-speed mixing. The resulting protein consists of millions of microscopic balls that slip and slide over one another, providing the slippery texture of fat.[16] Despite its "fatty" texture, Simplesse is made from protein and water and so contains a little more than 1 kcalorie per gram, compared with 9 kcalories per gram for fat.

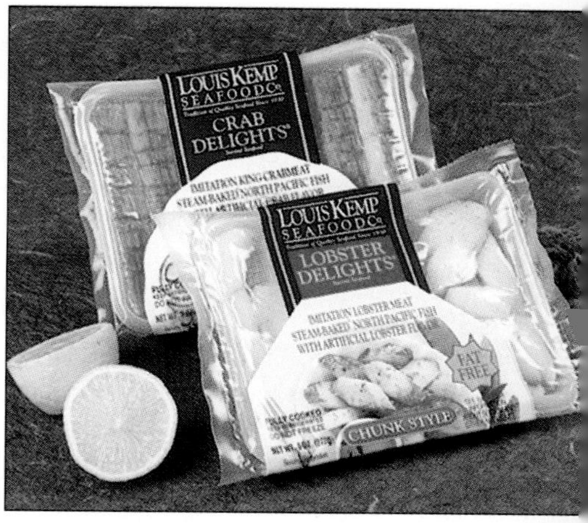

Figure 6.20
Fish proteins can be modified to give them the taste and texture of seafoods such as crab and lobster. (George Semple)

Protein hydrolysates or **hydrolyzed proteins** Mixtures of amino acids or amino acids and polypeptides produced when a protein is completely or partially broken down by treatment with acid or enzymes.

Amino Acids Added to Foods

The amino acid composition of foods is also sometimes changed by genetic engineering and food processing. For example, the amino acid composition of plant proteins can be modified by genetic engineering to produce a higher quality protein, such as a variety of corn that is higher in lysine than the usual variety. In processed foods, limiting amino acids can be supplemented to enhance the quality of vegetable protein. Amino acids are also added to provide flavor. Two examples are the low-kcalorie sweetener aspartame and the flavor enhancer monosodium glutamate (MSG).

Phenylketonuria (PKU) An inherited disease in which the body cannot metabolize the amino acid phenylalanine. If the disease is untreated, toxic by-products accumulate in the blood and cause mental retardation.

Aspartame Aspartame is a dipeptide composed of the amino acids aspartic acid and phenylalanine. Aspartame is used in a wide variety of foods, including carbonated beverages, gelatin desserts, and chewing gum (Figure 6.21). It cannot be used in cooked products because it breaks down when heated, losing its sweet taste. It has become popular in recent years, because both saccharin and cyclamates have been suggested to cause cancer in laboratory animals (see Chapter 4).

Aspartame contains the amino acid phenylalanine and therefore can be dangerous to individuals with a genetic disorder called **phenylketonuria (PKU).** In individuals with PKU, an enzyme needed to metabolize the amino acid phenylalanine does not function properly, leaving them unable to convert the essential amino acid phenylalanine to the semiessential amino acid tyrosine. Instead, phenylalanine is converted to compounds called phenylketones, which build up in the blood. High phenylketone levels can interfere with brain development causing mental retardation. To prevent mental retardation, infants and children with PKU must consume a diet with just enough phenylalanine to meet the body's need for protein synthesis but not so much that the buildup of phenylketones

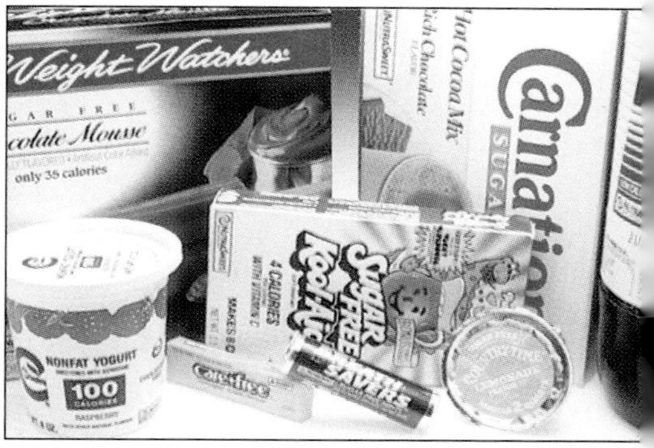

Figure 6.21
Aspartame is used to sweeten a variety of products. (Charles D. Winters)

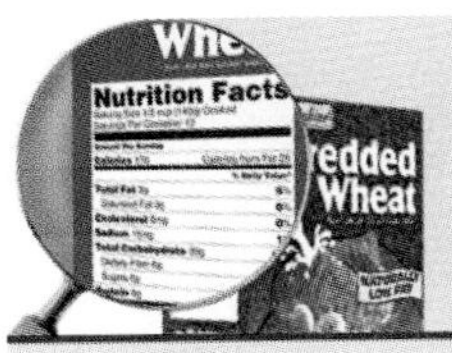

Off the Label

Identifying Protein Sources

Food labels provide information about the composition of foods and the contribution they make toward meeting daily nutrient intake recommendations. Since protein is a nutrient that is adequate in the diet of most Americans, the protein content of foods is listed but not emphasized on most food labels. For some individuals, however, such as those with allergies to certain proteins and those who wish to avoid specific foods for religious, ethical, or other reasons, food labels are an important source of information that can help identify foods appropriate for their diets.

Like other nutrients, information on protein is listed in the Nutrition Facts section of the food label as well as in the ingredient list. The Nutrition Facts section lists the number of grams of protein per serving. However, the percent Daily Value is required only on foods that contain protein of very low quality. When listed, the percent Daily Value is adjusted for protein quality. For example, a food that contains 10 grams of high-quality protein supplies 20% of the Daily Value for protein, whereas a food that contains 10 grams of a low-quality protein may indicate that it provides only 5% of the Daily Value for protein. Only the latter must list the percent Daily Value on the label.

The ingredient list indicates the source of protein in foods. For individuals who restrict their intake of certain proteins, this information can be invaluable. If an individual's religion prohibits the consumption of pork, the ingredient list is needed to determine if a packaged food, such as frozen egg rolls, contains pork. For a child who is allergic to peanut protein, the ingredient list can be lifesaving. Because peanut allergy can be so severe, even products that do not intentionally contain peanuts may include them at the end of the ingredient list if there is a potential for cross-contamination from equipment or foods made in the same facility. When foods contain isolated proteins such as the milk protein casein, determining the source of the protein is more challenging. For example, if someone who is allergic to casein wanted to use powdered creamer in his coffee, he might select a brand labeled nondairy creamer. Reading the ingredient list would show that the product does contain casein, along with the statement that casein is a milk derivative. If he selected a brand that does not claim to be nondairy, casein would be listed without the statement that it is a milk derivative.

Even products that typically contain little or no protein may have small amounts of protein hydrolysates added to them. To help individuals avoid specific proteins, foods containing protein hydrolysates are required to list the source of the hydrolysate. For example, the spaghetti sauce mix whose label is shown here contains so little protein that the Nutrition Facts section lists the grams of protein as zero. The ingredient list, however, shows that the product contains hydrolyzed corn gluten, soy protein, and wheat gluten protein. An individual with an allergy to soy should avoid this product and all products listing soy or hydrolyzed soy protein as an ingredient. This information is also helpful to vegetarians who restrict animal proteins.

Individual amino acids added to foods are also included in the ingredient list. For instance, some people try to avoid consuming the amino acid glutamate (glutamic acid) because they experience MSG symptom complex. Glutamate in the form of MSG is used as a flavor enhancer in foods such as potato chips and other snack foods; canned soups, meats, and fish; packaged meals such as frozen seafood, chicken, and other entrees; cured meats and lunch meats; and foods of many international cuisines. When added, it must appear on the label in the ingredient list as monosodium glutamate or potassium gluta-

occurs. The diet must also provide sufficient tyrosine, because the disease prevents conversion of phenylalanine to tyrosine. PKU afflicts about 1 in 12,000 newborn infants.[17] Infants are tested for this disorder at birth. Special low-phenylalanine or phenylalanine-free formulas are manufactured for infants with this disease. Pregnant women with PKU must be especially careful to consume a low-phenylalanine diet in order to protect their unborn children from high phenylketone levels and the mental retardation and other birth defects they cause.[18] Because these individuals must restrict their phenylalanine intake, warnings for individuals with PKU are included on the labels of all products containing aspartame, though few of them specify the actual amount of the sweetener contained in the product.

Monosodium Glutamate Monosodium glutamate (MSG) is a flavor enhancer best known for its use in Chinese cooking. It is added to a variety of packaged foods and sold as a powder for use in home cooking. It consists of the amino acid

mate, as shown in the figure. Seasonings that contain MSG include Accent, Ajinomoto, Zest, Vestin, Gourmet Powder, Subu, Chinese seasoning, Glutavene, Glutacyl, RL-50 Kombu extract, and Meijing or Wei-jing. Glutamate may also be added to food as a component of a protein hydrolysate. Foods containing ingredients that are sources of glutamate, such as hydrolyzed protein, may not state "no MSG" or "no added MSG" on the label.[1]

Food labels generally focus on providing information to help the population meet the current recommendations for maintaining health and preventing disease. In the case of protein, which is not a focus of public health guidelines in the United States, the information is helpful to individuals who have special needs.

[1]U.S. Food and Drug Administration. FDA and monosodium glutamate (MSG). FDA Backgrounder, August 31, 1995. Online at http://vm.cfsan.fda.gov/~lrd/msg.html

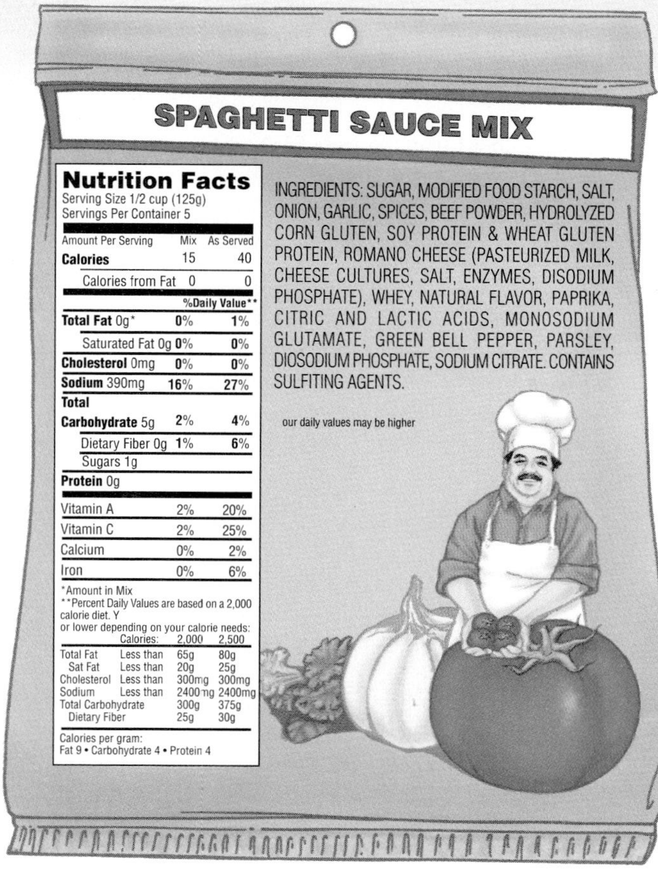
SPAGHETTI SAUCE MIX
Nutrition Facts
Serving Size 1/2 cup (125g)
Servings Per Container 5
Amount Per Serving Mix As Served
Calories 15 40
Calories from Fat 0 0
%Daily Value**
Total Fat 0g* 0% 1%
Saturated Fat 0g 0% 0%
Cholesterol 0mg 0% 0%
Sodium 390mg 16% 27%
Total Carbohydrate 5g 2% 4%
Dietary Fiber 0g 1% 6%
Sugars 1g
Protein 0g
Vitamin A 2% 20%
Vitamin C 2% 25%
Calcium 0% 2%
Iron 0% 6%
*Amount in Mix
**Percent Daily Values are based on a 2,000 calorie diet. Y
or lower depending on your calorie needs:
Calories: 2,000 2,500
Total Fat Less than 65g 80g
Sat Fat Less than 20g 25g
Cholesterol Less than 300mg 300mg
Sodium Less than 2400mg 2400mg
Total Carbohydrate 300g 375g
Dietary Fiber 25g 30g
Calories per gram:
Fat 9 • Carbohydrate 4 • Protein 4
INGREDIENTS: SUGAR, MODIFIED FOOD STARCH, SALT, ONION, GARLIC, SPICES, BEEF POWDER, HYDROLYZED CORN GLUTEN, SOY PROTEIN & WHEAT GLUTEN PROTEIN, ROMANO CHEESE (PASTEURIZED MILK, CHEESE CULTURES, SALT, ENZYMES, DISODIUM PHOSPHATE), WHEY, NATURAL FLAVOR, PAPRIKA, CITRIC AND LACTIC ACIDS, MONOSODIUM GLUTAMATE, GREEN BELL PEPPER, PARSLEY, DISODIUM PHOSPHATE, SODIUM CITRATE. CONTAINS SULFITING AGENTS.
our daily values may be higher

glutamic acid (or glutamate) bound to sodium. Some people report adverse reactions such as a flushed face, tingling or burning sensations, headache, rapid heartbeat, chest pain, and general weakness after consuming MSG.[19] These symptoms are referred to as MSG symptom complex, but have commonly been termed Chinese restaurant syndrome. They are most likely to occur within an hour after eating about 3 grams or more of MSG on an empty stomach. Individuals with asthma are more likely to experience symptoms at lower doses. When MSG is added to a food, it must appear in the label's ingredient list but the amount is not listed (see *Off the Label: Identifying Protein Sources*). A typical serving of foods containing MSG includes about 0.5 mg of MSG. Because glutamate is a neurotransmitter, some brain researchers are concerned that very high dietary intakes of glutamate could be toxic to nerves in humans. However, a review of scientific data has found no evidence that dietary MSG causes brain lesions or damages nerve cells in humans.[20] The FDA has therefore decided to keep glutamate on the list of substances generally recognized as safe (see Chapter 16).[20]

APPLICATIONS

These exercises are designed to help you apply your critical thinking skills to your own nutrition choices. Many are best performed using a diet analysis software program. If you do not have access to a computer program, the exercises can be hand-calculated using the information in this text and its appendices.

1. Calculate your average protein intake using the three-day food record you kept in Chapter 2.
   a. What is your average daily protein intake in grams?
   b. Is your intake higher or lower than the 1989 RDA for protein for someone of your weight, age, and life stage?
   c. If you consumed more than the 1989 RDA for protein, do you think you should decrease your protein intake? Why or why not?
   d. If you consumed less than the 1989 RDA for protein, modify one day of your diet to meet your protein needs. How did these changes affect the amount of fat in your diet?
2. Using the three-day record you kept in Chapter 2, compare your protein and fat intake for each day.

	Protein (g)	Fat (g)
Day 1		
Day 2		
Day 3		

   a. What is the relationship between the fat and protein in your diet?
   b. Look at the three foods that contribute the most protein to your diet each day. Are they animal or plant foods?
   c. What percentage of your total fat for that day do these provide?
3. Imagine that you have decided to become a lacto vegetarian. Make a list of the nondairy animal foods in your diet and then list plant foods you could substitute. Use protein complementation (see Figure 6.17) to be sure that you meet your need for essential amino acids.
   a. Does your modified diet meet the serving recommendations of the vegetarian pyramid in Figure 6.19? If not, what changes would you suggest?
   b. How much protein is in your lacto vegetarian diet? Does it meet the 1989 RDA for protein for someone in your age and gender group?
   c. If you already consume a lacto vegetarian diet, design a vegan diet by substituting plant sources of protein for dairy products. Make sure the diet includes at least 2 servings of calcium-rich foods.
4. Assume you are a vegetarian and you will be hosting Thanksgiving dinner for your family. Use a vegetarian cookbook or information on the Internet to design a vegetarian menu that will provide complementary proteins as well as provide a festive holiday meal.

Summary

1. Dietary protein comes from both animal and plant sources. In developed countries, protein intakes are usually well above needs.
2. Proteins are made of amino acid chains that fold over on themselves to create unique three-dimensional structures. The shape of a protein determines its function. Amino acids consist of a carbon atom with a hydrogen atom, a nitrogen-containing group, an acid group, and a unique side chain attached. The amino acids that the body is unable to make in sufficient amounts are referred to as essential amino acids.
3. Digestion breaks dietary protein into small peptides and amino acids, which are absorbed. Amino acids can be used for the synthesis of protein and other nitrogen-containing molecules and can be deaminated and used for energy.
4. The amino acids used by cells to synthesize proteins come from both dietary protein and the degradation of body proteins.
5. DNA in the nucleus of cells contains the information needed to make body proteins. These proteins then provide structure, regulate body functions as enzymes and hormones, transport molecules in the blood and in cells, function in the immune system, and aid in muscle contraction, fluid balance, and acid balance.
6. Protein-energy malnutrition is a public health concern, primarily in developing countries. Kwashiorkor occurs when the protein content of the diet is deficient. It is most common in children. Marasmus occurs when total energy intake is deficient.
7. For healthy adults, the 1989 RDA for protein is 0.8 gram per kilogram of body weight. Growth, pregnancy, lactation, and physical stress can increase requirements. Certain types of physical activity can also increase protein needs.
8. Animal proteins contain a pattern of amino acids that matches the needs of the human body more closely than the pattern of amino acids in plant proteins. Animal proteins are therefore said to be of higher quality than plant proteins.
9. Diets that include little or no animal protein can provide adequate protein if the sources of protein are complemented to supply enough of all the essential amino acids.
10. Proteins and amino acids can be used in the preparation of processed foods to enhance nutritional value and to change texture and flavor.

Review Questions

1. List some good sources of plant protein.
2. What are amino acids?
3. What is an essential amino acid?
4. What is the "amino acid pool"?
5. List six functions of proteins in the body.
6. Why is protein deficiency most common in infants and children?
7. How does the typical protein intake in North America compare to recommendations?
8. What effect does moderate exercise have on protein needs?
9. What does nitrogen balance suggest about the balance between protein synthesis and protein breakdown in the body?
10. What is protein quality?
11. What is protein complementation?
12. List some uses of proteins and amino acids in processed foods.

Nutrition Web Links

To further explore areas related to the material in this chapter go to the *Nutrition: Science and Applications* Web site at ***www.Wiley.com/college/Smolin*** and *click on* **Student Companion Site** for chapter-by-chapter links. Some Web sites related to the information in Chapter 6 include:

Sites that provide information on the recommendations for protein intake for the general population as well as those with special health concerns such as the American Dietetic Association and the National Institutes of Health.

Locations that provide information on the health and ecological benefits of vegetarian diets such as The Vegetarian Resource Group and the Tufts University Nutrition Navigator.

Sites that provide information on the risks and benefits of protein supplements such as the American College of Sports Medicine.

Sites that provide information on the availability of soy-based products such the U.S. Soyfoods Directory.

References

1. Kuhn, L. C. Iron and gene expression: molecular mechanisms regulating cellular iron homeostasis. Nutr. Rev. 56(II):S11–S19, 1998.
2. Williams, C. D. Kwashiorkor: nutritional disease of children associated with maize diet. Lancet 2:1151–1154, 1935.
3. National Research Council. *Diet and Health: Implications for Reducing Chronic Disease Risk.* Washington, D.C.: National Academy Press, 1989.
4. Maroni, B. J., and Mitch, W. E. Role of nutrition in prevention of the progression of renal disease. Annu. Rev. Nutr. 17:435–455, 1997.
5. Keys, T. J., Thorogood, M., Appleby, P. N., and Burr, M. L. Dietary habits and mortality in 11,000 vegetarian and health conscious people: results of a 17-year follow-up. British Med. J. 313:775–779, 1996.
6. Messina, M. J., and Messina, V. L. *The Dietitian's Guide to Vegetarian Diets: Issues and Applications.* Gaithersburg, Md.: Aspen Publishers, 1996.
7. Feskanich, D., Willet, W. C., Stampfer, M. J., and Colditz, G. A. Protein consumption and bone fractures in women. Am. J. Epidemiol. 143:472–479, 1996.
8. Food and Drug Administration, U.S. Department of Health and Human Services. FDA Talk Paper: Impurities confirmed in dietary supplement 5-hydroxy-L-tryptophan. August 31, 1998. Online at http://www.fda.gov/bbs/topics/ANSWERS/ANS00891.html.
9. Paul, G. L., Gautsch, T. A., and Layman, D. K. Amino acid and protein metabolism during exercise and recovery. In *Nutrition in Exercise and Sport*, 3rd ed. I. Wolinski, ed. Boca Raton, Fla.: CRC Press, 1998. 125–158.
10. Messina, V. K., and Burke, K. I. Position of the American Dietetic Association: vegetarian diets. J. Am. Diet. Assoc. 97:1317–1321, 1997.
11. Walter, P. Effects of vegetarian diets on aging and longevity. Nutr. Rev. 55(II):S61–S68, 1997.
12. Fonnebo, V. The healthy Seventh-Day Adventist. Am. J. Clin. Nutr. 59(suppl):1124S–1129S, 1994.
13. Snowdon, D. A. Animal product consumption and mortality because of all causes combined, coronary heart disease, stroke, diabetes, and cancer in Seventh-Day Adventists. Am. J. Clin. Nutr. 48(suppl):739S–748S, 1988.
14. Janelle, K. C., and Barr, S. I. Nutrient intakes and eating behavior scores of vegetarian and nonvegetarian women. J. Am. Diet. Assoc. 95:180–189, 1995.
15. Jacob, R. A., and Burri, B. J. Oxidative damage and defense. Am. J. Clin. Nutr. 63(suppl):985S–990S, 1996.
16. American Dietetic Association. Position paper of the American Dietetic Association: fat replacers. J. Am. Diet. Assoc. 98:463–468, 1998.
17. Seymour, C. A., Cockburn, F., Thomason, M. J., et al. Newborn screening for inborn errors of metabolism: a systematic review. Health Technol. Assess. I:1–95, 1997.
18. Levy, H. L., and Ghavami, M. Maternal PKU: a metabolic teratogen. Teratology 53:176–184, 1996.
19. Yang, W. H., Drouin, M. A., Herbert, M., et al. The monosodium glutamate symptom complex: assessment in a double-blind, placebo-controlled, randomized study. J. Allergy & Clin. Immunol. 99:757–762, 1997.
20. U.S. Food and Drug Administration. FDA and monosodium glutamate (MSG). FDA Backgrounder, August 31, 1995. Online at http://vm.cfsan.fda.gov/~lrd/msg.html

Chapter 7

Chapter Outline

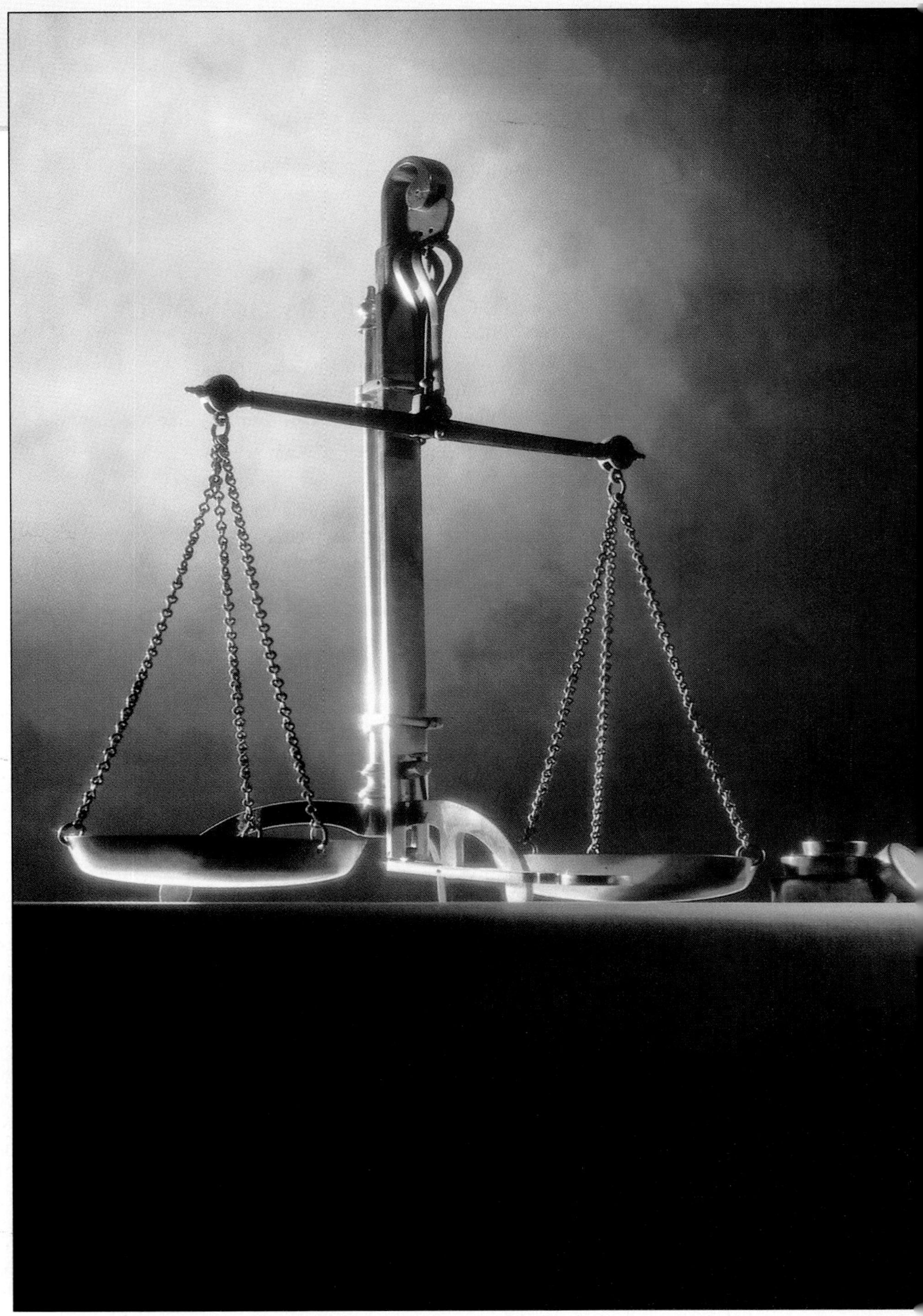

(© Gareth Trevor/Tony Stone Images, Inc.)

Energy Balance and Weight Management

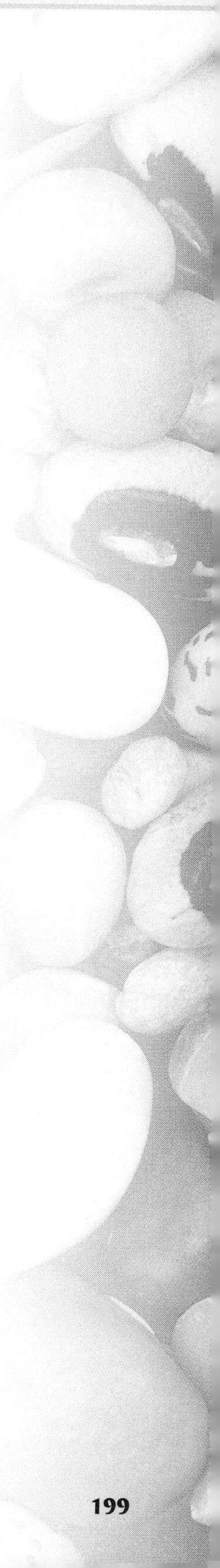

Chapter Concepts

1. Energy is the ability to do work. Energy in food and the body is measured in kcalories or kjoules.
2. Body weight is maintained by balancing energy intake with output—the principle of energy balance.
3. Carbohydrate, fat, protein, and alcohol provide energy that fuels the body.
4. Energy is needed for three major functions: maintaining basal metabolic rate, fueling physical activity, and processing the nutrients in food.
5. Energy consumed in excess of needs is stored primarily as fat.
6. Excess body fat, or obesity, is a disease that increases the risk of other chronic diseases and early death.
7. The amount and distribution of body fat is commonly evaluated using measures of weight, height, circumference, and skinfold thickness.
8. The propensity for storing excess body fat is determined by our genes, but environmental factors that influence our food intake and activity level affect what we actually weigh.
9. The overall goal of weight management is to reduce body fat to a healthy level and maintain that level throughout life.
10. There are hundreds of approaches to weight loss. All involve reducing food intake, increasing activity, and/or changing eating habits.
11. Eating disorders are psychological disorders that involve abnormal eating behaviors due to a pathological concern with body size and weight.

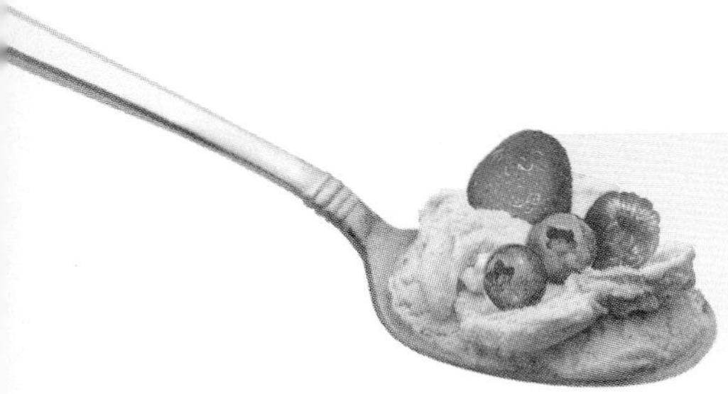

Just a Taste

Do overweight people consume more kcalories than thin people?

Is obesity inherited?

Are weight-loss drugs a safe approach to weight loss?

Our society puts a high value on physical appearance. Being thin is considered attractive and being fat is not. Overweight individuals face discrimination just about everywhere—in school, in the workplace, even on public transportation.[1] In addition to its social effects, excess body fat also increases the risk of developing chronic diseases such as diabetes, heart disease, and cancer. Nevertheless, more Americans are fatter every year; current estimates suggest that 35 to 55% of adults in the United States are overweight.[2] Why are we getting fatter when society and health promotion messages tell us to be thin?

It is not easy to lose weight. Although thousands of Americans diet every year, many never lose any weight at all, and most people who lose weight eventually regain it.[3] This creates a ready supply of customers for the thousands of weight-loss plans offered by commercial ventures, physicians, and support groups. Weight-loss centers in shopping malls and advertisements in newspapers, magazines, and on television push various weight-loss aids and programs. A tour of any bookstore will reveal a mind-boggling assortment of diet books. Weight-loss choices range from liquid diets and unusual food combinations to drug therapy and stomach bypass surgery.

The increasing prevalence of obesity and the failure of most attempts at weight loss have created a major public health problem. Estimates suggest that the health-care costs of obesity exceed $70 billion per year,[4] and another $30 to $50 billion is spent annually on weight-loss programs, special foods, and over-the-counter remedies.[5,6] Why are we overweight, and how can we reduce this growing trend?

What Is Energy?

Energy The capacity to do work.

Energy is the ability to do work. It exists in many forms that can be converted from one to another. For example, the energy in flowing water can be converted into electrical energy, which can then be converted into the light energy emitted by a lightbulb (Figure 7.1). In the human body, energy is obtained from the energy-containing nutrients in food. Once these nutrients have been consumed, cellular respiration converts the energy stored in carbohydrate, fat, protein, and alcohol into the high-energy compound ATP. The energy in ATP can be used to maintain the internal environment of the body, synthesize new molecules, and power activity. For example, the energy stored in the chemical bonds of a slice of bread can be converted into ATP, which then can be used for muscle contraction.

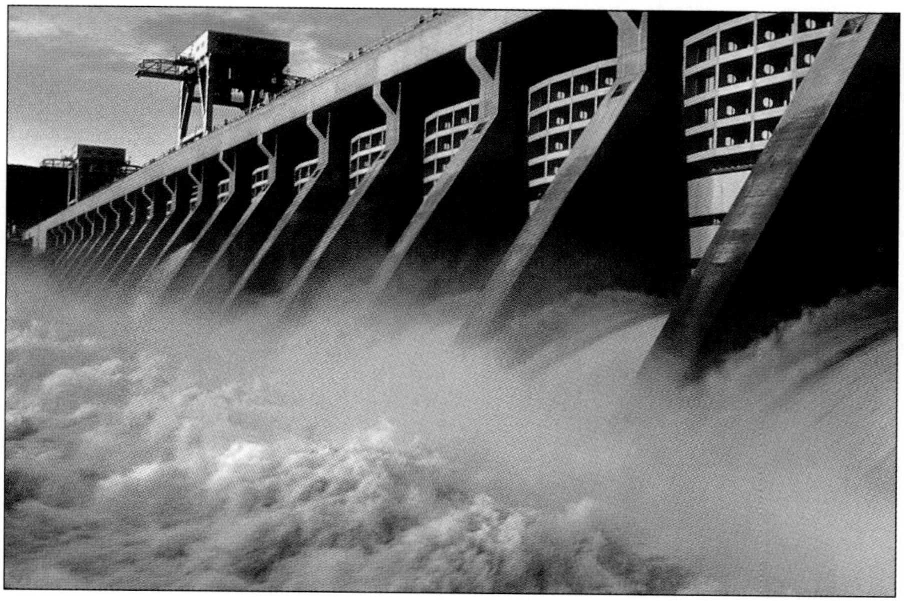

Figure 7.1
The energy in flowing water can be harnessed to produce electricity. In a similar way the energy in chemical bonds can be used by the body to produce ATP. (USDOE)

In the context of human activity, energy is measured in **kilojoules (kjoules),** which are units of work, and in **kilocalories (kcalories),** which are units of heat. A kjoule is the amount of work required to move an object weighing 1 kilogram a distance of 1 meter under the force of gravity. In Europe, the kjoule is the standard measure of energy in food and the body. Kcalories are the measure most commonly used in the United States and Canada. Technically, a kcalorie is the amount of heat required to raise the temperature of 1 kilogram of water 1 degree Celsius. In practical terms, a kcalorie is a measure of the amount of energy in food that can be supplied to the body. We don't eat kcalories; we eat food which provides energy measured in kcalories. Individuals who struggle with weight loss often think of kcalories as an enemy—something to be avoided. However, food and the energy it provides are essential to maintain life. Just as gasoline is necessary to run an engine, kcalories are necessary to run the body.

Kilojoule (kjoule) The amount of work required to move an object weighing 1 kilogram a distance of 1 meter under the force of gravity.

Kilocalorie (kcalorie) The amount of heat required to raise the temperature of 1 kilogram of water 1 degree Celsius.

The amount of energy consumed and the amount used are the critical components of **energy balance.** When the amount of energy—or number of kcalories—consumed is equal to the amount of energy that is used, body weight is maintained. If excess energy is consumed, the excess will be stored for later use, mostly as fat, and weight will increase. If too little energy is consumed, stored energy will be used to fuel the body and weight will be lost. This sounds very simple, but as anyone who has ever battled a weight problem can attest, balancing energy intake with output is not as simple as it sounds.

Energy balance A state in which body weight remains stable because the amount of energy consumed in the diet equals the amount expended.

Energy Intake

The energy needed to fuel the body comes from the carbohydrate, fat, protein, and alcohol in food (Figure 7.2). The amount of energy taken in depends on the total amount of food consumed and the nutrient composition of these foods.

Food: The Source of Energy

Food is the source of energy for our bodies. We eat in response to **hunger,** the physiological drive to consume food. What, when, and how much we eat are also affected by **appetite,** the drive to eat that is not necessarily related to hunger. Factors such as the time of day, cultural and social conventions, the appeal of the foods available, and one's emotional state can motivate eating.[7] Some people eat

Hunger Internal signals that stimulate one to acquire and consume food.

Appetite The desire to consume specific foods that is independent of hunger.

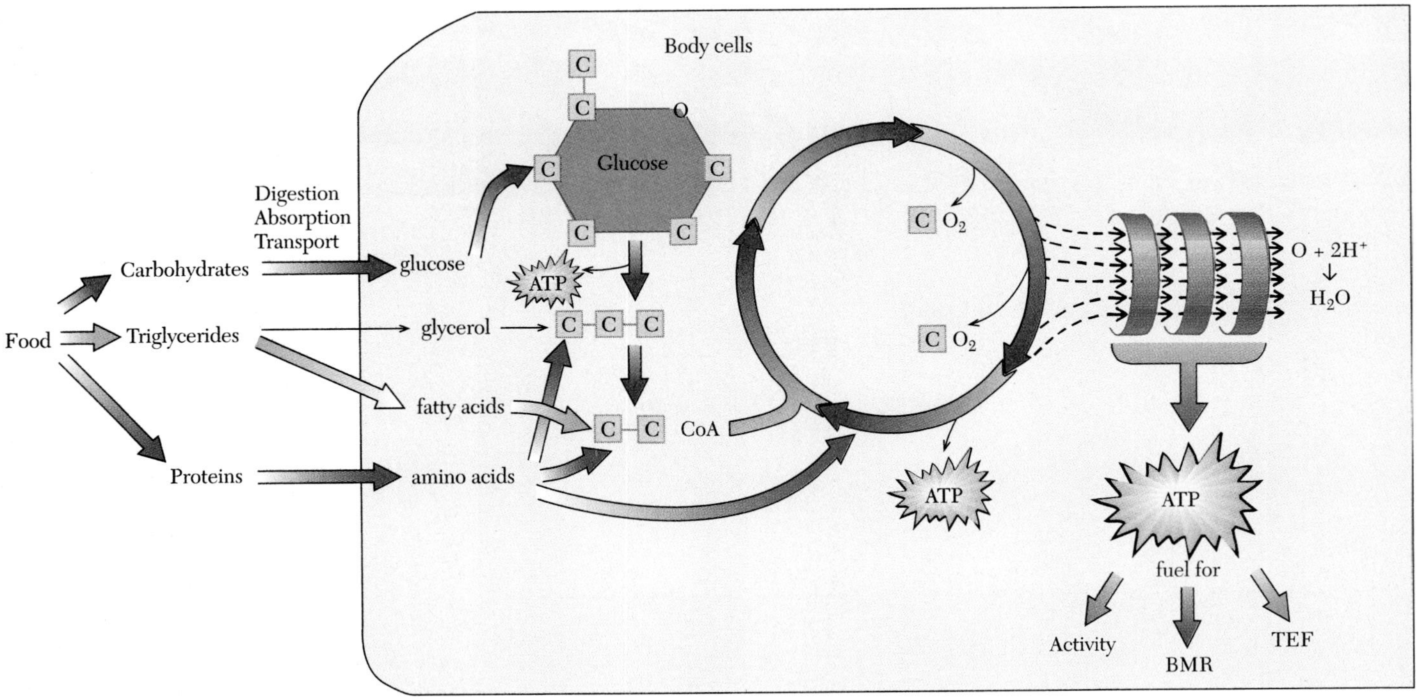

Figure 7.2
Energy is consumed in carbohydrates, triglycerides, and proteins, which can be metabolized to produce ATP.

lunch at noon out of social convention, not because they are hungry. We eat turkey on Thanksgiving because it is a tradition. We eat cookies or cinnamon rolls while walking through the mall because the smell entices us to buy them. The effect of emotions on appetite depends on the individual. Some people eat for comfort and to relieve stress. Others may lose their appetite when these same emotions are felt. We stop eating when we experience **satiety,** the feeling of fullness and satisfaction that follows food intake.

Satiety The feeling of fullness and satisfaction, caused by food consumption, that eliminates the desire to eat.

How Much Energy Is in Food?

The energy content of the food we eat can be measured precisely in the laboratory or estimated from its nutrient composition.

Measuring the Energy in Food In the laboratory, the energy content of food is determined by using a **bomb calorimeter,** which consists of a chamber surrounded by a jacket of water (Figure 7.3). Food is dried, placed in the chamber, and burned. As the food combusts, heat is released, raising the temperature of the water. The increase in water temperature can be used to calculate the amount of energy in the food based on the fact that 1 kcalorie is the amount of heat needed to increase the temperature of 1 kilogram of water by 1 degree Celsius. This method determines the total amount of energy contained in foods. However, because the body cannot completely digest, absorb, and utilize all of the nutrients in a food, bomb calorimeter values are slightly higher than the amount of energy the body can obtain from that food. For example, a bomb calorimeter can burn fiber, whereas the body cannot digest or absorb fiber; thus, its energy is not available for use by the body.

Bomb calorimeter An instrument used to determine the energy content of food. It measures the heat energy released when a food is combusted.

Estimating the Energy in Food Information on the energy content of foods can be found in food composition tables and databases and on food labels. The Nutrition Facts portion of food labels lists the total kcalories in a serving of food (see

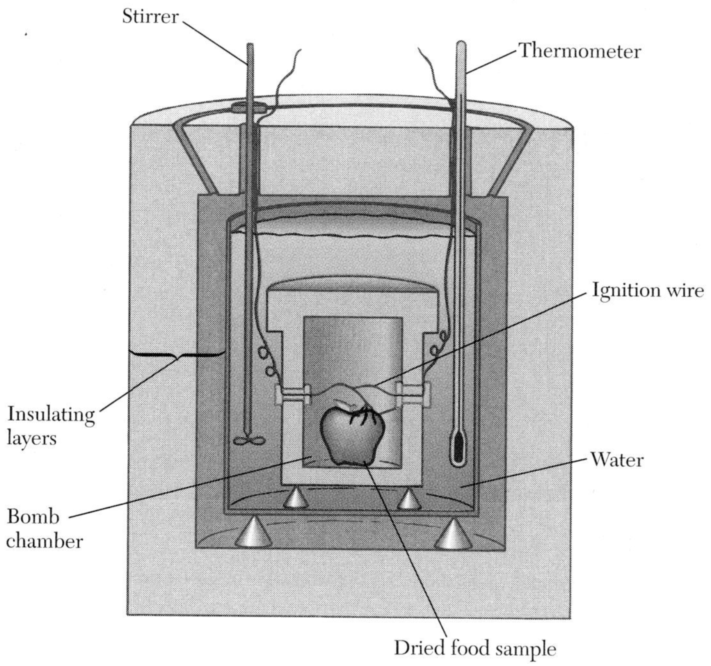

Figure 7.3
When dried food is combusted inside the chamber of a bomb calorimeter, the rise in temperature of the surrounding water can be used to determine the energy content of the food.

Off the Label: Low-Kcalorie Choices). The energy content of foods in a diet can also be estimated from the Exchange Lists shown in Table 7.1. For example, one starch exchange, whether a slice of bread, one-half cup (100 g) of cereal, or six saltines, provides about 80 kcalories.

Table 7.1 ***Using Exchange Lists to Calculate the Energy Content of a Diet***

Exchange Groups/Lists	Serving Size	Energy (kcal)
Carbohydrate Group		
Starch	1/2 cup rice, cereal, potatoes; 1 slice bread	80
Fruit	1 small apple, peach, pear; 1/2 banana; 1/2 cup canned juice-pack fruit	60
Milk	1 cup milk or yogurt	
Nonfat		90
Lowfat		110
Reduced fat		120
Whole		150
Other carbohydrates	Serving sizes vary	Varies
Vegetables	1/2 cup cooked vegetables, 1 cup raw	25
Meat/Meat Substitute Group	1 oz meat or cheese; 1/2 cup legumes	
Very lean		35
Lean		55
Medium fat		75
High fat		100
Fat Group	1 tsp butter, margarine, or oil; 1 Tbsp salad dressing	45

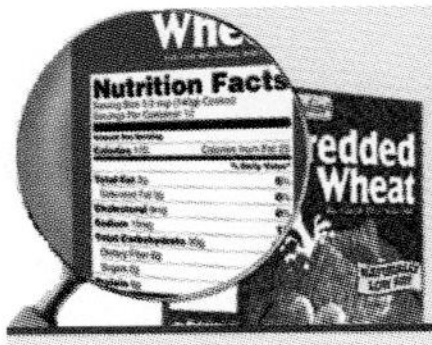

Off the Label

Low-Kcalorie Choices

If you are trying to lose weight by choosing foods that are low in kcalories, where should you start? When selecting packaged foods, start with the label. But be sure you know what the terms mean.

Descriptors such as "low calorie," "calorie free," and "light" on food labels may be the first thing a diet-conscious shopper sees. These terms all have standard definitions. A food labeled "low calorie" must have no more than 40 kcalories per serving. A product labeled "calorie free," must contain fewer than 5 kcalories in a serving. "Light" or "lite" may be used to describe foods that contain one-third fewer kcalories or half the fat of a comparable product. For example, the label on "lite" microwave popcorn or "light" corn chips must state both the number of kcalories per serving and that this is 30% fewer than the regular product. The terms "light" and "lite" are also used to describe food properties such as texture and color. For example, a label that says "light in texture" means just that; it does not mean that the kcalories are reduced. The term "light" may also appear without explanation on foods like brown sugar, cream, or molasses, which have traditionally included the term as part of their name.

Light foods that are reduced in fat compared to the original are a popular choice among dieters. Even though these products are reduced in fat they are not necessarily low in kcalories. When fat is removed, it must be replaced with something—most often with carbohydrates which contribute kcalories to the food. Compare the kcalories in a serving of lowfat cookies to the kcalories in regular cookies to be sure that substituting the lowfat variety will also decrease the energy content of your diet.

When checking the number of kcalories listed in the Nutrition Facts portion of a food label, be sure to check the serving size. Food labels are required to use standard serving sizes, but their standards may be different from yours. For instance, the standard serving of cookies is one ounce, or about three cookies. If you consume 12 cookies, you are consuming four times more energy than is listed on the label.

The bottom line on using food labels is to read and understand the entire label before assuming that you are making the best choice.

Regular Cookies

- **Low Cholesterol**
- **Low Saturated Fat**

CONTAINS 5g FAT AND 5mg CHOLESTEROL PER SERVING

Nutrition Facts
Serving Size 8 wafers (32g)
Servings Per Container About 11

Amount Per Serving	
Calories 140 Calories from Fat 40	
	% Daily Value*
Total Fat 5g	7%
Saturated Fat 1g	**4%**
Polyunsaturated Fat 0g	
Monounsaturated Fat 1.5g	
Cholesterol Less than 5 mg	1%
Sodium 100mg	4%
Total Carbohydrate 24g	**8%**
Dietary Fiber 0g	**0%**
Sugars 12g	
Protein 1g	
Vitamin A 0% • Vitamin C 0%	
Calcium 2% • Iron 4%	

*Percent Daily Values are based on a 2,000 calorie diet. Your daily values may be higher or lower depending on your calorie needs:

	Calories:	2,000	2,500
Total Fat	Less than	65g	80g
Sat Fat	Less than	20g	25g
Cholesterol	Less than	300mg	300mg
Sodium	Less than	2400mg	2400mg
Total Carbohydrate		300g	375g
Dietary Fiber		25g	30g

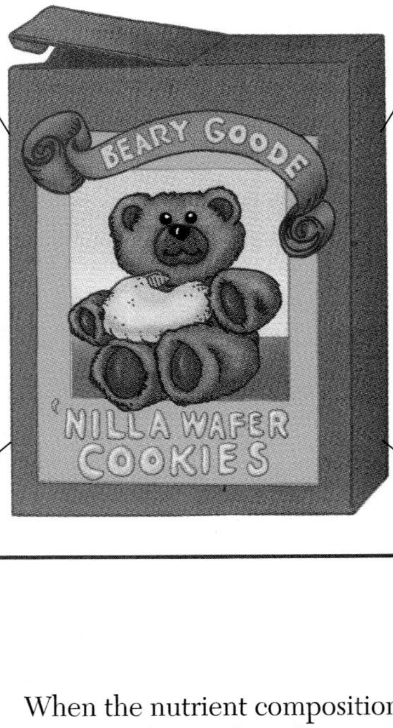

Reduced Fat Cookies

- **Low Cholesterol**
- **Low Saturated Fat**

50% Less Fat Than Original Nilla

Nutrition Facts
Serving Size 8 wafers (29g)
Servings Per Container About 11

Amount Per Serving	
Calories 120 Calories from Fat 20	
	% Daily Value*
Total Fat 2g	**3%**
Saturated Fat 0g	**0%**
Polyunsaturated Fat 0g	
Monounsaturated Fat 0.5g	
Cholesterol 0mg	**0%**
Sodium 105mg	**4%**
Total Carbohydrate 24g	**8%**
Dietary Fiber 0g	**0%**
Sugars 12g	
Protein 1g	
Vitamin A 0% • Vitamin C 0%	
Calcium 2% • Iron 4%	

*Percent Daily Values are based on a 2,000 calorie diet. Your daily values may be higher or lower depending on your calorie needs:

	Calories:	2,000	2,500
Total Fat	Less than	65g	80g
Sat Fat	Less than	20g	25g
Cholesterol	Less than	300mg	300mg
Sodium	Less than	2400mg	2400mg
Total Carbohydrate		300g	375g
Dietary Fiber		25g	30g

When the nutrient composition of a food is known, the energy content can be approximated by totaling the energy from the carbohydrate, fat, and protein in the food. Carbohydrate and protein provide about 4 kcalories per gram. So, 5 grams of sugar, which is almost pure carbohydrate, contains about 20 kcalories (5 g × 4 kcal/g). Fat, the most concentrated source of energy, provides 9 kcalories per gram, and alcohol provides 7 kcalories per gram. Five grams of corn oil, which is almost pure fat, contains about 45 kcalories (5 g × 9 kcal/g). Vitamins, minerals,

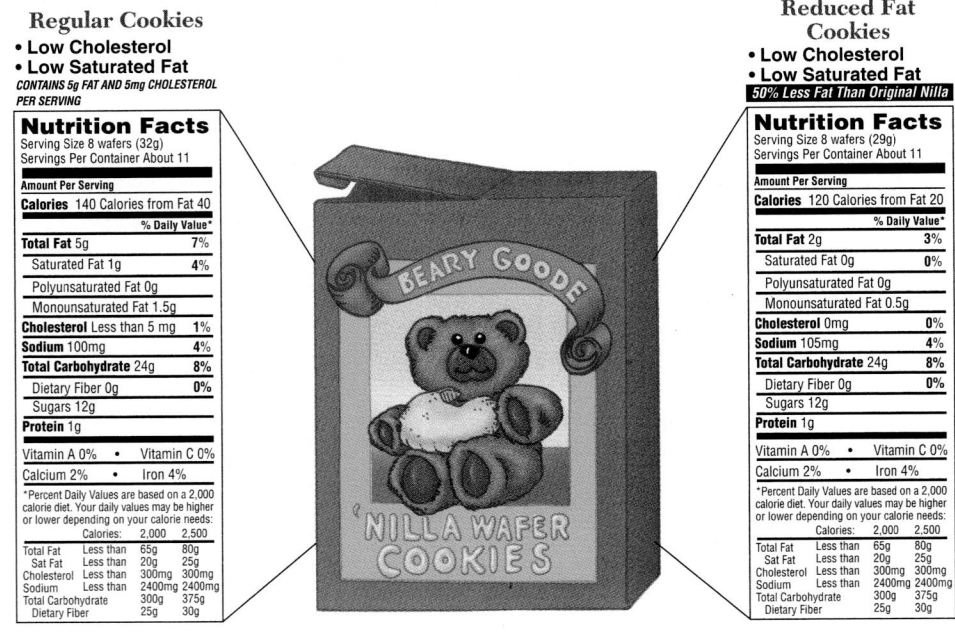

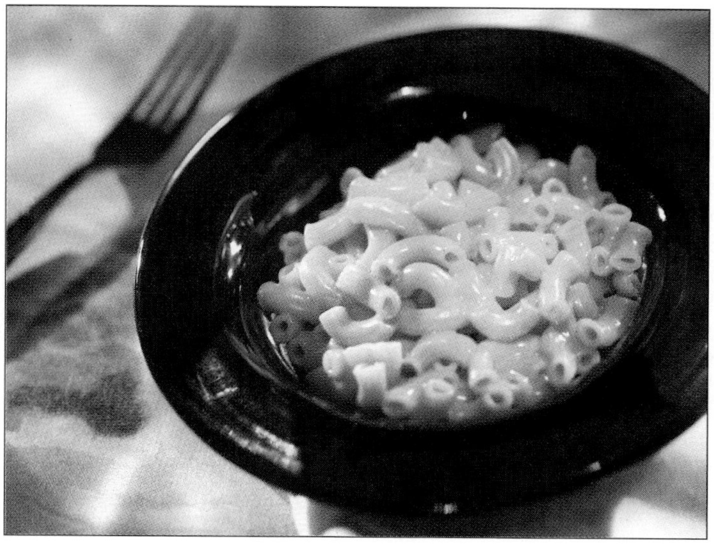

Figure 7.4
The carbohydrate, protein, and fat in macaroni and cheese contribute to its energy content. (Gary Bass/FPG International)

and water, though essential nutrients, do not provide energy to the body. Most foods are of mixed composition; for instance, a half-cup (100 g) serving of macaroni and cheese contains 8 grams of protein, 20 grams of carbohydrate, and 11 grams of fat (Figure 7.4). Its energy content is therefore:

$$(4 \text{ kcal/g} \times 8 \text{ g protein}) + (4 \text{ kcal/g} \times 20 \text{ g carbohydrate}) + (9 \text{ kcal/g} \times 11 \text{ g fat}) = 211 \text{ kcal}$$

Energy Output

The energy output of the body is the amount of energy used to maintain basic body functions, to fuel physical activity, and to process the nutrients consumed in food.

Basal Metabolic Rate (BMR)

About 60 to 75% of the body's total energy requirement is for the maintenance of basic body functions such as breathing, circulating blood, and maintaining a constant body temperature. This portion of the energy requirement is called the **basal metabolic rate (BMR).** It is the minimum amount of energy needed to keep an awake, resting body alive. The BMR includes the energy necessary for all essential metabolic reactions and life-sustaining functions, but it does not include the energy needed for physical activity or for the digestion and absorption of food. BMR is related to body weight, **lean body mass,** gender, growth rate, and age. BMR increases with increasing body weight, so is higher in heavier individuals. It also rises with increasing lean body mass; BMR is generally higher in men than in women because men have greater lean body mass. BMR is increased during periods of rapid growth because energy is required to produce new body tissue. It decreases with age, partly due to a decrease in lean body mass that usually occurs in older adults.

Basal metabolic rate (BMR) The minimum amount of energy that an awake resting body needs to maintain itself. It is measured after 12 hours without food or exercise.

Lean body mass Body mass attributed to nonfat body components such as bone, muscle, and internal organs. It is also called fat-free mass.

BMR can also be altered by certain abnormal conditions. An elevation in body temperature, such as that which occurs with a fever, increases BMR. It is estimated that for every 1 degree Fahrenheit above normal body temperature, there is a 7% increase in BMR. This extra energy use explains why weight loss can occur with fever. Abnormal levels of thyroid hormones can also affect BMR. Individuals with an overproduction of these hormones require more energy, and those with underproduction require less energy. The fact that thyroid hormones, produced by the thyroid gland, affect energy expenditure is the reason obesity was once explained as a glandular problem. It is now known that obesity due to a lack of thyroid hormone is rare.

BMR may also be affected by low-energy diets. Energy intake below needs may depress BMR by 10 to 20%, or the equivalent of 100 to 400 kcalories per day.[8] This drop in BMR decreases the amount of energy needed to maintain weight. It is a beneficial adaptation in starvation, but it makes intentional weight loss more difficult.

Physical Activity

Physical activity is the second major component of energy expenditure. It includes the energy needed for exercise as well as for performing the functions of daily life, such as sitting, standing, and walking. Since it takes more energy to move a heavier object, the amount of energy expended for many activities increases as body weight increases. In most cases, activity accounts for 15 to 30% of energy requirements, but this varies greatly among individuals. The energy required for an activity depends on how strenuous the activity is and the length of time it is performed. A professional athlete who may spend many hours a day training at a strenuous activity level uses a great deal more energy in her daily activities than does an office worker who spends most of her day sitting at a desk. Because technological advances have reduced the physical activity needed for daily tasks, people today need to consciously increase their physical activity. This does not mean you have to run marathons. Choosing to take the stairs rather than the elevator, walking rather than taking the bus, and riding a bike rather than driving to the store all increase activity (Figure 7.5). The energy costs of specific activities are listed in Appendix L.

The Thermic Effect of Food

Thermic effect of food (TEF) or **diet-induced thermogenesis** The energy required for the digestion, absorption, metabolism, and storage of food. It is equal to approximately 10% of daily energy intake.

The **thermic effect of food (TEF),** also called **diet-induced thermogenesis,** is the increase in energy expenditure that results from the digestion of food and the absorption, metabolism, and storage of nutrients. This causes body temperature to rise slightly for several hours after eating. The energy required for TEF is estimated to be about 10% of energy intake but can vary depending on the amounts and types of nutrients consumed. When a small amount of food energy is consumed, it is used immediately for fuel. When more is consumed, some is

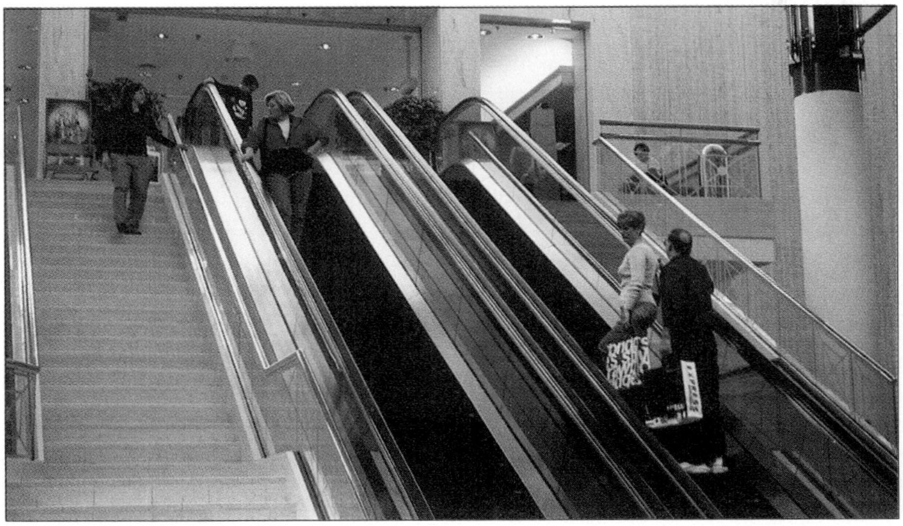

Figure 7.5
Even small increases or decreases in daily activity, such as the difference between riding the escalator and climbing the stairs, can affect energy balance. (George Semple)

stored for later use. Because it takes energy to store nutrients, TEF increases with the size of the meal. The composition of meals also affects TEF. A meal that is high in fat has a lower TEF than a meal high in carbohydrate or protein because dietary fat can be efficiently stored as body fat. This difference in the energy cost of storing energy means a diet high in fat may produce more body fat than a diet high in carbohydrate.[9]

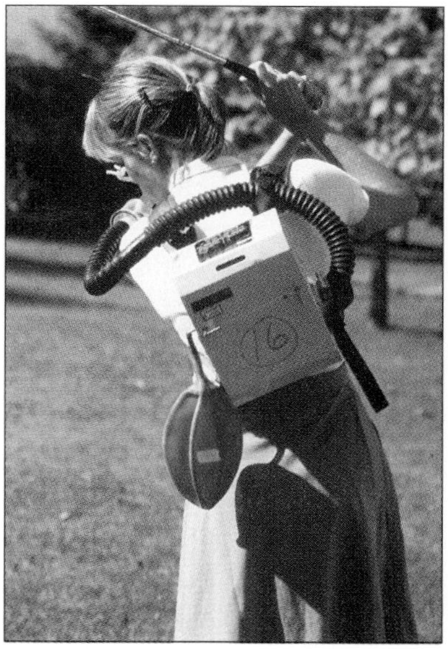

Figure 7.6
Indirect calorimetry can be used to estimate energy output during daily activities. (Dr. Frank Katch, Amherst, Mass.)

Determining Energy Needs

The energy requirements of the body are based on the sum of the needs for BMR, physical activity, and TEF. Energy requirements can be estimated in a variety of ways—some more precise than others.

Measuring Energy Expenditure The amount of energy used by the body can be measured in a process called calorimetry. **Direct calorimetry** measures heat production. Combusting food in a bomb calorimeter is a type of direct calorimetry. In humans, direct calorimetry measures the amount of heat generated by the metabolic reactions that both convert food energy into ATP and then use this ATP for various body processes. An individual's energy needs can be determined by measuring the amount of heat given off by the body; the heat produced is proportional to the amount of energy used by the individual. Direct calorimetry is an accurate method for measuring energy expenditure, but it is expensive and impractical because it requires that the individual being assessed remain in an insulated chamber throughout the evaluation.

The more commonly used method of estimating energy expenditure is **indirect calorimetry,** which measures the amounts of oxygen consumed and carbon dioxide expired by the body. The body's energy use can be calculated from these measures because cellular respiration uses oxygen and produces carbon dioxide. Oxygen use and carbon dioxide production can be measured by analyzing the difference between inhaled and exhaled air. Another indirect calorimetry method involves injecting or ingesting water labeled with **isotopes** of oxygen and hydrogen. The labeled oxygen and hydrogen are used by the body in metabolism. By measuring the amounts of labeled oxygen and labeled hydrogen that appear in body fluids, the amount of carbon dioxide produced by the energy-requiring reactions in the body can be estimated.[10] Both these methods are expensive but are more versatile than direct calorimetry. The equipment needed to measure inhaled and exhaled air is small enough to be carried in a backpack, so it can be used to measure the energy required for various activities (Figure 7.6). The labeled water method does not require the individual to carry any equipment and can be used to measure expenditure for periods up to several weeks.

Direct calorimetry A method of calculating energy use that measures the amount of heat produced by the body.

Indirect calorimetry A method of estimating energy use that compares the amount of oxygen consumed with the carbon dioxide expired.

Isotope An alternative form of an element that has a different atomic mass, which may or may not be radioactive.

Calorimetry can be used to measure the energy expended for BMR, activity, and TEF. BMR measurements must be done under very precise conditions to measure only the energy needed to stay alive and not that needed to process food or move about. Thus they are performed in a warm room in the morning before the subject rises, and at least 12 hours after the last food or activity. A modified BMR, called a **resting metabolic rate (RMR)** or **resting energy expenditure (REE),** is more often used. RMR is measured after only five to six hours without food or exercise. The difference between BMR and RMR is less than 10% in most cases.[11]

Resting metabolic rate (RMR) or **resting energy expenditure (REE)** An estimate of basal metabolic rate that is determined by measuring energy utilization after 5 to 6 hours without food or exercise.

Estimating Total Energy Expenditure Energy expenditure can be estimated by totaling the approximate amount of energy needed for RMR, activity, and TEF. Resting metabolic rates for individuals of the same age, sex, and weight are fairly consistent and can be calculated from body weight using the equations given in Appendix B. Some of these have been calculated for you in Table 7.2. Table 7.3 gives estimates of energy requirements for typical daily activities as

Table 7.2 *Resting Metabolic Rate Based on Body Weight*

Body Weight										
	(kg)	40	50	57	64	70	77	84	91	100
	(lb)	88	110	125	140	155	170	185	200	220
		Kcalories per 24 Hours								
Male										
Age (yr)										
10–18		1351	1526	1648	1771	1876	1998	2121	2243	2401
18–30		1291	1444	1551	1658	1750	1857	1964	2071	2209
30–60		1343	1459	1540	1621	1691	1772	1853	1935	2039
>60		1027	1162	1256	1351	1423	1526	1621	1716	1837
Female										
Age (yr)										
10–18		1234	1356	1441	1527	1660	1685	1771	1856	1966
18–30		1084	1231	1334	1437	1525	1628	1731	1833	1966
30–60		1177	1264	1325	1386	1438	1499	1560	1621	1699
>60		1016	1121	1195	1268	1331	1404	1478	1552	1646

Adapted from National Research Council, Food and Nutrition Board. *Recommended Dietary Allowances*, 10th ed. Washington, D.C.: National Academy of Sciences, 1989.

multiples of RMR; when calculated, these values include the energy needed for RMR plus activity. The energy needed for the thermic effect of food can be approximated as 10% of total energy intake. The sum of these factors equals the total daily energy requirement to maintain weight. See Table 7.4 for an example of how to calculate energy expenditure.

Table 7.3 *Factors for Estimating Energy Requirements of Various Activities in Relation to Resting Metabolic Rate*

Level of Activity	Activity Factor per Unit Time of Activity
Resting Sleeping, reclining	RMR × 1.0
Very light Seated and standing activities, painting, driving, laboratory work, typing, sewing, ironing, cooking, playing cards, playing musical instrument	RMR × 1.5
Light Walking on a level surface (2.5–3 mph), garage work, carpentry, housecleaning, child care, golf, sailing, table tennis	RMR × 2.5
Moderate Walking 3.5–4 mph, weeding and hoeing, carrying a load, cycling, skiing, tennis, dancing	RMR × 5
Heavy Walking with load uphill, tree felling, heavy manual digging, basketball, climbing, football, soccer	RMR × 7

National Research Council, Food and Nutrition Board. *Recommended Dietary Allowances*, 10th ed. Washington, D.C.: National Academy of Sciences, 1989.

Table 7.4 Calculating Energy Expenditure

1. Use Table 7.2 or the equations in Appendix B to determine RMR. For example, a 23-year-old female who weighs 125 lb has an RMR of 1334 kcal/day, or 1334 kcal/24 hours in a day = 55.6 kcal/hr.
2. The energy required for activity plus RMR can be estimated as a factor of her resting metabolic rate, as shown in Table 7.3. For example, if this individual spends 8 hours resting, 12 hours engaged in very light activity, and 4 hours engaged in light activity, her energy expenditure would be calculated as follows:

$$\text{8 hours of resting requires } 8 \text{ hr} \times (1 \times \text{RMR in kcal/hr}) = 8 \text{ hr} \times 1 \times 55.6 \text{ kcal/hr} = 445 \text{ kcalories}$$

$$\text{12 hours of very light activity requires } 12 \text{ hr} \times (1.5 \times \text{RMR in kcal/hr}) = 12 \text{ hr} \times 1.5 \times 55.6 \text{ kcal/hr} = 1001 \text{ kcalories}$$

$$\text{4 hours of light activity requires } 4 \text{ hr} \times (2.5 \times \text{RMR in kcal/hr}) = 4 \text{ hr} \times 2.5 \times 55.6 \text{ kcal/hr} = 556 \text{ kcalories}$$

$$\text{Total for RMR and activity} = 2002 \text{ kcalories}$$

3. The thermic effect of food is about 10% of daily energy intake. If the woman in this example consumes 2200 kcalories per day, 2200 kcalories × 10% = 220 kcalories.
4. Total energy expenditure = RMR + activity + TEF = 2002 + 220 = 2222 kcalories.

Recommended Energy Intakes

Energy expenditure calculations are used to determine recommended energy intakes. The 1989 RDAs for adults range from 30 to 40 kcalories per kilogram, depending on age and gender. For example, the 1989 RDA for a 51-year-old woman is about 30 kcalories per kilogram. The 1989 RDA for a 23-year-old man is about 40 kcalories per kilogram. These are calculated by averaging the amount of energy needed by individuals in the same age and gender category. In deriving these values, it is assumed that most individuals engage in only light to moderate activity. Since the 1989 RDA for energy is an average, about half of individuals will have an actual requirement that is above the RDA, and the other half will have a requirement that is below the RDA.

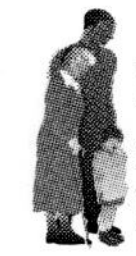

Energy requirements change throughout life. Energy needs per kilogram are higher during periods of rapid growth, such as infancy, adolescence, and pregnancy. The energy requirements for infants and children up to the age of ten are based on the amount needed for normal growth. From birth to six months of age, an intake of about 108 kcalories per kilogram of body weight is recommended. From one to three years, this decreases to about 102 kcalories per kilogram. Requirements per kilogram then drop off steadily until they reach the adult recommendations by about age 25. With aging, requirements continue to decrease slowly because lean body mass and physical activity generally decrease.

Beginning at about age ten, gender also affects energy requirements. The onset of puberty causes an increase in muscle mass in males and in body fat in females. From age ten into adulthood, males require more energy per kilogram than females.

Energy requirements also increase in pregnancy; an additional 300 kcalories per day is recommended after the first three months of pregnancy. This is to allow for the growth of the fetus, placenta, and added maternal tissues. Additional energy is also needed to support lactation. An individual's needs during lactation increase with the volume of milk produced.

Body Weight and Health

To maintain energy balance, energy intake must equal energy output. If excess energy is consumed, it will be stored, mostly as body fat. Some fat storage is essential and efficient. Individuals who have little stored fat have a greater risk for illness than individuals whose body fat is within the normal range. However, excess stored body fat also increases the risk of illness and can create psychological and social problems. Although we really are referring to overfat, we commonly call this condition overweight.

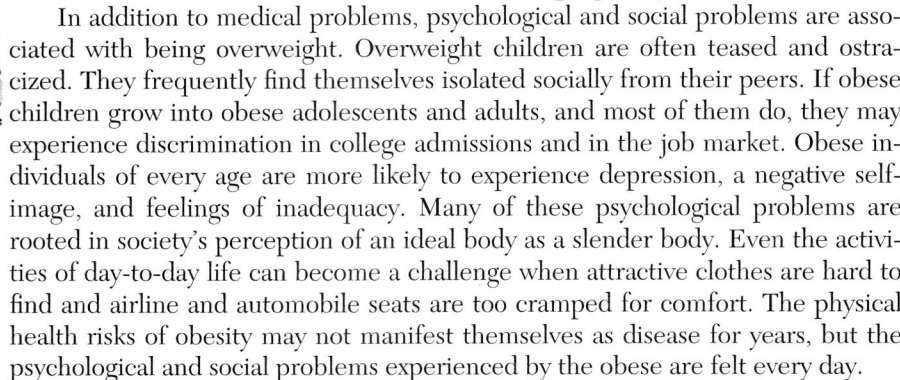

Excess body fat is a major public health problem in the United States. Over half of all adult Americans are considered overweight.[12] The prevalence is higher among minorities including Native Americans, Pacific Islanders, African Americans, and Hispanics.[13] Weight problems are also increasing among children and adolescents.[14] One quarter of U.S. children and adolescents are overweight (Figure 7.7).[15]

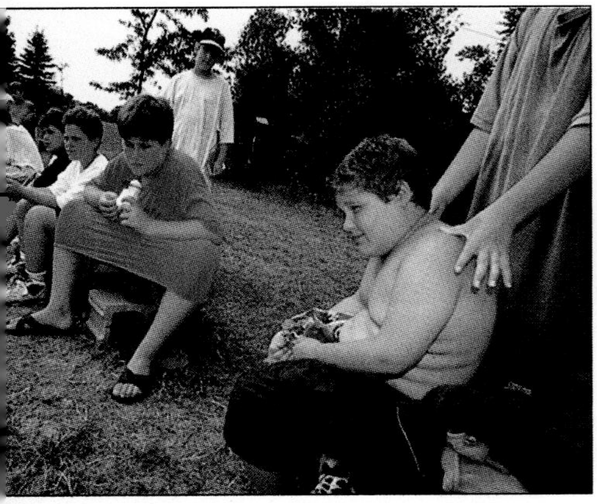

Figure 7.7
The number of children and teens who are overweight and obese has increased in recent years. (© Donna Binder/Impact Visuals)

What's Wrong With a Few Extra Pounds?

High blood pressure, heart disease, high blood cholesterol, diabetes, stroke, gallbladder disease, arthritis, sleep disorders, respiratory problems, and cancers of the breast, uterus, prostate, and colon all occur more frequently in overweight individuals.[2] People who gain excess weight at a young age and remain overweight throughout life have greater health risks. In addition to the amount of excess fat, the distribution of the fat affects the risk of developing many of these diseases.

In addition to medical problems, psychological and social problems are associated with being overweight. Overweight children are often teased and ostracized. They frequently find themselves isolated socially from their peers. If obese children grow into obese adolescents and adults, and most of them do, they may experience discrimination in college admissions and in the job market. Obese individuals of every age are more likely to experience depression, a negative self-image, and feelings of inadequacy. Many of these psychological problems are rooted in society's perception of an ideal body as a slender body. Even the activities of day-to-day life can become a challenge when attractive clothes are hard to find and airline and automobile seats are too cramped for comfort. The physical health risks of obesity may not manifest themselves as disease for years, but the psychological and social problems experienced by the obese are felt every day.

A Few Pounds Too Few?

If excess body fat is bad for you, what's wrong with being lean? Recent research has suggested that being on the low side of the body weight standard may reduce the risk of diabetes, and may even increase longevity.[16,17] However, some body fat is essential as an insulator and as a reserve for periods of illness. Substantial reductions in body weight have been shown to decrease the ability of the immune system to fight disease, and very low body weight is associated with an increased risk of early death.[18] In developed countries, socioeconomic conditions may create isolated pockets of undernutrition, but severe cases of wasting are usually a result either of self-starvation due to eating disorders such as anorexia nervosa or of a disease process such as AIDS or cancer.

Too little body fat causes problems at all stages of life. Low weight gains during pregnancy are correlated with an increase in low-birth-weight infants, who are at a higher risk of health complications and death (see Chapter 13). For teenage girls, too little body fat can delay sexual development. In healthy but very lean female athletes, menstrual irregularities are common, increasing the risk of developing osteoporosis (see Chapters 10 and 12).[19] Too little body fat in the elderly increases the risk of malnutrition.

Guidelines for Healthy Body Weight and Composition

Body mass index (BMI) An index of weight in relation to height that is used to compare body size with a standard.

Body weight includes the weight of body fat as well as lean body mass. There are many ways to evaluate desirable levels of body fat. Traditionally, weight is assessed in relation to height. **Body mass index (BMI)** is a calculation of body weight in relation to height. Although BMI is not actually a measure of body fat, it correlates well with body fat and has become the medical standard for assessing the degree of body fatness. More sophisticated measures that approximate the proportion of body weight that is fat are also available for assessing fatness.

Body Mass Index Body mass index is a means of expressing healthy body weight. BMI is calculated from the ratio of weight to height according to the following equation:

$$\text{BMI} = \frac{\text{body weight in kilograms}}{(\text{height in meters})^2}$$

$$\text{or, BMI} = \frac{\text{body weight in pounds}}{(\text{height in inches})^2} \times 704.5$$

For example, someone who is 6 feet (72 inches) tall and weighs 180 pounds has a body mass index of 24.5 kg/m^2 (180/72^2 $\times$ 704.5). Figure 7.8 can also be used to estimate body mass index.

Using BMI criteria, **underweight** is defined as a body mass index of less than 18.5 kg/m^2, normal weight is 18.5 to 24.9 kg/m^2, **overweight** is identified as 25 to 29.9 kg/m^2, and **obese** is 30 kg/m^2 or greater.[2] Statistically, the lowest health risks occur in people with body mass indexes between 19 and 25 kg/m^2.[20]

Underweight A body mass index of less than 18.5 kg/m^2 or a body weight 10% or more below the desirable body weight standard.

Overweight A body mass index of 25 to 29.9 kg/m^2 or a body weight 10 to 19% above the desirable body weight standard.

Obese A condition characterized by excess body fat. It is defined as a body mass index of 30 kg/m^2 or greater or a body weight that is 20% or more above the desirable body weight standard.

Weight Tables Weight tables list ranges of desirable or healthy weights based on height. Weight tables are convenient but less than ideal because they do not

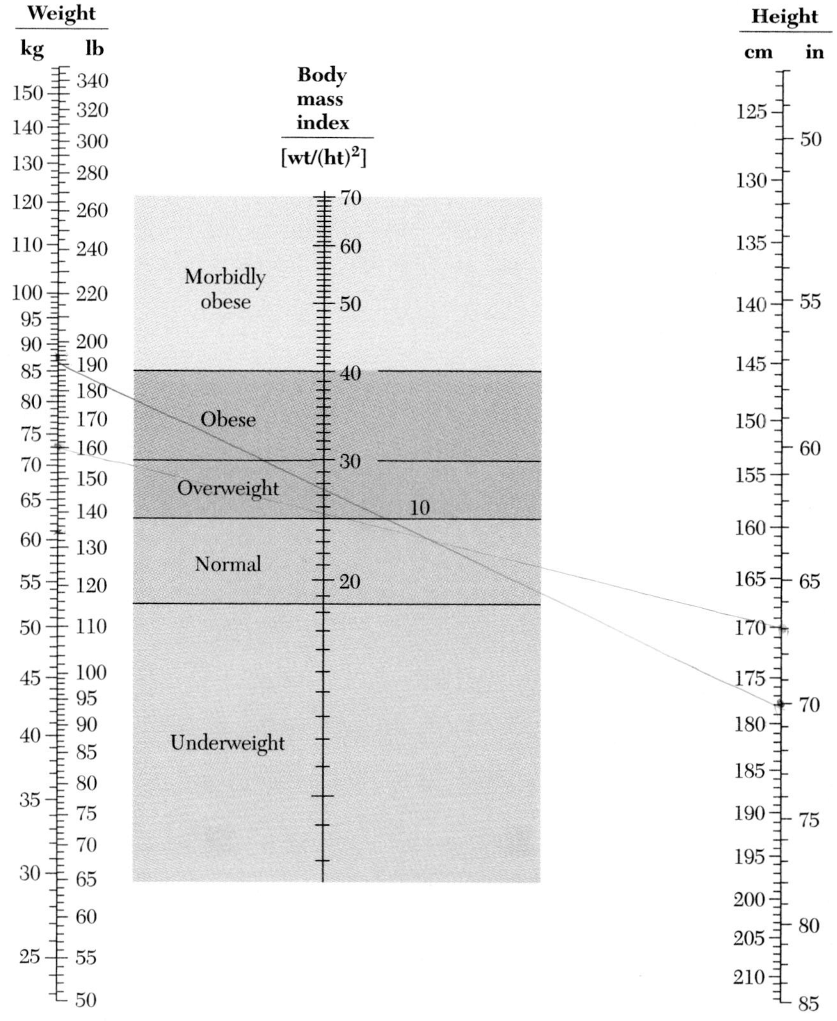

Figure 7.8
To determine body mass index using a nomogram, place a straightedge between your body weight in the left column and your height on the right. The point at which your line crosses the middle line is your body mass index. (Copyright © 1978, George A. Bray. Used with permission.)

distinguish excess body weight from excess body fat. This is important because health risks increase with increases in body fat but not necessarily with increases in body weight. For example, some people who exceed the weight for height standards, such as weight lifters, have a higher-than-average lean body weight but not excess body fat. If excess weight is due to a high lean body mass, there are no increased health risks. However, most people whose weight exceeds standards have excess body fat. Although measuring weight in relation to height does not consider the proportion of weight that is fat, it is an easy measure to use for comparison.

The most commonly used weight tables are the Metropolitan Life Insurance Company tables. These present desirable weight ranges based on height, sex, and **frame size,** which is an approximation of weight due to bone mass (see Appendix B). The Metropolitan Life tables were developed by determining the weight at which individuals of a given age, sex, and height live the longest. Longevity is a good measure of desirable weight; however, these tables were developed using weights recorded at the time individuals purchased insurance. Since there was no follow-up to determine if individuals' weights had changed by the time of death, the weights in the table may not represent the healthiest weights. In addition, since they are based on people who bought insurance, the values reflect only the segment of the population that can afford insurance. Lower socioeconomic groups and minorities are underrepresented.

Frame size An estimate of the proportion of body weight that is due to bone.

Another weight table, published along with the Dietary Guidelines for Americans and called Healthy Weight Ranges for Men and Women (see Appendix B), responds to some of these criticisms by giving a wider range of healthy weights. Unlike the Metropolitan Life Insurance tables, it does not differentiate for frame size or sex.

Body Fat Distribution The distribution of body fat affects the risks associated with being overfat. Fat that is located under the skin, called subcutaneous fat, carries less risk than fat that is deposited around the organs, called visceral fat (Figure 7.9). An increase in visceral fat is associated with a higher incidence of heart disease, high blood pressure, stroke, diabetes, and breast cancer. Fat in the hips and lower body is subcutaneous, whereas fat deposited around the waist in the abdominal region is primarily visceral fat. Therefore, people who carry their ex-

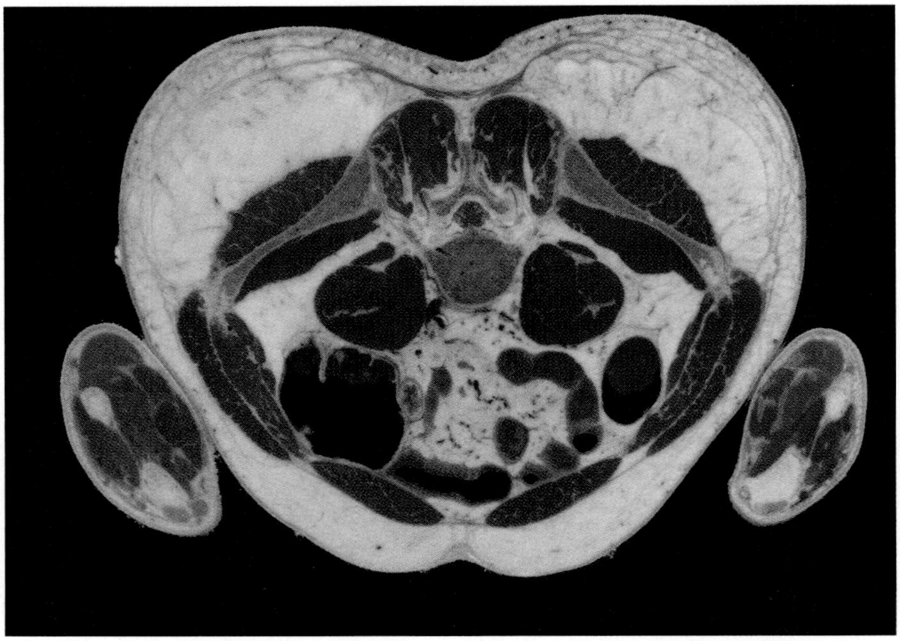

Figure 7.9
This cross section of the abdomen shows both subcutaneous and visceral fat. (Yuh-Jye Chang)

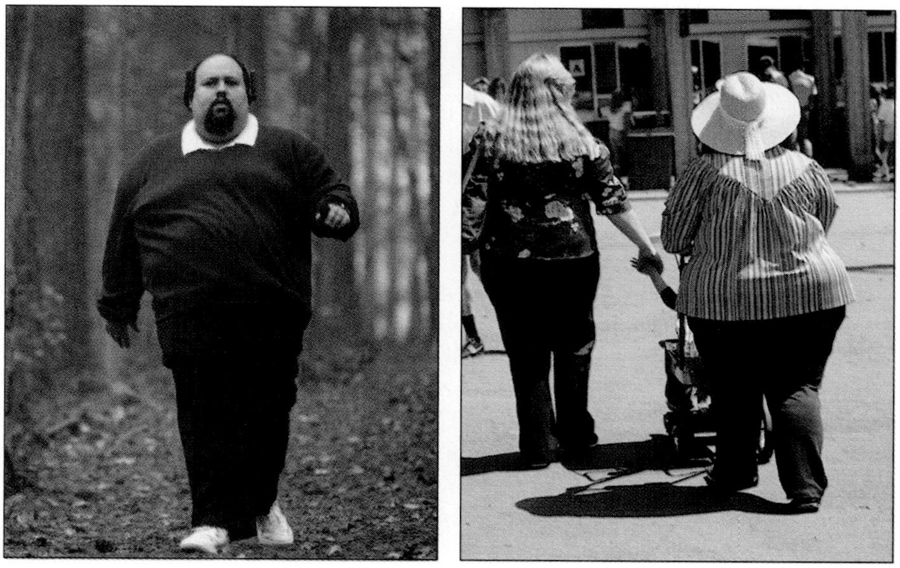

(a) (b)

Figure 7.10
(a) Overweight individuals with apple-shaped body types deposit fat in the abdominal region and are at greater risk of developing heart disease and diabetes. (b) Overweight individuals with pear-shaped body types deposit fat in the hips and thighs where it is primarily subcutaneous. (*a*, Corbis; *b*, © Tom McHugh/Photo Researchers, Inc.)

cess fat around and above the waist have more visceral fat. Those who carry their extra fat below the waist in the hips and thighs have more subcutaneous fat. These body types have been dubbed apples and pears, respectively, by the popular literature (Figure 7.10).

Distinguishing the relative amounts of visceral and subcutaneous fat requires sophisticated imaging techniques. However, visceral fat can be approximated by measuring waist circumference or by determining the ratio of waist to hip circumference. A waist measurement of greater than 40 inches (102 cm) in overweight men and greater than 35 inches (88 cm) in overweight women indicates more visceral fat and therefore an increased risk of developing obesity-related diseases.[2] When the waist-hip ratio is used, the waist circumference must be divided by the hip circumference. If this value is greater than 1.0 in men or 0.8 in women it indicates more visceral fat storage.[21]

Where an individual deposits body fat is determined primarily by genetics,[22] which includes ethnic background, but gender, age, and environment also influence where fat is stored.[23] African American women, who have an incidence of obesity that is 50% higher than that of Caucasian women, store less visceral fat.[13] Visceral fat storage is more common in men than women. But after menopause, visceral fat increases in women. Stress, tobacco, and alcohol consumption predispose people to visceral fat deposition, whereas activity reduces it.[24]

Body Composition Body composition—that is, the proportion of weight that is lean versus fat—is affected by gender and age. Women have more stored body fat than men, and body fat tends to increase with age. For adult women, the percent of body fat associated with the lowest health risk is between 20 and 30% of total weight; for adult men, it is between 12 and 20%.[20] Body fat of greater than 20% in men and 30% in women increases the risks of chronic disease. Body composition techniques measure fat mass (the proportion of weight that is fat) and the proportion that is lean or fat-free mass. Measures of body composition are more cumbersome than simply measuring height and weight, but these measures are important because it is the amount of fat, not weight, that correlates with the risk of chronic disease.

Underwater Weighing An accurate noninvasive technique for assessing body composition is **underwater weighing,** which involves weighing an individual both on land and in the water. The difference between these two weights can be

Underwater weighing A technique that uses the difference between body weight under water and body weight on land to estimate body composition.

used to determine body volume. The percentage of body fat can then be determined using standardized equations. To measure underwater weight, one must sit on a scale, expel the air from the lungs, and be lowered into a tank of water (Figure 7.11). Although this method is accurate, it requires special equipment and cannot be used for some groups such as small children or frail adults. A newer method for estimating body composition measures air displacement rather than water displacement to calculate body fat.

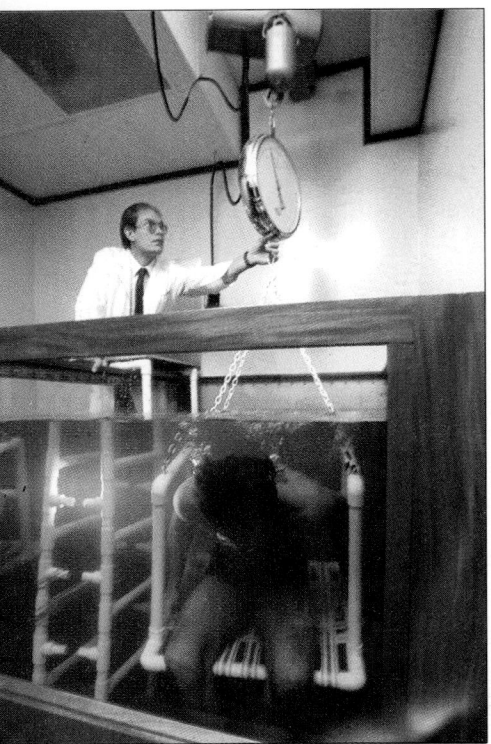

Figure 7.11
To determine the percent of body weight that is due to fat, body weight on land and weight in water (with all air expelled from his lungs) can be used. (© Jim Olive/Peter Arnold, Inc.)

Skinfold thickness A measurement of subcutaneous fat used to estimate total body fat.

Bioelectric impedance analysis A technique for estimating body composition that measures body water by directing electric current through the body and calculating resistance to flow.

Circumferences and Skinfold Thickness Measurements of circumference and **skinfold thickness** at various locations on the body can be used to assess body composition. Skinfold thickness measures the fat under the skin, or subcutaneous fat, and assumes that it is representative of the total body fat. It is measured at one or more locations using a caliper. The most common sites for skinfold measurements are triceps, the area over muscles on the back of the upper arm, and subscapular, the area just below the shoulder blade (Figure 7.12). Either a nomogram or mathematical equations are then used to estimate percent body fat from these measurements. These measurements provide accurate estimates of body fat in normal-weight individuals but are difficult to perform and less accurate in obese subjects.

Bioelectric Impedance Analysis **Bioelectric impedance analysis** estimates body fat by measuring the rate of current flow through the body. A painless, low-energy electrical current is directed through the body by electrodes placed on the hands and feet. The rate of current flow through the body is measured. Since fat is a poor conductor of electricity, it offers resistance to the current. The percentage of the body that is water and allows current flow is estimated and the remainder is assumed to be body fat. Bioelectric impedance techniques assume a standard amount of body water. Therefore, measurements should be done when the GI tract and bladder are empty and body hydration is normal. For example, measurements are not accurate if done within 24 hours of a strenuous bout of exercise because body water has been lost in sweat.

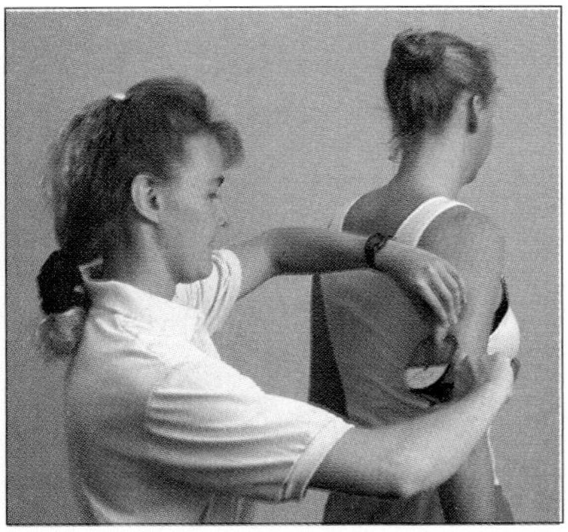

Figure 7.12
The triceps skinfold is measured at the midpoint of the back of the arm. This measure of the thickness of the fat layer under the skin can be used to estimate body fat. (David Young-Wolff/PhotoEdit)

High-Technology Methods Many other methods are available for measuring body composition, but for most, a laboratory or expensive equipment is required. One method relies on the principle of dilution. Since water is present primarily in lean tissue and not in fat, a water-soluble isotope can be ingested or injected into the bloodstream and allowed to mix in the water throughout the body. The amount of the isotope in a sample of body fluid, such as blood, can then be measured. The extent to which the isotope has been diluted can be used to calculate the amount of lean tissue, and body fat can then be calculated by subtracting lean weight from total body weight. Another technique measures a naturally occurring isotope of potassium. Since potassium is found primarily in lean tissue, measuring the amount of this isotope in the body can be used to determine the total amount of body potassium, which can then be used to estimate the amount of lean tissue.

Recently, a variety of newer technologies have been used to assess body composition. For example, computerized tomography (CT) uses low-dose x-rays to visualize fat and lean tissue. CT is more accurate than underwater weighing, skinfold measures, and total body potassium for evaluation of body composition, and is particularly useful for measuring the amount of abdominal adipose tissue.[25] Dual-energy x-ray absorptiometry (DEXA) is another method for assessing body composition that uses low-energy x-rays. In a single investigation it can determine with accuracy total body mass, bone mineral mass, and percent body fat, but it does not distinguish visceral and subcutaneous fat. Magnetic resonance imaging (MRI), on the other hand, can be used to accurately estimate the amount of abdominal fat by using magnetic fields to create an internal body image.

Changes in Body Composition Throughout Life Body composition changes throughout life. The percentage of body fat increases in the first year of life. During childhood, muscle mass increases and body fat decreases. During adolescence, females gain proportionately more fat and males gain more muscle mass. With aging, lean body mass decreases; between the ages of 20 and 50 to 60, body fat typically doubles even if body weight remains the same.[26] Some of this change may be prevented by physical activity.

Pregnancy also causes dramatic changes in body composition. An increase in blood volume and the production of amniotic fluid cause an increase in total body water. The amount of body fat increases to provide energy stores for the mother and fetus. There is also an increase in body protein due to the growth of the uterus and breasts, an increase in the number of blood cells in the mother, and an increase in fetal tissue.

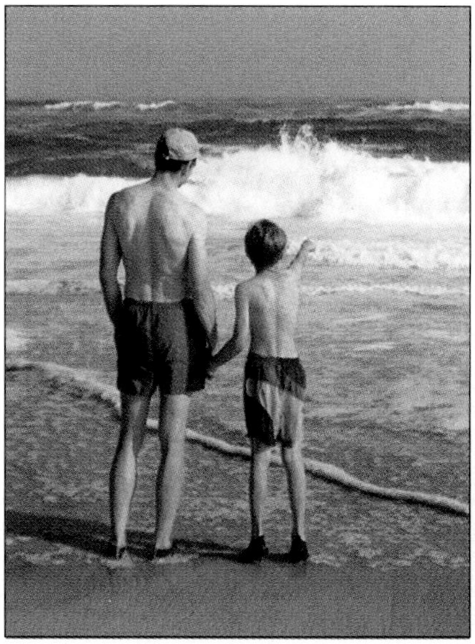

Figure 7.13
The genes we inherit from our parents are important determinants of our body size and shape. (Lori Smolin)

Why Are Some of Us Fat and Some of Us Not?

Excess body fat accumulates when energy intake exceeds energy output. Traditionally, the explanation for why some people are fat and others are not has been based on external factors such as excessive food intake or lack of exercise. However, this theory did not explain why children have body shapes, sizes, and compositions similar to their parents. Some of us inherit tall, slender bodies with long, thin bones (Figure 7.13). Others inherit stocky bodies with short bones, wide hips, and stubby fingers. Heredity also plays a role in how much body fat we accumulate and where it is deposited. Our understanding of how one's genetic background contributes to body fatness is expanding rapidly. A host of **genes** involved in the regulation of body weight have already been identified in rodents, and similar genes have been found in humans.[27,28] This is not to say that body fat and weight are determined purely by genetics; environmental and behavioral factors, such as what we eat and how much we exercise, are also involved.

Gene A length of DNA that contains the instructions for making a protein.

What Is Body Fat?

Body fat, or adipose tissue, lies under the skin and around internal organs. It insulates the body from changes in temperature, provides a cushion to protect against shock, and serves as an energy storage site. Adipose tissue is made up of fat cells or **adipocytes** (Figure 7.14). Adipocytes store triglycerides that they pick up from the blood with the help of the enzyme lipoprotein lipase (LPL).

Adipocytes Fat-storing cells.

Adipocytes grow in size as they accumulate more fat. The greater the number of adipocytes an individual has, the greater the ability to store fat. Most adipocytes are formed between infancy and adolescence. In adulthood, only excessive weight gain can cause the production of new fat cells. In mild obesity there is an increase in cell size as body fat accumulates, but severe obesity or obesity beginning in childhood involves an increase in fat-cell number as well.[28] Many of the health risks that come with increases in body fat are due to changes in fat cells that occur as they enlarge.[20] Even modest reductions in body fat will reduce fat-cell size and help normalize fat-cell function, improving blood lipid levels, blood glucose, and insulin levels.

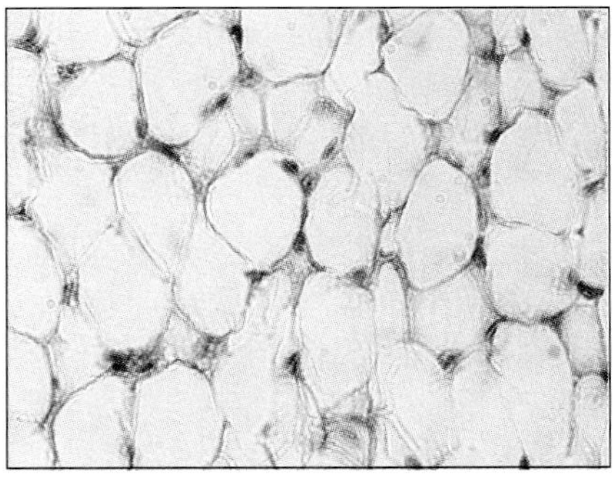

Figure 7.14
Adipocytes contain a droplet of fat surrounded by other cell components. As body fat is gained, the size of the fat droplet increases. (© Ed Reschke/Peter Arnold, Inc.)

What Determines Body Fatness?

The ability or tendency to store fat is affected by both genetic and lifestyle or environmental factors. We have no control over our genetic makeup but often can change the amount we eat or exercise.

How Do Genes Affect Body Weight? If one or both of your parents is obese, your risk of becoming obese is increased. Individuals with a family history of obesity are two to three times more likely to be obese, and the risk increases with the magnitude of the obesity.[29] In a study that overfed pairs of identical twins, some individuals in the study gained only 9 pounds, whereas others gained as much as 29 pounds, indicating that different people have different abilities to expend the extra energy taken in.[22] When the sets of identical twins were compared, it was found that each set of twins tended to gain the same amount of weight and that the fat was deposited in the same parts of their bodies. Because identical twins have the same genetic makeup, these results suggest that heredity affects the way we use energy and gain weight.

The reason that obesity is passed from parent to child is because the information that regulates energy balance, body size, and body shape is contained in genes. A gene is a segment of DNA that provides the code or blueprint for the synthesis of a protein. The proteins coded by these "obesity genes" are required to keep weight in the normal range. These proteins act by sending signals to the brain, particularly to a region called the **hypothalamus.** The hypothalamus monitors, integrates, and organizes these signals and then sends messages to other parts of the body to control food intake and energy expenditure. When a gene is defective, the protein it codes for is not made, or is made incorrectly. When an "obesity" gene is defective, the signals to decrease food intake and/or increase energy expenditure are not received, and weight gain results. Most human obesity is not likely to be due to a single abnormal gene but rather to variations in many genes that interact with one another and the environment to regulate body shape and size as well as energy intake and expenditure. An example of human obesity that clearly demonstrates a genetic link is the Pima Indians of the southwestern United States; more than 75% of this population is obese. Genetic analysis has identified a number of genes that may be responsible for this group's level of body fat.[30] Thus far, genes that are associated with obesity and body weight regulation have been identified in humans; but we do not know how all the proteins made by these genes affect body weight.[29]

Hypothalamus The region of the brain that monitors and regulates conditions and activities in the body, including food intake and energy expenditure.

How Does the Environment Affect Body Weight? Influences from our environment and our personal choices are also important determinants of body weight. An individual with a genetic predisposition to obesity who has a limited supply of food or who engages in strenuous physical labor may never be obese, but someone with no genetic tendency toward obesity who consumes a high-energy diet and gets little exercise may become obese.

The typical lifestyle in the United States today fosters increased food intake and discourages physical activity. This lifestyle has been proposed as a major reason for the increasing numbers of obese people in the United States.[31] Palatable, affordable food is available to the majority of the population. Supermarkets, fast-food restaurants, and all-night convenience marts provide ready access to food throughout the day and night. Bigger is marketed as better in terms of portion sizes. Super-size beverages often offer a liter of your favorite soft drink, which can contain over 600 kcalories. Along with the increase in food availability and portion sizes there has been a decrease in the amount of energy used in the activities of daily life. A farmer in 1900 did not have to plan an exercise program to increase his physical activity; his day-to-day life was active. Advances in technology have brought tractors, automobiles, elevators, and vacuum cleaners, which allow people to work without being as physically active; television, electronic games, and computers have given us sedentary ways to spend our leisure time.

The environment in the home can also influence energy balance. Having obese parents increases one's risk of obesity not only genetically but also because obese families typically consume more energy and expend less through exercise than leaner families.[32] Living in a household where high-kcalorie foods are always available and exercise is infrequent increases the likelihood of becoming overweight. Socioeconomic status can also affect body weight. Education, income, and occupation influence behaviors that affect energy consumption and expenditure.[33] Although genes seem to affect almost every behavior, including how much we exercise and what we eat,[23] the genes you inherit do not have the final say in whether you walk or take the bus, or in how much ice cream you have for dessert. A genetic predisposition to obesity makes maintaining desirable body weight more difficult, but not impossible.

How Is Body Fatness Regulated?

In most people, body fat and weight remain remarkably constant over long periods despite fluctuations in food intake and activity level. The reason is that body weight, like body temperature, is believed to be regulated to remain at a particular level or **set point.** When energy intake or activity level changes, the body compensates to prevent a significant change in weight or fat.[34]

Set point A level at which body fat or body weight seems to resist change despite changes in energy intake or output.

The set point for body fatness is determined by genetics. In an obese individual body fat is set to remain at a higher level or set point than it is in a lean individual. When people lose weight, regardless of whether they are lean or obese at the outset, metabolic signals are generated to decrease energy output and increase energy intake in order to return their weight to its set point.

Another example of set-point regulation is fat-cell size. Obese individuals have larger fat cells than normal weight people. With weight loss, fat cells shrink in size but rarely disappear. After they shrink, regulatory mechanisms act to increase their size to the preset level, whether that level is obese or normal. One factor that acts to increase fat-cell size is the fat-storing enzyme LPL. Higher levels of LPL allow more fat storage. Adipose tissue LPL is elevated in obese individuals and following weight loss it is elevated further. This suggests that enzyme activity is stimulated to replace lost fat stores and maintain the adipocyte size.[35]

The mechanisms that regulate the set point for body weight and fatness must respond both to changes in the intake of nutrients that occur over a short time frame as well as to more long-term changes in the amount of body fat. Signals related to food intake affect hunger or satiety over a short period of time—from meal to meal—whereas signals from the adipose tissue trigger the hypothalamus to adjust both food intake and energy expenditure for long-term regulation.

Short-Term Regulation: Signals Related to Food Intake The consumption of food sends signals to the brain to stop food intake. Some of these signals about the availability of nutrients are sent directly from the gastrointestinal tract, and some are relayed by hormones or changes in blood nutrient levels.[36]

The simplest type of signal about food intake occurs when the ingestion and digestion of food cause the stomach to stretch. Nerves in the stomach and small intestine sense pressure and send a "stop eating" message to the brain. The presence of glucose, fat, and/or amino acids in the gastrointestinal tract also sends information directly to the brain. In addition, the presence of these nutrients triggers the release of gastrointestinal hormones such as cholecystokinin that cause satiety. These satiety hormones help to limit the size of meals both by signaling the brain through peripheral nerves and by directly signaling control centers in the brain.[37] These signals can affect the amount of food consumed at individual meals but they do not control total body fat content.

After nutrients are absorbed, the brain continues to receive information that it uses to signal hunger or satiety. Circulating levels of nutrients, including glucose, amino acids, ketones, and fatty acids, are monitored by the brain and may stimulate signals for us to eat or not to eat.[36] Nutrients that are taken up by the brain may affect neurotransmitter concentrations, which then affect the amount and type of nutrients consumed. For example, when brain serotonin is low, carbohydrate is craved, but when it is high, protein is preferred.[36]

Other organs such as the liver and pancreas are also thought to be involved in signaling hunger and satiety. The liver is in a unique position to monitor changes in fuel metabolism because absorbed water-soluble nutrients go directly there. Changes in liver metabolism, in particular the amount of ATP, are believed to trigger food intake.[7] The pancreas is involved in food intake regulation because it releases insulin, which is involved in long-term body fat regulation.

Leptin A protein hormone produced by adipocytes that signals information about the amount of body fat.

Long-Term Regulation: Signals Related to Body Fatness To regulate body fatness at a set level the body must be able to monitor how much body fat is present. Some of this information comes from hormones such as insulin and **leptin,** that are secreted in proportion to the amount of body fat.[37] Insulin is secreted from the pancreas when blood glucose levels rise; its circulating concentration is proportional to the amount of body fat. Insulin's effect on the hypothalamus can reduce food intake and body weight, and insulin levels are believed to affect the amount of leptin produced and secreted. Leptin is produced by the adipocytes, and the amount of leptin produced is proportional to the size of adipocytes, so more leptin is released as fat stores grow. Leptin travels in the blood to the hypothalamus where it binds to proteins called leptin receptors. When leptin levels increase, mechanisms that cause an increase in energy expenditure and a decrease in food intake are stimulated. When fat stores shrink, less leptin is released. Low leptin levels in the hypothalamus act by a different mechanism to decrease energy expenditure and increase food intake.[27] Thus, leptin acts like a thermostat or lipostat to keep body fatness from changing (Figure 7.15).

Abnormalities in Body Fat Regulation Obesity can be thought of as a genetic abnormality in the regulation of body fat. The result of this abnormality is an increase in food intake, a decrease in energy expenditure, or a combination of both. Our understanding of how body fat is regulated is developing rapidly but is still in its early stages. For instance, we know that leptin is one signal involved in the long-term regulation of body fat, and that there are many steps that occur be-

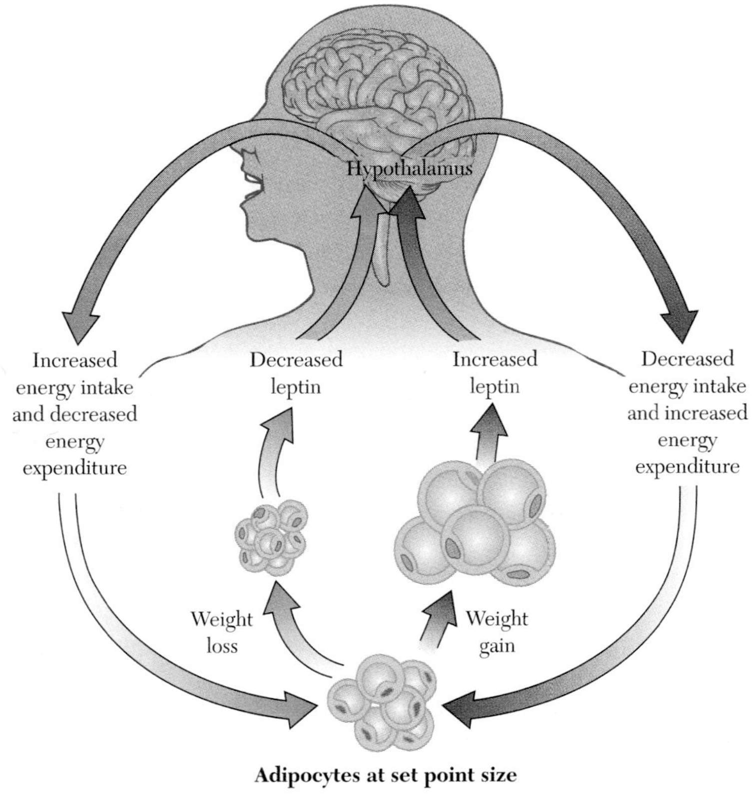

Figure 7.15
Leptin helps maintain body fat at a preset level. When adipocytes gain fat, more leptin is released, triggering events that decrease food intake and increase energy expenditure. When fat is lost, less leptin is released, causing an increase in food intake and a decrease in energy expenditure.

tween the production of leptin and alterations in food intake and energy expenditure. We know that a defect at any step along the way could interfere with the regulation of food intake, energy expenditure, and, ultimately, body weight. However, we do not know the exact defects that cause human obesity. A few cases of obesity have been linked directly to a defective leptin gene;[38] but mutations in this gene are not responsible for most human obesity. In fact, obese humans generally have high leptin levels in the blood.[39] This suggests a defect involving some step in the response to this hormone—for example, an abnormality in leptin receptors. If leptin receptors are defective, the leptin produced would have no place to bind. Thus far, however, no defects in the leptin receptor have been identified in humans.[40]

Do Obese People Eat More? It is clear that overweight individuals consume more energy than they burn, but whether they eat more than their lean counterparts has been controversial. Estimations from food intake records suggest that overweight populations do not consume more than lean ones. However, food records may not be accurate; studies suggest that obese individuals tend to underreport their food intake to a greater extent than nonobese individuals.[41] Measures of energy expenditure in weight-stable lean and obese individuals have shown that food intake is greater in obese than in lean individuals.[42]

Abnormalities in metabolic mechanisms, such as the level of insulin and leptin and the response to these hormones, may play a role in increasing food intake to keep body fat at an unhealthy level. The exact role such abnormalities play in the balance between intake and output is not well understood.

Another factor that may increase food intake in obese individuals is the extent to which they are affected by sensory and environmental stimuli. While we all eat in response to external cues such as the sight and smell of food, research suggests that overweight people respond more to these cues than their leaner counterparts. Obese individuals may be more influenced by cravings for specific foods, such as sweet or salty items,[43] and research has found that overweight individuals tend to choose high-fat foods.[44] Dietary fat is stored as body fat more efficiently than protein or carbohydrate, so fat kcalories can produce more body fat.

Do Obese Individuals Expend Less Energy? Although energy expenditure may be greater in obese individuals, they do not expend enough to keep their body fat in a healthy range. This may be due to mechanisms that regulate basal energy expenditure or to lifestyle factors that minimize physical activity.

In studies that control food intake, BMR decreases in both lean and obese subjects when food intake is restricted. BMR increases in both groups during overconsumption.[34] Changes in the amount of energy expended in response to changes in circumstance, such as over- or under-feeding, changes in temperature, or trauma, are referred to as **adaptive thermogenesis.** Increased energy expenditure through adaptive thermogenesis may prevent some of the weight gain that accompanies an increase in energy intake.[45,46]

Adaptive thermogenesis The change in energy expenditure induced by factors such as changes in ambient temperature and food intake.

Several biochemical mechanisms have been proposed to explain adaptive thermogenesis. The first is substrate cycling or futile cycling, which wastes energy by allowing opposing biochemical reactions to occur simultaneously. For example, a molecule is formed and then broken down; the result is that energy is consumed but there is no net change in the number of molecules in the body and therefore no storage of energy as fat. A second way that excess energy might be dissipated is by separating or uncoupling the electron transport chain from the production of ATP. When this occurs energy is lost as heat. For example, the increase in energy expenditure that occurs when mice are injected with leptin is hypothesized to be due to the stimulation of receptors on a specialized type of adipose tissue called **brown adipose tissue.** Brown adipose tissue can waste energy as heat. It contains many more mitochondria than other adipose tissue, and these mitochondria can be uncoupled from the electron transport chain to release

Brown adipose tissue A type of fat tissue that has a greater number of mitochondria than the more common white adipose tissue. It can waste energy by producing heat and is believed to be responsible for some of the change in energy expenditure in adaptive thermogenesis in rodents.

the energy in food as heat. In rats, brown adipose tissue generates heat to prevent weight gain during overfeeding and to provide warmth when the ambient temperature is low. Except for newborns, humans have only a very small amount of brown adipose tissue, but humans may be able to dissipate energy in other tissues. Several proteins that uncouple the electron transport chain from the production of ATP have been identified in human muscle, white adipose tissue, lung, spleen, white blood cells, bone marrow, and stomach.[47] It is hypothesized that these proteins may be involved in increasing energy output to regulate body weight in humans.

The amount of energy an individual expends depends primarily on metabolic rate and activity. Genetics determine our metabolic rate. Activity level is affected by genetics and individual choices. Both genetic factors and lifestyle choices that tend toward inactivity contribute to obesity. When the energy expended for physical activity is compared with the amount of body fat, it is found that individuals with the most body fat have the lowest levels of physical activity, supporting the hypothesis that obesity is associated with a lower level of physical activity.[48] This does not mean that reduced physical activity necessarily causes obesity. The reduction in activity may occur as a result of the obesity. Excess weight makes it more difficult to exercise or even to perform simple daily activities. The obese carry extra weight with every action. A 230-pound man walking a mile is carrying the same weight as a 200-pound man walking a mile carrying a 30-pound suitcase. This extra burden reduces the inclination to increase activity. In addition to the physical stress, obese individuals often shy away from exercise because they don't want to be compared with their leaner counterparts. Obese children may avoid athletic activities to escape being teased about their weight. Inactivity reduces energy expenditure regardless of whether it is a cause of obesity or the result of it (see *Critical Thinking: Is She Destined to Be Obese?*).

CRITICAL THINKING

Is She Destined to Be Obese?

April is unhappy about the 10 pounds she gained during her freshman year at college. Her parents are both obese, and she is worried that she too will become obese. She is 5 feet 4 inches tall, 23 years old, and weighs 140 pounds. She would like to weigh 130 pounds.

In analyzing why she gained weight, April realizes that, with her busy college schedule, she gets less exercise than she used to and often eats candy bars from the vending machine while studying late at night. By recording and analyzing her food intake for three days, she determines that she eats about 2650 kcalories per day. By keeping an activity log, she estimates that a typical day includes 8 hours of sleep, 14 hours of very light activity such as studying, and 2 hours of light activity such as walking. To determine her expenditure, she estimates the energy she needs for RMR, activity, and the thermic effect of the food.

What is her energy expenditure?

RMR + Activity =

Thermic Effect of Food =

Total Energy Needs =

April decides to increase her activity level. She loves to play tennis and so plans to try to add two hours of tennis a day to her schedule.

If she replaces two hours of her very light activity with two hours of tennis (a moderate activity), how much additional energy will this burn?

Answer:

Is this a reasonable plan?

Although April loves tennis, she probably won't play for two hours each day. A more reasonable approach might be to plan on playing tennis three days a week while also increasing daily activity by riding her bike to the store, using the stairs instead of the elevator, and going dancing some evenings with friends. She may not lose the weight as quickly as she would have with two hours of tennis every day, but she is more likely to keep up this schedule.

April's diet contains a number of high-kcalorie, high-fat foods such as cheese Danish, chicken nuggets, and macaroni and cheese. To decrease her energy intake by about 190 kcalories, she could have a bagel instead of a cheese Danish.

What other substitutions could she make to decrease her intake?

Answer:

Is she destined to become obese? What other recommendations would you give her about weight management?

Answer:

ACHIEVING AND MAINTAINING A HEALTHY WEIGHT

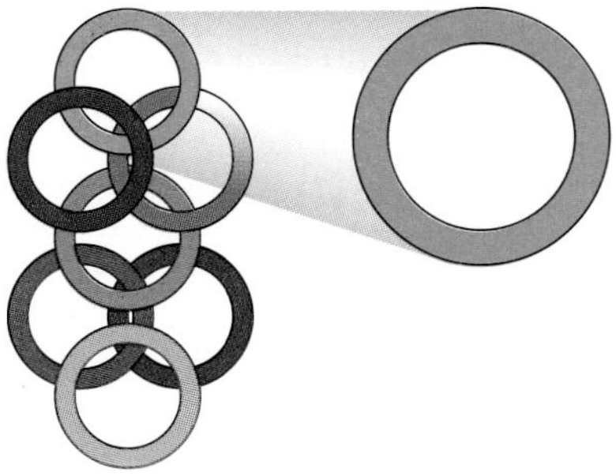
Balance the food you eat with physical activity; maintain or improve your weight

Figure 7.16
The Dietary Guidelines for Americans recommend that you balance the food you eat with physical activity to maintain or improve your weight. (USDA, DHHS, 1995)

Approximately 97 million American adults are overweight. Despite billions of dollars spent on medical research, weight-loss programs, and weight-loss medications, the percentage of overweight individuals is increasing in all segments of the population.[12] Even when individuals are successful at losing weight, they tend to regain the weight they have lost. The best solution to this problem is to prevent it in the first place (Figure 7.16). Healthy eating habits and active lives that promote the maintenance of a healthy weight should be developed in childhood and maintained throughout life. Just as a family history of heart disease or an increase in blood cholesterol should set in motion dietary and lifestyle changes to maintain health, a family history of obesity or an increase in body weight should trigger dietary and lifestyle changes that maintain weight at a healthy level. What about those who are already above their healthy weight range? If so much of our energy balance and body weight is determined by our genes, is there any hope for the fat to be thin?

How Can You Lose Weight?

The health problems associated with obesity and the alarming failure rate of long-term weight loss have caused researchers and physicians to reevaluate the way they think about this problem. They suggest that, rather than focusing on weight loss, which is unlikely to be successful in the long term, weight problems should be viewed in terms of weight management. The goal of weight management is to prevent excess body weight gain; for those who are already overweight, the goal is to reduce body fat to a healthy level that can be maintained over a lifetime.[49]

How Much Weight Should You Lose? If you are overweight, your goal for weight loss should be to achieve a healthy weight. A healthy weight is a reasonable upper limit for body weight that offers a reduction in disease risk and is within reach for most overweight adults.[50] A loss of 2 BMI units or about 10 to 16 pounds is considered sufficient to reduce disease risks and improve health problems related to being overweight.[50] This level of weight loss is considered achievable for most individuals and is easier to maintain than larger weight losses. Most individuals who lose large amounts of weight regain all that they have lost. Repeated cycles of weight loss and regain, referred to as **weight cycling** or **yo-yo dieting,** increase the proportion of body fat with each successive weight regain and cause a decrease in BMR, making subsequent weight loss more difficult (Figure 7.17).[3]

Weight cycling or **yo-yo dieting** The cycle of repeatedly losing and regaining weight.

The Mathematics of Weight Loss In order to decrease body weight or body fat, energy intake must be less than energy output. It is estimated that a pound of body fat provides 3500 kcalories. Therefore, to lose a pound of fat, one must decrease energy intake by this amount or increase energy output by this amount. To lose a pound in a week, one must shift energy balance by 500 kcalories per day ($3500 \div 7$ days $= 500$ kcal/day). This is the predicted average weight loss at this energy deficit. However, the actual amount of weight lost per week may vary over time. To promote the loss of fat and not lean tissue, a weight-loss program should encourage the loss of only 1/2 to 1 pound per week.[51] If weight is lost more rapidly, the loss is less likely to be maintained and the additional loss will be from fluid, muscle and liver glycogen, and muscle protein.

Although the arithmetic is simple, achieving a reduction in body weight is not easy. There are regulatory mechanisms at work to keep body weight stable. There are environmental and emotional motivators to increase food intake. And the inclination to exercise may be reduced in overweight individuals. Nonetheless, reductions in intake, increases in activity, and changes in behavior can promote weight loss and long-term weight management.

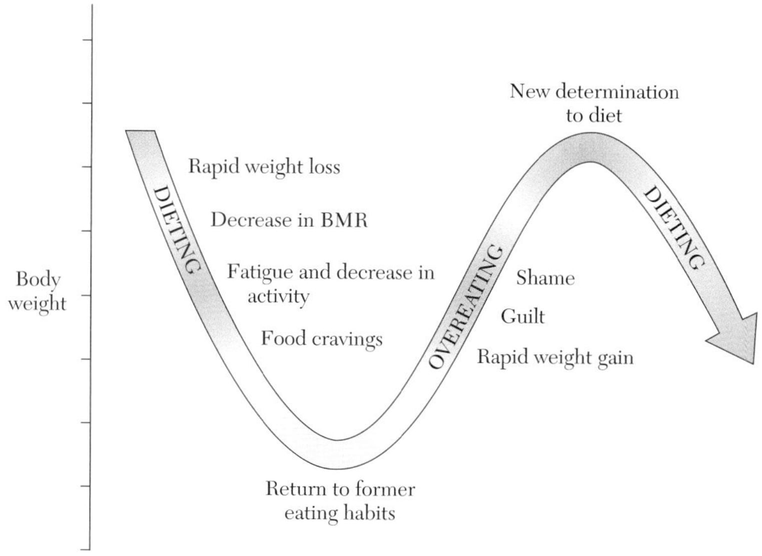

Figure 7.17
Weight cycling is the repeated loss and regain of body weight.

Choosing a Weight-Management Program When selecting an approach to weight management, people should be sure to choose one that fits their needs and that will promote lifestyle changes that can be maintained for a lifetime. Does the program offer a dietary pattern that suits your food preferences as well as your need for structure and social support? Consider whether the program has demonstrated safety and success in managing weight in individuals with similar medical and weight histories to your own. Cost, convenience, and the time commitment required by the program are also important considerations. If the program's approach is not one that you can follow for a lifetime, it is unlikely to promote successful weight management (Table 7.5).

Approaches to Weight Management

Weight reduction can be accomplished by reducing energy intake or increasing energy output. The rate of weight loss is increased when a reduction in kcalories

Table 7.5 ***What to Look for in a Weight-Loss/ Weight-Management Program***

Does the program take into consideration an individual's current eating habits and preferences?
Does the diet meet all nutrient needs?
Is the program based on sound scientific principles?
Does the program set realistic weight-loss goals? (It should promise a weight loss of one-half to one pound per week.)
Does the program include a nutrition education component to teach participants how to make healthy food choices?
Does the program stress the need to increase physical activity?
Does the program include some type of social support?
Does the program suit individual health needs (for example, if you are diabetic or have high blood cholesterol)?
Be skeptical of programs that require the purchase of special foods or other products, are sponsored by celebrities who look good but lack credentials, or promote the use of supplements or prescription drugs.

Adapted from the American Heart Association's online Web site at http://www.amhrt.org/Health/Risk_Factors/Overweight/Fad_Diets/fadguide.html

Table 7.6 *Examples of Commercial Approaches to Weight Management*

Program	Approach	Advantages	Disadvantages
Weight Watchers	Low energy, social support	Safe, inexpensive	—
Jenny Craig	Low energy	Safe, convenient	Expensive; relies on purchase of special foods
Slim Fast	Low-energy formula	Convenient, inexpensive	Relies on purchase of special products which do not promote long-term changes; no group support
Optifast	Low-energy formula	Rapid weight loss, medically supervised	Expensive; does not promote behavior change
Atkins Diet	Very low carbohydrate	Rapid weight loss	No group support; does not promote long-term weight management
Zone Diet	Low carbohydrate, low energy	Safe, inexpensive	No group support
Beverly Hills II	Low-energy food combinations	Inexpensive	Based on unsound principles, no group support
Fit or Fat	Increased exercise	Safe, inexpensive	No group support

is combined with regular exercise. In addition, exercise promotes the long-term maintenance of weight loss.[4] Applying techniques to change eating behaviors also improves success rates. An ideal weight-management program includes a reduction in energy intake along with education about meeting nutrient needs, an increase in energy expenditure, and relearning behaviors to change the patterns that led to weight gain. Prescription medications and surgery may also be acceptable weight-management tools for obese individuals when conventional methods fail. There are thousands of choices when looking for a weight-loss or weight-management program. Options vary in their approach, their intensity, the involvement of health-care practitioners, and cost. The best approach to weight management depends on the individual's physiological, psychological, and social needs (Table 7.6).

Decreasing Energy Intake For safe and effective weight loss, the diet must be low in energy but provide for all the body's nutrient needs. With energy intakes less than 1200 kcalories per day, it is difficult to meet the requirements for micronutrients. Therefore, medical supervision and a multivitamin and mineral supplement are recommended. The diet should take into account the individual's risk for obesity-related diseases, such as cardiovascular disease, and follow the recommendations of the Dietary Guidelines.

Decreasing energy intake does not require special foods or dramatic changes in eating habits. Programs that require unusual eating times and patterns are unlikely to promote permanent changes. The most realistic approach to changing one's diet is simply to reduce portion sizes and eliminate high-kcalorie foods.

Lowfat Diets for Weight Loss Because fat is high in kcalories, consuming a lowfat diet typically reduces energy intake. Lowfat diets provide more food for the same amount of energy than high-fat diets and seem to satisfy hunger after less energy is consumed. For example, when people are fed diets of differing fat composition, energy intake decreases as the percent of fat in the diet decreases.[52] Differences in the way dietary fat and dietary carbohydrate are used by the body also explain why lowfat diets are more effective for weight loss. Excess dietary fat kcalories are stored more efficiently than excess carbohydrate kcalories, so consuming excess energy from fat leads to a greater accumulation of body fat than consuming excess energy as carbohydrate.[9] Despite the advantages, even a diet low in fat will result in weight gain if energy intake exceeds energy output. This is illustrated by the fact that the percent of kcalories as fat in the typical American diet has decreased while at the same time the number of people who are overweight continues to increase.

Very-Low-Kcalorie Diets In response to a desire for rapid weight loss, **very-low-kcalorie diets**—those containing fewer than 800 kcalories per day—have become popular. These diets are generally a variation of the **protein-sparing modified fast,** a diet providing little energy and a high proportion of protein. The concept behind this is that the protein in the diet will be used to meet the body's protein needs and will, therefore, prevent excessive loss of body protein. Frequently, very-low-kcalorie diets are offered as a liquid formula. These formulas provide from 300 to 800 kcalories and 50 to 100 grams of protein per day and meet all other nutrient needs.

Very-low-kcalorie diet A weight-loss diet that provides fewer than 800 kcalories per day.

Protein-sparing modified fast A very-low-kcalorie diet of high protein content designed to maximize the loss of fat and minimize the loss of protein from the body.

Initial weight loss is rapid with very-low-kcalorie diets. This can provide a psychological boost and motivate the dieter to continue losing weight. In most cases almost 75% of this initial weight loss is water weight. Once the initial water loss occurs, weight loss slows. In addition, the dieter's BMR decreases to conserve energy. And energy expenditure typically decreases because people consuming so few kcalories often do not have the energy to continue their typical level of physical activity.

Very-low-kcalorie diets that provide less than about 50 grams of carbohydrate per day do not allow fat to be completely broken down (see Chapters 4 and 5), causing ketones to accumulate. If fluid intake is low, the kidneys cannot excrete the ketones and ketosis develops. At these low-energy intakes, body protein is broken down and potassium is excreted. Depletion of potassium can result in irregular heartbeats and is potentially deadly. Minor side effects include cold intolerance, fatigue, light-headedness, nervousness, constipation or diarrhea, anemia, hair loss, dry skin, and menstrual irregularities. Because these diets are not without risks, they are not recommended for people who are less than 30 to 40% above their desirable body weight. Since 1984, the FDA has required that all very-low-kcalorie diet formulas carry a warning that they can cause serious illness and should be used only under medical supervision.

Low-Carbohydrate Diets Low-carbohydrate diets have come and gone in popularity as a method of weight loss. Some of these severely restrict carbohydrate intake and promote the intake of high-protein foods such as eggs, red meat, fish, and poultry. They do not severely restrict energy but do restrict high-carbohydrate foods such as breads, grains, fruits, and vegetables.

There are several explanations as to why low-carbohydrate diets promote weight loss. First, when carbohydrate intake is low, glycogen stores, along with the water they hold, are lost, causing a rapid initial weight loss. Also, as fat is burned in the absence of carbohydrate, ketones are produced. Excretion of ketones causes additional water loss, and there is some evidence that ketones in the blood suppress appetite, making it easier to reduce food intake. One of the main reasons this type of diet results in weight loss is that boredom with the limited food choices causes a reduction in food intake. However, while these diets do cause weight loss in the short term, they are not palatable enough to be adhered to for long periods. The risks associated with severe carbohydrate restriction are dehydration, potassium depletion, and ketosis.

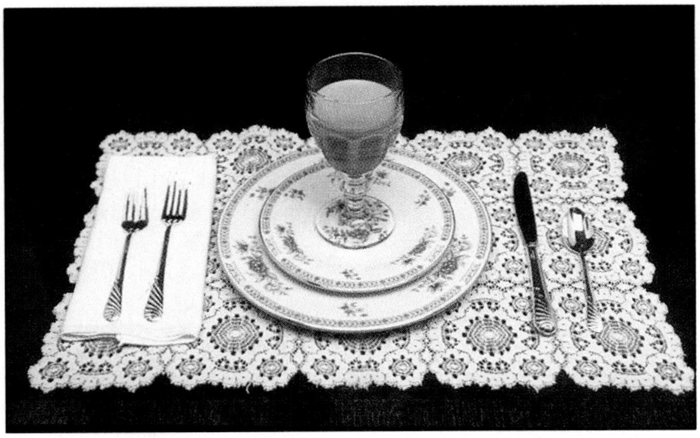

Figure 7.18
Liquid diets may result in weight loss but do nothing to change eating habits. (Gregory Smolin)

A less severe restriction in carbohydrate intake is promoted by the "Zone" diet.[53] This diet is based on the premise that excessive carbohydrate intake causes an increase in insulin, which promotes fat accumulation. Limiting carbohydrate intake to only about 40% of energy is claimed to reduce insulin levels to a particular zone, allowing fat stores to be broken down. In addition to promising weight loss, this diet claims to improve athletic performance and promote health. Blood insulin levels do rise when carbohydrate is consumed and insulin can promote fat storage, but the regulation of body fat stores involves more than a single hormone. The weight loss that occurs with this diet is really due to a reduction in the total amount of energy in the diet.

Liquid Weight-Loss Formulas Liquid diets can make dieting easier for some people because the problem of choosing a low-energy diet is eliminated. Liquid weight-loss diets that are available over the counter recommend a combination of food and formula to provide a daily energy intake of about 800 to 1200 kcalories. These formulas can be effective as long as the foods eaten with them are low in kcalories. But while over-the-counter formulas are easy to use and relatively inexpensive, they do little to change eating habits for life (Figure 7.18). Most diet programs that rely exclusively on liquid formulas have high dropout rates and poor long-term weight maintenance. Weight-loss regimens that rely exclusively on liquid formulas should not be used without medical supervision.

Other Fad and Novelty Diets Other diet fads have included everything from grapefruit to seaweed. Diets that emphasize eating primarily a single food such as rice or fruit rely on short-term energy deficits to promote weight loss. However, they do nothing to change long-term dietary habits. The limited food choices these diets offer can also result in nutrient deficiencies.

Some fads emphasize the supposed magical qualities of food. The grapefruit diet was based on the myth that grapefruit stimulates the breakdown of body fat. The Lecithin, B_6, Apple Cider Vinegar, and Kelp Diet was another combination that claimed to mobilize fat. In reality, weight loss on such diets is due to the reduction in energy intake and not the magical interaction of specific foods.

Another common diet approach focuses on food combinations and timing of intake. This approach is based on the faulty premise that certain foods should be eaten only in certain combinations (see Chapter 3) and that, if eaten in the wrong combination, they will not be not digested properly, resulting in weight gain and leading to disease.

Fad diets, in general, may promote weight loss over the short term, but since they are not nutritionally sound, they cannot be consumed safely for long periods. They do not encourage exercise or promote changes in eating behavior that will affect body weight over the long term (see *Critical Thinking: Do You Think This Diet Will Work?*).

CRITICAL THINKING

Do You Think This Diet Will Work?

FAT-AWAY DIET MEAL PROGRAM:
A Fast, Sensible, Three-Step Approach to Weight Loss

Step 1: Fat-Away's delicious and convenient reducing plan: Replace breakfast and lunch with a scrumptious, nutrient-dense chocolate, vanilla, peach, or strawberry shake. Each shake provides 200 kcalories, 15 grams of protein, and 50% of the Daily Value for vitamins and minerals.

Step 2: For dinner, eat a well-balanced meal, limiting kcalories to 500, including 3 ounces of lean meat, 1 cup of nonfat milk, and 1/2 to 1 cup each of starchy foods, fruits, and vegetables.

Step 3: Before going to bed, take Fat-Away's unique nighttime complex of amino acids. They help convert fat into energy, curb cravings for carbohydrate, and control appetite and satisfy hunger during the day.

Following these easy steps should result in a weight loss of 3 to 5 pounds per week and costs only $39.95 for one week's supply. You should consult your physician before trying this or any other diet.

Does this diet meet all nutritional needs except energy?

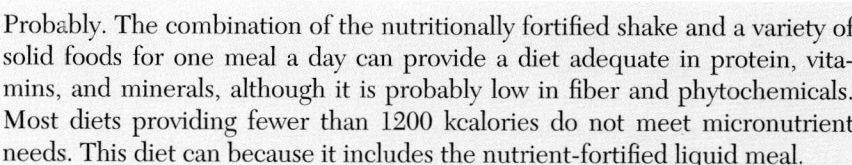

Probably. The combination of the nutritionally fortified shake and a variety of solid foods for one meal a day can provide a diet adequate in protein, vitamins, and minerals, although it is probably low in fiber and phytochemicals. Most diets providing fewer than 1200 kcalories do not meet micronutrient needs. This diet can because it includes the nutrient-fortified liquid meal.

Does the program provide a wide variety of obtainable foods with no special products to buy?

No. Although variety is encouraged in the one 500-kcalorie meal, the dieter is required to purchase the powdered meal formula as well as an amino acid supplement at a cost of about $5.70 per day.

Does the plan offer a reasonable rate of weight loss?

No. It promises a weight loss of 3 to 5 pounds per week. At this rate, muscle as well as fat will probably be lost.

Is the diet flexible enough to account for individual tastes, and is it adaptable to social settings?

Possibly. This plan allows some flexibility because individuals are free to choose what they will eat for one meal a day. However, it is not flexible enough for occasions such as holidays when traditional foods are served at more than one meal.

Is the diet based on scientifically sound principles?

Not entirely. Reducing energy intake below needs will result in weight loss, but an amino acid supplement will do little to curb appetite or convert fat into energy as you sleep.

Does this program include an exercise component?

No. The amino acid supplement is supposed to help convert fat into energy, but 30 minutes of aerobic exercise three to five times a week would be a more effective choice.

Does the program promote changes in eating habits and lifestyle that will encourage achieving and maintaining a healthy weight?

Answer:

Increasing Physical Activity Physical activity is an important component of any well-designed weight-management program. Exercise promotes fat loss and weight maintenance. It increases energy expenditure, so if intake remains the same, energy stored as fat is used for fuel. An increase in activity of 200 kcalories five times a week will result in the loss of a pound in about three and a half weeks. Exercise also promotes muscle development. This is important during weight loss because muscle is metabolically active tissue. Increasing muscle mass helps to prevent the drop in BMR that occurs as body weight decreases. Weight loss is also better maintained when physical activity is included in the weight-management program.[54] In addition to increasing energy expenditure and muscle mass, physical activity improves overall fitness and relieves boredom and stress. The benefits of exercise are discussed in Chapter 12.

Behavior modification A process used to gradually and permanently change habitual behaviors.

Behavior Modification A **behavior modification** approach to weight loss suggests that we eat in response to external cues. If these cues can be identified and altered, overconsumption can be reduced. The first step in a behavior modification program is to identify cues that lead to eating. This is usually done by keeping a log of all food consumed, where it was consumed, what other activities were involved, and what motivated the intake. The second step is to analyze these diaries to determine (1) what factors led to the eating (what were the antecedents of the behavior), (2) what the eating behaviors were, and (3) what the consequences of the eating were. These factors—antecedent, behavior, and consequence—are referred to as the ABCs of behavior modification. By keeping a log, eating patterns such as snacking or eating in response to emotional stresses can be identified. For instance, sitting down in front of the television and mindlessly demolishing a bag of potato chips leaves you feeling bad that you consumed these extra kcalories. In this case, the antecedent is watching TV, the behavior is mindlessly eating the chips, and the consequence is feeling remorse and gaining weight. The key to modifying this behavior is to recognize the antecedent, change the behavior, and replace the negative consequence with a positive one. For example, never taking food with you to the television, or taking only the portion of food you want to consume, eliminates the antecedent and the behavior. The consequence is that you have consumed only the food you planned, you do not gain weight, and you feel a sense of accomplishment. Thus, behavior modification can successfully reduce food intake by changing eating patterns and can promote maintenance of weight over the long term.

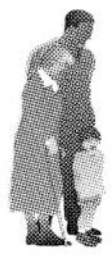

Weight Loss in Children About 25% of American children and adolescents are overweight and are likely to grow into overweight adults.[15] As with adults, this is due to excessive intake of foods high in fat and energy, and to inadequate physical activity. However, strict weight-loss diets are generally not recommended for children or adolescents because a reduction in intake can interfere with growth. The preferred technique is to encourage activity, provide a moderate energy restriction along with behavior modification, and then allow the child to grow into his weight (see Chapter 14).

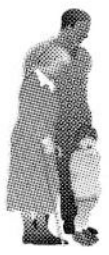

Weight Loss in the Elderly The risks associated with excess body fat are lower for older adults than for younger adults.[55] However, the decision to treat obesity should not be based on age alone. Weight loss can enhance day-to-day functioning and improve cardiovascular disease risk factors at all ages.[2] These benefits, however, must be balanced with the risk of restricting overall food intake in older individuals. A low-energy diet that is not carefully planned could result in deficiencies of protein or micronutrients. Also, involuntary weight loss is associated with disease and may be mistaken for successful voluntary weight loss. Therefore, older adults who want to lose weight should do so under the supervision of health professionals.

When Conventional Approaches Fail

There are thousands of conventional approaches to weight control. However, for some people, none of these approaches are effective at reducing body weight in the long term. For these individuals, when obesity greatly increases their risk for illness and death, drug therapy and surgery may be appropriate methods of weight reduction.

Drug Therapy As with other treatments for obesity, drug therapies are available in many forms. Some are well studied and offer legitimate aids to weight loss; others offer little more than water loss. An ideal drug treatment for obesity would permit an individual to lose weight and maintain the loss, be safe when used for long periods of time, have no side effects, and not be addictive. However, this ideal drug has not yet been developed. Currently, drug treatment is only recommended for those whose health is seriously compromised by their body weight. Drug therapy should be considered in individuals with a BMI greater than 30 with no risk factors or diseases, and in those with a BMI greater than or equal to 27 who have accompanying risk factors or diseases.[2]

Tried and Failed Treating obesity with drugs is not new. Extracts of thyroid hormone have been around for 100 years but were taken off the market because they caused deadly hyperthyroidism. Amphetamines, introduced for weight loss in the 1930s, were widely and often indiscriminately used in the 1950s and 1960s. The risk of addiction eventually stemmed their use. During the next 20 years, drug development continued but drug use for obesity declined.[56] In the 1990s, the recognition of obesity as a chronic disease increased interest in prescription weight-loss

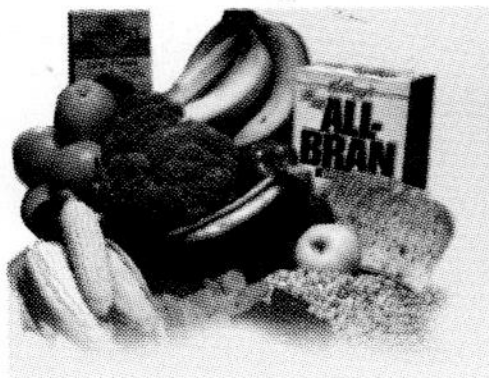

Off the Shelf

Weight-Loss Drugs: Are the Risks Too Great?

Fen-phen was a dream obesity treatment—a drug that reduced one's appetite to reduce eating. It made weight loss easy at last. Unfortunately, a few years after its release, fen-phen was found to be associated with a life-threatening heart valve defect. At that time, more than 18 million people had prescriptions for this diet drug.[1] Some of these individuals were obese, but many were only mildly overweight. The heart valve damage associated with taking fen-phen even for short periods of time could have affected millions. Would it have been better for many of these people to have simply stuck with diet and exercise? In the same year, a 13-year-old girl weighing 600 pounds died on her living room floor unable to move. Wouldn't drugs have been a better choice for her? As with any treatment, the risks must be weighed against the benefits.

The risks associated with obesity are well documented. Heart disease, hypertension, cancer, and diabetes all increase with this disease. Problems that limit mobility, such as arthritis, increase, as do social problems and isolation. It is estimated that obesity-related conditions contribute to 300,000 deaths per year. As weight increases, so does mortality, but not if you carry only a few extra pounds. The increase in mortality that accompanies an increase in body weight is small until body mass index reaches about 27 or 28 kg/m^2 (a 5′5″ woman who weighs 162 to 168 lbs). Age is also a factor. The correlation between body mass index and mortality decreases with age until it disappears at age 74.[2] So, the risk for overweight individuals depends on how overweight they are, how long they have been overweight, and how old they are.

The benefits of weight loss are clear. Even a reduction of 10 to 15 pounds reduces the risk of diseases associated with obesity. But should this loss be accomplished with drugs? Ideally, weight should be lost by reducing energy intake, increasing exercise, and changing long-term behavior. But for some obese people, these approaches chronically fail. For them, drugs may be an option. However, no perfect weight-loss drugs exist, nor are any likely to appear in the near future. Drugs may help people lose weight and maintain that loss, but they do not cure the disease. If people stop taking the drugs they will most likely regain the weight they have lost. Drug treatment would therefore need to continue for years—perhaps a lifetime. Over the short term, weight-loss drugs have been shown to reduce health risks by reducing blood pressure, blood lipid levels, and insulin resistance. But, there have been no long-term studies to indicate if weight loss accomplished by using drugs can improve health and decrease mortality.

Do the risks of obesity outweigh the risks of obesity drugs? It depends on the individual. For someone who is at significant medical risk due to obesity, or who has a medical condition such as cardiovascular disease (made worse by excess body fat), the benefits of these drugs outweigh the risks. On the other hand, for someone with 10 pounds to lose before the holidays the risks of drugs probably outweigh the benefits.

[1]Frackelmann, K. Diet drug debacle: how two federally approved weight-loss drugs crashed. Science News 152:252–253, 1997.

[2]Stevens, J., Cai, J., Pamuk, E. R., et al. The effect of age on the association between body mass index and mortality. N. Engl. J. Med. 338:1–7, 1998.

medications. New drugs and drug combinations have emerged, but safety continues to be a major concern with drug treatments for obesity. In 1997 a drug combination called fen-phen (fenfluramine and phentermine) that was being used to reduce food intake was linked to serious heart valve damage. As a result fenfluramine and the related drug dexfenfluramine were withdrawn from the market[57] (see *Off the Shelf: Weight-Loss Drugs: Are the Risks Too Great?*).

What's Currently Available Prescription obesity drugs work by one of four basic mechanisms. Some decrease food intake by affecting the activity of neurotransmitters in the brain that regulate food intake. Fenfluramine, dexfenfluramine, phentermine, and sibutramine work by these mechanisms. Others reduce the absorption of nutrients. For example, orlistat blocks fat-digesting enzymes in the intestine so fat absorption is reduced. Still others act by increasing energy expenditure through their effects on metabolism, or by stimulating fat mobilization or decreasing fat synthesis.[58] Most of these drugs are in the experimental stages and have shown only modest efficacy in reducing body weight when compared to a placebo; no long-term studies are available.[56] A significant problem with these drugs, however, is that unless eating habits change, weight is regained when the drugs are discontinued.

Over-the-Counter Medications In addition to prescription drug therapies, there are a variety of over-the-counter weight-loss pills and potions. Most of these con-

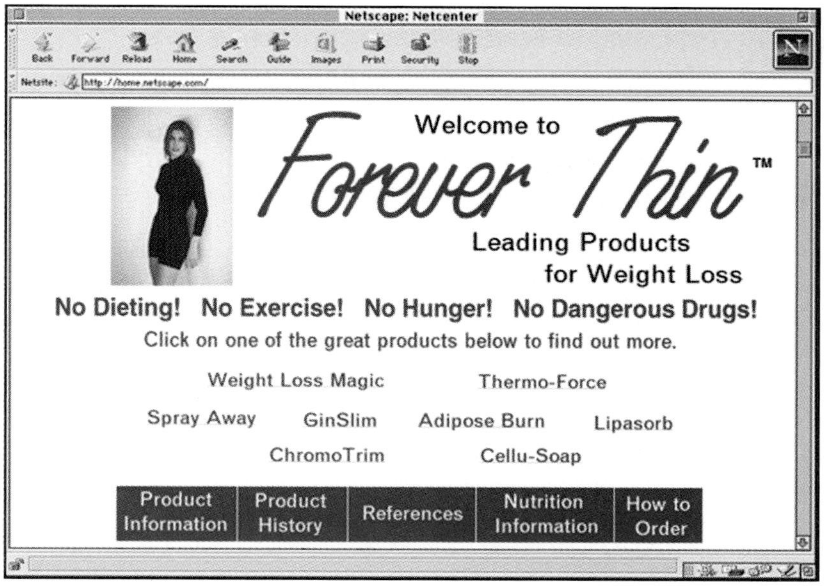

Figure 7.19
There are countless weight-loss products available, even online.

tain caffeine, phenylpropanolamine, benzocaine, or fiber. Caffeine is a popular ingredient because it is a stimulant and a diuretic. Stimulants tend to blunt the appetite and diuretics cause the kidneys to increase fluid excretion, resulting in weight loss from water loss. These same effects can be derived from caffeine-containing beverages like coffee, tea, and some soft drinks. Phenylpropanolamine is also a stimulant that depresses appetite and is approved by the FDA for weight loss. Benzocaine is an anesthetic that numbs the tongue, making eating a less pleasurable experience. Fibers such as methylcellulose and glucomannan absorb water to create a feeling of fullness; pills containing them claim to fill the stomach with indigestible bulk so that one feels sated. Some of these approaches are moderately effective and the side effects are minimal, but weight is usually regained when the pills or potions are stopped.

Amino acids are also common ingredients in weight-loss products. Those that claim to burn fat as you sleep usually contain the amino acids arginine and ornithine. These stimulate the release of growth hormone, which promotes fat loss and muscle growth, but research has not found any relationship between body weight and the levels of growth hormone. A number of supplements, such as chromium picolinate, claim to decrease body fat and increase the proportion of lean tissue. These products are not effective for weight loss (Figure 7.19). They generally target athletes and are discussed more thoroughly in Chapter 12.

Surgery A more drastic method of weight management is surgery. Surgical procedures are generally only recommended in cases of **morbid obesity,** defined as either greater than 100 pounds above desirable body weight, or a body mass index greater than or equal to 40. Currently, the most popular surgical approaches to treat obesity are gastroplasty and gastric bypass. Gastroplasty involves stapling off the top part of the stomach to make it smaller. Gastric bypass involves bypassing part of the stomach by connecting the intestine to the upper portion of the stomach. In both cases, food intake is reduced because the now smaller stomach becomes full with less food. Significant weight loss is usually achieved 18 to 24 months after surgery. Some weight regain is common after two to five years. The success rate is lower with gastroplasty because the staples can be broken by consumption of large meals. Both of these procedures have short-term surgical risks and a long-term risk of nutrient deficiencies, particularly of vitamin B_{12}, folate, and iron.[59] To be successful, even such surgical procedures must be accompanied by behavior modification, diet programs, and exercise.

Morbid obesity A condition in which body weight is 100 pounds (45.5 kg) above desirable body weight or body mass index is greater than 40.

Table 7.7 *Principles of Food Selection for Weight Loss, Weight Gain, or Weight Maintenance*

Starches are not high in energy. Remember, carbohydrate has only 4 kcalories per gram. It is usually the fats added to starches that add the energy.
Foods high in fat are high in energy. These include obvious fats, like butter and margarine, and hidden fats in fried foods and baked goods.
Foods high in fiber are relatively low in energy. Fiber cannot be absorbed, and fiber is filling, so high-fiber foods make us feel full longer.
Foods high in simple sugars, like soda, provide energy without many other nutrients.
All essential nutrients must be considered when designing a weight-loss diet.
When planning a diet, start by recording your typical food intake.
Start by making small, reasonable changes in your current diet.
Make changes that are likely to last a lifetime.

Another surgical approach, liposuction, is primarily a cosmetic procedure that will not significantly reduce overall body weight but may alter fat distribution. This procedure involves inserting a large hollow needle under the skin into a localized fat deposit and literally vacuuming out the fat. It is often advertised as a way to remove cellulite, which is just fat that has a lumpy appearance because of the presence of connections to the tissue layers below.

Suggestions for Weight Gain

As difficult as weight loss is for some people, weight gain can be equally elusive for underweight individuals (see Table 7.7). The first step toward weight gain is a medical evaluation to rule out medical reasons for low body weight. This is particularly important when weight loss occurs unexpectedly. If the low body weight is due to low intake or high expenditure, gradually increasing consumption of energy-dense foods is suggested. More frequent meals and high-kcalorie snacks such as peanut butter or milkshakes between meals can help increase energy intake. Replacing low-kcalorie fluids like water and diet beverages with fruit juices and milk may also help. Exercising to increase muscle mass is another way to increase weight. This approach requires extra kcalories to fuel the activity needed to build muscles. These recommendations, however, apply to individuals who are naturally thin and have trouble gaining weight on the recommended energy intake. This dietary approach will not result in weight gain in those who refuse to eat because of an eating disorder.

Eating Disorders

Princess Diana, Jane Fonda, Karen Carpenter—beautiful, successful women—all suffered from eating disorders. Eating disorders refer to a group of conditions that share a pathological concern with body weight and shape. According to mental health guidelines, there are three categories of eating disorders: anorexia nervosa, bulimia nervosa, and eating disorders not otherwise specified, including **binge-eating disorder** (see Table 7.8).[60] At the mild end of this spectrum is the individual with binge-eating disorder, who finds company in a box of donuts and cannot stop eating until they are gone. That person's weight may range from normal to obese. Individuals suffering from **bulimia nervosa** are more frequent **binge** eaters who are driven by compulsive behavior to consume extremely large

Binge-eating disorder An eating disorder characterized by recurrent episodes of binge eating in the absence of purging behavior.

Bulimia nervosa An eating disorder characterized by the consumption of large amounts of food at one time (bingeing), followed by purging behavior such as vomiting and the use of laxatives to eliminate food from the body.

Binge The rapid consumption of a large amount of food in a discrete period of time associated with a feeling that eating is out of control.

Table 7.8 *Diagnostic Criteria for Eating Disorders*

Anorexia Nervosa

Refusal to maintain body weight at or above 85% of normal weight for age and height.

Intense fear of gaining weight or becoming fat, even though underweight.

Disturbance in the way body weight or shape is experienced or denial of the seriousness of the current low body weight.

Absence of at least three consecutive menstrual cycles without other known cause.

Bulimia Nervosa

Recurrent episodes of binge eating.

Recurrent inappropriate compensatory behavior to prevent weight gain, such as self-induced vomiting; misuse of laxatives, diuretics, enemas, or other medications; fasting; or excessive exercise.

Occurrence, on average, of binge eating and inappropriate compensatory behaviors at least twice a week for three months.

Undue influence by body shape and weight on self-evaluation.

Disturbance does not occur exclusively during episodes of anorexia nervosa.

Eating Disorders Not Otherwise Specified

Criteria for anorexia nervosa are met except the individual menstruates regularly.

Criteria for anorexia nervosa are met except that, despite substantial weight loss, the individual's current weight is in the normal range.

Criteria for bulimia nervosa are met except binges occur at a frequency of less than twice a week and for a duration of less than three months.

Inappropriate compensatory behavior after eating small amounts of food in individuals of normal body weight.

Regularly chewing and spitting out, without swallowing, large amounts of food.

Binge-Eating Disorder

Recurrent episodes of binge eating in the absence of the regular use of inappropriate compensatory behaviors characteristic of bulimia.

From American Psychiatric Association. *Diagnostic and Statistical Manual,* 4th ed. Washington, D.C.: American Psychiatric Association, 1994.

amounts of high-kcalorie foods. They then experience depression and guilt, and initiate **purging,** such as self-induced vomiting. At the far end of the spectrum are individuals with **anorexia nervosa,** who engage in behaviors such as self-starvation and excessive exercise to reduce weight or prevent weight gain. If untreated, eating disorders can seriously affect health and even be fatal. Anorexia and bulimia affect about 3% of women, and the incidence of bulimia, the more common disorder, appears to be increasing.[61]

Purging Behaviors such as self-induced vomiting and misuse of laxatives and diuretics to rid the body of energy.

Anorexia nervosa An eating disorder characterized by self-starvation, a distorted body image, and low body weight.

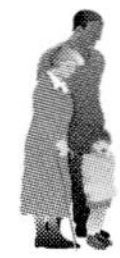

What Causes Eating Disorders?

In the search for the cause of eating disorders, sociocultural, psychological, and biological factors have been examined. Eating disorders most commonly begin in adolescence when physical, psychological, and social development is occurring rapidly. While they are more common in young women, males make up 5 to 10% of individuals with eating disorders; male athletes in weight-regulated activities like wrestling are at particular risk. Eating disorders are typically associated with Caucasians of higher socioeconomic class, but in reality they occur in all ethnic groups.[62] They are as common among Hispanic as Caucasian females, and are more frequent among Native Americans, and less frequent among African and Asian American females.[63]

Eating disorders are more prevalent in groups concerned with weight and body image.[64] The incidence is very low in underdeveloped countries and increases in certain subcultures in developed countries, such as professional dancers and models. In North America, young women in particular are concerned with body image. Being thin is associated with beauty, success, intelligence, and vitality. Being plump, on the other hand, is associated with ugliness, failure, stupidity, and clumsiness. What young woman would want to be plump? A young woman facing a future where she must be independent, have a prestigious job, maintain a successful love relationship, bear and nurture children, manage a household, and stay in fashion can become overwhelmed. Unable to master all these roles, she may look for some aspect of her life that she can control. Food intake and body weight are natural choices, since being thin brings the societal associations of success. The adage that you can never be too rich or too thin is too often followed by young women today.

Certain personality characteristics and psychological problems are also common among individuals with eating disorders. They feel ineffective and have low self-esteem and poor self-regulation.[65] A typical anorexic or bulimic can be described as an intelligent, adolescent female overachiever.

There is some evidence that biology may play a role. Much of the risk of developing anorexia and bulimia, as well as personality traits that predispose one to these disorders, appears to be inherited.[61] Abnormalities in the levels of neurotransmitters such as serotonin and their metabolites, and in levels of the hormone leptin, have been hypothesized to contribute to the behaviors typical of anorexia and bulimia.[61]

Anorexia Nervosa

Anorexia nervosa was originally described over a century ago. The name "anorexia," which means lack of appetite, is a misnomer because it is not a lack of appetite that causes individuals with this disorder to decrease their food intake, but rather a desire to remain thin (Figure 7.20).

A Profile of Anorexia Nervosa *For breakfast, I drank herbal tea with no sugar. For lunch, a few leaves of lettuce, and, for dinner, 2 ounces of broiled white-meat chicken without the skin and a carrot stick. . . . On this diet I was good. I was in control of the one thing I could control, my body. If I eat more than this, I might gain weight. I fear this more than anything else. Sometimes I lose control and eat too much. This must not happen. I must eat only what is allowed. I didn't let anyone see me eat this food; I didn't want them to see my weakness.*

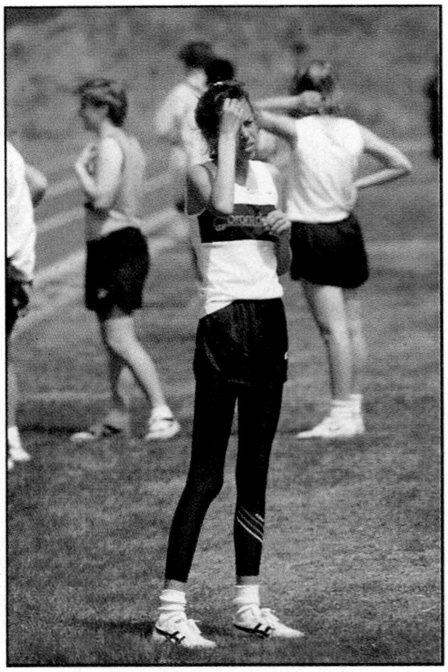

Figure 7.20
A person with anorexia nervosa may literally starve herself to death. (Tony Freeman/PhotoEdit)

Physiological State Anorexia nervosa is a life-threatening disorder in which mortality is 5% in the first two years and can reach 20% in untreated individuals.[66] Anorexia nervosa is relatively rare, affecting approximately 0.5% of women over their lifetime.[61]

Anorexia is characterized by excessive weight loss due to self-imposed starvation, an overwhelming fear of gaining weight, and use of body weight and shape as a means of self-evaluation. Disturbances in body image prevent anorexics from seeing themselves as underweight, so they continue to restrict food intake or exercise excessively.

Anorexics may use diets, exercise, or purging to remain thin. They often develop their own personal ritual about diet, limiting certain foods and eating them in specific ways. Anorexics spend an enormous amount of time thinking about food, talking about food, and preparing food for others. Instead of eating they move the food around the plate and cut it into tiny pieces. They may also use exercise to increase energy expenditure. But they do not stop when they are tired; instead, they train compulsively beyond reasonable endurance. Some may also binge and purge. As weight loss becomes severe, symptoms of starvation begin to appear.

Starvation affects mental function, causing anorexics to become apathetic, dull, exhausted, and depressed. Physical symptoms include fat-store depletion; muscle wasting; inflammation and swelling of lips; dry, peeling, flaking skin; abnormal hair growth on the body; and dry, thin, brittle hair on the head that may fall out. In females, estrogen levels drop and menstruation is irregular or stops. This affects sexual maturation and can have long-term effects on bone density. In males, testosterone levels decrease. In the final stages of starvation there is abnormal electrolyte balance, dehydration, edema, cardiac abnormalities, absence of ketones due to fat-store depletion, and finally infection, further increasing nutritional needs.

Treatment of Anorexia Nervosa Early treatment of anorexia is important because starvation may cause irreversible damage. The goal of treatment is to help resolve psychological and behavioral problems while providing for nutritional rehabilitation. The goal of nutrition intervention is to promote weight gain by increasing energy intake and expanding dietary choices.[67] Nutritional rehabilitation in mild cases involves learning about nutrition and meal planning in order to develop healthy eating patterns. In more severe cases, anorexics are hospitalized and their food intake and exercise behaviors are carefully controlled. Total parenteral nutrition (TPN) may be necessary to keep the individual alive. Some anorexics make full recoveries, but about half have poor long-term outcomes—remaining irrationally concerned about weight gain and never achieving normal body weight.

Bulimia Nervosa

Bulimia nervosa was not recognized as a separate eating disorder until the late 1970s. It is characterized by periodically recurring episodes of massive overeating, referred to as food binges, followed by inappropriate compensatory behaviors to prevent weight gain, such as vomiting, use of laxatives and enemas, fasting, and excessive exercise. During a food binge the individual experiences a sense of lack of control. While a normal teenager may consume 2000 to 3000 kcalories per day, a bulimic may consume over 3400 kcalories in under two hours, and some bulimics consume up to 20,000 kcalories in binges lasting as long as eight hours.[68] A binge usually occurs in secrecy and stops only when pain, fatigue, or an interruption intervenes.

A Profile of Bulimia Nervosa *I am alone in my dorm room. Alone with my self-disgust. I can't stand to live in this grotesque body any longer. Before I go on a diet, I decide on one last binge, but there is no food in my room. I walk the block and a half to the convenience store near campus and buy a pound package of chocolate chip cookies, a bag of corn chips, and a half gallon of ice cream. At the checkout, I am embarrassed by the foods that I am buying and don't look at the cashier. Once back in the secrecy of my own room, I start with the corn chips, then move through the bag of cookies. About halfway through the cookies, my stomach is feeling full, bulging out from under my rib cage, so I have several bowls of ice cream to make vomiting easier. I must then make sure the dorm bathroom is empty so no one can hear my vomiting. No one must know. When I return to my room, I finish the rest of the cookies, and I want more. To replenish my supply of binge foods, I must walk almost seven blocks in the other direction because I don't want the cashier in the convenience store to know. I buy doughnuts, brownies, and more cookies, which are all finished shortly after I return to my room. I again use the ice cream to make the vomiting easier. When the food is gone, I repeat the vomiting ritual. When done, I feel dizzy and weak. I straighten my room, take a shower, and go to bed. Tomorrow, like every day, I will start a diet.*

Physiological State Bulimia shares with anorexia the preoccupation with body weight and shape. As with anorexics, bulimics have a negative body image accompanied by an altered perception of their body size. They are preoccupied with the fear that once they start eating they will not be able to stop. Unlike anorexics, bulimics may maintain a normal body weight or even be overweight.

A diagnosis of bulimia is based on the frequency with which episodes of binge eating and inappropriate compensatory behaviors occur (see Table 7.8). Bulimia is subdivided into nonpurging and purging types. Nonpurging bulimics use behaviors such as fasting or excessive exercise to prevent weight gain. Purging bulimics regularly engage in behaviors that may include self-induced vomiting and misuse of enemas, laxatives, diuretics, or other medications. Despite the attractiveness of being able to eat all you want without gaining weight, purging rituals do not eliminate all the kcalories. Vomiting eliminates 70 to 80% of the ingested energy. The use of laxatives affects the colon, not the small intestine where food is absorbed. So water is lost, but most of the energy is not. Diuretics also result in the loss of water, not energy.

It is the purging of the binge-purge cycle that is most hazardous to health in bulimia nervosa. Purging by vomiting brings stomach acid into the mouth. Frequent vomiting affects the gastrointestinal tract by causing tooth decay, sores in the mouth and on the lips, swollen jaws and salivary glands, irritation of the throat, esophageal inflammation, and changes in stomach capacity and stomach emptying.[69] It also causes broken blood vessels in the face from the force of vomiting, electrolyte imbalance, dehydration, muscle weakness, and menstrual irregularities. Laxative and diuretic abuse can also cause dehydration and electrolyte imbalance. Rectal bleeding may occur from laxative overuse.

Treatment of Bulimia Nervosa The overall goal of therapy for people with bulimia nervosa is to separate eating from their emotions and from their perceptions of success, and to promote eating in response to hunger and satiety. Psychological issues related to body image and a sense of lack of control over eating must be resolved. Nutritional therapy must address physiological imbalances caused by purging episodes as well as providing education on nutrient needs and how to meet them. Antidepressant medications have also been shown to reduce the frequency of binge episodes. Treatment has been found to speed recovery, but for some women this disorder may remain a chronic problem throughout life.[70]

Other Eating Disorders

A third class of eating disorders, termed "eating disorders not otherwise specified," includes conditions such as weight loss that is less severe than the criteria dictate for anorexia (that is, 15% below desirable body weight) or binging and purging that is less frequent than the criteria for bulimia.

Binge-Eating Disorder Individuals who suffer from binge-eating disorder engage in recurrent episodes of binge eating but do not regularly engage in purging behaviors such as vomiting, fasting, or excessive exercise. These individuals are likely to have above-normal body weights and may seek help for treatment of obesity rather than for their binge-eating behavior.[71] About one quarter to one third of individuals who attend weight-loss clinics meet the criteria for binge-eating disorder.[61]

Fad Bulimia Because of the desire of some to have their cake and eat it too, bulimia is "catching on." To those who are concerned about being 10 pounds heavier than they were when they started college, but who don't want to miss out on the food at social gatherings, bulimia may seem like the perfect solution. This type of bulimia, often termed fad bulimia, takes place among friends and is common among female college students, particularly sorority members.[72] It is also common among male athletes who participate in sports with competitive weight categories, such as body building and wrestling.

The quantities of food consumed by fad bulimics are usually smaller than those in severe forms of bulimia, and the individuals engaged in these activities do not exhibit the serious emotional disturbances and shame about the bulimic practices that true bulimics do. Still, fad bulimia is dangerous. If an individual is predisposed to developing an eating disorder, this type of behavior may evolve into a more severe eating disorder. Even individuals not predisposed to an eating disorder may learn to use this behavior as a way of dealing with anxiety. The physical damage caused is the same in both fad bulimia and bulimia nervosa.

Organizations that provide information about eating disorders as well as support for victims and their families include:

American Anorexia/Bulimia Association, Inc.
418 E. 76th Street
New York, NY 10021
(212) 734–1114

National Association of Anorexia and Associated Disorders, Inc.
P.O. Box 7
Highland Park, IL 60035
(847) 831-3438

APPLICATIONS

These exercises are designed to help you apply your critical thinking skills to your own nutrition choices. Many are best performed using a diet analysis software program. If you do not have access to a computer program, the exercises can be hand-calculated using the information in this text and its appendices.

1. Using Appendix B, find your desirable body weight in the Metropolitan Life Insurance table and the table of Healthy Weight Ranges for Men and Women.
   a. There are differences between these tables. Does your actual body weight fall within the desirable range in both tables?
   b. Calculate your body mass index. How does it compare with standards?
2. Using the three-day food record you kept in Chapter 2, calculate your average energy intake.
   a. Determine your average energy expenditure using your RMR (see Table 7.2), activity factors (see Table 7.3), and the thermic effect of food based on the energy intake you just calculated (see Table 7.4).
   b. How does your energy expenditure compare with your calculated energy intake?
   c. If you consumed and expended these amounts of energy every day, would your weight increase, decrease, or stay the same?
   d. If intake does not equal output, how much would you gain or lose in a month?
   e. If your energy intake does not equal your energy expenditure, list some specific changes you could make in your diet or the amount of activity you get to make the two balance.
3. Use the Internet Web site for this book to locate anorexia and associated disorders. Can you locate information on how to approach a friend whom you suspect has an eating disorder?

Summary

1. Energy is the ability to do work. It is measured in kcalories or kjoules. A kcalorie is the amount of heat needed to raise the temperature of 1 kilogram of water 1 degree Celsius.
2. Energy intake from food is motivated by hunger and appetite. Protein and carbohydrate each provide 4 kcalories per gram, fat provides 9 kcalories per gram, and alcohol provides 7 kcalories per gram.
3. In the adult body energy is required for basal metabolism, activity, and the thermic effect of food. Basal metabolic rate (BMR) is the largest component of energy expenditure. It differs with body size, body composition, age, and gender. The energy needed for activity accounts for 15 to 30% of energy needs and depends on the individual. The thermic effect of food (TEF) is equal to about 10% of energy consumed.
4. The principle of energy balance states that for weight maintenance, energy intake must equal energy expenditure. If more energy is consumed than expended, weight gain results; and if more energy is expended than taken in, weight loss results. If the diet contains excess energy, it is stored in the body, primarily as fat.
5. Excess body fat increases the risk of chronic diseases such as diabetes, heart disease, high blood pressure, and certain types of cancer. Too little body fat is also unhealthy.
6. Desirable body weight and fat can be measured in many

ways. BMI is the currently accepted standard for assessing body fatness. It correlates better with body fat than does comparing weight for height. Techniques that measure body composition, including skinfold thickness, underwater weighing, isotope dilution techniques, and imaging can be used to assess the amount and distribution of body fat.

7. Excess body fat is the result of both genetics and environment. Genes have been identified that regulate body fatness in animals and there is evidence that similar mechanisms are at work in humans. Body fatness is regulated at a set point. Signals from the GI tract, hormones, and circulating nutrients regulate short-term hunger and satiety. Signals such as the release of leptin from fat cells regulate long-term energy intake and expenditure. Although much of the tendency to obesity is genetic, choices concerning the amount and type of food consumed and activity level also affect energy balance.
8. More than half of adult Americans are overweight. Most people succeed in short-term weight loss but, in the long term, regain all the weight they have lost.
9. Weight management involves adjusting energy intake and expenditure and modifying long-term behaviors. To lose a pound of fat, expenditure must be increased or intake decreased by approximately 3500 kcalories. Slow, steady weight loss of 1/2 to 1 pound per week is more likely to be maintained than rapid weight loss.
10. There are thousands of programs and techniques for weight management. All involve a decrease in energy intake and/or an increase in energy expenditure. An ideal program involves a decrease in intake, an increase in expenditure, and behavior modification to reduce body weight and maintain the loss.
11. When conventional therapies fail in certain obese individuals, drug therapy and surgery may be effective approaches to weight management. In cases of morbid obesity, surgery to reduce food intake and absorption may be appropriate. However, these methods do not foster development of long-term maintenance behaviors.
12. Eating disorders are psychological disorders in which the perception of body size is altered. Treatment involves supplying an adequate diet and psychological counseling to change body-image perceptions and improve eating habits.

Review Questions

1. What is energy balance?
2. What is a kcalorie?
3. Which nutrients provide energy?
4. What is basal metabolic rate?
5. What is the thermic effect of food?
6. List the three components of energy expenditure.
7. What health problems are associated with excess body fat?
8. List three ways that desirable body weight or composition can be measured. Explain the basic principle involved.
9. How does the distribution of body fat affect the risks of excess weight?
10. How is body fatness affected by genetics?
11. How is body fatness affected by environment?
12. Describe three approaches to weight management.
13. What is the best approach to weight management? Why?
14. How is nutrition involved in the treatment of eating disorders?

Nutrition Web Links

To further explore areas related to the material in this chapter go to the *Nutrition: Science and Applications* Web site at ***www.Wiley.com/college/Smolin*** and *click on* **Student Companion Site** for chapter-by-chapter links. Some Web sites related to the information in Chapter 7 include:

Sites that provide information on the risks associated with being overweight such as Healthy People 2010 and the American Heart Association.

Sites that provide information on weight management such as the Partnership for Healthy Weight Management.

Sites from companies in the business of weight management such as Weight Watchers International.

References

1. Cassell, J. A. Social anthropology and nutrition: a different look at obesity. J. Am. Diet. Assoc. 95:424–427, 1995.
2. National Institutes of Health; National Heart, Lung, and Blood Institute. Clinical guidelines on the identification, evaluation, and treatment of overweight and obesity in adults. Executive summary, June 1998. Online at: http://www.nhlbi.nih.gov/nhlbi/cardio/obes/prof/guide/ns/ob_home.htm
3. Jeffery, R. W. Does weight cycling present a health risk? Am. J. Clin. Nutr. 63(suppl):452S–455S, 1996.
4. Committee to Develop Criteria for Evaluating Outcomes of Approaches to Prevent and Treat Obesity, Food and Nutrition Board, Institute of Medicine, National Academy of Sciences. Criteria for evaluating outcomes and approaches to obesity. J. Am. Diet. Assoc. 95:1–10, 1995.
5. The painful business of losing weight. The Economist, August 30, 1997:45–7.
6. Kassirer, J. P., and Angell, M. A. Losing weight—an ill-fated New Year's resolution. New Engl. J. Med. 338:52–54, 1998.

7. Friedman, M. I. Control of energy intake by energy metabolism. Am. J. Clin. Nutr. 62(suppl):1096S–1100S, 1995.
8. Wadden, T. A., Foster, G. D., Letizia, K. A., and Muller, J. L. Long-term effects of dieting on resting metabolic rate in obese patients. J.A.M.A. 264:707–711, 1990.
9. Horten, T. S., Drougas, H., Brachey, A., et al. Fat and carbohydrate overfeeding in humans: different effects on energy storage. Am. J. Clin. Nutr. 62:19–29, 1995.
10. Seale, J. L. Energy expenditure measurements in relation to energy requirements. Am. J. Clin. Nutr. 62(suppl):1042S–1046S, 1995.
11. National Research Council, Food and Nutrition Board. *Recommended Dietary Allowances,* 10th ed. Washington, D.C.: National Academy Press, 1989.
12. Taubes, G. As obesity rates rise, experts struggle to explain why. Science 280:1367–1368, 1998.
13. Conway, J. M. Ethnicity and energy stores. Am. J. Clin. Nutr. 62(suppl): 1067S–1071S, 1995.
14. Troiano, R. P., Flegal, K. M., Kuczmarski, R. J., et al. Overweight prevalence and trends for children and adolescents: the National Health and Nutrition Examination surveys, 1963 to 1991. Arch. Pediatr. Adolesc. Med. 149:1085–1091, 1995.
15. Troiano, R. P., and Flegal, K. M. Overweight children and adolescents: description, epidemiology, and demographics. Pediatrics 101(suppl): 497–504, 1998.
16. Williamson, D. F. Intentional weight loss: patterns in the general population and its association with morbidity and mortality. Int. J. Obes. Relat. Metab. Disord. 21:(suppl) S14–S19, 1997.
17. Bosello, O., Armellini, S., Zamboni, M., and Fitchet, M. The benefits of modest weight loss in type II diabetes. Int. J. Obes. Relat. Metab. Disord. 21(suppl):S10–S13, 1997.
18. Casper, R. C. Nutrition and its relation to aging. Exp. Gerontol. 30:294–314, 1995.
19. Arena, B., Maffulli, N., Maffulli, F., and Morleo, M. A. Reproductive hormones and menstrual changes with exercise in female athletes. Sports Med. 19:278–287, 1995.
20. Abernathy, R. P., and Black, D. R. Healthy body weights: an alternative perspective. Am. J. Clin. Nutr. 63(suppl):448S–451S, 1996.
21. American Dietetic Association. Position of the American Dietetic Association: weight management. J. Am. Diet. Assoc. 97:71–74, 1997.
22. Bouchard, C., Tremblay, A., Després, J.-P., et al. The response to long term feeding in identical twins. N. Engl. J. Med. 322:1477–1482, 1990.
23. Albu, J., Allison, D., Boozer, C. N., et al. Obesity solutions: report of a meeting. Nutr. Rev. 55:150–156, 1997.
24. Dietz, W. H. Periods of risk in childhood for the development of adult obesity—what do we need to learn? J. Nutr. 127:1884S–1886S, 1997.
25. Plourde, G. The role of radiologic methods in assessing body composition and related metabolic parameters. Nutr. Rev. 55:289–296, 1997.
26. Snead, D. B., Birges, S. J., and Kohrt, W. M. Age-related differences in body composition by hydrodensitometry and dual-energy x-ray absorptiometry. J. Appl. Physiol. 74:770–775, 1993.
27. Friedman, J. M. The alphabet of weight control. Nature 385:119–120, 1997.
28. Spiegelman, B. M., and Flier, J. S. Adipogenesis and obesity: rounding out the big picture. Cell 87:377–389, 1996.
29. Bouchard, C. Genetics of human obesity: recent results from linkage studies. J. Nutr. 127:1887S–1890S, 1997.
30. Norman, R. A., Thompson, D. B., Foroud, T., et al. Genomewide search for genes influencing percent body fat in Pima Indians: suggestive linkage at chromosome 11q21-q22. Am. J. Human Genet. 60:166–173, 1997.
31. Hill, J. O., and Peters, J. C. Environmental contributions to the obesity epidemic. Science 280:1371–1374, 1998.
32. Moore, L. L., Lombardi, D. A., White, M. J., et al. Influence of parents' physical activity levels on activity levels of young children. J. Pediatr. 118:215–219, 1991.
33. Sobal, J. Obesity and socioeconomic status: a framework for examining relationships between physical and social variables. Med. Anthropol. 13:231–247, 1991.
34. Leibel, R. L., Rosenbaum, M., and Hirsch, J. Changes in energy expenditure resulting from altered body weight. N. Engl. J. Med. 332:622–628, 1995.
35. Kern, P. A. Potential role of TNFα and lipoprotein lipase as candidate genes for obesity. J. Nutr. 127:1917S–1922S, 1997.
36. Anderson, G. H. Regulation of food intake. In *Modern Nutrition in Health and Disease,* 8th ed. Shils, M. E., Olson, J. A., and Shike, M., eds. Philadelphia: Lea & Febiger, 1994. 524–536.
37. Woods, S. C., Seeley, R. J., Porte, D., and Schwartz, M. W. Signals that regulate food intake and energy homeostasis. Science 280:1378–1383, 1998.
38. Montague, C. T., Farooqi, I. S., Whitehead, J. P., et al. Congenital leptin deficiency is associated with severe early onset obesity in children. Nature 387:903–908, 1997.
39. Considine, R. V., Sinha, M. K., Heiman, M. L., et al. Serum immunoreactive-leptin concentrations in normal weight and obese humans. New Engl. J. Med. 334:292–295, 1996.
40. Considine, R. V., Considine, E. L., Williams, C. J., et al. The hypothalamic leptin receptor in humans. Diabetes 19:992–994, 1996.
41. Heymsfield, S. B., Darby, P. C., Muhlheim, L. S., et al. The calorie: myth, measurement, and reality. Am. J. Clin. Nutr. 62(suppl):1034S–1041S, 1995.
42. Platte, P., Pirke, K. M., Wade, S. E., et al. Physical activity, total energy expenditure, and food intake in grossly obese and normal weight women. Int. J. Eat. Disord. 17:51–57, 1995.
43. Drewnowski, A., Krahn, D. D., and Demitrack, M. A. Naloxone, an opiate blocker, reduces the consumption of high-fat foods in obese and lean binge eaters. Am. J. Clin. Nutr. 61:1201–1206, 1995.
44. Rolls, B. J., and Hammer, V. A. Fat, carbohydrate and the regulation of food intake. Am. J. Clin. Nutr. 62(suppl):1086S–1095S, 1995.
45. Tremblay, A., Després, J-P., Thriault, G., et al. Overfeeding and energy expenditure in humans. Am. J. Clin. Nutr. 56:857–862, 1992.
46. Diaz, E. O., Prentice, A. M., Goldberg, G. R., et al. Metabolic response to experimental overfeeding in lean and overweight healthy volunteers. Am. J. Clin. Nutr. 56:641–655, 1992.
47. Gura, T. Uncoupling proteins provide new clues to obesity's causes. Science 280:1369–1370, 1998.
48. Lisette, C. P., de Groot, G. M., and van Staveren, W. A. Reduced physical activity and its association with obesity. Nutr. Rev. 53:11–18, 1995.
49. Robison, J. I., Hoeer, S. L., Petersmarck, K. A., and Anderson, J. V. Redefining success in obesity intervention: the new paradigm. J. Am. Diet. Assoc. 4:422–423, 1995.
50. Meisler, J. G., and St. Jeor, S. Summary and recommendations from the American Health Foundation's Expert Panel on Healthy Weight. Am. J. Clin. Nutr. 63(suppl):474S–477S, 1996.
51. U.S. Department of Agriculture, U.S. Department of Health and Human Services. *Nutrition and Your Health: Dietary Guidelines for Americans,* 4th ed. Home and Garden Bulletin No. 232. Hyattsville, Md.: U.S. Government Printing Office, 1995.
52. Stubbs, R. J., Harbron, C. G., Murgatroyd, P. R., and Prentice, A. M. Covert manipulation of dietary fat and energy density: effect on substrate flux and food intake in men eating ad libitum. Am. J. Clin. Nutr. 62:316–329, 1995.
53. Sears, B. *The Zone.* New York: Regan Books, 1995.
54. Wilmore, J. H. Increasing physical activity: alterations in body mass and composition. Am. J. Clin. Nutr. 63(suppl):456S–460S, 1996.
55. Stevens, J., Cai, J., Pamuk, E. R., et al. The effect of age on the association between body mass index and mortality. N. Engl. J. Med. 338:1–7, 1998.
56. National Task Force on the Prevention and Treatment of Obesity. Long term pharmacotherapy in the management of obesity. J.A.M.A. 276:1907–1915, 1996.

57. Frackelmann, K. Diet drug debacle: how two federally approved weight-loss drugs crashed. Science News 152:252–253, 1997.
58. Campfield, L. A., Smith, F. J., and Burn, P. Strategies and potential molecular targets for obesity treatment. Science 280:1383–1387, 1998.
59. Flancbaum, L., and Choban, P. S. Surgical implications of obesity. Ann. Rev. Med. 49:214–234, 1998.
60. American Psychiatric Association. *Diagnostic and Statistical Manual,* 4th ed. Washington, D.C.: American Psychiatric Association, 1994.
61. Walsh, B. T., and Devlin, M. J. Eating disorders: progress and problems. Science 280:1387–1390, 1998.
62. Gard, M. C., and Freeman C. P. The dismantling of a myth: a review of eating disorders and socioeconomic status. Int. J. Eat. Disord. 20:1–12, 1996.
63. Crago M., Shisslak, C. M., and Estes, L. S. Eating disturbances among American minority groups: a review. Int. J. Eat. Disord. 19:239–248, 1996.
64. Hsu, L. K. Epidemiology of the eating disorders. Psychiatr. Clin. North Am. 19:681–700, 1996.
65. Leon, G. R., Keel, P. K., Klump, K. L., and Fulkerson, J. A. The future of risk factor research in understanding the etiology of eating disorders. Psychopharmacol. Bull. 33:405–411, 1997.
66. Foreyt, J. P., Poston, W. S. C., II, and Goodrick, G. K. Future directions in obesity and eating disorders. Addict. Behav. 21:767–778, 1996.
67. Rock, C. L., and Curran-Celentano, J. Nutritional management of eating disorders. Psychiatr. Clin. North Am. 19:701–713, 1996.
68. Farley, D. Eating disorders require medical attention. FDA Consumer 26:27–29, March 1992.
69. Anderson, L., Shaw, J. M., and McCargar, L. Physiological effects of bulimia nervosa on the gastrointestinal tract. Can. J. Gastroenterol. 11:451–459, 1997.
70. Keel, P. K., and Mitchell, J. E. Outcome in bulimia nervosa. Am. J. Psychiatry 154:313–321, March 1997.
71. American Dietetic Association. Position of the American Dietetic Association: nutrition intervention in the treatment of anorexia nervosa, bulimia nervosa, and binge eating. J. Am. Diet. Assoc. 94:902–907, 1994.
72. Crandall, C. S. Societal contagion of binge eating. J. Pers. Soc. Psychol. 55:589–599, 1988.

III

WATER AND THE MICRONUTRIENTS

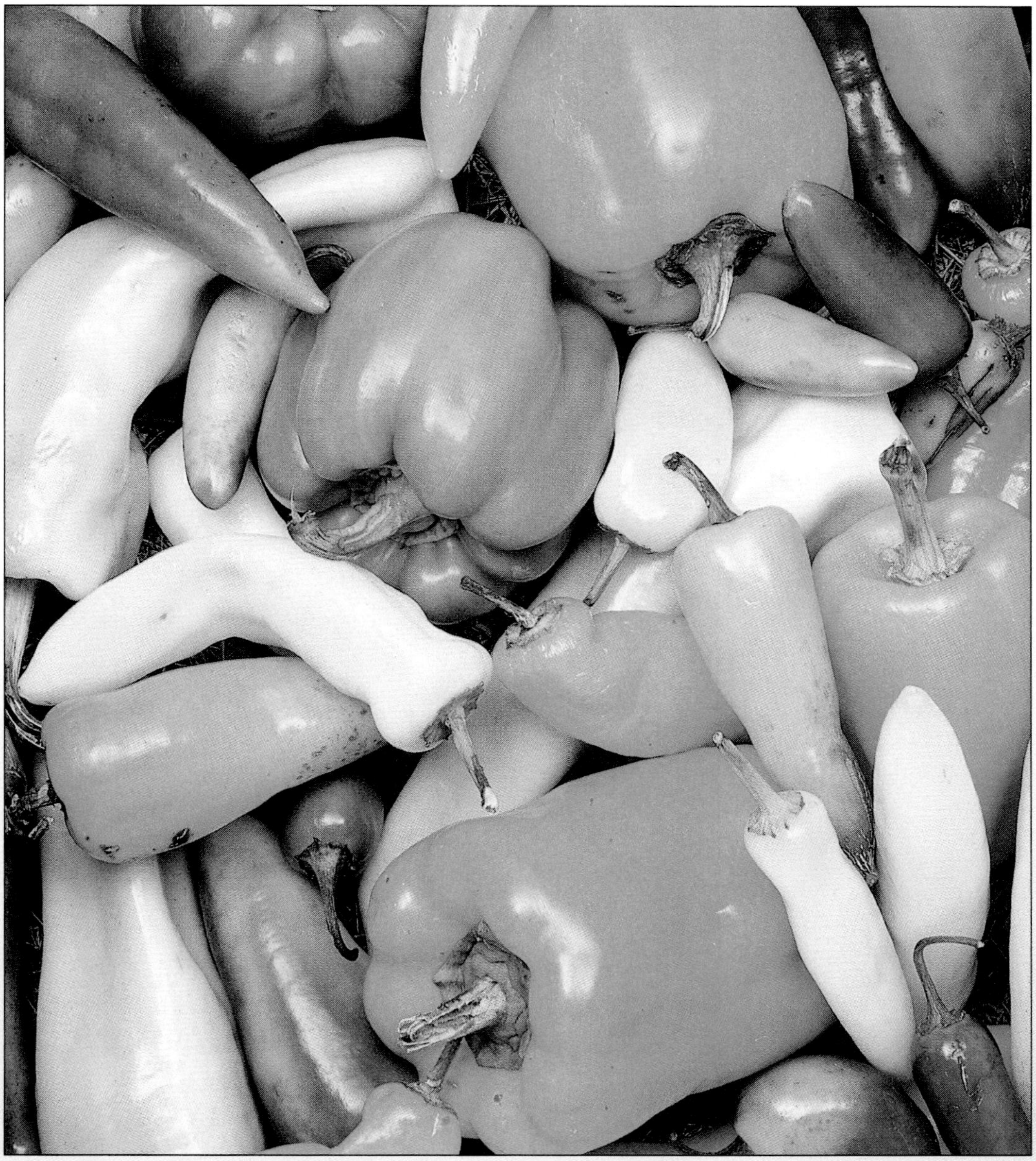

Chapter

8

Chapter Outline

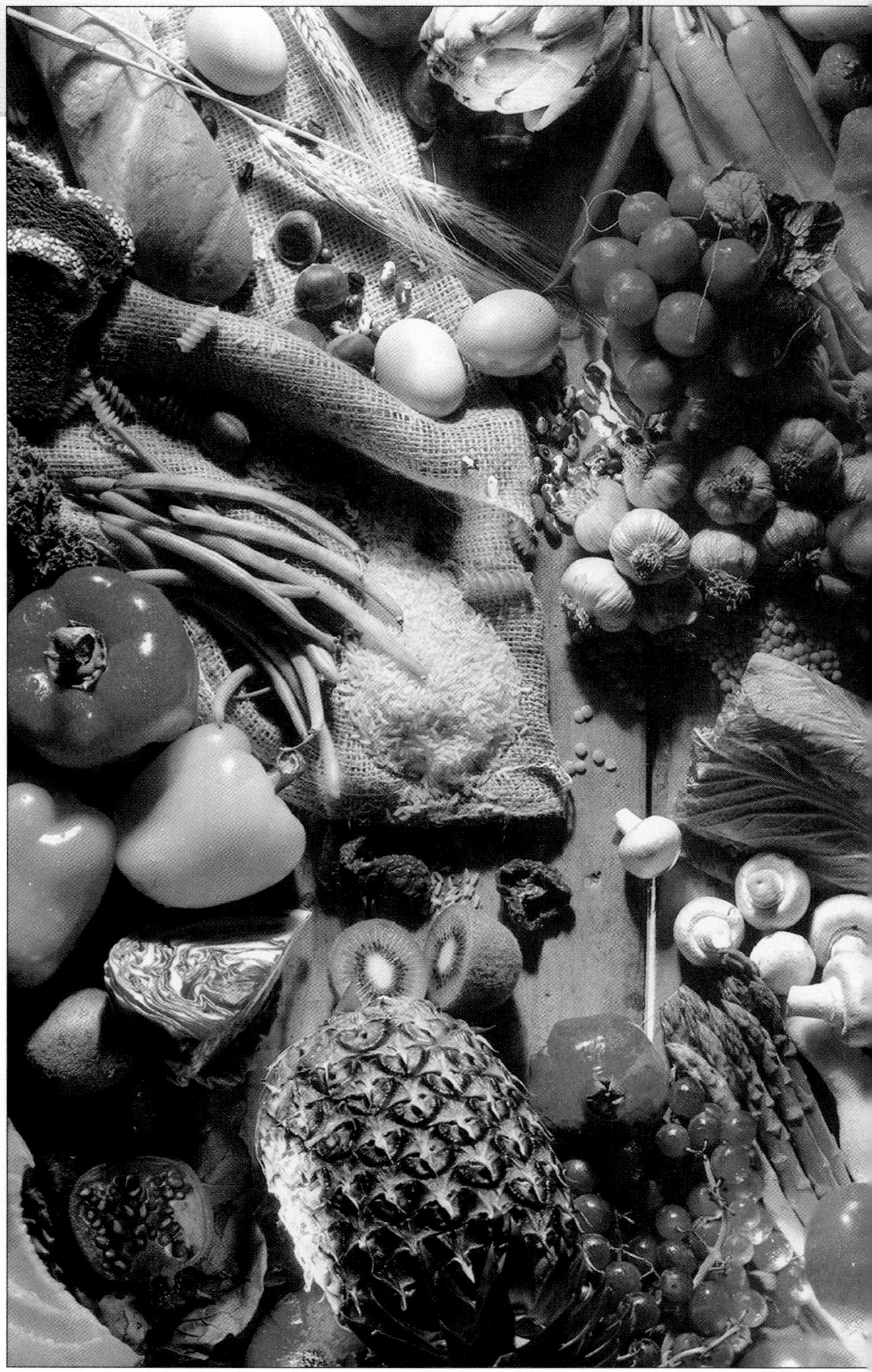

(© Rick Lance/Phototake)

A Vitamin Primer and the Water-Soluble Vitamins

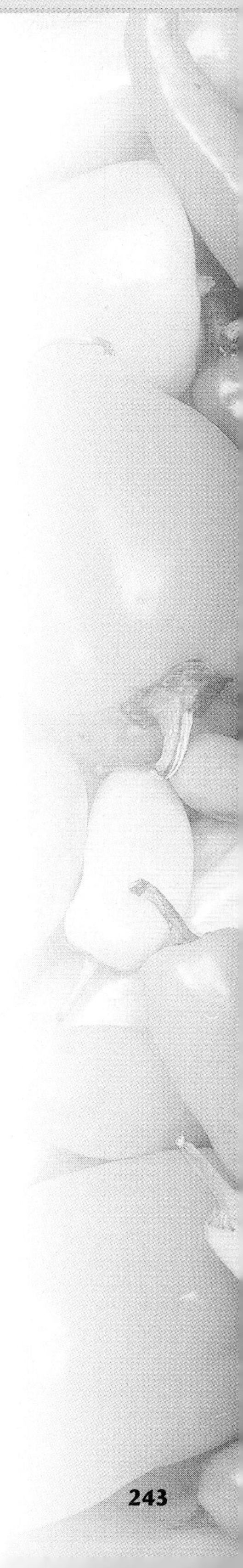

Chapter Concepts

1. Vitamins are essential organic nutrients that provide no energy but which are needed in small amounts in the diet to allow for growth, reproduction, and the maintenance of health. A lack of a vitamin results in deficiency symptoms that are relieved by the addition of the vitamin to the diet.
2. Vitamins are found naturally in almost all foods. Processing food can decrease its vitamin content or increase it through fortification and enrichment.
3. The amount of a vitamin that is available to the body depends on how much of it is consumed, absorbed, transported, activated, stored, and excreted.
4. For most individuals, a carefully planned diet can provide an adequate intake of vitamins.
5. Excess of some vitamins can be toxic.
6. Thiamin, riboflavin, niacin, biotin, and pantothenic acid function as coenzymes in reactions that produce energy from carbohydrate, fat, and protein, as well as alcohol.
7. Vitamin B_6 is a coenzyme essential for amino acid metabolism.
8. Folate is a coenzyme that is needed for cell division. It is particularly important for rapidly dividing cells.
9. Vitamin B_{12} is needed to maintain nerve cells and is a coenzyme for the metabolism of folate and methionine. It is found in animal products.
10. Vitamin C is needed for the synthesis of collagen, neurotransmitters, and hormones. It also functions as a general antioxidant that protects the water-soluble compartments of the cell from oxidative damage.
11. Choline is needed for the synthesis of cell membranes and may be essential at some stages of life.

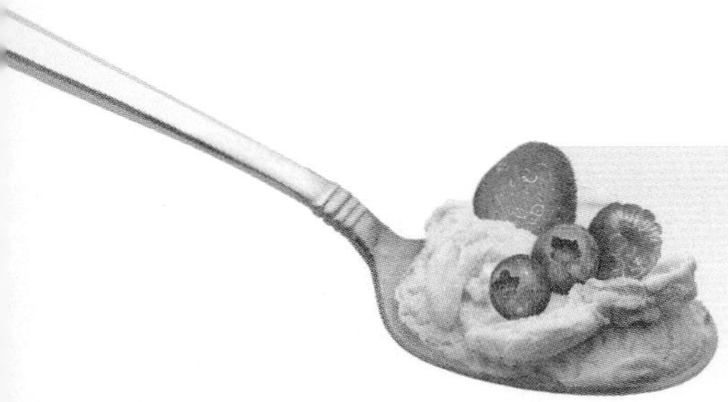

Just a Taste

Can vitamins give you extra energy?

Should everyone take folic acid supplements?

Does vitamin C cure the common cold?

Folic acid prevents birth defects! Vitamin E protects your heart! Vitamin A prevents cancer! As we enter the 21st century, the significance of vitamins in health promotion and disease prevention stimulates intrigue and excitement. A century ago, discoveries related to food, vitamins, and health were just as tantalizing. At that time, a number of diseases that seemed incurable, and that were often fatal, were cured by changes in diet. In 1885 it was discovered that beriberi, a disease that killed thousands of sailors in the Orient, could be prevented by adding meat and whole grains to the usual shipboard diet. In 1913, a fat-soluble factor that allowed animals to grow better was identified in butter, and in 1915, pellagra, a disease that filled psychiatric hospitals in the southern United States, was cured by adding meat to the diet. Discoveries such as these helped scientists connect specific diseases with dietary deficiencies. The existence of and need for vitamins were recognized because of the symptoms that occurred when they were absent. Even before the chemistry of these substances was determined, the civilized world was enchanted with the magic of vitamins. There was hope that incurable diseases could be remedied by simple dietary additions.

In the United States today, the vitamin deficiency diseases of the early 20th century are rare, but interest in vitamins as factors that protect against chronic disease, slow aging, and enhance performance is thriving. A knowledge of what vitamins do and how much of each we need is necessary to evaluate the information that promotes vitamins as magic bullets.

What Are Vitamins?

Vitamins Organic compounds needed in the diet in small amounts to promote and regulate the chemical reactions and processes needed for growth, reproduction, and maintenance of health.

Vitamins are organic compounds that are essential in the diet in small amounts to promote and regulate body functions necessary for growth, reproduction, and the maintenance of health. An organic compound is classified as a vitamin if a lack of the compound in the diet results in deficiency symptoms that are relieved by its addition to the diet. Although vitamins do not provide energy, many aid in the chemical reactions that produce energy from carbohydrate, fat, protein, and alcohol.

The term "vitamin" was coined in 1912 by Polish biochemist Casimir Funk, who originally used the word "vitamine" to refer to substances that are *amines* (compounds containing an amino group NH_2), and are vital to life (vital + amine). Today we know vitamins are vital to life, but they are not all amines, so the "e" has been dropped and the term "vitamin" refers to all these substances. Initially, the vitamins were named alphabetically in approximately the order in which they were identified: A, B, C, D, and E. The B vitamins were first thought to be one chemical substance but were later found to be many different substances, so the alphabetical name was broken down by numbers. Vitamins B_6 and B_{12} are the only ones that are still commonly referred to by their numbers. Thiamin, riboflavin, and niacin were originally referred to as vitamin B_1, B_2, and B_3, respectively.

Vitamins have traditionally been grouped based on their solubility in water or fat. This chemical characteristic allows generalizations to be made about how they are absorbed, transported, excreted, and stored in the body. The general properties of **water-soluble vitamins** and **fat-soluble vitamins** will be discussed at the beginning of this chapter, followed by a discussion of the functions of each of the water-soluble vitamins and choline, which may be essential at certain times of life but has not yet been classified as a vitamin. The fat-soluble vitamins will be discussed individually in Chapter 9.

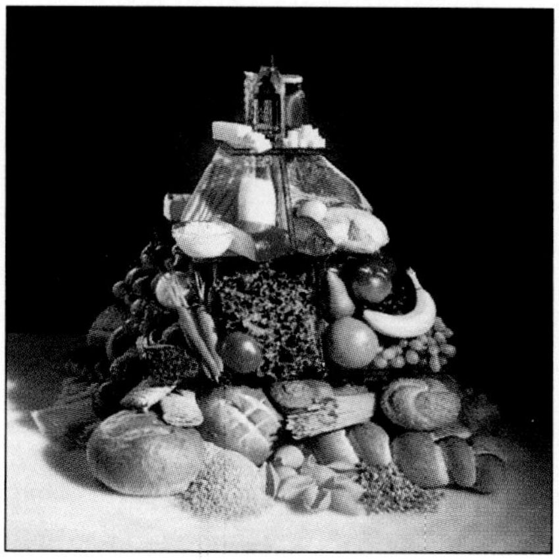

Figure 8.1
All the food groups contain choices that are good sources of vitamins. (© Gary Buss/FPG International)

Vitamins in the Diet

Water-soluble vitamins Vitamins that dissolve in water.

Fat-soluble vitamins Vitamins that dissolve in fat.

Almost all foods contain some vitamins (Figure 8.1). Grains are good sources of thiamin, niacin, riboflavin, pantothenic acid, and biotin. Meat and fish are good sources of all of the B vitamins. Milk provides riboflavin and vitamin D; leafy greens provide folate, vitamin A, vitamin E, and vitamin K; citrus fruit provides vitamin C; and vegetable oils are high in vitamin E (see *Off the Shelf: Maximizing the Vitamins in Your Vegetables*).

Food processing can affect the vitamin content of foods. The vitamins naturally found in foods can be washed away or destroyed by processing. But processing can also add nutrients to foods. The addition of nutrients to foods is called **fortification.** The added nutrients may or may not have been present in the original food. **Enrichment** is a type of fortification in which nutrients are added for the purpose of restoring those lost in processing to the same or a higher level than originally present. Enrichment of grain products adds back the vitamins thiamin, niacin, and riboflavin and the mineral iron, but not all the nutrients lost in processing are restored by enrichment. Figure 8.2 illustrates the effect of milling and enrichment on the nutrient content of wheat flour. Foods that are staples of the diet are often fortified to prevent vitamin or mineral deficiencies and promote health in the population. For example, milk is fortified with vitamin D to promote bone health, and grains are fortified with folate to reduce the incidence of birth defects. Some foods are fortified because they are used in place of other foods that are good sources of an essential nutrient. For example, margarine is fortified

Fortification A term used generally to describe the addition of nutrients to foods, such as the addition of vitamin D to milk.

Enrichment A term used to describe the addition of nutrients to a food in order to restore those lost in processing to a level equal to or higher than that originally present.

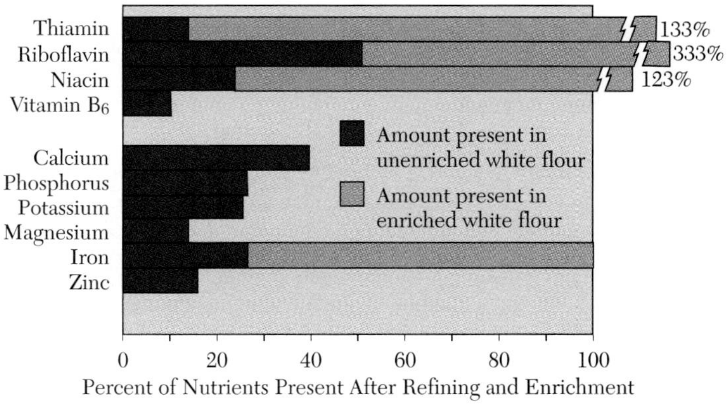

Figure 8.2
Many of the nutrients in whole grains are lost in refining, but only a few are added back in enrichment. This figure compares the amounts of some nutrients found in enriched and unenriched white flour with the amount in the whole wheat grain. The nutrients present in whole durum wheat are represented as 100%.

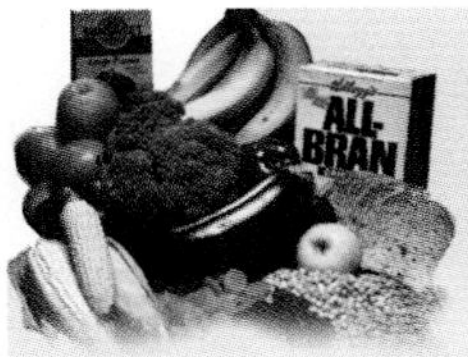

Off the Shelf

Maximizing the Vitamins in Your Vegetables

Heat, light, air, and the passage of time all cause vitamin loss from foods. Therefore, to optimize the nutrient content of your vegetables you should grow them yourself and pick them right before you are ready to eat them. This is probably not an option most of the time, but careful choices at the grocery store and proper storage and preparation techniques at home can significantly enhance the nutrient content of vegetables and other foods in your diet whether they are fresh, frozen, or canned.

When choosing fresh versus packaged foods, it is important to weigh the nutritional contribution the food makes to your diet against its convenience and availability. Fresh-picked vegetables are less available but provide more nutrients than frozen or canned vegetables. However, if the "fresh vegetable" has actually been a week in transport and another week in your refrigerator, frozen vegetables may actually supply more vitamins to your diet. Manufacturers of frozen vegetables often freeze their produce in the fields where it was grown, thereby maintaining most of the nutrients. The processing and heating of canned foods reduces their nutrient content. However, since canned foods keep for a long time, do not require refrigeration, and are often less expensive than fresh or frozen, they provide an available, affordable source of nutrients that may be the best choice in some situations.

Nutrients are lost with the passage of time, so where and how long foods are stored affect their nutrient content. Because heat increases losses, foods, whether canned or fresh, should be stored in a cool location. Even canned foods continue to lose vitamins on the shelf, especially at high temperatures. Fresh produce should be refrigerated and wrapped tightly to retain moisture and decrease exposure to air. For long storage, freezing is best. Fresh vegetables should be blanched before freezing to retain flavor and to stop enzyme activity that destroys vitamins.

Preparation techniques can also have a major impact on nutrient losses. Oxygen, light, and heat inactivate nutrients and water washes them away. To minimize exposure to oxygen and light, vegetables should not be cut up or cooked until the last minute. Also, the smaller the pieces into which they are cut before cooking, the greater the surface area exposed—and the

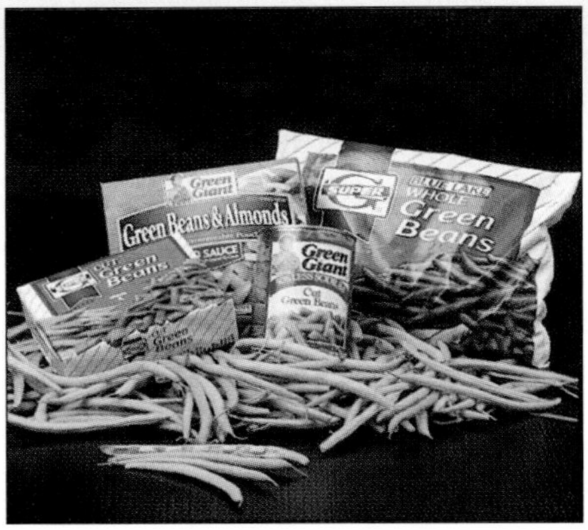

(George Semple)

greater the nutrient loss. To prevent water-soluble B vitamins and vitamin C from being washed down the drain, vegetables should not be soaked before cooking. Likewise, rice should not be washed before cooking because the water-soluble vitamins added in enrichment will be washed away. Frozen vegetables should not be thawed or washed before cooking.

Cooking technique, time, and temperature can also affect nutrient loss; the higher the temperature and the longer the

with vitamin A because it is often used instead of butter, which naturally contains vitamin A.

Supplements are another source of vitamins. While supplements provide specific nutrients, they do not provide all the benefits of foods. A pill that meets vitamin needs does not provide the energy, protein, minerals, fiber, or phytochemicals that would have been supplied by food sources of these vitamins (Figure 8.3). Supplements will be discussed with each nutrient and in greater depth at the end of Chapter 9.

Vitamins in the Digestive Tract

About 40 to 90% of the vitamins in food are absorbed, primarily in the small intestine (Figure 8.4). The composition of the diet and conditions in the body, however, may influence **bioavailability**—the amount of a nutrient that can be absorbed and utilized by the body. The bioavailability of a specific nutrient may also be affected by other foods and nutrients in the diet. For example, the amount of fat in the diet affects the bioavailability of fat-soluble vitamins because they are absorbed along with dietary fat. Fat-soluble vitamins are poorly absorbed when the diet is very low in fat. The mechanism by which vitamins are absorbed also determines the amount that enters the body. Fat-soluble vitamins are easily absorbed by simple diffusion. Many of the water-soluble vitamins depend on energy-requiring transport systems or binding molecules in the gastrointestinal tract

Bioavailability A general term that refers to how well a nutrient can be absorbed and used by the body.

heat is applied, the greater the loss. Cooking techniques that do not bring food into direct contact with water, such as steaming and pressure cooking, or dry heat such as roasting, grilling, stir-frying, or baking should be used. Vegetables should be cooked minimally so they remain slightly crisp. Pressure cookers can decrease cooking times for foods such as cabbage and beans that require longer cooking times. If foods are cooked in water, some of the vitamins can be retrieved by using cooking water to make soups and sauces. Microwave cooking is another option. Microwave cooking times are shorter and minimal water is used, both of which help preserve nutrients. For this reason, vitamin retention in microwaved vegetables is often higher than with conventional cooking.

To maximize your nutrient intake, use care in choosing, storing, and preparing vegetables and other foods. The choices you make at the store depend on availability, convenience, and economics. How you prepare foods depends on cooking facilities, taste preferences, time, and lifestyle. Even if fresh is best, it may not always be best for you.

Vitamin Losses in Handling

Vitamin	Causes of Loss
Thiamin	Exposure to heat, air, and neutral or low-acid conditions.
Riboflavin	Exposure to light, especially in moist and low-acid environments. Also destroyed by heat. When it is dry or in a food, it is more stable.
Niacin	Stable.
Biotin	Exposure to heat.
Pantothenic acid	Exposure to heat and low- or high-acid conditions.
Vitamin B_6	Exposure to heat and light.
Folate	Exposure to heat, air, light, and acid conditions.
Vitamin B_{12}	Exposure to air, light, and vitamin C.
Vitamin C	Exposure to light and heat, and contact with iron or copper cooking utensils. More stable in the presence of acid than in neutral or low-acid conditions, so citrus fruits maintain their vitamin C content longer than other sources. One of the most easily destroyed vitamins.
Vitamin A and beta-carotene	Exposure to air, light, and acid. Fairly stable in cooking.
Vitamin D	Exposure to air, light, heat, and low-acid conditions. Stable in cooking.
Vitamin E	High-temperature frying and exposure to light, air, and freezing.
Vitamin K	Exposure to light and low- or high-acid conditions.

in order to be absorbed. For example, thiamin and vitamin C are absorbed by energy-requiring transport systems, riboflavin and niacin require carrier proteins for absorption, and vitamin B_{12} must be bound to a protein produced in the stomach before it can be absorbed in the intestine.

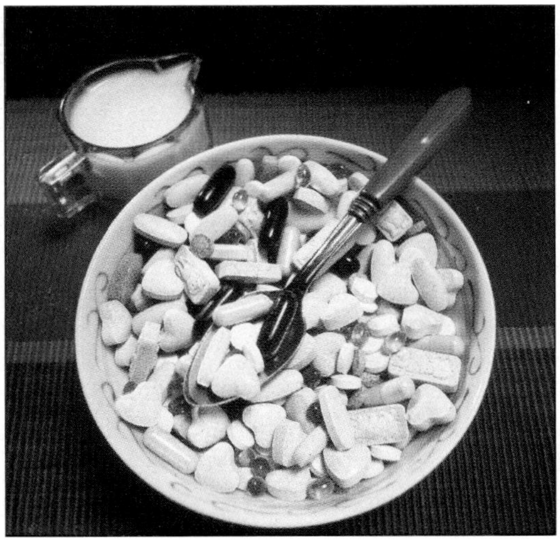

Figure 8.3
Vitamin supplements cannot take the place of a balanced diet. (Charles D. Winters)

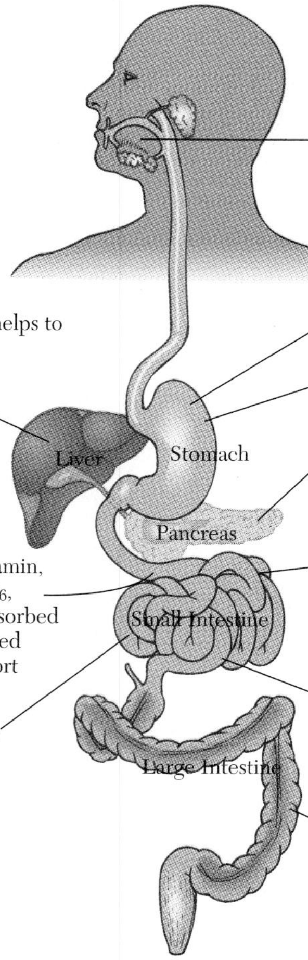

Chewing helps break apart fiber and release vitamins

Some niacin absorption

Digestive enzymes released by pancreas help to further release vitamins

Figure 8.4
An overview of vitamins in the digestive tract.

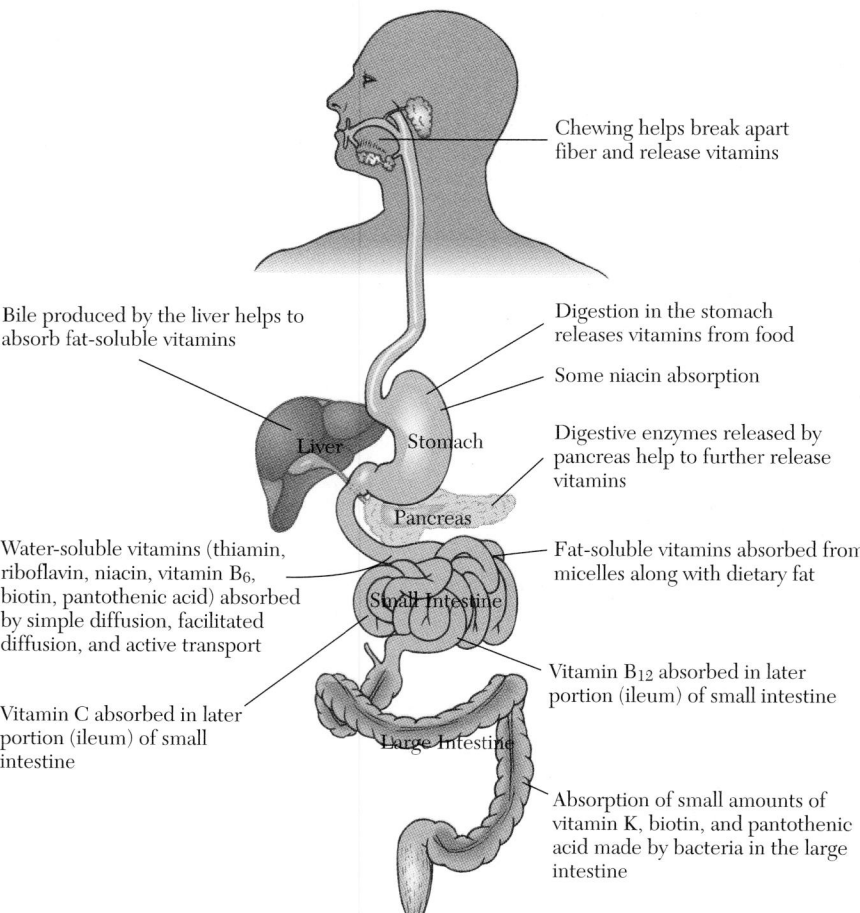

Provitamin or **vitamin precursor** A compound that can be converted into the active form of a vitamin in the body.

Some vitamins are absorbed in inactive **provitamin** or **vitamin precursor** forms that must be converted into active vitamin forms once inside the body. How much of each provitamin can be converted into the active vitamin and the rate at which this occurs determine the amount of a vitamin available to function in the body.

Vitamins in the Body

Coenzymes Small nonprotein organic molecules that act as carriers of electrons or atoms in metabolic reactions and are necessary for the proper functioning of many enzymes.

Vitamins promote and regulate body functions. For instance, vitamin C is essential for the synthesis of neurotransmitters, hormones, and a protein vital to the structure of connective tissue. Vitamin E functions as an antioxidant, vitamin A is needed for vision and affects cell maturation by altering how genes are expressed, vitamin D affects bone health, and vitamin K is needed for blood clotting. The B vitamins act as **coenzymes,** which are organic nonprotein substances that bind to enzymes to promote their activity (Figure 8.5). As coenzymes, B vitamins are essential to the proper functioning of numerous enzymes involved in the metabolism of the energy-containing nutrients.

Delivering Vitamins to Cells Once absorbed into the blood, vitamins must be transported to the cells. Despite their solubility in water, most of the water-soluble vitamins are bound to blood proteins for transport. Fat-soluble vitamins must be incorporated into lipoproteins or bound to transport proteins in order to be transported in the aqueous environment of the blood. For example, vitamins A, D, E, and K are all incorporated into chylomicrons for transport from the intestine. Vitamin A is stored in the liver, but it must be bound to a specific transport protein to be transported in the blood to other tissues; therefore, the amount delivered to the tissues depends on the availability of the transport protein. In protein deficiency, when sufficient amounts of the vitamin A transport protein are not available, vitamin A cannot be delivered to the cells where it is needed, even if it is adequate in the diet.

Excretion of the Vitamins The ability to store and excrete vitamins helps to regulate the amount present in the body. With the exception of vitamin B_{12}, the water-soluble vitamins are easily excreted from the body in the urine. Because they are not stored to any great extent, supplies of water-soluble vitamins are rapidly depleted and they must be consumed regularly in the diet. Nevertheless, it takes more than a few days to develop deficiency symptoms even when these vitamins are completely eliminated from the diet. Fat-soluble vitamins, on the other hand, are stored in the liver and fatty tissues and cannot be excreted in the urine. In general, because they are stored to a larger extent, it takes longer to develop a deficiency of fat-soluble vitamins when they are no longer provided by the diet.

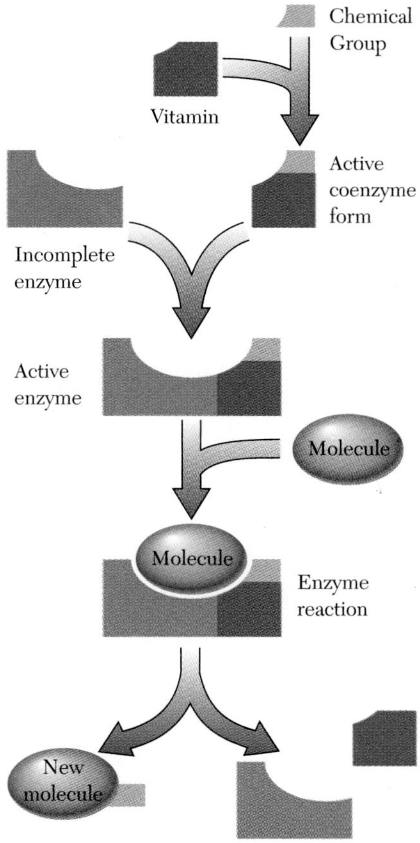

Figure 8.5
The B vitamins serve as coenzymes. The active coenzyme form of the vitamin is necessary for enzyme activity and acts as a carrier of chemical groups or electrons in the reaction.

How Much of Each Vitamin Do We Need?

As with other nutrients, the recommendations for vitamin intake for healthy populations in the United States and Canada are made by expert panels of the Dietary Reference Intake (DRI) committees (see Chapter 2). For each vitamin, these scientists review epidemiological data on current dietary intakes in North American populations and data from clinical trials, depletion-repletion studies, nutrient-balance studies, and biochemical and molecular biological studies.

Before an Estimated Average Requirement (EAR) and Recommended Dietary Allowance (RDA) or an Adequate Intake (AI) can be established, specific criteria upon which to base the adequacy of the nutrient are selected. These may include any parameter related to health and nutrient function, such as the amount of a nutrient or metabolite excreted in the urine, the level of a nutrient in the blood, or the activity of an enzyme dependent on that nutrient. The role of the nutrient in reducing disease risk is also taken into account. For example, the amount of a vitamin considered adequate may be defined as the amount that maintains normal blood levels and provides protection from a chronic condition such as cardiovascular disease. The requirements of each life stage and gender are considered separately.

The expert panels then use the criteria of adequacy and information about the vitamins' bioavailability to estimate the average requirement for the population—the EAR. The EAR value will meet the needs of 50% of the healthy population. This value is used to establish an RDA by increasing it to a level that will meet the needs of 97 to 98% of the healthy population. If sufficient information is not available to determine an EAR, an AI is set based on observed or experimentally determined estimates of the average intake in the healthy population. Therefore, for each vitamin and life stage, the DRIs include either an RDA value, when sufficient information is available, or an AI, when a recommendation is estimated from population data. Either of these values can be used as a goal for dietary intake by individuals.

The DRI subcommittees also establish Tolerable Upper Intake Levels (ULs) as a guide to the maximum amount of a vitamin that is unlikely to cause adverse health effects. For most vitamins the UL refers to total intake from foods, fortified foods, and nutrient supplements.

DRIs have not yet been finalized for some nutrients. For these, 1989 RDA values are available. When sufficient information was not available to establish a 1989 RDA, an **estimated safe and adequate daily dietary intake (ESADDI)** was set with the caution that the amounts at the upper level of the range should not be habitually exceeded. ESADDIs are not minimal requirements or optimal intakes, but rather recommended intakes that will prevent deficiencies in the majority of healthy individuals.

Estimated safe and adequate daily dietary intakes (ESADDIs) Recommended intakes of essential nutrients established when data were sufficient to estimate a range of requirements but insufficient to develop a 1989 RDA.

Vitamins and Health

Even though the last of the 13 compounds recognized as vitamins today was characterized in 1948, vitamin deficiencies remain a major public health problem in many parts of the world. Thousands of children in developing nations go blind due to vitamin A deficiency and have malformed bones from vitamin D deficiency. In industrialized countries, a more varied food supply, along with the fortification and enrichment of foods, has almost eliminated vitamin deficiency diseases in the majority of the population. Concern in these countries now focuses on meeting the needs of high-risk groups, evaluating the effects of marginal deficiencies, and assessing the risk of consuming toxic amounts from fortified foods and supplements.

Deficiency Groups at risk of deficiency include those whose requirements are increased, such as pregnant women and children, those whose intake is limited by financial or dietary restrictions, and those whose absorption or utilization is limited by a disease state. Mild deficiencies may also broadly impact public health. For example, mild deficiencies of vitamin B_6, folate, and vitamin B_{12} have been implicated as factors that increase the risk of cardiovascular disease and birth defects. Low intakes of fruits and vegetables that provide much of the vitamin C, vitamin E, beta-carotene, and phytochemicals in the diet may be increasing the rates of certain cancers and cardiovascular disease.

Toxicity The principle of "some is good so more must be better" does not universally apply in nutrition. Just as there is a minimum amount of a vitamin necessary to prevent deficiency, so is there a maximum level above which symptoms of toxicity are likely to occur. For years it was thought that only the fat-soluble vitamins could build up to toxic levels in the body and that excesses of water-soluble vitamins were merely excreted in the urine and could not reach toxic levels. However, as use of nutrient supplements became more popular, reports of toxicities of water-soluble vitamins, such as niacin and vitamin B_6, began to appear. If the popularity of vitamin supplements continues, toxicity symptoms are likely to become more common.

THE B VITAMINS AND ENERGY METABOLISM

Thiamin, riboflavin, niacin, pantothenic acid, and biotin all serve as coenzymes for reactions that release energy from carbohydrate, fat, and protein as well as alcohol (Figure 8.6). They are grouped together in this section because of this common role.

Thiamin

More than 4000 years ago, affluent members of Far Eastern societies began the practice of removing the outer hulls of rice to produce white or "polished" rice (Figure 8.7). As polished rice became the staple of the diet, the prevalence of the disease **beriberi** increased. A connection between diet and beriberi was not made until the late 19th century, when a surgeon in the Japanese navy demonstrated that shipboard beriberi could be prevented by the addition of meat and whole grains to the diet. These foods are now known to be good sources of thiamin.

Beriberi The disease resulting from a deficiency of thiamin.

Thiamin in the Diet Thiamin is widely distributed in foods. A large proportion of the thiamin consumed in the United States comes from enriched grains used in foods such as breakfast cereals and baked goods. Pork, whole grains, legumes,

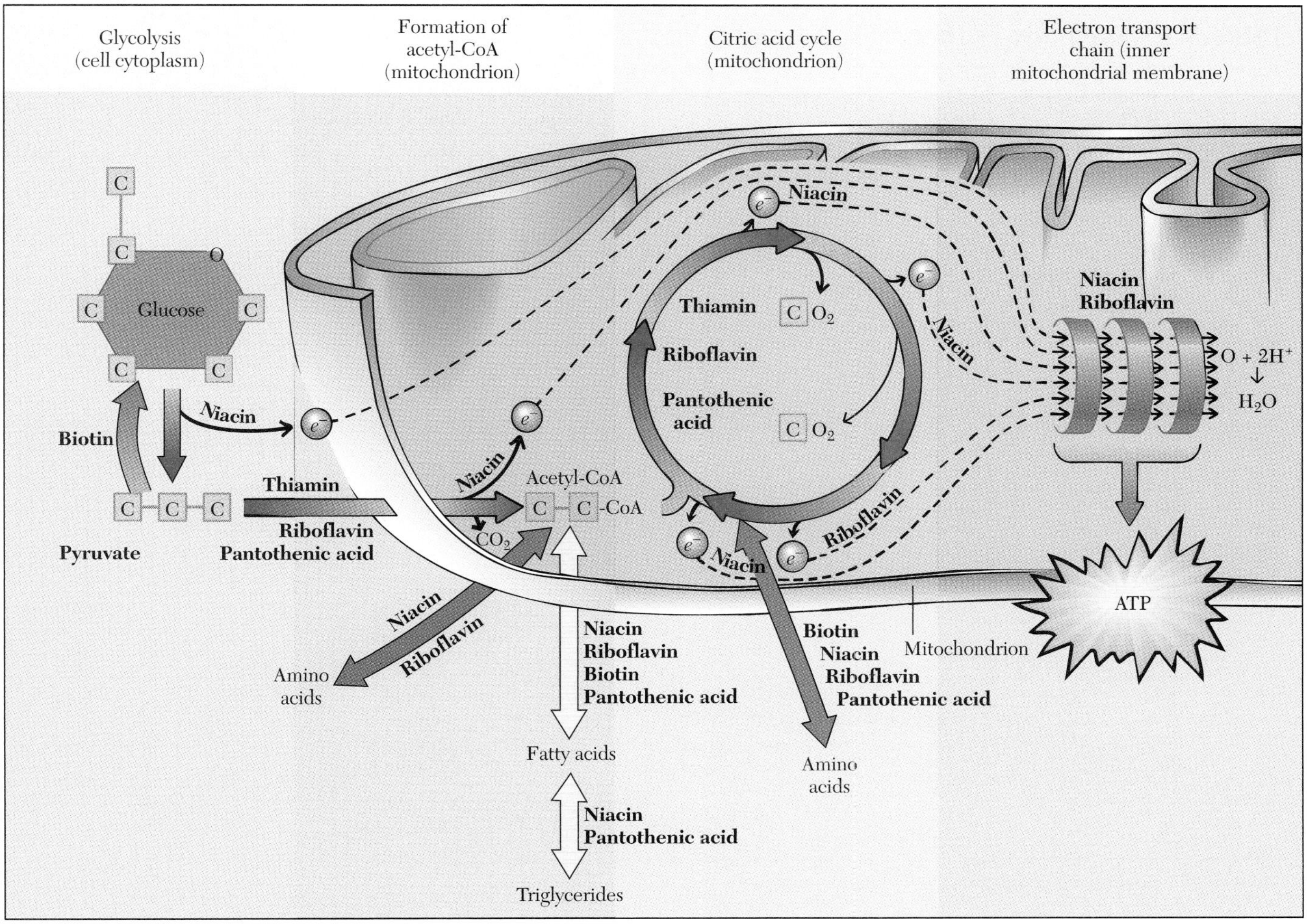

Figure 8.6
These are examples of metabolic reactions that require the vitamins thiamin, riboflavin, niacin, biotin, or pantothenic acid as coenzymes. These enzymes are particularly important for the production of energy from carbohydrate, fat, and protein.

nuts, seeds, and organ meats (liver, kidney, heart) are also good sources. The food groups that are good sources of dietary thiamin and the other B vitamins are summarized in Table 8.1.

Thiamin in foods may be destroyed during cooking or storage because it is sensitive to heat, oxygen, and low-acid conditions. Thiamin availability is also affected by the presence of antithiamin factors that destroy the vitamin. For instance, there are enzymes in raw shellfish and freshwater fish that degrade thiamin during food storage and preparation and during passage through the gastrointestinal tract. These enzymes are destroyed by cooking so they are only a concern in foods consumed raw. Other antithiamin factors that are not inactivated by cooking are found in tea, coffee, betel nuts, blueberries, and red cabbage. Because these make thiamin unavailable to the body, habitual consumption of foods containing antithiamin factors increases the risk of thiamin deficiency.[1]

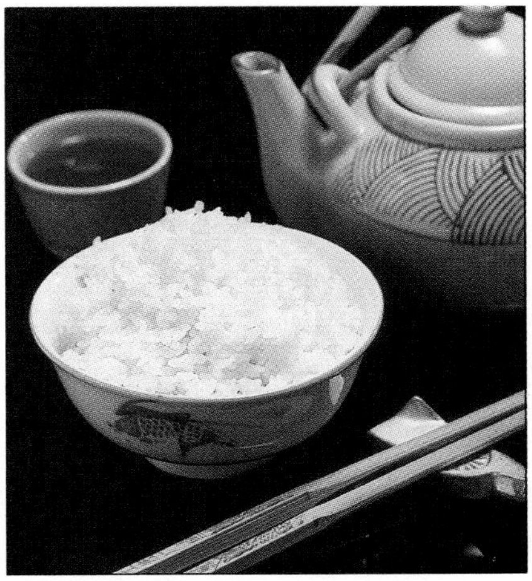

Figure 8.7
Unenriched white rice is a poor source of thiamin. (Charles D. Winters)

Thiamin in the Body Thiamin does not provide energy, but it is important in the energy-producing reactions in the body. The active form, thiamin pyrophosphate, is a coenzyme in reactions in which carbon dioxide is lost from larger molecules. For instance, the reaction that forms acetyl-CoA from pyruvate and one of the reactions of the citric acid cycle require thiamin pyrophosphate (see Figure 8.6). Thiamin is therefore essential to the production of energy from glucose.

Table 8.1 *Summary of Dietary Sources of B Vitamins**

Vitamin	Bread, Cereal, Rice, & Pasta Group	Vegetable Group	Fruit Group	Milk, Yogurt, & Cheese Group	Meat, Poultry, Fish, Dry Beans, Eggs, & Nuts Group			
					Meats	Dry Beans	Eggs	Nuts & Seeds
Thiamin	Whole and enriched grains				Pork, organ meats	Legumes		Sunflower seeds
Riboflavin	Whole and enriched grains	Mushrooms, asparagus, broccoli, leafy greens		Milk, cheeses	Liver, red meat, poultry, fish	Legumes	Eggs	
Niacin	Whole and enriched grains, wheat bran	Mushrooms, asparagus			Tuna, chicken, beef, turkey	Legumes, peanuts		Seeds
Biotin	Fortified cereals			Yogurt	Liver (muscle meats are poor sources)	Soybeans	Egg yolk	Nuts
Pantothenic acid	Whole grains	Mushrooms, broccoli, avocados			Meat	Legumes	Egg yolk	
Vitamin B_6	Whole wheat, brown rice	Broccoli, spinach	Bananas		Chicken, fish, pork, organ meats	Soybeans		Sunflower seeds
Folate	Fortified grains	Mushrooms, leafy greens, broccoli, asparagus, corn	Oranges (most fruits are poor sources)		Organ meats (muscle meats are poor sources)	Legumes		Nuts, sunflower seeds
Vitamin B_{12}				Milk products	Beef, poultry, fish, shellfish		Egg yolks	

*The colored boxes indicate food groups that provide a good source of each B vitamin.

Thiamin is also needed for the metabolism of other sugars and certain amino acids; the synthesis of the neurotransmitter acetylcholine; and the production of the sugar ribose, which is needed to synthesize RNA (ribonucleic acid).

How Much Thiamin Do We Need? The RDA for thiamin for adult men age 19 and older is set at 1.2 mg per day and for adult women 19 and older, at 1.1 mg per day. The RDA is based on the amount of thiamin needed to achieve and maintain normal activity of a thiamin-dependent enzyme found in red blood cells and normal urinary thiamin excretion.[2] For an average adult, half of the RDA can be obtained from 3 to 4 ounces (85 to 115 g) of pork or one-quarter cup of shelled sunflower seeds.

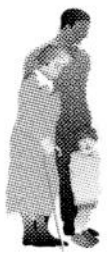

The requirement for thiamin is increased during pregnancy to accommodate the needs of growth and energy utilization, and during lactation to meet the need for both increased energy for milk production and to replace the thiamin secreted in milk. There is not enough information to establish an RDA for infants, so an AI has been set based on the thiamin intake of infants fed human milk.

Thiamin and Health In the United States today, neither thiamin deficiency nor toxicity is common in the general population. Thiamin deficiency is most often seen in chronic alcoholics.

Thiamin Deficiency Thiamin deficiency results in the disease beriberi. In Sri Lanka, the word "beriberi" literally means "I cannot," describing the extreme weakness and lassitude that occurs with this disease and reflecting the importance of this vitamin in energy metabolism.

Advanced beriberi also affects the nervous system and the cardiovascular system. Some, but not all, of these symptoms can be explained by the roles of thiamin in glucose metabolism and in the synthesis of the neurotransmitter acetylcholine. The earliest symptoms, depression and weakness, which occur after only about ten days on a thiamin-free diet, are probably related to the inability to completely use glucose. Since brain and nerve tissue rely on glucose for energy, the inability to form acetyl-CoA rapidly affects nervous system activity. Poor coordination, tingling in the arms and legs, and paralysis may also be caused by the lack of acetylcholine. It is not clear why thiamin deficiency causes cardiovascular symptoms such as heart failure.

Although overt beriberi is usually thought of as a disease of 19th-century Asia, there are population groups in North America today that are at a high risk for developing thiamin deficiency. Alcoholics are particularly vulnerable because thiamin absorption is decreased due to the effect of alcohol on the gastrointestinal tract. In addition, the liver damage that occurs with chronic alcohol consumption reduces conversion of thiamin to active coenzyme forms; thiamin intake also may be low due to a diet high in alcohol and low in nutrient-dense foods.[1] Thiamin-deficient alcoholics may develop a neurological condition known as the Wernicke-Korsakoff syndrome. It is characterized by mental confusion, psychosis, memory disturbances, and coma.

Thiamin Toxicity Since no toxicity has been reported when excess thiamin is consumed from either food or supplements, not enough information is available to establish a UL for thiamin intake.[2] This does not mean that high intakes are necessarily safe. Intakes of thiamin above the RDA have not been shown to provide health benefits.

Thiamin Supplements Thiamin supplements containing up to 50 mg per day are widely available and are marketed with the promise that they will provide "more energy." Although thiamin is needed to produce energy, it does not stimulate energy production. Unless thiamin is deficient, increasing thiamin intake does not increase the ability to produce energy. Because thiamin deficiency causes mental confusion and damages the heart, supplements often promise to improve mental function and prevent heart disease. However, in the absence of a deficiency, supplements do not have these effects.

A summary of the sources, recommended intakes, functions, deficiencies, and toxicities of thiamin and other water-soluble vitamins is provided in Table 8.2.

Riboflavin

While searching for a cure for beriberi, scientists also isolated riboflavin and several other B vitamins as well as thiamin. This occurred because the extracts they made from vegetables and grains could be separated into two components: One contained thiamin, the antiberiberi factor they sought, and cured beriberi; the other was a mix of B vitamins that was later determined to contain riboflavin along with vitamin B_6, niacin, and pantothenic acid.

Riboflavin in the Diet Milk is the best source of riboflavin in the North American diet. Other major sources include liver, red meat, poultry, fish, and whole grain and enriched breads and cereals. Vegetable sources include asparagus, broccoli, mushrooms, and leafy green vegetables such as spinach (see Table 8.1). Because riboflavin is destroyed by exposure to light, poor handling decreases a food's riboflavin content. This is a problem when milk is stored in clear containers

Table 8.2 *A Summary of the Water-Soluble Vitamins and Choline*

Vitamin	Sources	Recommended Intake for Adults	Major Functions	Deficiency	Groups at Risk	Toxicity	Tolerable Upper Intake Levels (UL)
Thiamin (vitamin B_1, thiamin mononitrate)	Pork, sunflower seeds, whole and enriched grains, legumes	**1.1–1.2 mg**	Coenzyme in glycolysis, citric acid cycle; nerve function	Beriberi: nerve tingling, poor coordination, weakness, heart changes	Alcoholics, those in poverty	None reported	ND
Riboflavin (vitamin B_2)	Milk, leafy greens, enriched grains	**1.1–1.3 mg**	Coenzyme in citric acid cycle, fat metabolism, electron transport chain	Inflammation of mouth and tongue	None	None reported	ND
Niacin (nicotinamide, nicotinic acid)	Enriched grains, peanuts, tuna, chicken, beef	**14–16 mg NE**	Coenzyme in glycolysis, electron transport chain, fat metabolism	Pellagra: dermatitis, diarrhea, dementia	Those consuming a limited diet high in corn products, alcoholics	Flushing, nausea, rash, tingling extremities	35 mg/d
Biotin	Liver, egg yolks, synthesized in the gut	30 μg*	Coenzyme in glucose production and fat synthesis	Dermatitis, nausea, depression, hallucinations	Those consuming large amounts of raw egg whites	Unknown	ND
Pantothenic acid (calcium pantothenate)	Meat, whole grains, legumes	5 mg*	Coenzyme in citric acid cycle, fat metabolism	Fatigue, rash	Alcoholics	Diarrhea, water retention	ND
Vitamin B_6 (pyridoxine, pyridoxine HCl, pyridoxal phosphate, pyridoxamine)	Meat, legumes, seeds, leafy greens, whole grains	**1.3–1.7 mg**	Coenzyme in protein metabolism, neurotransmitter and hemoglobin synthesis	Headache, neurologic symptoms, nausea, poor growth, anemia	Women, alcoholics	Nerve destruction	100 mg/d
Folate (folic acid, folacin)	Leafy greens, organ meats, legumes, orange juice	**400 μg DFE**	Coenzyme in RNA and DNA synthesis	Macrocytic anemia, inflammation of tongue, diarrhea, poor growth, neural tube defects	Pregnant women, alcoholics	Masks B_{12} deficiency	1000 μg/d
Vitamin B_{12} (cobalamin, cyanocobalamin)	Animal products	**2.4 μg**	Coenzyme in folate metabolism; nerve function	Pernicious anemia, macrocytic anemia, poor nerve function	Vegans, elderly, those with stomach or intestinal disease	None reported	ND
Vitamin C (ascorbic acid, sodium ascorbate, calcium ascorbate, magnesium ascorbate)	Citrus fruit, broccoli, strawberries, greens	60 mg†	Collagen synthesis, hormone and neurotransmitter synthesis, antioxidant	Scurvy: poor wound healing, bleeding gums	Alcoholics, elderly men	Diarrhea at intakes greater than 1–2 grams	NA
Choline	Egg yolks, organ meats, leafy greens, nuts	425–550 mg*	Synthesis of cell membranes and the neurotransmitter acetylcholine	Liver dysfunction	None	Sweating, reduced growth, low blood pressure, liver damage	3500 mg/d

Value in **bold** is a Recommended Dietary Allowance (RDA).
*Adequate Intake (AI).
†1989 RDA value.
ND—insufficient data to determine a UL.
NA—no UL established at time of publication.

and exposed to light. Cloudy plastic milk bottles block some light, partially protecting the riboflavin, but cardboard milk containers are better at preventing losses (Figure 8.8).[3]

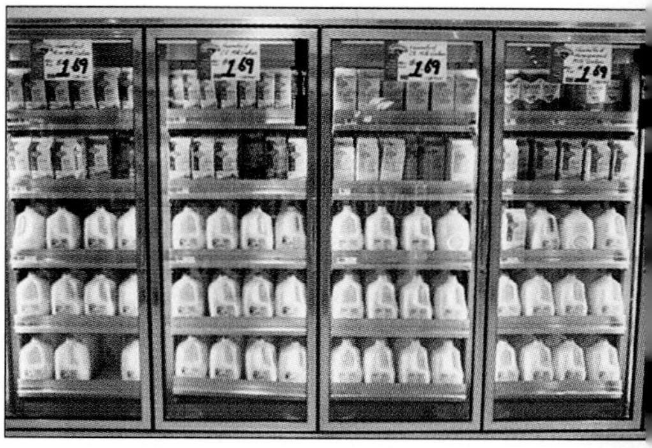

Figure 8.8
Milk in opaque containers is protected from riboflavin loss in lighted dairy cases. (Charles D. Winters)

Riboflavin in the Body Riboflavin forms the active coenzymes flavin mononucleotide (FMN) and flavin adenine dinucleotide (FAD). FAD functions in the citric acid cycle and is important for the breakdown of fatty acids. Both FMN and FAD function as electron carriers in the electron transport chain (see Figure 8.6). Therefore, adequate riboflavin is crucial in producing energy from carbohydrate, fat, and protein. Riboflavin is also involved directly or indirectly in converting a number of other vitamins, including folate, niacin, vitamin B_6, and vitamin K, into their active forms.

How Much Riboflavin Do We Need? The RDA for riboflavin for adult men age 19 and older is 1.3 mg per day and for adult women 19 and older, 1.1 mg per day. This recommendation is based on the amount of riboflavin needed to maintain normal activity of a riboflavin-dependent enzyme in red blood cells and normal riboflavin excretion in the urine.[2] Two cups of milk provide about half the amount of riboflavin recommended for a typical adult. The recommended intake can be met without milk if the daily diet includes two to three servings of meat and four to five servings of enriched grain products and high-riboflavin vegetables, such as spinach.

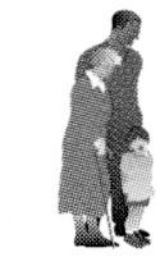

Additional riboflavin is recommended during pregnancy to support growth and increased energy utilization, and during lactation to allow for the riboflavin secreted in milk. There is not enough information to establish an RDA for infants, so an AI has been set based on the amount of riboflavin consumed by infants fed human milk.

Riboflavin and Health For the average healthy American, there is little risk of either riboflavin deficiency or toxicity. Worldwide, there are minor signs of deficiency, usually in combination with other deficiencies of water-soluble vitamins.[4]

Riboflavin Deficiency When riboflavin is deficient, injuries heal poorly because new cells cannot grow to replace the damaged ones. Tissues that grow most rapidly, such as the skin and the linings of the eyes, mouth, and tongue, are the first to be affected by a deficiency.[5] Symptoms of riboflavin deficiency, called **ariboflavinosis,** include inflammation of the eyes, lips, mouth, and tongue; scaly, greasy skin eruptions; cracking of the tissue at the corners of the mouth; and confusion. Deficiency symptoms may develop after approximately two months on a riboflavin-poor diet.

Ariboflavinosis The condition resulting from a deficiency of riboflavin.

A deficiency of riboflavin is rarely seen alone. It usually occurs in conjunction with deficiencies of other B vitamins. One reason is that the food sources of B vitamins are similar (see Table 8.1). Therefore, a deficiency due to poor diet will likely lead to multiple vitamin deficiencies. Because riboflavin is needed to convert other vitamins into their active forms, some of the symptoms seen with riboflavin deficiency are actually due to deficiencies of these other nutrients.

Riboflavin Toxicity No adverse effects have been reported from overconsumption of riboflavin from foods or supplements and there are not sufficient data to establish a UL for this vitamin. Large doses of riboflavin are not well absorbed and it is readily excreted in the urine.[6] A harmless side effect of high riboflavin intakes, such as may be obtained from over-the-counter supplements, is bright yellow urine.

Riboflavin Supplements As with thiamin, the role of riboflavin in energy production has led to claims that supplements containing riboflavin will provide an energy boost. Although riboflavin is needed for energy production, it does not provide energy. Since a deficiency causes skin and eye symptoms, riboflavin has also been suggested as a cure for eye diseases and skin disorders. However, in the absence of a deficiency, supplementation does not affect the eyes or skin.

Niacin

Pellagra The disease resulting from a deficiency of niacin.

In the early 1900s, psychiatric hospitals in the southeastern United States were filled with patients in the advanced stages of **pellagra,** the disease resulting from a deficiency of niacin. These individuals were institutionalized with dementia, a late symptom of pellagra, which led to a diagnosis of mental illness. In response to the pellagra epidemic, in 1909 the U.S. Public Health Service sent Dr. Joseph Goldberger to investigate. Goldberger believed that pellagra was due to a nutritional deficiency. To prove this, he conducted a study in which 12 convicts, promised pardons for their cooperation, were fed diets suspected of causing pellagra; 6 developed the disease. Proof that pellagra was not an infectious disease was provided by Goldberger and his coworkers, who tried to infect themselves with pellagra by ingesting blood, nasal secretions, feces, and urine from patients with the disease. None of them contracted pellagra. Goldberger was able to prevent and cure pellagra by improving the diets of patients in mental institutions. Nevertheless, pellagra remained a common problem among the southern poor who consumed a diet of primarily corn meal, molasses, and fatback or salt pork—all poor sources of niacin. A federally sponsored program was begun in 1941 to enrich grains, including corn meal, with niacin, thiamin, and riboflavin. This helped eliminate the pellagra epidemic in the United States.[7]

Niacin in the Diet Meat and fish are good sources of niacin. Other sources include legumes, mushrooms, wheat bran, asparagus, and peanuts. Niacin added to enriched flours and baked goods provides much of the usable niacin in the North American diet. Niacin can also be synthesized in the body from the essential amino acid tryptophan. In a diet that contains high-protein foods such as milk and eggs, which are poor sources of niacin but good sources of tryptophan, much of the need for niacin can be met by tryptophan. Tryptophan, however, is only used to make niacin if enough is available to first meet the needs of protein synthesis. When the diet is low in tryptophan, it is not used to synthesize niacin. Food composition tables and databases list only preformed niacin in a food, not the amount of niacin that can be made from tryptophan contained within the food.

Historically, the appearance of niacin deficiency has been associated with a predominantly corn diet. This has been attributed to the low-tryptophan content of corn and the fact that the niacin found naturally in corn (and to a lesser extent in other cereal grains) is bound to other molecules and therefore not well absorbed. The treatment of corn with lime water (water and calcium hydroxide), as is done in Mexico and Central America during the making of tortillas, enhances the availability of niacin (Figure 8.9). As a result, populations that consume corn treated with lime water rarely suffer from pellagra. Today, pellagra remains common in India and parts of China and Africa. Efforts to eradicate this deficiency include the development of new varieties of corn that provide more available niacin and more tryptophan than traditional varieties.

Niacin in the Body Niacin is important in the production of energy from the energy-containing nutrients as well as in reactions that synthesize other molecules. There are two forms of niacin: nicotinic acid and nicotinamide. Either form can be used by the body to make the two active coenzymes nicotinamide adenine dinucleotide (NAD) and nicotinamide adenine dinucleotide phosphate (NADP). NAD functions in glycolysis and the citric acid cycle, accepting released electrons and passing them on to the electron transport chain where ATP is formed (see Figure 8.6). NADP acts as an electron carrier in reactions that synthesize fatty acids and cholesterol. The need for niacin is so widespread in metabolism that a deficiency causes major changes throughout the body.

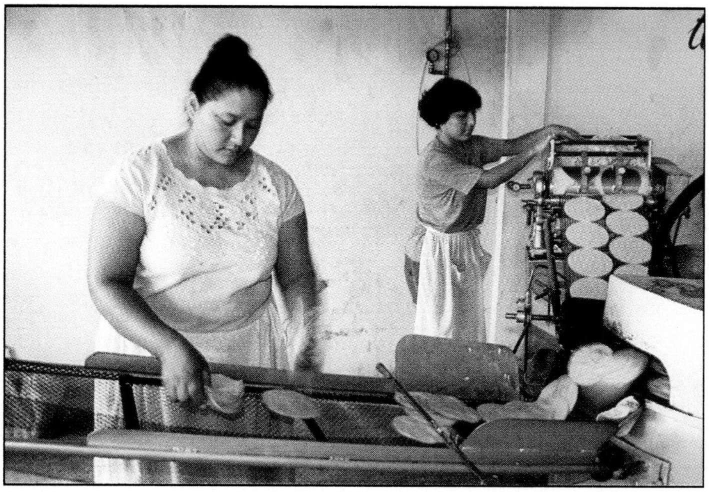

Figure 8.9
The treatment of corn with lime water during the preparation of tortillas makes niacin available and has prevented pellagra in Mexico and other Latin American countries. (© Jeff Greenberg/Photo Researchers, Inc.)

How Much Niacin Do We Need? The RDA for niacin is expressed as **niacin equivalents (NEs).** One NE is equal to 1 mg of niacin or 60 mg of tryptophan. This allows for the fact that some of the requirement for niacin can be met by the synthesis of niacin from tryptophan. Approximately 60 mg of tryptophan is needed to make 1 mg of niacin. To estimate the niacin contributed by high-protein foods, protein is considered to be about 1% tryptophan. The criterion used to estimate average niacin requirement is urinary excretion of niacin metabolites. The RDA for adult men and women of all ages is 16 and 14 mg NE per day respectively.[2] A meal of a medium chicken breast and a cup of steamed asparagus provides this amount.

Niacin equivalents (NEs) Used to express the amount of niacin present in food, including that which can be made from its precursor, tryptophan. One NE is equal to 1 mg of niacin or 60 mg of tryptophan.

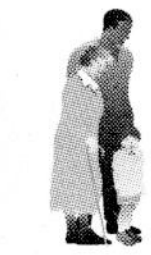

Niacin needs are increased in pregnancy to account for the increase in energy expenditure, and in lactation to account for both the increase in energy expenditure and the niacin secreted in milk. There is not enough information to establish an RDA for infants, so an AI has been set based on the amount of niacin found in human milk.

Niacin and Health Niacin deficiency is no longer of public health concern in the United States, but excessive intakes of niacin can be toxic. Despite this, niacin is a commonly used vitamin supplement.

Niacin Deficiency The early symptoms of pellagra include fatigue, decreased appetite, and indigestion, followed by the four Ds: dermatitis, diarrhea, dementia, and, ultimately, death. The dermatitis resembles sunburn and strikes parts of the body exposed to sunlight, heat, or injury. Gastrointestinal symptoms include a bright-red tongue and may include vomiting, constipation, or diarrhea. Mental symptoms begin with irritability, headaches, loss of memory, insomnia, and emotional instability and progress to psychosis, acute delirium, and eventually coma and death.

Niacin Toxicity There is no evidence of any adverse effects from consumption of niacin naturally occurring in foods, but supplements can be toxic. The adverse effects of high intakes of niacin include flushing of the skin, a tingling sensation in the hands and feet, a red skin rash, nausea, vomiting, diarrhea, high blood sugar levels, abnormalities in liver function, and blurred vision.[8] Since flushing is the first toxicity symptom to appear as the dose is increased, the UL for adults was set at 35 mg, the highest level that is unlikely to cause flushing in the majority of healthy people. This value applies to the forms of niacin contained in supplements and fortified foods, but does not include niacin naturally occurring in foods.

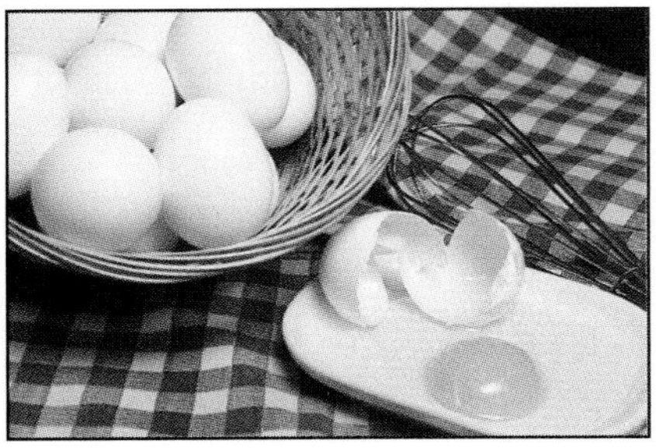

Figure 8.10
Egg yolks are a good source of biotin, but raw egg whites contain a protein that binds biotin, making it unavailable. (Gregory Smolin)

Niacin Supplements Unlike thiamin and riboflavin, which are touted for enhancing energy and mental capacity, high doses of niacin as supplements have been promoted to treat elevated blood cholesterol and to prevent or delay type 1 diabetes. When vitamins are taken in large doses to treat diseases that are not due to vitamin deficiencies, they are really being used as drugs rather than vitamins.

Doses of 50 mg per day or greater of the nicotinic acid form of niacin have been found to decrease blood levels of LDL cholesterol and triglycerides and increase HDL cholesterol. They are also associated with a reduction in recurrent heart attacks and deaths in individuals with cardiovascular disease[9] (see Chapter 5, *Off the Shelf: Are Supplements a Safe Way to Reduce Blood Cholesterol?*). Unfortunately, many people experience toxicity symptoms such as gastrointestinal distress, skin flushing, and liver abnormalities. Time-release niacin supplements have been developed to reduce these side effects. However, recent studies have shown that although these preparations slightly decrease skin flushing, they are still likely to cause gastrointestinal distress and abnormal liver function.[10] Supplements containing high doses of niacin should be used only with medical supervision.

Large doses (about 1–2 g/day) of the nicotinamide form of niacin are currently under investigation for preventing or delaying the onset of type 1 diabetes.[11] Type 1 diabetes is an autoimmune disease in which the body's immune system destroys the insulin-producing cells in the pancreas. Some but not all studies completed thus far have indicated that nicotinamide is beneficial in preserving pancreatic cell function, thus delaying the onset of type 1 diabetes.[12–14] Nicotinamide may also have beneficial effects in the treatment of type 2 diabetes.[15]

Biotin

Biotin was discovered when rats fed protein derived from raw egg white developed a syndrome of hair loss, dermatitis, and neuromuscular dysfunction. This deficiency of biotin was caused by a protein in raw egg white, called avidin, that tightly binds biotin and prevents its absorption (Figure 8.10).

Biotin in the Diet Good sources of biotin include liver, egg yolks, yogurt, and nuts. Fruit and meat are poor sources. Foods containing raw egg whites should be avoided not only because avidin binds biotin and prevents its absorption, but because raw eggs also may be contaminated with bacteria that can cause food-borne illness. Thoroughly cooking eggs destroys bacteria and denatures avidin so that it cannot bind biotin.

Biotin in the Body Biotin is a coenzyme for a group of enzymes that add the acid group COOH to molecules. It functions in energy production because it is needed to make a 4-carbon molecule necessary in the citric acid cycle and in glucose synthesis. It is also important in the metabolism of fatty acids and amino acids (see Figure 8.6).

How Much Biotin Do We Need? It is difficult to estimate a biotin requirement because some biotin is produced by bacteria in the gastrointestinal tract and absorbed into the body. No RDA could be determined for biotin, but an AI of 30 μg per day has been established for adult men and women based on the amount of biotin found in a typical North American diet (see Table 8.2).

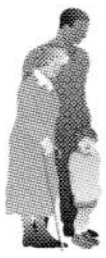

No additional biotin is recommended for pregnancy, but the AI is increased during lactation to account for the amount secreted in milk. The AI for infants is based on the amount of biotin consumed by infants fed human milk.

Biotin and Health Although biotin deficiency is uncommon, it has been observed in people with malabsorption or protein-energy malnutrition, those receiving tube feedings or total parenteral nutrition without biotin, those taking anticonvulsant drugs for long periods, and those frequently consuming raw egg whites.[16,17] When biotin intake is deficient, symptoms including nausea, thinning hair, loss of hair color, a red skin rash, depression, lethargy, hallucinations, and tingling of the extremities gradually appear.

No toxicity has been reported in patients given 200 mg per day of biotin to treat various disease states, and sufficient data are not available to establish a UL.[2]

Pantothenic Acid

Pantothenic acid, which gets its name from the Greek word *pantos* (meaning "from everywhere"), is widely distributed in foods.

Pantothenic Acid in the Diet Pantothenic acid is particularly abundant in meat, eggs, whole grains, and legumes. It is found in lesser amounts in milk, vegetables, and fruits.

Pantothenic Acid in the Body Pantothenic acid is part of coenzyme A (CoA), which is part of acetyl-CoA, a molecule formed during the breakdown of carbohydrates, fatty acids, and amino acids. Pantothenic acid is also needed to produce acyl carrier protein needed for the synthesis of cholesterol and fatty acids (see Figure 8.6).

How Much Pantothenic Acid Do We Need? There is no RDA for pantothenic acid, but an AI of 5 mg per day has been recommended for adult men and women.[2] This value is based on the intake of pantothenic acid sufficient to replace urinary losses. The AI is increased to 6 and 7 mg per day to meet the needs of pregnancy and lactation, respectively.

Pantothenic Acid and Health The wide distribution of pantothenic acid in foods makes deficiency rare in humans. A deficiency of this vitamin alone has not been reported, but it may occur as part of a multiple B vitamin deficiency resulting from malnutrition or chronic alcoholism.

Pantothenic acid is relatively nontoxic. No toxic symptoms were reported in a study that fed young men 10 grams of pantothenic acid per day for 6 weeks. Another study found that doses of 10 to 20 grams per day may result in diarrhea and water retention.[18] Data are not sufficient to establish a UL for pantothenic acid.

Vitamin B_6 and Protein Metabolism

Vitamin B_6 was identified only when a deficiency syndrome was discovered that did not respond to thiamin or riboflavin supplementation. It is essential for releasing energy from amino acids, so it—like thiamin, riboflavin, niacin, biotin, and pantothenic acid—can be considered an energy-releasing nutrient; but the important role of vitamin B_6 in amino acid metabolism distinguishes it from the other B vitamins.

Vitamin B_6 in the Diet

Vitamin B_6 is found in both animal and plant foods. Animal sources include chicken, fish, pork, and organ meats. Good plant sources include whole wheat products, brown rice, soybeans, sunflower seeds, and some fruits and vegetables such as bananas, broccoli, and spinach. Vitamin B_6 is easily destroyed in processing. It is not added back in the enrichment of grain products, but fortified breakfast cereals make an important contribution to vitamin B_6 intake.[19]

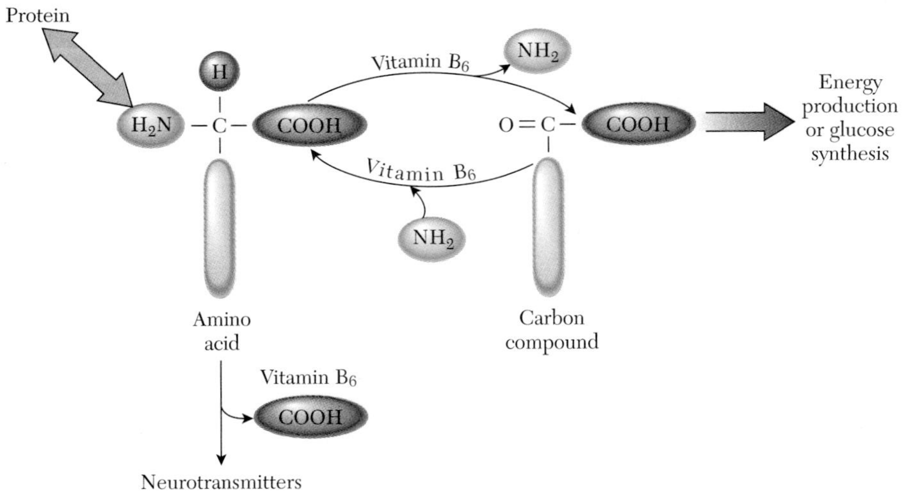

Figure 8.11
Vitamin B_6 is needed to synthesize nonessential amino acids by transamination, to remove the amino group so amino acids can be used to produce energy or to synthesize glucose, to remove the COOH group from amino acids for the synthesis of neurotransmitters, and for many other reactions of amino acid metabolism.

Vitamin B_6 in the Body

Pyridoxine The chemical term for vitamin B_6.

Vitamin B_6, also known as **pyridoxine,** comprises a group of compounds including pyridoxal, pyridoxine, and pyridoxamine. All three forms can be converted into the active coenzyme form, pyridoxal phosphate. Pyridoxal phosphate is needed for the activity of more than 100 enzymes involved in the metabolism of carbohydrate, fat, and protein. It is particularly important for protein and amino acid metabolism (Figure 8.11). Without pyridoxal phosphate, the nonessential amino acids cannot be synthesized and the semiessential amino acid cysteine cannot be synthesized from methionine. Pyridoxal phosphate is needed to synthesize hemoglobin, the oxygen-carrying protein in red blood cells. Pyridoxal phosphate is important for the immune system because it is needed to form white blood cells. It is also needed for the conversion of tryptophan to niacin, the metabolism of glycogen, the synthesis of certain neurotransmitters, and the synthesis of the lipids that are part of the myelin coating on nerves.

How Much Vitamin B_6 Do We Need?

The RDA for vitamin B_6 is 1.3 mg per day for both adult men and women 19 to 50 years of age.[2] This is the amount needed to maintain adequate blood concentrations of the active coenzyme pyridoxal phosphate. In adults 51 years and older, the RDA is increased to 1.7 mg per day in men and 1.5 mg per day in women to maintain normal blood pyridoxal phosphate. A 3-ounce (85-g) serving of chicken, fish, or pork, or half a baked potato, provides about a quarter of the RDA for an average adult; a banana provides about one third.

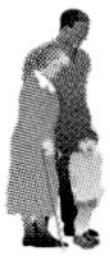

The RDA for vitamin B_6 is increased during pregnancy to allow for metabolic needs and growth of the mother and fetus. Because the vitamin B_6 concentration in breast milk is dependent on the mother's intake, the RDA is increased during lactation to assure adequate levels are supplied to the infant.[20] There is no RDA for infants, but an AI has been established based on the vitamin B_6 content of human milk.

Vitamin B_6 and Health

A vitamin B_6 deficiency syndrome was defined in 1954 when an infant formula was overheated in manufacture, destroying the vitamin B_6. The infants who consumed only this formula developed abdominal distress, convulsions, and other neurological symptoms.[21] No adverse effects have been associated with high intakes of vitamin B_6 from foods, but large doses found in supplements can cause serious toxicity symptoms.

Vitamin B_6 Deficiency Vitamin B_6 deficiency causes neurological symptoms including depression, headaches, confusion, numbness and tingling in the extremities, and seizures. These may be related to the the role of vitamin B_6 in neurotransmitter synthesis and myelin formation. Anemia also occurs in vitamin B_6 deficiency due to impaired hemoglobin synthesis; red blood cells are small (microcytic) and pale (hypochromic) due to the lack of hemoglobin. Other deficiency symptoms such as poor growth, skin lesions, and decreased antibody formation may occur because vitamin B_6 is important in protein and energy metabolism. Since vitamin B_6 is needed for amino acid metabolism, the onset of a deficiency can be hastened by a diet that is low in vitamin B_6 but high in protein.

Vitamin B_6 status in the body can be affected by a number of drugs, including alcohol and oral contraceptives. Alcohol decreases the formation of the active coenzyme pyridoxal phosphate and makes it more susceptible to breakdown. Oral contraceptive use has been associated with small decreases in blood levels of pyridoxal phosphate. But, vitamin B_6 supplements are not routinely recommended for women taking oral contraceptives.[2]

Vitamin B_6 Toxicity In the 1980s, there were reports of severe nerve impairment in individuals taking 2 to 6 grams of pyridoxine per day.[22] Some subjects were unable to walk. These symptoms improved when the pyridoxine supplements were stopped. The UL is based on an amount that will not cause nerve damage in the majority of healthy people. For adults it is set at 100 mg per day from food and supplements.[2] Since high-dose supplements of vitamin B_6 containing 100 mg per dose (5000% of the Daily Value) are available over the counter, it is easy to obtain a dose that exceeds the UL.

Vitamin B_6 Supplements Supplements of vitamin B_6 are marketed to help a wide variety of ailments ranging from cardiovascular disease and carpal tunnel syndrome to premenstrual syndrome (PMS) and poor immune function. Some of these marketing claims are founded in science, but others are exaggerated to sell products. Whatever the reason for considering vitamin B_6 supplements, one should use them with care to reduce the risk of toxicity.

A Consideration in Cardiovascular Disease? It has been hypothesized that vitamin B_6 affects the risk of heart disease through its role in the breakdown of homocysteine, an intermediate in methionine metabolism (Figure 8.12). Individuals with a rare genetic disorder that causes chronically high blood levels of homocysteine develop atherosclerosis at an early age. Large doses of vitamin B_6 (100–1000 mg/day) have been successfully used to reduce elevated homocysteine and the risk of atherosclerosis in these patients.[23]

In the normal population, a mild elevation in blood homocysteine has been shown to be a risk factor for cardiovascular disease.[24,25] It is estimated that about 10% of the risk of developing cardiovascular disease in the general population is due to high homocysteine levels.[26] It has been proposed that a deficiency of vitamin B_6, vitamin B_{12}, or folate, the latter two of which are also involved in homocysteine metabolism, may cause homocysteine accumulation and eventually lead to atherosclerosis. A study that examined the effect of folate and vitamin B_6 intake in women found that those with the highest levels of folate and vitamin B_6 in their diets (from food and supplements) had about half the risk of coronary heart disease as women with the lowest levels.[27] Supplements of all three of these vitamins have been used to reduce homocysteine levels in individuals with mild homocysteine elevation.[28] At this time however, the DRI panel believes that it is premature to conclude that increased intake of vitamin B_6, vitamin B_{12}, or folate could decrease the risk of cardiovascular disease.[2]

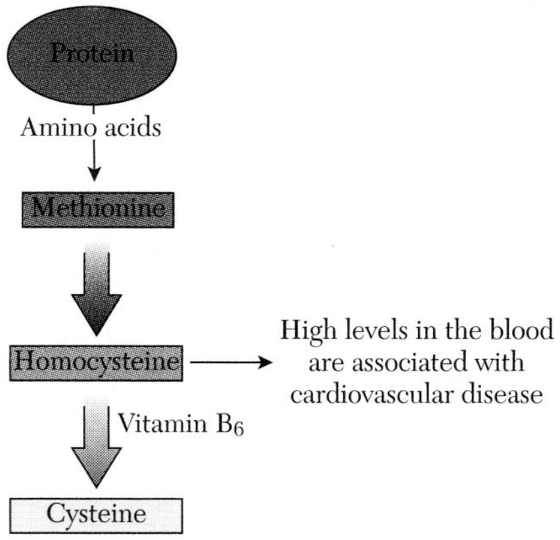

Figure 8.12
Vitamin B_6 is needed to convert homocysteine to cysteine. If vitamin B_6 is deficient, homocysteine can accumulate, increasing the risk of cardiovascular disease.

A Cure for Carpal Tunnel Syndrome? Vitamin B_6 has been suggested to be useful in treating a condition called carpal tunnel syndrome, in which pressure on the nerves in the hand causes pain and weakness. Studies have not found a relationship between carpal tunnel syndrome and vitamin B_6 status.[29] In some patients, supplements have been found to reduce pain, but there is little evidence to support the use of vitamin B_6 supplements as a treatment for carpal tunnel syndrome. Such treatment has the potential to be hazardous given the toxic effects of high doses of B_6.[30]

The PMS Promise? Premenstrual syndrome (PMS) causes mood swings, food cravings, bloating, tension, depression, headaches, acne, breast tenderness, anxiety, temper outbursts, and over 100 other symptoms. Supplements of vitamin B_6 are frequently taken in attempts to alleviate these symptoms. The proposed connection is the fact that vitamin B_6 is needed for the synthesis of the neurotransmitters serotonin and dopamine. Insufficient vitamin B_6 has been suggested to reduce levels of these neurotransmitters and cause the anxiety, irritability, and depression associated with PMS. Some studies have shown a reduction in PMS symptoms with vitamin B_6 supplements of 100 to 500 mg per day.[31] However, similar studies using approximately the same doses of vitamin B_6 have shown no effect. This inconsistency may be because studies did not use enough study subjects to ensure reliable results.[32]

Immune System Improver? Immune function can be impaired by a deficiency of any nutrient that hinders cell growth and division. Therefore, one of the most common claims for vitamin supplements in general is that they improve immune function. Vitamin B_6 is no exception. Vitamin B_6 supplements have been found to improve immune function in older adults.[33] However, since the elderly frequently have low intakes of vitamin B_6, it is unclear whether the beneficial effects of supplements are due to an improvement in vitamin B_6 status or immune system stimulation.

FOLATE, VITAMIN B_{12}, AND CELL DIVISION

The B vitamins folate and vitamin B_{12} have overlapping roles in the synthesis of DNA, which is required for cells to divide. Therefore, some of the same symptoms are seen in severe deficiency of either vitamin—most notably anemia. This type of anemia occurs because developing red blood cells cannot divide. Marginal deficiencies of these nutrients are a modern concern, particularly for two life-stage groups—women of childbearing age and the elderly.

Folate or Folic Acid

It has been known for over a hundred years that anemia often occurs during pregnancy. In 1937, anemia in a pregnant woman was successfully treated with a yeast preparation named Wills Factor, after the Dr. Wills who treated this patient. The Wills Factor was later isolated from spinach and named folate, after the Latin word for foliage. Folate is a general term for the many chemical forms of this vitamin. Folic acid is a stable form of folate that rarely occurs naturally in food but is used in vitamin supplements and fortified foods. An increased intake of folic acid is recommended before and during early pregnancy, to reduce the incidence of **neural tube defects.**[34]

Neural tube defects Abnormalities in the brain or spinal cord that result from errors that occur during prenatal development.

Folate in the Diet Excellent food sources of folate include liver, yeast, asparagus, oranges, legumes, and fortified grain products. Fair sources include vegetables such as corn, snap beans, mustard greens, and broccoli, as well as some nuts. Small amounts are found in meats, cheese, milk, fruits, and other vegetables (Figure 8.13).

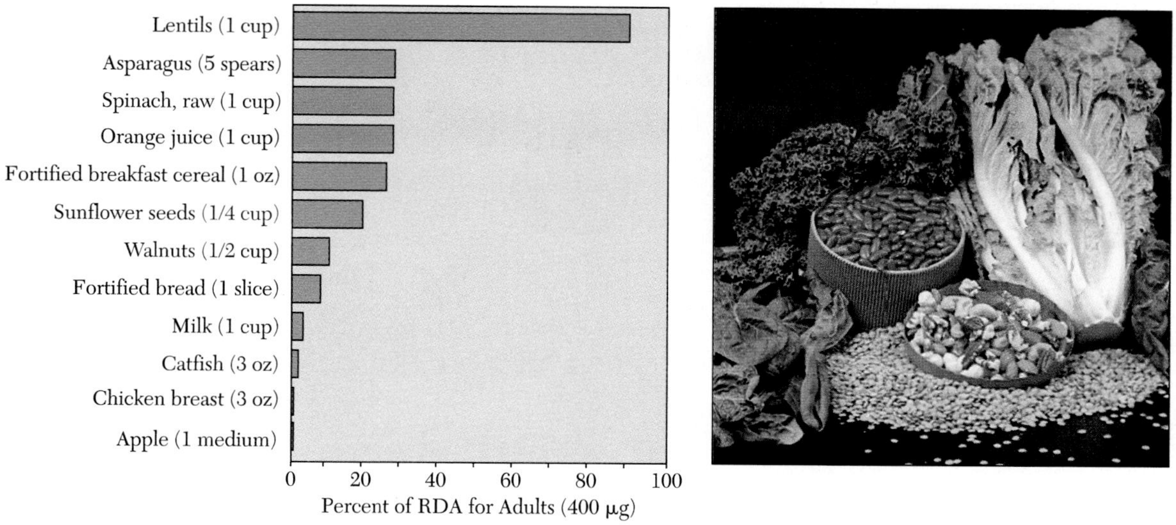

Figure 8.13
The folate content of foods as a percent of the RDA for adults (400 μg). (*right,* George Semple)

The bioavailability of folate found naturally in food is only about half that of the synthetic folic acid added to fortified grain products and used in supplements. The fortification of grain products, including enriched breads, flours, corn meal, pasta, grits, and rice, with folic acid has been required since January 1998. Fortified foods provide 140 μg of folic acid per 100 grams of flour used in the product.[2]

Folate in the Body There are a number of different active coenzyme forms of folate that are involved in reactions that transfer chemical groups containing a single carbon atom. Folate coenzymes are needed for the synthesis of DNA and RNA and the metabolism of some amino acids. Before a cell divides, its DNA must replicate. Therefore, the role of folate in DNA synthesis makes it particularly important during periods of rapid growth, such as early in embryonic life, and in tissues where cells are rapidly dividing, such as bone marrow, where red blood cells are made, intestines, and skin.

How Much Folate Do We Need? The adult RDA for folate is set at 400 μg **dietary folate equivalents (DFEs)** per day for adult men and women. One DFE is equal to 1 μg of food folate, 0.6 μg of synthetic folic acid from fortified food or supplements consumed with food, or 0.5 μg of synthetic folic acid consumed on an empty stomach. These distinctions are made because of the differences in absorption between folate naturally present in foods and synthetic folic acid. The RDA of 400 μg DFE can be obtained from a diet that contains a cup of fortified breakfast cereal, 1/2 cup of orange juice, 1/2 cup of cooked lentils, and 1 cup of raw spinach.

Dietary folate equivalents (DFEs) Used to express the amount of folate present in food. One DFE is equivalent to 1 μg of folate naturally occurring in food, 0.6 μg of synthetic folic acid from fortified food or supplements consumed with food, or 0.5 μg of synthetic folic acid consumed on an empty stomach.

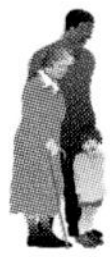

The RDA for folate during pregnancy is increased to 600 μg per day due to the increase in cell division. Although this level can be met by a carefully selected diet, folate is typically supplemented during pregnancy. The RDA is increased during lactation to account for folate secretion in milk. Needs are higher for infants and children than for adults because of their rapid growth. Human and cow's milk provide enough folate to meet infant needs, but goat's milk does not. Infants and children given goat's milk may not receive adequate folate unless it is provided from other sources.

In order to reduce the risk of neural tube defects, a special recommendation is made for women capable of becoming pregnant. A daily intake of 400 μg of

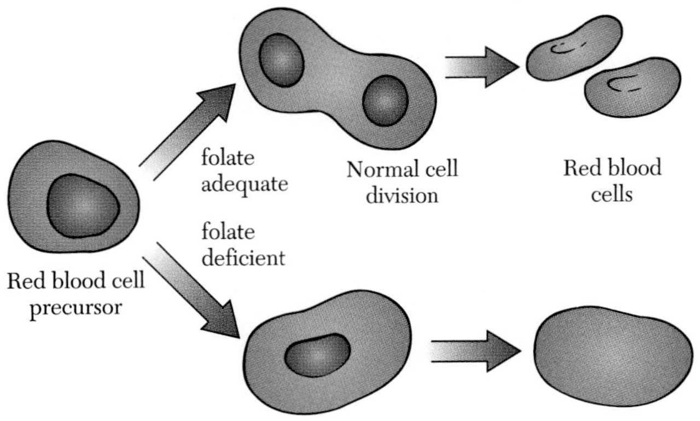

Figure 8.14
Macrocytic anemia occurs when blood cells are unable to divide, leaving large immature red blood cells (megaloblasts) and large mature red blood cells (macrocytes).

synthetic folic acid from fortified foods and/or supplements is recommended in addition to the food folate consumed in a varied diet. Therefore, the total folate intake of this group should exceed the RDA.

Folate and Health A severe deficiency of folate results in anemia, but low intakes of folate have been associated with an increased risk of neural tube defects, heart disease, and certain types of cancer. An excess of folate can mask the symptoms of vitamin B_{12} deficiency.

Folate Deficiency A deficiency of folate leads to a drop in blood folate levels and a rise in blood homocysteine followed by changes that affect rapidly dividing cells. Deficiency symptoms include poor growth, problems in nerve development and function, diarrhea, inflammation of the tongue, and anemia. Anemia results when folate is deficient because the bone marrow cells that develop into blood cells cannot duplicate their DNA, and so cannot divide. Instead, they just grow bigger. These large immature cells are known as **megaloblasts** and can be converted into large red blood cells called **macrocytes.** The result is that fewer mature red cells are produced, and the oxygen-carrying capacity of the blood is reduced. This condition is called **megaloblastic** or **macrocytic anemia** (Figure 8.14).

Megaloblasts Large, immature red blood cells that are formed when developing red blood cells are unable to divide normally.

Macrocytes Larger-than-normal mature red blood cells that have a shortened life span.

Megaloblastic or **macrocytic anemia** A condition in which there are abnormally large immature and mature red blood cells and a reduction in the total number of red blood cells.

Groups at risk of folate deficiency include pregnant women and premature infants because of their rapid rate of cell division and growth; the elderly because of their limited intake of foods high in folate; alcoholics because alcohol inhibits folate absorption; and tobacco smokers because smoke inactivates folate in the cells lining the lungs.[35]

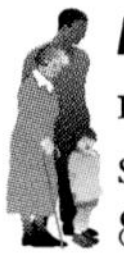

Folate and Neural Tube Defects In the United States each year about 4000 pregnancies result in a baby with a neural tube defect. Neural tube defects, such as spina bifida and other birth defects that affect the brain and spinal cord (Figure 8.15), are not true folate deficiency symptoms because not every pregnant woman with inadequate folate levels will give birth to a child with a neural tube defect. Instead, neural tube defects are probably due to a combination of factors that include low folate levels and a genetic predisposition. The exact role of folate in neural tube development is not known, but it is necessary for a critical step called neural tube closure. Neural tube closure occurs only 28 days after conception; therefore, folate status should be adequate even before a pregnancy begins (see Chapter 13). Studies in which supplemental folic acid was given to women before and during early pregnancy showed that 360 to 800 μg per day of synthetic folic acid in addition to food folate was associated with a reduced incidence of neural tube defects.[2,28] Because it is not known whether a diet naturally rich in folate offers the same protection as supplements, and because folate must be adequate

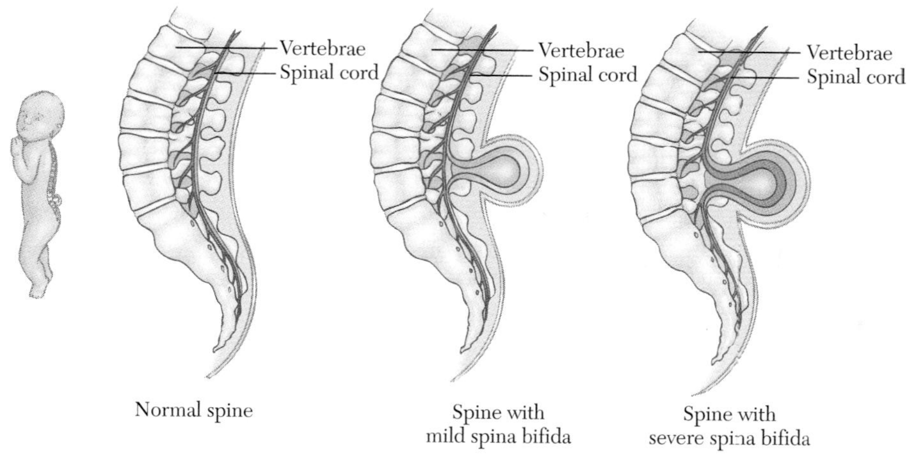

Figure 8.15
The neural tube develops into the brain and spinal cord. If folate is inadequate during neural tube closure, neural tube defects such as spina bifida, shown here, occur more frequently.

before most women are aware that they are pregnant, synthetic folic acid from supplements or fortified foods is recommended for all women of childbearing age.

Folate and Heart Disease Folate's effect on heart disease risk is related to its role in the metabolism of the amino acid methionine. When folate is lacking, homocysteine, produced during methionine metabolism, accumulates because it cannot be converted back to methionine (Figure 8.16). The risk of cardiovascular disease increases with elevated homocysteine levels and homocysteine level increases with folate deficiency (see preceding discussion of vitamin B_6 and cardiovascular disease).[28] Homocysteine levels and the risk of cardiovascular disease are reduced by increasing intakes of folate.[27,28]

Folate and Cancer Folate status has been found to affect the risk of developing forms of cancer that affect epithelial tissues such as the uterus, cervix, lung, stomach, esophagus, and colon. Although folate deficiency does not cause cancer, it has been hypothesized that low folate intake enhances an underlying predisposition to cancer. Data supporting the effects of folate intake on cancer risk are strongest for colon cancer. Epidemiological studies support an inverse relationship between folate intake and colon cancer.[36] Also, alcohol consumption greatly increases the cancer risk associated with a low folate diet. It is still not clear how much folate is needed to minimize cancer risk and whether food folate and supplemental folic acid are equally effective. Over a 15-year period, women who consumed greater than 400 μg of folate per day were found to have a reduced colon

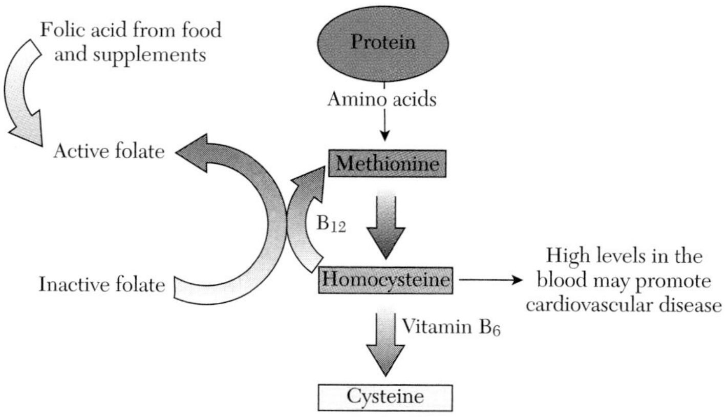

Figure 8.16
Folate and vitamin B_{12} are needed to convert homocysteine to methionine. This reaction converts folate into a form that is active for DNA synthesis. This form can also be supplied by supplements. A deficiency of either folate or vitamin B_{12} can lead to the accumulation of homocysteine, which is associated with an increased risk of cardiovascular disease.

cancer risk compared to women who consumed 200 μg per day or less. The reduction in risk was greatest among women who took vitamin supplements containing folic acid.[37]

Folate Toxicity Although there is no known folate toxicity, a high intake may mask the early symptoms of vitamin B_{12} deficiency, allowing irreversible nerve damage to occur. The UL for folic acid for adults is set at 1000 μg per day from supplements and/or fortified foods. This value was determined based on the progression of neurological symptoms seen in patients who are deficient in vitamin B_{12} and taking folic acid supplements.

Meeting Folate Needs With Food and Supplements It is estimated that adult women in the United States consume an average of 400 μg DFE of folate from natural and fortified foods daily. This level of intake meets the RDA but falls short of the recommendation for women of childbearing age to consume 400 μg DFE from fortified foods and supplements in addition to food folate. Women should be educated to increase the folate content of their diets by consuming foods that are naturally rich in folate as well as grain products fortified with folic acid. Depending on food choices, including 400 μg DFE of synthetic folic acid from fortified foods would mean eating about 4 to 8 servings of fortified grain products each day.

Because the fortification of grain products with folic acid is relatively recent, food composition databases may not provide the fortified folate value for all products (Appendix A includes fortified values for all nonbrand name items). For many products made with fortified grains, food labels list the folate content as a percent of the Daily Value. For example, a serving of pasta provides about 30% of the Daily Value or 133 μg DFE; a serving of bread provides 10% or 40 μg DFE. Labels on foods and supplements that are good sources of folate may include the health claim that consumption of folate has been linked to a decreased risk of a neural-tube-defect-affected pregnancy. If it is not possible to consume 400 μg DFE of folic acid from fortified foods, supplements should be used (see *Critical Thinking: Four Hundred of Fortified Folate*).

Vitamin B_{12}

Pernicious anemia An anemia resulting from vitamin B_{12} deficiency that occurs when dietary vitamin B_{12} cannot be absorbed due to a lack of intrinsic factor. If not treated with vitamin B_{12} injections, the condition will result in nerve damage.

In 1820, **pernicious anemia,** a fatal form of anemia that did not respond to iron supplementation, was described. Pernicious anemia is caused by an inability to absorb sufficient vitamin B_{12}. In 1926, Drs. Minot and Murphy were awarded the Nobel Prize for curing the disease with a diet containing large quantities of liver, which is a good source of vitamin B_{12}. The vitamin itself was not isolated until 1948. Today, concern focuses on the effects of marginal deficiencies of this vitamin and the potential masking of B_{12} deficiency by high intakes of folic acid.

Vitamin B_{12} in the Diet Vitamin B_{12} can be made by bacteria, fungi, and algae but not by plants and animals. Vitamin B_{12} is produced by the microorganisms in the human colon, but it cannot be absorbed. Animals acquire the vitamin indirectly from bacteria. In our diet, vitamin B_{12} is found almost exclusively in animal products. Meats, such as beef and poultry, are excellent sources. Vitamin B_{12} is not supplied by plant-based foods unless they have been contaminated with bacteria, soil, insects, or other sources of B_{12}, or have been fortified with vitamin B_{12}. Vegans seeking nonanimal sources of vitamin B_{12} sometimes consume spirulina algae or miso and tempeh, which are soybean products fermented by microorganisms, but these foods contain almost no usable vitamin B_{12}.[38] Diets that do not include animal products must include supplements or foods fortified with vitamin B_{12} in order to meet needs.[39]

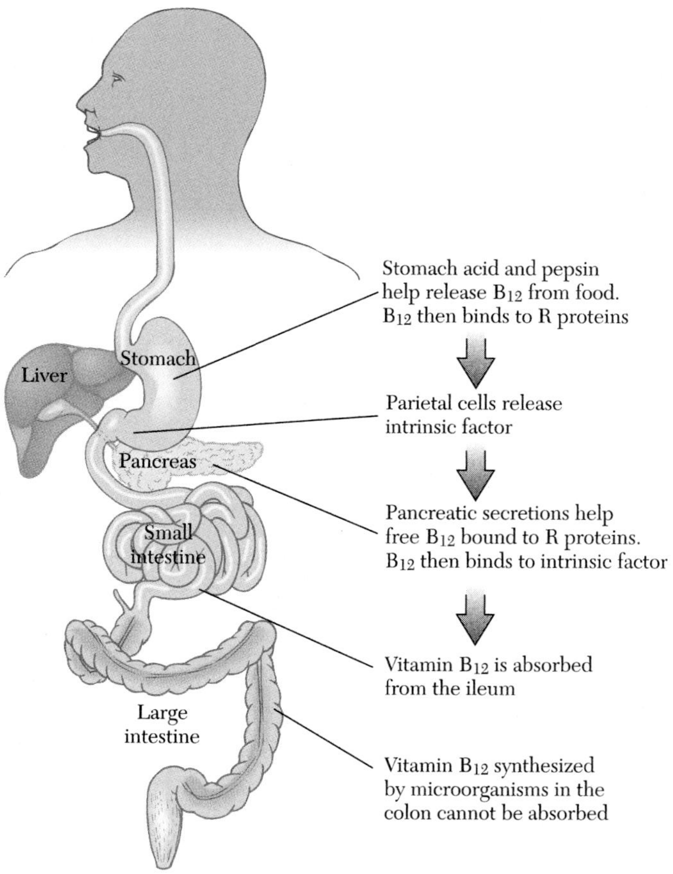
Stomach acid and pepsin help release B12 from food. B12 then binds to R proteins
Parietal cells release intrinsic factor
Pancreatic secretions help free B12 bound to R proteins. B12 then binds to intrinsic factor
Vitamin B12 is absorbed from the ileum
Vitamin B12 synthesized by microorganisms in the colon cannot be absorbed
Liver
Stomach
Pancreas
Small intestine
Large intestine

Figure 8.17
The absorption of vitamin B_{12} involves the stomach, pancreas, and small intestine.

Vitamin B_{12} in the Digestive Tract Naturally occurring vitamin B_{12} is bound to protein in food and must be released before it can be absorbed. It is released in the stomach by stomach acid and pepsin. The released vitamin B_{12} then binds to special proteins called R proteins secreted by the salivary glands and stomach mucosa. The R protein–bound vitamin B_{12} travels to the small intestine where pancreatic enzymes free it from the R proteins so it can bind to **intrinsic factor.** Intrinsic factor is a protein secreted by the **parietal cells** in the lining of the stomach. It binds to vitamin B_{12} and allows the vitamin to be absorbed in the ileum of the small intestine (Figure 8.17). Vitamin B_{12} absorption can be disrupted by reduced stomach acid, insufficient pancreatic secretions, and low levels of intrinsic factor. If the ileum or stomach is damaged or removed, vitamin B_{12} must be injected to prevent pernicious anemia.

Intrinsic factor A protein produced in the stomach that is needed for the absorption of adequate amounts of vitamin B_{12}.

Parietal cells Large cells in the stomach lining that produce and secrete intrinsic factor and hydrochloric acid.

Vitamin B_{12} in the Body The terms vitamin B_{12} and **cobalamin** refer to members of a group of cobalt-containing compounds. Vitamin B_{12} is necessary for the maintenance of myelin, which insulates nerves and is necessary for nerve transmission. Vitamin B_{12} can be converted into either of two active cobalamin coenzyme forms that function in several reactions. One B_{12}-dependent reaction rearranges carbon atoms so that the breakdown products of fatty acids can be used to generate energy via the citric acid cycle. A second reaction synthesizes the amino acid methionine from homocysteine. This reaction also regenerates the active coenzyme form of folate that functions in DNA synthesis (see Figure 8.16). Because of the need for vitamin B_{12} in folate metabolism, a deficiency of vitamin B_{12} can cause a secondary folate deficiency and, consequently, megaloblastic anemia. If individuals with vitamin B_{12} deficiency consume enough folate, they will not develop anemia but will develop more serious symptoms, such as permanent

Cobalamin The chemical term for vitamin B_{12}.

nerve damage. The fortification of grain products with folate has raised concern that additional folate in the food supply could delay diagnosis of vitamin B_{12} deficiency in some individuals.[40]

How Much Vitamin B_{12} Do We Need? The RDA for adults of all ages for vitamin B_{12} is 2.4 μg per day.[2] This is the amount needed to maintain normal red blood cell parameters and blood vitamin B_{12} concentrations. It is assumed that only 50% of the vitamin B_{12} ingested is absorbed. Average intake in the U.S. population exceeds the RDA for both adult men and women.

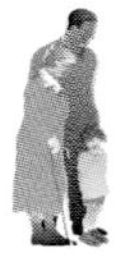

The RDA for vitamin B_{12} is increased during pregnancy, even though absorption is increased. The RDA during lactation is increased to account for the amount secreted in milk. Pregnant and lactating vegans, like anyone who does not eat animal products, are advised to take a supplement or consume fortified foods to provide the recommended intake for vitamin B_{12}.

Vitamin B_{12} and Health Blatant deficiencies of vitamin B_{12} are rare because the body stores and reuses it. However, marginal vitamin B_{12} status is of public health concern particularly for older adults and vegetarians who consume no animal products.

Vitamin B_{12} Deficiency Vitamin B_{12} is secreted into bile, and most of it is reabsorbed. Because of this efficient recycling, it can take many years of a deficient diet before the symptoms of vitamin B_{12} deficiency appear. Deficiency symptoms occur more rapidly when absorption is impaired because vitamin B_{12} recycling is reduced.

Early symptoms of vitamin B_{12} deficiency include an increase in blood homocysteine levels and a macrocytic, megaloblastic anemia that is indistinguishable from that seen in folate deficiency. Later symptoms include degeneration of the myelin that coats the nerves, spinal cord, and brain, eventually causing paralysis and death. Pernicious anemia, a disease in which the parietal cells that produce intrinsic factor are destroyed, is the major cause of severe B_{12} deficiency. Without parietal cell production of intrinsic factor, vitamin B_{12} cannot be absorbed normally. This anemia must be treated with injections of the vitamin.

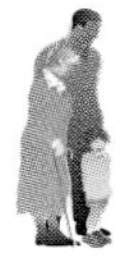

Groups at Risk About 10 to 30% of individuals over 50 years of age are unable to absorb food-bound vitamin B_{12} normally because they have a condition that reduces stomach acid secretion and allows microbial overgrowth in the stomach and small intestine.[2,41] When stomach acid is reduced, the enzymes that release protein-bound vitamin B_{12} cannot function properly and the bound vitamin B_{12} cannot be released and absorbed. In addition, microbes in the gut reduce absorption by competing for available vitamin B_{12}. It is recommended that individuals over the age of 50 meet their RDA for vitamin B_{12} by consuming fortified foods such as fortified breakfast cereals or soy-based products or by taking a vitamin B_{12}–containing supplement.[2] The vitamin B_{12} in fortified foods and supplements is not bound to proteins so it is absorbed even when stomach acid is low.

Vitamin B_{12} deficiency is also a concern among vegan vegetarians since vitamin B_{12} is only found in foods of animal origin. Severe deficiency has been observed in breast-fed infants of vegan women, but marginal deficiency in vegetarians of all ages is a concern if supplements or fortified foods are not included in the diet.

Vitamin B_{12} Toxicity No toxic effects have been reported with vitamin B_{12} intakes of up to 100 μg per day. There are not sufficient data to establish a UL for vitamin B_{12}.

Vitamin B_{12} Supplements Supplements of vitamin B_{12} are available as cyanocobalamin in both oral and injectable forms. Because vitamin B_{12} deficiency causes anemia, supplements of the vitamin, particularly as injections, have been promoted as a pick-me-up for tired, run-down individuals. However, there are no proven benefits of vitamin B_{12} supplementation in individuals who are not vitamin B_{12} deficient. Oral supplements may be of benefit for those at risk for vitamin B_{12} deficiencies, such as vegans and individuals over 50 who may poorly absorb vitamin B_{12} from foods.

CRITICAL THINKING

Four Hundred of Fortified Folate

Marcia is considering having a child and wants to be sure she is in the best shape possible before trying to conceive. She consults her physician who gives her a clean bill of health but suggests she evaluate the amount of folate in her diet.

Why do women capable of becoming pregnant need so much folate?

Research has shown that adequate folate reduces the risk of a type of birth defect called a neural tube defect that affects the brain or spinal cord. For folate to be beneficial, an adequate amount must be consumed for at least a month before conception and continued for a month after. Since many pregnancies are not planned, it is recommended that this amount be included routinely in the diets of women of childbearing age.

Marcia records her food intake for one day to determine her folate intake:

Food	Servings	Total Folate (μg)
Breakfast		
Corn flakes	1 cup	100
Milk, reduced fat	1 cup	12
Banana	1 medium	22
Orange juice	8 oz (240 ml)	75
Coffee	1 cup	0
Lunch		
Hamburger	1	11
Hamburger bun	1	32
French fries	20 pieces	24
Coke	12 oz	0
Apple	1 medium	4
Dinner		
Chicken	3 oz	4
Refried beans	1/2 cup	106
Rice	1 cup	80
Roll	1	60
Margarine	2 tsp	1
Salad	1 cup	64
Salad dressing	1 Tbsp	1
Milk, reduced fat	1 cup	12
Cake	1 piece	32
Total		**640**

Does her folate intake meet the RDA?

Yes. She consumes 640 μg of folate, which is greater than the RDA of 400 μg DFE, but her doctor reminds her that women who are capable of becoming pregnant should consume 400 μg of folic acid from fortified foods or supplements each day in addition to the folate found in a varied diet.

Why not set the RDA at 800 μg DFE?

Prevention of neural tube defects was not used as a criterion of adequacy for the RDAs for several reasons. First of all, only women who actually become pregnant would benefit from this amount. In addition, the period of time that this intake is beneficial is short (about one month before to one month after conception). Finally, the studies that showed a reduced risk of neural tube defects were done using folic acid supplements in addition to other dietary folate. It is uncertain whether folate found naturally in foods will have the same effect.

What foods in Marcia's diet are natural sources of folate? Which are fortified with folic acid?

The best sources of naturally occurring folate are the orange juice and the beans. Other fruits, vegetables, and dairy products contribute smaller amounts. Meats contribute little folate. Together, these foods provide 336 μg of folate. The grain products in her diet, including the cereal, hamburger bun, roll, rice, and cake, are all fortified and together contribute about 304 μg of folate. Some of this is from the folate naturally found in these grains but most is from folic acid added in fortification. Fortified foods can be identified because folic acid is included on food labels in the ingredient list. Many products also list the amount of folate as a percent of the Daily Value, which can be used to calculate the μg of folate per serving (see Table 9.3).

List some substitutions that would increase Marcia's intake of naturally occurring folate and of folic acid from fortified foods.

Answer:

Would you recommend Marcia take a folate supplement?

Answer:

VITAMIN C

Vitamin C deficiency has been the scourge of armies, navies, and explorers throughout history. This deficiency, known as **scurvy,** was described by ancient Greeks, Egyptians, and Romans. In the mid-1500s, the Indians of eastern Canada knew that an extract from white cedar needles would cure the disease. In the 17th century, Sir Richard Hawkins observed on his voyage to the South Seas that this sickness could be cured by including citrus fruit in the diet. Despite his observation, 10,000 British sailors died of scurvy that same year. Over 100 years later, James Lind, a Scottish physician serving in the British navy, tested various agents for their effectiveness at curing scurvy and reported that two patients given citrus fruits recovered within six days. However, it was another 48 years before it was required that lime or lemon juice be included in the rations of the mercantile service, earning British sailors the name *limeys.* Unfortunately, the rest of the world did not heed the lesson of the limeys. In the mid-19th century, during the American Civil War, scurvy was rampant.

Scurvy A vitamin C deficiency disease.

Vitamin C in the Diet

Citrus fruits, such as oranges, lemons, and limes, are an excellent source of vitamin C. Other fruits that are high in vitamin C include strawberries and cantaloupe. Vegetables in the cabbage family, such as broccoli, cauliflower, bok choy, and brussels sprouts, as well as green leafy vegetables, green and red peppers, okra, tomatoes, and potatoes, are good sources (Figure 8.18). Meat, fish, poultry, eggs, dairy products, and grains are poor sources. The amount of vitamin C in packaged foods must be listed on food labels as a percentage of the Daily Value. Vitamin C is unstable and is destroyed by oxygen, light, and heat, so it is readily lost in cooking. This loss is accelerated by contact with copper or iron cooking utensils and by low-acid conditions.

Vitamin C in the Body

Vitamin C, known as **ascorbic acid,** is a water-soluble vitamin that donates electrons in biochemical reactions, including those needed for the synthesis and

Ascorbic acid The chemical term for vitamin C.

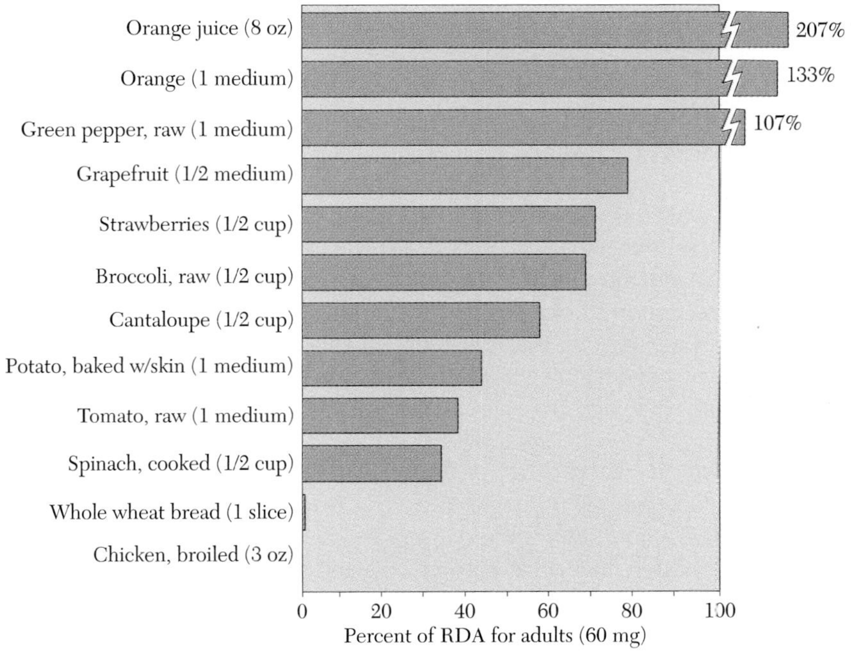

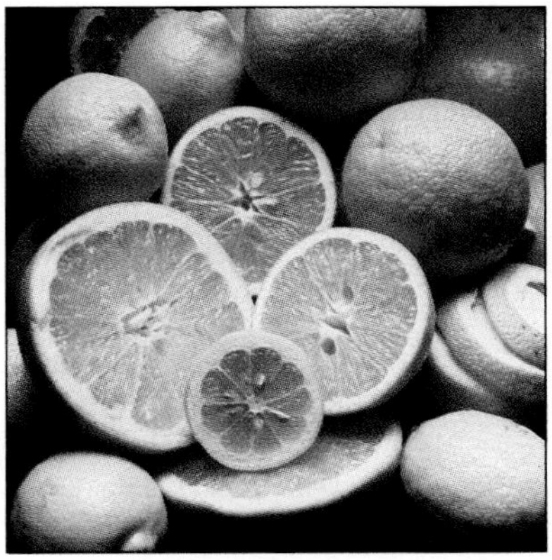

Figure 8.18
The vitamin C content of foods as a percent of the 1989 RDA for adults. (*right,* Charles D. Winters)

Figure 8.19
Vitamin C is needed for the formation of chemical bonds that link collagen molecules together to give connective tissue strength and stability.

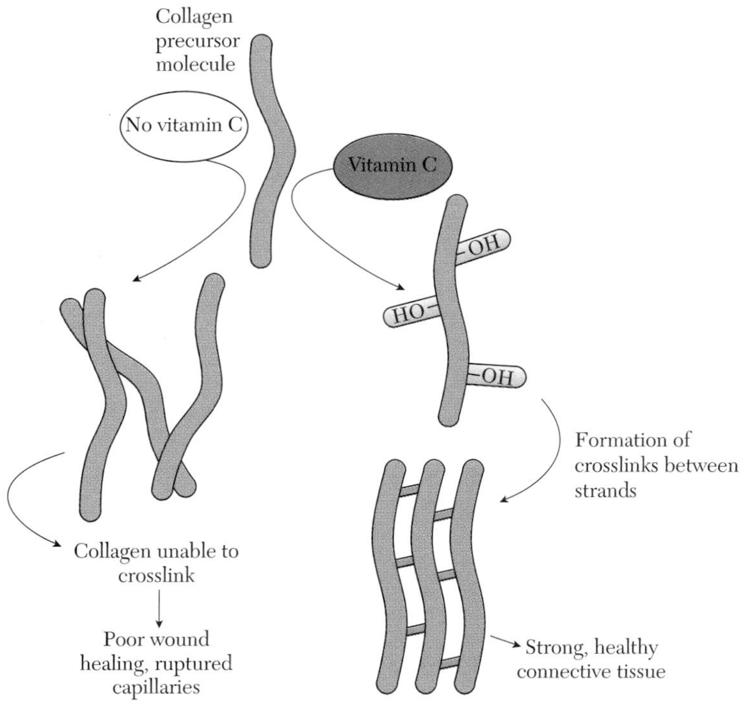

maintenance of connective tissue. Vitamin C also has a more general role as an antioxidant that protects the body from reactive oxygen molecules, helps maintain the immune system, and aids in the absorption of iron.

Reactions Requiring Vitamin C: Connective Tissue Many of the reactions requiring vitamin C add a hydroxyl group (OH) to other molecules. Two such reactions are essential for the formation of **collagen,** the protein that forms the base of all connective tissue in the body. The hydroxyl groups are necessary for the formation of chemical bonds that crosslink strands of collagen to give it strength (Figure 8.19). Vitamin C also serves in reactions needed for the synthesis of other cell compounds, including neurotransmitters, hormones such as the thyroid and steroid hormones, bile acids, and carnitine needed for fatty acid breakdown.

Collagen The major protein in connective tissue.

Vitamin C as a General Antioxidant Vitamin C also functions as an **antioxidant.** Antioxidants are substances that protect against **oxidative damage,** which is damage caused by reactive oxygen molecules. Reactive oxygen molecules can be generated by normal oxygen-requiring reactions inside the body or can come from environmental sources such as air pollution or cigarette smoke. **Oxidative stress** refers to a serious imbalance between the amounts of reactive oxygen molecules generated and the amounts of antioxidant defenses available. Oxidative stress has been related to the aging process as well as to the development of cancer and heart disease. Agents that can induce oxidative stress by causing an increase in reactive oxygen molecules, a decrease in antioxidant defenses, or an increase in oxidative damage are called **pro-oxidants.**

Antioxidant A substance that is able to neutralize reactive oxygen molecules.

Oxidative damage Damage caused by highly reactive oxygen molecules that steal electrons from other compounds, causing changes in structure and function.

Oxidative stress A condition that occurs when there are more reactive oxygen molecules than can be neutralized by available antioxidant defenses. It occurs either because excessive amounts of reactive oxygen molecules are generated or because antioxidant defenses are deficient.

Pro-oxidant A substance that promotes oxidative damage.

How Do Antioxidants Work? Most of the oxygen we inhale is used in the mitochondria to produce energy, but some can form reactive oxygen molecules such as **free radicals.** Free radicals cause damage by snatching electrons from DNA, proteins, or unsaturated fatty acids, causing changes in the structure and function of these molecules. DNA damage is hypothesized to be a major reason for the increase in cancer incidence that occurs with age. Damage to proteins can result in

Free radical One type of highly reactive molecule that causes oxidative damage.

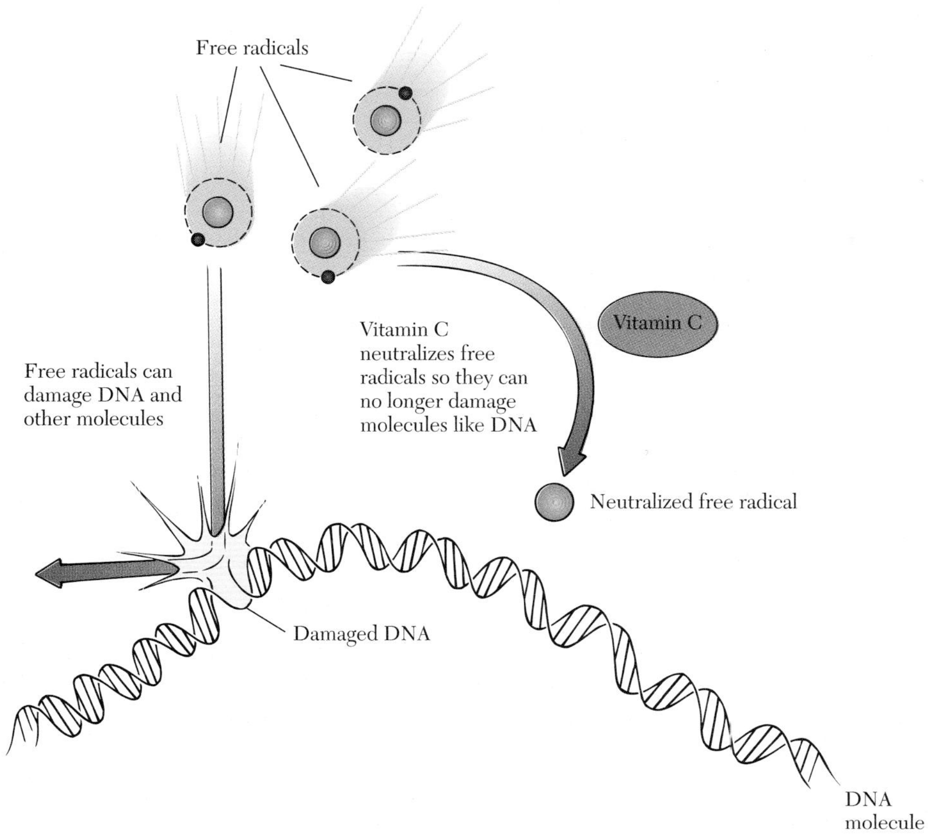

Figure 8.20
Vitamin C functions as an antioxidant, neutralizing free radicals so that they are no longer damaging.

inactivation of enzymes. And free radical damage to lipoproteins and lipids in membranes is implicated in the development of atherosclerosis.[42]

Antioxidants act by destroying reactive oxygen molecules before they can do damage. Some directly destroy free radicals while others neutralize superoxide radicals or hydrogen peroxide, which are other reactive molecules, before they can form free radicals. Some antioxidants are produced in the body; others are dietary constituents such as vitamin E, vitamin C, and certain phytochemicals (see *Off the Shelf: Will Antioxidant Supplements Keep Us Healthy?*). Many of the antioxidant enzymes produced in the body require dietary minerals (see Chapter 11).

The Role of Vitamin C Vitamin C acts as an antioxidant in the blood and other body fluids.[43] It can destroy superoxide radicals and free radicals before they can damage lipids and DNA (Figure 8.20). Vitamin C also helps protect the immune system from reactive oxygen molecules. The antioxidant properties of vitamin C also affect other nutrients. It regenerates the active antioxidant form of vitamin E, helps keep the active form of folate in the reduced state, and enhances iron absorption by keeping iron in its more readily absorbed reduced form (Fe^{+2}). When about 50 mg of vitamin C—the amount contained in 3.5 ounces (100 ml) of orange juice—is consumed in a meal containing iron, iron absorption is enhanced (see Chapter 11).

Vitamin C may also act as a pro-oxidant by converting iron and copper to reduced forms that can then generate free radicals. In a study which gave 500 mg of supplemental vitamin C to healthy adults, the supplement showed a protective effect by decreasing one type of oxidative DNA damage, but at the same time it had a detrimental effect by increasing a second type of DNA damage.[44] It is not known what factors determine whether the antioxidant or pro-oxidant properties of vitamin C predominate.

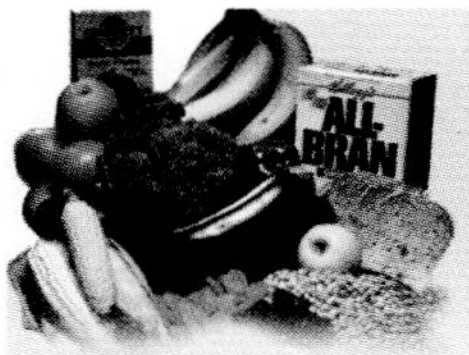

Off the Shelf

Will Antioxidant Supplements Keep Us Healthy?

Many vitamins, minerals, and enzymes are marketed as antioxidant supplements. These are suggested to boost our antioxidant defenses and keep us healthy. Although antioxidant nutrients are an important part of our defense system, they are not the only source of antioxidant protection, and more is not always better.

The rationale for needing extra antioxidants is based on the fact that we are constantly bombarded with damaging reactive oxygen molecules, such as free radicals, peroxides, and superoxides, that come from reactions inside our body or from environmental sources such as air pollution or cigarette smoke. If the body's antioxidant defense mechanisms become overwhelmed, oxidative stress occurs. Sometimes a cell in oxidative stress adapts and increases the production of antioxidant defenses, making it more resistant. If the stress is too great or lasts too long, oxidative damage to DNA, proteins, and lipids occurs and cell death can result. The cumulative effect of oxidative stress is believed to play a role in the aging process and in the development of chronic diseases.

To protect us from oxidative damage, the body is equipped with many types of antioxidant defenses. Some of these are vitamins or vitamin precursors—vitamin C, vitamin E, and beta-carotene. Others are enzymes—catalase, glutathione peroxidase, and superoxide dismutase. These enzyme systems rely on minerals, including zinc, copper, manganese, iron, and selenium, for activity.

Can supplements of nutrients or enzymes boost our antioxidant defenses? Each antioxidant in the body acts under specific conditions to destroy particular types of reactive oxygen compounds. Vitamin C can inactivate free radicals, superoxide, and hydrogen peroxide. Vitamin E and beta-carotene can inactivate lipid free radicals in membranes. Selenium is a part of the antioxidant enzyme glutathione peroxidase, which neutralizes peroxides before they can form dangerous free radicals. The molecule glutathione, which is made of three amino acids, plays an antioxidant role by participating in this reaction and by helping to regenerate vitamin C. Catalase is an iron-containing enzyme that can also destroy peroxides. Zinc, copper, and manganese are necessary for forms of the enzyme superoxide dismutase, which destroys superoxide free radicals.

Each antioxidant also acts at a specific location inside the body or cell. Antioxidant enzymes are located primarily inside cells, where each patrols a specific cellular compartment. For example, zinc/copper-superoxide dismutase and glutathione peroxidase police the cytoplasm, along with vitamin C. Glutathione peroxidase also acts inside the mitochondria, along with manganese-superoxide dismutase. Catalase acts inside another organelle, the peroxisome. Vitamin E and beta-carotene are fat-soluble nutrients that protect cell membranes. Vitamin C, vitamin E, and the copper-containing protein ceruloplasmin function outside the cells by inactivating free radicals circulating in the blood and body fluids (see figure).

Although scientific evidence confirms the role of certain nutrients as antioxidants, we do not know the optimum dose of each for maximum antioxidant protection. The amounts needed will vary depending on environmental conditions and the health and genetic makeup of the individual. In addition, many of the antioxidant nutrients interact. Therefore a deficiency of one of these nutrients could increase the need for another, and an excess of one may create a deficiency of another. For instance, vitamin C is necessary to regenerate the active form of vitamin E, and vitamin E in turn can spare beta-carotene by protecting it from oxidation. Vitamin E can also help prevent selenium deficiency and vice versa. And excesses of zinc can cause copper deficiency. Some antioxidants such as vitamin C and beta-carotene can also act as pro-oxidants under certain conditions. Therefore it is possible for the wrong amounts to promote rather than prevent oxidative damage.

How Much Vitamin C Do We Need?

Humans are one of only a few animal species that require vitamin C in the diet. Most animals can synthesize vitamin C in their bodies. For example, a pig makes 8 grams a day. The 1989 RDA for adult humans is 60 mg per day. This amount is easily obtained by drinking a 4-ounce (120 ml) glass of orange juice or eating an orange.

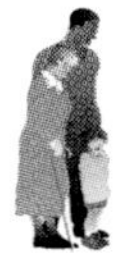

The 1989 RDA for vitamin C is increased during pregnancy and lactation. For infants, it is based on the vitamin C content of human milk. The recommended intake for vitamin C is not increased in older adults, but this is a population that may be at risk of deficiency because their intake of fresh fruits and vegetables is often marginal.

Cigarette smoking increases the requirement for vitamin C because vitamin C is used to break down compounds in cigarette smoke. Studies have shown that even an intake of 100 mg per day may not maintain normal blood vitamin C levels in cigarette smokers.[45]

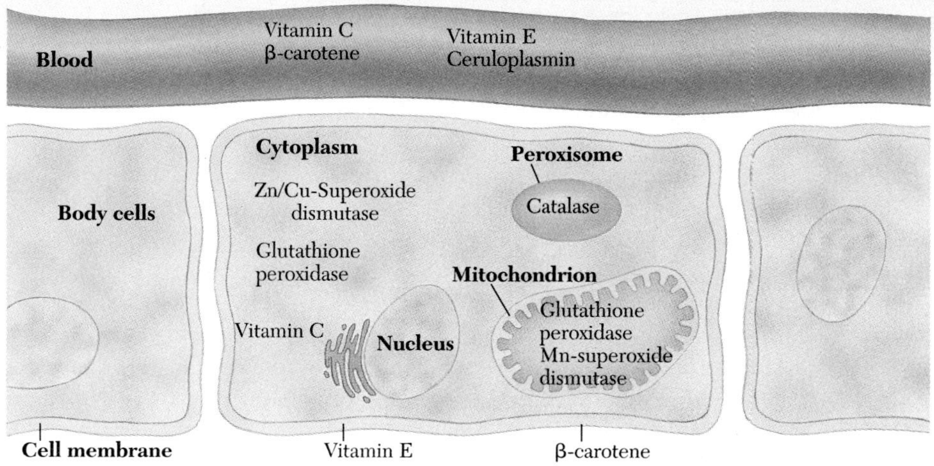

Each of the antioxidant defenses functions in specific locations in the body and protects against specific types of damaging reactions.

If antioxidant vitamins and minerals are deficient in the diet, increasing their intake will enhance antioxidant defenses. But whether consumption of these nutrients above the recommended intake will further improve the body's antioxidant defenses is still under investigation. Taking a supplement that contains an antioxidant enzyme like catalase, superoxide dismutase, or glutathione peroxidase will not boost antioxidant defenses because it will not increase the amount of enzyme in the body. Enzymes supplied in the diet, whether in food or in supplements, are broken down to amino acids and peptides in the gastrointestinal tract before they can be absorbed.

The total diet is probably more important in health promotion than any of these nutrients alone. Some of the antioxidants present in foods are phytochemicals with no vitamin activity. Other components of the diet, such as total fat and fiber intake, may be just as important as vitamins and minerals at protecting us from chronic disease. Based on our current understanding, it is best to boost antioxidant nutrients by eating more fruits and vegetables that are high in beta-carotene, vitamin C, vitamin E, and phytochemicals, and by including foods containing iron, copper, selenium, manganese, and zinc in your diet.

Vitamin C and Health

Two centuries ago, fruits containing vitamin C saved the lives of thousands of sailors. In the United States today scurvy is rare, but vitamin C is the most frequently consumed vitamin supplement.

Vitamin C Deficiency When vitamin C intake is below 10 mg per day, the symptoms of scurvy may appear. These symptoms reflect the role of vitamin C in the maintenance of collagen and blood-vessel integrity. Without vitamin C, the bonds holding adjacent collagen molecules together cannot be formed and maintained, resulting in poor wound healing, the reopening of previously healed wounds, bone and joint aches, bone fractures, and improperly formed and loose teeth. Due to weakened blood vessels and ruptured capillaries, small skin discolorations appear, the gums bleed, and bruising occurs easily. Anemia may also occur from impaired iron absorption. The psychological manifestations of scurvy include depression and hysteria.

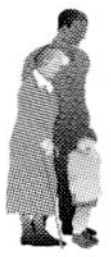

Worldwide, vitamin C deficiency goes hand in hand with poverty. In the United States, marginal vitamin C deficiency is a concern for individuals who consume few fruits and vegetables. Severe vitamin C deficiency leading to scurvy is uncommon. Scurvy can occur in infants fed diets consisting exclusively of cow's milk and in alcoholics and elderly individuals consuming nutrient-poor diets.

Vitamin C Toxicity Vitamin C is generally considered nontoxic. Large increases in intake do not cause large increases in the amount of vitamin C in body fluids. This is because the percentage of the dose absorbed decreases as the size of the dose increases and because vitamin C absorbed in excess of need is excreted by the kidney.[46] The most common symptoms that occur with consumption of vitamin C doses of 1 gram or more are diarrhea, nausea, and abdominal cramps. These are caused when unabsorbed vitamin C draws water into the intestine. Another concern with vitamin C supplements is damage to tooth enamel. Vitamin C is an acid that is strong enough to dissolve tooth enamel when vitamin C tablets are chewed.

Although high doses of vitamin C are relatively nontoxic in healthy individuals, they can cause problems in individuals prone to kidney stones or iron overload. A restriction of vitamin C is recommended in the diets of individuals who have metabolic defects that lead to kidney stone formation. In individuals who are unable to regulate iron absorption, too much vitamin C should be avoided because it increases the absorption of nonheme iron and may therefore contribute to iron overload (see Chapter 11). Other potential problems associated with vitamin C intakes greater than 3 grams per day include interference with drugs prescribed to slow blood clotting and promotion of symptoms in individuals with sickle-cell anemia. Since the structure of vitamin C is similar to that of glucose, it may also interfere with urine tests used to monitor glucose levels in diabetics.

Vitamin C Supplements Vitamin C is often taken in gram quantities, doses 15 to 30 times the 1989 RDA. One third of the population of the United States takes supplements of vitamin C in the hope that it will prevent or reduce symptoms of the common cold. More recently, however, the role of vitamin C as an antioxidant has been used to promote vitamin C supplements as protection against cardiovascular disease and cancer.

Vitamin C and the Common Cold Studies examining the relationship between vitamin C and the common cold date back to the 1930s; however, its effectiveness is still a matter of debate. A review of placebo-controlled trials that used amounts greater than or equal to 1 gram per day found that vitamin C did not reduce the incidence of colds but did cause a reduction in the duration and severity of cold symptoms.[47] The effect of vitamin C on cold symptoms may be due to its direct antiviral effect, its antioxidant effect, its role in stimulating various aspects of immune function, its ability to increase the breakdown of histamine (a molecule that causes inflammation), or a combination of these.[48,49]

Vitamin C and Cardiovascular Disease Vitamin C supplements have been suggested to reduce the risk of cardiovascular disease by reducing blood pressure, blood cholesterol levels, and the formation of oxidized LDL cholesterol. Several studies have suggested that blood pressure is inversely related to vitamin C status; however, the data are not conclusive.[50] It has been hypothesized that vitamin C reduces blood cholesterol because it is involved in the synthesis of bile acids from cholesterol in the liver. Adequate vitamin C allows cholesterol to be used for bile synthesis and therefore may reduce the amount of cholesterol in the blood. Animal studies have demonstrated that low vitamin C status increases LDL cholesterol and decreases HDL cholesterol and that this effect is reversed by feeding the animals vitamin C.[50] Similar studies on the effect of vitamin C on blood cholesterol are not available in humans. It has been proposed that vitamin C and other antioxidants delay atherosclerosis by preventing the oxidation of LDL cholesterol (see Chapter 5). Vitamin C is an important plasma antioxidant that can prevent the oxidation of lipids. Many studies done in cell culture show that vitamin C protects LDL cholesterol from oxidation, but this effect has been difficult to investigate inside a living human.[50] Despite these important roles of vitamin C in modulating blood cholesterol levels and protecting LDL cholesterol from oxidation, data thus far from epidemiology and human intervention trials have provided little evidence to support the use of vitamin C supplements in preventing atherosclerosis in humans.[51]

Vitamin C and Cancer It has been suggested that high doses of vitamin C both treat and prevent cancer. Although controlled trials have not found any benefits of vitamin C in the treatment of patients with advanced cancer,[52] there is evidence supporting a role for vitamin C in cancer prevention. Epidemiological studies have found inverse relationships between dietary vitamin C intake and cancers of the cervix, breast, rectum, lungs, stomach, mouth, and pancreas.[53] As an antioxidant, vitamin C may protect against cancers caused by oxidative damage. In the case of gastrointestinal cancers, vitamin C may prevent cancer by inhibiting the formation of carcinogenic nitrosamines (see Chapter 16). Despite the association between higher intakes of vitamin C and a lower incidence of various cancers, these studies cannot rule out factors other than vitamin C found in fruits and vegetables that might be responsible for the protective effect.[54]

Choline: Is It a Vitamin?

Choline is needed to synthesize a number of important molecules, including a phospholipid found in cell membranes, the neurotransmitter acetylcholine, and the methyl donor betaine. It is also an important source of carbon atoms in biochemical reactions. Choline can be synthesized to a limited extent by humans and is not currently classified as vitamin. However, there is evidence that it is essential in healthy men.[55] There is not enough information to determine if choline is also essential in the diets of women, infants, children, and older adults.[2]

Choline is widely distributed in foods. Particularly good sources include egg yolks, organ meats, spinach, nuts, and wheat germ. Average daily choline intake is estimated to be about 600 to 1000 mg per day. An AI of 550 mg per day for men and 425 mg per day for women has been established based on the amount needed to prevent liver damage. There are few data to assess whether dietary choline is needed at all stages of life. At some stages, requirements may be met by synthesis in the body. Choline deficiency causes liver abnormalities. Deficiency is unlikely in healthy humans, but it has been observed in individuals fed a choline-deficient diet and in those receiving total parenteral nutrition without choline.[56] Choline is required by human cells grown in culture, and prolonged deficiency in animals leads to fat accumulation in the liver and may contribute to liver cancer.

Intakes of choline that are much higher than can be obtained from foods can cause body odor, sweating, reduced growth rate, low blood pressure, and liver damage. A UL for adults of 3.5 g per day has been set based on the occurrence of low blood pressure.

APPLICATIONS

These exercises are designed to help you apply your critical thinking skills to your own nutrition choices. Many are best performed using a diet analysis software program. If you do not have access to a computer program, the exercises can be hand-calculated using the information in this text and its appendices.

1. Use your food intake record from Chapter 2 to answer the following:
   a. How much folate does your diet contain?
   b. How does your intake compare with the RDA?
   c. If your diet doesn't meet recommendations, modify it to meet the RDA for folate.
   d. List sources of folate in your diet that are natural and from fortification.
2. Evaluate each of the following supplements:

   Pyridoxine: 100 mg dose

   Stress tab: pyridoxine, 35 mg; thiamin, 1 mg; riboflavin, 1.1 mg; niacin, 30 mg; choline, 500 mg

   Folic acid: 800 μg dose

   a. Do any of them create a risk for toxicity? Which ones and why?
   b. Would you recommend them for everyone? For a specific group? Why or why not?
3. Using the Web page for this book, find a link to a nutritional supplement manufacturer. What is the highest dose of pyridoxine that you see included in one of its products? Is this a safe dose? What advertising promises are included with supplements containing pyridoxine? Evaluate these claims for accuracy. What forms of niacin are in supplements marketed by this company? How much niacin is included per dose? Is this a safe level of intake?

Summary

1. Vitamins are essential organic nutrients that do not provide energy and are required in small quantities in the diet to promote and regulate body activities needed for growth, reproduction, and tissue maintenance. They are classified by their solubility in either water or fat.
2. We consume vitamins that are naturally present in foods, added to foods by fortification and enrichment, and contained in supplements.
3. The amount of a vitamin that is available to the body is regulated by vitamin absorption, transport, activation, storage, and excretion.
4. Vitamin deficiencies remain a major health problem worldwide. In industrialized countries, marginal dietary deficiencies and toxicities from supplements are a growing concern.
5. Recommended intakes for vitamins are established by evaluating the results from many different kinds of research. Currently these are expressed as RDAs or AIs established by the DRI committee, and, for some vitamins as 1989 RDAs.
6. The active forms of thiamin, riboflavin, niacin, biotin, and pantothenic acid function as coenzymes in reactions involved in the metabolism of carbohydrate, fat, and protein.
7. Thiamin is required for the generation of energy from carbohydrate, fat, and protein and for the synthesis of the neurotransmitter acetylcholine. The best food sources are lean pork, legumes, and whole or enriched grains. Thiamin deficiency, or beriberi, causes nervous system abnormalities. Deficiencies are common in alcoholics. No toxicity has been identified.
8. Riboflavin coenzymes are needed for the generation of energy. Riboflavin deficiency is rarely seen alone because food sources of riboflavin are also sources of other B vitamins and because riboflavin is needed for the utilization of several other vitamins. Milk, meat, and enriched grain products are the best food sources. No toxicity has been identified.
9. Niacin coenzymes are important in the breakdown of carbohydrate, fat, and protein and in the synthesis of fatty acids and sterols. A deficiency results in pellagra, which is characterized by dermatitis, diarrhea, dementia, and, finally, death. Beef, chicken, turkey, fish, and enriched grain products are the best food sources. The amino acid tryptophan can be converted into niacin, so dietary tryptophan can meet some of the niacin requirement. Supplements of the nicotinic acid form of niacin can lower elevated blood cholesterol but frequently cause toxicity symptoms such as flushing, tingling sensations, nausea, and a red skin rash.
10. Biotin is needed for the synthesis of glucose, fatty acids, and the metabolism of certain amino acids. An RDA has not been established because some of our biotin need is met by bacterial synthesis in the gastrointestinal tract. However, an AI has been set. Liver and egg yolks are good sources. Toxicity has not been reported.
11. Pantothenic acid is part of coenzyme A (CoA), which is required for the production of energy from carbohydrate, fat, and protein and the synthesis of cholesterol and fat. It is abundant in the food supply, and deficiency is rare. There is no RDA, but an AI has been established.
12. Pyridoxal phosphate, the coenzyme form of vitamin B_6, is needed for the activity of more than 100 enzymes involved in the metabolism of carbohydrate, fat, and protein. Vitamin B_6 is particularly important for amino acid metabolism. Food sources include chicken, fish, liver, eggs, and whole grains. Large doses of vitamin B_6 can cause nervous system abnormalities.
13. Folate is necessary for the synthesis of DNA, so it is especially important for rapidly dividing cells. Folate deficiency results in macrocytic anemia. Low levels of folate before and during early pregnancy are associated with an increased incidence of neural tube defects in the offspring. It is recommended that women of childbearing age consume 400 μg of folic acid from fortified foods and supplements in addition to the folate found in a varied diet. Food sources include liver, legumes, oranges, leafy green vegetables, and fortified grains. A high intake of folate can mask the early symptoms of vitamin B_{12} deficiency.
14. Vitamin B_{12} is needed for the metabolism of folate and fatty acids and to maintain the insulating layer of myelin surrounding nerves. Deficiency results in anemia and permanent nerve

damage. The inability to absorb vitamin B_{12} due to lack of intrinsic factor results in a form of anemia called pernicious anemia. If not treated with B_{12} injections, it can be fatal. Vitamin B_{12} is found almost exclusively in animal products. The absorption of vitamin B_{12} from food requires adequate levels of stomach acid, intrinsic factor, and pancreatic secretions. Marginal deficiency is a concern in vegans, who consume no animal products, and in older individuals in whom stomach acid secretion is reduced.

15. Vitamin C is necessary for the synthesis and maintenance of connective tissue and for the synthesis of hormones and neurotransmitters. Vitamin C deficiency, called scurvy, is characterized by poor wound healing, bleeding, and other symptoms related to the improper formation and maintenance of collagen. The best food sources are citrus fruits. Vitamin C supplements are the most commonly taken vitamin supplements and are usually used to reduce the symptoms of the common cold.
16. Vitamin C is also a water-soluble antioxidant. Antioxidants protect the body from reactive oxygen molecules such as free radicals. These molecules are generated from normal body reactions and come from the environment. They cause damage by stealing electrons from DNA, proteins, and unsaturated fatty acids.
17. Choline is a substance necessary for metabolism and is not currently classified as a vitamin. It may be required in the diet at certain stages of life so an AI has been established.

Review Questions

1. What is a vitamin?
2. List four factors that affect how much of a vitamin is available to the body.
3. What do enrichment and fortification mean?
4. List a function common to all of the B vitamins.
5. In what population groups is thiamin deficiency a concern?
6. Why should milk be packaged in opaque containers?
7. What is pellagra?
8. How is vitamin B_6 involved in protein metabolism?
9. Why is low folate intake of particular concern for women of childbearing age?
10. Why would someone who has had his stomach removed (or had gastric bypass surgery) need to receive injections of vitamin B_{12} to meet his needs?
11. Why are vegans and the elderly at risk for vitamin B_{12} deficiency?
12. Why does vitamin C deficiency cause poor wound healing?
13. What are reactive oxygen molecules and how do they cause damage?
14. What is the role of antioxidants and pro-oxidants in oxidative stress?
15. Does choline fit the definition of a vitamin? Why or why not?

Nutrition Web Links

To further explore areas related to the material in this chapter, go to the *Nutrition: Science and Applications* Web site at ***www.Wiley.com/college/Smolin*** and *click on* **Student Companion Site** for chapter-by-chapter links. Some sites related to information in Chapter 8 include:

Food companies such as Dole that provide information on fruit and vegetable sources of vitamins.

Agencies such as the FDA, the CDC, and the NIH Office of Dietary Supplements that provide information on the recommendations for and safety of vitamins.

Sites that provide information on vitamins and health promotion, such as the Women's Health Group of America, the American Academy of Family Physicians, and the Spina Bifida Association of America.

References

1. Tanphaichitr, V. Thiamin. In *Modern Nutrition in Health and Disease*, 9th ed. Shils, M. E., Olson, J. A., Shike, M., and Ross, A. C., eds. Baltimore: Williams & Wilkins, 1999, 381–389.
2. Institute of Medicine, Food and Nutrition Board. *Dietary Reference Intakes for Thiamin, Riboflavin, Niacin, Vitamin B-6, Folate, Vitamin B-12, Pantothenic Acid, Biotin, and Choline.* Washington, D.C., National Academy Press, 1998.
3. Potter, N. N., and Hotchkiss, J. H. *Food Science*, 5th ed. New York: Chapman & Hall, 1995.
4. McCormick, D. B. Riboflavin. In *Modern Nutrition in Health and Disease*, 9th ed. Shils, M. E., Olson, J. A., Shike, M., and Ross, A. C., eds. Baltimore: Williams & Wilkins, 1999, 391–399.
5. Roe, D. A. Riboflavin deficiency: mucocutaneous signs of acute and chronic deficiency. Semin. Dermatol. 10:293–295, 1991.
6. Zempleni, J., Galloway, J. R., and McCormick, D. B. Pharmacokinetics of orally and intravenously administered riboflavin in healthy humans. Am. J. Clin. Nutr. 63:54–66, 1996.
7. Syndenstricker, V. P. The history of pellagra, its recognition as a disorder of nutrition and its conquest. Am. J. Clin. Nutr. 6:409–441, 1958.
8. McKenney, J. M., Proctor, J. D., Harris, S., and Chinchili, V. M. A comparison of the efficacy and toxic effects of sustained- vs immediate-release niacin in hypercholesterolemic patients. J.A.M.A. 271:672–677, 1994.
9. Ginsberg, H. N. Update on the treatment of hypercholesterolemia, with a focus on HMG-CoA reductase inhibitors and combination regimens. Clin. Cardiol. 18:307–315, 1995.

10. Gibbons, K. W., Gonzales, V., Gordon, N., and Grundy, S. The prevalence of side effects with regular and sustained release nicotinic acid. Am. J. Med. 99:378–385, 1995.
11. Pozzilli, P. Prevention of insulin-dependent diabetes mellitus. Diabetes Metab. Rev. 14:69–84, 1998.
12. Gale, E. A., Molecular mechanisms of beta-cell destruction in IDDM: the role of nicotinamide. Horm. Res. 45(suppl 1):39–43, 1996.
13. Lampeter, E. F., Klinghammer, A., Scherbaum, W. A., et al. The Deutsche Nicotinamide Intervention Study: an attempt to prevent type 1 diabetes. DENIS Group. Diabetes 47:980–984, 1998.
14. Pozzilli, P., Brown, P. D., and Kolb, H. Meta-analysis of nicotinamide treatment in patients with recent-onset IDDM: The Nicotinamide Trialists. Diabetes Care 19:1357–1363, 1996.
15. Polo, V., Saibene, A., and Pontiroli, A. E., Nicotinamide improves insulin secretion and metabolic control in lean type 2 diabetic patients with secondary failure to sulphonylureas. Acta Diabetol. 35:61–64, 1998.
16. Velazquez, A., Teran, M., Baez, A., et al. Biotin supplementation affects lymphocyte carboxylases and plasma biotin in severe protein energy malnutrition. Am. J. Clin. Nutr. 61:385–391, 1995.
17. Mock, N. I., Malik, M. I., Stumbo, P. J., et al. Increased urinary excretion of 3-hydroxyisovaleric acid and decreased urinary excretion of biotin are sensitive to early indicators of decreased biotin status in experimental biotin deficiency. Am. J. Clin. Nutr. 65:951–958, 1997.
18. Food and Nutrition Board, National Research Council. *Recommended Dietary Allowances*, 10th ed. Washington, D.C.: National Academy Press, 1989.
19. USDA Agricultural Research Service. *Results From USDA 1994–1996 CSFII*. 1997.
20. Borschel, M. W. Vitamin B_6 in infancy: requirements and current feeding practices. In *Vitamin B-6 Metabolism in Pregnancy, Lactation and Infancy.* Raiten, D. J., ed. Boca Raton: CRC Press, 1995, 109–124.
21. Bessey, O. A., Adam, D. J., and Hansen, A. E. Intake of vitamin B_6 and infantile convulsions: a first approximation of requirements of pyridoxine in infants. Pediatrics 20:33–44, 1957.
22. Schaumburg, H., Kaplan, J., Windebank, A., et al. Sensory neuropathy from pyridoxine abuse. N. Engl. J. Med. 309:445–448, 1983.
23. Wilcken, D. E., and Wilcken, B. The natural history of vascular disease in homocystinuria and the effects of treatment. J. Inherit. Metab. Dis. 20:295–300, 1997.
24. Mayer, E. L., Jacobsen, D. W., and Robinson, R. Homocysteine and coronary atherosclerosis. J. Am. Coll. Cardiol. 27:517–527, 1996.
25. Graham, I. M., Daly, L. E., Reefsum, H. M., et al. Plasma homocysteine as a risk factor for vascular disease. The European Concerted Action Project. J.A.M.A. 227:1775–1781, 1997.
26. Boushey, C. J., Beresford, S. A. A., Omenn, G. S., and Motulsky, A. G. A quantitative assessment of plasma homocysteine as a risk factor for vascular disease. J.A.M.A. 274:1049–1057, 1995.
27. Rimm, E. B., Willett, W. C., Hu, F. B., et al. Folate and vitamin B_6 from diet and supplements in relation to risk of coronary heart disease among women. J.A.M.A. 279:359–364, 1998.
28. Refsum, H., Ueland, P. M., Nygard, O., and Vollset, S. E. Homocysteine and cardiovascular disease. Annu. Rev. Med. 49:31–62, 1998.
29. Franzblau, A., Rock, C. L., Werner, R. A., et al. The relationship of vitamin B_6 status to median nerve function and carpal tunnel syndrome among active industrial workers. J. Occup. Environ. Med. 38:485–491, 1996.
30. Jacobson, M. D., Plancher, K. D., and Kleinman, W. B. Vitamin B_6 (pyridoxine) therapy for carpal tunnel syndrome. Hand. Clin. 12:253–257, 1996.
31. Diegoli, M. S., da Fonseca, A. M., Diegoli, C. A., and Pinotti, J. A. A double-blind trial of four medications to treat severe premenstrual syndrome. Int. J. Gynaecol. Obstet. 62:63–67, 1998.
32. Kleijnen, J., Ter Riet, G., and Knipschild, P. Vitamin B_6 in the treatment of the premenstrual syndrome—a review. Br. J. Obstet. Gynecol. 98:329–330, 1991.
33. Lesourd, B. M., Mazari, L., and Ferry, M. The role of nutrition in immunity in the aged. Nutr. Rev. 56(II):S113–S125, 1998.
34. Czeizel, A. E., and Dudas, I. Prevention of the first occurrence of neural tube defects by periconceptional vitamin supplementation. N. Engl. J. Med. 327:1832–1835, 1992.
35. Bailey, L. B. Evaluation of a new Recommended Dietary Allowance for folate. J. Am. Diet. Assoc. 92:463–468, 1992.
36. Mason, J. B., and Levesque, T. Folate: effects on carcinogenesis and the potential for cancer chemoprevention. Oncology (Huntingt) 10:1727–1736, 1742–1743, 1996.
37. Giovannucci, E., Stampfer, M. J., Colditz, G. A., et al. Multivitamin use, folate, and colon cancer in women in the Nurses' Health Study. Ann. Intern. Med. 129:517–524, 1998.
38. Miller, D. R., Specker, B. L., Ho, M. L., and Norman, E. J. Vitamin B_{12} status in a macrobiotic community. Am. J. Clin. Nutr. 53:524–529, 1991.
39. Messina, V. K., and Burke, K. I. Position of the American Dietetic Association: vegetarian diets. J. Am. Diet. Assoc. 97:1317–1321, 1997.
40. Bower, C. Folate and neural tube defects. Nutr. Rev. 53:S33–S38, 1995.
41. van Asselt, D. Z., van den Broek, W. J., Lamers, C. B., et al. Free and protein-bound cobalamin absorption in healthy middle-aged and older subjects. J. Am. Geriatr. Soc. 44:949–953, 1996.
42. Halliwell, B. Antioxidants and human disease: a general introduction. Nutr. Rev. 55:(II)S44–S52, 1997.
43. Padh, H. Vitamin C: newer insights into its biochemical functions. Nutr. Rev. 49:65–70, 1991.
44. Podmore, I. D., Griffiths, H. R., Herbert, K. E., et al. Vitamin C exhibits pro-oxidant properties. Nature 392:559, 1998.
45. Schectman, G., Byrd, J. C., and Hoffman, R. Ascorbic acid requirements for smokers, analysis of a population survey. Am. J. Clin. Nutr. 53:1466–1470, 1991.
46. Blanchard, J., Tozer, T. N., and Rowland, M. Pharmacokinetic perspectives on megadoses of ascorbic acid. Am. J. Clin. Nutr. 66:1165–1171, 1997.

47. Hemilä, H. Does vitamin C alleviate the symptoms of the common cold? A review of current evidence. Scand. J. Infect. Dis. 26:1–6, 1994.
48. Jari, R. J., and Harakeh, S. Antiviral and immunomodulatory activities of ascorbic acid. In *Subcellular Biochemistry*, vol. 25: *Ascorbic Acid: Biochemistry and Biomedical Cell Biology*. Harris, J. R., ed. New York: Plenum Press, 1996, 215–231.
49. Johnston, C. S. The antihistamine action of ascorbic acid. In *Subcellular Biochemistry*, vol. 25: *Ascorbic Acid: Biochemistry and Biomedical Cell Biology*. Harris, J. R., ed. New York: Plenum Press, 1996, 189–213.
50. Lynch, S. M., Gaziano, M., and Frei, B. Ascorbic acid and atherosclerotic cardiovascular disease. In *Subcellular Biochemistry*, vol. 25: *Ascorbic Acid: Biochemistry and Biomedical Cell Biology*. Harris, J. R., ed. New York: Plenum Press, 1996, 331–367.
51. Lonn, E. M., and Yusuf, S. Is there a role for antioxidant vitamins in the prevention of cardiovascular diseases? An update on epidemiological and clinical trials data. Can. J. Cardiol. 13:957–965, 1997.
52. Shklar, G., and Schwartz, J. L. Ascorbic acid and cancer. In *Subcellular Biochemistry*, vol. 25: *Ascorbic Acid: Biochemistry and Biomedical Cell Biology*. Harris, J. R., ed. New York: Plenum Press, 1996, 233–247.
53. Barja, G. Ascorbic acid and aging. In *Subcellular Biochemistry*, vol. 25: *Ascorbic Acid: Biochemistry and Biomedical Cell Biology*. Harris, J. R., ed. New York: Plenum Press, 1996, 157–188.
54. van Poppel, G., and van den Berg, H. Vitamins and cancer. Cancer Lett. 19:195–202, 1997.
55. Zeisel, S. H., Da Costa, K. A., Franklin, P. D., et al. Choline, an essential nutrient for humans. FASEB J. 5:2093–2098, 1991.
56. Zeisel, S. H. Choline and phosphatidylcholine. In *Modern Nutrition in Health and Disease*, 9th ed. Shils, M. E., Olson, J. A., Shike, M., and Ross, A. C., eds. Baltimore: Williams & Wilkins, 1999, 513–523.

Chapter 9

Chapter Outline

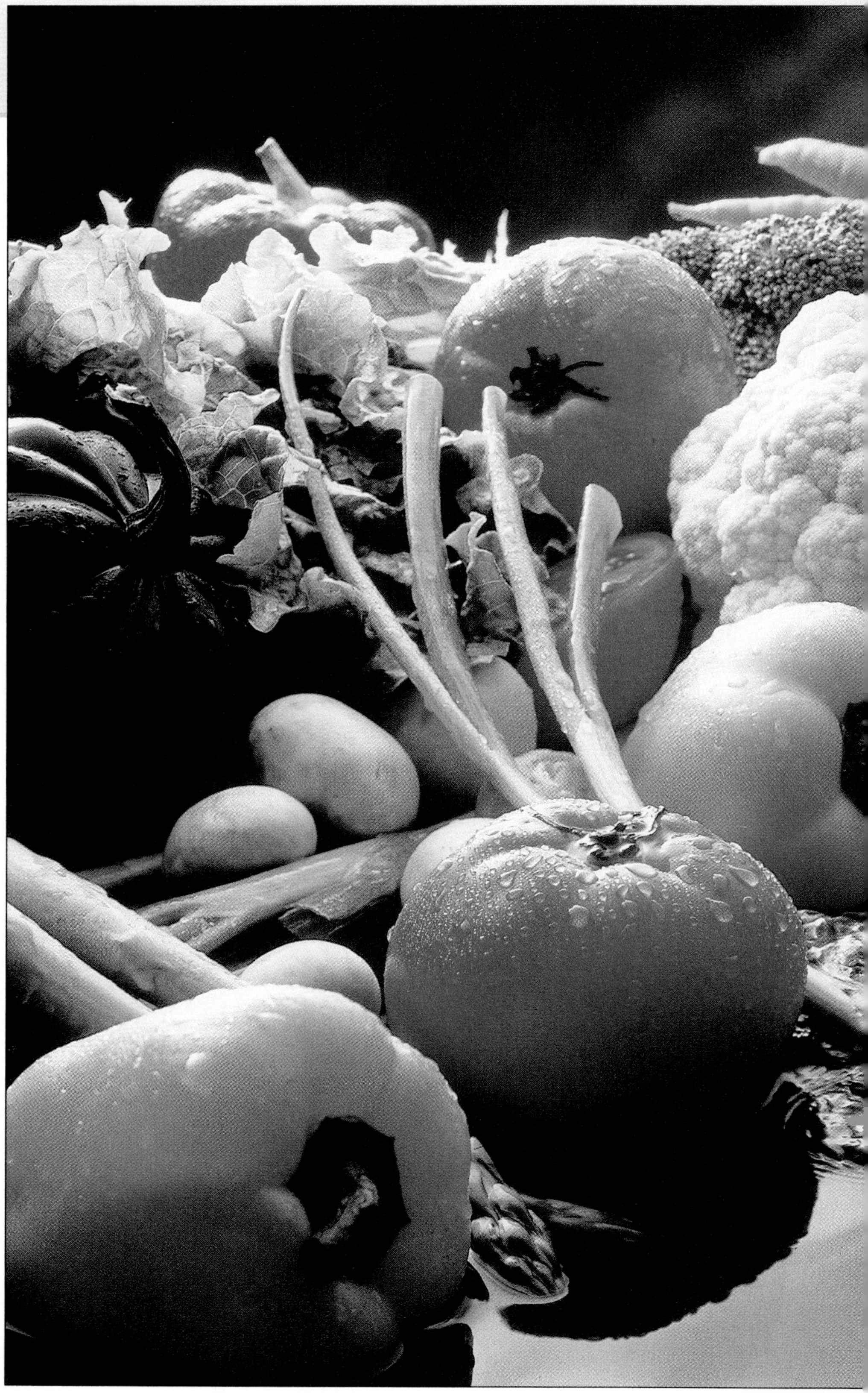

(© Myers Photography Inc./The Stock Market)

Fat-Soluble Vitamins and Meeting Your Vitamin Needs

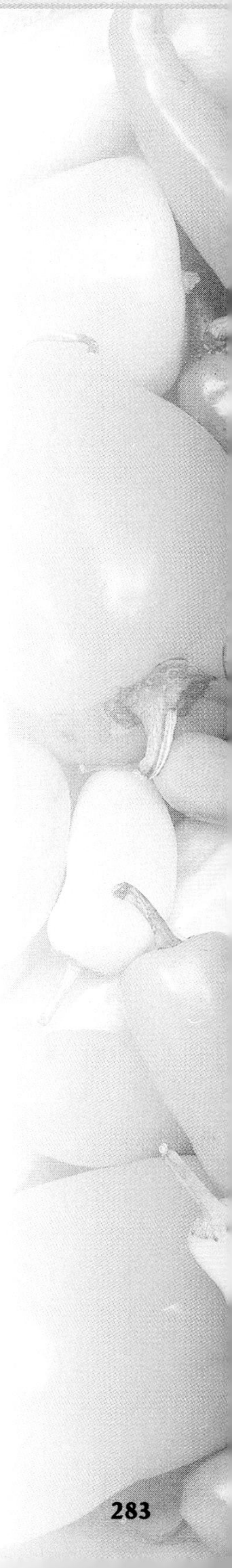

Chapter Concepts

1. The fat-soluble vitamins are grouped together because of their solubility, but each has unique functions.
2. Vitamin A exists in preformed and precursor forms. It is essential for vision and it regulates cell differentiation and growth by affecting gene expression.
3. Beta-carotene and some other carotenoids are vitamin A precursors and also act as antioxidants.
4. When exposure to sunlight is limited, vitamin D is a dietary essential. It acts by affecting gene expression and is necessary for the formation and maintenance of bone.
5. Vitamin E is an antioxidant that protects lipid membranes.
6. Vitamin K is necessary for blood clotting.
7. Vitamin needs can be met by consuming a balanced diet from a variety of food sources.
8. In addition to essential nutrients, food also provides other health-promoting substances such as phytochemicals, which are not essential nutrients.
9. Dietary supplements can be a source of nutrients. Supplements of nonessential substances are also available. When taking supplements, consumers should be aware that more is not always better and too much can be toxic.

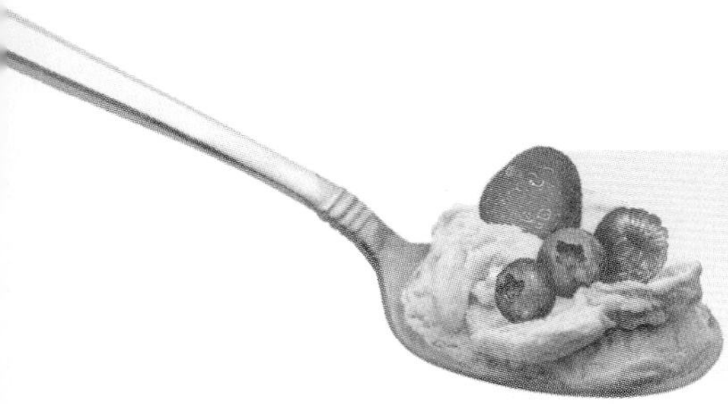

Just a Taste

Does eating carrots improve your vision?

Will vitamin E prevent heart disease?

Can dietary supplements improve your health and extend your life?

In the early 20th century, micronutrient discoveries led to cures for deficiency diseases. As the vitamins were identified and chemically isolated, they were concentrated into pills and potions. As long ago as the 1920s, products ranging from health elixirs to chocolate bars were promoted as vitamin-rich cure-alls. As the century turns, we are still studying micronutrients and their role in health—but the emphasis has switched from preventing deficiency diseases to protecting us from chronic diseases.

The concept of nutrients as a defense against chronic disease has fueled enthusiasm for nutrient supplementation. People swallow a cornucopia of supplement pills hoping to protect themselves from cardiovascular disease, reduce the risk of cancer, and stay young. There is scientific evidence that some micronutrients may reduce the risk of developing cardiovascular disease and cancer, delay the changes associated with aging, and affect immune function. However, epidemiologists are finding that supplements do not provide all the benefits that foods do. Studies show that people who eat more fruits and vegetables have a lower incidence of a host of chronic diseases. These same benefits are not duplicated by taking nutritional supplements. Fruits and vegetables provide antioxidant nutrients, but they also contain other substances that are not nutrients but that have health-promoting properties. The identification of a number of these phytochemicals has led scientists to reexamine the importance of foods and dietary patterns, rather than just essential nutrients, in maintaining health and preventing chronic disease. Nonetheless, supplements are big business. They are marketed to improve athletic performance, prevent depression, enhance memory, boost energy level, change body composition, and more. Many of the supplements available are not nutrients and have effects that have not been carefully studied. Since we do not yet know all there is to know about nutrition, consumers must not ignore the importance of a wholesome diet or overuse supplements.

Vitamin A: A Vitamin That Turns On Our Genes

Are carrots really good for your eyes? Carrots are high in a precursor of vitamin A, and vitamin A is important for vision. This connection between vision and foods that we now know are high in vitamin A has been known for centuries. In ancient times, the Egyptians knew that eating liver could treat night blindness, a difficulty in adjusting from bright light to dim light, such as when a bright light strikes your eyes at night. In 1968, George Wald earned the Nobel Prize in medicine for identifying the mechanism by which vitamin A is involved in vision. Although this is a key function of vitamin A, attention today is focused more on how vitamin A interacts with genes to regulate growth and **cell differentiation.** Despite our expanding understanding of the functions of vitamin A, deficiency remains a world health problem.

Cell differentiation Structural and functional changes that cause cells to mature into specialized cells.

Vitamin A in the Diet

Vitamin A is found preformed and in precursor or provitamin forms in our diet. Preformed vitamin A compounds are known as **retinoids.** The retinoids include retinal, retinol, and retinoic acid. They are found in animal foods such as liver, fish, egg yolks, and dairy products. Margarine and nonfat and reduced-fat milk are fortified with vitamin A because they are often consumed in place of butter and whole milk, which are good sources of this vitamin.

Retinoids The chemical forms of preformed vitamin A: retinol, retinal, and retinoic acid.

Plant sources of vitamin A, including carrots, cantaloupe, apricots, mangoes, and sweet potatoes, contain yellow-orange pigments called **carotenoids.** About 50 of the 600 carotenoids that have been isolated provide vitamin A activity. **Beta-carotene (β-carotene),** the most potent precursor, is plentiful in carrots, squash, and other red and yellow vegetables and fruits as well as in leafy greens where the yellow pigment is masked by green chlorophyll (Figure 9.1). Other carotenoids that provide some provitamin A activity include alpha-carotene found in leafy green vegetables, carrots, and squash; beta-cryptoxanthin found in corn, green peppers, and lemons; and lutein and zeaxanthin found in corn, green peppers, peaches, and tomatoes. Lycopene, the carotenoid that gives the red color to tomatoes, cannot be converted to vitamin A.[1,2]

Carotenoids Natural pigments synthesized by plants and many microorganisms. They give yellow and red-orange fruits and vegetables their color.

Beta-carotene (β-carotene) A carotenoid that has more provitamin A activity than other carotenoids. It also acts as an antioxidant in the body.

To help consumers identify food sources of vitamin A, labels on packaged foods must list the vitamin A content as a percentage of the Daily Value. All forms of vitamin A in the diet are fairly stable when heated but may be destroyed by exposure to light and oxygen.

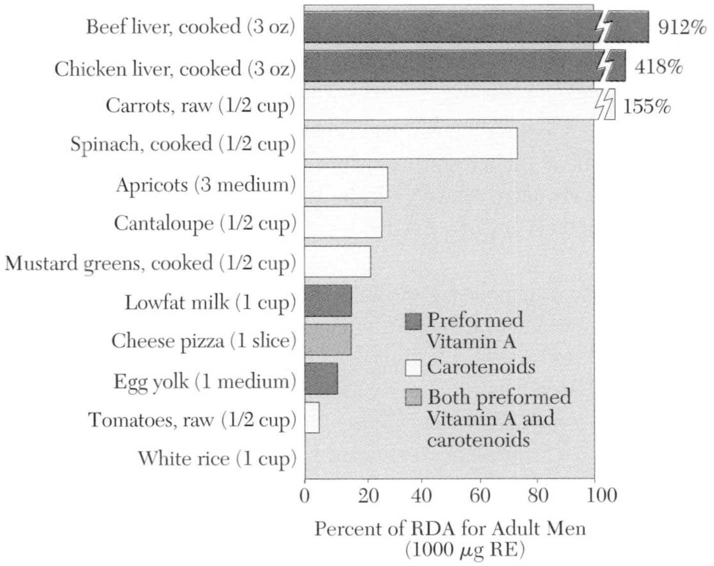

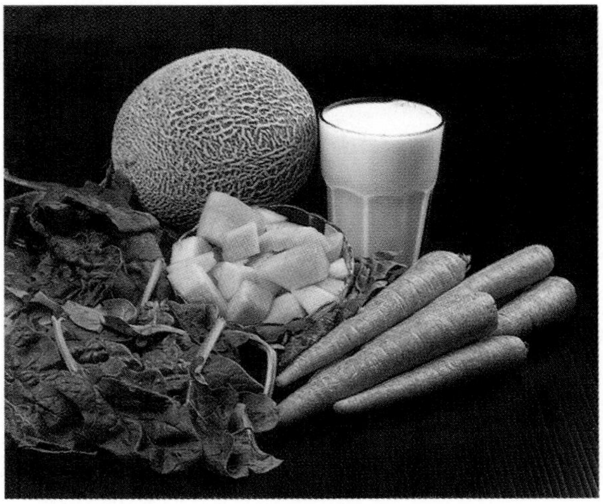

Figure 9.1
The vitamin A content of foods as a percent of the 1989 RDA for adult men. (*right,* George Semple)

Vitamin A in the Digestive Tract

Both retinoids and carotenoids are bound to proteins in foods. To be absorbed, they must be released from the protein by pepsin and other protein-digesting enzymes. Then the released carotenoids and retinoids must combine with bile acids and other fat-soluble food components to form micelles, which facilitate their diffusion into mucosal cells.[2] Insufficient fat intake (less than 10 g/day) can reduce vitamin A absorption. This is rarely a problem in industrialized countries, where typical fat intake ranges from 50 to 100 grams per day. However, in populations with low dietary fat intakes, vitamin A deficiency may occur due to poor absorption. Diseases that cause fat malabsorption can also interfere with vitamin A absorption and cause a deficiency.

Consumption of large amounts of the artificial fat Olestra (sucrose polyester) interferes with vitamin A absorption. Olestra cannot be digested and absorbed in the human digestive tract. As it passes through the intestine it takes fat-soluble substances with it. It therefore decreases the absorption of the fat-soluble vitamins A, D, E, and K, as well as beta-carotene and other carotenoids. Foods containing Olestra are fortified with vitamins A, D, E, and K, but not with carotenoids.

Carotenoid absorption decreases as intake increases, so large amounts are not absorbed. Once in the mucosal cells, much of the beta-carotene is converted into retinol, but up to 30% may leave the intestine unchanged. It is estimated that 6 μg of beta-carotene are needed to produce 1 μg of retinol.

Vitamin A in the Body

Retinol-binding protein A protein that is necessary to transport vitamin A in the blood.

Retinoids and carotenoids are transported from the intestine in chylomicrons. These lipoproteins deliver the retinoids and carotenoids to body tissues such as bone marrow, blood cells, spleen, muscles, kidney, and liver. In the liver, some carotenoids can be converted into retinol. To move from liver stores to the tissues, preformed vitamin A must be bound to **retinol-binding protein.** There is no specific blood transport protein for carotenoids, but since they are fat soluble, they must be incorporated into lipoproteins to travel in the bloodstream.

The different forms of vitamin A have different functions. Retinol and retinal can be interconverted from one to the other. Retinal is the form that is important for vision. Retinoic acid, which is made from retinol or retinal, cannot be used in the visual cycle (see below) but is the form that affects gene expression and is responsible for vitamin A's role in cell differentiation, growth, and reproduction.[3] Carotenoids that are not converted to retinoids function as antioxidants.

Rhodopsin A light-sensitive compound found in the retina of the eye that is composed of the protein opsin loosely bound to retinal.

The Visual Cycle Vitamin A is involved in the perception of light (Figure 9.2). In the eye, the retinal form of the vitamin combines with the protein opsin to form the visual pigment **rhodopsin.** Rhodopsin helps transform the energy from light into a nerve impulse that is sent to the brain. This nerve impulse allows us to see.

The visual cycle begins when light passes into the eye and strikes rhodopsin. The light changes retinal in rhodopsin from a curved molecule to a straight one by converting a *cis* double bond in retinal to a *trans* double bond. This change in shape initiates a series of events causing a nerve signal to be sent to the brain and retinal to be released from opsin. After the light stimulus has passed, the *trans* retinal is converted back to its original *cis* form and recombined with opsin to regenerate rhodopsin. Each time this cycle occurs, some retinal is used up and must be replaced by retinol from the blood. The retinol is converted into retinal in the eye. When vitamin A is deficient, there is a delay in the regeneration of rhodopsin, which causes difficulty in adapting to dim light after experiencing a bright light—a condition called night blindness. Night blindness is one of the first and more easily reversible symptoms of vitamin A deficiency.

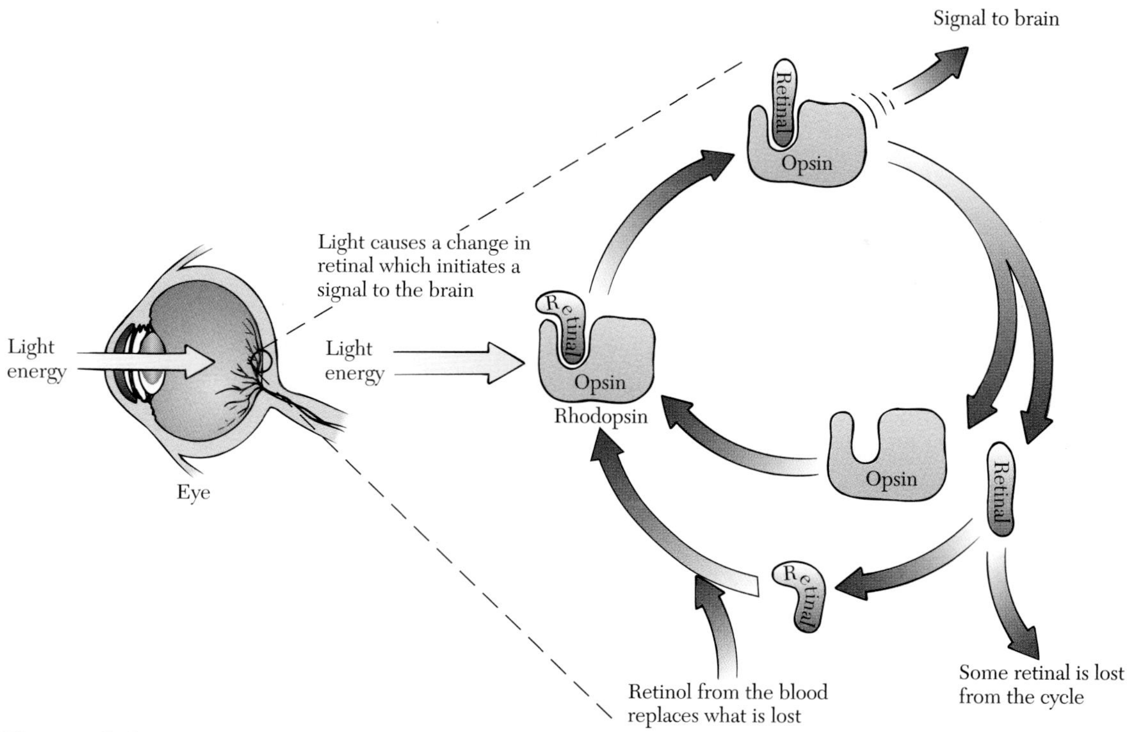

Figure 9.2
The visual cycle. In the eye, retinal binds to the protein opsin to form rhodopsin. When light strikes rhodopsin, it causes a change in retinal that sends a nerve signal to the brain and causes retinal to be released from opsin. Some retinal returns to its original form and binds opsin to begin the cycle again. Some retinal is lost, and retinol from the blood must be converted to replace it.

Regulating Gene Expression: Cell Differentiation Cell differentiation is the process whereby immature cells change in structure and function to become specialized. For instance, in the bone marrow, some cells differentiate into white blood cells, whereas others differentiate to form red blood cells. Vitamin A affects cell differentiation through its effect on gene expression. This means that it can turn on or turn off the production of certain proteins that regulate functions within cells and throughout the body. By affecting gene expression, vitamin A can also determine what type of cell an immature cell will become.

In order to affect gene expression, the retinoic acid form of vitamin A enters specific target cells. Inside the nucleus of these target cells, retinoic acid binds to protein receptors; this retinoic acid–protein receptor complex then binds to regulatory regions of DNA. This binding changes the amount of messenger RNA (mRNA) that is made by the gene. The change in mRNA changes the amount of the protein that is produced (Figure 9.3). This turning on (or turning off) of the gene increases (or decreases) the production of proteins and thereby affects various cellular functions. For example, vitamin A turns on a gene that makes an enzyme in liver cells which enables the liver to make glucose by gluconeogenesis.

Maintenance of Epithelial Tissue Vitamin A is necessary for the maintenance of epithelial tissue. This type of tissue covers external body surfaces and lines internal cavities and tubes. It includes the skin and the linings of the eyes, intestines, lungs, vagina, and bladder. When vitamin A is deficient, epithelial cells do not differentiate normally because vitamin A is not there to turn on or turn off the production of particular proteins. For example, the epithelial tissue on many body surfaces contains cells that produce mucus for lubrication. When mucus-secreting

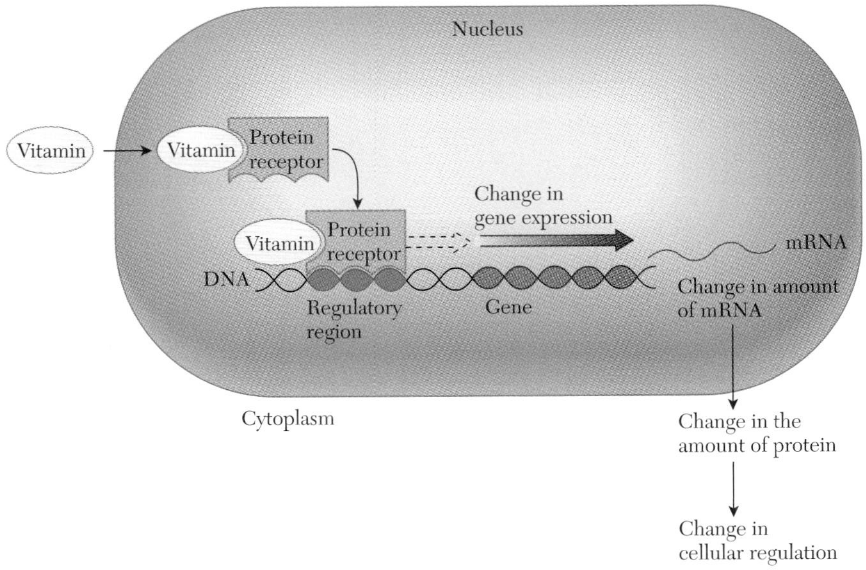

Figure 9.3
The retinoic acid form of vitamin A functions by entering the nucleus and binding to a protein receptor. The complex then binds to a regulatory region of DNA to change the expression of a gene and hence the amount of a protein synthesized as well as the cellular functions and body processes that the protein affects.

Keratin A hard protein that makes up hair and nails.

Xerophthalmia A spectrum of eye conditions resulting from vitamin A deficiency. It is characterized by a lack of mucus, which leaves the eye dry and vulnerable to cracking and infection. Xerophthalmia may lead to blindness.

cells die, new cells differentiate into mucus-secreting cells to replace them. When vitamin A is deficient, the new cells do not differentiate properly and instead become cells that produce a protein called **keratin.** Keratin is the hard protein that makes up hair and fingernails. As the mucus-secreting cells die and are replaced by keratin-producing cells, the epithelial surface becomes hard and dry. This process is known as keratinization. The hard, dry surface does not have the protective capabilities of normal epithelium and increases the likelihood of infection. The risk of infection is compounded by the fact that vitamin A deficiency also decreases the activity of the immune system.

All epithelial tissues are affected by vitamin A deficiency, but the eye is particularly susceptible to damage. The mucus in the eye normally provides lubrication, washes away dirt and other particles, and also contains a protein that helps destroy bacteria. When vitamin A is deficient, the lack of mucus and the buildup of keratin cause the cornea to dry and leave the eye open to infection. This condition, known as **xerophthalmia,** can be treated by increasing vitamin A intake. If left untreated, it can result in a softening of the cornea (keratomalacia) and permanent blindness.

Reproduction, Growth, and Immunity The ability of vitamin A to regulate the growth and differentiation of cells makes it essential throughout life for normal reproduction, growth, and immune function. In reproduction, vitamin A is hypothesized to play a role during early embryonic development by directing cells to form the shapes and patterns needed for a completely formed organism.[4] Poor overall growth is an early sign of vitamin A deficiency in children. Vitamin A affects the activity of cells that form and break down bone, and a deficiency early in life can cause abnormal jawbone growth, resulting in crooked teeth and poor dental health. In the immune system, vitamin A is needed for the differentiation that produces the different types of immune cells. When vitamin A is deficient, the activity of specific immune cells cannot be stimulated. This impaired immune function increases the risk of illness and infection due to defective epithelial tissue barriers.

Beta-Carotene: A Vitamin A Precursor and an Antioxidant Some carotenoids, particularly beta-carotene, can be converted to vitamin A in the intestinal mucosa. Unconverted carotenoids also reach the blood and tissues where they function as antioxidants, a role independent of any conversion to vitamin A. Beta-carotene and other carotenoids are fat-soluble antioxidants that are important in protecting cell membranes from damage by free radicals. The antioxidant properties of carotenoids have stimulated interest in their ability to protect against diseases in which oxidative processes play a role, such as cancer, heart disease, and impaired vision due to macular degeneration and cataracts.

How Much Vitamin A Do We Need?

The recommended intake of vitamin A is expressed in **retinol equivalents (REs)**—the amount of any form of vitamin A that provides the function of 1 μg of retinol. For example, 6 μg of beta-carotene or 12 μg of other provitamin A carotenoids provide 1 RE. The 1989 RDA for vitamin A is 1000 μg RE for adult men and 800 μg RE for adult women. This amount can be supplied by one carrot or a third of an ounce of beef liver.

Retinol equivalents (REs) A unit of measure for vitamin A equal to the amount of any form of vitamin A that provides the function of 1 μg of retinol.

Although the RDA has been expressed in REs since 1980, many food tables and vitamin supplement labels still use the older measure of international units (IUs). Ten IU of beta-carotene or 3.3 IU of preformed vitamin A are equal to 1 RE.

Vitamin A and Health

Vitamin A deficiency is a world health problem responsible for growth failure, increased susceptibility to infection, blindness, and death. Consumption of too much preformed vitamin A, however, can also be deadly (see Toxicity, below). A low intake of carotenoids is not associated with any specific deficiency disease as long as sufficient preformed vitamin A is supplied in the diet.

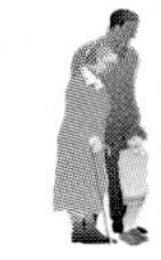

Vitamin A Deficiency: A World Health Problem Vitamin A deficiency is a threat to the health, sight, and lives of millions of children in the developing world.[5] Children deficient in vitamin A grow poorly, have poor appetites, have more infections, are more anemic, are more likely to go blind, and are more likely to die in childhood than their peers. Vitamin A deficiency increases the risk of death from common childhood infections such as diarrheal diseases and measles.[6] It is estimated that over 3 million children worldwide have clinical signs of vitamin A deficiency such as keratomalacia and xerophthalmia, and that approximately 250 million children are at risk of vitamin A deficiency.[7] It is most common in India, Africa, Latin America, and the Caribbean (Figure 9.4).

Vitamin A deficiency can be caused by insufficient intakes of vitamin A, fat, protein, or the mineral zinc. Without fat, vitamin A cannot be absorbed, so a diet very low in fat can cause a deficiency by reducing vitamin A absorption. Protein deficiency can cause vitamin A deficiency because the retinol-binding protein needed to transport vitamin A cannot be made in sufficient quantities. The importance of zinc for vitamin A utilization is believed to be due to its role in protein synthesis. When zinc is deficient, proteins needed for vitamin A transport and metabolism are lacking.

Vitamin A deficiency is not common in developed countries, but intakes below the RDA may be caused by poor food choices. In the United States the intake of fresh fruits and vegetables, many of which are excellent sources of provitamin A, does not meet recommendations. A typical fast-food meal of a hamburger and french fries provides almost no vitamin A.

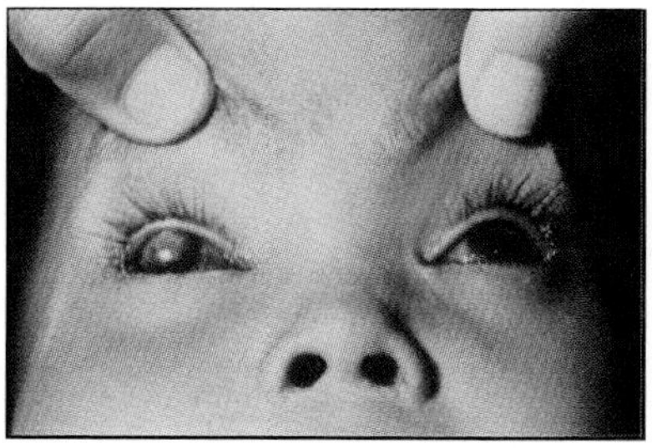

Figure 9.4
Vitamin A deficiency is a major cause of blindness worldwide. (L.V. Bergman/The Bergman Collection)

Toxicity Preformed vitamin A can be toxic. Acute toxicity occurs with doses of 100 times the RDA and can result in coma and death. This has been reported in Arctic explorers who consumed polar bear liver, which contains about 60,000 μg RE of vitamin A in just 3 ounces. Although polar bear liver is not a common dish at most dinner tables, supplements of preformed vitamin A also have the potential to deliver a toxic dose. Signs of acute toxicity include nausea, vomiting, headache, dizziness, blurred vision, and a lack of muscle coordination. Chronic toxicity occurs when preformed vitamin A doses as low as ten times the RDA are consumed for a period of months to years. The symptoms of chronic toxicity include weight loss, muscle and joint pain, liver damage, bone abnormalities, visual defects, dry scaling lips, and skin rashes.

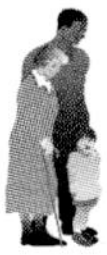

Birth defects are also associated with high dietary intakes of preformed vitamin A. One study found that women who consumed more than 3000 µg RE (about four times the RDA) of preformed vitamin A as supplements were about five times more likely to have a baby with birth defects than women who consumed 1500 µg RE or less.[8] Since 3000 µg RE of vitamin A is easily obtained from supplements, it is recommended that if supplements are taken during pregnancy, they contain only carotenoids, which have not been found to cause birth defects. Vitamin A derivatives, used to treat acne, can also cause birth defects (see Chapter 14).

Unlike preformed vitamin A, provitamin A carotenoids are nontoxic. This is because their absorption from the diet decreases at high doses, and once in the

Table 9.1 *A Summary of the Fat-Soluble Vitamins*

Vitamin	Sources	Recommended Intake for Adults	Major Functions	Deficiency	Groups at Risk	Toxicity	Tolerable Upper Intake Level (UL)
Vitamin A (vitamin A acetate, vitamin A palmitate, retinol, retinal, retinoic acid, retinyl palmitate, provitamin A, carotene, β-carotene, carotenoids)	Liver, carrots, peaches, leafy greens, fortified milk, sweet potatoes, broccoli	800–1000† µg RE	Vision, growth, cell differentiation, reproduction, immune function	Night blindness, xerophthalmia, poor growth, dry skin, impaired immunity	Those who live in poverty (particularly children and pregnant women), those consuming very lowfat or low-protein diets	Headache, vomiting, hair loss, liver damage, skin changes, birth defects, bone pain	NA
Vitamin D (cholecalciferol, ergocalciferol)	Egg yolk, liver, fish oils, tuna, salmon, fortified margarine and milk, sunlight	5 µg (200 IU)°	Absorption of calcium and phosphorus, maintenance of bone	Rickets in children, osteomalacia in adults	Breast-fed infants, children and elderly (especially with dark skin and little sun exposure), people with kidney disease	Calcium deposits in the soft tissues, growth retardation, kidney damage	50 µg/day (2000 IU)
Vitamin E (alpha-tocopherol acetate, alpha-tocopherol, mixed tocopherols)	Vegetable oils, leafy greens, nuts, peanuts	8–10 mg α-TE†	Antioxidant, protects cell membranes	Hemolyzed red blood cells, nerve damage	Those with poor fat absorption, premature infants	Inhibition of vitamin K activity	NA
Vitamin K (phylloquinone, menaquinone)	Beef liver, leafy greens, intestinal bacteria	65–80 µg†	Blood clotting	Hemorrhage	People on long-term antibiotics, newborns (especially premature)	Anemia, brain damage	NA

°Adequate Intake (AI).
†1989 RDA value.
NA—No UL established at time of publication.

body, their conversion to active vitamin A is limited. Large daily intakes of carotenoids—usually in the form of carrot juice or beta-carotene supplements—do, however, lead to a condition known as **hypercarotenemia.** In this condition, the carotenoids stored in the adipose tissue make the skin look yellow-orange. This is particularly apparent on the palms of the hands and the soles of the feet. It is not known to be dangerous, and when intake decreases, the skin returns to its normal color.

Hypercarotenemia A condition caused by an accumulation of carotenoids in the adipose tissue, causing the skin to appear yellow-orange.

Vitamin A Supplements Most supplements contain beta-carotene in order to avoid any risk of vitamin A toxicity. Epidemiological evidence showing a relationship between diets high in beta-carotene–containing foods and a reduction in cancer and heart disease risk has prompted studies on the benefits of beta-carotene supplements.

Intervention studies that supplement beta-carotene have not consistently shown a reduction in cancer risk. Only one intervention trial showed a decrease in cancer incidence with supplemental beta-carotene.[9] Others, including a trial that lasted 12 years, found no effect of beta-carotene on overall cancer risk,[10] and two trials found that beta-carotene supplements increased the incidence of lung cancer in people who smoke cigarettes.[11,12] Even though other trials have not shown this effect, until more information is available, smokers are advised to avoid beta-carotene supplements and rely on food sources to obtain carotenoids in their diet.

Some studies evaluating cardiovascular disease and beta-carotene supplements have found a beneficial effect.[13] In one trial, men known to have cardiovascular disease had a reduction in heart attacks when supplemented with beta-carotene.[14] However, in another trial no reduction in cardiovascular risk was found, and men receiving beta-carotene supplements actually accounted for more cardiovascular deaths.[12] Another study showed no effect at all, either beneficial or harmful.[10]

Table 9.1 provides a summary of the fat-soluble vitamins.

CRITICAL THINKING

Evaluating Vitamin Supplements

Miguel is halfway through his freshman year at college. He has been feeling run down and tired and has had two colds already this semester. When he describes his concerns to the clerk at a local health food store, she recommends several supplements to keep him healthy and help him withstand the stresses of school. These include a vitamin C supplement, a stress formula B vitamin supplement called B50, Prevention Plus, and Brain Booster. After enrolling in a nutrition class, he begins to wonder if he really needs all these and if some could actually be harmful. He decides to evaluate their benefits and risks.

Is Miguel consuming more than the recommended intake or UL of any nutrients in these supplements?

Using information from the Supplement Facts label, he compiles the following table. He then looks up the recommended intakes (RDAs, AIs, and 1989 RDAs) and UL values in his nutrition book. For some of these nutrients, no UL has been established because no toxicity symptoms have been identified. For others, no UL is available because the DRI values have not been completed.

Supplement	Frequency	Nutrient	Dose	Recommended Intake	UL
Vitamin C	1/day	Vitamin C	500 mg	60 mg	NA
B50	2/day	Thiamin	50 mg	1.2 mg	ND
		Niacin	50 mg	16 mg	35 mg
		Vitamin B_6	60 mg	1.3 mg	100 mg
		Riboflavin	50 mg	1.3 mg	ND
		Biotin	50 μg	30 μg	ND
		Pantothenic acid	50 mg	5 mg	ND
		Folic acid	50 μg	400 μg	1000 μg
		Vitamin B_{12}	50 μg	2.4 μg	ND
Prevention Plus	1/day	Vitamin E	400 IU	400 mg α-TE	NA
		Beta-carotene	5000 μg RE		NA
		Vitamin C	1000 mg	60 mg	NA
Brain Booster	2/day	Choline	100 mg	550 mg	3500 mg
		Niacin	50 mg	16 mg	35 mg

NA—no UL established at time of publication.
ND—not determined due to lack of data on adverse effects.

When he totals the amounts of nutrients in all the supplements, Miguel finds that he is exceeding the recommended intake for vitamin C and all the B vitamins except folate. His intake exceeds the UL for niacin and vitamin B_6.

Niacin: The B50 and Brain Booster both contribute niacin. If he takes the doses recommended by the manufacturers, he will be consuming 200 mg daily. This is well in excess of the UL of 35 mg.

Vitamin B_6: By taking two tablets of B50 a day as directed, his intake will be 120 mg and will exceed the UL of 100 mg.

Will any of these vitamins cause toxicity symptoms?

Miguel's intake of vitamin C is 1500 mg (500 mg + 1000 mg from Prevention Plus), 25 times the 1989 RDA. It is unlikely that this amount will cause symptoms other than possibly some GI upset. His niacin intake well exceeds the UL and may cause a rash and flushing. His intake of vitamin B_6 exceeds the UL and puts him at risk for nerve damage. The ULs are set at a level that will not cause an adverse reaction in the majority of healthy people. However, there is no known benefit to consuming an amount of a nutrient above the RDA.

Will any of these prevent Miguel from getting sick or help boost his energy level?

Answer:

Would you suggest that Miguel stop taking any of these supplements?

Answer:

Vitamin D: The Sunshine Vitamin

Vitamin D is known as the sunshine vitamin because it can be produced in the skin by exposure to ultraviolet light. Because vitamin D can be made in the body, there is a long-standing debate as to whether vitamin D is a vitamin or a hormone. By definition, vitamins are dietary essentials. However, vitamin D can be formed in the skin, so it is only essential in the diet when exposure to sunlight is limited or the body's ability to synthesize the vitamin is reduced. Vitamin D acts like a hormone because it is produced in one organ, the skin, and affects other organs, primarily the intestine and bone.

Vitamin D in the Diet

Only a few foods are natural sources of vitamin D. These include liver, fatty fish such as salmon, and egg yolks (Figure 9.5). These foods contain **cholecalciferol,** or vitamin D_3. Cholecalciferol is the form of vitamin D that is made in the skin of animals by the action of sunlight on a cholesterol compound called

Cholecalciferol The chemical name for vitamin D_3. It can be formed in the skin of animals by the action of sunlight on a form of cholesterol called 7-dehydrocholesterol.

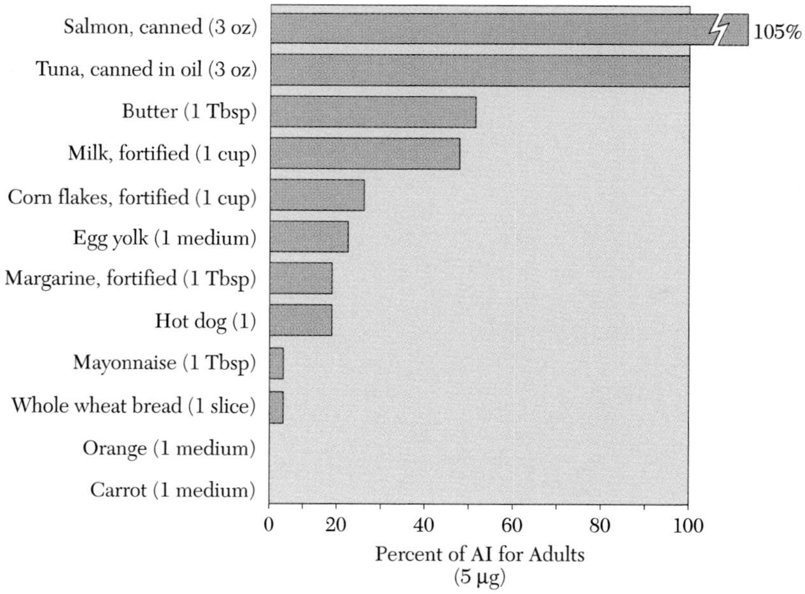

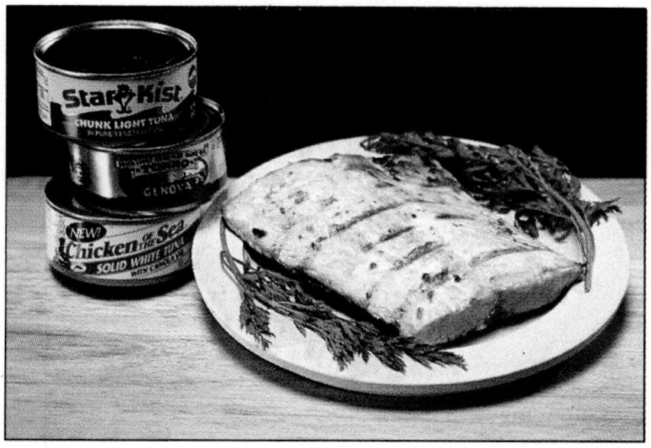

Figure 9.5
The vitamin D content of foods as a percent of the AI for adults. (*right,* Charles D. Winters)

7-dehydrocholesterol. Foods fortified with vitamin D include milk and margarine. These may contain vitamin D_3 or vitamin D_2, another active form of the vitamin.

Vitamin D in the Body

Vitamin D from the diet and from synthesis in the skin is inactive until it is chemically altered in the liver and then the kidney. In the liver, a hydroxyl group (OH) is added to vitamin D to form 25-hydroxy vitamin D_3, which then travels to the kidney where another hydroxyl group is added to make the active form of vitamin D: 1,25-dihydroxy vitamin D_3 (Figure 9.6).

The principal function of vitamin D is to maintain normal blood levels of calcium and phosphorus. When blood calcium levels drop too low, the parathyroid

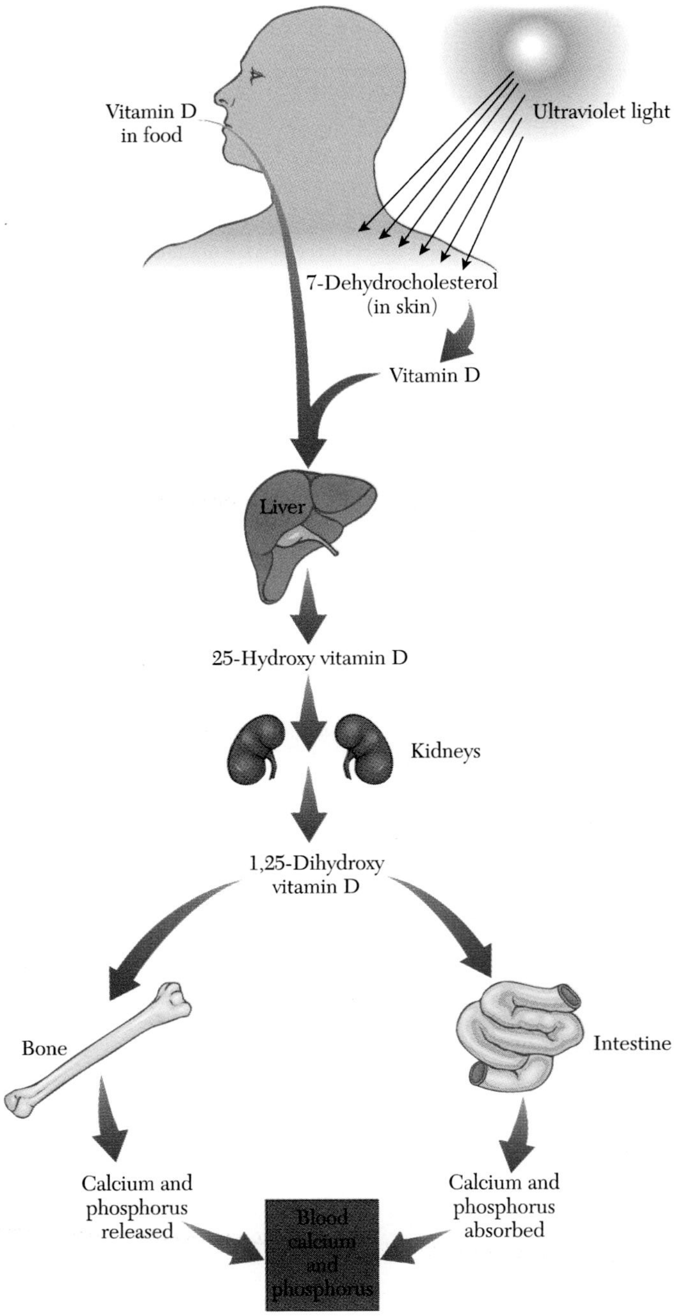

Figure 9.6
Vitamin D comes from food and from synthesis in the skin. In order to function, it must have hydroxyl groups (OH) added at the liver and kidney. Active vitamin D then functions in maintaining calcium and phosphorus balance by stimulating the release of these minerals from bone and their absorption from the intestine.

gland releases **parathyroid hormone (PTH).** PTH release stimulates enzymes in the kidney to convert 25-hydroxy vitamin D_3 to the active form of the vitamin.

Parathyroid hormone (PTH) A hormone released by the parathyroid gland that acts to increase blood calcium levels.

Active vitamin D regulates calcium and phosphorus balance by altering gene expression in cells at the intestine and bone. At the intestine, vitamin D increases the absorption of calcium and phosphorus. This occurs because vitamin D increases the expression of genes that code for intestinal calcium transport proteins (see Figure 9.3). At the bone, vitamin D works in conjunction with PTH to increase bone breakdown, releasing calcium and phosphorus into the blood. This occurs because vitamin D causes precursor cells in the bone to differentiate into cells that break down bone.[15] Vitamin D also acts with PTH to increase the amount of calcium retained by the kidneys. In addition to bone, intestine, and kidney, receptors for active vitamin D have been found in the pancreas, parathyroid gland, cells of the immune system, reproductive organs, and skin.[16] The effect of vitamin D in these tissues is under investigation.

How Much Vitamin D Do We Need?

The recommended intake of vitamin D is based on the amount needed in the diet to maintain normal blood levels of 25-hydroxy vitamin D_3. The AI for adult men and women is set at 5 μg per day.[17] The AI is expressed in μg, but the vitamin D content of foods and supplements may also be given as International Units (IUs); one IU is equal to 0.025 μg of vitamin D_3 (40 IU = 1 μg of vitamin D). The AI for vitamin D for adults is contained in about 2 cups of vitamin D–fortified milk (see Table 9.1).

The AI is based on the assumption that no vitamin D is synthesized in the skin. This assumption is made because of the variation in the extent to which synthesis from sunlight meets the requirement. If there is sufficient sun exposure, dietary vitamin D is not needed. The amount synthesized in the skin is affected by skin pigmentation, climate, season, clothing, the presence of pollution and tall buildings that block sunlight, and the use of sunscreens. Although sunscreens prevent the formation of vitamin D in the skin, children and active adults usually spend enough time outdoors without sunscreens to provide for their vitamin D requirement.

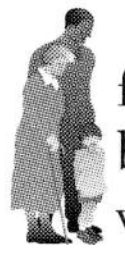

Despite the smaller body size of infants and children, the AI for vitamin D for this age is the same as that for adults. This is to allow sufficient vitamin D for bone development during periods of rapid growth. Although breast milk is low in vitamin D, infants who are exposed to sunlight for about half an hour per day do not require supplemental vitamin D. The AI for adults 50 to 70 years of age is 10 μg per day to prevent bone loss during periods of low sun exposure. In adults 70 and older the AI is 15 μg per day to maintain blood levels of vitamin D and prevent skeletal fractures. The AI is not increased for pregnancy and lactation.

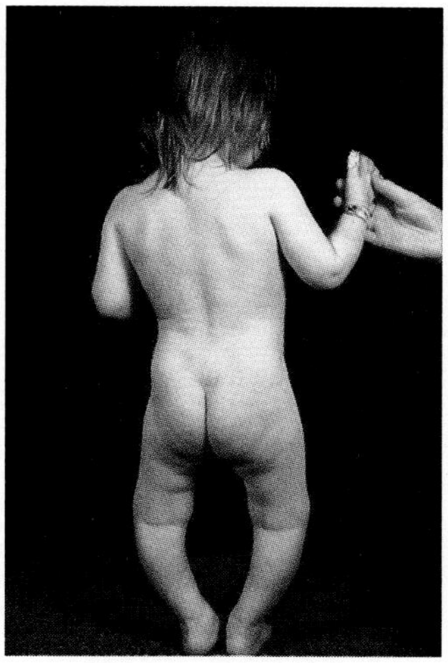

Figure 9.7
Bowed legs are characteristic of rickets. (© Biophoto Associates/Photo Researchers, Inc.)

Vitamin D and Health

Vitamin D is essential for bone health. A deficiency causes improper bone development in children and weakened bones in adults. However, too much vitamin D can be toxic.

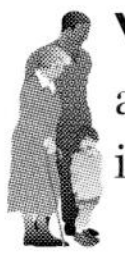

Vitamin D Deficiency When vitamin D is deficient, dietary calcium cannot be absorbed efficiently. As a result, calcium is not available for proper bone mineralization and abnormalities in bone structure occur.

In children who are deficient in vitamin D, bones are weak because they do not contain enough calcium and phosphorus. This syndrome, called **rickets,** is characterized by bone deformities such as narrow rib cages known as pigeon breasts, and bowed legs (Figure 9.7). The legs bow because the bones are too weak to support the weight of the body. Rickets was common in 17th- to 19th-century Europe. The incidence increased during the Industrial Revolution when large numbers of poorly nourished children lived under a layer of smog in the

Rickets A vitamin D deficiency disease in children that is characterized by poor bone development because of inadequate calcium deposition.

newly industrialized cities. Even though the fortification of milk with vitamin D has helped to greatly reduce rickets in most developed countries, it is still a problem in inner-city children who have a poor diet and whose exposure to sunlight is limited by tall buildings and smog. Dark-skinned children are more likely to be vitamin D deficient than those with lighter skin because dark skin pigment prevents the UV light rays from penetrating into the dermis of the skin, thereby reducing the formation of vitamin D. Rickets is also seen in children with disorders that affect fat absorption and in vegetarian children who do not drink milk.

Osteomalacia A vitamin D deficiency disease in adults that causes weak bones and an increase in bone fractures.

In adults, the vitamin D deficiency disease comparable to rickets is called **osteomalacia.** It results in the weakening of bones because not enough calcium is available to form the mineral deposits needed to maintain healthy bone. Insufficient bone mineralization leads to fractures of the weight-bearing bones such as those in the hips and spine. Osteomalacia is common in adults with kidney failure because the conversion of vitamin D from inactive to active forms is reduced. The elderly are at risk for vitamin D deficiency because the ability to produce vitamin D in the skin decreases with age and older adults typically cover more of their skin with clothing and spend less time in the sun than their younger counterparts.[18] In addition, the elderly tend to have a lower intake of dairy products. Bones may also become weakened and fracture easily because of a condition called osteoporosis (see Chapter 10).

Vitamin D Toxicity and Supplements Consumption of unfortified foods does not cause vitamin D toxicity. And, synthesis of vitamin D from exposure to sunlight does not produce toxic amounts because vitamin D formation is carefully regulated. However, oversupplementation and overfortification do pose a risk. One case of accidental overfortification of milk resulted in the hospitalization of 56 individuals and the death of 2.[19] Symptoms of vitamin D toxicity include high blood and urine calcium concentrations, deposition of calcium in soft tissues such as the blood vessels, and kidney and cardiovascular damage. A UL of 50 μg has been established for adults.

VITAMIN E: AN ANTIOXIDANT VITAMIN

Vitamin E is a fat-soluble vitamin with an antioxidant function. It was first identified as a fat-soluble component of grains that was necessary for fertility in laboratory rats. It took almost 30 years to isolate this vitamin and to determine that it is also necessary for reproduction in humans. The chemical name for vitamin E, **tocopherol,** is from the Greek *tos,* meaning childbirth, and *phero,* to bring forth. Vitamin E has been promoted as a cure for infertility, an antiscar medication, a defense against air pollution, and a fountain of youth. Today we continue to explore the role of this antioxidant in protecting us from chronic disease.

Tocopherol The chemical name for vitamin E.

Vitamin E in the Diet

Alpha-tocopherol (α-tocopherol) The form of tocopherol that is most common and has the greatest biological activity.

There are several forms of vitamin E. The most common one is **alpha-tocopherol (α-tocopherol),** which provides more than twice the amount of vitamin E activity of other tocopherols. Dietary sources of vitamin E include nuts and peanuts; plant oils, such as soybean, corn, and sunflower oils; leafy green vegetables; wheat germ; and fortified breakfast cereals (Figure 9.8).

Because vitamin E is sensitive to destruction by oxygen, metals, light, and heat, some is lost during food processing, cooking, and storage. Although it is relatively stable at normal cooking temperatures, the high temperatures used in deep-fat frying and the repeated use of the same oil tend to destroy most of the vitamin E.

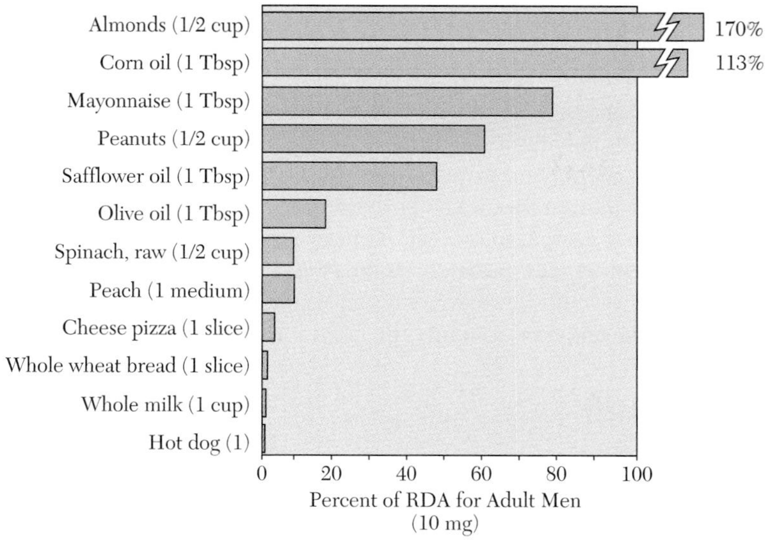

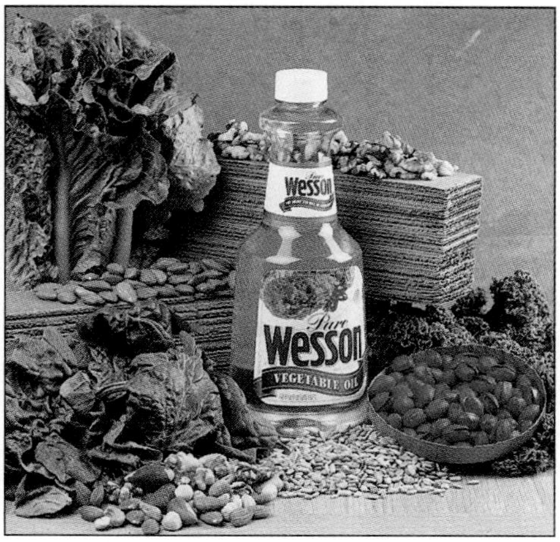

Figure 9.8

The vitamin E content of foods as a percent of the 1989 RDA for adult men. (*right,* George Semple)

Vitamin E in the Body

Vitamin E functions primarily as an antioxidant. It neutralizes reactive oxygen compounds before they damage unsaturated fatty acids in cell membranes (Figure 9.9). By protecting cell membranes, vitamin E is important in maintaining the integrity of red blood cells, cells in nervous tissue, and cells of the immune system. Vitamin E can also defend cells from damage by heavy metals, such as lead and mercury, and toxins, such as carbon tetrachloride, benzene, and a variety of drugs. It also protects against some environmental pollutants such as ozone. After vitamin E is used to eliminate free radicals, its antioxidant function can be restored by vitamin C.

How Much Vitamin E Do We Need?

The recommended intake for vitamin E is expressed in ***α*-tocopherol equivalents (*α*-TEs).** The 1989 RDA is 8 mg *α*-TE for adult women and 10 mg *α*-TE for adult men (see Table 9.1). This amount is contained in about a tablespoon of

***α*-tocopherol equivalents (*α*-TEs)** A unit of measure for vitamin E, equal to the amount of any form of tocopherol that provides the function of 1 mg of alpha-tocopherol.

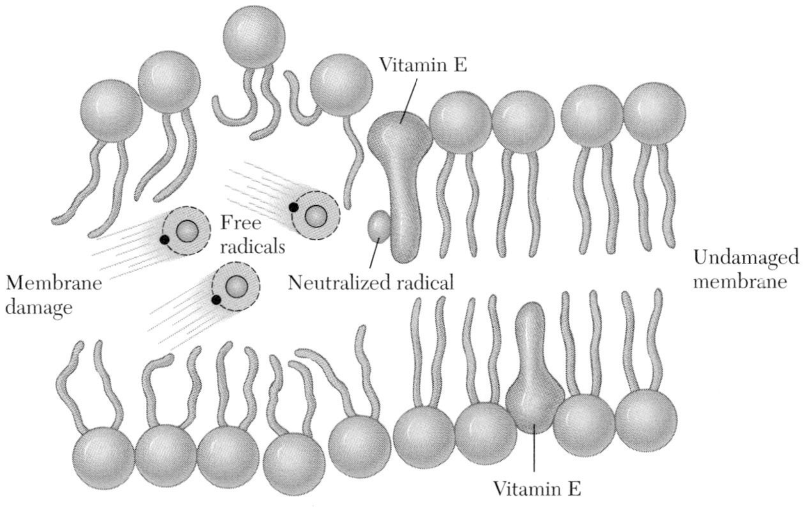

Figure 9.9

Vitamin E functions as an antioxidant that protects the unsaturated fatty acids in cell membranes by neutralizing free radicals.

corn oil. One α-TE is equal to 1 mg of α-tocopherol or the amount of any tocopherol that provides the function of 1 mg of α-tocopherol. Vitamin supplement labels often express vitamin E content in IUs. One IU is equal to 1 mg of synthetic vitamin E or about 0.74 mg of natural α-tocopherol. The need for vitamin E increases as the polyunsaturated fat content of the diet increases. This is because a diet high in polyunsaturated fats increases the polyunsaturated fatty acid content of cell membranes, making them more susceptible to oxidative damage. More vitamin E is needed to protect them. Foods high in polyunsaturated fats are usually good sources of vitamin E. Increasing the intake of foods such as greens and fortified cereals increases vitamin E intake without increasing polyunsaturated fat intake and consequently the need for vitamin E.[20]

Vitamin E and Health

Although vitamin E deficiency is uncommon, supplements are promoted to grow hair; restore, maintain, or increase sexual potency and fertility; alleviate fatigue; maintain immune function; enhance athletic performance; reduce the symptoms of PMS and menopause; slow aging; prevent heart disease and cancer; and treat a host of other medical problems.

Vitamin E Deficiency Vitamin E protects membranes; therefore a deficiency can cause membrane changes. Red blood cells and nerve tissue are particularly susceptible.[21] For example, when vitamin E is deficient, red blood cell membranes are damaged and may rupture. Vitamin E deficiency is rare because vitamin E is plentiful in the food supply and is stored in many of the body's tissues. Deficiencies have been identified in premature infants, in individuals consuming very lowfat diets for long periods, and in individuals with fat malabsorption. In individuals with cystic fibrosis, a condition that reduces fat absorption, deficiency can develop rapidly, causing serious neurological problems, which, if untreated, can become permanent.

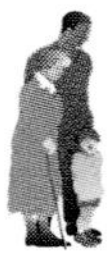

All newborn infants have low blood tocopherol levels because there is little transfer of vitamin E from mother to fetus until the last weeks of pregnancy. The levels are lower in premature infants who are born before much vitamin E is transferred from the mother. In these infants, ruptured red blood cells may cause a type of anemia called hemolytic anemia. Infant formula for premature newborns is supplemented with higher amounts of vitamin E than formula for full-term infants.

Vitamin E Toxicity Vitamin E is relatively nontoxic. Few side effects have been seen even with doses as high as 3200 mg α-TE per day (320 times the 1989 RDA).[22] Large doses of vitamin E can inhibit blood clotting by interfering with the action of vitamin K. Therefore, vitamin E supplements should not be taken by individuals taking blood-thinning medications that also interfere with the action of vitamin K.

Vitamin E Supplements: Do They Improve Antioxidant Protection? Vitamin E has been suggested to reduce the risk of both cancer and heart disease. Although there is evidence that diets high in vitamin E and supplements of vitamin E reduce the risk of certain types of cancer, the link between vitamin E and heart disease is stronger. Intakes of vitamin E greater than 100 IU per day or 70 mg α-TE per day have been associated with a reduced risk of heart disease in both men and women,[23,24] and animal studies have shown that vitamin E supplements can inhibit the formation of atherosclerotic plaque.[25] Although increasing vitamin E intake may provide some protection from heart disease, most of the data are based on epidemiological studies which show a relationship between diets high in vitamin E–containing foods and a reduced risk. Because these foods may contain other substances that protect against heart disease, additional studies are needed before vitamin E supplements can be recommended to the general public to decrease the risk of heart disease.

VITAMIN K: KOAGULATION

Vitamin K is one of the few vitamins about which extravagant claims are not made. Like the other fat-soluble vitamins, it was discovered inadvertently by feeding animals a fat-free diet. In this case, researchers in Denmark noted that chicks fed this diet developed a type of bleeding disorder that was cured by feeding them a fat-soluble extract from green plants. Vitamin K was named for *koagulation,* the Danish word for **coagulation,** or blood clotting.

Coagulation The process of blood clotting.

Vitamin K in the Diet

As with all the fat-soluble vitamins, vitamin K is found in several forms. **Phylloquinones** are the vitamin K forms found in plants. Another group of vitamin K compounds, called **menaquinones,** are found in fish oils and meats and are synthesized by bacteria, including those in the human intestine. Menaquinones are the form found in supplements. The best sources of dietary vitamin K are liver and leafy green vegetables such as spinach, broccoli, brussels sprouts, kale, and turnip greens. Milk, meats, eggs, and cereals contain smaller amounts (Figure 9.10). Some of the vitamin K produced by bacteria in the human gastrointestinal tract is also absorbed. Since the exact vitamin K content of foods has been technically difficult to determine, vitamin K values are not included in most food composition tables.

Phylloquinones The forms of vitamin K found in plants.

Menaquinones The forms of vitamin K synthesized by bacteria and found in animals.

Vitamin K in the Body

Unlike other fat-soluble vitamins, vitamin K is used rapidly by the body, so a constant supply is necessary. Vitamin K is needed for the production of the blood-clotting protein **prothrombin** and other specific blood-clotting factors. These proteins are needed to produce fibrin, the protein that forms the structure of a

Prothrombin A blood protein required for blood clotting.

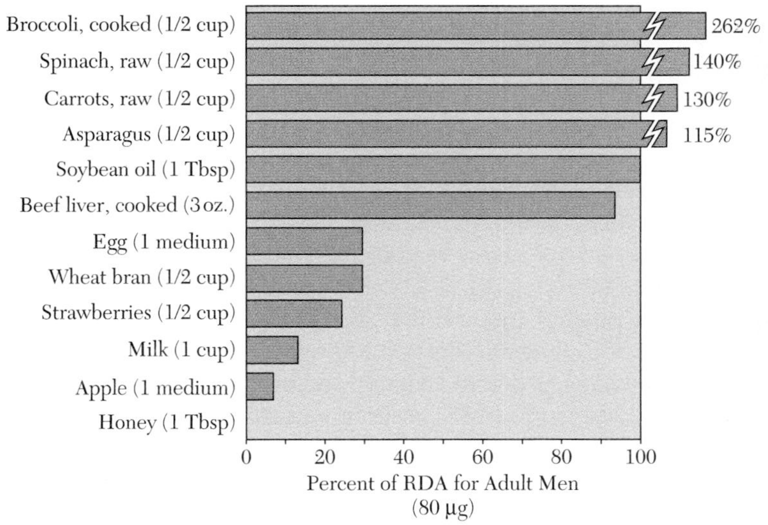

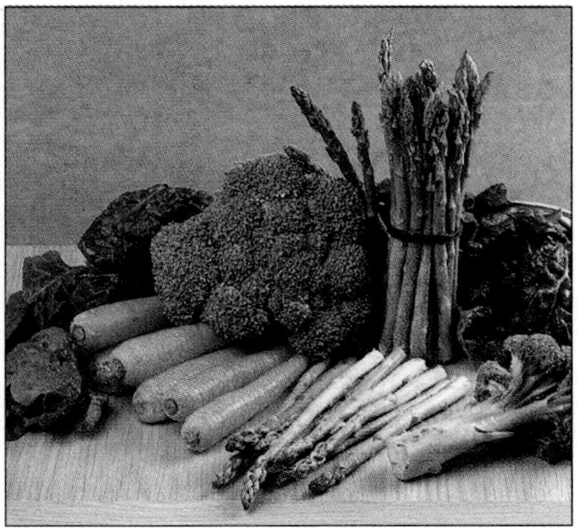

Figure 9.10
The vitamin K content of foods as a percent of the 1989 RDA for adult men. (*right,* George Semple)

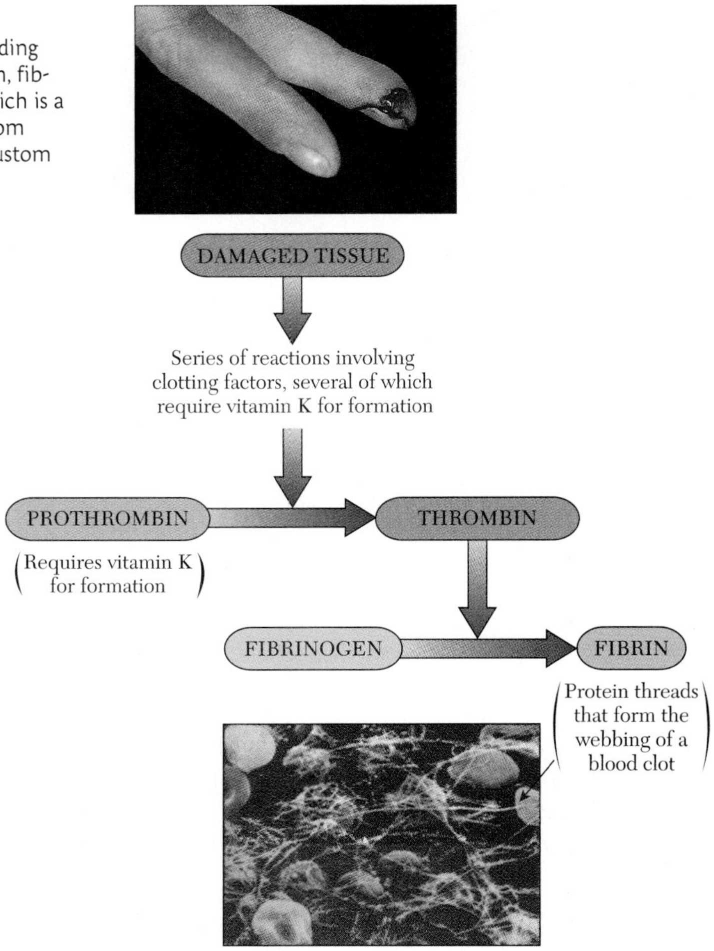

Figure 9.11
The formation of a blood clot. Several clotting factors, including prothrombin, require vitamin K for synthesis. Without them, fibrinogen cannot be converted into its active form, fibrin, which is a structural component of blood clots. (*top*, © Amethyst/Custom Medical Stock Photo; *bottom*, CNRI/Science Photo Library/Custom Medical Stock Photo)

blood clot (Figure 9.11). Injuries as well as the normal wear and tear of daily living produce micro tears in blood vessels. To prevent blood loss, these tears must be repaired with blood clots. Other roles for vitamin K are less well understood. For example, there are several vitamin K–dependent proteins in bone that may be involved in bone mineralization and demineralization.[26]

How Much Vitamin K Do We Need?

The 1989 RDA for vitamin K is set at about 1 μg per kilogram of body weight per day (see Table 9.1). Typical intakes in North America are well above this.[27] Additional vitamin K is provided by bacteria in the gastrointestinal tract. Although the form produced by intestinal bacteria is less well absorbed than that from plant sources, it is an important source of this vitamin.

Vitamin K and Health

The inability to form blood clots due to vitamin K deficiency or drugs that interfere with vitamin K activity can cause death from excess blood loss. Conversely, blood clots causing heart attacks and strokes are responsible for killing about a half-million Americans annually.

Vitamin K Deficiency Abnormal blood coagulation is the major symptom of vitamin K deficiency. A deficiency is very rare in the healthy adult population, but it may result from the long-term use of antibiotics. The antibiotics kill the bacteria in the gastrointestinal tract that are a source of the vitamin. In combination with an illness that reduces the dietary intake of vitamin K, this may precipitate a deficiency. Injections of vitamin K are typically administered before surgery to aid in blood clotting.

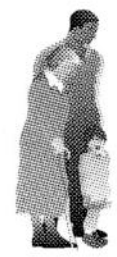

Vitamin K deficiency is most common in newborns. There is little transfer of this vitamin from mother to fetus, and because the infant gut is free of bacteria, none is made there. Further, breast milk is low in vitamin K. Therefore, to prevent uncontrolled bleeding, infants are typically given a vitamin K injection at birth.

Of Cows and Clover: The Value of Medically Induced Vitamin K Deficiency In 1933, a disgruntled farmer delivered a bale of moldy clover hay, a pail of unclotted blood, and a dead cow to the laboratory of Dr. Carl Link at the University of Wisconsin. Six years and many bales of moldy clover later, Link and colleagues had isolated the **anticoagulant** dicumarol from moldy clover. Dicumarol is a derivative of coumarin, which gives clover its sweet scent; mold converts coumarin to dicumarol. Cows fed moldy clover consume dicumarol, which interferes with vitamin K activity. It inhibits their blood from clotting, and they bleed to death from minor cuts and scratches. Within a few years of its discovery, dicumarol was widely used to treat heart attack victims and others at risk for blood clots. Further work with this anticoagulant led Link to propose the use of a more potent derivative, called warfarin, as rat poison. When rats consume the odorless, colorless warfarin, their blood fails to clot, and they bleed to death. Warfarin is now also used as a blood thinner to save the lives of heart attack victims.

Anticoagulant A substance that delays or prevents blood coagulation.

Vitamin K Toxicity and Supplements Vitamin K toxicity occurs only as a result of supplement overuse. Excessive doses result in the clotting and breaking of blood cells. This causes anemia and releases the yellow pigment bilirubin into the circulation. Bilirubin can cause brain damage at high levels. Treatment for vitamin K toxicity involves the administration of dicumarol, which interferes with vitamin K activity and prevents blood from clotting.

Meeting Your Vitamin Needs and Staying Healthy

All that science has learned about vitamin functions, chemical structures, and nutrient interactions helps us understand our needs—but it doesn't always help us meet them. Vitamins are needed in small amounts, but when we don't consume enough of them we may suffer debilitating deficiencies and in some cases increase our risk for chronic disease. It would be a daunting task to calculate the amount of each vitamin in every food we eat each day to determine if we are meeting our requirements. But, this is not really necessary to meet our needs.

Almost every food contains some vitamins—in varying amounts and combinations. We do not need to consume our exact requirement every day in order to meet our needs. It is the average intake, consumed over a period of days or weeks, that is important. By consuming a balanced, varied diet, most people can meet their nutrient needs. A varied diet also provides other food components that may be important to health but have not been determined to be dietary essentials. For those who cannot meet their needs with food, vitamin and mineral supplements can help. In addition to nutrient supplements, there are many other types of dietary supplements available.

Meeting Your Vitamin Needs With Food

Nutritionists have been saying it for years and mothers for even longer—"eat your vegetables." But vegetables are not the only foods that help us meet our micronutrient needs. Each food group provides vitamins: Meat contains thiamin, vitamin

B_6 and B_{12}; leafy green vegetables contain vitamin A and vitamin K; fruits contain vitamin C; grains contain many of the B vitamins, including folate; milk contains riboflavin and vitamins A and D; and oils contain vitamin E. How do we put this all together to make a healthy diet? One simple way is to follow the recommendation of the Food Guide Pyramid. In addition, food labels provide a source of information about vitamins in food.

Vitamins and the Food Guide Pyramid The Food Guide Pyramid is designed as a guide to the selection of a diet that meets nutrient needs. Up to this point we have focused on the macronutrients in the Food Guide Pyramid, but it also takes into account micronutrients. A diet that meets the serving recommendations of the Food Guide Pyramid and consists of a variety of nutrient-dense choices from within each group will meet vitamin needs. Following the serving recommendations is important because no one food group provides all the vitamins you need. For example, whole grains are good sources of vitamin E and most of the B vitamins but are poor sources of vitamin C. Fruits and vegetables are excellent sources of vitamins A, C, K, and folate but provide no vitamin B_{12}. Animal products are plentiful in vitamins B_6 and B_{12} but lack vitamin E (Figure 9.12).

The food choices made from within each group also affect the micronutrient content of the diet. The Food Guide Pyramid provides selection tips on food choices from within each group (see Table 2.2). Many of these suggestions are based on nutrient density—the amounts of essential nutrients in a food relative to the energy provided. For instance, a slice of white bread and a slice of whole wheat bread are both choices from the grain group that provide about 70 kcalories, but white bread provides less vitamin B_6 because it is lost during refining. Similarly, you can get 50% of your RDA for thiamin and niacin from a Big Mac or from a turkey sandwich. But choosing the turkey sandwich, which is more nutrient dense (the Big Mac contains over 500 kcalories, whereas the turkey sandwich contains about 300 kcalories), allows you to eat more of other foods, which contain other nutrients, without exceeding your energy requirements. Because vitamin losses can occur through food processing, storage, and cooking, the vitamin-conscious consumer must also consider these factors when purchasing and preparing food (see Chapter 8, *Off the Shelf: Maximizing the Vitamins in Your Vegetables*).

Vitamins on Food Labels Food labels can be helpful in determining vitamin intake from packaged foods. Any vitamin that is added in processing must be listed in the ingredient list, although the amounts are not included. The Nutrition Facts section must list the amount of vitamin A and vitamin C as a percent of the Daily Value. Listing of other vitamins is voluntary, but many foods such as fortified breakfast cereals provide this information. The % Daily Values on labels help consumers determine whether a food makes a significant contribution to their needs. Table 9.2 illustrates how the actual amount of a vitamin or mineral in a food can

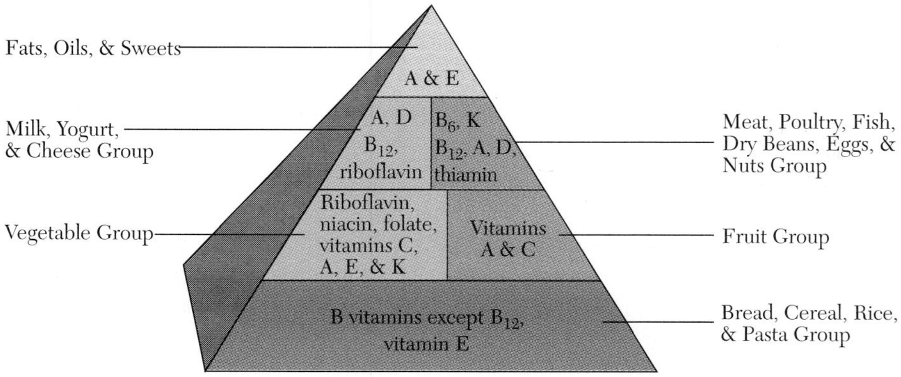

Figure 9.12
A diet that follows the recommendations of the Food Guide Pyramid provides many sources of vitamins.

Table 9.2 *Calculating Vitamin and Mineral Content From Food Labels*

1. Look up the RDI for the nutrient of interest (see Table 2.4).
2. Find the % Daily Value for that nutrient on your food label.
3. Multiply the % Daily Value by the RDI to determine the amount of the nutrient in a serving.
   Example: The RDI for vitamin C is 60 mg
   A fruit snack has 2% of the Daily Value for vitamin C
   60 mg × 2% of Daily Value = 60 × 0.02 = 3 mg vitamin C
4. Be sure to consider how many servings you plan to eat.

be calculated by multiplying the % Daily Value by the RDI for that nutrient (see Table 2.4 for RDI values). Fresh vegetables and fruits rarely come with labels, but nutritional information about these foods is usually provided at the produce counter.

Other Benefits of Food: Phytochemicals

Food provides nutrients in infinite combinations and with unlimited variety. In addition to nutrients, food contains factors that affect absorption and nutrient utilization and offer disease protection. Foods that may prevent disease or promote health are often referred to as **functional foods.**[28] Although this is a relatively new term, interest in the therapeutic properties of foods is not new. Early medicine relied on many food prescriptions to treat disorders, and Eastern cultures have long used foods for their medicinal benefits. Until recently most of this was based on beliefs and tradition rather than scientific evidence. During the last decade, however, many studies have examined the relationship between the consumption of specific foods, typical dietary patterns, and health. Most of this research has focused on phytochemicals (Figure 9.13).

Functional foods Foods that provide health benefits.

What Are Phytochemicals? The term "phytochemical" literally means plant chemical—*phyto* is derived from the Greek word for plant. The term refers to the hundreds, perhaps thousands, of biologically active non-nutritive chemicals found in plants. In plants, phytochemicals serve as protection. For example, the allium compounds in onions and garlic serve as natural pesticides, protecting plants from insects. In our diet, we ingest hundreds of these plant chemicals. Some can make plants toxic to humans. For instance, chemicals in some wild mushrooms can cause symptoms ranging from stomach upset, dizziness, and hallucinations to liver and kidney failure, coma, and death (see Chapter 16). Others have no effect on human health, and many provide health benefits. Generally, we use the term "phytochemical" to refer to those substances found in plants that have health-promoting properties. Phytochemicals can be classified by their chemical structure (see Table 9.3). Most classes are found in more than one type of plant food and many have multiple actions within the body.

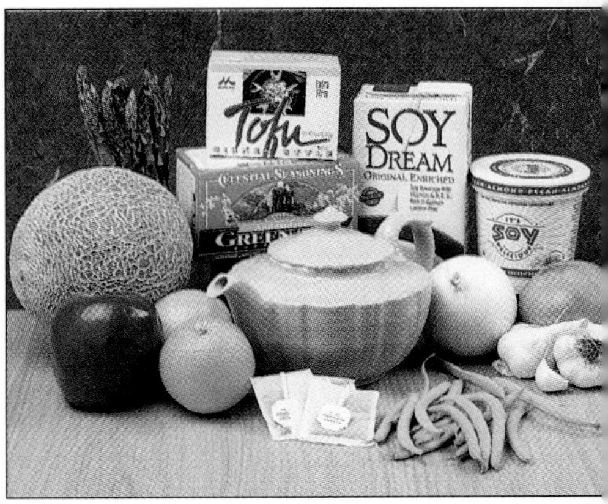

Figure 9.13
These plant foods contain a vast assortment of phytochemicals. (George Semple)

Phytochemicals and Health Epidemiological observations that identified a relationship between diets high in fruits and vegetables and reduced cancer incidence led researchers to experiment with supplemental doses of the nutrients in these foods.[29,30] The results of many of these studies found that the foods have a greater protective effect than do supplements of an individual nutrient. Research continues to expand our knowledge of the health benefits of phytochemicals, but our understanding is still in its infancy. Of the hundreds of plant chemicals we ingest, we fully understand the functions of only a few. Most research to date has focused on cancer prevention, and most of the classes of phytochemicals thus far identified have anticancer and antioxidant activities.

Table 9.3 *Some Classes of Phytochemicals*

Phytochemical Class	Food Source
Carotenoids	Yellow/orange vegetables and fruits and dark-green leafy vegetables
Dithiolthiones	Cruciferous vegetables—broccoli, cauliflower, brussels sprouts, etc.
Glucosinolates/indoles	Cruciferous vegetables—broccoli, cauliflower, brussels sprouts, etc.
Isothiocyanates/thiocyanates	Cruciferous vegetables—broccoli, cauliflower, brussels sprouts, etc.
Coumarins	Vegetables and citrus fruits
Flavonoids	Most fruits and vegetables
Phenols	Most fruits and vegetables, green tea, wine
Protease inhibitors	Seeds and legumes, particularly soy
Plant sterols	Vegetables
Isoflavones	Soybeans
Saponins	Plants, particularly soybeans
Inositol hexaphosphate	Plants, particularly soybeans and cereals
Allium compounds	Onions, garlic, leeks, chives
Limonene	Citrus fruits

From: Hasler, C. M. Functional foods: the Western perspective. Nutr. Rev. 54(II):S6–S10, 1996.

Phytochemicals as Cancer Protection In the last five years, the National Cancer Institute has spent over $20 million researching the anticancer properties of plant foods. Foods with significant anticancer activity include garlic, soybeans, cruciferous vegetables, legumes, onions, citrus fruits, tomatoes, whole grains, and a variety of herbs and spices. The chemicals in these foods that seem to be responsible for this effect are allium compounds, phenols, isoflavones, saponins, indoles, isothiocyanates, flavonoids, carotenoids, phytates, lignans, glucarates, phthalides, and terpenoids.[31] The health and anticancer benefits of many of the phytochemicals may be due to their role as antioxidants.[32] Others are anticarcinogens due to their ability to inhibit the metabolic activation of carcinogens, stimulate enzymes that help eliminate carcinogens, maintain DNA repair, or act at some other stage of cancer development such as cell differentiation or cell proliferation.[30]

Antioxidant phytochemicals include carotenoids, flavonoids, and phenols.[33] The intake of carotenoids has been associated with a reduced risk of cancer, cardiovascular disease, and age-related eye diseases such as cataracts and macular degeneration.[13] The antioxidant properties of carotenoids are believed to play a role in these effects. Beta-carotene is the best known carotenoid but it may be a less effective antioxidant than others.[34] The carotenoids lutein and zeaxanthin are most strongly associated with reduced risk of macular degeneration. Lycopene, the carotenoid that gives tomatoes their color, is a more potent scavenger of oxygen radicals than other dietary carotenoids.[35] Flavonoids are also antioxidant pigments. They include the anthocyanins that give the blue and red colors to blueberries, raspberries, and red cabbage, as well as the anthoxanthins that give the pale yellow color to potatoes, onions, and orange rinds. Phenolics, which are antioxidant phytochemicals found in tea, wine, soybeans, and other legumes, act as antioxidants by binding metals such as iron and preventing them from acting as pro-oxidants.

Other phytochemicals with anticancer properties function by other mechanisms. The phytochemicals in green tea inhibit an enzyme crucial for cancer growth.[36] Sulforaphane, an isothiocyanate found in broccoli, cauliflower, brussels sprouts, and cabbage, boosts the activity of enzyme systems that detoxify carcinogens and has been shown to protect animals from breast cancer.[37] Allyls in onions, garlic, scallions, leeks, and chives can induce enzymes that detoxify carcinogens and also act in the gastrointestinal tract to decrease the formation of cancerous nitrosamines.[30] Isoflavones in soybeans compete with estrogen and therefore inhibit estrogen-promoted breast cancer (see Chapter 6, *Off the Shelf: Is Soy the Perfect Protein?*).

Phytochemicals as Pro-Oxidants Phytochemicals can have both antioxidant and pro-oxidant activity. For example, carotenoids provide antioxidant protection but they may also promote oxidation depending on the particular carotenoid as well as the amount of oxygen present, the amount of the carotenoid, and interactions with other antioxidants. Some studies show that when beta-carotene is added to a vitamin E-deficient diet, it acts as a pro-oxidant.[38] But in the presence of vitamin E, beta-carotene acts as an antioxidant. One explanation for the increase in the incidence of lung cancer among smokers supplemented with beta-carotene is that pro-oxidant activity prevails over antioxidant activity. Phenolics are another class of phytochemical that has both pro-oxidant and antioxidant activity. There is evidence that in certain tissues and under certain conditions phenolics could be more of a pro-oxidant risk than an antioxidant benefit.[39] Pro-oxidant activity, however, is not always harmful. The pro-oxidant activity of carotenoids may be involved in blocking the growth of cancerous cells.[38]

Phytochemicals: How Much Do We Need? The concept that dietary recommendations should be made for substances in foods that are not essential nutrients is relatively new. A set of DRIs that will include a recommendation for phytochemical intake has been proposed. To date, however, the 1989 RDAs do not give specific recommendations for the amounts of phytochemicals consumed in the diet.

Recommendations for a healthy diet such as those of the Food Guide Pyramid suggest that at least 5 servings of fruits and vegetables be consumed daily.[40] The Dietary Guidelines support this with the recommendation that the diet contain plenty of grain products, vegetables, and fruits (Figure 9.14). Despite these recommendations, the average American eats only about 1.5 servings of vegetables and 1 serving of fruit each day; only 1 in 11 Americans meets the recommendations of at least three vegetables and two fruits daily.[31] As a result, there are numerous public education campaigns designed to promote "Five A Day"—that is, consuming at least five fruit and vegetable servings daily. Table 9.4 includes some suggestions for increasing fruit and vegetable intake.

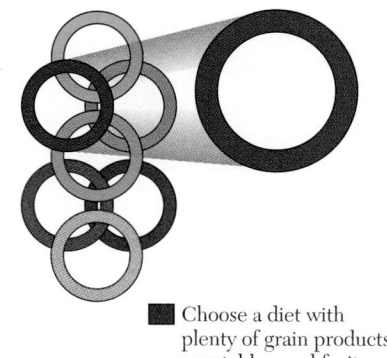

Figure 9.14
The Dietary Guidelines for Americans recommend choosing a diet with plenty of grain products, vegetables, and fruits. A diet that follows this recommendation will be rich in vitamins and phytochemicals. (USDA, DHHS, 1995)

Table 9.4 *Suggestions for Increasing Fruit and Vegetable Intake*

Try a new fruit or vegetable each week.
Eat fruits and vegetables for snacks.
Put fruit on your cereal in the morning or vegetables in your eggs.
Try dried fruit instead of candy.
Drink fruit or vegetable juices instead of soft drinks.
Try baked fruit for dessert.
Eat a vegetarian dinner at least once a week.
Add vegetables to your favorite entrees.

Off the Label

What's in a Dietary Supplement?

Until recently, nutritional supplements were not classified as either foods or drugs. There was no consistency in their labeling and the content of advertising claims was up to the manufacturer. After years of debate, the Dietary Supplement Health and Education Act of 1994 defined dietary supplements and established regulations for their labeling and advertising.[1]

The content of labels on dietary supplement packages is regulated by the FDA. The name of the product must state that it is a dietary supplement. For example, a bottle of ginseng capsules must be labeled "Ginseng, a Dietary Supplement." These products must carry a "Supplement Facts" panel similar to the "Nutrition Facts" panel found on most processed foods. This panel lists the recommended serving size and the name and quantity of each ingredient per serving. The source of the ingredient may be given with its name in the "Supplement Facts" panel or in the ingredient list below the panel. The 14 nutrients for which Daily Values have been established are listed first. The Daily Value is based on the Reference Daily Intakes (see Table 2.4). Other dietary ingredients for which no Reference Daily Intakes have been established are listed next.[2]

Dietary supplements must meet certain criteria to use the terms "high potency" and "antioxidant." When describing an individual vitamin or mineral, high potency means that 1 serving provides 100% or more of the Daily Value. For multinutrient products it means that 1 serving provides more than 100% of the Daily Value for two thirds of the vitamins and minerals present. A supplement may use the term antioxidant if it is "a good source of" or "high in" a nutrient for which there is an established Daily Value and the nutrient is shown by scientific evidence to inactivate free radicals or prevent free radical–initiated reactions. For example, a supplement containing 60 mg of vitamin C could be labeled as an antioxidant supplement.

The types of health claims that can be made on supplement labels are also regulated. Three types of claims are allowed: nutrient content claims, disease claims, and nutrition support claims.[3] Nutrient content claims describe the level of a nutrient in a supplement. For example, a supplement containing at least 20% of the Daily Value (12 mg) of vitamin C per serving can state that it is an "excellent source of vitamin C." Disease claims point out a link between a supplement and a disease or health-related condition. Supplement labels are permitted to mention only the FDA-approved claims linking a food or substance with the risk of a specific disease or health-related condition (see Chapter 2). Nutrition support claims describe the relationship between a nutrient and a deficiency disease that can result if the nutrient is lacking in the diet. For example, a vitamin C supplement could state "vitamin C prevents scurvy." Nutrition support claims can also include structure-function claims. These refer to the effect of a supplement on body structure or function. For example, a calcium supplement might say that "calcium builds strong bones." The ginseng supplement shown here claims that ginseng improves performance by stating that "when you need to perform your best, take ginseng." These structure-function claims are based on the manufacturer's review and interpretation of the scientific literature and do not require FDA approval. But, they must be accompanied by the disclaimer: "This statement has not been evaluated by the Food and Drug Administration. This product is not intended to diagnose, treat, cure, or prevent any disease." Although the Dietary Supplement Health and Education Act limits the claims manufacturers can use on labels, products may still be promoted by using information in the form of articles, book chapters, and scientific abstracts that are displayed separately from the products. This information must not be false or misleading or promote a particular brand of supplement, and it must be presented in a balanced fashion.

Dietary Supplements: What Is Their Role?

Dietary supplements are big business. They are available from the shelves of health food stores, grocery stores, and drug stores, as well as through mail-order catalogs, TV advertisements, and the Internet. A recent survey found that more than half of the adults in the United States use dietary supplements. In 1996, Americans spent more than $6.5 billion on these products.[41]

If food provides all the nutrients we need as well as phytochemicals, why then are dietary supplements such big sellers? People take supplements to energize themselves, to protect themselves from disease, to cure their illnesses, to enhance what they get in food, and simply to ensure against deficiencies. Can dietary supplements provide these benefits? Are they safe?

What Are Dietary Supplements? By definition, a dietary supplement is a product intended for ingestion as a supplement to the diet. Supplements may contain one or more of the following ingredients: vitamins; minerals; herbs, botanicals, or other plant-derived substances; amino acids; enzymes; concentrates; and extracts. Dietary supplements come as pills, tablets, capsules, gelcaps, liquids, powders, and more.

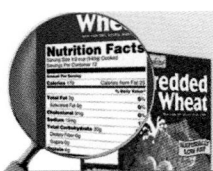

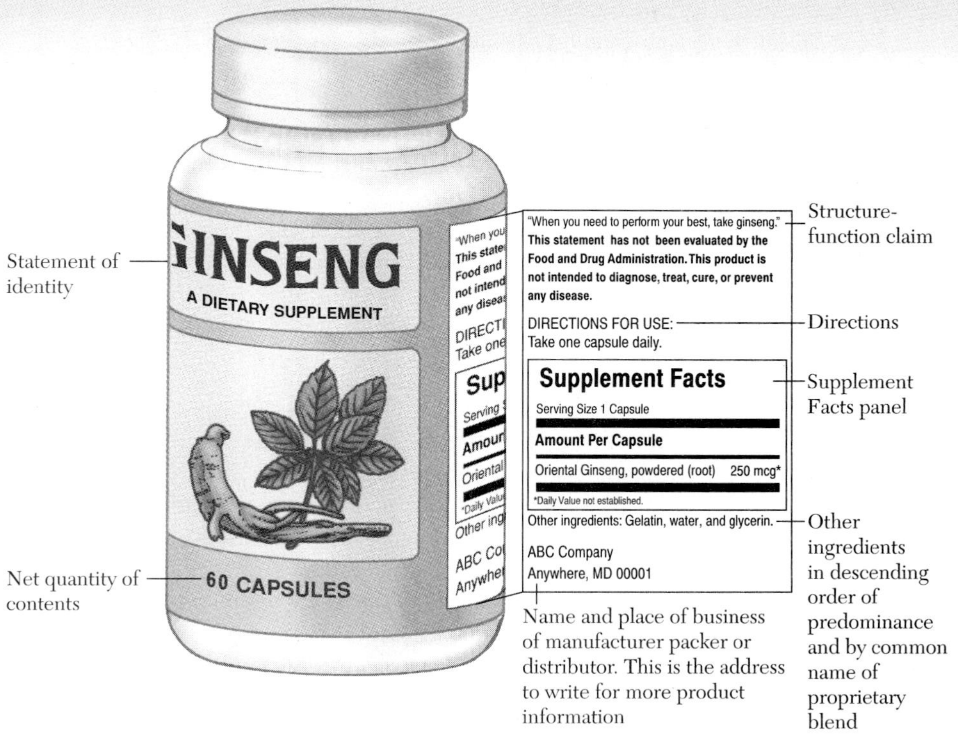
Statement of identity
GINSENG
A DIETARY SUPPLEMENT
Net quantity of contents
60 CAPSULES
"When you need to perform your best, take ginseng."
This statement has not been evaluated by the Food and Drug Administration. This product is not intended to diagnose, treat, cure, or prevent any disease.
Structure-function claim
DIRECTIONS FOR USE:
Take one capsule daily.
Directions
Supplement Facts
Serving Size 1 Capsule
Amount Per Capsule
Oriental Ginseng, powdered (root) 250 mcg*
*Daily Value not established.
Supplement Facts panel
Other ingredients: Gelatin, water, and glycerin.
Other ingredients in descending order of predominance and by common name of proprietary blend
ABC Company
Anywhere, MD 00001
Name and place of business of manufacturer packer or distributor. This is the address to write for more product information

Supplement labels provide important information. Before purchasing a supplement, consumers should know what they are purchasing and why. When consuming supplements, consumers should follow dosage recommendations to avoid toxicities.

[1]Dietary supplements: recent chronology and legislation. Nutr. Rev. 53:31–36, 1995.

[2]New FDA labeling rules for dietary supplements. FDA Consumer 32:2, Jan./Feb., 1998.

[3]Kurtzweil, P. An FDA guide to dietary supplements. FDA Consumer 32:28–35, Sept./Oct., 1998.

How Are Dietary Supplements Regulated? The Dietary Supplement Health and Education Act of 1994 set up a framework for the regulation of dietary supplements. This law requires that any product intended for ingestion as a supplement to the diet must include the words "dietary supplement" on the label and that these products carry a standardized label similar to food labels (see *Off the Label: What's in a Dietary Supplement?*). The Federal Trade Commission regulates advertising of dietary supplements and the FDA oversees product claims made on labels and in package inserts and literature.

Under the Dietary Supplement Health and Education Act, the FDA also oversees the safety and manufacturing of dietary supplements. Since dietary supplements are considered foods, not drugs, supplements are not bound by the strict laws that regulate drug manufacture. For instance, before a drug can be marketed, the FDA requires that the manufacturer prove its safety and effectiveness for the prescribed use. Supplements require FDA approval only if they contain an ingredient that was not marketed in the United States before October 15, 1994. In addition, the manufacturing of supplements is not standardized, so the concentration and solubility may vary from dose to dose. Solubility is important—if it takes a supplement several hours to dissolve, only a small percentage of the compounds it contains may be available for absorption when it reaches the small intestine. In response to concerns about supplement safety and nutritional value, the U.S. Pharmacopoeial (USP) Convention, which sets the standards for drug manufacture, is setting standards for supplements. These standards will not be mandatory, but many companies will adopt them. Such standards will protect the consumer from inconsistencies in supplement composition but may also increase the cost of dietary supplements.

Types of Dietary Supplements There are thousands of types of dietary supplements. Some contain essential nutrients, some are designed to affect the macronutrient content of the diet, some provide substances that are found in the body but are not essential nutrients, some contain herbs and other plant preparations. Their uses are as varied as their composition. Some are taken to enhance athletic performance (see Chapter 12), some to prevent deficiencies, some to promote weight loss, some to alleviate existing symptoms and conditions, and some to promote a longer life and prevent chronic disease. Supplements containing vitamins and minerals as well as those containing substances that are not essential nutrients are discussed below.

Vitamin and Mineral Supplements Vitamin and mineral supplements are available as multivitamins and minerals, individual nutrients, and special combinations for target groups such as women, children, men, and older adults, as well as for special situations such as pregnancy, stress, or weight loss. Are these necessary? Should you be taking vitamin and mineral supplements to assure that you are meeting your needs? Can supplements provide additional benefits even if the diet is carefully planned?

Who Needs Vitamin and Mineral Supplements? Most healthy adults who consume a reasonably good diet do not need supplements. However, individuals who cannot meet their requirements with food, either because they have increased needs or excess losses, benefit from vitamin and mineral supplements. Groups who typically need vitamin and mineral supplements include dieters, vegans, and groups who are nutritionally vulnerable because of chronic disease; use of medications, cigarettes, or alcohol; or life stage (Figure 9.15).

Dieters Individuals following weight-loss diets restrict the amount of energy in their diet and consequently reduce their intake of micronutrients. It is difficult to consume the recommended amounts of all vitamins and minerals if energy intake is less than 1200 kcalories per day, no matter how well planned the diet is. Therefore, it is important to supplement diets that contain fewer than 1200 kcalories (see Chapter 7).

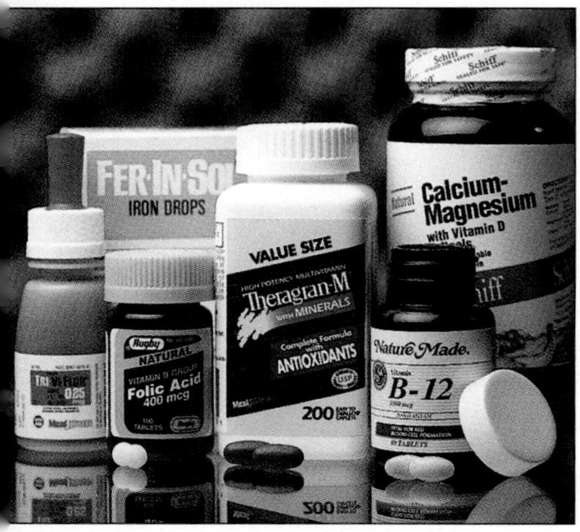

Figure 9.15
Many vitamin and mineral supplements are targeted to groups with increased needs of certain nutrients. (George Semple)

Vegans Although vegetarian diets are generally high in micronutrients, a vegan diet, which excludes all animal food products, will be deficient in vitamin B_{12}. Vegans need to obtain vitamin B_{12} from fortified foods or from supplements (see Chapters 6 and 8).

Nutritionally Vulnerable Populations Individuals with chronic diseases that affect nutrient utilization, or those taking certain medications, may require vitamin and mineral supplements. For instance, individuals with pernicious anemia require injections of vitamin B_{12} to meet their needs. Individuals who are lactose-intolerant may not be able to consume enough dairy products to meet their need for calcium and vitamin D and may therefore benefit from fortified foods and supplements. Individuals who take certain blood pressure medications (thiazide diuretics) may require supplemental potassium (see Chapter 10). Individuals who routinely take medications should discuss nutrient–drug interactions and the need for specific vitamin and mineral supplementation with their doctor or pharmacist (see Chapter 15).

The use of cigarettes and alcohol also affects vitamin requirements. Heavy cigarette smokers, for instance, require more vitamin C to maintain the blood concentrations of vitamin C found in nonsmokers.[42] Individuals who consume more than two alcoholic beverages per day may require supplemental thiamin, niacin, vitamin B_6, and folate because alcohol inhibits their absorption and may affect their metabolism (see Chapters 14 and 15).

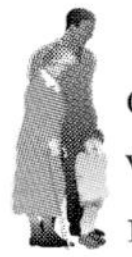

Pregnant women and older adults may need supplements to meet their micronutrient needs. Although a well-planned diet can meet the needs of pregnant women, supplements of iron and folate are recommended, and multivitamin and mineral supplements are usually prescribed (see Chapter 13). In addition, women who are planning a pregnancy should consume supplemental folic acid in fortified foods or supplements (see Chapter 8). A vitamin and mineral supplement may also benefit elderly individuals because the capacity to absorb or utilize vitamins may decrease with aging. For example, many individuals over 50 do not absorb vitamin B_{12} bound in food. Food fortified with B_{12} or supplements are recommended for this age group (see Chapters 8 and 15).

If You Choose to Take a Supplement It is unclear whether supplements are beneficial for the population at large. Eating a variety of foods is the best way to meet nutrient needs, but for individuals with limited dietary intakes, a multivitamin and mineral supplement that supplies no more than 100% of the Daily Values may provide some benefit. However, an argument against the use of supplements is that it gives people a false sense of security, causing them to pay less attention to the nutrient content of the foods they choose. Individuals who are concerned about their nutrient intake should have their diet and nutritional status assessed by a dietitian and a physician.[43]

If you decide to take a micronutrient supplement, choose with care. To evaluate the possibility of toxicity, compare the amounts of nutrients in the supplement with the Daily Values and ULs. The pros and cons of specific vitamin supplements and the risks of toxicity have been reviewed for each vitamin in this and the preceding chapter and for the minerals in Chapters 10 and 11 (see *Critical Thinking: Evaluating Vitamin Supplements*, p. 291). Even if you choose to take a supplement, select the food you eat wisely.

Other Dietary Supplements A survey of supplement shelves reveals that there are many products other than vitamin and mineral supplements. Some of these are nutrients, such as protein and amino acids (see Chapters 6 and 12) and carbohydrates (see Chapters 4 and 12). Some are compounds that are found in the body but are not considered essential in the diet, and others are compounds found in plants. Although many of these are not nutrients, they are all classified as dietary supplements (Figure 9.16).

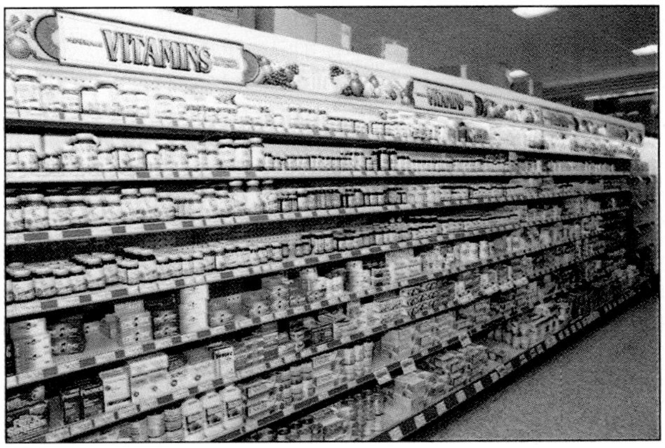

Figure 9.16
There are thousands of different types of dietary supplements available on the shelves of health food stores, drug stores, and grocery stores. (George Semple)

Supplements Containing Compounds Found in the Body Some of the ingredients in supplements are substances that are found in the body or that are their precursors or metabolites. These are not dietary essentials because they are made in the body in sufficient quantities to meet needs and no deficiency symptoms occur when they are absent form the diet. However, some consumers take these supplements because they believe that body levels may not be sufficient for optimal health. Substances that fit into this category include enzymes, hormones, and vitamin-like substances that function in metabolism. Although unnecessary, in moderate doses they are unlikely to be harmful.

Supplements of enzymes and hormones frequently do not reach the target organs they are supposed to affect. Because enzymes are proteins, they will be digested into amino acids before they reach cells inside the body (see Chapter 6). Some hormones are lipids rather than proteins and may reach the bloodstream intact and affect function. For example, the hormones DHEA and melatonin are taken in the hope that they will delay aging (see Chapter 15).

Supplements also contain other structural or regulatory molecules. Glucosamine sulfate and chondroitin sulfates provide substances needed for the formation of healthy joints and are sold to alleviate the pain and progression of arthritis (see Chapter 15).[44] Inositol is a component of phospholipids in cell membranes where it plays a role in relaying messages to the inside of the cell. Inositol can be synthesized from glucose and has not been shown to be essential in the human diet, but it may have some clinical value in treating diseases such as diabetes and kidney failure.[45] Para-aminobenzoic acid (PABA) is a part of the folate molecule but has no vitamin activity on its own and cannot be used by humans to make folate. Although topical PABA is used as a sunblock, there is no evidence that oral PABA offers protection from the sun or anything else, and in large doses it may cause liver damage. Carnitine is needed to transport fatty acids into the mitochondria for ATP production (see Chapters 5 and 12).

Some supplements contain substances with coenzyme activity. Lipoic acid is a coenzyme needed for the conversion of pyruvate into acetyl-CoA and for a reaction of the citric acid cycle. Although essential to energy production, lipoic acid can be synthesized in adequate amounts by human cells. Ubiquinone, or coenzyme Q, is important for the production of energy from carbohydrate, fat, and protein because it is one of the electron carriers in the electron transport chain. As its name implies, it is present ubiquitously, in animals, plants, and microorganisms, and it is made in the human body. Supplements of ubiquinone have been reported to improve reproductive performance in rats fed a diet deficient in vitamin E, but there is no evidence that it is needed in the diet of healthy humans.

Herbs, Botanicals, and Other Plant-Derived Substances Many supplements contain compounds extracted from plants, parts of the plants, and even the whole plant itself. As already discussed, plants contain hundreds of phytochemicals. Some products try to bottle the health-promoting properties of phytochemicals by extracting them and pressing them into pills or capsules. Popular phytochemical supplements include flavonoids, such as rutin, hesperidin, and pycnogonol. Flavonoids and bioflavonoids are antioxidants advertised as cures for arthritis, heart disease, high blood pressure, and colds. Although this type of supplement may provide the benefits of the phytochemicals that have been extracted, they contain only a few of the hundreds of compounds found in the whole foods.

Herbal supplements include leaves, flowers, stems, roots, seeds, or any other part of a plant. Throughout human history herbs have been used as medicine. This

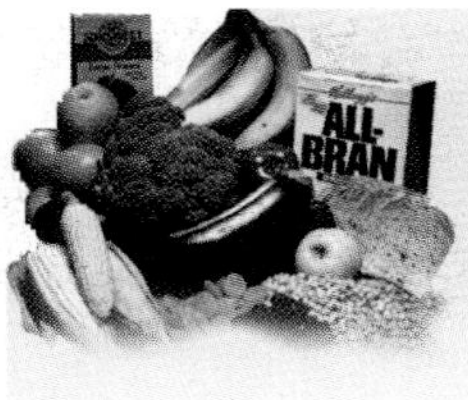

Off the Shelf

Herbal Risk or Herbal Benefit?

Herbal remedies are becoming increasingly popular. They are taken to cure a variety of ailments such as arthritis, depression, and menopausal symptoms, as well as to slow aging, improve memory, and enhance well-being. Many herbs have been used medicinally for thousands of years. Because they are "natural"—that is, they are not processed or altered from their original plant sources—herbs are often viewed as harmless. Natural, however, is no guarantee of safety. Why are herbs so popular? How can you tell whether you are choosing an herbal risk or an herbal benefit?

Herbs and herbal supplements are readily available and relatively inexpensive. They can be purchased without a trip to the doctor or a prescription. While these factors may be viewed as beneficial by consumers who want to manage their own health, they also increase risks. When a drug is prescribed to treat an ailment, we assume that the pill prescribed will have a beneficial effect on our ailment, that each dose will contain the same amount of drug, that the physician or pharmacist has considered other medications we are taking and other medical conditions that affect us, and that the drug itself will not cause a severe side effect. These assumptions cannot be made with herbs. Because their manufacture is not strictly regulated, not all pills provide the same dose. Because consumers can decide what to treat, herbal remedies can be used inappropriately or can cause a delay in medical intervention. And there is no guarantee that the herb will not be toxic, either alone or in combination with other drugs and herbs being consumed.

Consumers who choose to use herbal remedies should use them with care. The first step before taking any dietary supplement is to consult your physician or dietitian; often, however, these individuals may not be trained in the use of herbal medicines. What about the clerk in the health food store? Sometimes these individuals are knowledgeable, but for many, selling supplements is just an after-school job. The safest advice is to do your own research. Know what you are taking and why. Go beyond the label on the bottle.

Use the suggestions for judging nutrient claims discussed in Chapter 1 of this text to evaluate herbs before you take them. Does the information you have on the herb make sense? Is it too outrageous to believe? For example, a product advertised to cure arthritis overnight is unlikely to fulfill its promise. Where does the information come from? Is it in the ad for the product or a suggestion from the clerk who is selling the herbs? Or did it come from a source not involved in the sale of the product? Is the claim based on scientific research? Who did the research studies? Were the studies done correctly? Were the results interpreted correctly? Can the results be applied to people with your condition or in your life stage? Vague claims that are hard to measure, such as "energize," "detoxify," or "purify," are unlikely to be backed up by scientific research. Check out the product's safety record. Many studies have been done to assess the safety and effectiveness of herbs.

Do a risk-benefit analysis before you buy. For example, echinacea is an herbal immune enhancer often taken to prevent or treat cold symptoms. Should you use it? The proposed benefit is prevention of colds or a reduction in cold symptoms. There is research in humans that shows this herb enhances the immune response. And research has shown it to be relatively nontoxic in healthy adults. A bottle of capsules costs about $5.00. So for most people, the risks are small and the benefits may be real.

This is not the case for all herbs. For some, the risks outweigh the benefits. Serious side effects from excessive doses or unusual combinations of herbs and medications are not uncommon. The accompanying table lists some of the risks associated with popular herbal supplements.

Potential Risks Associated With Various Herbal Supplements

Product	Suggested Benefit	Side Effects
St. John's Wort	Promotes mental well-being	Contains same ingredients as the antidepressant drug Prozac and should not be used by people taking these drugs
Dong Quai	Increases energy	Teratogen during pregnancy
Echinacea	Cold remedy	Allergy possible
Comfrey	As a poultice for wounds and sore joints; as a tea for digestive disorders	Do not take orally; liver failure possible
Willow Bark	Pain and fever relief	Reye's syndrome, allergies
Lobelia (Indian Tobacco)	Relaxation; respiratory remedy	Breathing problems, rapid heartbeat, low blood pressure
Wormwood	Relieves digestive ailments	Numbness or paralysis of legs
Ephedra (Ma Huang)	Relieves cold symptoms	High blood pressure, irregular heartbeat, heart attack

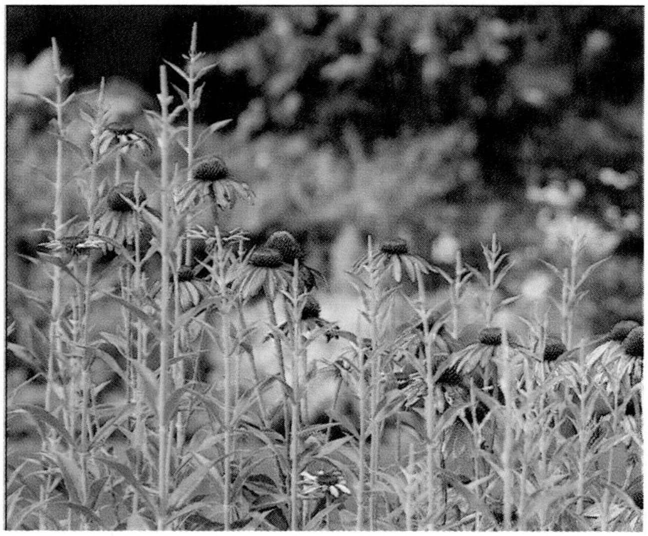

Figure 9.17
Just because herbs such as this echinacea are natural doesn't mean they are safe. (Larry Le Fever/Grant Heilman)

herbal or phyto medicine is an ancient art based in folklore and culture. Herbal products available today, such as Dong Quai, Indian Tobacco, and St. John's wort, borrow from the traditional medicine of many cultures (see *Off the Shelf: Herbal Risk or Herbal Benefit?*). These herbal supplements are offered to improve general well-being as well as for their specific medicinal functions. The physiological effects of some of these are rooted in tradition and anecdote. For others, scientific research has determined that the plant has an effect on human physiology. Supplements that are currently popular include garlic, ginseng, gingko biloba, St. John's wort, and echinacea.

Garlic has been used medicinally for centuries, and recent research has shown that it may lower blood cholesterol (see Chapter 5, *Off the Shelf: Are Supplements a Safe Way to Reduce Blood Choleterol?*).[46] Garlic supplements allow consumers to increase garlic intake without eating the spice at every meal; some preparations contain a deodorized form. Ginseng has been used in Asia for centuries for its energizing, stress-reducing, and aphrodisiac properties. High doses may cause nervousness and heart palpitations. Gingko biloba, also called "maiden hair," is an herb that has been used to enhance memory and to treat a variety of circulatory ailments. Consumption of the leaves may cause side effects such as headaches, GI upset, and dizziness. Consumption of other parts of the plant can cause allergic skin reactions. Other herbs such as comfrey and camomile are consumed in tea; in high doses these can be toxic (see Chapter 16, *Off the Shelf: Herbal Tea: Healthful or Hazardous?*). St. John's wort is an herb taken to promote mental well-being. Analysis reveals that it contains low doses of the chemical found in the antidepressant drug Prozac. Petals of the echinacea plant were used by Native Americans as a treatment for colds, flu, and infections. Today, it is a popular herbal cold remedy. Studies have documented that it is an immune system stimulant. Although side effects have not been reported, allergies are possible.[47] In Germany, echinacea is available from pharmacists in prescription doses (Figure 9.17).

When using herbal or any other dietary supplements, read product labels, follow directions, and heed all warnings. If you suffer a harmful effect or illness that you think is related to the use of a supplement, seek medical attention and report the incident to FDA MedWatch by calling 1-800-FDA-1088 or going into the MedWatch Web site.

APPLICATIONS

These exercises are designed to help you apply your critical thinking skills to your own nutrition choices. Many are best performed using a diet analysis software program. If you do not have access to a computer program, the exercises can be hand-calculated using the information in this text and its appendices.

1. Using the three-day food intake record you kept in Chapter 2:
   a. Calculate your average daily intake of vitamin A.
   b. How does your vitamin A intake compare to the 1989 RDA for someone of your age and sex?
   c. What are three major food sources of vitamin A in your diet?
   d. Do the major food sources of vitamin A in your diet contain preformed vitamin A or provitamin A carotenoids?
2. Using the food intake record you kept in Chapter 2:
   a. Calculate your average intake of vitamin E.
   b. How does your intake of vitamin E compare with the 1989 RDA?
   c. If your diet does not meet the 1989 RDA, make modifications that will add enough vitamin E to your diet to meet the RDA without increasing your energy intake.
3. Use the Internet to identify several supplements on the market that contain phytochemicals.
   a. What health promises are made about these supplements?
   b. Do they contain a single compound or are they an extract of a whole plant containing multiple compounds?
   c. What are the advantages and disadvantages of these supplements? Would you recommend them to a friend? Why or why not?

Summary

1. The fat-soluble vitamins A, D, E, and K each have unique functions in the body.
2. Vitamin A is needed for vision and for the growth and differentiation of cells. It affects epithelial tissue, reproduction, and immune function by altering gene expression. It is found in the diet both preformed as retinoids and in precursor forms. Preformed vitamin A can be toxic at doses as low as ten times the 1989 RDA and increases the risk of birth defects at doses only four times the 1989 RDA. The major food sources of preformed vitamin A include liver, eggs, fish, and fortified dairy products.
3. Some carotenoids are precursors of vitamin A. The most potent is beta-carotene. Carotenoids are found in fruits and vegetables such as mangoes and carrots. Beta-carotene functions as an antioxidant, a role that is independent of its conversion to vitamin A. Carotenoids are not toxic, but a high intake can give the skin a yellow appearance.
4. Vitamin D can be made in the skin by exposure to sunlight, so dietary needs vary depending on the amount synthesized. Vitamin D is found in fish oils and fortified milk. It is essential for maintaining proper levels of calcium and phosphorus in the body. It promotes calcium and phosphorus absorption from the intestines and release from bone. A deficiency in children results in a condition called rickets; in adults, vitamin D deficiency causes osteomalacia.
5. Vitamin E functions primarily as a fat-soluble antioxidant. It is necessary for reproduction and protects cell membranes from oxidative damage. Since polyunsaturated fats are particularly susceptible to oxidative damage, the requirement for vitamin E increases as the polyunsaturated fat content of the diet increases. It is found in nuts, plant oils, green vegetables, and fortified cereals.
6. Vitamin K is essential for blood clotting. Since vitamin K deficiency is a problem in newborns, they are routinely given vitamin K injections at birth. Dicumarol, a substance that inhibits vitamin K activity, is used medically as an anticoagulant. Vitamin K is found in plants and is synthesized by bacteria in the gastrointestinal tract.
7. Our needs for vitamins can be met by a carefully selected diet that follows the recommendations of the Food Guide Pyramid.
8. Phytochemicals are chemicals found in plants. Some have health-promoting properties as antioxidants and via other mechanisms. Dietary recommendations advise us to increase our consumption of fruits and vegetables because these foods are sources of phytochemicals.
9. Over half the adult population in the United States takes some form of dietary supplements. Dietary supplements may contain vitamins; minerals; herbs, botanicals, or other plant-derived substances; amino acids; enzymes; concentrates or extracts. These are regulated by the FDA, but since they are classified as foods and not drugs, regulations are not as strict.
10. Vitamin supplements are recommended for some groups of individuals such as dieters, vegetarians, and nutritionally vulnerable groups.
11. Many substances that are not nutrients are available as supplements. Some dietary supplements contain compounds that are already present in the body but are not essential in the diet. Many contain plant extracts and herbs. These products may have beneficial physiological actions, but they can also be dangerous.

Review Questions

1. List two food sources of preformed vitamin A and two of provitamin A.
2. List three functions of preformed vitamin A.
3. What is the function of beta-carotene?
4. Is vitamin A deficiency a common problem? Why or why not?
5. Is vitamin A toxic? Is beta-carotene toxic?

6. Why is vitamin D called the sunshine vitamin?
7. Name two sources of vitamin D in the diet.
8. What is the function of vitamin D?
9. Explain how vitamin A and vitamin D can increase the amount of a protein produced.
10. What is the function of vitamin E?
11. Name two sources of vitamin E in the diet.
12. What is the main function of vitamin K?
13. What do phytochemicals do in plants and what do they do in people?
14. Is there a dietary recommendation for phytochemical intake?
15. Are vitamin and mineral supplements necessary? Why or why not?
16. Are dietary supplements safe? Why or why not?

Nutrition Web Links

To further explore areas related to the material in this chapter, go to the *Nutrition: Science and Applications* Web site at ***www.Wiley.com/college/Smolin*** and *click on* **Student Companion Site** for chapter-by-chapter links. Some Web sites related to the information in Chapter 9 include:

Organizations that offer information on micronutrients, health promotion, and disease prevention, such as the National Cancer Institute.

Sites that provide information on meeting micronutrient needs with food, such as food manufacturers and the National Five-A-Day program.

Sites that provide information on dietary supplements, such as the Office of Alternative Medicine, the U.S. Pharmacopoeia, and companies that grow and market herbs.

References

1. Clinton, S. K. Lycopene: chemistry, biology, and implications for human health and disease. Nutr. Rev. 56(I):35–51, 1998.
2. Furr, H. C., and Clark, R. M. Intestinal absorption and tissue distribution of carotenoids. Nutr. Biochem. 8:364–377, 1997.
3. Mangelsdorf, D. J. Vitamin A receptors. Nutr. Rev. 52:S32–S44, 1994.
4. Maden, M. Vitamin A in embryonic development. Nutr. Rev. 52:S3–S12, 1994.
5. Ross, D. A. Vitamin A and public health. Proc. Nutr. Soc. 57:159–165, 1998.
6. Underwood, B. A. Micronutrient malnutrition: is it being eliminated? Nutr. Today 33:121–129, 1998.
7. Underwood, B. A. From research to reality: the micronutrient story. J. Nutr. 128:145–151, 1998.
8. Rothman, K. J., Moore, L. L., Singer, M. R., et al. Teratogenicity of high vitamin A intake. N. Engl. J. Med. 333:1369–1373, 1995.
9. Blot, W. J., Li, J-Y., Taylor, P. R., et al. Nutrition intervention trials in Linxian, China: supplementation with specific vitamin/mineral combinations, cancer incidence, and disease-specific mortality in the general population. J. Natl. Cancer Inst. 85:1483–1491, 1993.
10. Hennekens, C. H., Buring, J. E., Manson, J. E., et al. Lack of effect of long-term supplementation with beta-carotene on the incidence of malignant neoplasms and cardiovascular disease. N. Engl. J. Med. 334:1145–1149, 1996.
11. Omenn, G. S., Goodman, G. E., Thornquist, M. D., et al. Effects of a combination of beta-carotene and vitamin A on lung cancer and cardiovascular disease. N. Engl. J. Med. 334:1150–1155, 1996.
12. The Alpha-Tocopherol, Beta-Carotene Cancer Prevention Study Group. The effect of vitamin E and beta-carotene on the incidence of lung cancer and other cancers in male smokers. N. Engl. J. Med. 330:1029–1035, 1994.
13. Mayne, S. T. Beta-carotene, carotenoids, and disease prevention in humans. FASEB J. 10:690–701, 1996.
14. Gaziano, J. M. Antioxidant vitamins and coronary artery disease risk. Am. J. Med. 97:(Suppl. 3A):18S–21S, 1994.
15. Holick, M. F. Vitamin D. In *Modern Nutrition in Health and Disease*, 9th ed. Shils, M. E., Olson, J. A., Shike, M., and Ross, A. C., eds. Baltimore: Williams & Wilkins, 1999. 329–345.
16. DeLuca, H. F., and Zierold, C. Mechanisms and functions of vitamin D. Nutr. Rev. 56(II):S4–S10, 1998.
17. Food and Nutrition Board, Institute of Medicine. *Dietary Reference Intakes: Calcium, Phosphorus, Magnesium, Vitamin D, and Fluoride.* Washington, D.C.: National Academy Press, 1997.
18. Gloth, F. M., and Tobin, J. D. Vitamin D deficiency in older people. J. Am. Geriatr. Soc. 43:822–828, 1995.
19. Blank, S., Scanlon, K. S., Sinks, T. H., and Falk, H. An outbreak of hypervitaminosis D associated with the overfortification of milk from a home-delivery dairy. Am. J. Public Health 85:656–659, 1995.
20. Murphy, S. P., Subar, A. F., and Block, G. Vitamin E intakes and sources in the United States. Am. J. Clin. Nutr. 52:361–367, 1990.
21. Howard, L. J. The neurologic syndrome of vitamin E deficiency: laboratory and electrophysiologic assessment. Nutr. Rev. 48:169–177, 1990.
22. Bendich, A., and Machlin, L. J. Safety of oral intake of vitamin E. Am. J. Clin. Nutr. 48:612–619, 1988.
23. Rimm, E. B., Stampfer, M. J., Ascherio, A., et al. Vitamin E consumption and the risk of heart disease in men. N. Engl. J. Med. 328:1450–1456, 1993.
24. Stampfer, M. J., Hennekens, C. H., Manson, J. E., et al. Vitamin E consumption and the risk of heart disease in women. N. Engl. J. Med. 328:1487–1489, 1993.
25. Abbey, M. The importance of vitamin E in reducing cardiovascular risk. Nutr. Rev. 53:S28–S32, 1995.
26. Olson, R. E. Vitamin K. In *Modern Nutrition in Health and Disease*, 9th ed. Shils, M. E., Olson, J. A., Shike, M., and Ross, A. C., eds. Baltimore: Williams & Wilkins, 1999. 363–380.
27. Harris, J. E. Interaction of dietary factors with oral anticoagulants: review and applications. J. Am. Diet. Assoc. 95:580–584, 1995.
28. Hasler, C. M. Functional foods: the Western perspective. Nutr. Rev. 54(II):S6–S10, 1996.
29. Fund, W. C. R. Food, nutrition and the prevention of cancer: a global perspective. Washington, D.C.: American Institute for Cancer Research, 1997.
30. Steinmetz, K. A., and Potter, J. D. Vegetables, fruit, and cancer prevention: a review. J. Am. Diet. Assoc. 96:1027–1039, 1996.
31. Craig, W. J. Phytochemicals: guardians of our health. J. Am. Diet. Assoc. 97:199–204, 1997.
32. Decker, E. A. The role of phenolics, conjugated linoleic acid, carnosine, and pyrroloquinoline quinone as nonessential dietary antioxidants. Nutr. Rev. 53:49–58, 1995.

33. Dreosti, I. E. Bioactive ingredients: antioxidants and polyphenols in tea. Nutr. Rev. 54 (II):S51–S58, 1996.
34. Halliwell, B. Antioxidants and human disease: a general introduction. Nutr. Rev. 55:(II)S44–S52, 1997.
35. Miller, N. J., Sampson, J., Candeias, L. P., et al. Antioxidant activities of carotenes and xanthophylls. FEBS Lett. 384:240–246, 1996.
36. Jankun, J., Selman, S. H., and Swiercz, R. Why drinking green tea could prevent cancer. Nature 387:561, 1997.
37. Fehey, J. W., Zhang, Y., and Talalay, P. Broccoli sprouts: an exceptionally rich source of inducers of enzymes that protect against carcinogens. Proc. Natl. Acad. Sci. USA 94:10367–10372, 1997.
38. Palozza, P. Prooxidant actions of carotenoids in biologic systems. Nutr. Rev. 56:257–265, 1998.
39. Decker, E. A. Phenolics: prooxidants or antioxidant? Nutr. Rev. 55:396–407, 1997.
40. American Dietetic Association. Position paper on phytochemicals and functional foods. Am. J. Diet. Assoc. 95:493–496, 1995.
41. Kurtweil, P. An FDA guide to dietary supplements. FDA Consumer 28–35, 32:Sept./Oct.,1998.
42. Bui, M. H., Sauty, A., Collet, F., and Leuenberger, P. Dietary vitamin C intake and concentrations in the body fluids and cells of male smokers and nonsmokers. J. Nutr. 122:312–316, 1992.
43. American Dietetic Association. Position paper of the American Dietetic Association: vitamin and mineral supplementation. J. Am. Diet. Assoc. 96:73–77, 1996.
44. Kelly, G. S. The role of glucosamine sulfate and chondriotin sulfates in the treatment of degenerative joint disease. Altern. Med. Rev. 3:27–39, 1998.
45. Aukema, H. M., and Holub, B. J. Inositol and Pyrroloquinoline Quinone. In *Modern Nutrition in Health and Disease*, 8th ed. Shils, M. E., Olson, J. A., and Shike, M., eds. Philadelphia: Lea & Febiger, 1994. 449–458.
46. Milner, J. A. Garlic: its anticarcinogenic and antitumorigenic properties. Nutr. Rev. 54:(II)S82–S86, 1996.
47. Bartels, C. L., and Miller, S. L. Herbal and related remedies, NCP 13:3–18, 1998.

Chapter 10

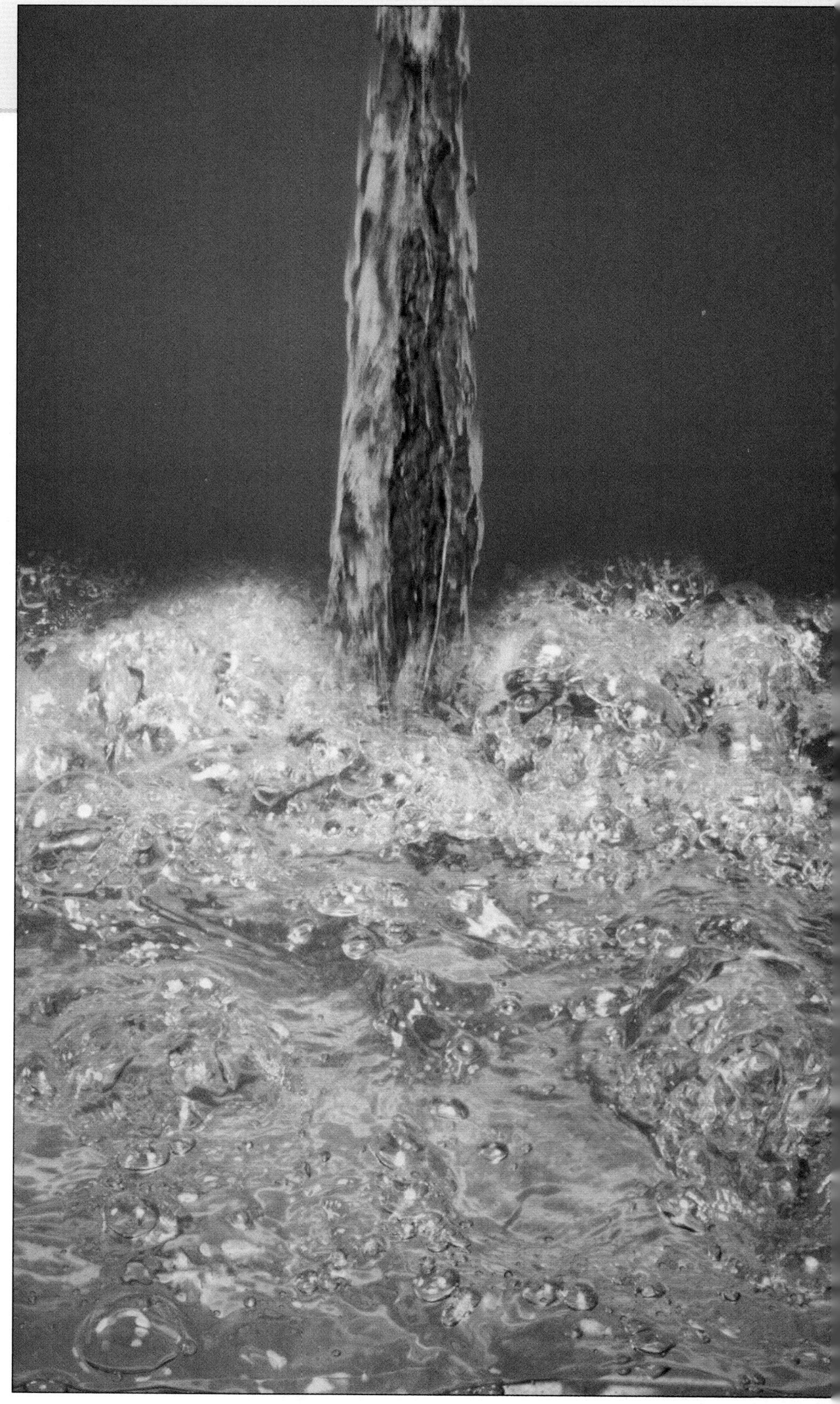

(© Corbis/Tecmap Corporation)

Chapter Outline

The Internal Sea: Water and the Major Minerals

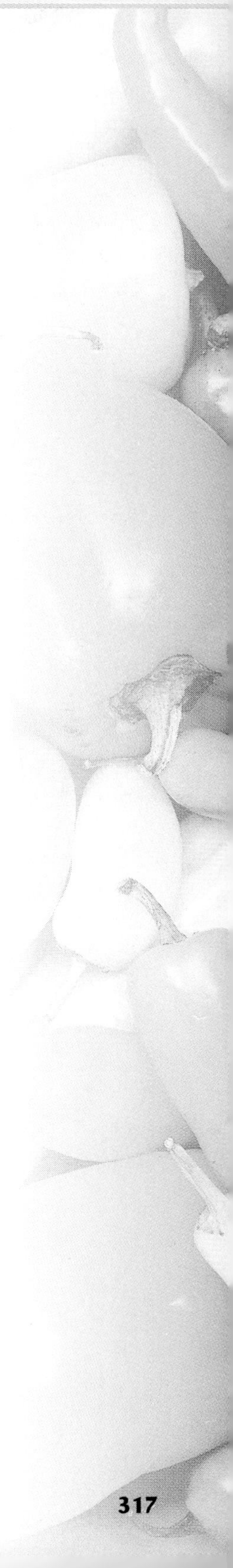

Chapter Concepts

1. Water is an essential macronutrient needed in the body as a transport fluid, a protector and lubricator, a regulator of body temperature, a solvent, and a biochemical reactant.
2. Water cannot be stored; to maintain fluid balance, intake from fluid and food must equal loss through urine, feces, and evaporation.
3. Nutritionally, minerals are inorganic molecules needed in the diet that function as structural components and regulators of the chemical reactions and body processes needed to maintain health.
4. The absorption and functions of many minerals are interrelated, so that a deficient or excessive intake of one affects the levels and functions of others.
5. In nutrition, sodium, chloride, and potassium are referred to as the electrolytes. They regulate fluid balance and function in nerve conduction and muscle contraction.
6. Hypertension, or high blood pressure, is a major public health problem in the United States. Blood pressure can be affected by the amount of sodium, chloride, potassium, and calcium in the diet as well as the dietary pattern as a whole.
7. Bone is a metabolically active tissue that is constantly being broken down and reformed. With age, bone breakdown exceeds bone formation, and this imbalance can result in osteoporosis, a disease characterized by reduced bone mass and an increased risk of bone fractures.
8. Calcium provides structure to bones and teeth. Calcium in body fluids is essential for nerve conduction, muscle contraction, blood clotting, and blood pressure regulation.
9. Phosphorus provides structure to bones and teeth and is important in acid-base balance. It is a component of cell membranes, ATP, and DNA.
10. Magnesium is important to bone structure and functions as a cofactor in many enzymatic reactions. It is important in energy production and the proper functioning of the nerves and muscles.
11. Sulfur is important in the structure of some proteins and vitamins and in the regulation of acid-base balance.

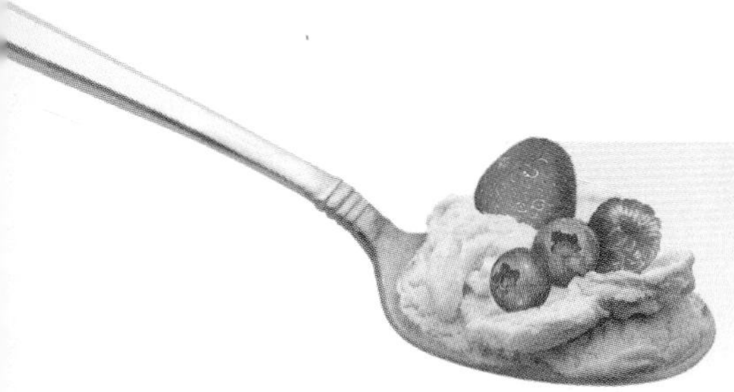

Just a Taste

How long can a person survive without water?

Does reducing salt intake reduce blood pressure?

Does drinking milk build strong bones?

The complex molecules necessary for the emergence of life were forged in the earth's first seas. These primordial seas supported life because they were rich in inorganic minerals as well as organic substances. As organisms grew in complexity, the chemicals critical to their survival were incorporated into an internal sea of water and dissolved substances. As creatures grew bigger, an internal skeleton was necessary for support. This internal support was comprised of an organic framework which incorporated inorganic minerals for strength and rigidity. These minerals also played an essential role in the internal sea.

Just as the right combination of water, organic molecules, and minerals was necessary for the beginning of life, the right combination is necessary in the body for the maintenance of life. Scientists are still researching the exact mixture of minerals and other substances necessary for this internal sea to sustain life. We understand the function of some minerals, such as the importance of calcium in bone, but our understanding of the amount needed for optimal health is still evolving. For other minerals, such as nickel and arsenic, essentiality is just now being established and there is not enough information to determine recommended intakes.

In the next two chapters, we will discuss the sources, functions, and requirements of the inorganic components of the internal sea—water and minerals. In Chapter 10 we discuss water as a nutrient and introduce minerals. This general discussion is followed by specific information about the electrolytes sodium, potassium, and chloride; the minerals calcium, phosphorus and magnesium, which play important roles in calcified tissues; and finally, sulfur, a major mineral that is a component of amino acids. The trace elements and their roles in oxygen transport, antioxidant defenses, and other aspects of metabolism are discussed in Chapter 11.

Water: The Internal Sea

Water is essential to survival. Without food, an average individual can live for about eight weeks, but a lack of water reduces survival to only a few days. Although the amount and distribution of body water are regulated, water cannot be stored. Even minor changes in the amount and distribution of body water can be life threatening. When water losses are increased, as they are in hot weather and with exercise, intake must increase to maintain homeostasis.

Water in the Diet

Most of the water in the body comes from the diet—not only as water we drink but from other liquids and solid food (Figure 10.1). Milk is 90% water, apples are about 85% water, and roast beef is about 50% water. A small amount of water is generated inside the body by metabolism, but this is not significant in meeting body water needs (see *Off the Shelf: Is Bottled Water Better?*).

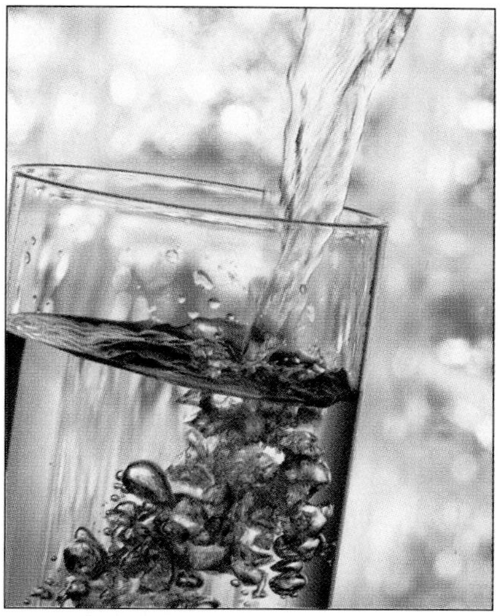

Figure 10.1
The body's need for water is met by the water consumed in fluids and food. (© Charles Thatcher/Tony Stone Images)

Water in the Body

In adults, about 60% of body weight is water. The percentage is higher in infants and generally decreases with age. Water is found in varying proportions in all the tissues of the body; blood is about 90% water, muscle about 75%, and bone about 25%. The proportion of water distributed among body compartments also varies. About two thirds of body water is found inside cells; this is known as **intracellular fluid.** The remaining one third is outside cells, as **extracellular fluid.** Extracellular fluid includes that in the blood and lymph as well as between cells, called **interstitial fluid.**

Not only does the amount of water differ among body compartments, but the concentration of substances dissolved in the water, or **solutes,** also varies. The concentration of protein is highest in intracellular fluid, lower in extracellular fluid, and even lower in interstitial fluid. Extracellular fluid has a higher concentration of sodium and chloride and a lower concentration of potassium, and intracellular fluid is higher in potassium and lower in sodium and chloride.

The amount of water in each compartment depends on the concentration of solutes in the water. When the concentration of solutes in one compartment is higher than in another, water will move in to equalize the solute concentration. This diffusion of water across a membrane from an area with a lower solute concentration to an area with a higher solute concentration is called **osmosis.** Osmosis occurs when there is a selectively permeable membrane, such as a cell membrane, which allows water to pass freely but regulates the passage of other substances. Water moves across this membrane in a direction that will equalize the concentration of solutes on both sides. For example, when sugar is sprinkled on fresh strawberries, the water inside the strawberries moves across the skin of the fruit to try to equalize the sugar concentration on each side, causing the fruit to shrink (Figure 10.2). The body controls the amount of water in each compartment by regulating the concentration of solutes and relying on osmosis to move water in response to concentration changes.

Intracellular fluid The fluid located inside cells.

Extracellular fluid The fluid located outside cells. It includes fluid found in the blood, lymph, gastrointestinal tract, spinal column, eyes, and joints, and that found between cells and tissues.

Interstitial fluid The portion of the extracellular fluid located in the spaces between cells and tissues.

Solutes Dissolved substances.

Osmosis The passive movement of water across a membrane to equalize the concentration of dissolved solutes on both sides.

Regulating Water Intake The essential functions of water in the body require that there be a constant supply without excess or deficiency. Water intake must equal water loss in order to maintain water balance. The need to consume water or other fluids is signaled in a number of ways. A decrease in the amount of water in the body decreases saliva secretion, making the mouth dry and stimulating thirst. In addition, a decrease in body water causes a decrease in total blood volume and a drop in blood pressure. This is sensed by the brain, signaling the need to drink. These signals to consume water are not perfect regulators. The sensation of thirst often lags behind the need for water. For example, athletes exercising in hot weather lose water rapidly but do not experience intense thirst until they have lost so much body water that their physical performance is compromised.[1] A person with fever, vomiting, or diarrhea may also be losing water rapidly and thirst mechanisms may not be adequate to replace the fluid. In the elderly, the thirst

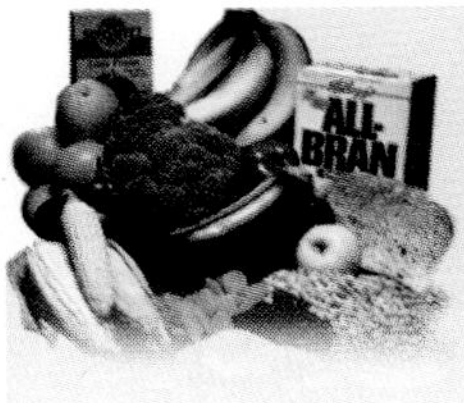

Off the Shelf

Is Bottled Water Better?

We need to consume water to survive. We want it to be safe and taste good. In general the water supply in the United States is safe; but, water is not risk free. Our drinking water is potentially exposed to hundreds of different contaminants including pesticides, nitrates from fertilizers, microorganisms, metals such as lead and iron, and radioactive compounds. Sometimes a problem arises because contamination has entered a municipal water supply, and sometimes the source of contamination is an individual well or household. For example, in one community, *Cryptosporidium*, a parasite that is commonly found in rivers and lakes, found its way into a municipal water supply and caused an outbreak of gastrointestinal illness.[1] Well water can be contaminated with pesticides and fertilizers from agricultural runoff, and lead, leaching from old household plumbing, can contaminate water after it enters the home. Although water contamination is rare, stories such as these have created concern about the safety of the water supply and prompted many consumers to purchase bottled water. But is bottled better?

Bottled water comes in many forms—spring water, drinking water, purified water, well water. There are over 700 different brands of bottled water available in the United States. Consumers who assume that buying water in a bottle is a guarantee of purity may be wasting their money. In reality, the jug at the water cooler and the Evian that you guzzle at the gym may not be any safer than tap water. Standards for the purity of municipal water systems are set by the EPA. These standards are used by the FDA to ensure that the minimum quality of bottled water is comparable with that of tap water.[2] Because the standards that regulate bottled water are no more rigid than those regulating tap water, it is not surprising that some bottled water actually is tap water.

About 75% of bottled water comes from protected wells and springs, but the other 25% is from municipal water supplies. To help consumers identify the source of their bottled water and make labeling consistent from state to state, the FDA established standard definitions for all bottled water products.[3] Under these regulations, bottled water that comes from tap water must be clearly labeled as such. Water that has been taken from a municipal water supply and then treated to remove minerals need not indicate that it is tap water, but is labeled as "distilled" or "purified," depending on the treatment. If you want water that did not come from the tap, select artesian water, spring water, well water, or mineral water. These come from underground water sources.

Water from all of these sources, as well as the water used in certain types of flavored bottled waters, must comply with the bottled water standards set by the FDA. Products labeled as carbonated water, seltzer water, soda water, and tonic water are considered soft drinks and so are exempt from bottled water regulations.

Individuals who are concerned about their tap water, but who do not want to carry water home from the grocery store, may choose a home water-treatment system. There are many different kinds. Faucet filters remove chlorine and other substances that make the water taste bad. More elaborate filter units, distillation units, and water softeners remove contaminants but may also change the mineral content of the water. For example, an ion exchange unit, or water softener, removes some minerals, mainly calcium and magnesium, from water and replaces them with sodium. Since minerals in hard water stain tubs, clog water heaters, and cause soap to form a film that is difficult to remove from laundry, softened water makes life easier at home. But, there may be health benefits to hard water. The incidence of heart attacks is lower in areas of the country that have hard water.[4] In addition, softened water has about twice the amount of sodium—about 94 mg per liter. If you are following a sodium-restricted diet, you may need to bypass the water softener when it comes to drinking water.

When choosing your water you must weigh the benefits against the risks. Bottled water and water-treatment systems cost money and whether you are drinking your tap water straight, filtering it with a home water-treatment system, or buying bottled water off the shelf, contamination is possible. The safest alternative is to buy distilled water. In the distillation process chemicals are removed and the heat destroys bacteria and other biological contaminants. The resulting water is probably free of contaminants, but it is tasteless and lacking in essential dietary minerals that water usually supplies. Before making a choice, take a look at the results of water-monitoring tests your water company is required to perform and compare them with the legal limits of contaminants set by the EPA. This should help you decide. For information, call the FDA, the International Bottled Water Association, or the EPA Hotline or look for their sites on the World Wide Web.

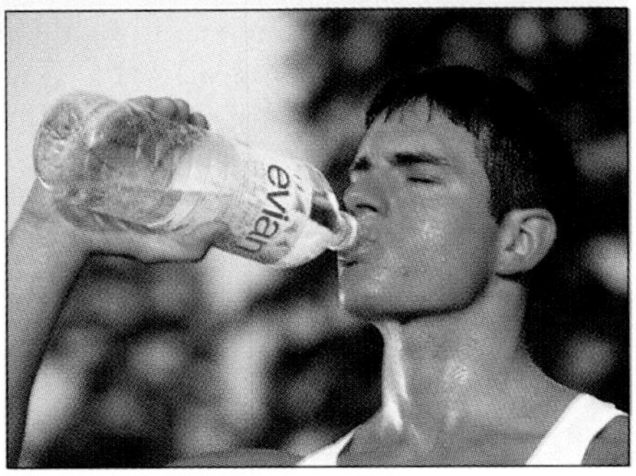

(© Nadine Markova/The Stock Market)

[1]EPA and CDC Office of Ground Water and Drinking Water. Guidance for people with severely weakened immune systems. June 17, 1998. Online at http://www.epa.gov/safewater/crypto.html

[2]Notebook. FDA Consumer 29:27, March 1995.

[3]FDA Talk. Paper No. 2 (T95–59), November 7, 1995.

[4]Rubenowitz, E., Axelsson, G., and Rylander, R. Magnesium in drinking water and death from acute myocardial infarction. Am. J. Epidemiol. 143:456–462, 1996.

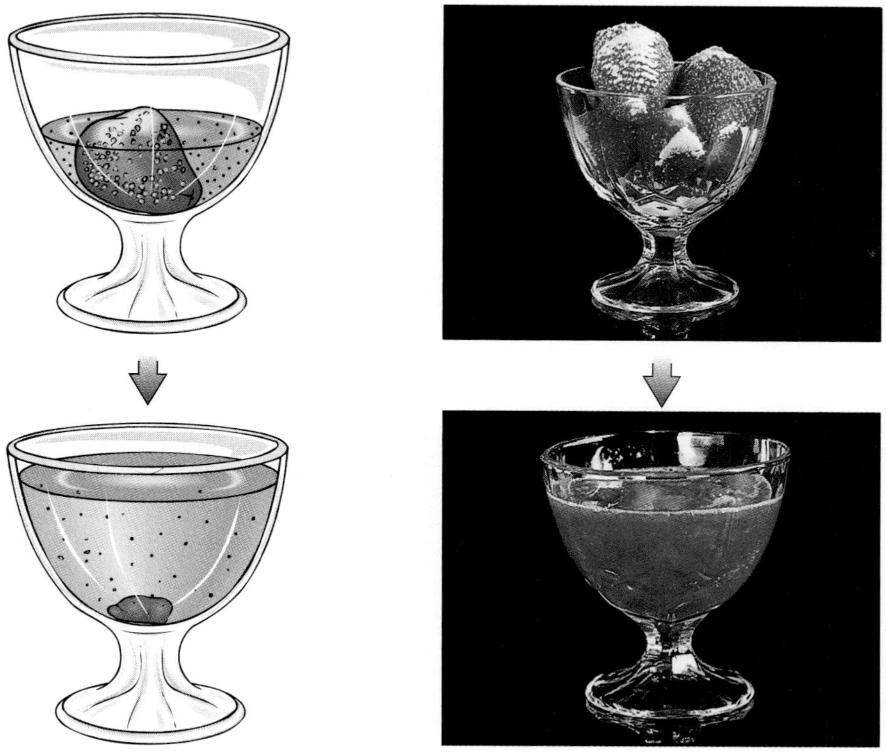

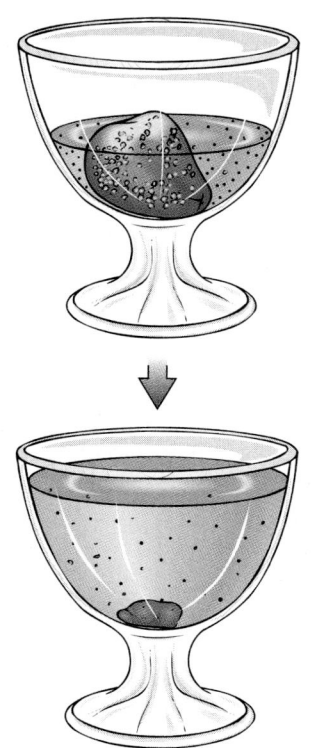

Figure 10.2
Osmosis is the process by which water moves across a membrane from an area of lower solute concentration to an area of higher solute concentration. When sugar is sprinkled on strawberries, osmosis draws water out of the strawberries to dilute the concentrated sugar solution on the surface. (Photos, Dennis Drenner)

mechanism often becomes unreliable, so an individual may not be thirsty even though body water is depleted. Also, being thirsty does not mean that the individual will take a drink. Since people cannot and do not always respond to thirst, water loss from the body is regulated to prevent dehydration.

Water Loss From the Body Water is lost from the body in urine, in feces, and through evaporation from the lungs and skin. As shown in Figure 10.3, a typical young man loses 2.75 liters of water daily through urine, feces, and evaporation. This amount must be replaced through consumption of food and fluids in order to maintain water balance.

Typical urine output is 1 to 2 liters per day, but this varies depending on the amount of fluid consumed and the amount of waste to be excreted. The waste products that must be excreted in urine include urea and other nitrogen-containing products from protein breakdown, ketones from fat breakdown, phosphates, sulfates, and other minerals. The amount of urea that must be excreted is increased when dietary or body protein breakdown is increased. Ketone excretion is increased when body fat is broken down. In both cases, the need for water increases in order to produce more urine to excrete the extra wastes.

The amount of water lost in the feces is usually small, only about 200 ml per day (less than a cup). This is remarkable because more than 4 liters of fluid enter the gastrointestinal tract via food, water, and secretions. Under normal conditions, more than 95% is reabsorbed before the feces are eliminated. However, in cases of severe diarrhea, large amounts of water can be lost through the gastrointestinal tract.

Water loss due to evaporation from the skin and lungs occurs without the individual being aware that it is occurring; such losses are therefore referred to as **insensible losses.** An inactive person at room temperature may lose less than 1 ml per minute, or about 1.1 liters per day. Insensible losses increase as environmental temperature and activity increase. For example, with strenuous exercise in a hot environment, water used to cool the body by evaporation of sweat may increase insensible losses tenfold. Humidity also affects insensible losses. A very dry

Insensible losses Fluid losses that are not perceived by the senses, such as evaporation of water through the skin and lungs.

Figure 10.3
To maintain water balance, intake must equal output. This figure approximates the sources of water intake and output in a 70-kg adult who is not losing water in sweat.

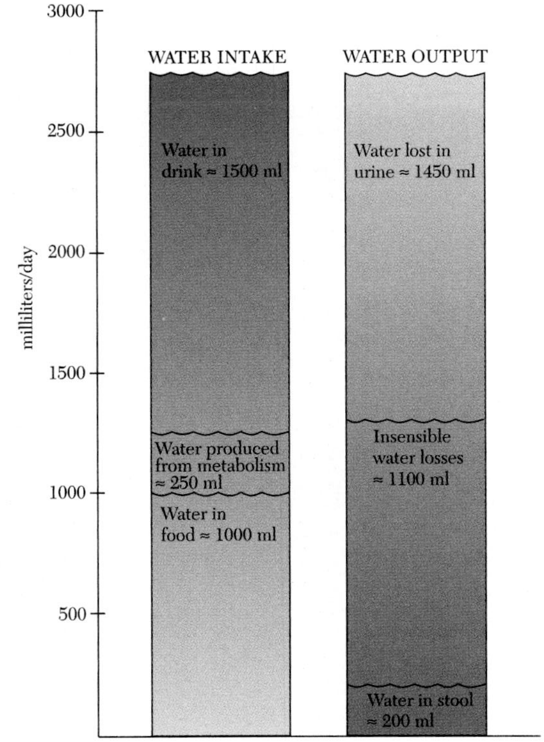

environment, such as in an airplane or in the desert, increases evaporative losses. Adequate water intake is essential to compensate for these losses. Endurance athletes can estimate water loss by weighing themselves before and after exercise. Lost weight should then be replaced by consuming the equivalent weight in fluids. For instance, an athlete who loses 2 pounds during a workout should consume an extra 2 pints or a liter of fluid (1 lb = 1 pint = 1/2 liter) (see Chapter 12).

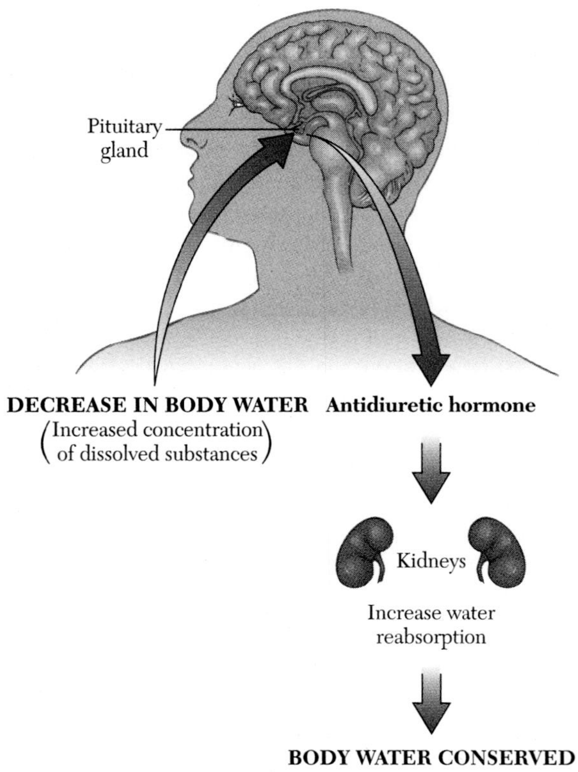

Figure 10.4
When body water decreases, the increased solute concentration signals the pituitary gland to secrete antidiuretic hormone, which acts on the kidneys to decrease water losses.

Table 10.1 *A Summary of Water and the Major Minerals*

Nutrient	Sources	Recommended Intake for Adults	Major Functions	Deficiency	Groups at Risk	Toxicity	Tolerable Upper Intake Levels (UL)
Water	Food and beverages	1 ml/kcal	Solvent, reactant, protector, transporter, temperature regulator	Thirst, weakness, poor endurance, confusion, disorientation	Infants, those with fever and diarrhea, elderly, athletes	Unlikely, confusion, coma, convulsions	NA
Sodium	Table salt, processed foods	500–2400 mg	Major extracellular ion, nerve transmission, regulates fluid balance	Muscle cramps	Those consuming a severely sodium-restricted diet	High blood pressure in sensitive individuals	NA
Potassium	Fruits, vegetables, grains	At least 1600–3500 mg	Major intracellular ion, nerve transmission	Irregular heartbeat, fatigue, muscle cramps	Those consuming diets high in processed foods, those taking thiazide diuretics	Abnormal heartbeat	NA
Chloride	Table salt	750–3400 mg	Major extracellular ion	Unlikely	None	None likely	NA
Calcium	Dairy products, bony fish, leafy green vegetables	1000–1200 mg*	Bone and tooth structure, nerve transmission, muscle contraction, blood clotting	Increased risk of osteoporosis	Postmenopausal women, teenage girls, those with kidney disease	Kidney stones in susceptible individuals	2500 mg
Phosphorus	Meat, dairy, cereals, and baked goods	**700 mg**	Structure of bones, teeth, membranes, ATP and DNA, buffer	Bone loss, weakness, lack of appetite	Premature infants, alcoholics, elderly	Calcium resorption from bone	4000 mg
Magnesium	Nuts, greens, whole grains, seeds	**310–420 mg**	Bone structure, ATP reactions, nerve and muscle function	Nausea, vomiting, weakness, heat changes	Alcoholics, those with kidney and gastrointestinal disease	Nausea, vomiting, low blood pressure	350 mg nonfood
Sulfur	Protein foods, preservatives	None specified	Part of amino acids and vitamins, buffer	None when protein needs are met	None	None likely	NA

Value in **bold** is a Recommended Dietary Allowance (RDA).
*Adequate Intake (AI).
NA—No UL established at time of publication.

Kidneys Regulate Water Excretion The kidneys serve as a filtering system that regulates the amount of water and dissolved substances retained in the blood and excreted in urine. As blood flows through the kidneys, water and small molecules are filtered out of the blood vessels. Some of the water and molecules are reabsorbed and the rest are excreted in the urine. The amount of water that is reabsorbed depends on conditions in the body. When the concentration of solutes in the blood is high, **antidiuretic hormone (ADH),** which is secreted from the pituitary gland, signals the kidneys to reabsorb water to reduce the amount lost in the urine. This reabsorbed water is returned to the blood, decreasing the solute concentration in the blood to normal (Figure 10.4). When the solute concentration in the blood is low, ADH levels decrease so less water is reabsorbed and more is excreted in the urine, allowing blood solute concentration to increase to normal. The amount of sodium in the blood, blood volume, and blood pressure also play a role in regulating body water.

Antidiuretic hormone (ADH) A hormone secreted by the pituitary gland that increases the amount of water reabsorbed by the kidney and therefore retained in the body.

Functions of Water in the Body In the body, water transports nutrients, provides protection, helps regulate temperature, participates in reactions, and provides the medium in which chemical reactions take place (Table 10.1).

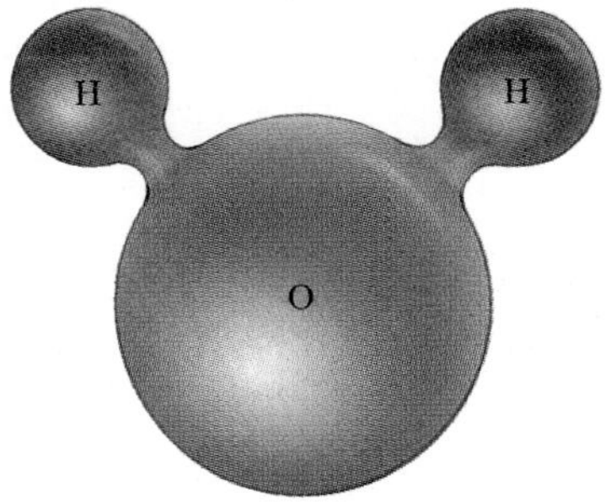

Figure 10.5
Two hydrogen atoms share electrons with one oxygen atom to form a molecule of water. The electrons spend more time around the oxygen atom, giving it a slightly negative charge, while the side of the molecule with the two hydrogens has a slightly positive charge. When salt (sodium chloride) is added to water the positive sodium ion is attracted to the negative pole of the water molecule and the negative chloride ion is attracted to the positive pole.

Water as Transport Blood, which is 90% water, transports oxygen and nutrients to cells. It then carries carbon dioxide and waste products away from the cells. Water in urine transports waste products, such as urea and ketones, out of the body.

Water as Protection Water functions as a lubricant and cleanser. Watery tears lubricate the eyes and wash away dirt, synovial fluid lubricates the joints, and saliva lubricates the mouth, making it easier to chew and swallow food. Water inside the eyeballs and spinal cord acts as a cushion against shock. Similarly, during pregnancy, water in the amniotic fluid provides a protective cushion for the fetus.

Water as a Regulator of Temperature Body temperature is closely regulated to maintain a normal level of around 98.6°F (37°C). If the body temperature rises above 108°F or falls below 80°F, death is likely. The fact that water changes temperature slowly in response to changes in the external environment helps the human body resist temperature change when the outside temperature fluctuates. The water in blood actively regulates body temperature. When body temperature starts to rise, the blood vessels in the skin dilate, causing blood to flow close to the surface of the body and release some of the heat to the environment. This occurs with fevers as well as when environmental temperature rises. In a cold environment, blood vessels in the skin constrict, restricting the flow of blood near the surface and conserving body heat. The most obvious way that water helps regulate body temperature is through the evaporation of sweat. When body temperature increases, the sweat glands in the skin secrete this watery substance. As the sweat evaporates from the skin, heat is lost.

Water in Chemical Reactions Water is involved in chemical reactions in the body. Hydrolysis reactions break large molecules into smaller ones by the addition of water. For example, water is added in the reaction that breaks a molecule of maltose into two glucose molecules. Water is also involved in reactions that join two molecules. These reactions are referred to as condensation reactions. The formation of a dipeptide from two amino acids requires the removal of a water molecule.

Solvent A fluid in which one or more substances dissolve.

Polar Used to describe a molecule that has a positive charge at one end and a negative charge at the other.

Electrons Negatively charged particles.

Ion An atom or group of atoms that carries a negative or a positive electrical charge.

Dissociate To separate two charged ions.

Electrolytes Substances that separate in water to form positively and negatively charged ions. In nutrition this term refers to sodium, potassium, and chloride.

Water as a Solvent One of the key functions of water in the body is as a **solvent,** which is a fluid in which solutes can dissolve to form a solution. Water is an ideal solvent for some substances because it is **polar;** that is, the two sides or poles of the water molecule have different electrical charges. The polar nature of water comes from its structure, which consists of two hydrogen atoms and one oxygen atom. These atoms, like all atoms, are made up of a positively charged central core, or nucleus, with negatively charged **electrons** orbiting around it. To form a water molecule, the two hydrogen atoms move close enough to share their electrons with an atom of oxygen. But the sharing is not equal. The shared electrons spend more time around the oxygen atom than around the hydrogen atoms, giving the oxygen side of the molecule a slightly negative charge and the hydrogen side a slightly positive charge. This polar nature of water allows it to surround other charged molecules and disperse them. Table salt, which dissolves in water, consists of a positively charged sodium **ion** bound to a negatively charged chloride ion. When placed in water, the sodium and chloride ions move apart, or **dissociate,** because the positively charged sodium ion is attracted to the negative pole of the water molecule and the negatively charged chloride ion is attracted to the positive pole (Figure 10.5). Substances like sodium chloride that dissociate in water to form positively and negatively charged ions are known as **electrolytes.** Electrolytes got their name because they are capable of conducting an electrical current when dissolved in water.

How Much Water Do We Need?

Adults need about 1 ml of water per kcalorie of energy requirement, or about 2 to 3 liters per day. This amount is sufficient under average conditions, but needs can be increased by variations in activity, environment, and diet. For instance, a man doing physical labor in a hot climate can require an additional 4 liters or more per day to replace water lost through evaporation (Figure 10.6). Water needs are also affected by the composition and adequacy of the diet. For example, a low-energy diet increases water needs because water losses increase to excrete the ketones produced by fat breakdown. A high-protein diet increases the amount of nitrogenous waste that must be excreted. A high-sodium diet increases water needs because the excess salt must be excreted in the urine. Caffeine is a diuretic, so a diet that is high in caffeine increases water loss from the kidneys and therefore increases water needs. A high-fiber diet also increases water needs because more fluid is retained in the gastrointestinal tract.

Water needs also increase during pregnancy and lactation. In pregnancy, water is needed to increase blood volume, produce amniotic fluid, and nourish the fetus. During lactation, the fluid secreted in milk, about 750 ml or 3 cups per day, must be restored by the mother's fluid intake.

The fluid requirements for infants are higher than those for adults. One reason is that the infant's kidneys cannot concentrate urine as efficiently as adult kidneys, so water loss is greater. Moreover, insensible losses are greater in infants and children because body surface area relative to body weight is much greater than in adults. In addition to having greater water needs, infants are susceptible to dehydration because they cannot ask for a drink when they are thirsty. An intake of 1.5 ml per kcalorie of energy expenditure, or about 3 cups (750 ml) a day for a six-month-old infant, is recommended. This is the water-to-energy ratio in human milk.

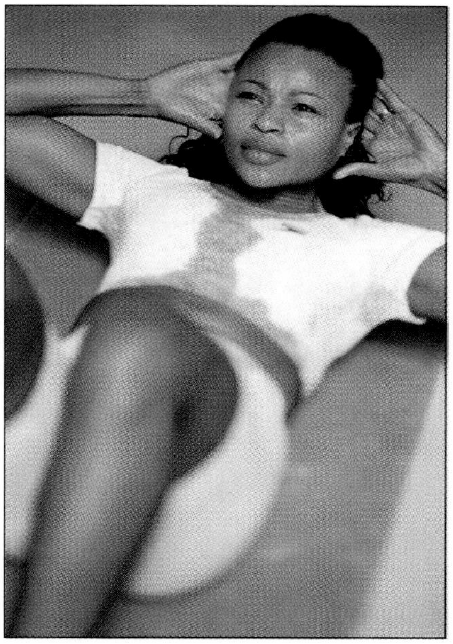

Figure 10.6
Exercise in a hot environment can dramatically increase water losses from sweat. (© Lori Adamski Peek/Tony Stone Images)

Water and Health

When water loss exceeds water intake, dehydration results. A loss of about 3% of the body's water will cause a decrease in blood volume. When this occurs, oxygen and nutrients cannot be efficiently delivered to tissues and waste products cannot be removed. A 5% loss will cause confusion and disorientation. A loss of about 10 to 20% can result in death.

Young athletes involved in sports with weight classes, such as wrestling and boxing, sometimes use dehydration to reduce their body weight so they can compete in a lower weight class. Being at the high end of the lower weight class is thought to provide an advantage over smaller opponents in that class.[2] However, when this is accomplished through even mild dehydration, such as a water loss of 1% of body weight, exercise performance can be impaired (see Chapter 12).

An excess of water, or water toxicity, is rare because of the kidneys' ability to regulate how much water is excreted. However, it can occur due to illness or improper administration of intravenous fluids. Symptoms of water toxicity include mental dulling, confusion, coma, convulsions, and even death.

WHAT ARE MINERALS?

Minerals are inorganic elements needed by the body as structural components and regulators of chemical reactions and body processes. Minerals have traditionally been divided into **major minerals,** or those needed in the diet in amounts greater than 100 mg per day or present in the body in amounts greater than 0.01% of body weight, and **trace elements,** which are minerals required by the body in an amount of 100 mg or less per day or present in the body in an amount of 0.01% or less of body weight (Figure 10.7).

Major minerals Minerals needed in the diet in amounts greater than 100 mg per day or present in the body in amounts greater than 0.01% of body weight.

Trace elements Minerals required in the diet in amounts 100 mg or less per day or present in the body in amounts 0.01% of body weight or less.

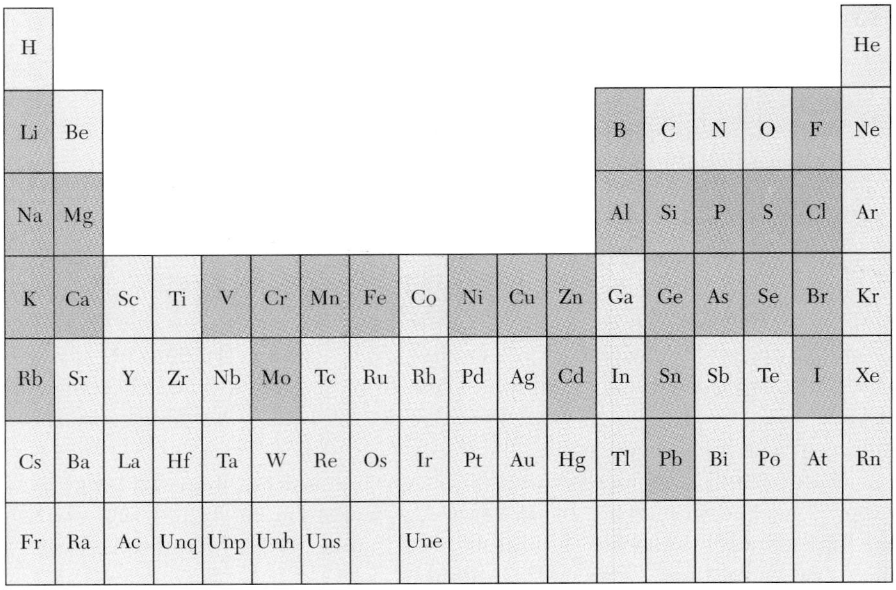

Figure 10.7
Minerals are chemical elements found in the periodic table. The major minerals are shown in purple and the trace elements are shown in blue.

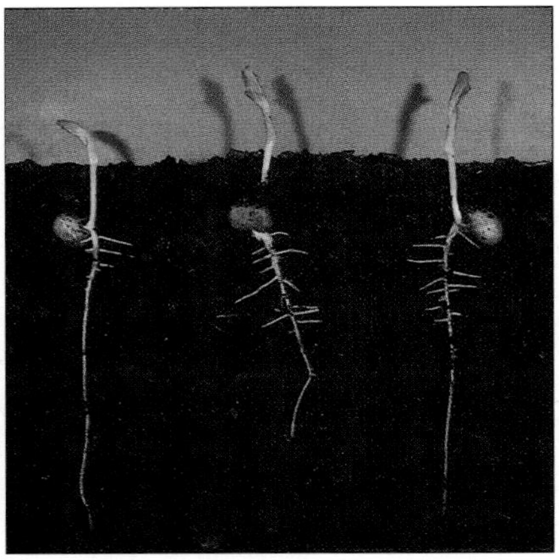

Figure 10.8
The mineral content of some plants varies with the mineral content of the soil in which they are grown. (Stephen J. Krasemann/Peter Arnold, Inc.)

Minerals in the Diet

Minerals in the diet come from both plant and animal sources. In some foods, the amounts of minerals are predictable because the minerals are regulated components of the plant or animal. For instance, iron is a component of muscle tissue; therefore it is found in consistent amounts in meat. Magnesium is a component of chlorophyll, so is found in consistent amounts in leafy greens. The amounts of some trace minerals in food vary depending on the mineral concentration in the soil and water at the food's source (Figure 10.8). For example, the soil content of iodine is high near the ocean but usually quite low in inland areas. Therefore, foods grown near the ocean are better sources of iodine than those grown inland. In developed countries, modern agriculture and transportation systems make foods produced in many locations available, so the diet is unlikely to be deficient in trace elements. In countries where the diet consists predominantly of locally grown foods, individual trace element deficiencies and excesses are more likely to occur.

Food processing and refining also affect the mineral content of foods. When the skins of produce and the bran and germ of grains are removed, trace elements are lost. For example, iron, selenium, zinc, and copper are lost when flour is refined. But only iron is replaced by enrichment. Processing tends to decrease the potassium content of foods and increase the sodium content. Some minerals are inadvertently added to food through processing and handling. For example, the iodine content of dairy products is increased when contaminated with the cleaning solutions used in milking machines. The mineral content of the diet can be maximized by eating a variety of foods, including many unprocessed or less processed foods such as fresh fruits, vegetables, and whole grains and cereals (Figure 10.9).

Minerals in the Digestive Tract

Phytic acid, or phytate An inorganic phosphorus storage compound found in seeds and grains that can bind minerals and decrease their absorption.

The absorption of minerals is affected by other nutrients and food components in the diet. For example, vitamin C in the diet enhances the absorption of the trace element iron. **Phytic acid,** or **phytate**—an organic compound containing phosphorus that is found in whole grains, bran, and soy products—binds calcium, zinc, iron, and magnesium, limiting their absorption. Phytic acid can be broken down by yeast, so the bioavailability of minerals is increased in yeast-leavened foods

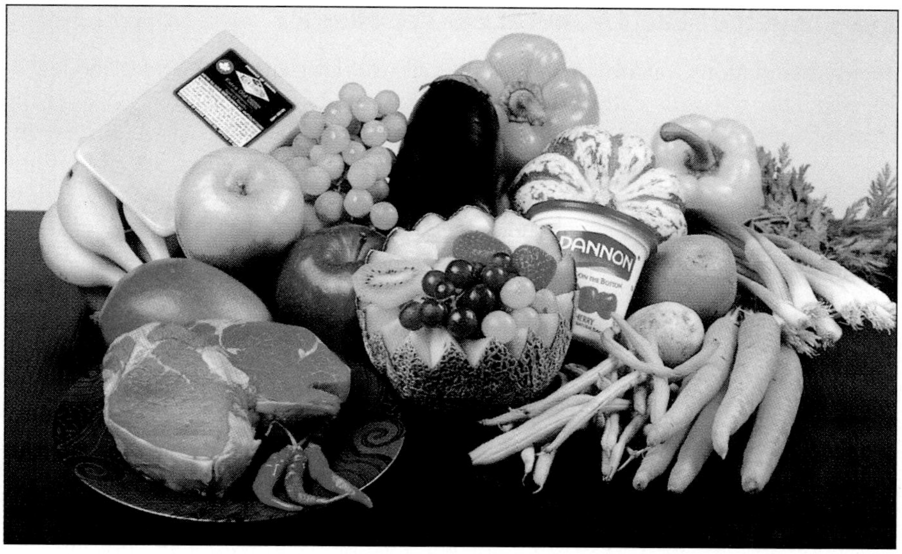

Figure 10.9
The trace element content of the diet can be maximized by eating a variety of nutrient-dense foods. (George Semple)

such as breads. **Tannins,** found in tea and some grains, can interfere with iron absorption, and **oxalates,** which are organic acids found in spinach, rhubarb, beet greens, and chocolate, have been found to interfere with calcium and iron absorption (Figure 10.10). Dietary fiber also interferes with mineral absorption. Although North Americans generally do not consume enough of any of these components to cause trace element deficiencies, problems may occur in developing countries. For example, in some populations the intake of phytate (which decreases zinc absorption) is high enough to increase the requirement for zinc.

Tannins Substances found in tea and some grains that can bind certain minerals and decrease their absorption.

Oxalates Organic acids found in spinach, rhubarb, and other leafy green vegetables that can bind certain minerals and decrease their absorption.

Interaction among the minerals can affect their absorption and transport. Mineral ions that carry the same charge compete for absorption in the gastrointestinal tract. Calcium, magnesium, zinc, copper, and iron all carry a 2+ charge and compete with one another for absorption. Therefore, a high intake of one, such as might be consumed in a supplement, may decrease the absorption of the others. Some interactions are significant enough to affect requirements. For example, a high intake of zinc reduces copper absorption, so copper requirements are affected by the amount of zinc in the diet.

Nutritional status and life stage can also affect mineral bioavailability. For example, when iron stores are low, the ability of the body to transport iron from mucosal cells to body tissues increases, but when iron stores are high, iron stays in the mucosal cells and is lost when they die. During pregnancy, increased calcium needs are met by an increase in absorption.

Minerals in the Body

Minerals perform a wide range of vital structural and regulatory roles in the body. For example, calcium, phosphorus, magnesium, and fluoride affect the structure and strength of bones. Iodine is a component of the thyroid hormones which regulate metabolic rate, chromium plays a role in regulating blood glucose levels, and zinc plays an important role in gene expression. Many of the minerals serve as **cofactors** necessary for enzyme activity. Selenium, copper, zinc, iron, and manganese each function as a cofactor for antioxidant enzyme systems.

Cofactor An inorganic ion or coenzyme required for enzyme activity.

Some minerals interact in their structural and regulatory functions. For example, calcium and phosphorus are both needed to mineralize bone, and blood levels of one can influence how the other is used. Sodium and potassium ions, which both carry a 1+ charge, are exchanged across cell membranes to regulate fluid balance and the electrical charge of the membrane.

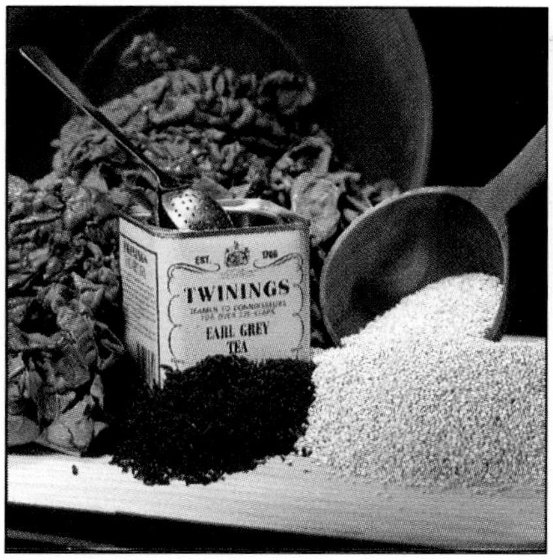

Figure 10.10
Compounds such as phytic acid, oxalates, and tannins found in these foods decrease mineral absorption. (Charles D. Winters)

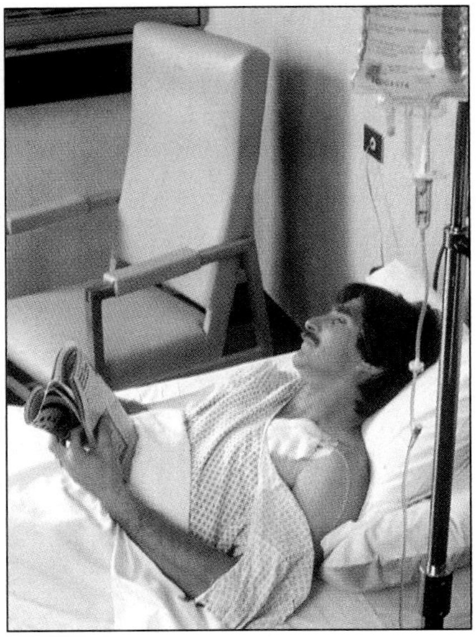

Figure 10.11
Trace element deficiencies can occur if incomplete TPN solutions are administered long-term. (© W. L. Steinmark/Custom Medical Stock Photo)

How Much of Each Mineral Do We Need?

Recommendations for the intake of minerals are determined by expert review of the available scientific data and selection of criteria of adequacy that consider the amounts needed to prevent deficiency as well as to reduce the risk of chronic disease. Many types of data are reviewed, including epidemiological data describing the intake of healthy populations, balance studies, depletion-repletion studies, and studies using biochemical and molecular biological techniques. Because of the many potential interactions among minerals and other dietary components, the need for any one mineral must be examined within the context of the total diet, and thus studied along with known amounts of other dietary components that interact with it.

Experiments to determine trace element needs are particularly difficult. Nutrients are considered essential if a deficiency consistently results in less than optimal biological function and is preventable or reversible by supplementation of that nutrient at levels similar to those found normally in the diet. Because trace elements already in the body can meet requirements for months or even years, depletion studies are very costly and may take years to complete. Because the amounts needed are so small, contamination from the environment may supply enough of a trace element to meet needs. Therefore, when studying trace elements in animals, everything that comes in contact with the animals, including food, water, air, cages, and keepers, must be kept cleansed of the elements. Similarly, balance studies in humans must consider interactions with other dietary components and all potential sources of a nutrient, including drinking water, medications, and toothpaste.

In addition to planned experiments, information about trace element needs has come from the study of deficiency symptoms in individuals fed solely by total parenteral nutrition (TPN) solutions for long periods of time. The nutrient intake of an individual receiving TPN is entirely dependent on the composition of the TPN solution (Figure 10.11). Only elements known to be essential are provided. Occasionally, deficiency has occurred inadvertently when elements were not included because at the time they were not known to be essential. For example, selenium was determined to be essential after a patient was given TPN without selenium. The patient developed symptoms that resolved when selenium was added to the solution.

Information about trace element needs has also been obtained by studying diseases that affect trace element utilization. For example, much of our knowledge about copper comes from studying Menkes' kinky hair syndrome, an inherited condition in which copper absorption and metabolism are abnormal. The symptoms of this syndrome are manifestations of a copper deficiency.

As with other nutrients, when no other data are available, mineral needs can be estimated by evaluating the intake in a healthy population. It is assumed that if there are no deficiency symptoms, the diet must meet the requirement for that nutrient. One problem with this approach, however, is that deficiency symptoms may become apparent only when the deficiency is severe. Subtle signs of a mineral deficiency in a population may be difficult to detect.

Minerals and Health

The right amount of each mineral is needed in the correct proportion in order to maintain health. Both deficiencies and excesses cause changes in body function. For some minerals, too much or too little causes obvious symptoms that impact short-term health. For others, underconsumption or overconsumption has few immediate symptoms but may affect the risk of chronic disease later in life.

Deficiency Deficiencies of the minerals iron and iodine are world health problems. Only a few months of inadequate iron intake can cause a decrease in the number and size of red blood cells, reducing the blood's capacity to deliver oxygen. Iron deficiency affects people in both the developed and the developing world. Iodine deficiency disorders are a problem primarily in developing countries, where they impact individuals at every stage of life.

Deficiencies of other minerals are rare, occurring only when the food supply is particularly limited. For example, in certain rural areas of China, selenium deficiency is common because the selenium content of the soil is extremely low and the diet is based on locally grown food. Calcium is an exception. Intake is below recommended levels in the diets of many people in the United States, particularly women. Too little dietary calcium has no short-term consequences, but it can reduce bone density and impact bone health later in life.

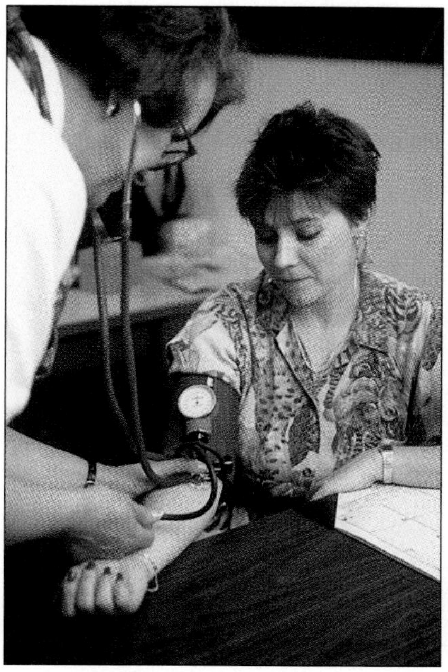

Figure 10.12
Everyone should have blood pressure monitored regularly since high blood pressure has no obvious symptoms. (Charles D. Winters)

Toxicity Mineral toxicity occurs most often as a result of environmental pollution or excessive use of supplements. For example, environmental lead from old chipped lead paint, lead pipes, and soil and air contamination is a risk to small children. Chronic exposure can cause growth retardation and learning disabilities (see Chapter 14). Trace element supplements may pose a risk of toxicity because elements that are essential in small doses may be toxic when consumed in larger amounts. For instance, iron is essential yet can be deadly at high doses.

Mineral supplements may also cause problems because of the complex interactions among minerals. Taking high doses of one can compromise the bioavailability of others, creating a mineral imbalance that can interfere with functions essential to human health. The body's regulatory mechanisms control the absorption and excretion of minerals but have evolved to deal with the amounts of these elements that occur naturally in the diet. Large doses of mineral supplements may override this regulation, causing toxicity.

Electrolytes: Salts of the Internal Sea

Electrolytes are elements that conduct electricity. In nutrition, the term is used to refer to the minerals sodium, potassium, and chloride. The modern diet is typically low in potassium and high in sodium and chloride, which are generally consumed together as sodium chloride, or table salt. This is a change from the diets of prehistoric hunter-gatherers, which consisted of plant foods such as nuts, berries, roots, and greens that are high in potassium and low in salt. Most of this change is due to the use of salt as a food additive. Salt is used as a preservative in food because it inhibits bacterial growth; it is also used to add flavor and to heighten existing flavors. It was highly prized by ancient cultures in Asia, Africa, and Europe, where it was used in rituals as well as in the preservation of food. Roman soldiers were paid in *sal*, the Latin word for salt from which we get our word *salary*.

Today, rather than a prized commodity, salt is a substance we attempt to limit in the diet. The reason for restricting salt is that diets high in salt have been implicated as a risk factor for **hypertension.** Approximately 50 million Americans are at increased risk of illness and early death because of hypertension[3] (Figure 10.12).

Hypertension Blood pressure that is consistently elevated to 140/90 mm of mercury or greater.

Electrolytes in the Diet

The typical American diet contains about 9 grams of salt. Salt is 40% sodium and 60% chloride by weight, so 9 grams contains 3.6 grams of sodium ($9 \times 40\% = 3.6$ g) and 5.4 grams of chloride. Most of the salt in the Western diet comes from processed foods. Only 10% comes from salt found naturally in food; 15% is from that added in cooking and at the table, and 75% is from that added during processing and manufacturing. Most of the sodium in processed foods is from

Table 10.2 *Sodium and Potassium in Fresh and Processed Foods*

Food	Amount	Sodium (mg)	Potassium (mg)
Roast pork	3 oz (85 g)	55	333
Ham	3 oz	1010	243
Milk (2%)	1 cup (240 ml)	122	376
American cheese	1 oz	405	46
Whole wheat bread	1 slice	185	88
Biscuit from mix	1	271	53
Potato, baked	1 medium	6	477
Potato chips	1 oz	168	362
Fresh tomato	1 medium	11	273
Spaghetti sauce	1/2 cup	657	565
Orange juice	1 cup	2.5	473
Orange drink	1 cup	8	0

sodium chloride, but other sodium salts, such as sodium bicarbonate, sodium citrate, and sodium glutamate, are used as food additives and contribute to the sodium content of the diet. These sodium-containing additives are used as preservatives and leavening agents. Drinking water from community water supplies contributes less than 10% of our sodium intake.[4] Softened water or mineral water is often higher in sodium than tap water and, if consumed in large quantities, can contribute significantly to daily sodium intake.

In contrast to sodium and chloride, the richest sources of potassium are unprocessed foods such as fruits, vegetables, whole grains, and fresh meats. Bananas, oranges, potatoes, and tomatoes are some of the best sources. Processed foods are generally low in potassium (see Table 10.2).

Electrolytes in the Digestive Tract

Almost all of the sodium, chloride, and potassium consumed in the diet is absorbed. Despite large variations in dietary intake, homeostatic mechanisms act to regulate the concentrations of these electrolytes in the body. For example, in northern China, sodium chloride intake is greater than 13.9 grams per day; in the Kalahari Desert, it is less than 1.7 grams per day; and in an Indian population in Brazil, consumption may be less than 0.06 gram of salt per day. However, blood levels of sodium are not significantly different among these groups.[4]

Electrolytes in the Body

In the body, electrolytes help regulate fluid balance and are important for nerve conduction and muscle contraction.

Electrolytes and Fluid Balance Electrolytes and other solutes cannot move freely back and forth across cell membranes, but water can. The movement of water between intracellular and extracellular compartments therefore depends on the concentrations of sodium and potassium and other solutes in these compartments. For example, if the concentration of electrolytes is high in the blood, water is drawn into the blood by osmosis to dilute the electrolytes, reducing their concentration.

Electrolytes and Nerve Conduction and Muscle Contraction Sodium and potassium are important for the conduction of nerve impulses (see Table 10.1). Nerve impulses are created by a change in the electrical charge across cell membranes. In the extracellular fluid, sodium is the most abundant positively charged electrolyte and chloride is the principal negatively charged ion. Potassium is the principal positively charged ion inside cells, where it is 30 times more concentrated than outside the cell. An electrical charge, or membrane potential, exists across cell membranes because the number of negative ions just inside the cell membrane is greater than the number outside. Stimuli, such as neurotransmitters, change the cell membrane's permeability to sodium, allowing it to rush into the cells. This reverses, or depolarizes, the charge of the cell membrane at that location, and an electrical current is generated. The nerve impulse travels as an electrical current. Once the nerve impulse passes, the original membrane potential is rapidly restored by another change in cell membrane permeability; then the original distribution of sodium and potassium ions across the cell membrane is restored by a sodium-potassium pump in the cell membrane (the sodium-potassium ATPase). A similar mechanism causes the depolarization of the muscle cell membranes, leading to muscle contraction.

Regulation of Electrolyte Balance Sodium and chloride homeostasis is regulated to some extent by the intake of both water and salt. When salt intake is high, thirst is stimulated to increase water intake. When salt intake is very low, a salt appetite causes the individual to seek out the mineral. These mechanisms help ensure that appropriate proportions of salt and water are taken in. The kidneys, however, are the primary regulator of sodium and chloride concentration in the body.

Excretion of sodium in the urine is decreased when sodium intake is low and increased when intake is high. Because water follows sodium by osmosis, the ability of the kidneys to conserve sodium provides a mechanism to conserve body water. When the concentration of sodium in the blood increases, water follows, causing an increase in blood volume. Changes in blood volume can change **blood pressure,** the pressure of the blood against the arterial walls. Changes in blood pressure trigger the production and release of proteins and hormones that affect the amount of sodium, and hence water, retained by the kidneys. For example, when blood pressure decreases, the kidneys release the enzyme **renin,** beginning a series of events leading to the production of **angiotensin II** (Figure 10.13).

Blood pressure The amount of force exerted by the blood against the artery walls.

Renin An enzyme produced by the kidney that aids in the conversion of angiotensin to its active form, angiotensin II.

Angiotensin II A compound that causes blood vessel walls to constrict and stimulates the release of the hormone aldosterone.

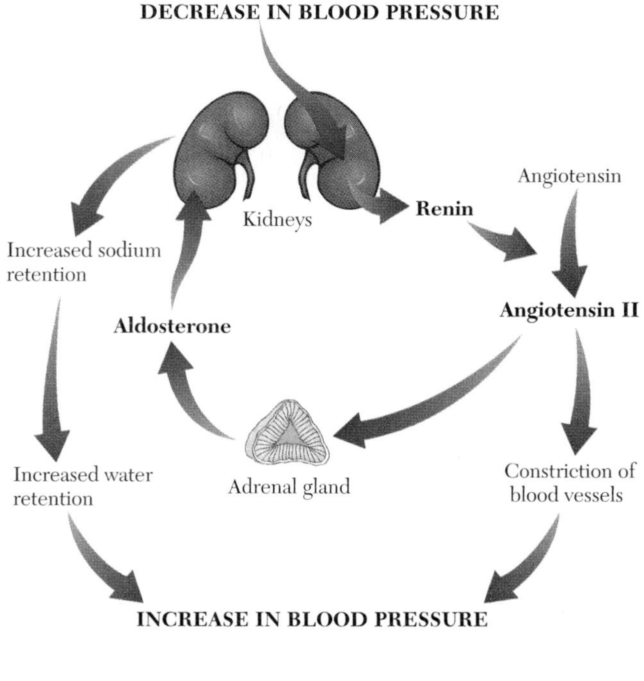

Figure 10.13
When blood pressure decreases, a series of events returns blood pressure to normal by constricting blood vessels and increasing sodium and water retention by the kidney.

Aldosterone A hormone that increases sodium reabsorption and therefore enhances water retention by the kidney.

Angiotensin II increases blood pressure both by causing the blood vessel walls to constrict and by stimulating the release of the hormone **aldosterone,** which acts on the kidneys to increase sodium reabsorption. Water follows the reabsorbed sodium, resulting in an increase in blood volume and, consequently, blood pressure. The increase in blood pressure then inhibits the release of renin and aldosterone so that blood pressure does not continue to rise.

As with sodium and chloride, the kidneys regulate potassium excretion to maintain a relatively constant amount of potassium in the body. If blood levels begin to rise, aldosterone is released, causing the kidney to excrete potassium and retain sodium. Most excess potassium is excreted by the kidney. Some is lost in the secretions of the gastrointestinal tract, and a very small amount is lost in sweat.

Electrolytes: How Much Do We Need?

Although there is no 1989 RDA for sodium, the National Research Council has estimated a minimum requirement of 500 mg of sodium per day for healthy adults.[4] The Daily Reference Value used to determine a Daily Value for food labels recommends consuming no more than 2400 mg of sodium per day. This is below the typical intake in the United States of about 3600 mg per day of sodium. Because of the effect of sodium on blood pressure in some individuals, the Dietary Guidelines for Americans recommend that salt and sodium be consumed in moderation.

There is no 1989 RDA for chloride. The estimated minimum requirement is 750 mg per day for adults. The Daily Value used on food labels is 3400 mg.

No 1989 RDA has been established for potassium either, but the National Research Council has recommended a minimum intake of 1600–2000 mg per day to maintain normal body stores and fluid concentrations. The Daily Reference Value recommends at least 3500 mg per day of potassium for adults. Potassium intakes vary greatly depending on food selection. Diets containing few fruits and vegetables provide about 2000 mg of potassium per day, and those high in fruits and vegetables provide 8000 to 11,000 mg.[5]

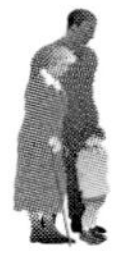

Pregnancy slightly increases sodium needs because the extracellular fluid volume increases. Pregnant women are advised to follow the recommendation for the general population for sodium intake (see Chapter 13).[6] At one time, a dietary salt restriction was common during pregnancy to prevent a syndrome known as pregnancy-induced hypertension. The cause of pregnancy-induced hypertension is not known, but salt restriction is no longer recommended. During lactation, sodium needs are increased to replace the amount secreted in milk. This is equal to about 135 mg per day. In infants, sodium needs are estimated from the amount consumed in human milk, which contains more chloride than sodium. This same chloride-to-sodium ratio has been recommended for infant formulas.

Potassium is needed to build new cells, so its requirement increases during times of growth. In pregnancy, extra potassium is needed to build new tissue. During lactation, the increased need is to replace losses in milk. In children, potassium is needed for growth; required amounts can be met by following the recommendations of the Food Guide Pyramid.

Electrolytes and Health: Hypertension

Electrolytes in the body are carefully regulated and, in turn, regulate fluid volume. As the extracellular fluid volume increases, blood pressure increases. A certain level of blood pressure is necessary to ensure that blood is delivered to all tissues. A healthy blood pressure is 120/80 mm of mercury or less. However, an increase in blood volume or a narrowing of the blood vessels can cause high blood pressure, or hypertension, generally defined as a blood pressure of 140/90 mm of mercury or greater. Hypertension has been called the silent killer because it has no outward symptoms but can lead to atherosclerosis, heart attack, stroke, kidney disease, and early death.

Causes of Hypertension Most people with high blood pressure have essential hypertension—hypertension with no obvious external cause. It is a complex disorder, most likely resulting from disturbances in one or more of the mechanisms that control body fluid and electrolyte balance. High blood pressure that occurs as a result of other disorders is referred to as secondary hypertension.

There is a genetic predisposition to hypertension, so a family history of high blood pressure increases one's risk of developing this disorder. It is more common in African Americans, Puerto Ricans, and Cuban and Mexican Americans than in non-Hispanic whites.[7] The increased incidence among African Americans is reflected in their 80% higher rate of death from stroke, 50% higher rate of death from heart disease, and 320% greater rate of hypertension-related kidney failure compared to Caucasians.[8] The risk of hypertension increases with age regardless of ethnicity or race. Hypertension occurs more frequently in individuals who have diabetes. Risk increases with obesity, particularly when the excess body fat is visceral fat. The risk of hypertension decreases with weight loss.[9]

Lifestyle factors also contribute to hypertension. A lack of physical activity, heavy alcohol consumption, and stress can increase blood pressure.[9] Blood pressure is also affected by diet. Diets high in salt are associated with a higher incidence of hypertension, whereas diets high in potassium, calcium, and magnesium are associated with a lower incidence of hypertension. Higher intakes of omega-3 fatty acids lower blood pressure.[10] A dietary pattern that incorporates a moderate sodium intake and larger amounts of these other nutrients has a greater impact than that of any single nutrient.[11]

Sodium, Salt, and Blood Pressure The Intersalt study, which examined the incidence of hypertension in different populations, found that in populations consuming less than 4.5 grams of salt per day, average blood pressure was low and hypertension was rare or absent. In populations consuming 5.8 grams of salt or more per day, blood pressure increased with sodium intake.[12] As a result of epidemiological studies such as this one, a restriction of dietary sodium was commonly prescribed to reduce blood pressure in all hypertensive individuals. In addition, to decrease the incidence of hypertension in the population as a whole, moderate sodium intake was recommended by the Dietary Guidelines for Americans.

Recent research, however, suggests that the intake of sodium or salt does not affect blood pressure in all individuals.[13,14] The impact of sodium intake on blood pressure depends on whether or not the individual is salt sensitive. Of individuals with hypertension, about half are salt sensitive—that is, their hypertension is aggravated by a high-salt diet. In the other half, dietary salt does not affect blood pressure.[15] In individuals who are salt sensitive, sodium has been shown to have little effect on blood pressure unless it is consumed with chloride as salt.[16]

The failure of research to consistently support the benefits of sodium or salt restriction for reducing blood pressure has caused some to question the justification for the population-wide recommendation of moderate salt intake made by the Dietary Guidelines.[17] However, the level of salt consumption recommended by the Dietary Guidelines and the Daily Values used on food labels is not harmful and may be beneficial because it encourages the consumption of fresh fruits, vegetables, grains, meats, and dairy products that are low in sodium.

Other Dietary Components Recently nutrients other than sodium and chloride, and the dietary pattern as a whole, have received more recognition for their role in reducing America's blood pressure. Epidemiology has shown that dietary patterns with high intakes of fiber and the minerals potassium, magnesium, and

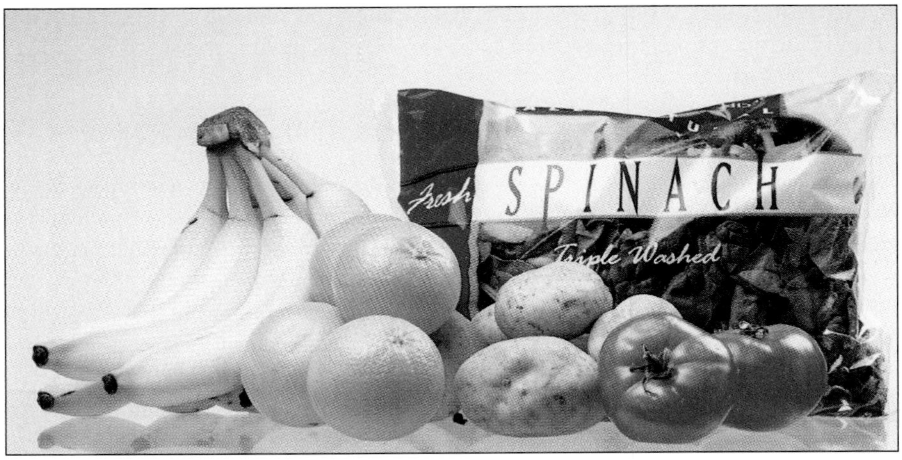

Figure 10.14
These foods are rich in potassium. (George Semple)

calcium are associated with lower blood pressure. For example, populations and individuals consuming vegetarian diets, which are high in these nutrients, generally have lower blood pressure than nonvegetarians.[18]

Potassium Intake Primitive cultures worldwide and vegetarians in industrialized countries whose diets are high in potassium have a low incidence of hypertension, whereas groups that have low potassium intakes have a high incidence of hypertension.[19] In addition, a 20-year study of middle-aged men found that those with greater intakes of fruits and vegetables, which are high in potassium, were at a lower risk of developing strokes.[20] Because populations that have high intakes of sodium generally have low intakes of potassium, it is difficult to tell if the hypertension associated with a high-sodium diet is due to the high sodium or the low potassium. The fact that a high dietary sodium intake increases the excretion of potassium suggests that low levels of potassium in the body affect hypertension. Potassium supplements have been shown to decrease blood pressure.[21] Since excessive potassium intakes can cause an irregular heartbeat, potassium supplements are not recommended unless supervised by a physician. Increasing consumption of potassium-rich foods such as bananas, oranges, and potatoes is a safer way to increase potassium intake (Figure 10.14).

Calcium and Magnesium Epidemiology also supports a role for calcium and magnesium in regulating blood pressure. Numerous studies have found that individuals with low calcium intakes are more likely to have hypertension.[22] Calcium supplementation has been shown to lower blood pressure slightly in individuals with hypertension, and some analyses have also shown an effect in those with normal blood pressure.[23,24] Low dietary magnesium has also been associated with hypertension, with dietary magnesium inversely correlated with blood pressure.[25,26]

The Total Dietary Pattern: The DASH Diet The results of the wide variety of studies on mineral intake and hypertension have been equivocal. This may be because the impact of each individual nutrient is small and a significant effect is seen only when several components of the diet are modified simultaneously. The Dietary Approaches to Stop Hypertension (DASH) trial examined the effect of dietary patterns on blood pressure.[11] Three diets were used, all containing 3000 mg of sodium per day, an amount somewhat greater than the Daily Value of 2400 mg per day. The first, a control diet, was a typical American dietary pattern—low in potassium, magnesium, calcium, and fiber, and high in fat and protein. One of the experimental diets was high in fruits and vegetables, providing 8 to 10 servings per day, making it high in potassium, magnesium, and fiber, but otherwise similar to the control diet. The other experimental diet was not only high in fruits

Table 10.3 *Serving Recommendations for the DASH Diet*

Food Group	Number of Servings*			
Kcalorie level	**1600**	**2000**	**2600**	**3100**
Grains	6–7	7–8	10–11	12–13
Vegetables	3–4	4–5	5–6	6–7
Fruits	3–4	4–5	5–6	6–7
Lowfat dairy	2–3	2–3	3–4	3–4
Meats, fish, poultry	1–2	1–2	2	2–3
Beans, nuts, and seeds	1/3	1/2	2/3	3/4
Limit fats and sweets				

*Serving sizes correspond to the serving sizes recommended by the Food Guide Pyramid.

and vegetables but also contained lowfat dairy products, whole grains, and lean meat, fish, and poultry, making it higher in potassium, magnesium, calcium, and fiber, and lower in fat, saturated fat, and cholesterol than the control diet (see Table 10.3). Both experimental diets lowered blood pressure in individuals both with hypertension and normal blood pressure. However, the effect was most dramatic in the diet that emphasized fruits and vegetables as well as lowfat dairy products, whole grains, and lean meats.[11] The reduction in blood pressure occurred after only two weeks of consuming the diet and persisted throughout the trial. Reductions were similar to that seen with drug therapy or diets that restrict sodium to very low levels of 1100 to 1800 mg per day.[27] A follow-up study called DASH2 is examining the impact of this pattern at various sodium intakes.

The results of the DASH trial suggest that a modification of the total diet is more effective in lowering blood pressure than changing any single nutrient. The importance of this finding goes beyond the treatment and prevention of hypertension. This dietary pattern, referred to as the **DASH diet,** may also reduce cancer risk, prevent osteoporosis, and protect against heart disease (see *Critical Thinking: A Diet for Health*).

DASH diet A dietary pattern that is plentiful in fruits and vegetables and lowfat dairy products and therefore high in potassium, magnesium, calcium, and fiber, and low in saturated fat and cholesterol.

Electrolyte Deficiency and Toxicity Deficiencies of sodium and chloride are rare in healthy individuals. Although the taste for salt that triggers your desire to plunge into a bag of salty chips is a learned preference rather than a response to physiological need, humans with very low salt intakes do have a true physiological drive to consume salt (Figure 10.15). Conditions that cause sodium and chloride depletion include heavy and persistent sweating, chronic diarrhea or vomiting, and kidney disease. A sodium or chloride imbalance can cause disturbances in acid-base and electrolyte balance.

Toxicities are also rare in healthy individuals. Excessive sodium intake has been related to hypertension in salt-sensitive individuals, but, for individuals without salt-sensitive hypertension, no toxic level of sodium intake has been documented as long as water needs are met and the kidneys are functioning properly. However, a high sodium intake increases calcium excretion and has been related to an increased risk of osteoporosis.[28]

Symptomatic potassium deficiency is also uncommon. It occurs as a result of vomiting, diarrhea, increased urinary losses, and excessive sweating. Individuals at risk include those with eating disorders who may vomit frequently or abuse laxatives, those consuming very-low-energy diets, and those taking diuretic medications, known as thiazide diuretics, to treat hypertension. Generally, potassium supplements are prescribed along with or incorporated into medications that cause potassium loss. Potassium deficiency results in poor appetite, muscle cramps, confusion, apathy, constipation, and, eventually, an irregular heartbeat.

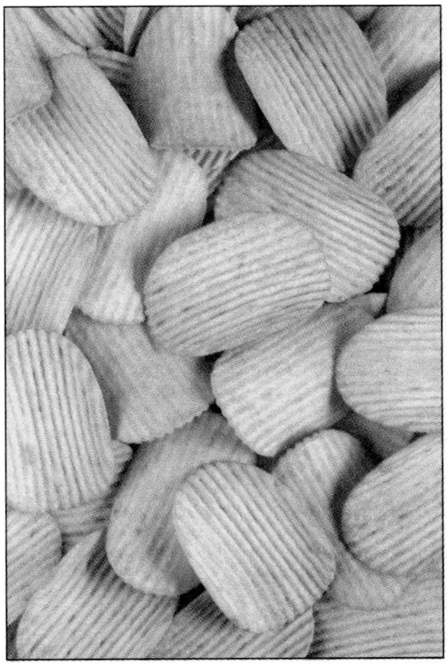

Figure 10.15
Many snack foods are high in salt. (© 1999 Photo Disc, Inc.)

Table 10.4 *Tips for Reducing Your Sodium Intake*

1. Reduce the salt in your diet gradually so that you learn to enjoy the unsalted flavors in foods.
2. When shopping:
   - Use food labels to select foods low in sodium.
   - Choose unprocessed foods—they have less sodium than processed foods.
   - Choose fresh or frozen vegetables rather than canned.
3. When cooking:
   - Prepare meals from scratch so you control the amount of salt added.
   - Do not add salt to the water when cooking rice, pasta, and cereals.
   - Flavor foods with ingredients such as lemon juice, onion or garlic powder (not salt), pepper, curry, dill, basil, oregano, or thyme rather than salt.
4. When eating:
   - Limit use of salt at the table.
   - Limit salted snack foods like potato chips, salted nuts, salted popcorn, and crackers, and replace them with fresh fruits and vegetables.
   - Limit cured, salted, or smoked meats such as bologna, corned beef, hot dogs, and smoked turkey to a few servings a week or less. Substitute sliced roasted turkey, chicken, or beef.
   - Limit salty or smoked fish such as sardines, anchovies, or smoked salmon (lox).
   - Limit foods prepared in salt brine such as pickles, olives, and sauerkraut.
   - Cut down on cheeses, especially processed cheeses.
   - Limit the amounts of soy sauce, Worcestershire sauce, barbecue sauce, ketchup, and mustard you add to food.
5. When eating out:
   - Choose foods without sauces, or ask for them to be served on the side.
   - Ask that food be prepared without added salt.

Potassium toxicity from the diet is rare because urinary excretion is proportional to intake when kidney function is normal. If supplements are consumed in excess or kidney function is compromised, blood levels of potassium can increase and can eventually cause death due to an irregular heartbeat.

Choosing a Diet to Prevent Hypertension and Stay Healthy A diet that promotes healthy blood pressure provides plenty of potassium, calcium, and magnesium; is moderate in sodium chloride; and maintains a healthy weight. This DASH diet pattern can be achieved by using the Food Guide Pyramid as a guide and aiming toward the high end of the recommended number of servings of vegetables, fruits, dairy products, and grains. Dry beans and nuts should be frequent choices from the Meat, Poultry, Fish, Dry Beans, Eggs, & Nuts Group. Nutrient-dense choices from each group will ensure that the energy content of the diet does not exceed needs. Table 10.3 gives the number of servings recommended for several different energy levels.

Moderate Sodium Intake To moderate sodium intake, be aware of the sources of salt in the diet. Limit the use of salt added in cooking and at the table as well as that contained in processed foods (see Table 10.4). Read food labels. All the sodium-containing additives are itemized in the ingredient list and the total sodium content per serving is included in the Nutrition Facts section. To help assess how the amount of sodium in a food fits into the recommended diet, food labels also give the sodium content of a serving as a percent of the Daily Value. The Daily Value for sodium is 2400 mg, which is considered the upper limit that is desirable in the diet. For example, the Nutrition Facts on the label in Figure 10.16 indicates that a serving of spaghetti sauce contains 250 mg, or 10% of the sodium that should be included in the daily diet. Additional information can be obtained from nutrient claims relating to the salt or sodium content of a product. Products

Nutrition Facts

Serving Size 1/2 cup (125g)
Servings Per Container about 3½

Amount Per Serving	
Calories 50	Calories from Fat 10
	%Daily Value**
Total Fat 1g	**2%**
Saturated Fat 0g	**0%**
Cholesterol 0mg	**0%**
Sodium 250mg	**10%**
Potassium 530mg	**15%**
Total Carbohydrate 9g	**3%**
Dietary Fiber 1g	**4%**
Sugars 7g	
Protein 2g	
Vitamin A 10% •	Vitamin C 25%
Calcium 2% •	Iron 10%

*Percent Daily Values are based on a 2,000 calorie diet. Your daily values may be higher or lower depending on your calorie needs.

	Calories:	2,000	2,500
Total Fat	Less than	65g	80g
Sat Fat	Less than	20g	25g
Cholesterol	Less than	300mg	300mg
Sodium	Less than	2,400mg	2,400mg
Potassium		3,500mg	3,500mg
Total Carbohydrate		300g	375g
Dietary Fiber		25g	30g

Light Spaghetti Sauce, 250 milligrams (mg) per serving
Regular Spaghetti Sauce, 500mg per serving

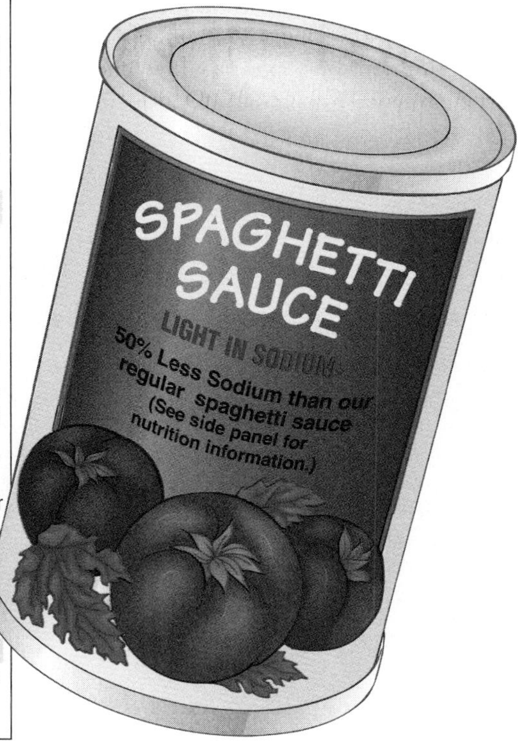

Figure 10.16
Food labels help determine how much sodium a food contributes to the diet.

with reduced salt content may be labeled as "low salt," "less salt," or "unsalted." Over-the-counter medications such as cough medicine and laxatives can also contain large amounts of sodium, but many are now available in low-sodium formulas.

Maintain a Healthy Weight and Lifestyle Guidelines for preventing high blood pressure recommend reducing body weight if overweight, limiting alcohol intake to 24 ounces of beer or 10 ounces of wine daily for men and half that for women, increasing aerobic physical activity to 30 to 45 minutes most days, and, for overall cardiovascular health, stopping smoking and reducing dietary saturated fat and cholesterol.

Critical Thinking

A Diet for Health

Rashamel is a 43-year-old father of three children. His father died of a stroke at the age of 54 as a result of undiagnosed and untreated high blood pressure. Rashamel wants to live to see his grandchildren, so he exercises as often as he can, about three times a week, quit smoking, and watches his diet and weight. Despite these efforts, at his recent physical his blood pressure was elevated to 144/92. Rather than start him on medication, his doctor suggested a dietary approach and referred him to a dietitian. A 24-hour recall reveals that Rashamel is maintaining a normal body weight of 175 pounds by consuming about 2500 kcal per day. After evaluating his current diet, the dietitian recommends he follow the DASH diet to reduce his blood pressure. The modified diet shown here illustrates the dietitian's recommendations.

Current Diet		Modified Diet	
Breakfast		**Breakfast**	
Orange juice	3/4 cup	Orange juice	3/4 cup
1% lowfat milk	1 cup	1% lowfat milk	1 cup
Wheaties w/ 1 tsp sugar	1 cup	Wheaties w/1 tsp sugar	1 cup
		Banana	1 medium
Whole wheat bread w/ jelly	1 slice	Whole wheat bread w/jelly	2 slices
Margarine	1 tsp	Margarine	1 tsp
Lunch		**Lunch**	
Tuna salad	3/4 cup	Tuna salad	3/4 cup
Wheat bread	2 slices	Wheat bread	2 slices
		Carrot sticks	1/2 cup
		Bell pepper strips	1/2 cup
~~Chips~~	1 oz	Fruit cocktail (light syrup)	1/2 cup
~~Cola~~	1 can	1% lowfat milk	1 cup
Dinner		**Dinner**	
~~Baked chicken~~	3 oz	Chicken stir fry	3 oz
		Almonds	10
		Broccoli	1/2 cup
		Mushrooms	1/2 cup
Rice	1 cup	Rice	1-1/2 cup
Salad	1 cup	Salad	1 cup
Light salad dressing	1 Tbsp	Light salad dressing	1 Tbsp
Dinner roll	1	Dinner roll	1
Margarine	2 tsp	Margarine	2 tsp
Cantaloupe	1/2 cup	Cantaloupe	1/2 cup
~~Iced tea (sweetened)~~	12 oz	1% lowfat milk	1 cup
Snacks		**Snacks**	
~~Cookies~~	2 large	Frozen yogurt	1/2 cup
Dried apricots	5	Dried apricots	5
~~Milky Way candy bar~~	1	Graham crackers	2
Cola	1 can		

How does the modified diet compare to the recommendations of the Food Guide Pyramid? To Rashamel's current diet?

Answer:

How do these changes affect the sodium and potassium content of Rashamel's diet?

His original diet was not high in sodium, containing about 2500 mg, which is slightly above the Daily Value of 2400 mg. The diet changes reduce his sodium slightly but increase his potassium intake from 2870 mg to 5000 mg. The amount of magnesium is also increased slightly.

Rashamel's wife Yuka is 42 years old. Although she is not concerned about her blood pressure her mother was recently hospitalized with a hip fracture. Yuka is concerned about preventing osteoporosis and wants to make sure she is consuming adequate calcium. She is mildly lactose intolerant.

If she consumed the modified diet would it meet her AI for calcium?

Yes, her AI is 1000 mg and the modified diet contains 1320 mg of calcium. Because of her lactose intolerance Yuka has difficulty drinking milk. She can tolerate a small amount on her morning cereal and can consume yogurt and cheese in moderate amounts. If the milk consumed at lunch and dinner is eliminated from her diet she would not meet the AI.

What changes would increase the amount of calcium from low lactose sources?

To increase calcium Yuka could substitute canned salmon for tuna in the salad at lunch. She could also include more tofu in her diet—a food she ate frequently while growing up in Japan. Including a serving of miso soup with tofu, or using tofu instead of chicken in the stir fry at dinner would increase calcium by about 130 mg. She can also replace the milk with amounts of yogurt and lowfat cheeses that are tolerable. She might also consider adding a daily calcium supplement.

Yuka only weighs 110 pounds and requires about 1800 kcal to maintain her body weight.

How could this diet be changed to reduce the energy content without reducing the calcium?

Answer:

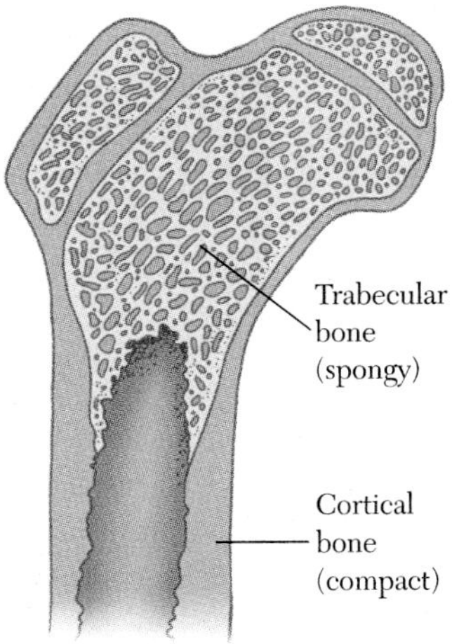

Figure 10.17
The compact bone that forms the outer layer of bone is called cortical bone and the spongy interior is called trabecular bone.

Minerals Involved in Bone Health

Bone is composed of a protein framework that is hardened by deposits of minerals. There are two types of bone: cortical or compact bone, which forms the sturdy, dense outer surface layer, and trabecular or spongy bone, which forms an inner spongy lattice that supports the cortical shell (Figure 10.17). Healthy bone requires adequate dietary protein and vitamin C to maintain collagen—the most abundant protein in bone matrix—and a sufficient supply of minerals to ensure solidity. The mineral deposits of bone consist primarily of calcium and phosphorus but also include magnesium, fluoride, and other trace minerals (see Chapter 11). Adequate vitamin D (discussed in Chapter 9) is necessary to maintain appropriate levels of calcium and phosphorus in the body.

Bone: A Living Tissue

Bone remodeling The process whereby bone is continuously broken down and reformed to allow for growth and maintenance.

Peak bone mass The maximum bone density attained at any time in life, usually occurring in young adulthood.

Osteoporosis A bone disorder characterized by a reduction in bone mass, increased bone fragility, and an increased risk of fractures.

Bone is a living, metabolically active tissue that is constantly being broken down and reformed in a process called **bone remodeling.** Bone is formed by cells called osteoblasts and broken down or resorbed by cells called osteoclasts. During bone formation the activity of the bone-building osteoblasts exceeds that of the osteoclasts. When bone is being broken down, the osteoclasts resorb bone more rapidly than the osteoblasts can rebuild it.

Most bone is formed early in life. In the growing bones of children, bone formation occurs more rapidly than breakdown. Even after growth stops, bone mass continues to increase into young adulthood when **peak bone mass** is achieved, somewhere between the ages of 16 and 30.[29] In healthy adults, bone breakdown and formation are in balance, so bone mass remains constant. After about age 35 to 45, the amount of bone broken down begins to exceed that which is formed. Although both types of bone are lost with age, the loss of spongy trabecular bone begins earlier than does cortical bone loss.[30] If enough bone is lost, the skeleton is weakened and fractures occur easily. This is known as **osteoporosis,** a condition which generally has no symptoms until the fifth or sixth decade of life. In the United States today, about 28 million people have osteoporosis or are at risk due to low bone mass, and 80% of them are women.[31]

Osteoporosis: Bone Loss

Menopause The physiological changes that mark the end of a woman's capacity to bear children.

Osteoporosis is caused by a loss in both the protein matrix and the mineral deposits of bone, resulting in a decrease in the total amount of bone (Figure 10.18). As bone mass decreases, the likelihood of fractures increases. In the United States, 1.5 million fractures per year are associated with osteoporosis.[32] The mechanisms that lead to osteoporosis are not fully understood, but the risk depends on the level of peak bone mass and the rate at which bone is lost.

Peak bone mass and the rate of bone loss are affected by gender, race, and age as well as lifestyle. The risk of osteoporosis increases progressively with age. It is lower in African Americans because they typically achieve a greater peak bone mass.[33] This greater peak bone mass reduces the risk of osteoporosis because more bone can be lost before fractures are likely. Risk is greater in women than men because men have a higher peak bone mass and because women have an acceleration of bone loss for about five years after **menopause.**[34] This **post-**

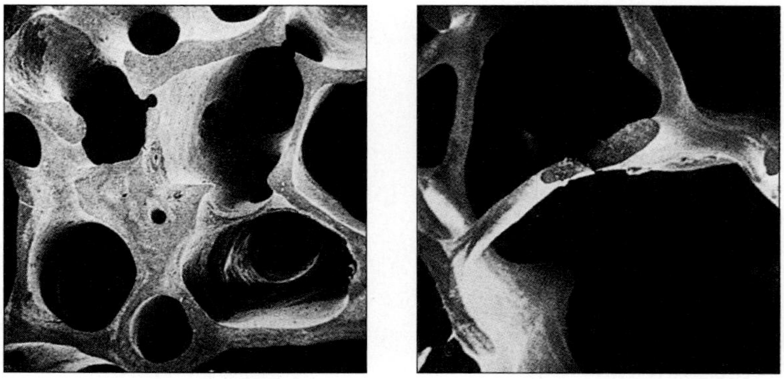

Figure 10.18
Osteoporosis causes a decrease in bone density and increases the risk of fractures. Normal bone (*left*). Bone weakened by osteoporosis (*right*). (Courtesy of Wyeth-Ayerst Laboratories)

menopausal bone loss is related to a drop in levels of the hormone estrogen which then affects bone cells and decreases intestinal calcium absorption. During this period, women lose a disproportionate amount of trabecular bone. This pattern of bone loss can cause postmenopausal, or type I, osteoporosis.[35] After the postmenopausal period, women continue to lose bone but more slowly. This age-related bone loss, which also occurs in men, involves the loss of both the compact cortical bone and the spongy trabecular bone. If too much bone is lost, age-related, or type II, osteoporosis may occur, usually in men and women over 75 years of age. Osteoporosis-related fractures occur in one out of every two women over age 50 and in about one in every eight men over 50[31] (Figure 10.19).

Lifestyle factors that affect bone mass include smoking, alcohol consumption, exercise, and diet. Smoking and alcohol consumption can decrease bone mass, whereas weight-bearing exercise, such as walking and jogging, increases bone mass.[36] Having more body fat decreases the risk of osteoporosis because adipose tissue produces estrogen, which helps maintain bone mass and enhances calcium absorption. A greater body weight also increases the amount of weight-bearing exercise that the individual gets in day-to-day activities, which increases bone mass.[37] Minerals that affect bone mass and bone health include sodium, calcium, phosphorus, magnesium, and several of the trace minerals. A high sodium intake increases calcium excretion and has been related to an increased incidence of osteoporosis.[28] The importance of calcium, phosphorus, and magnesium in the diet and the body, and their roles in bone formation and general health, are discussed separately in the following sections.

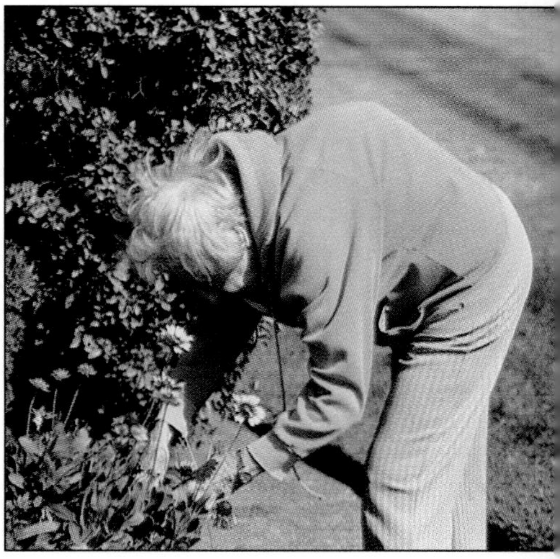

Figure 10.19
The bone loss due to osteoporosis can cause a stooped posture and a decrease in stature. (© Larry Mulvehill/Science Source/Photo Researchers, Inc.)

Postmenopausal bone loss The accelerated bone loss that occurs in women for about five years after estrogen production decreases.

Calcium

Calcium is the most abundant mineral in the body. It accounts for 1 to 2% of adult body weight. Over 99% of the calcium in the body is found in the solid mineral deposit in bones and teeth.[38] The remaining 1% is present in blood and intracellular and extracellular fluid, where it plays vital roles in nerve transmission, muscle contraction, blood pressure regulation, and the release of hormones.

Calcium in the Diet The main source of calcium in the North American diet is dairy products such as milk, cheese, and yogurt. Fish, such as sardines, that are consumed in their entirety, including the bones, are also a good source, as are some green vegetables such as broccoli, Chinese cabbage, and kale. Calcium is poorly absorbed from foods high in oxalic acid such as spinach, sweet potatoes, and rhubarb. For example, only about 5% of the calcium in spinach is absorbed;[39] the rest is bound by oxalates and excreted in the feces. Chocolate also contains oxalates, but chocolate milk is still a good source of calcium because the amount of chocolate added is small. Phytic acid found in seeds, nuts, and grains also reduces calcium absorption. Even though grains are not rich sources of calcium, they are consumed in such large quantities that they make a significant contribution to dietary calcium.

Some of the calcium in the diet is added during food processing. Baked goods such as breads, rolls, and crackers, to which nonfat dry milk powder has been added, provide calcium. Tortillas that are treated with lime water (calcium hydroxide) provide calcium. Tofu is a good source when calcium is used in its processing. In addition, there are products on the market, such as orange juice, that are fortified with calcium.

Calcium in the Digestive Tract The bioavailability of calcium is affected by a number of dietary factors, including the presence of lactose, which enhances calcium absorption, and tannins, fiber, phytates, and oxalates, which decrease calcium absorption. Absorption is also decreased by a form of phosphorus, found in many processed foods, which prevents absorption by binding calcium in the gastrointestinal tract. Despite these interactions, the efficiency of calcium absorption is fairly similar for most foods; therefore, the calcium content of the food is generally of greater significance than the presence of factors that affect bioavailability.[38]

Calcium is absorbed by both active transport and passive diffusion. Active transport depends on the active form of vitamin D and accounts for most absorption when intakes are low to moderate. At high intakes, passive transport becomes more important. As calcium intake increases, the percentage that is absorbed declines. When vitamin D is deficient, absorption decreases dramatically.

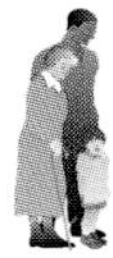

The efficiency of calcium absorption varies with life stage. During infancy, about 60% of calcium consumed is absorbed. In a young adult, absorption is about 25%. Absorption declines gradually with age due to a decrease in blood levels of the active form of vitamin D.[40] An additional decrease in calcium absorption occurs in women after menopause due to the decrease in estrogen. During pregnancy, when calcium need is high, elevated estrogen helps increase calcium absorption.

Calcium in the Body Calcium is important in the maintenance of bones and teeth (see Table 10.1), where it is primarily found with phosphorus as solid mineral crystals known as hydroxyapatite. It also plays extremely important roles in cell communication and the regulation of body processes. Calcium helps regulate enzymes and is necessary in blood clotting. It is involved in transmitting chemical and electrical signals along nerves and muscles, and it is necessary for the release of neurotransmitters, which allow nerve impulses to pass from one nerve to another and from nerves to other tissues. Calcium plays a role in blood pressure regulation, possibly by controlling the contraction of muscles in the blood vessel walls and signaling the secretion of substances that regulate blood pressure.[22] Inside the muscle cells, calcium allows the two muscle proteins, actin and myosin, to interact to cause muscle contraction.

Parathyroid hormone (PTH) A hormone secreted by the parathyroid gland that increases blood calcium levels.

Calcitonin A hormone secreted by the thyroid gland that reduces blood calcium levels.

The roles of calcium are so vital to survival that powerful regulatory mechanisms ensure that constant intracellular and extracellular concentrations are maintained. Slight changes in blood calcium levels trigger responses that quickly raise or lower them back to normal levels. This homeostasis is maintained by the hormones **parathyroid hormone (PTH),** which raises blood calcium, and **calcitonin,** which lowers blood calcium (Figure 10.20). If the level of blood calcium

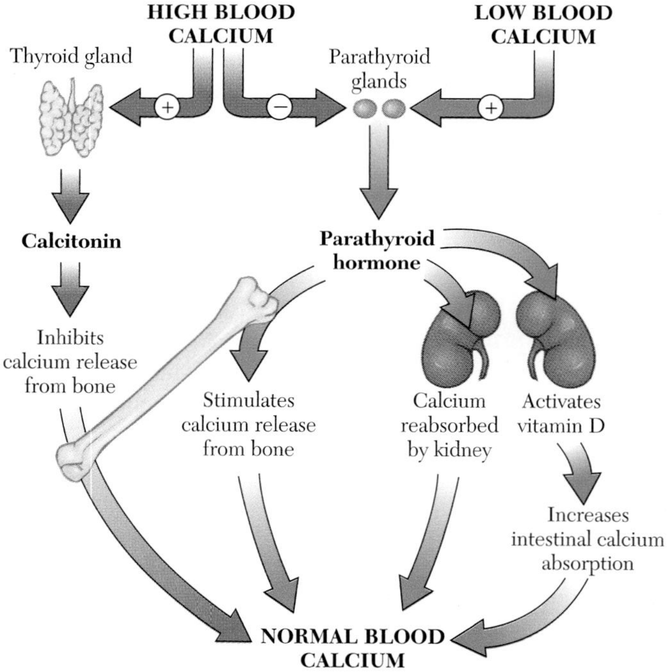

Figure 10.20
Levels of calcium in the blood are very tightly regulated by parathyroid hormone and calcitonin.

falls too low, parathyroid hormone is released, stimulating the release of calcium from bone, reducing calcium excretion by the kidney, and activating vitamin D. Activated vitamin D increases the amount of calcium absorbed from the gastrointestinal tract and, with parathyroid hormone, stimulates calcium release from the bone. The overall effect is to rapidly increase blood calcium levels. If blood calcium levels become too high, the secretion of parathyroid hormone is shut off and calcitonin is secreted. Calcitonin acts primarily on bone to inhibit the release of calcium, resulting in a decrease in blood calcium levels. The ability to maintain blood calcium levels by removing calcium from bone is beneficial over the short term, but if continued over the long term, it results in progressive loss of bone mass and bone weakening.

How Much Calcium Do We Need? Ideally, calcium intake should be adequate to maintain bone and prevent fractures from osteoporosis later in life. However, it has not been possible to determine how much is needed at each life stage to prevent osteoporosis in older adults. Therefore, recommended calcium intakes have been set at the amount that allows maximum calcium retention. Increasing dietary calcium above this level will not increase the amount of calcium retained in the body. Adults may continue to lose bone mass at this intake level due to other causes such as loss of estrogen, smoking, and a sedentary lifestyle, but this loss is not due to inadequate calcium intake.

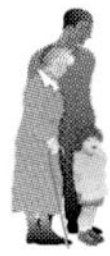

Rather than an RDA, an AI has been determined for calcium because it was not possible to precisely estimate the dietary intake needed for maximum retention. The AI for adults age 19 through 50 years is 1000 mg per day.[38] The value for older adults is set at a level above which calcium retention cannot be further increased by increasing dietary calcium. Since absorption decreases with age, the AI for men and women age 51 and older is increased to 1200 mg per day. Postmenopausal bone loss cannot be prevented by increasing calcium intake, so the AI is not higher in women. For adolescents the AI is higher than for adults—1300 mg per day for boys and girls age 9 through 18. In children and adolescents the AI is set at a level that will support bone growth.

Infants thrive on the amount of calcium they obtain from human milk. For infants, an AI is set based on the mean intake of infants fed principally with human milk. Because calcium is not as well absorbed from infant formulas, formula-fed infants require more. There is no special AI for formula-fed infants, but formulas are higher in calcium than breast milk to compensate for the reduced absorption.

The AI for calcium during pregnancy is not increased above nonpregnant levels. This is because there is an increase in maternal calcium absorption during pregnancy that helps to supply the calcium needed for the fetal skeleton. In addition, since there is no correlation between the number of pregnancies and bone mineral density, the maternal skeleton does not appear to be used as a supply of calcium for the fetus. However, during lactation, calcium is secreted in milk, and the source of this calcium does appear to be the maternal skeleton.[41] This bone resorption occurs regardless of calcium intake.[42] Since the loss of maternal skeleton is not prevented by increasing dietary calcium, and since the calcium lost appears to be regained following weaning, the AI is not increased during lactation.

Calcium and Health Osteoporosis is the major health problem associated with calcium status. Osteoporosis occurs because bone acts as a calcium reservoir inside the body. If calcium intake is not adequate to maintain normal blood levels, calcium will be resorbed from bone to maintain blood levels.

Calcium Deficiency: A Role in Osteoporosis Low calcium intake during the years of bone formation results in a lower peak bone mass. If calcium intake continues to be low after peak bone mass has been achieved, the rate of bone loss may be increased and, along with it, the risk of osteoporosis.

Although low dietary calcium is the most significant dietary factor contributing to osteoporosis, calcium intake alone does not predict the risk of osteoporosis. Genetics as well as other dietary and lifestyle factors also affect calcium status and bone mass. Diets high in phytates, oxalates, and tannins reduce calcium absorption, as does low vitamin D status. High sodium chloride intake increases calcium loss in the urine.[43,44] Increasing dietary protein and phosphorus intake also increases urinary calcium and there is a correlation between calcium-to-phosphorus and calcium-to-protein ratios and bone mineral density.[29] The risk of developing osteoporosis can be reduced by consuming a diet adequate in vitamin D and calcium and not excessive in phosphorus, protein, or sodium; by maintaining an active lifestyle that includes weight-bearing exercise; and by limiting smoking and alcohol consumption.[45]

Preventing and Treating Osteoporosis The best treatment for osteoporosis is to prevent it in the first place by following dietary and lifestyle patterns that reduce risk. Once osteoporosis has occurred it is difficult to restore lost bone.

Individuals who do not meet their calcium needs with diet alone can benefit from calcium supplementation. However, because high calcium intake can interfere with the absorption of other minerals, supplements should be taken with care. In young individuals who do not meet their calcium needs with food, supplemental calcium can increase peak bone mass. Calcium supplements have been found to be helpful in reducing bone loss in postmenopausal women, but are not effective at increasing bone mass.[46] The effect of calcium supplements in decreasing calcium losses in postmenopausal women is greatest after the first five years of menopause and has more of an effect on cortical than on trabecular bone loss.[38] Benefits increase when calcium supplementation is combined with other therapies. For example, treatment with calcium and vitamin D has been shown to prevent bone loss, increase bone density, and decrease the frequency of bone fractures.[47] Replacing the estrogen lost in menopause—known as hormone replacement therapy—also has been shown to reduce bone loss and restore some lost bone, and the effectiveness of this therapy is enhanced by taking calcium supplements.[48,49] Other treatments for osteoporosis include the hormone calcitonin and drugs known as bisphosphonates. Calcitonin injections or nasal spray can reduce bone resorption, and its effects are also enhanced by calcium supplementation.[50] Bisphosphonates act by inhibiting bone resorption and have been shown to prevent postmenopausal bone loss and increase bone mineral density in patients with osteoporosis.[51,52] Exercise can also be helpful in treating osteoporosis.[36] Minerals other than calcium that have been used to prevent and treat bone loss include magnesium, fluoride, and boron, but results with these have been equivocal (see *Off the Shelf: Calcium Supplements: Do You Need One? Which Should You Choose?*).

Calcium Toxicity Adverse effects associated with high calcium consumption focus on intake from supplements. Too much calcium from supplements may cause kidney stone formation and kidney insufficiency, and may interfere with the absorption of other minerals. Calcium interacts with iron, zinc, magnesium, and phosphorus. Although calcium supplements inhibit iron absorption, there is no evidence that the long-term use of calcium supplements with meals affects iron status.[53] High intakes of calcium from supplements have also been found to reduce zinc absorption and thereby increase zinc needs in the diet.[54] There is no evidence of depletion of phosphorus or magnesium associated with calcium intake. A UL of 2500 mg per day has been set for adults age 19 to 70 years.

Meeting Calcium Needs Americans do not currently consume enough calcium. Estimates of typical intakes in the United States suggest that the average calcium intake for teenage girls is about 770 mg per day, and few consume the AI of 1300 mg per day.[55] Adequate calcium intake can be achieved by following the Food

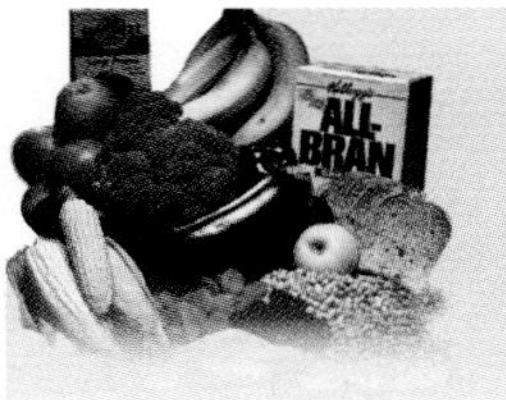

Off the Shelf

Calcium Supplements: Do You Need One? Which Should You Choose?

Do you need a calcium supplement? The AI for calcium for adults is 1000 mg per day. This is the amount in a little more than three glasses of milk, 10 cups of cooked kale, or 24 ounces of canned salmon with the bones. While 1000 mg of calcium can be obtained from a carefully planned varied diet, many people choose to use a supplement to ensure that they meet their AI on a daily basis. Do supplements provide the same benefits as calcium from foods? Are there any risks? If you choose to take a calcium supplement, which one should you take?

The calcium in most supplements is absorbed as well as that from a mixed diet. The calcium in calcium carbonate is absorbed as well as the calcium from milk.[1] As with calcium in foods, the absorption of calcium from supplements is affected by other food components and nutrients consumed with it. Acidic foods, lactose, and fat, which prolongs transit time, increase calcium absorption from supplements. Oxalate, phytates, and fiber inhibit calcium absorption. Absorption is lower when a large amount (400 mg or more) is taken in a single dose.[2] Absorption also depends on how quickly the supplement dissolves in the stomach.

When selecting a supplement, choose one that contains a calcium compound alone, such as calcium carbonate. Multivitamin and mineral supplements typically contain only a small portion of the Daily Value for calcium—they would have to be the size of a marble to contain 1000 mg of calcium plus other nutrients. Avoid supplements containing magnesium or iron because these minerals compete with calcium for absorption. And if supplements containing vitamin D are used, consumers should monitor the amount of vitamin D they are consuming since it is toxic in large doses.

The most common and least expensive form of calcium used in supplements is calcium carbonate. This form provides the greatest concentration of calcium per gram but it is not the best choice for everyone. In individuals with low stomach acid, it dissolves very slowly so absorption is decreased.[3] Other common calcium compounds such as calcium citrate, gluconate, lactate, citrate-malate, and phosphate are better absorbed when stomach acid is low but contain less calcium per gram of supplement. The calcium in preparations such as bone meal, powdered bone, dolomite (limestone), and oyster shell are not different from other supplements in terms of calcium, but they may contain enough lead to be a health hazard if consumed routinely.[4]

Calcium-containing antacids are popular as calcium supplements. For instance, Tums, which contain calcium carbonate, are often used as a calcium supplement because they are inexpensive and taste good. Antacids that contain aluminum and magnesium may negatively affect calcium status. These minerals bind phosphorus, preventing its absorption. As a result, phosphorus is released from bone to maintain blood levels, and in the process, calcium is also released and excreted in the urine. Excessive use of any antacid may cause gastrointestinal problems and is not recommended.

[1]Mortensen, L., and Charles, P. Bioavailability of calcium supplements and the effect of vitamin D: comparisons between milk, calcium carbonate, and calcium carbonate plus vitamin D. Am. J. Clin. Nutr. 63:354–357, 1996.

[2]Heaney, R. P., Weaver, C. M., and Fitzsimmons, M. L. Influence of calcium load on absorption fraction. J. Bone Miner. Res. 5:1135–1138, 1990.

[3]Whiting, S. J., Wood, R., and Kim, K. Calcium supplementation. J. Am. Acad. Nurse Pract. 9:187–192, 1997.

[4]Bourgoin, B. P., Evans, D. R., Cornett, J. R., et al. Lead content in 70 brands of dietary calcium supplements. Am. J. Public Health 83:1155–1160, 1993.

Guide Pyramid recommendation of 2 to 3 servings of milk, yogurt, or cheese daily plus 3 to 5 servings of vegetables a day (Figure 10.21). Ice cream, puddings, and soups made with milk are also good calcium sources. Sources of calcium that are low in lactose include dark-green leafy vegetables such as kale, broccoli, turnip and mustard greens; soy products processed with calcium; and fish consumed

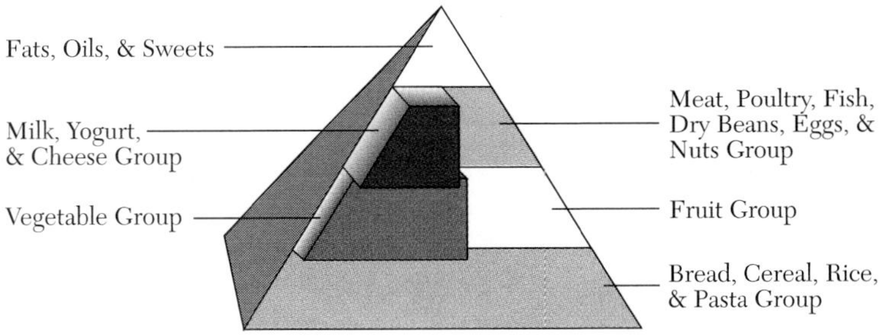

Figure 10.21
The food groups that are sources of calcium are raised and colored purple. The darker the shade, the more calcium-rich foods the group contains.

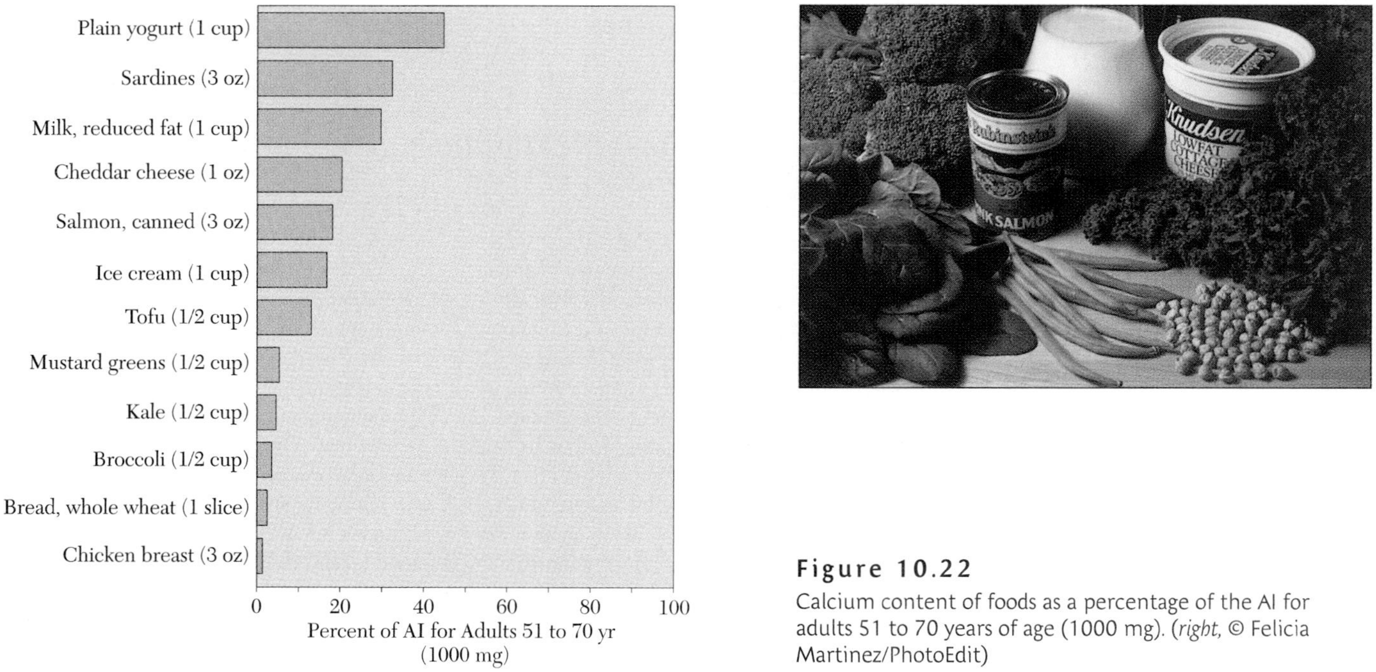

Figure 10.22
Calcium content of foods as a percentage of the AI for adults 51 to 70 years of age (1000 mg). (*right*, © Felicia Martinez/PhotoEdit)

with the bones (Figure 10.22). For packaged foods, the Nutrition Facts section of the label must provide the percent Daily Value of calcium in a serving (refer again to *Critical Thinking: A Diet for Health*).

Phosphorus

Phosphorus makes up about 1% of the adult body by weight and 85% of this is found as a structural component of bones.[38] The phosphorus in soft tissues has both structural and regulatory roles. In nature, phosphorus is most often found in combination with oxygen as phosphate.

Phosphorus in the Diet Phosphorus is more widely distributed in the diet than calcium. Like calcium, it is found in dairy products such as milk, yogurt, and cheese, but meat, cereals, bran, eggs, nuts, and fish are also good sources. Food additives used in baked goods, cheeses, processed meats, and soft drinks also provide phosphorus.

Phosphorus in the Digestive Tract Phosphorus is more readily absorbed than calcium. There is no evidence that the efficiency of absorption is affected by the amount in the diet. Vitamin D does aid phosphorus absorption via an active mechanism, but most absorption occurs by diffusion. Therefore when vitamin D is deficient, phosphorus can still be absorbed but its absorption is reduced.

Phosphorus in the Body. Phosphorus has important structural roles. The phosphorus and calcium in hydroxyapatite form the structure of bones. Phosphorus is a component of phospholipids, which form the structure of cell membranes. It is a major constituent of DNA and RNA. Phosphorus is also involved in regulating enzyme activity because the addition of a phosphate can activate or deactivate certain enzymes. The high-energy bonds of ATP are formed between phosphate groups. Phosphorus as phosphate is an important **buffer** that helps regulate the level of acidity or **pH** in the cytoplasm of all cells. This is important because the efficiency of most biological functions is best when pH is nearly neutral (pH 7)

Buffer A substance that reacts with an acid or base by picking up or releasing hydrogen ions to prevent changes in pH.

pH A measure of the level of acidity or alkalinity of a solution compared to neutrality.

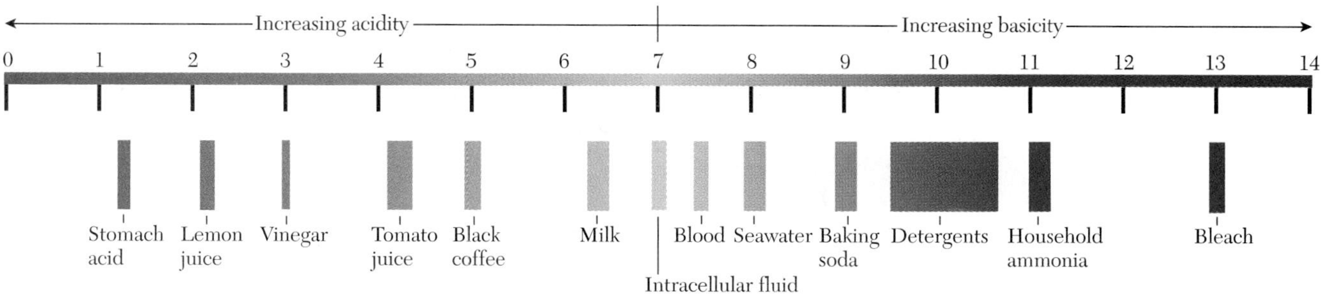

Figure 10.23
The pH values for some common fluids.

(Figure 10.23). Buffers such as phosphate are important for maintaining this neutral pH so that chemical reactions can proceed normally.

Blood levels of phosphorus are not as strictly controlled as those of calcium, but the level is maintained in a ratio with calcium that allows bone mineralization. When blood levels of phosphorus are low, the active form of vitamin D is synthesized. This increases the absorption of both phosphorus and calcium from the intestine and increases their release from bone. With high-phosphorus intakes, more is lost in the urine so plasma levels rise only slightly. A rise in serum phosphorus indirectly stimulates parathyroid hormone release, causing phosphorus excretion and calcium retention by the kidney as well as calcium release from bone. When parathyroid hormone is not secreted (such as when calcium levels rise), phosphorus is retained by the kidney and calcium is excreted.

How Much Phosphorus Do We Need? For men and women 19 to 50 years of age the RDA for phosphorus is set at 700 mg.[38] This is the amount needed to maintain normal blood phosphorus levels. Since neither phosphorus absorption nor urinary losses change significantly with age, the same RDA is adopted for older adults.

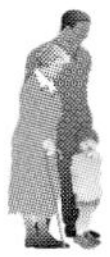

For growing children and adolescents, the accumulation of body phosphorus was used to determine recommended intakes. An RDA was established based on the phosphorus intake necessary to meet the needs for bone and soft tissue growth. There is no evidence that phosphorus requirements are increased during pregnancy; intestinal absorption increases by about 10%, which is sufficient to provide the additional phosphorus needed by the mother and fetus. The RDA is not increased during lactation because the phosphorus in milk is provided by an increase in bone resorption and a decrease in urinary excretion that are independent of dietary intake of either phosphorus or calcium.

Phosphorus and Health Because phosphorus is so widely distributed in food, dietary deficiencies are rare. Marginal phosphorus deficiencies are most common in premature infants, vegans, alcoholics, and the elderly. Causes of marginal phosphorus status include chronic diarrhea and chronic use of aluminum-containing antacids, which prevent phosphorus absorption.

Toxicity from high phosphorus intake is rare in healthy adults. Increased consumption of phosphorus-containing food additives has caused some to be concerned about its impact on bone health.[56] Diets high in phosphorus and low in calcium cause PTH to rise, resulting in an increase in bone resorption.[38] But, since the same effect occurs when the diet is low in calcium and not high in phosphorus, the effect is not believed to be due to high phosphorus levels. A study that monitored bone resorption found that it did not increase when phosphorus intake was doubled from 800 to 1600 mg per day.[57] Levels of phosphorus intake typical in the United States are not believed to affect bone health as long as calcium intake is adequate.[38] Based on the upper level of normal serum phosphate, a UL for phosphorus of 4.0 grams per day has been set for adults age 19 to 70.

Magnesium

There are approximately 25 grams of magnesium in the adult human body. Magnesium is a mineral that affects the metabolism of calcium, sodium, and potassium.

Magnesium in the Diet Magnesium is found in leafy greens such as spinach and kale because it is a component of chlorophyll. The germ and bran of whole grains, nuts, seeds, and bananas are also good sources, but fruits, fish, meat, and milk are poor sources. In areas with hard water, the water supply may provide a significant amount of magnesium.

Magnesium in the Digestive Tract About 50% of the magnesium in the diet is absorbed and the percentage decreases as intake increases. The active form of vitamin D can enhance magnesium absorption to a small extent, and the presence of phytate and fiber decrease absorption. As calcium in the diet increases, the absorption of magnesium decreases, so the use of calcium supplements can reduce the absorption of magnesium.

Magnesium in the Body About 50 to 60% of the magnesium in the body is in bone where it is essential for the maintenance of structure. Magnesium is also involved in regulating calcium homeostatis and is needed for the action of vitamin D and many hormones including parathyroid hormone.[58]

Magnesium is a cofactor for over 300 enzymes. It is necessary for the generation of energy from carbohydrate, lipid, and protein (see Table 10.1). In some of these reactions it is involved indirectly as a stabilizer of ATP, and in some, directly as an enzyme activator. Magnesium is needed for the activity of sodium-potassium ATPase responsible for active transport of sodium and potassium across membranes. It is therefore essential for maintenance of electrical potentials across membranes and proper functioning of the nerves and muscles, including those in the heart. It is important for maintaining a supply of nucleotides for DNA and RNA synthesis, and so is particularly important in dividing growing cells.

Blood levels of magnesium are closely regulated by the kidney. When magnesium intake is low, excretion in the urine is decreased. As intake increases, urinary excretion increases to maintain normal blood levels. This efficient regulation permits homeostasis over a wide range of dietary intakes.

How Much Magnesium Do We Need? The RDA for magnesium is 400 mg per day for young men and 310 mg per day for young women.[38] This is based on the maintenance of total body magnesium balance over time. Slightly higher RDAs were set for men and women age 31 and older because more magnesium was needed in these age groups to maintain balance. Magnesium requirements in children and adolescents are also based on balance data.

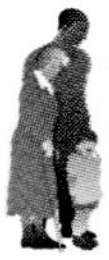

The requirement for pregnancy is increased by 35 mg per day to account for the addition of lean body mass. No increase is provided for lactation because magnesium is released when bone is resorbed and urinary excretion is decreased. An AI is set for infants based on the magnesium content of human milk. A serving of whole-grain breakfast cereal, spinach, or legumes contains about 100 mg of magnesium.

Magnesium and Health Magnesium deficiency is rare in the general population. However, it does occur in those with alcoholism, malnutrition, kidney disease, and gastrointestinal disease, as well as in those who use diuretics that increase magnesium loss in the urine. Deficiency symptoms include nausea, muscle weakness and cramping, irritability, mental derangement, and changes in blood pressure and heartbeat. Low blood magnesium levels affect levels of blood calcium and potassium, therefore some of these symptoms may be due to alterations in the levels of these other minerals.

Low intakes of magnesium have been associated with a number of chronic diseases. Oral magnesium supplements given to postmenopausal women with osteoporosis caused an increase in bone density and a decrease in fracture rate, suggesting that magnesium status is related to osteoporosis.[58] Epidemiological evidence suggests that humans with good magnesium status are at a lower risk of atherosclerosis, and supplements improve blood lipid levels.[59] Areas with hard water which is high in calcium and magnesium tend to have lower rates of death from cardiovascular disease.[60] Magnesium may also be involved in blood pressure regulation and dietary magnesium has been found to be inversely correlated with blood pressure.[26]

No adverse effects have been observed from ingestion of magnesium in foods, but toxicity may occur from concentrated sources such as magnesium-containing drugs and supplements. Toxicity has been reported in elderly patients with impaired kidney function who frequently use magnesium-containing laxatives and antacids such as milk of magnesia. Magnesium toxicity is characterized by nausea, vomiting, low blood pressure, and other cardiovascular changes. The UL for adults and adolescents over nine years of age is 350 mg of nonfood magnesium. There is no evidence that large intakes of magnesium are harmful to people with normal kidney function.

SULFUR

Sulfur in the diet comes from organic molecules such as the sulfur-containing amino acids in proteins and the sulfur-containing vitamins. It is also found in some inorganic food preservatives such as sulfur dioxide, sodium sulfite, and sodium and potassium bisulfite, which are used as antioxidants. In the body, the sulfur-containing amino acids methionine and cysteine are needed for protein synthesis. Cysteine is also part of the compound glutathione, which is important in detoxifying drugs and protecting cells from oxidative damage. The vitamins thiamin and biotin, essential for energy production, also contain sulfur. Sulfur-containing ions are a part of an important buffer system that regulates acid-base balance.

There is no recommended intake for sulfur, and no deficiencies are known when protein needs are met (see Table 10.1).

APPLICATIONS

These exercises are designed to help you apply your critical thinking skills to your own nutrition choices. Many are best performed using a diet analysis software program. If you do not have access to a computer program, the exercises can be hand-calculated using the information in this text and its appendices.

1. Use one day of the food record you kept in Chapter 2 to see how your diet compares to the DASH diet.
   a. Compare the number of servings from each of the food groups to the recommended servings for your energy intake as shown in Table 10.3.
   b. Modify your diet to meet DASH guidelines.
   c. What difficulties or inconveniences do you see with following this dietary pattern?
   d. What other dietary or lifestyle changes might you make if you are at high risk of hypertension?
2. Keep a log of all the fluids you consume in one day.
   a. Calculate your fluid intake by totaling the volume of water,

beverages, and foods that are liquid at room temperature, such as soup and ice cream, that you consumed.
   b. How does your intake on this day compare with your estimated requirement?
3. a. Using food labels, estimate the amount of sodium you consume from processed foods each day.
   b. Make a list of the processed foods that contain more than 10% of the Daily Value for sodium (2400 mg) per serving.
4. Using the food record you kept in Chapter 2, calculate your average calcium intake.
   a. How does your intake compare with the AI for calcium for someone of your age and sex?
   b. If your calcium intake is below the AI, modify your diet to increase your calcium consumption without significantly increasing your energy intake.
5. Using the Web site for this book, link to the Web site for the DASH diet. What is DASH2? How is the study being designed and what new information is expected to be gained from it?

Summary

1. Water is an essential nutrient that constitutes about 60% of the adult human body. It is consumed in beverages and food, and a small amount is produced by metabolism. Fluid intake is stimulated by the sensation of thirst, which occurs in response to a decrease in body water.
2. Body water is distributed between intracellular and extracellular compartments. The amount in each compartment depends largely on the concentration of solutes. Since water will diffuse by osmosis from a compartment with a lower concentration of solutes to one with a higher concentration, the body regulates the distribution of water by adjusting the concentration of electrolytes and other solutes in each compartment.
3. Water helps to transport other nutrients and waste products within the body and to excrete wastes from the body. It also helps to protect the body, regulate body temperature, and lubricate areas such as the eyes and the joints. Its polar structure allows it to function as a solvent for the molecules involved in metabolism.
4. Water is lost from the body in urine and feces and through evaporation from the skin and lungs. The kidney is the primary regulator of water output. If water intake is low, antidiuretic hormone will cause the kidney to conserve water. If water intake is high, more water will be excreted in the urine. The amount of water required by the body, about 1 ml per kcalorie of intake, may vary depending on environmental conditions and activity level. Dehydration can occur if water intake is too low or output is excessive.
5. Minerals are elements needed by the body to regulate chemical reactions and provide structure. They come from plant and animal sources, and their bioavailability is affected by interactions with other minerals, vitamins, and other dietary components such as fiber, phytates, oxylates, and tannins. For some minerals, bioavailability is affected by body need.
6. The minerals sodium, chloride, and potassium are electrolytes important in the maintenance of fluid balance and the formation of membrane potentials. The North American diet is abundant in sodium and chloride from processed foods and table salt but generally low in potassium, which is high in unprocessed foods such as fruits and vegetables.
7. Electrolyte and fluid homeostasis is regulated primarily by the kidneys. A decrease in blood pressure or blood volume signals the release of the enzyme renin, which helps form angiotensin II. Angiotensin II causes blood vessels to constrict and the hormone aldosterone to be released. Aldosterone causes the kidneys to reabsorb sodium and hence water, thereby increasing blood volume. Failure of these regulatory mechanisms may be a cause of hypertension.
8. Hypertension is common in the United States. Although the causes of most hypertension are not known, some individuals have a form that is sensitive to salt intake. For these individuals, a reduction in salt intake helps reduce blood pressure. Other nutrients, including potassium, magnesium, and calcium, also affect blood pressure.
9. There are no 1989 RDAs for sodium, chloride, or potassium. To reduce the risk of hypertension, public health recommendations suggest a moderate intake of salt and sodium, adequate dietary potassium, weight loss in overweight individuals, limited alcohol consumption, and increased exercise. The adoption of the DASH diet—a dietary pattern high in fruits, vegetables, lowfat dairy products, whole grains, and lean meat, fish, and poultry—is also recommended. This diet is rich in potassium, magnesium, calcium, and fiber, and low in fat, saturated fat, and cholesterol.
10. Bone is a living tissue that is constantly being broken down and reformed in a process known as bone remodeling. Early in life, bone formation occurs more rapidly than bone breakdown to allow bone growth and an increase in bone mass. Peak bone mass occurs in young adulthood. With age, bone breakdown begins to outpace formation causing a decrease in bone mass; this is accelerated in women at menopause.
11. Osteoporosis is a condition in which loss of bone mass increases the risk of bone fractures. The risk of osteoporosis is related to the level of peak bone mass and the rate of bone loss. These are affected by race and sex as well as diet and exercise.
12. Most of the calcium and phosphorus in the body is in bone as hydroxyapatite. Calcium not found in bone is essential for nerve transmission, muscle contraction, blood clotting, and blood pressure regulation. Blood levels of calcium are regulated by parathyroid hormone and calcitonin. Parathyroid hormone stimulates the release of calcium from bone, decreases calcium excretion by the kidney, and activates vitamin D to increase the amount of calcium absorbed from the gastrointestinal tract and released from bone. Calcitonin blocks calcium release from bone.
13. The AI for calcium ranges from 1000 to 1200 mg per day for adults and is 1300 mg per day in adolescents. Sources of calcium in the American diet include dairy products, fish consumed with bones, and leafy green vegetables.
14. In addition to its structural role in bones and teeth, phospho-

rus is part of a buffer system that helps prevent changes in pH. It is an essential component of phospholipids, ATP, and DNA. Good sources of phosphorus include dairy products, meats, and grains. The RDA is 700 mg per day.

15. Magnesium is important for bone health and it is needed as a cofactor for numerous reactions throughout the body. In reactions involved in energy production it acts as an enzyme activator and stabilizer of ATP. It is also needed to maintain membrane potentials; thus it is essential for nerve and muscle conductivity. Homeostasis is regulated by the kidney. Deficiency is rare, and the best dietary sources are whole grains and green vegetables.
16. Sulfur is needed in the diet as preformed organic molecules such as the amino acids methionine and cysteine, which are needed to synthesize proteins and glutathione, and the vitamins thiamin and biotin, needed for energy metabolism. Sulfur is also part of a buffer system that regulates acid-base balance. A dietary deficiency is unknown in the absence of protein malnutrition.

Review Questions

1. How is the amount of water in the body regulated?
2. Describe the functions of water in the body.
3. What is the recommended water intake for adults?
4. List three factors that increase water needs.
5. How do sodium, potassium, and chloride function in the body?
6. What types of foods contribute the most sodium to the North American diet?
7. What types of foods are good sources of potassium?
8. What is the relationship between dietary sodium and blood pressure?
9. What is the DASH diet and how does it affect blood pressure?
10. What is the major source of calcium in the North American diet?
11. How are blood calcium levels regulated?
12. How is calcium intake related to the risk of osteoporosis?
13. What factors other than calcium are related to the risk of osteoporosis?
14. What is the function of phosphorus in the body?
15. Name some food sources of phosphorus.
16. What is the function of magnesium in the body?
17. Where is sulfur found in the body?

Nutrition Web Links

To further explore areas related to the material in this chapter, go to the *Nutrition: Science and Applications* Web site at ***www.Wiley.com/college/Smolin*** and *click on* **Student Companion Site** for chapter-by-chapter links. Some Web sites related to information in Chapter 10 include:

Government agencies that give water safety guidelines such as the Environmental Protection Agency.

Groups that answer questions related to hypertension such as the American Heart Association and the DASH diet.

Health organizations that provide information about bones and osteoporosis prevention and treatment such as the National Resource Center for Osteoporosis and Related Bone Diseases.

References

1. Askew, E. W. Nutrition and performance in hot, cold, and high altitude environments. In *Nutrition in Exercise and Sport,* 3rd ed. Wolinsky, I., ed. Boca Raton, Fla: CRC Press, 1998, 597–619.
2. Oppliger, R. A., Case, H. S., Horswill, C. A., et al. American College of Sports Medicine position statement: weight loss in wrestlers. Med. Sci. Sports Exerc. 28:ix–xii, 1996.
3. Burt, V. L., Whelton, P., Roccella, E. J., et al. Prevalence of hypertension in the U.S. adult population: results from the third National Health and Nutrition Examination Survey, 1988–1991. Hypertension 25:305–313, 1995.
4. National Research Council, Food and Nutrition Board. *Recommended Dietary Allowances,* 10th ed. Washington, D.C.: National Academy Press, 1989.
5. National Research Council. *Diet and Health: Implications for Reducing Chronic Disease Risk.* Washington, D.C.: National Academy Press, 1989.
6. Committee on Nutritional Status During Pregnancy and Lactation, National Academy of Sciences. *Nutrition During Pregnancy.* Washington, D.C.: National Academy Press, 1990.
7. American Heart Association. High Blood Pressure Statistics. Online at http://www.amhrt.org/Heart_and_Stroke_A_Z_Guide/hbps.html
8. The Sixth Report of the Joint National Committee on Prevention, Detection, Evaluation, and Treatment of High Blood Pressure. Arch. Intern. Med. 157:2413–2446, 1997.
9. Hennekens, C. H. Lessons from hypertension trials. Am. J. Med. 104: 50S–53S, 1990.

10. Nurminen, M. L., Korpela, R., and Vapaatalo, H. Dietary factors in the pathogenesis and treatment of hypertension. Ann. Med. 30:143–150, 1998.
11. Appel, L. J., Moore, T. J., Obarzanek, E., et al. A clinical trial of the effects of dietary patterns on blood pressure. N. Engl. J. Med. 336: 1117–1124, 1997.
12. Carvalho, J. J., Baruzzi, R. G., Howard, P. F., et al. Blood pressure in four remote populations in the Intersalt study. Hypertension 14:238–246, 1989.
13. Graudal, N. A., Galloe, A. M., and Garrod, P. Effects of sodium restriction on blood pressure, renin, aldosterone, catacholamines, cholesterols, and triglyceride: a meta-analysis. J.A.M.A., 279:1383–1391, 1998.
14. Effects of weight loss and sodium reduction intervention on blood pressure and hypertension incidence in overweight people with high-normal blood pressure. The trials of Hypertension Prevention Collaborative Research Group. Arch. Intern. Med. 157:657–667, 1997.
15. Luft, L. C., and Weinberger, M. H. Heterogeneous responses to changes in dietary salt intake: the salt sensitivity paradigm. Am. J. Clin. Nutr. 65(suppl):612S–617S, 1997.
16. Kotchen, T. A., and Kotchen, J. M. Dietary sodium and blood pressure: interactions with other nutrients. Am. J. Clin. Nutr. 65(suppl): 708S–711S, 1997.
17. McCarron, D. A. Diet and blood pressure—the paradigm shift. Science 281:933–934, 1998.
18. Beilin, L. J., and Burke, V. Vegetarian diet components, protein and blood pressure: which nutrients are important? Clin. Exp. Pharmacol. Physiol. 22:195–198, 1995.
19. Young, D. B., Lin, H., and McCabe, R. D. Potassium's cardiovascular protective mechanisms. Am. J. Physiol. 268:R825–837, 1995.
20. Gillman, M. W., Cupples, A., Gagnon, D., et al. Protective effect of fruits and vegetables on development of stroke in men. J.A.M.A. 273:1113–1117, 1995.
21. Whelton, P. K., He, J., Cutler, J. A., et al. Effects of oral potassium on blood pressure: meta-analysis of randomized controlled clinical trials. J.A.M.A. 227:1624–1632, 1997.
22. Hamet, P. The evaluation of the scientific evidence for a relationship between calcium and hypertension. J. Nutr. 125(suppl):311S–400S, 1995.
23. Allender, P. S., Cutler, J. A., Follmann, D., et al. Dietary calcium and blood pressure: a meta-analysis of randomized clinical trials. Ann. Intern. Med. 124:825–831, 1996.
24. Dwyer, J. H., Dwyer, K. M., Scribner, R. A., et al. Dietary calcium, calcium supplementation, and blood pressure in African American adolescents. Am. J. Clin. Nutr. 68:648–655, 1998.
25. Singh, R. B., Niaz, M. A., Moshiri, M., et al. Magnesium status and risk of coronary artery disease in rural and urban populations with variable magnesium consumption. Magnes. Res. 10:205–213, 1997.
26. Ma, J., Folsom, A. R., Melnick, S. L., et al. Associations of serum and dietary magnesium with cardiovascular disease, hypertension, diabetes, insulin, and carotid arterial wall thickness: the ARIC study. Atherosclerosis Risk in Community Study. J. Clin. Epidemiol. 48:927–940, 1995.
27. Zemel, M. B. Dietary pattern and hypertension: the DASH diet. Nutr. Rev. 55:303–305, 1997.
28. Antonios, T. F., and MacGregor, G. A. Salt intake: potential deleterious effects excluding blood pressure. J. Hum. Hypertens. 9:511–515, 1995.
29. Teegarden, D., Lyle, R. M., McCabe, G. P., et al. Diet and bone mineral measure in young women. Am. J. Clin. Nutr. 68:749–754, 1998.
30. Groff, J. L., Gropper, S. S., and Hunt, S. M. *Advanced Nutrition and Human Metabolism,* 2nd ed. St. Paul, Minn.: 1995. West Publishing Company.
31. Osteoporosis Overview. Osteoporosis and Related Bone Diseases National Resource Center. Online at http://www.osteo.org/osteo.html
32. Riggs, B. L., and Melton, L. J. III. The worldwide problem of osteoporosis: insights afforded by epidemiology. Bone 17:505S–511S, 1995.
33. Gasperino, J. Ethnic differences in body composition and their relation to health and disease in women. Ethn. Health 1:337–347, 1996.
34. Reeker, R. R., Davies, K. M., Hiners, S. M., et al. Bone gain in young adult women. J.A.M.A. 268:2403–2408, 1992.
35. Riggs, B. L., Khosla, S., and Melton, L. J. 3rd., A unitary model for involutional osteoporosis: estrogen deficiency causes both type I and type II osteoporosis in postmenopausal women and contributes to bone loss in aging men. J. Bone Miner. Res. 13:763–773, 1998.
36. Ernst, E. Exercise for female osteoporosis: a systematic review of clinical trials. Sports Med. 25:359–368, 1998.
37. Melton, L. J. Epidemiology of spinal osteoporosis. Spine 22:2S–11S, 1997.
38. Institute of Medicine, Food and Nutrition Board. *Dietary Reference Intakes for Calcium, Phosphorus, Magnesium, Vitamin D, and Fluoride.* Washington, D.C.: National Academy Press, 1997.
39. Heaney, R. P., Weaver, C. M., and Recker, R. R. Calcium absorption from spinach. Am. J. Clin. Nutr. 47:707–709, 1988.
40. Bouillon, R., Carmeliet, G., and Boonen, S. Ageing and calcium metabolism. Baillieres Clin. Endocrinol. Metab. 11:341–365, 1997.
41. Affinito, P., Tommaselli, G. A., DiCarlo, C., et al. Changes in bone mineral density and calcium metabolism in breast-feeding women: a one year follow-up study. J. Clin. Endocrinol. Metab. 81:2314–2318, 1996.
42. Cross, N. A., Hillman, L. S., Allen, S. H., and Krasue, G. F. Changes in bone mineral density and markers of bone remodeling during lactation and postweaning in women consuming high amounts of calcium. J. Bone Miner. Res. 10:1312–1320, 1995.
43. O'Brian, K. O., Abrams, S. A., Stuff, J. E., et al. Variables related to urinary calcium excretion in young girls. J. Pediatr. Gastroenterol. Nutr. 23:8–12, 1996.
44. Dawson-Hughes, B., Fowler, S. E., Dalsky, G., and Gallagher, C. Sodium excretion influences calcium homeostasis in elderly men and women. J. Nutr. 126:2107–2112, 1996.
45. Bunker, V. W. The role of nutrition in osteoporosis. Br. J. Biomed. Sci. 51:228–240, 1994.
46. Riggs, B. L., O'Fallon, W. M., Muhs, J., et al. Long-term effects of calcium supplementation on serum parathyroid hormone level, bone turnover, and bone loss in elderly women. J. Bone Miner. Res. 13:168–174, 1998.
47. Reid, I. R. The roles of calcium and vitamin D in the prevention of osteoporosis. Endocrinol. Metab. Clin. North Am. 27:389–398, 1998.
48. Mizunuma, H., Okano, H., Soda, M., et al. Calcium supplements increase bone mineral density in women with low serum calcium levels during long-term estrogen therapy. Endocr. J. 43:411–415, 1996.
49. Devine, A., Dick, I. M., Heal, S. J., et al. A 4-year follow-up study of the effects of calcium supplementation on bone density in elderly postmenopausal women. Osteoporos. Int. 7:23–28, 1997.
50. Nieves, J. W., Komar, L., Cosman, F., and Lindasya, R. Calcium potentiates the effect of estogen and calcitonin on bone mass: review and analysis. Am. J. Clin. Nutr. 67:18–24, 1998.
51. McClung, M., Clemmesen, B., Daifotis, A., et al. Alendronate prevents postmenopausal bone loss in women without osteoporosis. A double-blind, randomized, controlled trial. Alendronate Osteoporosis Prevention Study Group. Ann. Intern. Med. 128:253–261, 1998.
52. Wimalawansa, S. J. A four-year randomized controlled trial of hormone replacement and bisphosphonate, alone or in combination, in women with postmenopausal osteoporosis. Am. J. Med. 104:219–226, 1998.
53. Minihane, A. M., and Fairweather-Tait, S. J. Effect of calcium supplementation on daily nonheme-iron absorption and long-term iron status. Am. J. Clin. Nutr. 68:96–102, 1998.
54. Wood, R. J., and Zheng, J. J. High dietary calicum intakes reduce zinc absorption and balance in humans. Am. J. Clin. Nutr. 65:1803–1809, 1997.
55. U.S. Department of Agriculture, Agricultural Research Service. Data Tables: Results from USDA's 1994–1996 Continuing Survey of Food Intakes by Individuals and 1994–1996 Diet and Health Knowledge

Survey (Online), ARS Food Surveys Research Group. Online (under Releases) at http://www.barc.usda.gov/bhnrc/foodsurvey/home.htm
56. Calvo, M. S., and Park, Y. K. Changing phosphorus content of the U.S. diet: potential for adverse effect on bone. J. Nutr. 126:1168S–1180S, 1996.
57. Bizik, B. K., Ding, W., and Cerklewski, F. L. Evidence that bone resorption of young men is not increased by high dietary phosphorus obtained from milk and cheese. Nutr. Res. 16:1143–1146, 1996.
58. Sojka, J. E., and Weaver, C. M. Magnesium supplementation and osteoporosis. Nutr. Rev. 53:71–74, 1995.
59. Dreosti, I. E. Magnesium status and health. Nutr. Rev. 53:S23–S27, 1995.
60. Rubenowitz, E., Axelsson, G., and Rylander, R. Magnesium in drinking water and death from myocardial infarction. Am. J. Epidemiol. 143:456–462, 1996.

Chapter 11

Chapter Outline

TRACE ELEMENTS THAT INTERACT WITH OXYGEN
Iron (Fe)
Copper (Cu)
Zinc (Zn)
Manganese (Mn)
Selenium (Se)

MINERALS WITH UNIQUE FUNCTIONS
Iodine (I): Regulating Metabolism
Chromium (Cr): Insulin Action
Fluoride (F): Strong Teeth
Molybdenum (Mo)

OTHER TRACE ELEMENTS
Boron (B)
Arsenic (As)
Nickel (Ni)
Silicon (Si)
Aluminum (Al) , Bromine (Br), Cadmium (Cd), Germanium (Ge), Lead (Pb), Lithium (Li), Rubidium (Rb), Tin (Sn), and Vanadium (V)

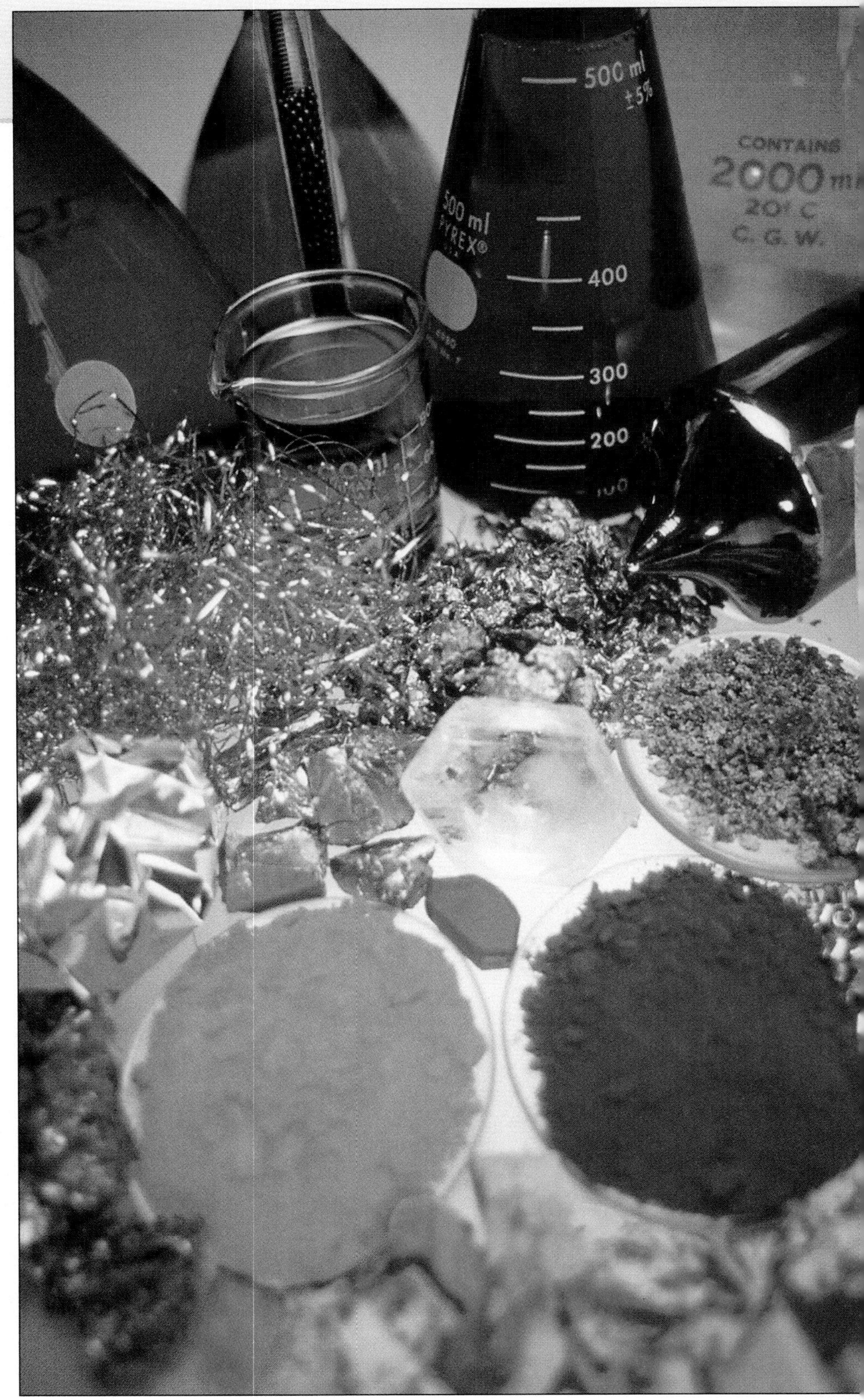

(Charles D. Winters)

The Trace Minerals: Our Elemental Needs

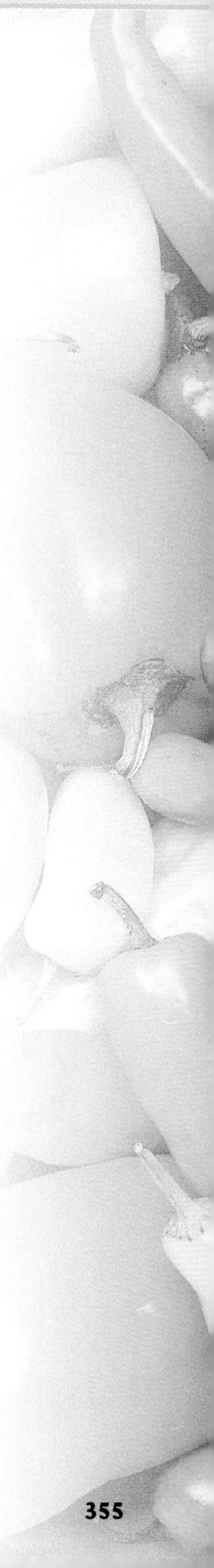

Chapter Concepts

1. Trace elements are required in the diet in small amounts but have important functions in regulating body processes.
2. Iron is a component of the oxygen transport protein hemoglobin, found in red blood cells.
3. Iron deficiency anemia is the most common nutritional deficiency worldwide, but too much iron can be toxic.
4. Copper is needed to transport iron; therefore, a deficiency can cause anemia. Copper is also involved in the synthesis of connective tissue, lipid metabolism, and antioxidant protection.
5. High intakes of zinc can interfere with copper absorption.
6. Zinc is a cofactor for many enzymes and also affects protein synthesis through gene expression. It is needed for tissue growth and repair, sexual development, and immune function.
7. Manganese is a component of the antioxidant enzyme superoxide dismutase.
8. Selenium is an essential part of the antioxidant enzyme glutathione peroxidase. Adequate dietary selenium can reduce the need for vitamin E.
9. Iodine is essential for the synthesis of the thyroid hormones, which regulate basal metabolic rate and other body functions.
10. Iodine deficiency is a problem in developing countries, but the use of iodized salt has virtually eliminated iodine deficiency in North America.
11. Chromium is needed for insulin to transport glucose into cells.
12. Fluoride is important for healthy bones and teeth. An adequate intake reduces dental caries.
13. Molybdenum is needed for the activity of several enzymes involved in uric acid production.
14. There are many other trace elements found in the body which have not been determined to be dietary essentials.

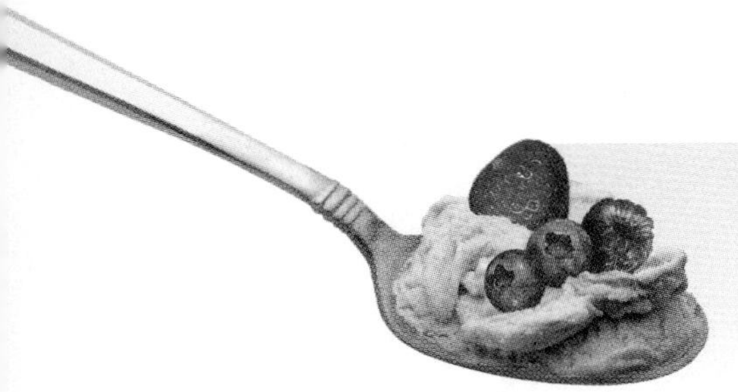

Just a Taste

Can taking a supplement of one mineral cause a deficiency of another?

Are iron supplements dangerous?

Can taking chromium supplements change body composition?

Trace elements are the most recently recognized of the essential nutrients. By definition, trace elements are minerals that are required by the body in an amount of 100 mg or less per day or that are present in the body in an amount of 0.01% or less of body weight. The methods traditionally used to establish the essentiality of substances and to determine requirements for nutrients have not been effective for studying many of the trace elements. The requirements for some of these elements are so small and interactions among the elements and other dietary components so great that isolated deficiencies of trace elements have not always been possible to create, even in the laboratory. This has caused researchers to focus not only on the needs for individual nutrients, but on the balanced interactions of nutrients within the whole diet.

Determining the health impact of trace mineral deficiencies presents a mixture of old challenges and new frontiers. Deficiencies of iron and iodine have been public health concerns for generations. It is estimated that more than 2 billion people worldwide suffer from iron deficiency, including 8.5 million women, adolescent girls, and children in the United States.[1,2] Iodine deficiency, although virtually eradicated in the United States, is a major health problem in developing countries. While eliminating these deficiencies is a continuing challenge, new concerns have arisen about marginal deficiencies of some of the trace elements. Such deficiencies are an important focus of international public health agendas. For example, is zinc deficiency a widespread public health problem or a rare condition? How important is selenium to cancer prevention? Is marginal selenium deficiency an important public health concern? There are no good ways to diagnose these marginal deficiencies and there is still much to learn about the breadth of function of these trace elements.

In the discussion that follows, iron, copper, zinc, manganese, and selenium are discussed sequentially because they function in oxygen transport and in antioxidant enzymes. These discussions are followed by presentation of minerals that serve other unique functions. The final section presents some of the other trace elements—those for which we are just unraveling their role in health and nutrition.

Trace Elements That Interact With Oxygen

Oxygen is essential for life, but it can also be poisonous. Many of the trace elements interact with oxygen—some by assuring it is delivered to cells and some by preventing oxidative damage. Minerals can also catalyze the formation of dangerous free radicals. To prevent this, the body stores, transports, and uses these minerals in forms that are bound to proteins and therefore unable to cause free radical formation. A number of enzymes that contain trace elements are able to destroy reactive oxygen molecules and protect cells from oxidative damage. Iron, copper, zinc, manganese, and selenium all serve as components of antioxidant enzyme systems. In addition to these parallel roles, each trace element has additional unique functions.

Iron (Fe)

Iron was identified as a major constituent of blood in the 18th century. By 1832, iron tablets were used to treat young women in whom "coloring matter" was lacking in the blood. Today we know that the red color in blood is due to the iron-containing protein **hemoglobin,** and that a deficiency of iron decreases hemoglobin production. Despite the fact that iron is one of the best understood of the trace elements, iron deficiency remains the most common nutritional deficiency in North America and worldwide.[1,2]

Hemoglobin An iron-containing protein in red blood cells that binds and transports oxygen through the bloodstream to cells.

Iron in the Diet Iron in the diet comes from both plant and animal sources. Much of the iron in animal products is **heme iron**—iron that is part of a chemical complex found in proteins, such as **myoglobin** in muscle and hemoglobin in blood. Heme iron is absorbed more than twice as efficiently as nonheme iron. Meat, poultry, and fish are good sources of heme iron. Heme iron accounts for about 10 to 15% of the dietary iron in industrialized countries.[3]

Leafy green vegetables, legumes, and whole or enriched grains are good sources of **nonheme iron** (Figure 11.1). Another source of nonheme iron in the diet is iron cooking utensils, from which iron leaches into food. Leaching is enhanced by acidic foods. For example, spaghetti sauce cooked in a glass pan con-

Heme iron A readily absorbed form of iron found in animal products that is chemically associated with proteins such as hemoglobin and myoglobin.

Myoglobin An iron-containing protein in muscle cells that binds oxygen.

Nonheme iron A poorly absorbed form of iron found in both plant and animal foods that is not part of the iron complex found in hemoglobin and myoglobin.

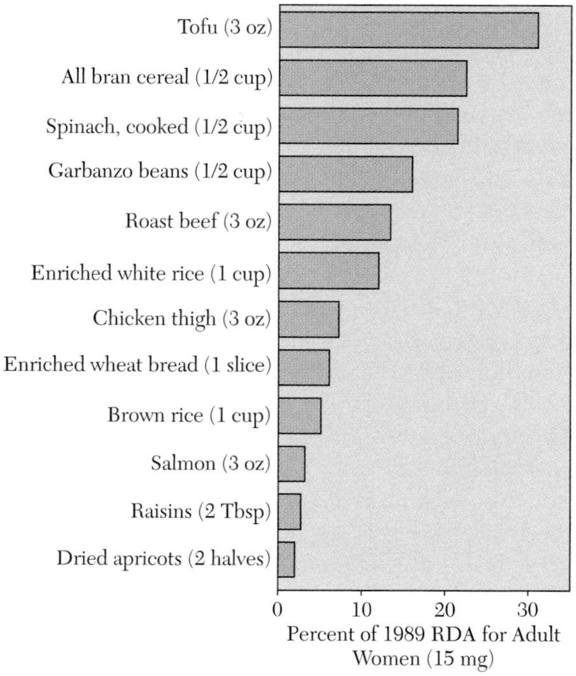

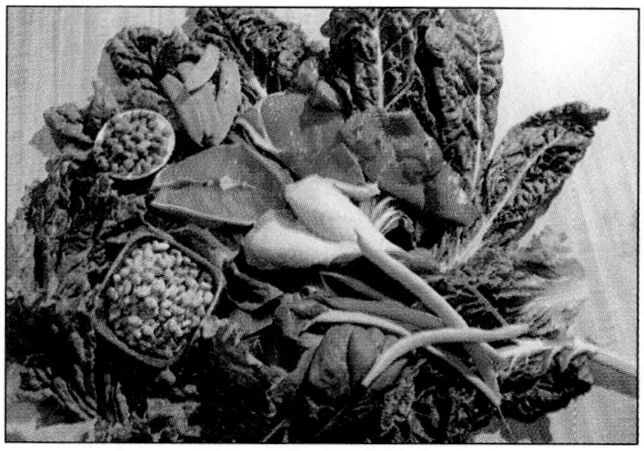

Figure 11.1
The iron content of foods as a percentage of the 1989 RDA for adult women. (*right,* © Tony Freeman/PhotoEdit)

tains about 3 mg of iron, but the same sauce cooked in an iron skillet may contain more than 80 mg, depending on how long it is cooked. The bioavailability of nonheme iron is determined by overall meal composition. Some dietary components enhance absorption. The presence of acids such as ascorbic acid (vitamin C), citric acid, lactic acid, and others enhance iron absorption by helping to keep iron in the ferrous (Fe^{2+}) form, which is better absorbed than the ferric (Fe^{3+}) form. The best studied of these acids is vitamin C, which enhances the absorption of iron for two reasons: First, as an acid, it keeps iron in its more absorbable form; and second, it forms a complex with iron that remains soluble and bioavailable, preventing iron from forming unabsorbable complexes in the gastrointestinal tract.[4] To have this effect, the vitamin C must be consumed in the same meal as the iron; it can then enhance nonheme iron absorption up to sixfold.[3] Consuming meats such as beef, fish, or poultry that are sources of heme iron also increases the absorption of nonheme iron. For example, a small amount of hamburger in a pot of chili will enhance the body's absorption of iron from the beans.

Dietary factors that interfere with the absorption of nonheme iron include fiber, phytates found in cereals, tannins found in tea, and oxalates found in some leafy greens such as spinach. These prevent absorption by binding iron in the gastrointestinal tract. The presence of other minerals may also decrease iron absorption. For instance, calcium supplements decrease iron absorption, particularly when both are consumed at the same meal.[5]

Iron in the Gastrointestinal Tract The amount of iron in the body is controlled primarily by how much is absorbed. Iron from the diet is absorbed into the intestinal mucosal cells. The amount of iron transported from the mucosal cells to the rest of the body depends on need. If body stores of iron are high, less iron is transported from the mucosal cells. If iron stores are low, a greater percentage of the iron that has been absorbed into the mucosal cells is transported to other tissues. The transport and delivery of iron is regulated by several proteins: The copper-containing protein **ceruloplasmin** is needed to convert absorbed iron to the form that binds to the iron transport protein **transferrin** and the iron storage protein **ferritin** (Figure 11.2).

Ceruloplasmin A copper-containing protein that converts iron to the ferric form, which can bind to iron storage and iron transport proteins.

Transferrin An iron transport protein in the blood.

Ferritin The major iron storage protein.

Iron in the Body Iron that has entered the mucosal cells of the small intestine can be bound to ferritin or picked up and transported in the blood to the liver, bones, and other body tissues by transferrin. Transferrin receptors on cell membranes bind to the transferrin-iron complex allowing it to enter the cell, where the iron is released for use. When iron is in short supply, less of the iron storage protein ferritin is made and the number of transferrin receptors increases, allowing more iron to be transported into the cells.[6] When iron is plentiful, more ferritin is made to increase storage capacity and the number of transferrin receptors decreases, so the capacity to pick up iron from the mucosal cells and transport it into body cells is reduced. Iron that is not picked up from mucosal cells is excreted in the feces along with mucosal cells when they die and are sloughed off into the intestinal lumen.

Iron that is absorbed in excess of immediate needs can be stored in the protein ferritin primarily in the liver, spleen, and bone marrow. Levels of ferritin in the blood can be used to estimate iron stores. When ferritin concentrations in the liver become high, some is converted to an insoluble storage protein called hemosiderin. Iron can be mobilized from body stores as needed, and deficiency signs will appear only after stores are depleted.

Iron is not readily excreted. Even when red blood cells die, the iron in their hemoglobin is not lost from the body. The cells are removed from the blood by the spleen and liver and degraded; the iron is then attached to transferrin for transport back to the bone where it can be incorporated into new red blood cells. Most iron loss even in healthy individuals occurs through blood loss, including

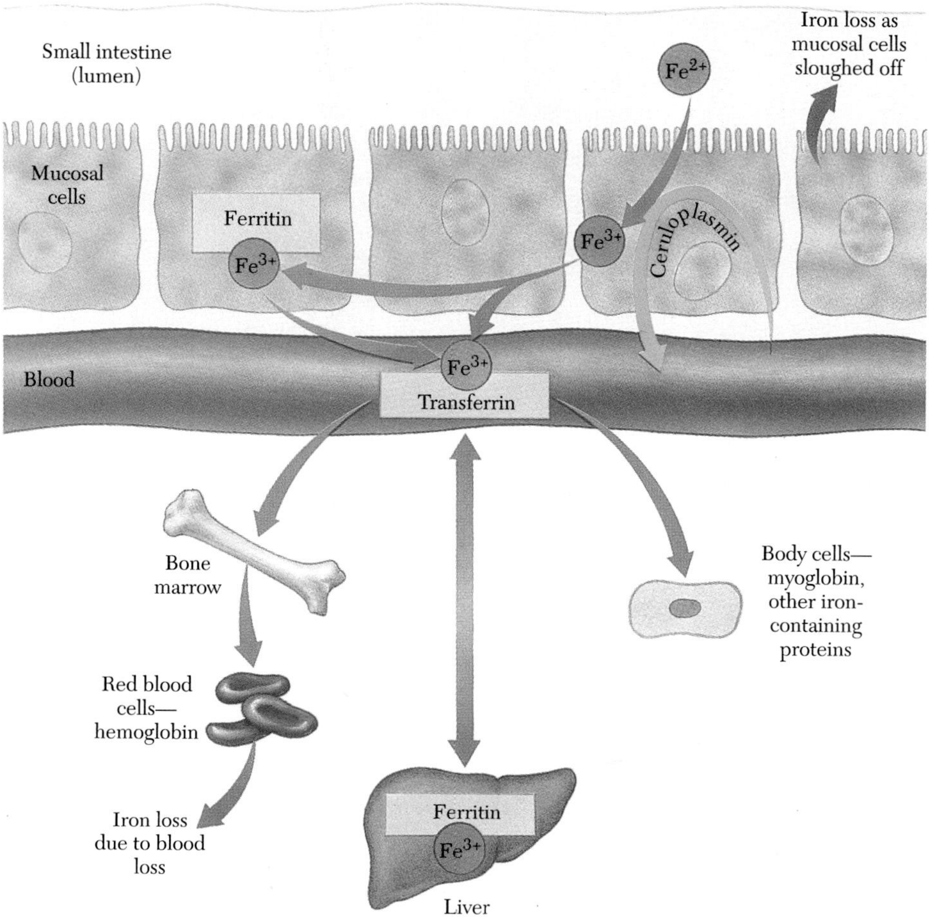

Figure 11.2
Ferrous iron (Fe^{2+}) is absorbed and converted to ferric iron (Fe^{3+}) by ceruloplasmin. The excess remains in mucosal cells bound to ferritin and is excreted when the cells die. Iron is transported in the blood bound to transferrin. It is delivered to bone, where it is needed to synthesize hemoglobin for red blood cells, and to other body cells, where it is used to synthesize myoglobin and other iron-containing proteins. Excess iron is stored primarily in the liver, bound to ferritin.

that lost during menstruation and the small amounts lost from the gastrointestinal tract. Some iron is also lost through the shedding of cells from the intestine, skin, and urinary tract.[4]

Iron in the body is essential for the delivery of oxygen to cells. It is a component of two oxygen-carrying proteins, hemoglobin and myoglobin. Most of the iron in the body is part of hemoglobin. Hemoglobin in red blood cells transports oxygen to body cells and carries carbon dioxide away from cells for elimination by the lungs. Myoglobin is found in the muscle, where it stores oxygen for use in muscle contraction. Iron is also a part of several proteins involved in the electron transport chain, drug metabolism, and the immune system, and it is part of the enzyme catalase, which protects the cell from oxidative damage by destroying hydrogen peroxide before it can form free radicals.

How Much Iron Do We Need? The 1989 RDA for iron is 10 mg per day for adult men. This recommendation is based on the fact that the average man loses approximately 1 mg of iron per day. Since only about 10% of the iron consumed in a typical diet is absorbed, an intake of 10 mg per day will replace the 1 mg lost.

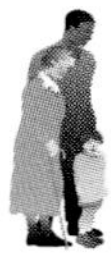

Iron is the only nutrient for which the requirement for adult women is greater than that for adult men. The 1989 RDA for women of childbearing age is 15 mg per day. The additional 5 mg is recommended to make up for menstrual losses. For adolescent males, the 1989 RDA is 12 mg, and for females, 15 mg. The recommended intake during pregnancy is increased to 30 mg per day. There is no additional requirement during lactation because little iron is lost in milk and menstruation is usually absent during lactation. To meet the needs of rapid growth, infants require 1 mg of iron per kilogram of body weight. Children older

Figure 11.3
Iron deficiency anemia is diagnosed when levels of red blood cells or proteins containing iron are low. It causes the red blood cells to become small and pale. (a) Normal red blood cells. (b) Iron deficiency anemia. (*a*, © B & B Photos/ Custom Medical Stock Photo; *b*, © Custom Medical Stock Photo)

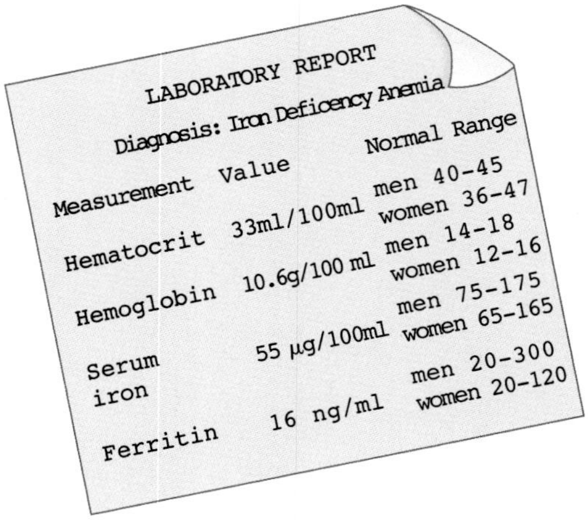
LABORATORY REPORT
Diagnosis: Iron Deficiency Anemia
Measurement Value Normal Range
Hematocrit 33ml/100ml men 40-45 women 36-47
Hemoglobin 10.6g/100 ml men 14-18 women 12-16
Serum iron 55 µg/100ml men 75-175 women 65-165
Ferritin 16 ng/ml men 20-300 women 20-120

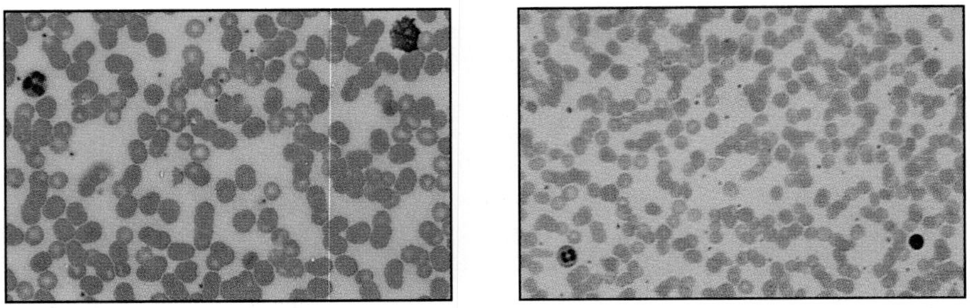

(a) (b)

than three years of age need about 10 mg per day until adolescence. The recommended intake in older men is not different from that in younger men, but in older women the recommended intake is decreased because iron loss due to menstruation ceases.

Iron and Health Iron deficiency and toxicity are both health concerns. Iron deficiency is the most common nutritional deficiency in the United States, affecting 7.8 million adolescent girls and women of childbearing age and 700,000 children aged one to two years.[2] But, when iron accumulates in the body it can damage tissues, and a single large dose can poison a child.

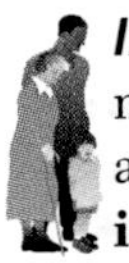

Iron Deficiency When iron is deficient, hemoglobin cannot be produced. When not enough hemoglobin is available, the red blood cells that are formed are small and pale and unable to deliver adequate oxygen to the tissues. This is known as **iron deficiency anemia** (Figure 11.3). It is estimated that about 10% of women of childbearing age have insufficient iron stores and 3 to 5% have iron deficiency anemia. Among children aged one to three years, 9% are iron deficient and 3% have iron deficiency anemia.[2] Among low-income and minority women and children, the incidence is even greater. Only about one fourth of adolescent girls and women of childbearing age meet the RDA for iron through their diet.[2]

Symptoms of iron deficiency anemia include fatigue, weakness, headache, decreased work capacity, an inability to maintain body temperature in a cold environment, changes in behavior, decreased resistance to infection, impaired development in infants, and an increased risk of lead poisoning in young children. One strange symptom thought to be related to iron deficiency is **pica.** This is a compulsion to eat nonfood items such as clay, ice, paste, laundry starch, paint chips, and ashes. Pica can cause the consumption of substances containing toxic minerals, such as lead-based paints, and it can introduce substances into the diet that inhibit mineral absorption (see Chapter 13).

Iron deficiency anemia A condition that occurs when the oxygen-carrying capacity of the blood is decreased because there is insufficient iron to make hemoglobin. It is diagnosed in adults when hemoglobin concentration is less than 11 grams per 100 ml of blood.

Pica The compulsive ingestion of nonfood substances such as clay, laundry starch, and paint chips.

Women of reproductive age are at risk for iron deficiency anemia because of iron loss due to menstruation. The need for iron is also increased during pregnancy because of the increase in maternal blood volume and the growth of other maternal tissues and the fetus. Iron deficiency is common among pregnant women even in industrialized countries and can lead to premature delivery and greater risk to the mother.[7] Iron deficiency is common in infants and children from four months to six years of age because their rapid growth increases iron needs. Iron stores at birth are sufficient to meet iron needs for the first four to six months of life; after this, infants should consume formula or cereal fortified with iron to ensure an adequate intake. Toddlers with finicky eating habits should be monitored to ensure they are consuming adequate iron from foods such as meats, leafy green vegetables, and fortified cereals (see Chapters 13 and 14).

Adolescents are also at risk for iron deficiency anemia. In adolescent boys, rapid growth and an increase in muscle mass and blood volume increase iron need. In adolescent girls, iron needs are increased because weight gain is almost as great as in boys and iron losses are increased by the onset of menstruation (see Chapter 14).

Athletes are another group susceptible to iron deficiency. This may be due to a low iron intake, greater iron losses in sweat, and increased needs for the production of hemoglobin and other iron-containing proteins.[8] If the deficiency progresses to anemia, it can impair performance (see Chapter 12 and *Critical Thinking: Increasing Iron Intake*).

Iron Toxicity Iron toxicity can be acute, resulting from ingestion of a single large dose at one time, or chronic, due to the accumulation of iron in the body over time. Chronic iron overload can result from the chronic consumption of large but nontoxic doses of iron over a long period, but generally occurs only in individuals with hereditary abnormalities in iron absorption (the most common cause), diseases requiring frequent blood transfusions, or a deficiency in folate or vitamin B_{12}.[9]

Acute Toxicity Iron is toxic in large amounts. Even a single large dose can be life-threatening. Iron toxicity from supplements is one of the most common forms of poisoning among children under age six. Iron poisoning may cause damage to the intestinal lining, abnormalities in body pH, shock, and liver failure. Iron supplement overdose is the leading cause of liver transplants in children. To protect children from accidental poisoning from iron-containing drugs and supplements, these products display a warning on the label (Figure 11.4). In addition, since

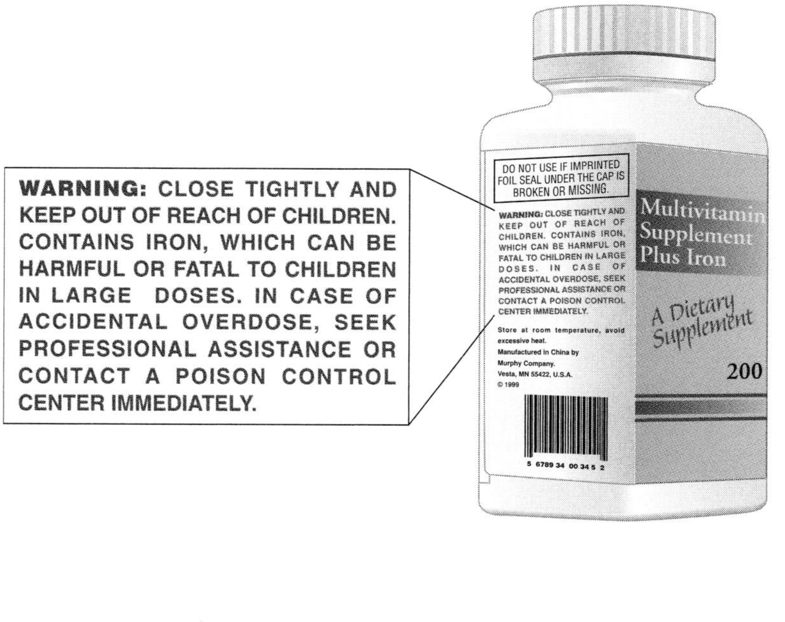
WARNING: CLOSE TIGHTLY AND KEEP OUT OF REACH OF CHILDREN. CONTAINS IRON, WHICH CAN BE HARMFUL OR FATAL TO CHILDREN IN LARGE DOSES. IN CASE OF ACCIDENTAL OVERDOSE, SEEK PROFESSIONAL ASSISTANCE OR CONTACT A POISON CONTROL CENTER IMMEDIATELY.
DO NOT USE IF IMPRINTED FOIL SEAL UNDER THE CAP IS BROKEN OR MISSING.
WARNING: CLOSE TIGHTLY AND KEEP OUT OF REACH OF CHILDREN. CONTAINS IRON, WHICH CAN BE HARMFUL OR FATAL TO CHILDREN IN LARGE DOSES. IN CASE OF ACCIDENTAL OVERDOSE, SEEK PROFESSIONAL ASSISTANCE OR CONTACT A POISON CONTROL CENTER IMMEDIATELY.
Store at room temperature, avoid excessive heat.
Manufactured in China by Murphy Company.
Vesta, MN 55422, U.S.A.
© 1999
5 6789 34 00 34 5 2
Multivitamin Supplement Plus Iron
A Dietary Supplement
200

Figure 11.4

Labels on iron-containing supplements and medications must carry a toxicity warning.

most cases of serious iron poisoning have occurred with products containing 30 mg or more per dose, these products are packaged in individual doses to make consumption of many pills difficult for a young child.[10]

Chronically Elevated Iron Stores Iron stores that are above normal but below toxic levels have been hypothesized to be associated with a greater risk of both heart disease and cancer. The relationship between iron and heart disease was originally suggested because heart disease occurs less frequently in premenopausal women, who lose iron monthly, than in postmenopausal women and men. Because iron can act as a pro-oxidant, too much iron is hypothesized to increase the formation of oxidized LDL cholesterol, which then leads to atherosclerosis.[11] Excess iron is suggested to increase cancer incidence by boosting the formation of free radicals, suppressing the activity of the immune system, and promoting cancer cell multiplication. Some studies have found a relationship between iron storage and cancer risk, but it is not clear what types of cancers may be involved.[9]

Hemochromatosis An inherited condition that results in increased iron absorption.

Hemochromatosis The most common cause of chronic iron overload is the genetic disorder **hemochromatosis,** which is a condition that allows increased iron absorption. Hemochromatosis afflicts about 1.5 million Americans. It is the most common inherited disease in Caucasian populations in North America, Australia, and Europe, occurring in about 1 in 300 individuals.[12] Although more frequent in Caucasian populations, it is also seen in African Americans and Hispanics.[13] The accumulation of excess iron that occurs in hemochromatosis causes oxidative changes resulting in heart and liver damage, diabetes, and certain types of cancer. Iron deposits also darken the skin. To have these symptoms, an individual must inherit the hemochromatosis gene from both parents. The one in ten people who inherit the gene from only a single parent don't have these serious symptoms but do absorb iron better than people who do not have the gene at all.

The public health impact of hemochromatosis is potentially significant. The availability of red meat and the prevalence of iron-fortified foods in the American diet virtually assures that individuals with two genes for hemochromatosis will eventually accumulate damaging levels of iron. Individuals with only one gene may also be at risk. If individuals with hemochromatosis can be identified, treatment is simple: regular blood withdrawal, the equivalent of the ancient treatment of bloodletting. Regular blood withdrawal will prevent the complications of iron overload. To be effective it must be begun before organs are damaged, so screening to identify and treat young healthy individuals is essential in preventing complications.[14] The gene for this disease has been identified, so screening and early diagnosis for this disorder may soon become common.[15]

Meeting Iron Needs: Consider the Total Diet To meet iron needs, both the amount and the bioavailability of iron from the diet should be considered. The best sources of iron are red meats and organ meats such as liver and kidney. Good vegetable sources are leafy greens such as spinach and kale, although the nonheme iron in plants is less well absorbed than the heme iron in animal sources (Figure 11.5). Iron absorption can be enhanced by including meat, fish, poultry, and foods rich in vitamin C in meals containing iron, while decreasing the consumption of dairy products, which are high in calcium, at these meals.[16]

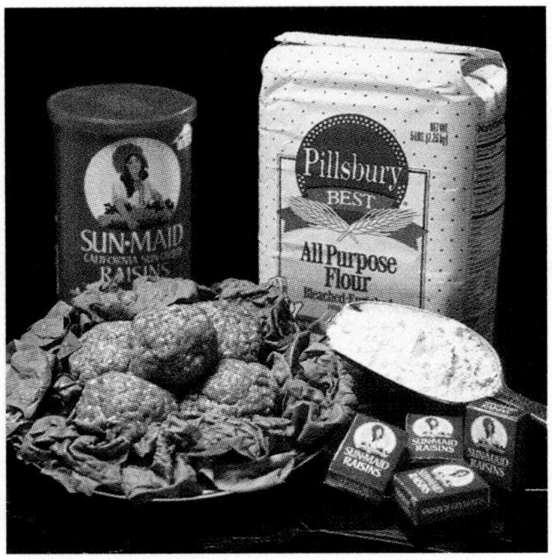

Figure 11.5
Iron in our diets comes from both animal and plant sources, but bioavailability from plant sources is often low. (Charles D. Winters)

Because iron is a nutrient at risk for deficiency in the American diet, the iron content of packaged foods must be listed on food labels. It is given as a percent of the Daily Value for iron, which is 18 mg for adults. Therefore, if your breakfast cereal provides 10% of the Daily Value for iron, it contains about 1.8 mg of iron per serving.

Although diet is the ideal way to meet iron needs, supplements are often recommended for groups at risk for deficiency such as small children, women of childbearing age, and pregnant women. Iron is commonly available as an individual supplement or as part of multivitamin and mineral supplements. These contain nonheme iron. As with nonheme iron in the diet, to enhance the absorption of iron in a supplement, it should be consumed with foods containing vitamin C,

Table 11.1 *A Summary of the Trace Elements*

Mineral	Sources	Recommended Intake for Adults	Major Functions	Deficiency	Groups at Risk	Toxicity
Iron	Red meats, leafy greens, dried fruits, whole or enriched grains	10–15 mg†	Part of hemoglobin, which delivers oxygen to cells, and myoglobin, which stores oxygen in muscle	Iron deficiency anemia, weakness, lethargy	Infants and preschool children, adolescents, women of childbearing age, pregnant women, athletes	Liver damage
Copper	Organ meats, nuts and seeds, whole grains, seafood	1.5–3.0 mg‡	Functions in proteins in iron and lipid metabolism, SOD, nerve and immune function, collagen synthesis	Anemia, poor growth	Those who over-supplement zinc	Vomiting
Zinc	Meat, seafood, milk, whole grains, eggs	12–15 mg†	Regulates protein synthesis; functions in growth, development, wound healing, immunity, and SOD	Poor growth and development, dermatitis, decreased immune function	Vegetarians, low-income children, elderly	Decreased copper absorption
Manganese	Nuts, whole grains	2.0–5.0 mg‡	Functions in carbohydrate and lipid metabolism, SOD	Growth retardation	None	Nerve damage
Selenium	Organ meats, eggs, and seafood	55–70 μg†	Antioxidant as part of glutathione peroxidase, spares vitamin E	Muscle pain and weakness, Keshan disease	Populations in areas with low-selenium soil	Nausea, diarrhea, vomiting, fatigue, hair changes
Iodine	Iodized salt, saltwater fish, and seafood	150 μg†	Needed for synthesis of thyroid hormones	Goiter, cretinism	Populations living where soil is iodine deficient and iodized salt is not used	Enlarged thyroid
Chromium	Liver, brewer's yeast, nuts, grains	50–200 μg‡	Glucose tolerance	Impaired glucose metabolism	Malnourished children	None reported
Fluoride§	Fluoridated water, tea, fish, toothpaste	3.1–3.8 mg°	Strengthens tooth enamel	Increased risk of dental caries	Populations in areas with unfluoridated water	Mottled teeth, kidney damage, abnormal bones
Molybdenum	Milk, organ meats, grains, legumes	75–250 μg‡	Cofactor for many enzymes	Unknown in humans	None	Arthritis and joint inflammation

° Adequate Intake (AI).
† 1989 RDA value.
‡ ESADDI value.
§ The Tolerable Upper Intake Level for fluoride is 10 mg.

such as orange juice; taken with a meal containing meat, fish, or poultry; and not taken with dairy products or substances that bind iron. Iron from supplements that contain the ferrous form (Fe^{2+}) of iron, such as ferrous sulfate, is more readily absorbed than iron from those with the ferric form (Fe^{3+}). Iron supplements should not be taken at the same meal as calcium supplements. Large intakes of iron from supplements can interfere with the absorption of zinc and copper (Table 11.1). Iron-containing supplements should be taken only as suggested on the label and stored out of the reach of children or others who may consume them in excess.

CRITICAL THINKING

Increasing Iron Intake

Odelia is a twenty-three-year-old college sophomore. She has been feeling tired and run down all semester. She recently read an article about iron deficiency in young women and became concerned about her iron status. She decides to go to the health center where she has blood drawn. Her lab values, shown in Figure 11.3, indicate that she has iron deficiency anemia.

A review of her typical diet shows that Odelia's iron intake is less than the recommended amount. She decides to try to increase the amount of iron she gets from her diet before considering iron supplements. Odelia is originally from Ghana. She enjoys many native foods and consumes a primarily vegetarian diet. At home in Ghana her mother prepared meals in iron cookware. Since moving to the United States, Odelia has used stainless steel cookware and she believes that this may have contributed to her anemia.

Typical Diet

Food	Amount	Iron (mg)
Breakfast		
Grits with	1 cup	0.5
butter	1 tsp	0
Plantain	1	0.9
Whole wheat toast	1 slice	1.2
Apple juice	3/4 cup	0.7
Tea with	1 cup	0
sugar	1 tsp	0
Lunch		
Apple	1 medium	0.2
Cornbread with	1 piece	1.5
butter	1 tsp	0
Yogurt	1 cup	0.2
Tomato	1 medium	0.5
Tea with	1 cup	0
sugar	1 tsp	0
Dinner		
Rice	1 cup	2.4
Peanuts	1/3 cup	0.9
Kale	1 cup	1.2
Yams	1 cup	1.1
Apple juice	3/4 cup	0.7
Tea with	1 cup	0
sugar	1 tsp	0
Total		**12.0**

What dietary factors could contribute to Odelia's poor iron status?

1. Her total iron intake is marginal at 12 mg per day compared with the 1989 RDA of ______________________.
2. The iron in her diet comes from plant sources that contain only nonheme iron, which ______________________.
3. The diet is low in vitamin C-rich foods, which ______________________.
4. The switch to stainless steel cookware ______________________.

How could Odelia's breakfast and lunch be modified to increase her iron intake?

Odelia is a vegetarian, so her iron sources are limited to plant foods, which are generally lower in iron and contain only the less-well-absorbed nonheme form of iron. There are, however, good plant sources of naturally occurring iron as well as sources fortified with iron. For instance, switching from the half cup of grits, containing about 0.5 mg of iron, to a fortified cereal will greatly increase her intake. Adding 2 tablespoons of raisins to the hot cereal contributes another 0.4 mg. Another good vegetarian source of iron is beans. A bowl of chili with beans at lunch will add 8 mg of iron.

What modifications could Odelia make to increase the iron content of her dinner?

Answer:

Does Odelia's diet meet the recommendations of the Food Guide Pyramid for vegetarians? Are there other nutrient deficiencies for which she may be at risk?

Answer:

Copper (Cu)

A deficiency of copper can result in iron deficiency anemia because copper is needed for the transport of iron and the maintenance of red blood cell membranes. The ability of copper to treat certain types of anemia helped establish the essentiality of copper in human nutrition.[17] Further understanding of the impact of copper deficiency in humans came from studying individuals who were inadvertently fed intravenous (TPN) solutions deficient in copper and those with a rare genetic disease in which there is a defect in copper utilization.

Copper in the Diet The richest dietary sources of copper are organ meats such as liver and kidney. Seafood, nuts and seeds, whole grain breads and cereals, and chocolate are also good sources. As with many other trace elements, soil content affects the amount of copper in plant foods.

Copper in the Gastrointestinal Tract About 30 to 40% of the copper in a typical diet is absorbed.[18] The absorption of copper is affected by the presence of other minerals and vitamins in the diet. The zinc content of the diet can have a major impact on copper absorption. When zinc intake is high, it stimulates the synthesis of the protein **metallothionein** in the mucosal cells. Metallothionein helps regulate zinc absorption; however, metallothionein preferentially binds copper rather than zinc. Therefore, when metallothionein is synthesized, it binds copper, preventing it from being moved out of mucosal cells into the blood.[19] The antagonism between copper and zinc is so great that phytates, which inhibit zinc

Metallothionein A protein that binds zinc and copper in intestinal cells and limits their absorption into the blood.

absorption, actually increase the absorption and utilization of copper. Copper absorption is also reduced by high intakes of iron, manganese, and molybdenum. Other factors that affect copper absorption include vitamin C, which decreases absorption,[18] and large doses of antacids, which inhibit copper absorption and, over the long term, can cause copper deficiency.

Copper in the Body Once absorbed, copper binds to albumin, a protein in the blood, and travels to the liver, where it binds to the protein ceruloplasmin for delivery to other tissues. Copper can be removed from the body by secretion in the bile and subsequent elimination in the feces.

Copper functions in a number of important proteins and enzymes that are involved in iron and lipid metabolism, connective tissue synthesis, maintenance of heart muscle, and function of the immune and central nervous systems.[20] The copper-containing protein ceruloplasmin converts iron into a form that can bind to transferrin for transport. Copper is also an essential component of the antioxidant enzyme **superoxide dismutase (SOD).** Copper plays a role in cholesterol and glucose metabolism, and elevated blood cholesterol levels have been reported in copper deficiency. It is also needed for the synthesis of the neurotransmitters norepinephrine and dopamine, and may be involved in the synthesis of myelin, which is necessary for transmission of nerve signals.

Superoxide dismutase (SOD) An enzyme that protects the cell from oxidative damage by neutralizing superoxide free radicals. One form of the enzyme requires zinc and copper for activity and another form requires manganese.

How Much Copper Do We Need? There is no 1989 RDA for copper. The ESADDI is 1.5 to 3.0 mg per day for adults. The American Academy of Pediatrics recommends that formula-fed newborns consume about 0.4 mg of copper per day. Needs increase throughout childhood until they reach adult levels. Specific recommendations have not been made for pregnancy, lactation, or the elderly.[21]

Copper and Health The amount of copper in Western diets is below or in the low range of the ESADDI.[20] In addition, the consumption of foods such as breakfast cereals that are commonly fortified with iron and zinc—minerals that interfere with copper absorption—may have an impact on copper status.[22] Despite this, severe copper deficiency is relatively rare, occurring most often in preterm infants. Marginal copper deficiency may be more prevalent but has been difficult to diagnose.[23]

Copper Deficiency The most common manifestation of copper deficiency is anemia. This is due primarily to the fact that the copper-containing protein ceruloplasmin is needed for iron transport. In copper deficiency, even if iron is sufficient in the diet, iron cannot be transported out of the intestinal mucosa. In addition, when copper is deficient the copper-containing antioxidant enzyme superoxide dismutase is not available to protect red blood cell membranes from oxidative damage further contributing to anemia. A third connection between copper and anemia is copper's role in the synthesis of the connective tissue protein collagen. Connective tissue cannot form properly when copper is deficient. Because connective tissue strengthens blood vessels, vessels are weakened and may rupture when copper is deficient, causing blood loss and, consequently, anemia. Copper's role in the synthesis of connective tissue may also explain the skeletal changes that occur due to deficiency. These mimic the skeletal abnormalities observed with vitamin C deficiency (scurvy), and include osteoporosis and bone fractures.[20] Copper deficiency has also been associated with impaired growth, degeneration of the heart muscle, degeneration of the nervous system, and changes in hair color and structure. Because of copper's role in the development and maintenance of the immune system, a diet low in copper decreases the immune response and increases the incidence of infection.[24,25]

Copper Toxicity Copper toxicity from dietary sources is extremely rare. No toxicity has been reported from intakes up to 0.5 mg per kilogram of body weight, or

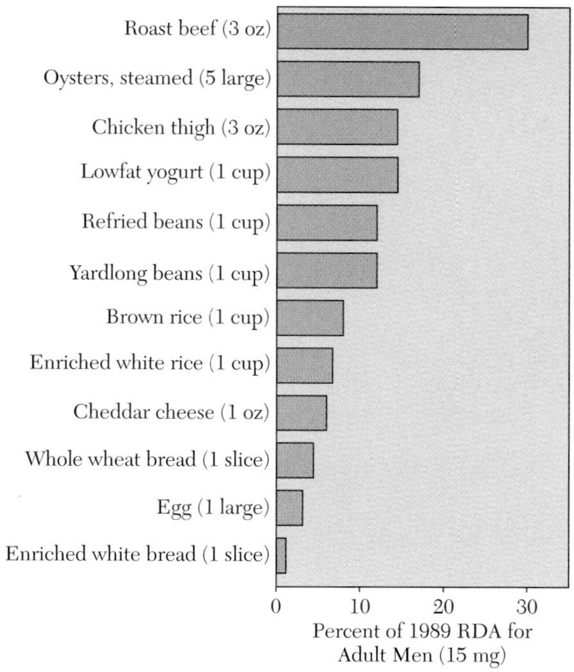

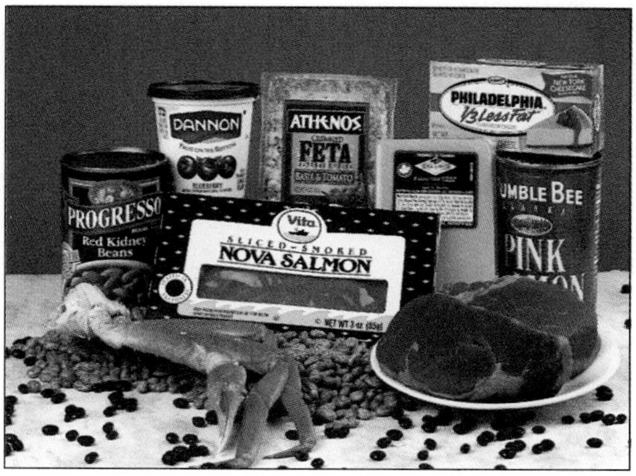

Figure 11.6
The zinc content of foods as a percentage of the 1989 RDA for adult men. (*right,* George Semple)

about 3.5 mg per day. An occasional intake of up to 10 mg per day is probably safe, but acute doses of greater than 10 to 15 mg may cause vomiting.[21]

Zinc (Zn)

Dietary zinc interacts with both iron and copper. A diet high in iron can decrease zinc absorption, while a high-zinc diet decreases copper absorption. Zinc and copper both function in the antioxidant enzyme superoxide dismutase.

Zinc in the Diet Zinc is found in foods from both plant and animal sources. Zinc from animal sources is better absorbed than that from plants, because the zinc in plant foods is often bound by phytates. Zinc is abundant in red meat, liver, eggs, dairy products, vegetables, and some seafood (Figure 11.6). Whole grains are a good source but refined grains are not, because zinc is lost in milling and not added back in enrichment. Grain products leavened with yeast provide more zinc than unleavened products because the yeast leavening of breads reduces the phytate content.[26]

Zinc in the Gastrointestinal Tract The amount of zinc in the body is regulated in part by the amount that is absorbed. Zinc entering the mucosal cells of the intestine may be used by the mucosal cell itself, pass through the cell into the blood, or be bound by the protein metallothionein, which helps regulate the amount of zinc that reaches body tissues. Zinc in the mucosal cell stimulates the synthesis of metallothionein, and when zinc intake is high more metallothionein is made. Zinc bound to metallothionein is not easily transported out of the muscosal cell and is lost when the cells die (Figure 11.7). Conversely, when zinc intake is low, metallothionein synthesis is not stimulated, so concentrations drop and zinc is readily transferred from the mucosal cells to the blood. Since metallothionein does not completely prevent zinc transfer, high intakes can override this regulatory mechanism.

Zinc in the Body Once zinc has been absorbed, homeostasis can be maintained to some extent by regulating excretion. Zinc is contained in pancreatic juice,

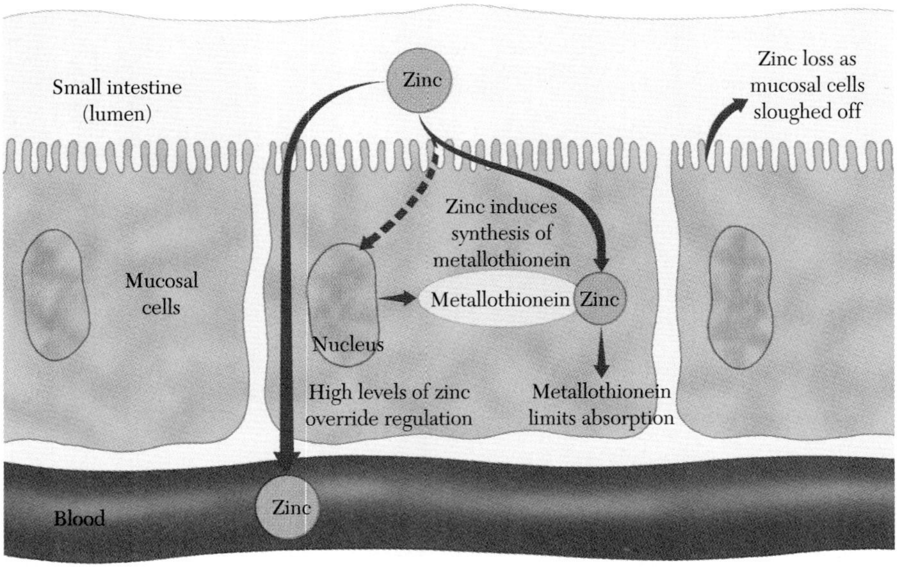

Figure 11.7
Zinc absorption is regulated by the protein metallothionein in intestinal mucosal cells.

which is secreted into the intestine. When zinc levels are low, the zinc lost in pancreatic juice can be reabsorbed and recycled. When levels are high, it is not reabsorbed and is therefore eliminated in the feces.

Many of the functions of zinc can be traced to its role in gene expression. Zinc is needed for the activity of vitamin A, vitamin D, and a number of hormones. Without zinc, these nutrients and hormones cannot bind to DNA to increase or decrease gene expression, and, hence, the synthesis of certain proteins. Zinc is therefore needed for the growth and repair of tissues, the activity of the immune system, and the development of sex organs and bone. In addition to this role in gene expression, zinc is involved in the functioning of at least 70 different enzymes, including a form of superoxide dismutase, which is vital for protecting cells from free radical damage. Zinc is essential for enzymes needed for DNA and RNA synthesis and it also plays a role in the storage and release of insulin, the mobilization of vitamin A from the liver, and the stabilization of cell membranes.

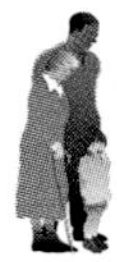

How Much Zinc Do We Need? The 1989 RDA for zinc is 15 mg per day for men and 12 mg per day for women. During pregnancy, the recommendation for zinc is increased to meet the needs of maternal and fetal tissues. During lactation, the increase in zinc requirement is calculated from the amount of zinc secreted in breast milk. The 1989 RDA for formula-fed infants has been set at 5 mg per day. Breast-fed infants need less zinc than formula-fed infants because the protein in human breast milk enhances the bioavailability of zinc. The recommended intake for children is 10 mg of zinc per day. Although zinc requirements do not appear to change with age, the elderly population may be at risk for zinc deficiency because of low intake.[27]

Zinc and Health Zinc, like iron and copper, is important in providing antioxidant protection to the body. The symptoms of zinc deficiency reflect its importance in protein synthesis and gene expression. Because it is needed for the proper functioning of vitamins A and D and the activity of numerous enzymes, deficiency symptoms can resemble deficiencies of other essential nutrients.

Zinc Deficiency The essentiality of zinc in the human diet was first recognized about 30 years ago, when a syndrome of growth depression and delayed sexual development, seen in Iranian and Egyptian men consuming diets based on vegetable protein, was alleviated by supplemental zinc.[28] Although the diet was not low in zinc, it was high in grains containing phytates, which interfered with zinc absorption, causing a deficiency. The symptoms of zinc deficiency include growth retardation, loss of appetite, taste changes, delayed sexual maturation, dermatitis, hair loss, skeletal abnormalities, malabsorption, night blindness, and depressed immunity.[29] Because zinc is required for vitamin A transport, a deficiency can affect vitamin A status.[30] The risk of zinc deficiency is greater in individuals who consume diets low in animal foods, including the elderly, low-income children, and vegetarians—particularly female vegans—and when diets high in phytates, fiber, tannins, and oxalates are consumed, as in developing countries. Although uncommon in North America, in developing countries zinc deficiency has important health and developmental consequences.[31,32]

Zinc Toxicity Zinc can be toxic when consumed in excess of recommendations. Acute zinc toxicity occurs with intakes of 2 grams or more, which can cause gastrointestinal irritation and vomiting. Intakes of 50 to 300 mg per day have been shown to cause decreased immune function and a reduction in HDL cholesterol, the type of cholesterol that has a protective effect against heart disease.[33] Supplements providing 50 mg per day of zinc have been shown to interfere with the absorption of copper.[19] Supplements providing more than 15 mg of zinc are not recommended.

Zinc Supplements Zinc is often marketed as a supplement to improve immune function, enhance fertility and sexual performance, and cure the common cold. For individuals consuming adequate zinc, there is no evidence that extra is beneficial. In individuals with a mild zinc deficiency, supplementation may result in improved wound healing, immunity, and appetite; in children it can result in improved growth and learning. In healthy older adults, supplements of zinc have been shown to improve the immune response (see Chapter 15).[34] Oversupplementation may result in toxicity and can also contribute to copper deficiency. Evidence to support the effectiveness of zinc lozenges as a cold treatment is equivocal—some studies find a benefit while others do not (see *Off the Shelf: Will Zinc Cure the Common Cold?*).[35]

Manganese (Mn)

Manganese, like copper and zinc, protects against oxidative damage by functioning in superoxide dismutase. The form of the enzyme that requires manganese is located inside the mitochondria.

The best dietary sources of manganese are whole grains and nuts. Fruits and vegetables are fair sources; meat, fish, and poultry are poor sources (Table 11.2).

Manganese homeostasis is maintained by regulating both absorption and excretion. As with iron, manganese absorption increases when intake is low and decreases when intake is high. Manganese is eliminated by excretion into the intestinal tract in bile. Manganese is involved in carbohydrate and lipid metabolism and brain function, and is needed as a constituent of some enzymes and an activator of others.

How Much Manganese Do We Need? The ESADDI for manganese is 2 to 5 mg per day for adults. This was established based on the typical intake of manganese, since deficiency does not appear to be a nutritional problem in the United States.

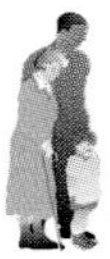

Breast-fed infants consume about 2 mg per day of manganese during the first months of life. This level of intake results in decreases in tissue levels of manganese, but no deficiency symptoms have been reported. Once solid foods are introduced into the infant diet, manganese intake increases.

It is not known if the manganese requirement is increased by pregnancy, but absorption of manganese triples during pregnancy. Since very little manganese is lost in breast milk, it is unlikely that lactation increases needs.[21]

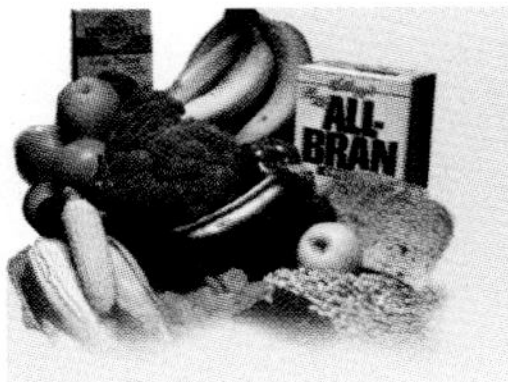

Off the Shelf

Will Zinc Cure the Common Cold?

Despite advances in modern medical science, the common cold remains as common as ever. Adults in the United States develop two to four colds per year, and children get six to eight.[1] Colds make you feel miserable and decrease productivity—and are responsible for 15 million sick days each year.

It is likely that man has been trying to cure the common cold for as long as viruses have been causing coughs and sneezes. Your great grandmother may have had nothing to offer but a bowl of chicken soup, or maybe honey with lemon, for your cough. Today there are a multitude of over-the-counter medications to relieve symptoms. They will lower your fever, clear your nose, and suppress your cough, but they won't make your cold go away. Since folk remedies and pharmaceuticals are unable to cure the common cold and people are unwilling to take time out of their busy lifestyles to rest and drink plenty of fluids, many have turned to dietary supplements that promise to make colds go away. Vitamin C has been promoted as a cold cure for many years. And although it can't cure a cold, there is some evidence that it reduces a cold's duration and symptoms (see Chapter 9).

A more recent addition to the medicine cabinet is zinc lozenges, which promise to reduce the duration and severity of the common cold. Do they keep their promise? Of the double-blind placebo-controlled clinical trials that have been completed to assess the efficacy of zinc lozenges, half have shown them to be effective while the other half found no difference between the placebo and zinc groups. Analyses of these trials concluded that any benefit is maximized if the lozenges are started immediately after the onset of cold symptoms.[2] One reason for the difference between trial results is speculated to be the difference in the formulation of the lozenges used. To have an effect, the zinc needs to be delivered as Zn^{2+} ions to the mucosal surfaces. Lozenges that released Zn^{2+} ions into the saliva shortened colds, but lozenges that released negatively charged zinc ions actually lengthened colds.[3] The lozenges found to release the most Zn^{2+} ions contained zinc acetate. Zinc gluconate also released Zn^{2+} ions and is the form that has been used most frequently in over-the-counter preparations. The zinc in your daily vitamin and mineral supplement will not have any effect because this zinc goes to your stomach and doesn't contact the mucosal surfaces affected by cold viruses. The addition of citric acid or tartaric acid to the lozenge will bind zinc and decrease the amount available.

Thus far there is little information regarding the mechanism whereby zinc might affect cold symptoms. It has been suggested that zinc may block the inflammatory response by complexing with proteins on the cold virus and on human cells.[4]

Should you take zinc lozenges? They are certainly not a cure, and the evidence supporting their benefits is not conclusive, but anything that shows promise in making the sniffles go away faster is irresistible to many. However, zinc is toxic at high doses. Too much zinc can suppress the immune system, lower HDL levels, and impair copper absorption. The lozenges each contain about 11–14 mg of elemental zinc, and the dosage instructions say to take no more than 6 lozenges in 24 hours. This dose is almost six times the 1989 RDA for zinc. If you try zinc lozenges, try cautiously. Use them only when you have a cold, not to prevent colds. And it can't hurt to also have a bowl of chicken soup.

[1]Mossad, S., Macknin, M., Mendendorp, S., and Mason, P. Zinc gluconate lozenges for treating the common cold: a randomized, double-blind, placebo-controlled study. Ann. Intern. Med. 125:81–88, 1996.

[2]Garland, M. L., and Hagmeyer, K. O. The role of zinc lozenges in treatment of the common cold. Ann. Pharmacother. 32:63–69, 1998.

[3]Eby, G. A. Zinc ion availability—the determinant of efficacy in zinc lozenge treatment of common colds. J. Antimicrob. Chemother. 40:483–493, 1997.

[4]Novick, S. G., Godfrey, J. C., Pollack, R. L., and Wilder, H. R. Zinc-induced suppression of inflammation in the respiratory tract caused by infection with human rhinovirus and other irritants. Med. Hypotheses 49:347–357, 1997.

Manganese and Health Manganese deficiency in animals results in growth retardation, reproductive problems, congenital malformations in the offspring, and abnormalities in brain function, bone formation, glucose regulation, and lipid metabolism.

Although a naturally occurring manganese deficiency has never been reported in humans, a man participating in a study of vitamin K was inadvertently fed a diet deficient in manganese for 17 weeks. He lost weight, his black hair turned a red color, and he developed dermatitis. Manganese deficiency was further studied in young male volunteers fed a manganese-deficient diet for 39 days. These men developed dermatitis and had altered blood levels of cholesterol, calcium, and phosphorus.[21]

Toxic levels of manganese result in damage to the nervous system. In humans, toxicity has been reported in manganese mine workers exposed to high

Table 11.2 *A Summary of Good Dietary Sources of Trace Elements**

Mineral	Bread, Cereal, Rice, & Pasta Group	Vegetable Group	Fruit Group	Milk, Yogurt, & Cheese Group	Meat, Poultry, Fish, Dry Beans, Eggs, & Nuts Group				Other
					Meats	Dry Beans	Eggs	Nuts & Seeds	
Iron	Whole and enriched grains	Leafy greens	Dried fruit		Meat, poultry, fish	Tofu, kidney beans			Iron cookware
Copper	Whole grains				Organ meats, seafood			Nuts and seeds	Chocolate
Zinc	Whole grains	Vegetables		Yogurt, cheese	Red meat, liver	Legumes	Eggs		
Manganese	Whole grains							Nuts and seeds	
Selenium					Seafood, organ meats		Eggs		
Iodine				Dairy products	Fish, seafood				Iodized salt
Chromium	Whole grains				Organ meats			Nuts and seeds	Brewer's yeast
Fluoride					Fish with bones				Water, tea, toothpaste
Molybdenum	Whole grains			Dairy products	Organ meats	Legumes			

*The colored boxes indicate food groups that provide a good source of each mineral.

concentrations of inhaled manganese dust. Dietary intakes of up to 10 mg per day are considered safe.[21]

Selenium (Se)

Although selenium was discovered about 180 years ago, its essential role in human nutrition was not recognized until the 1970s. Selenium functions in an important antioxidant enzyme that works in concert with vitamin E to protect the body from oxidative damage. Because of the similar roles of selenium and vitamin E, it has been difficult to separate symptoms of selenium deficiency from those of vitamin E deficiency.

Selenium in the Diet Seafood, kidney, liver, and eggs are excellent sources of selenium (see Table 11.2). Fruits, vegetables, and drinking water are generally poor sources of selenium. Grains and seeds can be good sources depending on the selenium content of the soil where they were grown. For example, wheat grown in Kansas has a different selenium content from wheat grown in Michigan. Soil selenium content can have a significant impact on the selenium intake of populations consuming primarily locally grown food.

Selenium in the Body Once selenium is absorbed, homeostasis is maintained by regulating its excretion in the urine. Selenium is an essential part of the enzyme **glutathione peroxidase.** Glutathione peroxidase neutralizes peroxides so they no longer form free radicals, which cause oxidative damage. By reducing free radical formation, selenium can spare some of the requirement for vitamin E, because vitamin E is used to stop the action of free radicals once they are produced (Figure 11.8). Selenium is also needed for the synthesis of the thyroid hormones, which regulate basal metabolic rate.

Glutathione peroxidase A selenium-containing enzyme that protects cells from oxidative damage by neutralizing peroxides.

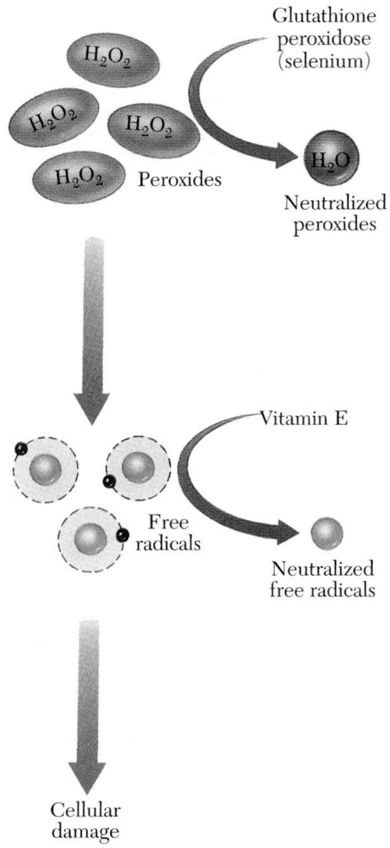

Figure 11.8
Selenium is a part of the enzyme glutathione peroxidase, which neutralizes peroxides before they form free radicals. This can spare some of the need for vitamin E.

How Much Selenium Do We Need? The 1989 RDA for selenium is 55 μg per day for women and 70 μg per day for men. The estimated average intake of selenium in the United States meets or nearly meets this recommendation for all age groups.[36]

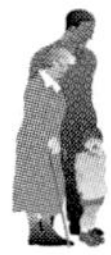

An increase in selenium intake is recommended during pregnancy and lactation. The1989 RDA for infants is 10 μg per day for the first six months of age and 15 μg per day after six months.

Selenium and Health Selenium intake has been suggested to be related to the incidence of both heart disease and cancer, probably through its antioxidant function. Epidemiological studies have shown that a low selenium intake is associated with an increased risk of developing heart disease.[37] The mechanism is not known. The hypothesis that selenium protects against cancer was developed based on the increased incidence of certain human cancers in regions where selenium intake is low. A clinical study that provided supplements of 200 μg per day to skin cancer patients found that, in the selenium-supplemented group, skin cancer recurrence was not reduced but total cancer incidence, cancer mortality, and cases of lung, prostate, and colon cancer all decreased compared to the placebo group.[38] The mechanism of cancer protection is believed to be selenium's ability to turn on the self-destruct mechanism in cancer cells and therefore eliminate cancers before they spread.[39]

Selenium Deficiency A role for selenium was first recognized by studying animals deficient in vitamin E. Selenium deficiency was not identified in humans until the late 1970s when it was observed in patients fed TPN solutions inadvertently deficient in selenium and in individuals living in a region of China where the soil is selenium deficient. Symptoms of deficiency include muscular discomfort and weakness. A form of heart disease called Keshan disease may also occur with selenium deficiency. Selenium supplements relieve most of the symptoms of Keshan disease and reduce its incidence, but selenium deficiency is not the only cause of this disease.[40] It is hypothesized to be due to several interacting factors which include selenium deficiency, other nutritional factors, and an infectious agent.[41] Selenium deficiency is not likely to be a problem when the diet includes foods grown in many different locations.

Selenium Toxicity Adverse effects occur at levels of 910 μg of selenium per day and may occur with intakes as low as 600 μg per day, but intakes of 200 μg per day have been shown to be safe.[42] At levels of about 1000 μg per day, symptoms such as hair loss, fingernail loss, and gastrointestinal problems occur. In a region of China with very high selenium in the soil, an intake of 5 mg per day resulted in fingernail changes and hair loss. Selenium toxicity has also been reported in the United States because of a manufacturing error that created mineral supplements containing a dose of 27 mg of selenium per day. The individuals who used these supplements had symptoms which included nausea, diarrhea, abdominal pain, fingernail and hair changes, nervous system abnormalities, fatigue, and irritability.[21]

Selenium Supplements Selenium supplements are marketed with claims that they will protect against environmental pollutants, prevent cancer and heart disease, slow the aging process, and improve immune function. Although selenium does play a role in these processes, supplements of selenium have not been shown to be of additional benefit except perhaps in the case of cancer, where supplements have been shown (see the study mentioned above) to reduce cancer incidence. If you decide to protect yourself from cancer by increasing selenium intake, it may be difficult to do with diet because the selenium content depends on where the food is grown. If you decide to take a supplement, be cautious and select one that contains no more than 200 μg per day.

Minerals With Unique Functions

Although many minerals serve complementary and interdependent roles, others have separate unique roles. For example, as a component of the thyroid hormones, iodine helps regulate metabolic rate. Chromium is part of a complex that is important for getting glucose into cells, and fluoride helps strengthen tooth enamel. Finally, molybdenum serves a cofactor role, but is distinguished from the nutrients discussed above because it is not part of the antioxidant defenses. Despite their unique roles, these minerals are still found within the total diet, and their function depends on adequate levels of all other nutrients.

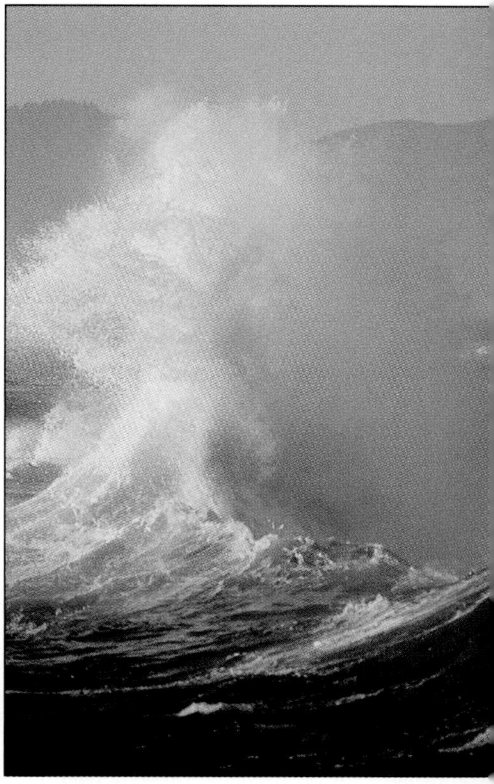

Figure 11.9
Most of the iodine in our diet comes from the sea. (© Darrell Gulin/Tony Stone Images)

Iodine (I): Regulating Metabolism

Iodine is needed for the synthesis of thyroid hormones. One hundred years ago, iodine deficiency was common in the central United States and Canada, but it has virtually disappeared due to the addition of iodine to table salt. Iodine deficiency, however, remains a world health problem.

Iodine in the Diet Most of the iodine in our diets comes from the sea. There are high concentrations of iodine in seawater and seafood (Figure 11.9). Plants grown close to the sea are high in iodine. The amount of iodine in plants grown inland depends on the iodine content of the soil.

Iodine in our diet also comes from contaminants and additives in foods. Dairy products may contain iodine because of the iodine-containing additives used in cattle feed and the use of iodine-containing disinfectants on cows, milking machines, and storage tanks. Iodine-containing sterilizing agents are also used in fast-food restaurants, and iodine is used in dough conditioners and some food colorings. Most of the iodine in the North American diet comes from salt fortified with iodine, referred to as iodized salt. It is commonplace in the United States, and only iodized salt is sold in Canada. Iodized salt should not be confused with sea salt, which is a poor source of iodine because the iodine is lost in the drying process.

Iodine in the Body Iodine is an essential component of the thyroid hormones, which regulate basal metabolic rate, growth and development, and promote protein synthesis. Iodine, along with selenium, is essential for the synthesis of thyroid hormones. If blood levels of the thyroid hormones drop, thyroid-stimulating hormone is released. This hormone signals the thyroid gland in the neck to take up iodine and synthesize thyroid hormones. When the supply of iodine is adequate, thyroid hormones can be made and their presence turns off the synthesis of thyroid-stimulating hormone (Figure 11.10).

How Much Iodine Do We Need? The 1989 RDA for iodine in adult men and women is 150 μg per day. The current intake of iodine in North America exceeds this amount but is considered safe.[36]

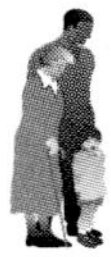

Iodine needs are increased during pregnancy and lactation. The recommended intake for infants is 40 μg, an amount that is easily obtained from breast milk or formula. The recommended intake is not different for older adults.

Iodine and Health Enlargement of the thyroid gland occurs with too little and too much iodine. In terms of world health, deficiency is of greater impact than toxicity, and programs to fortify the food supply with iodine or to supplement individuals in the population are used to reduce the incidence of iodine deficiency (see *Off the Label: Should You Choose Iodized Salt?*).

Iodine Deficiency Iodine deficiency reduces the production of thyroid hormones. Metabolic rate slows with insufficient thyroid hormones, causing fatigue and

Off the Label

Should You Choose Iodized Salt?

When selecting a box of salt for the kitchen cupboard, you can choose one that just says "salt" or one that is labeled "iodized salt." Iodized salt is salt to which the trace element iodine has been added. Which should you choose?

Iodine is an essential nutrient. The amount we consume in our diet depends as much on where foods are grown as on which foods we choose. Foods produced in regions where the soil is rich in iodine are better sources of iodine than foods produced in regions where the soil is iodine-poor. The iodine content of plants grown in iodine-deficient soil may be 100 times less than those grown in iodine-rich soil.[1] When the earth was formed, all soils were high in iodine, but today iodine is most plentiful in areas close to the sea. Mountainous areas and river valleys have little iodine left in the soil because it has been washed out by glaciers, snow, rain, and flood waters. The iodine washed from the soil has accumulated in the oceans, where it is present as iodide ions. When these ions come in contact with sunlight, they are oxidized to form iodine, which can escape into the air. Every year approximately 400,000 tons of iodine escapes into the atmosphere from the ocean surface. The iodine in the atmosphere is returned to the soil in rain, but the return is slow and the amounts returned to the soil are small. In areas where the forces of nature have resulted in iodine-deficient soil, the iodine deposited from rain will be washed away again by these same forces. Therefore, iodine-deficient soil will remain deficient.

Iodine-depleted soil is not new to the planet's ecology. Its effect on human health has become a part of history in many areas of the world. In Europe the presence of iodine deficiency was recorded by classical art, which portrayed even the wealthy with goiter and cretinism. Leonardo da Vinci is said to have been more knowledgeable about goiter than medical professors of his time.[2] A century ago goiter was endemic in the central regions of North America. And in parts of Asia today, iodine deficiency is a major public health problem.

In the United States, Switzerland, and some other European countries, iodine deficiency was virtually eliminated in the early part of the 20th century by the iodinization of salt. And today, developing nations, where iodine deficiency is still a public health problem, have experimented with iodized salt[3,4] as well as iodine-fortified fish sauce, sugar, and drinking water as ways to add iodine to the diet.[5,6]

Why fortify salt? The Dietary Guidelines for Americans recommend that we consume salt in moderation. If we follow that guideline or choose plain salt, will we get enough iodine? Salt was selected as the vehicle for added iodine because it is a food item consistently consumed by the majority of the population at risk. People did not need to change their eating habits to include the fortified product in their diet. The iodine also could be added to salt uniformly, inexpensively, and in a form that was well utilized by the body. It could be added in amounts that would eliminate deficiency when typical quantities of salt were consumed by the population, but would not cause toxicity in those consuming larger amounts of iodized salt or in those who already meet their iodine needs from other sources.

In the United States today, iodine deficiency is rare. Iodized salt is available and the typical diet includes foods from many sources across the country and around the world. In addition to iodine from seafood and plants grown in iodine-rich soils, we get iodine from food additives and food processing. Does this mean that we are getting enough iodine from the foods we eat? Do we still need iodized salt? In Canada there is no choice; all salt is iodized. In the United States, both are available. If you live inland where the soil is deficient in iodine, and you eat little seafood and consume primarily foods grown locally, iodized salt is the best choice. If you live on the coast and buy your food in a supermarket, you are unlikely to be iodine deficient even if you choose plain salt. But because there are few risks associated with consuming the amounts of iodine added to salt, choose iodized if you are not sure.

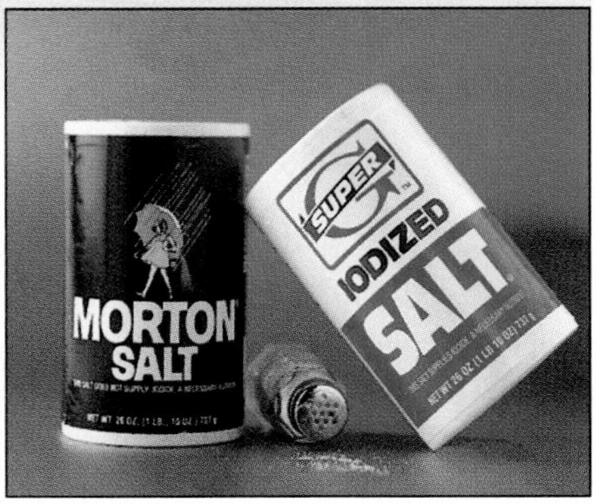

(George Semple)

[1]Hertzel, B. S., and Clugston, G. A. Iodine. In *Modern Nutrition in Health and Disease,* 9th ed. Shils, M. E., Olson, J. A., Shike, M., and Ross, A. C. Baltimore: Williams & Wilkins, 1999, 253–264.

[2]Underwood, B. A. Micronutrient malnutrition: is it being eliminated? Nutr. Today 33:121–129, 1998.

[3]Melse-Boonstra, A., Rozendaal, M., Rexwinkel, H., et al. Determination of discretionary salt intake in rural Guatemala and Benin to determine the iodine fortification of salt required to control iodine deficiency disorders: studies using lithium-labeled salt. Am. J. Clin. Nutr. 68:636–641, 1998.

[4]Ranganathan, S., and Reddy, V. Human requirements of iodine and safe use of iodized salt. Indian J. Med. Res. 102:227–232, 1995.

[5]Eltom, M., Elnagar, B., Sulieman, E. A., et al. The use of sugar as a vehicle for iodine fortification in endemic iodine deficiency. Int. J. Food Sci. Nutr. 46:281–289, 1995.

[6]Saowakhontha, S., Sanchaisuriya, P., Pongpaew, P., et al. Compliance of population groups of iodine fortification in endemic areas of goiter in northeast Thailand. J. Med. Assoc. Thai. 77:449–454, 1994.

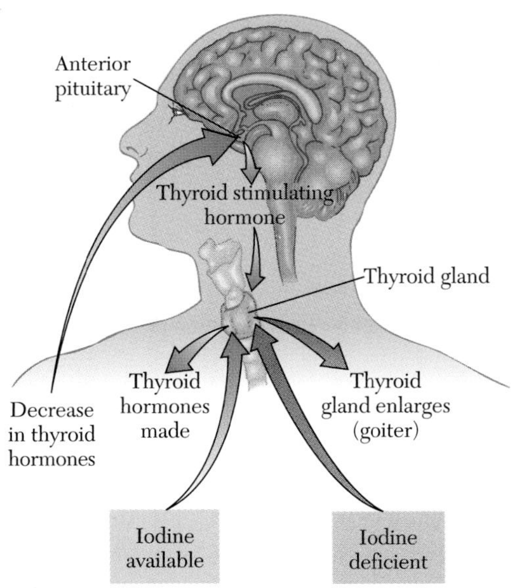

Figure 11.10
When thyroid hormone levels drop too low, thyroid-stimulating hormone stimulates the thyroid gland to take up iodine and synthesize more hormones. If iodine is not available, the stimulation continues and the thyroid enlarges, forming a goiter.

weight gain. The most obvious outward sign of deficiency is an enlarged thyroid gland called a **goiter** (Figure 11.11). A goiter forms when reduced thyroid hormone levels cause thyroid-stimulating hormone to be released, stimulating the thyroid gland to make more thyroid hormones. Because iodine is unavailable, the hormones cannot be made and the stimulation continues causing the thyroid gland to enlarge. In milder cases of goiter, treatment with iodine causes the thyroid gland to return to normal size, but this result is not consistent in more severe cases.

Goiter An enlargement of the thyroid gland caused by a deficiency of iodine.

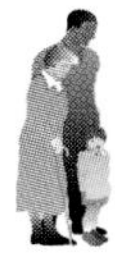

A number of other iodine deficiency disorders occur because of the effect of iodine on growth and development. If iodine is deficient during pregnancy, it increases the risk of stillbirth and spontaneous abortion. Deficiency also can cause a condition called **cretinism** in the offspring. There are a number of forms of cretinism characterized by symptoms such as mental retardation, deaf mutism, and growth failure. Iodine deficiency during childhood and adolescence can also result in goiter and impaired mental function.

Cretinism A condition resulting from poor maternal iodine intake during pregnancy that causes stunted growth and poor mental development in offspring.

The risk of iodine deficiency is increased by consuming **goitrogens,** substances in food that interfere with the utilization of iodine or with thyroid function. Goitrogens are found in turnips, rutabaga, cabbage, and cassava. Most are destroyed in cooking or are present in foods that do not play an important role in human diets. However, in African countries where cassava is a dietary staple, high goitrogen intake may play a role in the development of iodine deficiency disorders.[43]

Goitrogens Substances that interfere with the utilization of iodine or the function of the thyroid gland.

Iodine Fortification Since it was first used in Switzerland in the 1920s, iodized salt has been the major means of combating iodine deficiency. Because of the fortification of table salt with iodine, cretinism and goiter are now rare in North America, but worldwide, 600 million people have goiter and 1.5 billion people are at risk for iodine deficiency.[44] At the recommendation of the United Nations Joint Committee on Health Policy, salt iodinization is now being applied in most countries with an iodine deficiency disease problem of public health significance.[45] For groups who do not have access to iodized salt or who will not use it, other forms of iodine supplementation, such as injections or oral doses of iodized oil may be effective for control of iodine deficiency.[46]

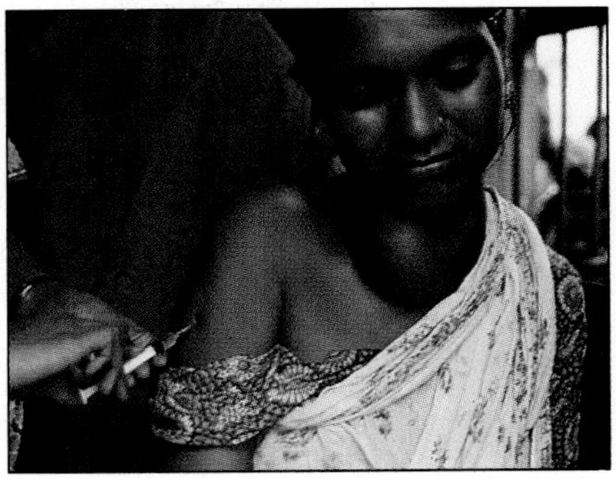

Figure 11.11
Iodine deficiency causes enlargement of the thyroid gland, a condition called goiter. (John Paul Kay/Peter Arnold, Inc.)

Iodine Toxicity Acute toxicity can occur with very large doses of iodine. Intakes between 200 and 500 mg per kilogram of body weight have caused death in laboratory animals.[21] Chronically high intakes of iodine can cause an enlargement of the thyroid gland that resembles goiter. This can also occur if iodine intake changes drastically. For example, in a population with a marginal intake, a large increase in intake due to supplementation can cause thyroid enlargement even at levels that would not be toxic in a healthy population.[47] Generally, doses of 2 mg or less per day have no toxic effects.

Chromium (Cr): Insulin Action

Chromium is essential for insulin to function normally. Currently it is recognized by many as the popular supplement chromium picolinate, promoted to increase lean body mass.

Chromium in the Diet Dietary sources of chromium include liver, brewer's yeast, nuts, and whole grains. Milk, vegetables, and fruit are poor sources. Refined carbohydrates such as white breads, pasta, and white rice are also poor sources because chromium is lost in milling and not added back in the enrichment process. Chromium intake can be increased by cooking in stainless steel cookware because chromium leaches from the steel into the food.

Chromium in the Body In general, chromium is poorly absorbed; however, absorption increases when chromium intake is low.

Chromium is involved in carbohydrate and lipid metabolism. It is part of a glucose tolerance factor necessary for insulin action and hence the transport of glucose into cells, but the exact mechanism is not known. Deficient dietary chromium has been suggested to play a role in glucose intolerance and the development of type 2 diabetes.[48] Chromium supplementation at levels that exceed the upper limit of the ESADDI have been shown to have beneficial effects on blood glucose, insulin, and cholesterol levels in individuals with type 2 diabetes.[49]

How Much Chromium Do We Need? The ESADDI for chromium is 50 to 200 μg per day for adults.[21] This level is recommended because no deficiency signs have been reported in American populations consuming around 50 μg and no adverse affects have been reported in studies of subjects with daily intakes of 200 μg.

Chromium and Health Chromium deficiency is not a problem in the U.S. population, but marginal deficiency may play a role in the development of type 2 diabetes.

Chromium Deficiency Current dietary intake of chromium is often below the minimum suggested intake of 50 μg per day.[49] Deficiencies have been reported in patients receiving long-term TPN not containing chromium and in malnourished children. Deficiency symptoms include impaired glucose tolerance with diabetes-like symptoms, such as elevated blood glucose levels and increased insulin levels. Chromium deficiency may also cause elevated blood cholesterol and triglyceride levels, but the role of chromium in lipid metabolism is not fully understood.[50]

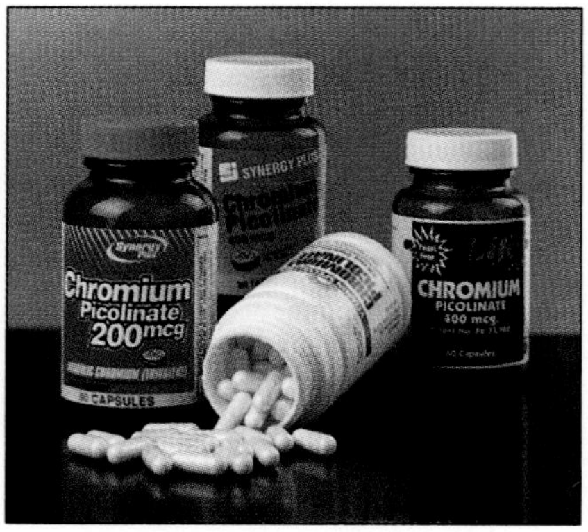

Figure 11.12
Chromium supplements are marketed to increase lean body mass and decrease body fat. (George Semple)

Chromium Toxicity Despite widespread use of chromium supplements among athletes, no dietary toxicity has been reported in humans, and oral chromium picolinate at doses containing 1.0 mg of chromium per day has produced no adverse effects.[42]

Chromium Supplements Chromium supplements, marketed as chromium picolinate, have been promoted recently to reduce body fat and increase lean body tissue. This appeals to individuals wanting to lose weight as well as to athletes trying to build muscle (Figure 11.12). Because chromium is needed for insulin action and insulin promotes protein synthesis, it is likely that adequate chromium is necessary to increase lean body mass. However, research in humans has not consistently shown chromium picolinate supplements to affect muscle strength or body composition.[51,52]

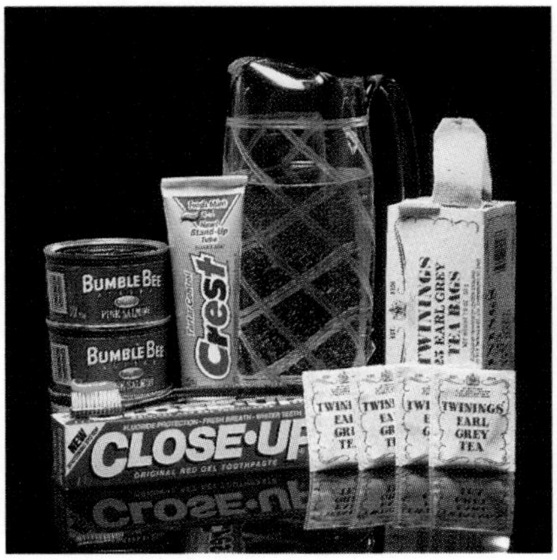

Figure 11.13
Dietary sources of fluoride include water, tea, fish eaten with bones, and toothpaste. (Charles D. Winters)

Fluoride (F): Strong Teeth

The importance of fluoride for dental health has been recognized since the 1930s, when an association between the fluoride content of drinking water and the prevalence of dental caries was noted.

Fluoride in the Diet Fluoride is present in small amounts in almost all soil, water, plants, and animals. The richest dietary sources of fluoride are fluoridated water, tea, and marine fish consumed with their bones (Figure 11.13). Tea contributes significantly to total fluoride intake in countries that consume large amounts of the beverage. Brewed tea contains 1 to 6 mg of fluoride per liter depending on the amount of dry tea used, the brewing time, and the fluoride content of the water.[53] In the United States, most of the fluoride in the diet comes from toothpaste and from fluoride added to the water supply—usually 0.7 to 1.2 mg per liter (Water companies often report fluoride levels in parts per million [ppm], 1 mg/liter = 1 ppm). Because food readily absorbs the fluoride in cooking water, the fluoride content of food can be significantly increased when it is handled and prepared using fluoridated water. Cooking utensils also affect food fluoride content. Foods cooked with Teflon utensils can pick up fluoride from the Teflon, whereas aluminum cookware can decrease fluoride content. Fluoride is absorbed into the body in proportion to its content in the diet.

Fluoride in the Body Fluoride has a high affinity for calcium and so is usually associated with calcified tissues such as bones and teeth. Fluoride is incorporated into the tooth enamel crystals, where it forms the compound fluorhydroxyapatite, which is more resistant to acid than the hydroxyapatite crystals it replaces.

How Much Fluoride Do We Need? The criterion used to establish an AI for fluoride was the estimated intake shown to reduce the occurrence of dental caries maximally without causing unwanted side effects. Epidemiology has confirmed the effectiveness of fluoridated water in reducing dental cavities.[54] The AI for fluoride from all sources is set at 0.05 mg per kg per day for all ages six months and older because it protects against dental caries with no adverse effects.[53] Thus, for children age four through eight years, the AI is set at 1.1 mg per day using a reference weight of 22 kg. For adult men age 19 and older, the AI is 3.8 mg per day based on a weight of 76 kg, for women, it is 3.1 mg per day based on a weight of 61 kg. The AI is not increased in pregnancy or lactation.

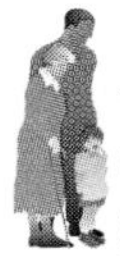

Breast milk is low in fluoride, and ready-made infant formulas are prepared with unfluoridated water. Unless infant formula is prepared at home with fluoridated water, it contains little fluoride. The American Academy of Pediatrics suggests a supplement of 0.25 mg per day for children 6 months to 3 years of age, 0.5 mg per day for ages 3 to 6 years, and 1.0 mg per day for ages 6 to 16 who are receiving less than 0.3 mg per liter of fluoride in the water supply.[55] These supplements are available by prescription for children living in areas with low water fluoride concentrations. Swallowed toothpaste is estimated to contribute about 0.6 mg per day of fluoride in young children.[53]

Fluoride and Health Adequate dietary fluoride is important for bone and dental health. Fluoride has its greatest effect on dental caries prevention early in life, during maximum tooth development up to the age of thirteen, but it has been shown to have some effect in adults.[56] In addition to making tooth enamel more acid resistant, fluoride protects teeth in other ways. Fluoride in saliva reduces

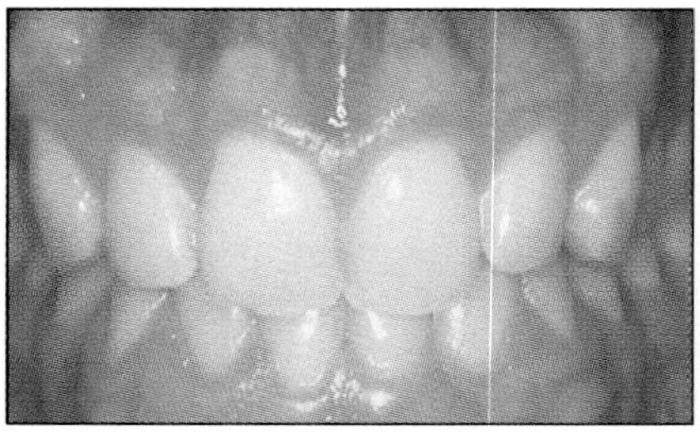

(a)

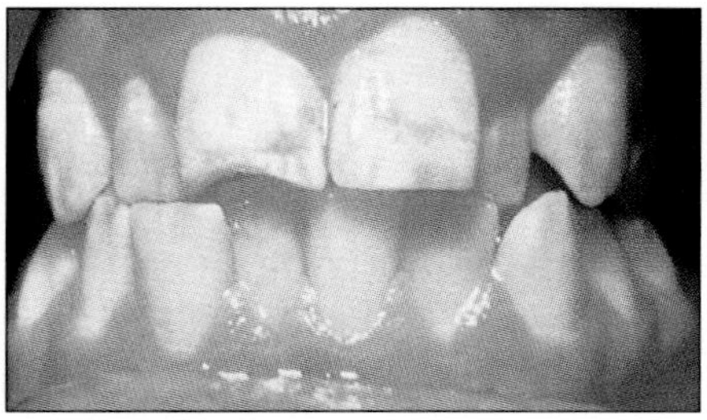

(b)

Figure 11.14
Too much dietary fluoride causes the teeth to appear mottled (enamel fluorosis). (a) Normal teeth. (b) Teeth showing enamel fluorosis. (*a,* © Edward H. Gill/Custom Medical Stock Photo; *b,* © NIH/Custom Medical Stock Photo)

cavities by reducing acid produced by bacteria and by increasing enamel remineralization after acid exposure.[57] Fluoride seems to stimulate new bone formation and has therefore been suggested to strengthen bones in adults with osteoporosis. Slow-release fluoride supplements have been shown to increase bone mass and prevent new fractures.[58]

Fluoride Toxicity Fluoride can cause adverse effects in high doses. Fluoride intakes of 2 to 8 mg per day can cause mottled teeth in children (Figure 11.14). A recent increase in the prevalence of this condition in the United States has occurred due to the chronic ingestion of toothpaste containing fluoride. In adults doses of 20 to 80 mg per day can result in changes in bone health that can be crippling, as well as changes in kidney function and possibly nerve and muscle function. Death was reported with an intake of 5 to 10 grams per day. Due to concern over excess fluoride intake, a new warning is now required on fluoride-containing toothpastes. The label must state, "If you accidentally swallow more than used for brushing, seek professional help or contact a poison control center immediately."

The UL for fluoride is set at 0.1 mg per kg per day for infants and children less than 9 years of age, and at 10 mg per day for people ages 9 through 70.[53]

Fluoridated Water The fluoridation of public drinking water to prevent dental caries began in Grand Rapids, Michigan, in 1945. Today, over half of the U.S. population lives in communities with fluoridated drinking water.[54] Some people believe that water fluoridation represents a public health hazard and increases the risk of cancer. These beliefs are not supported by scientific facts. Based on epidemiological data and available evidence related to the adverse effects of fluoride, the small amounts consumed in drinking water do not pose a risk for health problems such as cancer, kidney failure, or bone disease.[59,60]

Molybdenum (Mo)

Like many other trace elements, molybdenum is needed to activate enzymes. The molybdenum content of food varies with the molybdenum content of the soil where the food is produced. The most reliable sources include milk, milk products, organ meats, breads, cereals, and legumes.

Molybdenum is readily absorbed from foods. The amount in the body is regulated by excretion in the urine and bile. Molybdenum is a cofactor for enzymes necessary for the metabolism of sulfur-containing amino acids and nitrogen-containing compounds present in DNA and RNA, the production of uric acid, and the oxidation and detoxification of various other compounds.

Although molybdenum deficiency in humans has been reported as a result of long-term TPN, a naturally occurring deficiency has never been reported. Deficiency has been induced in laboratory animals by feeding them high doses of the element tungsten, which inhibits molybdenum absorption. The resulting deficiency caused growth retardation, decreased food intake, impaired reproduction, and decreased life expectancy.

Based on estimates of molybdenum intake in the American diet, the ESADDI has been set at 75 to 250 μg per day for adults.[24]

Toxicity has been reported in a region with high environmental molybdenum. Intakes of 10 to 15 mg per day have been associated with goutlike symptoms such as arthritis and inflammation of the joints. Molybdenum also interacts with copper, and levels of 500 μg per day have been associated with increased excretion of copper in the urine.[24]

Other Trace Elements

During the past 25 years animal experiments have provided evidence of the essentiality of many other trace elements.[61] These include aluminum, arsenic, boron, bromine, cadmium, germanium, lead, lithium, nickel, rubidium, silicon, tin, and vanadium. In the case of boron, studies in humans have confirmed the original reports of its role in animals,[62] and the evidence that arsenic, nickel, and silicon are essential in humans is more compelling than it is for many of the others.[63]

Boron (B)

Boron in the forms of borax and boric acid was used as a preservative in fish, meats, and ham from the 1870s until the 1950s. It has been known to be essential in plants for almost 70 years, but only since the early 1980s has boron been recognized as an essential element in the human diet. Foods of plant origin such as fruits, leafy vegetables, nuts, and legumes are rich sources of boron. Cider, wine, and beer are also high in boron, whereas meat, fish, and dairy products are poor sources. Drinking water can also contribute significant amounts of boron, depending on the geographical location.

Although the biochemical function of boron is unknown, studies suggest that it is involved in vitamin D metabolism and affects calcium and magnesium homeostasis. It has also been hypothesized to be involved in the maintenance of cell membranes and in cell communication. Boron deficiency has been demonstrated in animals and humans.[62] In the young, a deficiency retards growth. In adults, boron deficiency increases urinary excretion of calcium and magnesium and affects the levels of certain steroid hormones.

Surveys indicate that the average daily intake of boron is in the range of 1 to 2 mg per day.[62] Despite our limited understanding of boron, several brands of nutritional supplements containing boron are marketed to protect against osteoporosis. Since our understanding of the role of boron in bone formation and breakdown is in its infancy, a balanced diet, rather than supplements, is a safer way to ensure adequate boron intake.

Arsenic (As)

Although we usually think of arsenic as a poison, the organic forms of arsenic that occur in foods are nontoxic. Fish, meats, grains, cereal products, and starchy vegetables contribute to the arsenic content of the diet. Arsenic is hypothesized to affect the conversion of the amino acid methionine into compounds that affect heart function and cell growth.[63] A deficiency of arsenic depresses growth and impairs reproduction in several species of animals, and in humans it has been correlated with nervous system disorders, blood vessel diseases, and cancer.[64] The arsenic needs of humans are estimated to be in the range of 12 to 25 μg per day.[63]

Nickel (Ni)

Good dietary sources of nickel include chocolate, nuts, legumes, and grains. Diets high in fat and foods of animal origin may be low in nickel. Nickel is thought to function in enzymes involved in the metabolism of certain fatty acids and amino acids, and it may play a role in folate metabolism.[65] It also affects the distribution and functioning of a number of other nutrients, including calcium, iron, zinc, folate, and vitamin B_{12}. Nickel deficiency has been shown in a number of animal species and results in depressed growth, impaired reproductive performance, and decreased plasma glucose levels.[66] Human intakes of dietary nickel are generally less than 150 μg per day.[66]

Silicon (Si)

Silicon is involved in the synthesis of collagen and the calcification of bone, possibly by aiding in collagen cross-linking and in the initiation of bone mineralization.[63] Dietary silicon sources include whole grain products and root vegetables. Silicon deficiency has been reported in chickens and rats and results in abnormalities in bone and connective tissue.

Aluminum (Al) , Bromine (Br), Cadmium (Cd), Germanium (Ge), Lead (Pb), Lithium (Li), Rubidium (Rb), Tin (Sn), and Vanadium (V)

Specific functions for aluminum, bromine, cadmium, germanium, lead, lithium, rubidium, tin, and vanadium have not been defined; however, growth depression and impaired reproduction have been demonstrated in animals fed diets lacking in these elements. Since deficiencies can be produced only under laboratory conditions with the strictest precautions to prevent contamination, requirements, if they exist, are likely to be very low and easily met by amounts normally consumed in the diet (Figure 11.15). For some of these elements, a defined biochemical function and essentiality may ultimately be established; for others, presence in the human body may be the result of environmental exposure.

For all of the essential trace elements, there is a range of intake that is safe and compatible with good health. When either too much or too little is consumed, health is adversely affected.[67] All the minerals, both those known to be essential and those that are still being assessed for their role in human health, can be obtained by choosing a variety of foods from each of the groups of the Food Guide Pyramid (Figure 11.16).

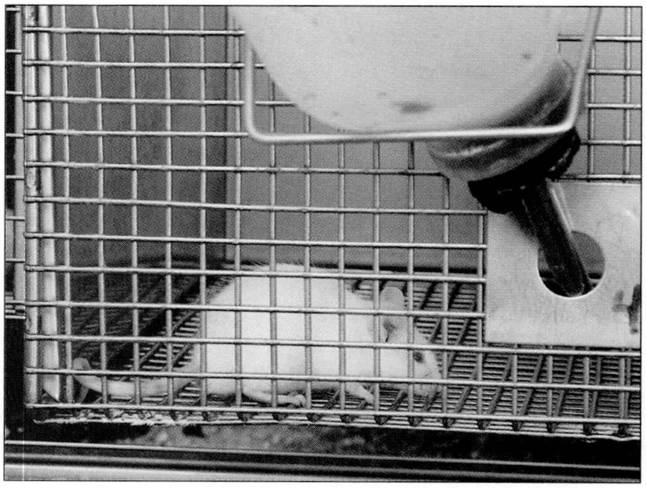

Figure 11.15
Some trace elements are required in such small amounts that deficiencies are found only under strictly controlled laboratory conditions. (Matt Meadows/Peter Arnold, Inc.)

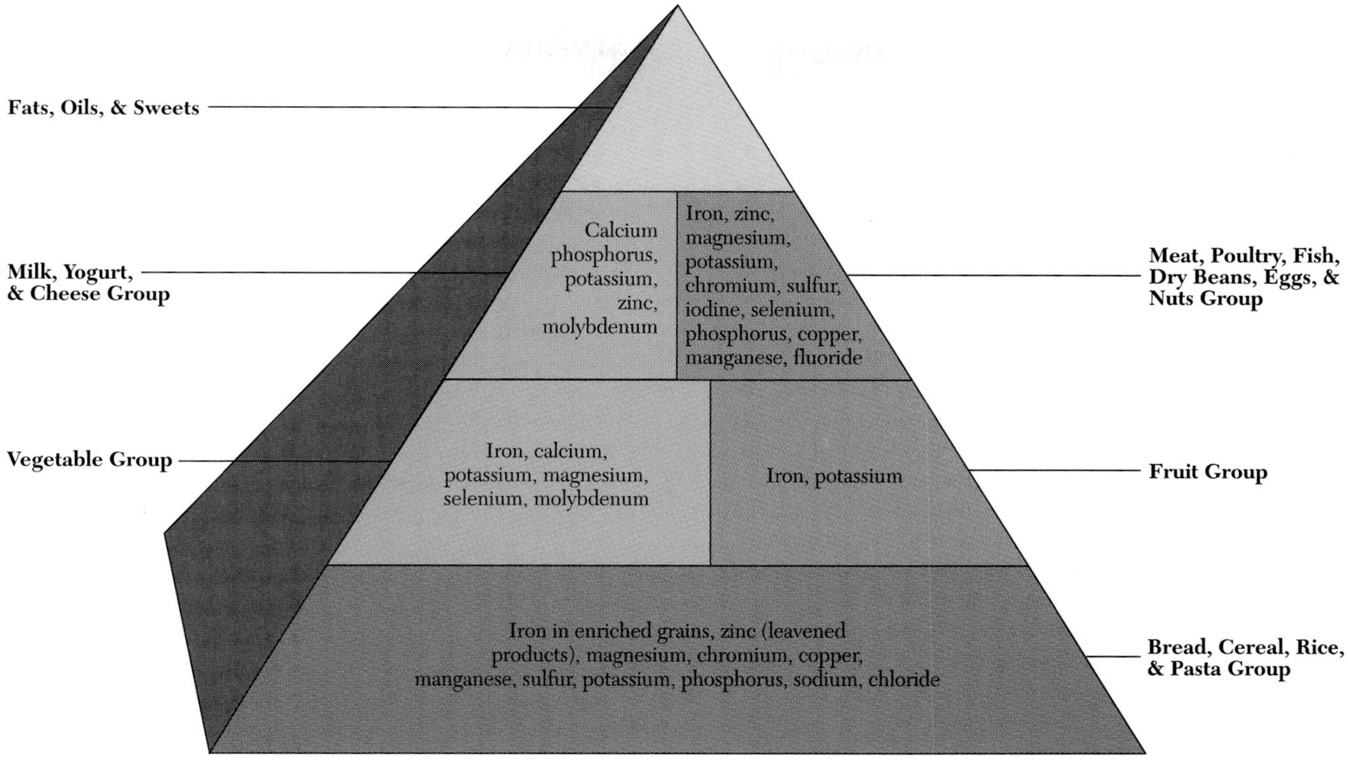

Figure 11.16
Each group of the Food Guide Pyramid includes foods that are good sources of minerals; good sources of all minerals are not found within any one group. The Meat, Poultry, Fish, Dry Beans, Eggs, & Nuts Group contributes the most variety of minerals because of the diverse types of foods—ranging from beef to legumes and nuts—found in this group.

APPLICATIONS

These exercises are designed to help you apply your critical thinking skills to your own nutrition choices. Many are best performed using a diet analysis software program. If you do not have access to a computer program, the exercises can be hand-calculated using the information in this text and its appendices.

1. Using the three-day food intake record you kept in Chapter 2:
   a. Calculate your average daily intake of iron.
   b. How does your iron intake compare with the recommendation for someone of your age and sex?
   c. If your intake is low, modify your diet to meet the 1989 RDA for iron for someone your age and sex.
   d. If your diet already meets the recommendations for iron, make a list of foods you like that are good sources of iron.
   e. Identify the major food sources of iron in your diet and indicate whether they contribute heme iron.
2. Using your food record, calculate your zinc intake.
   a. If you eliminated meat from your diet, would you meet the 1989 RDA for zinc?
   b. What foods could you substitute for meat that would allow you to meet the 1989 RDA?
3. Using the Internet, search for information on a supplement discussed in this chapter—for instance, zinc lozenges or chromium picolinate.
   a. How does the information compare to the discussion in the text?
   b. Who provided the information? Does it promote the sale of a product?
   c. Is the information supported by scientific studies?

Summary

1. Trace elements are required in the diet in small amounts. Although, iron, zinc, copper, manganese, and selenium each have unique roles, they are also all involved in either transporting oxygen in the body or in protecting us from its damaging effects.
2. Iron functions as part of hemoglobin, which transports oxy-

gen in the blood, and myoglobin, which stores oxygen for use during muscle contraction. When iron is deficient, adequate hemoglobin cannot be made, resulting in iron deficiency anemia—the most common nutritional deficiency worldwide. Iron is also a component of many enzymes, including some in the electron transport chain and the antioxidant enzyme catalase.

3. The amount of iron that is absorbed from the diet depends on the type of iron, other dietary components, and the body's need for the element. Much of the iron in animal-based food products is heme iron, an easily absorbable form. Nonheme iron, which is not well absorbed, comes from both animal and plant sources. If body iron stores are low, more iron is transported from the intestinal mucosa to body cells. When body stores are adequate, less iron is transported from the mucosa.
4. Iron can be toxic. Ingestion of a single large dose can be fatal. The accumulation of iron in the body over time causes heart and liver damage and contributes to diabetes and certain types of cancer. The most common cause of chronic iron overload is hemochromatosis, a genetic disorder in which too much iron is absorbed.
5. Copper functions in a number of important proteins that affect iron and lipid metabolism, synthesis of connective tissue, and antioxidant protection. The copper-containing protein ceruloplasmin is needed for iron transport. The richest sources of copper in the diet are organ meats. A copper deficiency can cause anemia and bone abnormalities.
6. Zinc absorption is regulated by metallothionein, a protein that binds zinc in the mucosal cells and limits how much can enter the blood. Since copper binds the same protein, an excess of zinc can stimulate metallothionein synthesis and trap copper in the mucosal cells, causing a copper deficiency.
7. Zinc is needed for the activity of many enzymes, including a form of the antioxidant enzyme superoxide dismutase that also requires copper. Many of the functions of zinc are believed to be related to its role in gene expression. Zinc is needed for tissue growth and repair, development of sex organs and bone, proper immune function, storage and release of insulin, mobilization of vitamin A from the liver, and stabilization of cell membranes. Good sources of zinc include red meats, eggs, dairy products, and whole grains. Zinc deficiency results in poor growth, delayed sexual maturation, skin changes, hair loss, skeletal abnormalities, and depressed immunity.
8. Manganese is necessary for the activity of some enzymes, including a form of the antioxidant enzyme superoxide dismutase. Manganese is involved in carbohydrate and lipid metabolism and brain function. Good dietary sources include whole grains and nuts.
9. Selenium protects against oxidative damage as an essential part of the enzyme glutathione peroxidase. Glutathione peroxidase destroys peroxides before they can form free radicals. Adequate dietary selenium reduces the need for vitamin E. Dietary sources include seafood, eggs, organ meats, and plant foods grown in selenium-rich soils. Severe selenium deficiency is rare except in regions with very low soil selenium content and limited diets. In China, selenium deficiency is associated with a heart condition known as Keshan disease. Low selenium intake has been linked to increased cancer risk.
10. Iodine is an essential component of thyroid hormones, which control basal metabolic rate, growth, and development. The best sources of iodine in the diet are seafood, foods grown near the sea, and iodized salt.
11. When iodine is deficient, continued release of thyroid-stimulating hormone causes the thyroid gland to enlarge, forming a goiter. Iodine deficiency during pregnancy causes a condition in the offspring known as cretinism, which is characterized by growth failure and mental retardation. Iodine deficiency during childhood and adolescence can impair mental function. Although iodine deficiency is a world health problem, it has been virtually eliminated in North America through the use of iodized salt.
12. Chromium is needed for normal insulin action and glucose utilization. It is found in liver, brewer's yeast, nuts, and whole grains.
13. Fluoride is necessary for the maintenance of bones and teeth. Adequate dietary fluoride helps prevent dental caries. Most of the fluoride in the diet in the United States comes from fluoridated drinking water and toothpaste.
14. Molybdenum is a cofactor for enzymes involved in the metabolism of the amino acids methionine and cysteine and nitrogen-containing compounds such as DNA and RNA.
15. There is evidence that boron is essential in humans and that arsenic, nickel, and silicon may be essential in humans as well as animals. Specific functions for aluminum, bromine, cadmium, germanium, lead, lithium, rubidium, tin, and vanadium have not been established. They may be necessary in small amounts but can be toxic if consumed in excess.

Review Questions

1. Why does iron deficiency cause red blood cells to be small and pale?
2. List three life stage groups at risk for iron deficiency anemia.
3. List several good sources of iron in the diet and indicate if they contain heme iron.
4. Discuss three factors that affect iron absorption.
5. What is hemochromatosis?
6. Give two reasons why a deficiency of copper can contribute to anemia.
7. Why does excess zinc cause a deficiency of copper?
8. How does zinc affect the synthesis of proteins?
9. What is the role of selenium in the body?
10. Why does selenium decrease the need for vitamin E?
11. What is a goiter and what causes it?
12. What is the role of chromium in the body?
13. How does fluoride function in dental health?
14. How are needs estimated for trace elements when traditional measures of nutrient balance and function are not available?

Nutrition Web Links

To further explore areas related to the material in this chapter, go to the *Nutrition: Science and Applications* Web site at ***www.Wiley.com/college/Smolin*** and *click on* **Student Companion Site** for chapter-by-chapter links. Some Web sites related to the information in Chapter 11 include:

Sites that provide information about diseases related to iron overload and iron deficiency such as the Iron Disorders Institute and the Iron Overload Diseases Association.

Sites that provide information about the role of fluoride in dental health such as the American Dental Association and National Center for Fluoridation Policy and Research.

Sites that provide information on iodine deficiency such as the International Council for the Control of Iodine Deficiency Disorders.

Sites that provide information on dietary supplements such as the Office of Dietary Supplements at the National Institutes of Health, and the FDA.

References

1. Underwood, B. A. Micronutrient malnutrition: is it being eliminated? Nutr. Today 33:121–129, 1998.
2. Centers for Disease Control and Prevention. Recommendations to prevent and control iron deficiency in the United States. MMWR Morb. Mortal. Wkly. Rep. 47:1–29, 1998. Online at http://www.cdc.gov/epo/mmwr/mmwr_rr.html
3. Lynch, S. R. Interaction of iron with other nutrients. Nutr. Rev. 55:102–110, 1997.
4. Bothwell, T. H. Overview and mechanisms of iron regulation. Nutr. Rev. 53:237–245, 1995.
5. Whiting, S. J. The inhibitory effect of dietary calcium on iron bioavailability: a cause for concern? Nutr. Rev. 53:77–80, 1995.
6. Kuhn, L. C. Iron and gene expression: molecular mechanisms regulating cellular iron homeostasis. Nutr. Rev. 56:S11–S19, 1998.
7. Allen, L. H. Pregnancy and iron deficiency: unresolved issues. Nutr. Rev. 55:91–101, 1997.
8. Clarkson, P. M., and Haymes, E. M. Exercise and mineral status of athletes: calcium, magnesium, phosphorus, and iron. Med. Sci. Sports Exerc. 27:831–843, 1995.
9. Guthrie, J. F., and Schwenk, N. E. Current issues related to iron status: implications for nutrition education and policy. USDA, Family Economics and Nutrition Review 9:2–19, 1996.
10. Iron-containing supplements and drugs: label warning statements and unit-dose packaging requirements. Federal Register, January 1997.
11. Corti, M. C., Gaxiano, M., and Hennekens, C. H. Iron status and risk of cardiovascular disease. Ann. Epidemiol. 7:62–68,1997.
12. Halliday, J. W. Hemochromatosis and iron needs. Nutr. Rev. 56(II): S30–S37, 1998.
13. Iron overload disorders among Hispanics—San Diego, California, 1995. MMWR Morb. Mortal. Wkly. Rep. 45:991–993, 1996.
14. Edwards, C. Q., Griffin, L. M., Ajioka, R. S., and Kushner, J. P. Screening for hemochromatosis: phenotype versus genotype. Semin. Hematol. 35:72–76, 1998.
15. Hollan, S. Iron overload in light of the identification of a haemochromatosis gene. Haematologia (Budap) 28:109–116, 1997.
16. Whiting, S. J. The inhibitory effect of dietary calcium on iron bioavailability: a cause for concern? Nutr. Rev. 53:77–80, 1995.
17. Mills, E. S. The treatment of idiopathic (hypochromic) anemia with iron and copper. Can. Med. Assoc. J. 22:175–178, 1930.
18. Wapnir, R. A. Copper absorption and bioavailability. Am. J. Clin. Nutr. 67(suppl):1054S–1060S, 1998.
19. Turnlund, J. R. Copper. In *Modern Nutrition in Health and Disease,* 9th ed. Shils, M. E., Olson, J. A., Shike, M., and Ross, A. C., eds. Baltimore: Williams & Wilkins, 1999, 241–252.
20. Uauy, R., Olivares, M., and Gonzales, M. Essentiality of copper in humans. Am. J. Clin. Nutr. 67(suppl):952S–959S, 1998.
21. National Research Council, Food and Nutrition Board. *Recommended Dietary Allowances,* 10th ed. Washington, D.C.: National Academy Press, 1989.
22. Johnson, M. A., Smith, M. M., and Edmonds, J. T. Copper, iron, zinc, and manganese in dietary supplements, infant formulas, and ready-to-eat breakfast cereals. Am. J. Clin. Nutr. 67(suppl):1035S–1040S, 1998.
23. Milne, D. B. Copper intake and assessment of copper status. Am. J. Clin. Nutr. 67(suppl):1041S–1045S, 1998.
24. Kelley, D. S., Daudu, P. A., Taylor, P. C., et al. Effects of low-copper diets on human immune response. Am. J. Clin. Nutr. 62:412–416, 1995.
25. Percival, S. S. Copper and immunity. Am. J. Clin. Nutr. 67(suppl): 1064S–1068S, 1998.
26. King, J. C., and Keen, C. L. Zinc. In *Modern Nutrition in Health and Disease,* 9th ed. Shils, M. E., Olson, J. A., Shike, M., and Ross A. C., eds. Baltimore: Williams & Wilkins, 1999, 223–239.
27. Leonard, B. M. Nutrition and immunity in the elderly: modification of immune responses with nutritional treatments. Am. J. Clin. Nutr. 66(suppl):478S–484S, 1997.
28. Prasad, A. S. Discovery of human zinc deficiency and studies in an experimental human model. Am. J. Clin. Nutr. 53:403–412, 1991.
29. Shankar, A. H., and Prasad, A. S. Zinc and immune function: the biological basis of altered resistance to infection. Am J. Clin. Nutr. 68(suppl):447S–463S, 1998.
30. Christina, P., and West, K. P. Interactions between zinc and vitamin A: an update. Am. J. Clin. Nutr. 68(suppl.):435S–441S, 1998.
31. Aggett, P. J., and Comerford, J. G. Zinc and human health. Nutr. Rev. 53:S16–S22, 1995.
32. Black, R. E. Preface: zinc for child health. Am J. Clin. Nutr. 68(suppl): 409S, 1998.
33. Sandstead, H. H. Requirements and toxicity of essential trace elements, illustrated by zinc and copper. Am. J. Clin. Nutr. 61(suppl): 621S–624S, 1995.
34. Bogden, J. D. Studies on micronutrient supplements and immunity in older people. Nutr. Rev. 53:S59–S65, 1995.
35. Jackson, J. L., Peterson, C., and Lesho, E. A meta-analysis of zinc salts lozenges and the common cold. Arch. Intern. Med. 157:2373–2376, 1997.
36. Pennington, J. A., and Schoen, S. A. Total diet study: estimated dietary intakes of nutritional elements, 1982–1991. Int. J. Vitam. Nutr. Res. 66:350–362, 1996.
37. Huttunen, J. K. Selenium and cardiovascular disease. Biomed. Environ. Sci. 10:220–225, 1997.

38. Clark, L. C., Combs, G. F. Jr., Turnbull, B. W., et al. Effect of selenium supplementation for cancer prevention in patients with carcinoma of the skin. J. Am. Med. Assoc. 276:1957–1968, 1996.
39. Harrison, P. R., Lanfear, J., Wu, L., et al. Chemopreventive and growth inhibitory effects of selenium. Biomed. Environ. Sci. 10:235–245, 1997.
40. Xu, G. L., Wang, S. C., Gu, B. Q., et al. Further investigation on the role of selenium deficiency in the aetiology and pathogenesis of Keshan disease. Biomed. Environ. Sci. 10:316–326, 1997.
41. Levander, O. A., and Beck, M. A. Interacting nutritional and infectious etiologies of Keshan disease: insights from coxsackie virus B–induced myocarditis in mice deficient in selenium or vitamin E. Biol. Trace Elem. Res. 56:5–21, 1997.
42. Hathcock, J. N. Vitamins and minerals: efficacy and safety. Am. J. Clin. Nutr. 66:427–437, 1997.
43. Rao, P. S., and Lakshmy, R. Role of goitrogens in iodine deficiency disorders and brain development. Indian J. Med. Res. 102:223–226, 1995.
44. Underwood, B. A. From research to global reality: the micronutrient story. J. Nutr. 128:145–151, 1998.
45. van der Haar, F. The challenge of the global elimination of iodine deficiency disorders. Eur. J. Clin. Nutr. 51(suppl):S3–S8, 1997.
46. Furnee, C. A. Prevention and control of iodine deficiency: a review of a study on the effectiveness of oral iodized oil in Malawi. Eur. J. Clin. Nutr. 51(suppl):S9–S10, 1998.
47. Stanbury, J. B., Ermans, A. E., Bourdoux, P., et al. Iodine-induced hyperthyroidism: occurence and epidemiology. Thyroid 8:83–100, 1998.
48. Anderson, R. A. Chromium as an essential nutrient for humans. Regul. Toxicol. Pharmacol. 26:S35–S41, 1997.
49. Anderson, R. A., Cheng, N., Bryden, N. A., et al. Elevated intakes of supplemental chromium improve glucose and insulin variables in individuals with type 2 diabetes. Diabetes 46:1786–1791, 1997.
50. Anderson, R. A. Recent advances in the clinical and biochemical manifestations of chromium deficiency in human and animal nutrition. J. Trace Elem. Exp. Med. 11:241–250, 1998.
51. Lukaski, H. C., Bolonchuk, W. W., Siders, W. A., and Milne, D. B. Chromium supplementation and resistance training: effects on body composition, strength, and trace element status of men. Am. J. Clin. Nutr. 63:954–965, 1996.
52. Anderson, R. A. Effects of chromium on body composition and weight. Nutr. Rev. 56:266–270, 1998.
53. Institute of Medicine, Food and Nutrition Board. *Dietary Reference Intakes for Calcium, Phosphorus, Magnesium, Vitamin D, and Fluoride.* Washington, D.C.: National Academy Press, 1997.
54. Horowitz, H. S. The effectiveness of community water fluoridation in the United States. J. Pub. Hlth. Dent. 56:253–258, 1996.
55. ADA (American Dental Association Council on Dental Therapeutics). New fluoride guidelines proposed. J. Am. Dent. Assoc. 125:366, 1994.
56. American Dental Association. Fluoridation facts. Online at http://www.ada.org/consumer/fluoride/facts/ff-menu.html
57. Marquis, R. E. Antimicrobial actions of fluoride for oral bacteria. Can. J. Microbiol. 41:955–964, 1995.
58. Pak, C. Y., Sakhaec, K., and Zerwekh, J. E. Sustained-release sodium fluoride in the management of established menopausal osteoporosis. Am. J. Med. Sci. 313:23–32, 1997.
59. National Research Council. The health effects of ingested fluoride. Report of the Subcommittee on the Health Effects of Ingested Fluoride, Committee on Toxicology, Board of Environmental Studies and Toxicology, Commission on Life Sciences. Washington, D.C.: National Academy Press, August 16, 1993.
60. Government assesses fluoride. FDA Consumer 25:4, May 1991.
61. Mertz, W. Risk assessment of essential trace elements: new approaches to setting recommended dietary allowances and safe limits. Nutr. Rev. 53:179–185, 1995.
62. Hunt, C. D., and Stoecker, B. J. Deliberations and evaluations of the approaches, endpoints and paradigms for boron, chromium, and fluoride dietary recommendations. J. Nutr. 126:2441S–2451S, 1996.
63. Uthus, E. O., and Seaborn, C. D. Deliberations and evaluations of the approaches, endpoints and paradigms for dietary recommendations of other trace elements. J. Nutr. 126:2452S–2459S, 1996.
64. Mayer, D. R., Kosmus, W., Beyer, W., et al. Serum arsenic and selenium concentrations in hemodialysis patients: correlations to associated diseases. In *Trace Elements in Nutrition and Health.* Abdulla, M., Vohora, S. B., and Athar, M., eds. New Delhi: Wiley Eastern Limited, 1995, 41–48.
65. Uthus, E. O., and Poellot, R. A. Dietary folate affects the response of rats to nickel deprivation. Biol. Trace Elem. Res. 52:23–35, 1996.
66. Nielsen, F. H. Other trace elements. In *Present Knowledge in Nutrition*, 7th ed. Ziegler, E. E., and Filer, L. J. Jr., eds. Washington D.C.: ILSI Press, 1996, 353–377.
67. Mertz, W., Abernathy, C. O., and Olin, S. S., eds. *Risk Assessment of Essential Elements.* Washington, D.C.: ILSI Press, 1994.

IV

Applying Nutrition to Life

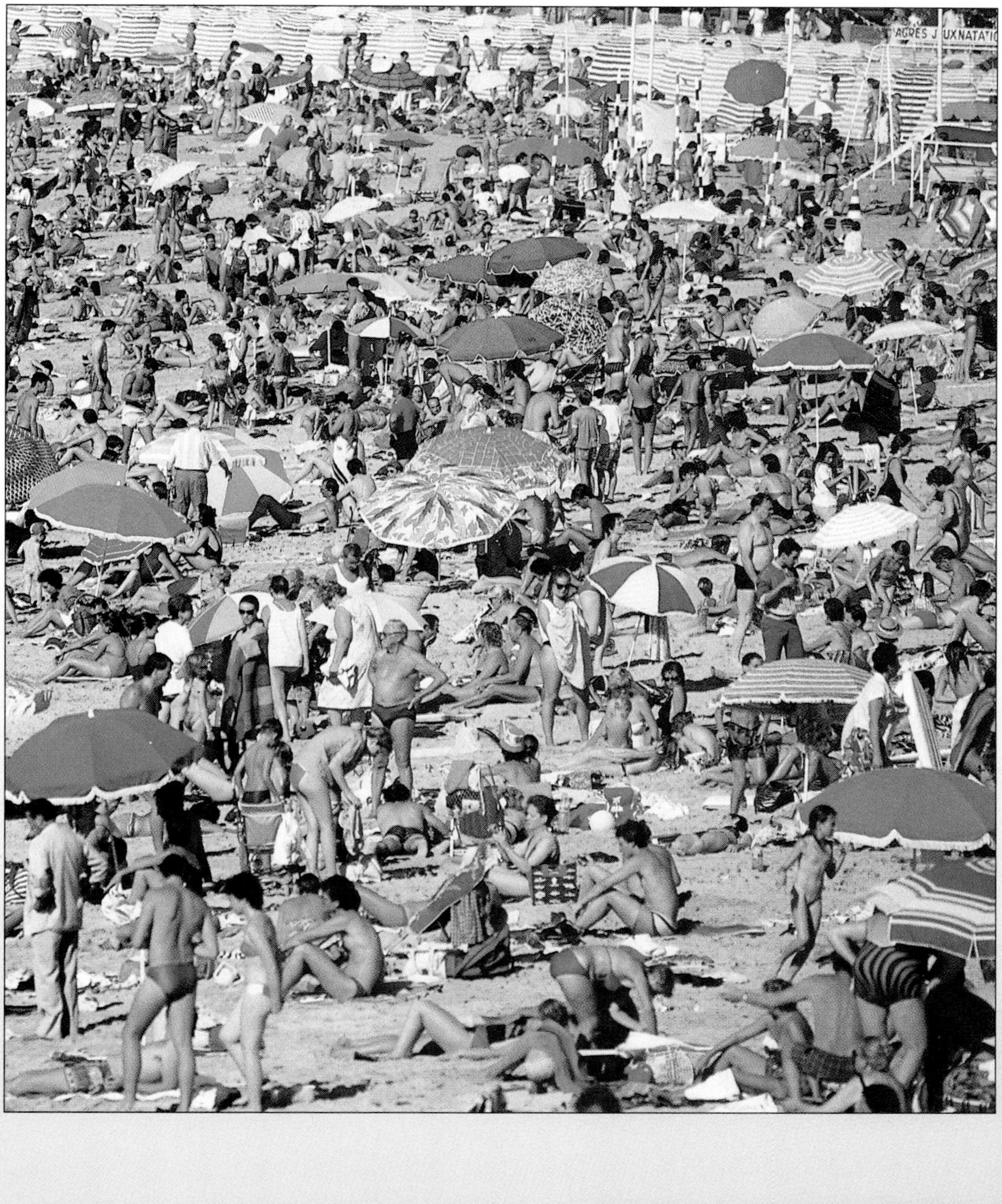

Chapter 12

Chapter Outline

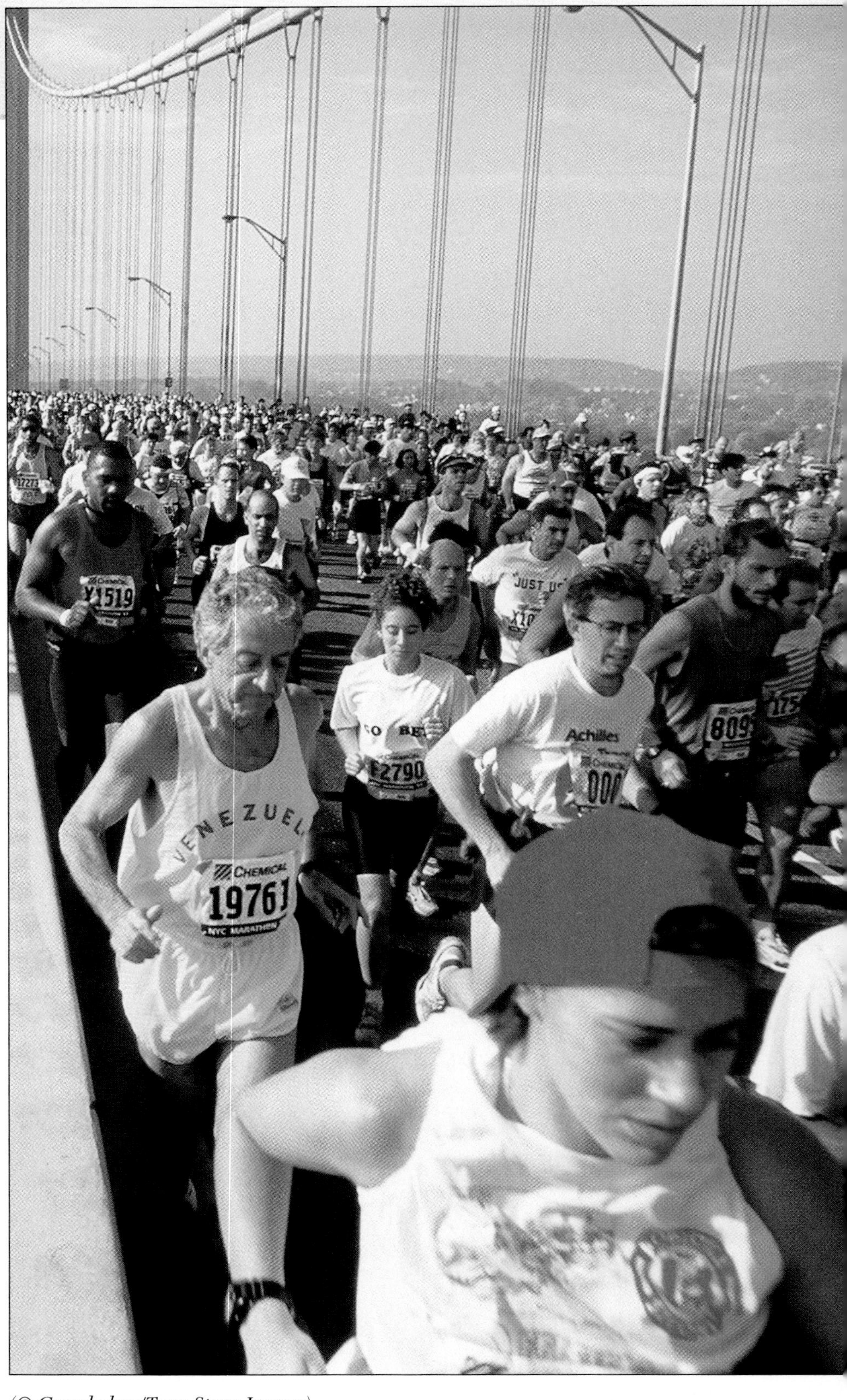

(© Grandadam/Tony Stone Images)

Fueling Fitness: Nutrition and Exercise

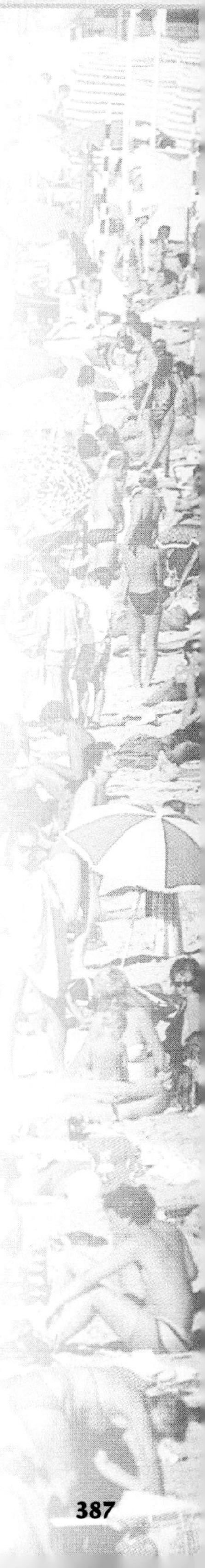

Chapter Concepts

1. Enhancing fitness through regular exercise can improve overall health and reduce the risk of chronic disease. Despite this, most Americans get little exercise.
2. An active lifestyle includes exercise that is part of everyday life as well as planned exercise activities. A well-designed exercise program includes aerobic exercise, stretching, and strength training.
3. Activity requires ATP generated from the breakdown of carbohydrate, fat, and protein.
4. The availability of oxygen affects which nutrients can be used to produce ATP and how much is produced.
5. The fuel used by the body to power activity depends on the intensity and duration of the exercise and the physical conditioning of the exerciser.
6. Diets for physically active individuals should provide adequate energy and the same proportions of carbohydrate, fat, and protein that are recommended for the general population.
7. Athletes may be at risk for deficiencies of iron and calcium.
8. Sufficient water is essential during all types of exercise to transport nutrients, eliminate wastes, and cool the body.
9. Nutrient intake before, during, and after competition may affect athletic performance.
10. The popularity of performance-enhancing (ergogenic) supplements continues to increase among athletes. Before they are used, the risks should be weighed against the benefits.

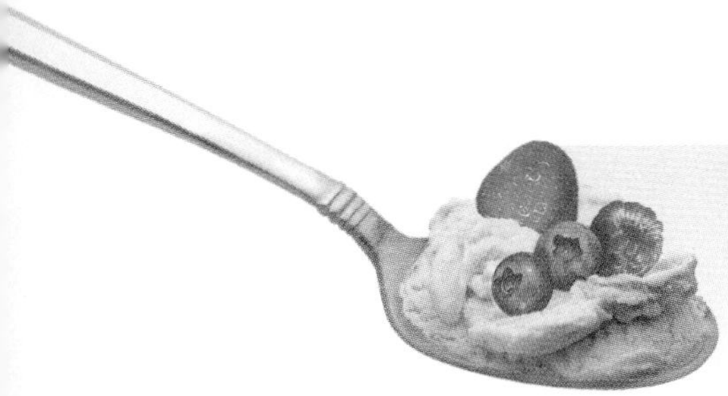

Just a Taste

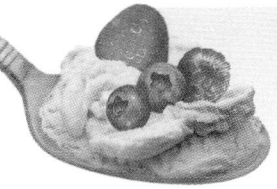

How much exercise is enough?

Does exercise increase protein needs?

Can dietary supplements enhance athletic performance?

Good nutrition is important throughout life, and specific nutrient needs vary with stage of life, gender, and activity level. In the previous chapters of this book, the principles of nutrition have been presented; in this chapter, these principles will be applied to a special condition—exercise. Exercise influences nutritional status and overall health, and nutrition has an impact on exercise ability. Both sound nutrition and physical activity are essential to good health.

Although many of us think of exercise as running marathons and competing in the Olympic Games, even moderate exercise can improve health and fitness. For some, fitness means being able to easily walk around the block, mow the lawn, or play with their children. For more seasoned athletes, fitness means optimal performance of strenuous exercise. For everyone, fitness reduces the risk of chronic diseases such as cardiovascular disease and obesity. In turn, diet and nutritional status can influence exercise performance. Whether your goal is maintaining your health or competing in athletic events, nutrition provides a launching pad from which physical fitness can be improved. The right mixture of the energy-containing nutrients—carbohydrate, fat, and protein—along with adequate micronutrients and water enhances the performance of the body "machine."

To understand the nutritional needs for activity—whether the activity is a brisk walk through the park or a 100-mile bicycle tour—the principles of nutrition must be applied to the special context of activity.

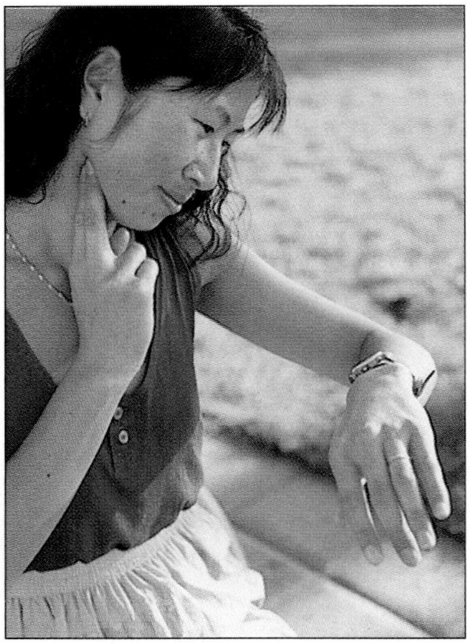

Figure 12.1
Heart rate can be estimated by feeling the pulse at the side of the neck just below the jaw bone. A pulse is caused by the heart beating and forcing blood through the arteries. The number of pulses per minute equals heart rate. (© Michael Newman/PhotoEdit)

Fitness in Your Life

Exercise improves **fitness.** You don't need to run 10-kilometer races or swim the English Channel to be physically fit. Even a small amount of exercise is better than none, and, within reason, more exercise is better than less. Whether you are 16 or 60, fitness through regular exercise can improve your overall health.

The Many Faces of Fitness

Fitness involves cardiorespiratory endurance, muscle strength and endurance, flexibility, and desirable body composition. These components of fitness are important for athletes but also extend to every aspect and task of daily life.

Cardiorespiratory Endurance Cardiorespiratory endurance determines how long you can continue a task, whether it is climbing stairs, raking leaves, or running a race. It requires muscle strength but also involves the cardiovascular and respiratory systems, referred to jointly as the **cardiorespiratory system.** Endurance is increased by **aerobic exercise,** the type of exercise that increases the heart rate and uses oxygen. To be aerobic, an activity should be performed at an intensity low enough to allow you to carry on a conversation but high enough that you cannot sing while exercising. Aerobic activities include walking, dancing, jogging, cross-country skiing, cycling, and swimming.

Regular aerobic exercise strengthens heart muscle and increases **stroke volume,** which is the amount of blood pumped with each beat of the heart. This in turn decreases **resting heart rate,** which is the rate at which the heart must beat to supply blood to the tissues at rest. Resting heart rate can be estimated by measuring the pulse (Figure 12.1). The more fit people are, the lower their resting heart rate and pulse are and the more activity they can perform before reaching **maximum heart rate.** Maximum heart rate is the maximum number of beats per minute that the heart can attain. It is dependent on age and can be estimated by subtracting one's age from 220. Aerobic exercise should be performed at a heart rate of 60 to 90% of maximum heart rate. For example, a 40-year-old individual would have a maximum heart rate of 180 beats per minute and should exercise at a pace that keeps the heart rate between 108 and 162 beats per minute (see Figure 12.2).

Fitness The ability to perform routine physical activity without undue fatigue.

Cardiorespiratory system The circulatory and respiratory systems which together deliver oxygen and nutrients to cells.

Aerobic exercise Exercise such as jogging, swimming, or cycling that increases heart rate and requires oxygen in metabolism. This type of exercise improves cardiovascular fitness.

Stroke volume The volume of blood pumped by each beat of the heart.

Resting heart rate The number of times that the heart beats per minute while a person is at rest.

Maximum heart rate The maximum number of beats per minute that the heart can attain. It declines with age and can be estimated by subtracting age in years from 220.

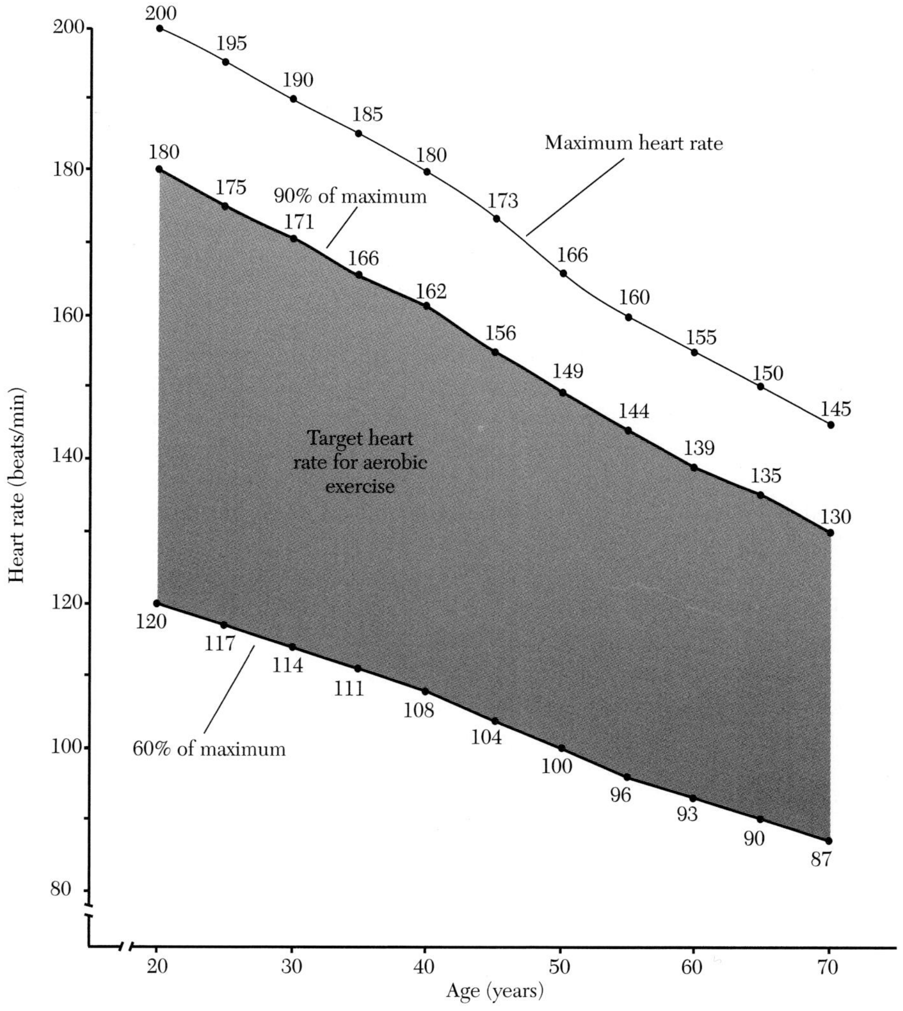

Figure 12.2

The orange area represents the target heart rate for aerobic exercise—between 60 and 90% of maximum heart rate. Exercise performed at this level will benefit cardiovascular health. (Adapted from McArdle, W. D., Katch, F. I., and Katch, V. L. *Exercise Physiology: Energy, Nutrition, and Human Performance*, 3rd ed. Philadelphia: Lea & Febiger, 1991.)

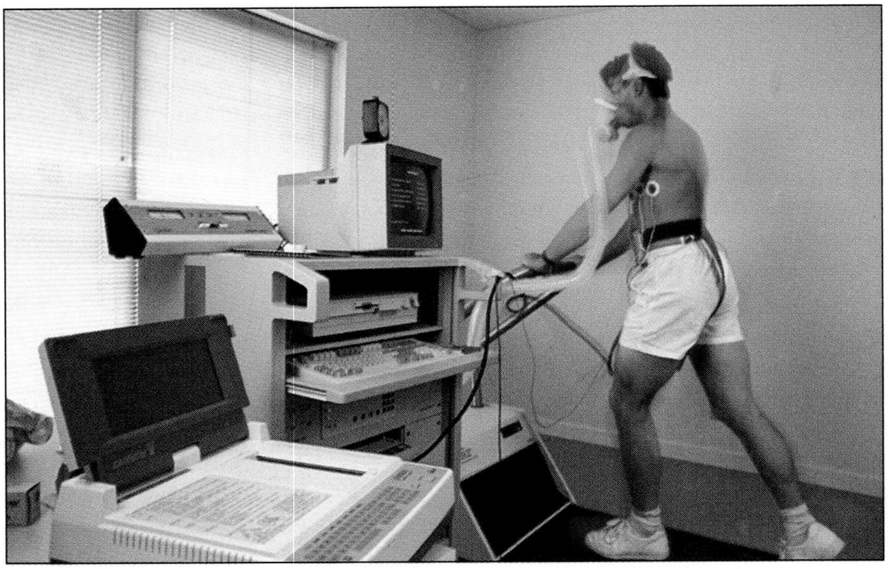

Figure 12.3
Maximal oxygen consumption can be estimated by measuring oxygen uptake while running to exhaustion on a treadmill. (© Jon Love/The Image Bank)

Maximal oxygen consumption or **VO_2 max** The maximum amount of oxygen that can be consumed by the tissues during exercise.

Aerobic exercise also increases **maximal oxygen consumption,** or **VO_2 max,** which is the maximum amount of oxygen that can be consumed by the body's cells during exercise. VO_2 max is dependent on the ability of the cardiorespiratory system to deliver oxygen to the cells and the ability of the cells to use oxygen to produce energy. The greater the VO_2 max, the more intense activity a person can perform before a lack of oxygen affects performance. VO_2 max can be determined in an exercise laboratory by measuring oxygen uptake during exercise using the following equation:

$$\text{Oxygen inhaled} - \text{Oxygen exhaled} = \text{Oxygen uptake}$$

To measure VO_2 max, an individual may be asked to run on a treadmill. The workload is then increased by increasing the speed and/or grade of the treadmill until the individual can no longer continue (Figure 12.3). The amount of oxygen consumed at the highest workload achieved is the VO_2 max. A trained athlete will have a greater VO_2 max than an untrained individual.

Muscle Strength and Endurance Muscle strength and endurance enhance the ability to perform tasks such as pushing or lifting. In daily life, this could mean lifting a bag of groceries, unscrewing the lid of a jar, or shoveling snow from your driveway. Muscle strength and endurance are increased by repeatedly using muscles in activities that require moving against a resisting force. This type of exercise is called strength-training or resistance-training exercise and includes activities such as weight lifting.

Flexibility Flexibility determines range of motion—how far one can bend and stretch muscles and ligaments. If flexibility is poor, you cannot easily bend to tie your shoes or stretch to remove packages from the car. Regularly moving the limbs, neck, and torso through their full ranges of motion helps increase and maintain flexibility (Figure 12.4).

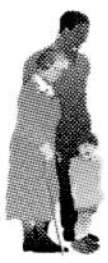

Desirable Body Composition A regular program of balanced physical activity helps to limit or reduce body fat and maintain or increase lean tissue. Individuals who are physically fit have a greater proportion of lean body tissue than unfit individuals of the same body weight. In general, women have more stored body fat than men. During adolescence, females gain proportionately more fat and males gain more muscle mass. For adult women, the desirable percent of body fat is 20 to 30% of total weight; in adult men, the desirable percent is about 12 to 20%.[1]

With aging, lean body mass decreases in both men and women, and there is an increase in the percentage of body fat even if body weight remains the same. Some of this change may be prevented by physical activity. Because lean body tissue is more metabolically active than adipose tissue, the more lean body mass a person has, the greater the energy requirement. Too much body fat—greater than 20% in men and 30% in women—is associated with an increased risk of chronic disease.

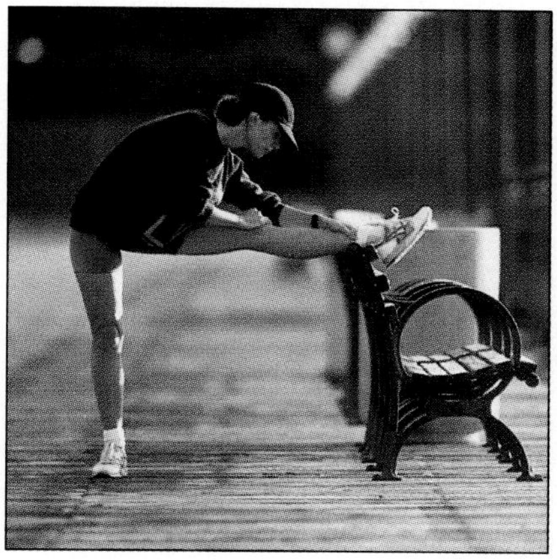

Figure 12.4
Stretching muscles to increase and maintain flexibility is an important component of any exercise regimen. (© David Madison/Tony Stone Images)

The Health Benefits of Exercise

In addition to making the tasks of everyday life easier, fitness through regular activity offers many health benefits. A regular exercise program makes it easier to maintain a healthy body weight, helps maintain muscles, bones, and joints, and reduces the risk of osteoporosis. It can also help to prevent or delay the onset of cardiovascular disease, hypertension, diabetes, and colon cancer. And, it can improve mood and prevent depression.[2]

Preventing and Treating Obesity Exercise makes weight maintenance easier. Regular exercise increases the amount of energy expended for activity. It also increases the proportion of lean tissue in the body, which in turn increases the energy needed for basal metabolic rate (BMR). In addition, basal metabolic rate rises for a number of hours after a bout of exercise. While in the short term the increase in BMR after light to moderate exercise is too small to have a significant effect on energy balance or weight loss,[3] the increase in lean body mass has a long-term, and significant, effect on metabolic rate.

Exercise is an essential component of any weight-reduction program. It promotes the loss of body fat and slows the loss of lean tissue that occurs with energy restriction as well as increasing energy needs.[4]

Cardiovascular Disease Exercise reduces the risk of cardiovascular disease.[5] Aerobic exercise strengthens the heart muscle, thereby reducing resting heart rate and decreasing the heart's workload. Exercise may also lower blood pressure and increase HDL cholesterol levels in the blood, both of which reduce the risk of cardiovascular disease.[6]

Diabetes People with excess body fat are more likely to develop diabetes. By keeping body fat within the normal range, aerobic exercise can decrease one's risk of developing diabetes. Aerobic exercise also benefits individuals who already have diabetes, since exercise and the reduction in body fat it promotes increase the sensitivity of tissues to insulin.[7] This may reduce or eliminate the need for medication to maintain normal blood glucose levels. People with diabetes should develop exercise programs with the help of physicians and dietitians, because exercise can affect dietary and medication needs.

Osteoporosis and Joint Disorders Exercise reduces the risk of osteoporosis. One of the causes of bone loss, like muscle loss, is lack of use; therefore, weight-bearing exercise such as walking, running, and aerobic dance can increase peak bone mass and also prevent bone loss (see Chapter 10). Exercise can also benefit individuals with arthritis because the strength and flexibility promoted by exercise help arthritic joints move more easily.

Cancer Individuals who exercise regularly may be reducing their cancer risk. There is some evidence that exercise reduces breast cancer risk, but it is not clear whether risk reduction is related to exercise intensity, duration, or the age at which the exercise is performed.[8] The evidence that exercise reduces colon cancer risk is stronger; active individuals are less likely to develop colon cancer than their sedentary counterparts.[9] When evaluating the impact of exercise on cancer risk, diet and other lifestyle factors also must be carefully considered. It is possible that some of the effect is due to the fact that people who exercise regularly are more likely to have healthier overall diets and lifestyles.

Exercise Can Slow the Changes That Occur With Age Many physiological changes occur with increasing age, including a decrease in lean body mass, muscle strength and endurance, and cardiorespiratory endurance (see Chapter 15). Regular physical activity can prevent or slow some of these changes.[6] For example, a program of regular exercise that includes strength training can prevent some of the reduction in lean body mass and maintain muscle strength and endurance, and regular aerobic exercise can increase or maintain cardiorespiratory endurance.

Exercise Benefits Children The health of our children tomorrow may depend on their fitness today, because children who are inactive are likely to have sedentary lifestyles as adults. Children who learn to enjoy physical activity are more likely to be active adults who maintain a healthy body weight and have a lower risk of cardiovascular disease, diabetes, osteoporosis, and certain types of cancer (Figure 12.5).

Psychological Benefits of Exercise In addition to its other benefits, exercise can improve sleep patterns and overall outlook on life. Exercise stimulates the release of chemicals called endorphins, which are thought to be natural tranquilizers that play a role in triggering what athletes describe as an "exercise high." In addition to causing this state of exercise euphoria, endorphins are thought to aid in relaxation; improve mood, pain tolerance, and appetite control; and reduce anxiety.

An Exercise Program for You

Most Americans include very little activity in their daily lives.[5] Based on the evidence that increasing exercise reduces the incidence of chronic disease, many public health organizations are recommending that Americans increase their activity level. Recommendations on how much exercise is enough vary depending on who is making the recommendation. Some recommendations are based on the number of kcalories expended. For instance, the Surgeon General's Report on Physical Activity and Health recommends that Americans expend at least 150 kcalories a day or 1000 kcalories a week being active.[2] Other recommendations are based on the amount of time spent in activity. For example, the Centers for Disease Control and Prevention and the American College of Sports Medicine recommend that Americans engage in 30 minutes or more of moderate activity on most if not all days of the week. Healthy People 2010 recommends 30 minutes of vigorous activity daily and suggests that for most people this will increase energy expenditure by about 1050 kcalories per week.[10] No matter how the recommendation is worded, each acknowledges that there is a significant health benefit to including a moderate amount of physical activity on most if not all days of the week. Despite this, about two thirds of Americans do not spend 30 minutes or expend 150 kcalories per day engaged in activity.[11]

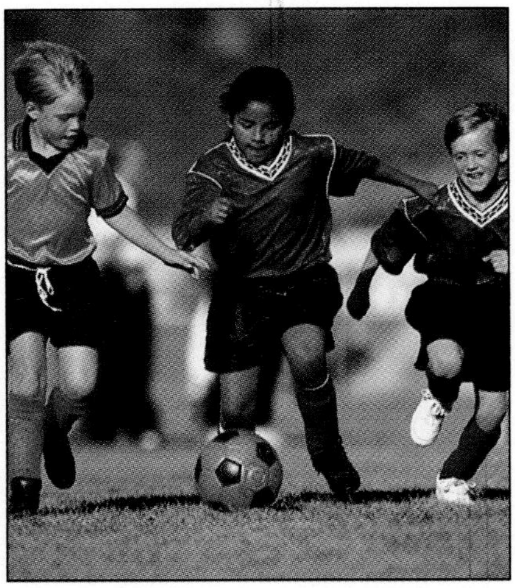

Figure 12.5
Children who participate and enjoy exercise are more likely to have active lifestyles as adults. (© Lori Adamski Peek/Tony Stone Images)

Components of a Good Exercise Regimen What type of exercise offers the greatest health benefit? The American College of Sports Medicine suggests that a good exercise regimen include aerobic exercise, which raises heart rate and therefore improves cardiorespiratory fitness; stretching, which promotes and maintains flexibility; and strength training, which enhances the strength and endurance of specific muscles.[4]

Aerobic exercise, such as walking, bicycling, skating, swimming, or jogging, should be performed for about 20 to 60 minutes three to five days per week. For optimal benefit, aerobic activity should be performed at a level that raises the heart rate to 60 to 90% of its maximum (see Figure 12.2). For a sedentary individual beginning an exercise program, mild exercise such as walking can raise the heart rate into this range. As fitness improves, exercisers must perform more intense activity to raise their heart rates to this level.

Stretching exercises should be done at least three days a week. Muscles should be stretched to a position of mild discomfort and held for 10 to 30 seconds. Each stretch should be repeated three to five times. Muscle groups that are particularly important to stretch are those in the lower back and thighs.

Strength training, such as weight lifting, should be done two to three days a week at the start of an exercise program, and two days a week after the desired strength has been achieved. This can be done with weights or with resistance-exercise machines. Each session should include a minimum of 8 to 10 exercises that train the major muscle groups. Each exercise should be repeated 8 to 12 times. The weights should be heavy enough to cause the muscle to be near exhaustion after the 8 to 12 repetitions. As fitness improves, increasing the amount of weight lifted will increase muscle strength, whereas increasing the number of repetitions will improve endurance.

Getting Started These recommendations may seem intimidating for someone currently getting little or no exercise. How the recommendations are applied depends on who you are and what your goals are. What is best for a middle-aged man trying to reduce his risk of chronic disease is different from what is best for an 18-year-old college basketball player, and different still from that for an octogenarian trying to continue living independently. Almost everyone can participate in some form of exercise, no matter where they live, how old they are, or what physical limitations they have. Exercise classes are taught in nursing homes. Heart patients, amputees, the blind, and those confined to wheelchairs compete in athletic events. You are never too old to exercise, and it is never too late to start.

Changing Behavior Incorporating exercise into day-to-day life requires a behavior change, and changing behavior is not easy. The first step in beginning an exercise program is to recognize the reasons for not exercising and identify ways to overcome them. Many people avoid exercise because they do not enjoy it, feel they have to join an expensive health club, have little motivation to do it alone, or find it inconvenient and uncomfortable. Finding a type of exercise that is enjoyable, a time that is realistic and convenient, and a place that is appropriate and safe are important first steps in adopting a pattern of increased exercise. Special clothes and large amounts of time and money are not needed. Riding your bike to class or work rather than driving or taking the bus, taking a walk on your lunch break, and enjoying a game of catch or tag with your children are all effective ways to increase your everyday activity level. Behavioral strategies such as those listed in Table 12.1 may help promote regular exercise.

Building an Activity Pyramid A good way to organize your daily activity is to use a pyramid, similar to that used to make dietary selections (Figure 12.6).[12] The goal is to gradually make lifestyle changes that increase physical activity. The base of the pyramid includes activities that you should do every day, or as much as possible. It includes small, everyday activities like walking the dog, parking farther away to increase the distance you walk to the office or grocery store, or taking the stairs rather than the elevator. At the next level of the pyramid are aerobic and recreational activities that should be layered on top of your activity base. These focus on improving heart and lung function and include walking, running, swimming, or biking, or aerobic recreational activities such as basketball, soccer, or hiking. These should be done three to five times a week for 20 minutes or longer. The third level of the pyramid includes activities to build flexibility and strength.

Table 12.1 *Suggestions for Beginning and Maintaining an Exercise Program*

1. **Start slowly**—Instead of planning to run 3 miles a day five days a week, plan to start with a 20-minute walk three days a week.
2. **Make it fun**—Choose activities you enjoy and find a partner with whom to exercise.
3. **Set specific attainable goals**—"I will walk for 20 minutes on Mondays, Wednesdays, and Fridays."
4. **Make it convenient**—Plan to walk early in the morning, during your lunch hour at work, or after dinner.
5. **Record your progress**—Keep a record of your activity so you can track your progress and keep yourself motivated.
6. **Reward yourself**—Plan to reward yourself when you succeed at your goal: a new book, a movie.

It focuses on strengthening muscles throughout the body and emphasizes the importance of stretching exercises. The exercise at this level should take place two to three times a week and include such leisure activities as golf or bowling and such flexibility and strength activities as yoga and weight lifting. As with the Food Guide Pyramid, the very top level of the Activity Pyramid focuses on things you should do less of, such as sitting, watching TV, and playing computer games. You should make a conscious effort to break up long periods of sitting (more than 30 minutes) by getting up and moving for a few minutes. While sitting at your desk or in the library, get up and walk around every half hour, if possible. While talking on the phone, stand up and move around. While sitting in traffic, move your shoulders to relieve tension. In general, any activity is better than none at all. Even a little exercise has health benefits, and more, within reason, is better.

Exercising Safely Safety should be a concern in planning any exercise regimen. Before beginning, everyone should check with their physician to be sure that their plans are safe in relation to their medical history. In particular, individuals who are over age 45, have been inactive, have a personal or family history of heart disease, or have any risk factors for heart disease should consult their physician before beginning an exercise program that includes activities from the second level of the Activity Pyramid. To decrease the risk of injury, each exercise session should begin with a warm-up to increase blood flow to the muscles. This might include a few minutes of mild stretching and some easy walking or jogging.

A safe, well-lit location should be found for exercise. Busy work schedules often force people to exercise in the dark early-morning or evening hours. Exercisers who use the street for walking or jogging should wear light-colored, reflective clothing so they can be seen by motorists. Exercising with a partner is safer and more enjoyable.

Temperature is also a concern. Extreme heat or cold can cause problems for exercisers. Physical activity produces heat, which normally is dissipated to the environment, partly by the evaporation of sweat. When the environmental temperature is high, heat is not efficiently transferred to the environment, and when humidity is high, sweat evaporates slowly, making it difficult to cool the body. Thus, exercise should be reduced or curtailed in hot and humid conditions. Cold environments can also pose problems for the outdoor exerciser. In general, cold does not impair exercise capacity, but the numbing of exposed flesh and the bulk of extra clothing can cause problems for joggers and bicyclists. Because exercise

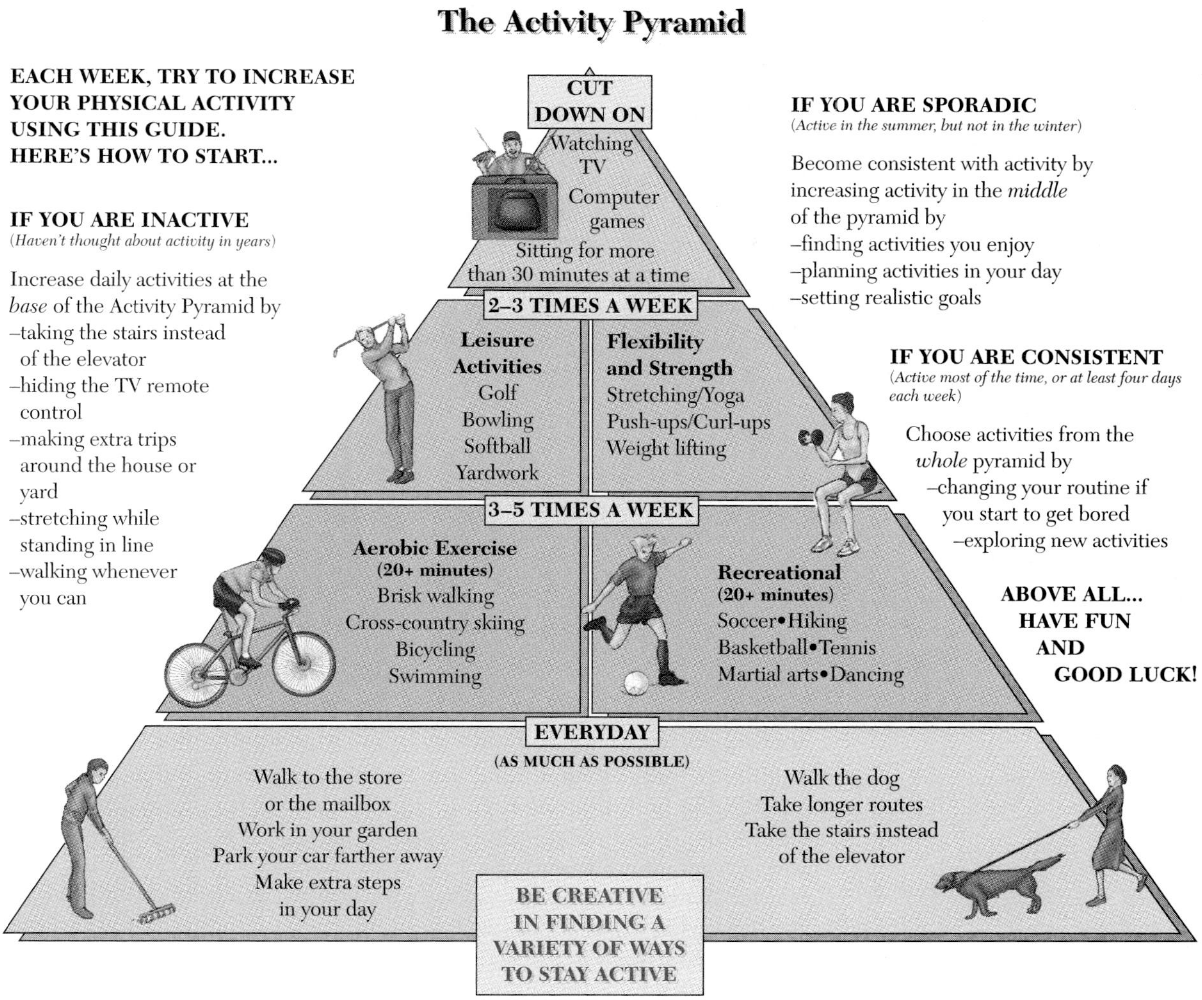
The Activity Pyramid
EACH WEEK, TRY TO INCREASE YOUR PHYSICAL ACTIVITY USING THIS GUIDE. HERE'S HOW TO START...
IF YOU ARE INACTIVE
(Haven't thought about activity in years)
Increase daily activities at the base of the Activity Pyramid by
–taking the stairs instead of the elevator
–hiding the TV remote control
–making extra trips around the house or yard
–stretching while standing in line
–walking whenever you can
CUT DOWN ON
Watching TV
Computer games
Sitting for more than 30 minutes at a time
IF YOU ARE SPORADIC
(Active in the summer, but not in the winter)
Become consistent with activity by increasing activity in the middle of the pyramid by
–finding activities you enjoy
–planning activities in your day
–setting realistic goals
2–3 TIMES A WEEK
Leisure Activities
Golf
Bowling
Softball
Yardwork
Flexibility and Strength
Stretching/Yoga
Push-ups/Curl-ups
Weight lifting
IF YOU ARE CONSISTENT
(Active most of the time, or at least four days each week)
Choose activities from the whole pyramid by
–changing your routine if you start to get bored
–exploring new activities
3–5 TIMES A WEEK
Aerobic Exercise
(20+ minutes)
Brisk walking
Cross-country skiing
Bicycling
Swimming
Recreational
(20+ minutes)
Soccer•Hiking
Basketball•Tennis
Martial arts•Dancing
ABOVE ALL... HAVE FUN AND GOOD LUCK!
EVERYDAY
(AS MUCH AS POSSIBLE)
Walk to the store or the mailbox
Work in your garden
Park your car farther away
Make extra steps in your day
Walk the dog
Take longer routes
Take the stairs instead of the elevator
BE CREATIVE IN FINDING A VARIETY OF WAYS TO STAY ACTIVE

Figure 12.6

The Activity Pyramid. A pyramid shape can be used to build an active lifestyle. At the base are activities that you do every day. Layered over this base are aerobic exercise, recreational activities, and strength and flexibility exercises. At the very top are sitting activities that should be reduced.

produces heat, clothing must allow for evaporation of sweat while providing protection from the cold. For swimmers, cold water can cause a deterioration in performance.

Environmental conditions can pose particular risks for young exercisers.[13] Hot environments are of concern because children produce more heat, are less able to transfer heat from muscles to the skin, and sweat less than adults. To reduce risks, children should rest periodically in the shade, consume fluids frequently, and limit the intensity and duration of activities on hot days. Also, children lose more heat in cold environments than adults because they have a greater surface area per unit of body weight. Therefore, they are more prone to **hypothermia** (see *Critical Thinking: Incorporating Exercise Sensibly*).

Hypothermia A condition in which body temperature drops below normal. Hypothermia depresses the central nervous system, resulting in the inability to shiver, sleepiness, and eventually coma.

Exercise Recommendations for Children Healthy children should be encouraged to engage in regular physical activity with the goal of adopting appropriate lifelong exercise behaviors. The National Association for Sports and Physical Education recommends that preadolescent children spend a minimum of 60 minutes per day in developmentally appropriate exercise.[14] Activity for young children should be intermittent, with periods of moderate to vigorous activity lasting 10 to 15 minutes or more along with periods of rest and recovery. To promote this amount of exercise, a variety of enjoyable activities should be stressed and competition de-emphasized. Learning by example is always best. Children who have physically active parents are the leanest and the fittest.

Television is an important cause of inactivity among children. Studies have found that children who watch 4 or more hours of television per day have more body fat and a greater body mass index than those who spend fewer than 2 hours watching TV.[15] Watching television takes time away from more strenuous activities and, because of the type of advertising included in children's programming, may promote the consumption of foods high in fat, salt, and refined sugars. As a result, the American Academy of Pediatrics recommends that children watch no more than 2 hours of television daily[16] (see Chapter 14).

CRITICAL THINKING

Incorporating Exercise Sensibly

Nicole recently turned 45 years old. Her promise to herself was to get back in shape. She is 5 feet 4 inches tall and weighs 140 pounds. Although her weight is still within the healthy weight range suggested by the Dietary Guidelines, she is about 5 pounds above her usual weight. Currently Nicole exercises about once a month and then suffers from a few days of sore muscles. When the family goes on outings, she finds that she tires long before her husband and children. She would like to lose a few pounds, but more importantly she would like to increase her strength and endurance.

Before beginning her exercise program she checks with her physician, who agrees that she should increase her exercise and recommends that she do stretching and strength-training exercise as well as aerobic activities that increase her heart rate to 60 to 90% of her maximum.

What is 60 to 90% of Nicole's maximum heart rate?

Maximum heart rate = 220 − age = 220 − 45 = 175 beats per minute

60% of maximum = 175 × 0.6 = 105 beats per minute

90% of maximum = 175 × 0.9 = 158 beats per minute

She should exercise at a heart rate of at least 105 but no more than 158 beats per minute.

Nicole's fitness plan

Nicole decides she will exercise for 90 minutes a day, 5 days a week. Her plan is to join a gym and stretch and lift weights for 30 minutes, followed by an hour of aerobic exercise outdoors, either jogging or riding a bicycle in the park.

After three days on her new schedule, a rainy day keeps Nicole indoors. She realizes that her family is angry and feels abandoned. She hasn't been able to do an hour of aerobics without exceeding her maximum heart rate. She is tired, sore, and ready to give up and accept the fact that she is just not an athletic person.

Where did she go wrong?

It is unrealistic to go from exercising one day a month to five days a week. She needs an exercise program that will fit easily into her daily routine, without drastically changing her schedule. It is unnecessary to lift weights five days a week to gain muscle strength, and she can reach 60 to 90% of her maximum heart rate by walking quickly. A more achievable goal might be a stretching routine at home, three days of walking for 20 to 60 minutes at a moderate rate, and two weight-lifting sessions per week. She can increase the frequency and duration of her exercise as her strength and endurance improve. She also needs to make alternative plans for bad weather and allow time for warming up and cooling down in order to exercise safely.

Nicole's new fitness plan

She continues her gym membership but only goes to lift weights two evenings a week, when her husband can watch the children. As a treat afterwards she relaxes in the whirlpool before showering and returning home. She shares her story with a friend at work, and they decide to walk during their lunch hour three days a week. As their fitness improves, they walk faster to keep their heart rate between 60 and 90% of maximum to improve cardiovascular fitness.

How has this change in activity affected Nicole's energy needs for the day?

On the three days a week when she walks, she replaces 1 hour of sitting with 1 hour of walking, increasing her energy expenditure by 175 kcalories (see Table 12.2).

$$1 \text{ hour of walking} = 244 \text{ kcal}$$

$$1 \text{ hour of sitting} = 69 \text{ kcal}$$

$$\text{Increase in energy expenditure} = 244 \text{ kcal} - 69 \text{ kcal} = 175 \text{ kcal}$$

On days that Nicole goes to the gym she spends 15 minutes weight lifting (323 kcal per hour $\times$ 0.25 hour = 81 kcal). This replaces 15 minutes of very light activity at only about 17 kcalories, so she expends an extra 64 kcalories. During the week she therefore expends an extra 653 kcalories (175 kcal $\times$ 3 days of walking + 64 kcal $\times$ 2 days of weight lifting).

If Nicole's food intake does not increase, how long will it take for her to lose 5 pounds?

Answer:

As Nicole's fitness level improves, she finds she has more energy for other activities. By spending more time gardening and joining the kids for bike rides and occasional hikes she finds that she is getting about 30 minutes of exercise almost every day, as recommended by public health guidelines.

FUELING ACTIVITY

Just as an automobile engine runs on energy from gasoline, the body machine runs on energy from the carbohydrate, fat, and protein in food and body stores. These fuels are needed whether you are writing a letter, walking around the block, or running a marathon. But the amount of each of these nutrients that is used depends on the type of activity that is performed, how long it is performed, and the physical conditioning of the exerciser.

Energy for Activity

Carbohydrate, fat, and protein are the fuel sources for the body. But before they can be used to fuel activity, their energy must be converted into the high-energy compound ATP. ATP is the immediate source of energy for all body functions. In a resting muscle, there is enough stored ATP to sustain activity for a few seconds. As the ATP in muscle is used, enzymes break down another high-energy compound, **creatine phosphate,** to replenish the ATP supply. As with ATP, the amount of creatine phosphate stored in the muscle at any time is small. During the first 10 to 15 seconds of exercise, the muscles use energy from the ATP and creatine phosphate that is stored there. But activity of longer duration requires that the body replenish ATP from the metabolism of the energy-containing nutrients (Figure 12.7).

Creatine phosphate A compound found in muscle that can be broken down to make ATP.

Converting Fuels Into Energy

Carbohydrate, fat, and protein all can be used to produce ATP when oxygen is available. When no oxygen is available, only carbohydrate can be used, and although it produces ATP rapidly it is not used efficiently. The ability to deliver oxygen to muscle cells is determined both by how quickly the heart can pump blood from the lungs—where it picks up oxygen—to the muscle cells, and by the amount of hemoglobin available to transport oxygen in the blood.

Producing Energy From Carbohydrate The carbohydrate fuel used for exercise is glucose. It can be used as a fuel source whether or not oxygen is available at the cells. The glucose used to power muscle activity may come from glycogen inside the muscle or from glucose delivered via the bloodstream. The glucose delivered in the blood comes from that released by the liver or absorbed from the diet.

The first step of glucose metabolism does not require oxygen and is referred to as **anaerobic metabolism** or **anaerobic glycolysis.** It breaks down glucose to form the three-carbon compound pyruvate, releases electrons, and produces

Anaerobic metabolism or **anaerobic glycolysis** Metabolism in the absence of oxygen. In glycolysis, two molecules of ATP are produced from each molecule of glucose. Glucose is metabolized in this way when the blood cannot deliver oxygen to the tissues quickly enough.

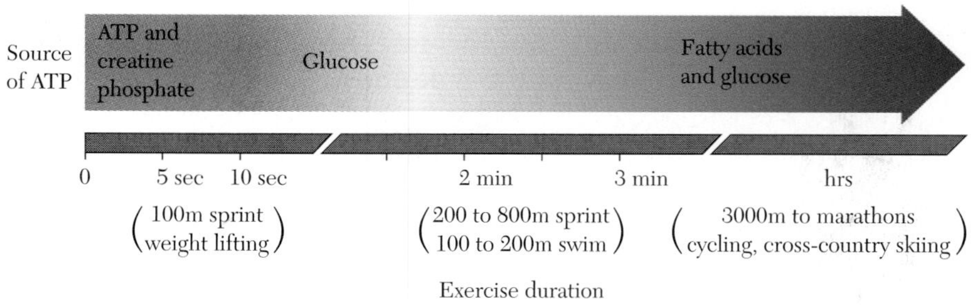

Figure 12.7
When exercise begins, ATP and creatine phosphate stored in the muscle provide ATP for muscle contraction. As creatine phosphate stores become depleted, anaerobic glycolysis, which breaks down glucose from the blood or from muscle glycogen, becomes the predominant source of ATP. After about 3 minutes, aerobic metabolism, which uses fatty acids and glucose to produce ATP, begins to predominate.

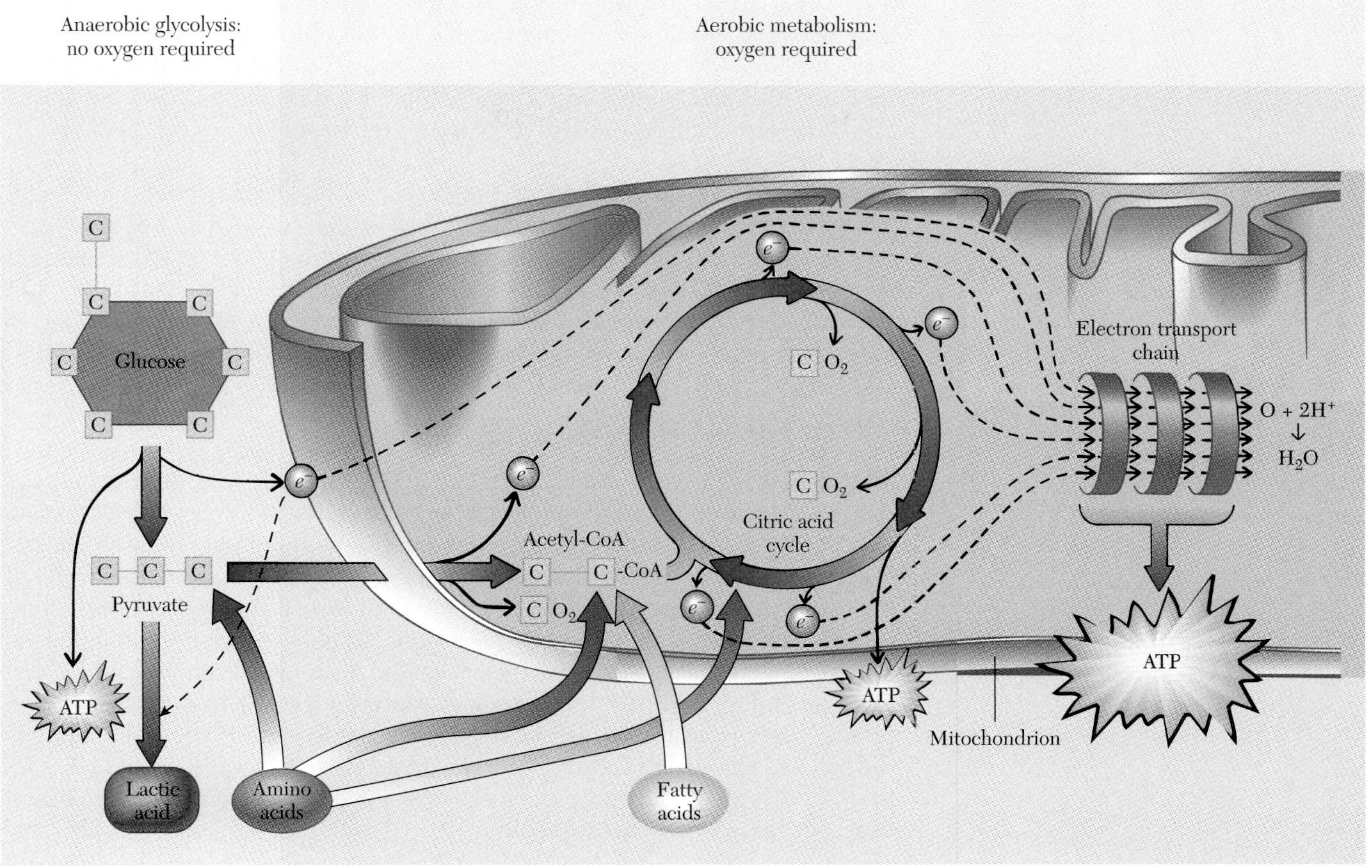

Figure 12.8
In the absence of oxygen, ATP is produced by the anaerobic glycolysis of glucose. When oxygen is present, ATP is produced by aerobic metabolism of glucose, fatty acids, and amino acids.

two molecules of ATP. When oxygen is unavailable, the pyruvate and released electrons combine to form **lactic acid.** When oxygen is available, the pyruvate and electrons proceed through **aerobic metabolism,** producing carbon dioxide, water, and more ATP. Aerobic metabolism includes (1) the conversion of pyruvate to acetyl-CoA; (2) the citric acid cycle, which breaks down acetyl-CoA, producing some ATP and releasing electrons; and (3) the electron transport chain, which passes electrons down a chain of molecules to oxygen, releasing energy to make ATP. Aerobic metabolism produces ATP more efficiently than anaerobic metabolism. The same molecule of glucose that produces two molecules of ATP in anaerobic glycolysis can produce about 36 to 38 molecules of ATP when metabolized aerobically (Figure 12.8).

Lactic acid A compound produced from the breakdown of glucose in the absence of oxygen.

Aerobic metabolism Metabolism in the presence of oxygen. In aerobic metabolism, the citric acid cycle and the electron transport chain break down carbohydrates, fatty acids, and amino acids into carbon dioxide and water to produce ATP.

Producing Energy From Fat Fatty acids from the diet and from body stores can be used for fuel, but oxygen must be present. Stored fat accounts for 90% of stored energy in a typical adult. It provides a lightweight, energy-dense fuel supply.

To produce ATP, triglycerides in fat stores are broken down into fatty acids and glycerol, and released into the blood. Fatty acids enter muscle cells and are transported into the mitochondria, where they are broken into two-carbon units to form acetyl-CoA. Acetyl-CoA is metabolized via the citric acid cycle and electron transport chain to produce ATP, carbon dioxide, and water.

The rate at which fatty acids can be used by the muscle depends on how quickly they can be released from fat deposits and delivered to muscle-cell mitochondria, where ATP is produced. To enter the mitochondria, fatty acids must be activated with the help of **carnitine.** Carnitine supplements are marketed to athletes with the promise that they will enhance the utilization of fat during exercise.

Carnitine A molecule synthesized in the body that is needed to transport fatty acids and some amino acids into the mitochondria for metabolism. Supplements of carnitine are marketed to athletes to enhance performance.

This would spare carbohydrate and thereby allow athletes to exercise for a longer time before exhaustion. Carnitine is made by the cells, so it does not need to be supplied in the diet to ensure the efficient use of fatty acids. Studies that examined the effect of carnitine supplements found that they did not affect the utilization of fat as fuel during exercise or improve exercise endurance.[17]

Producing Energy From Protein Protein can be broken down into amino acids which can also be used to produce ATP when oxygen is available. For most exercise, protein contributes only a small percentage of the energy used. It becomes an important source of energy only when exercise continues for many hours. Endurance exercise increases the use of amino acids both as an energy source as well as for glucose production via gluconeogenesis to maintain blood glucose levels.

Which Fuels Are Used?

The amount of oxygen available at the cells determines the proportions and sources of fuels used for different activities. At rest, the blood can deliver enough oxygen for aerobic metabolism, so muscles derive most of their energy from fatty acids and only a small proportion from glucose.[18] During exercise, the ability of the cardiorespiratory system to deliver oxygen to tissues affects the contributions of carbohydrate and fat to energy production. High-intensity exercise relies on anaerobic metabolism because oxygen is limited. Less intense exercise allows aerobic metabolism to proceed. For example, during a friendly basketball game you probably rely primarily on aerobic metabolism. If, however, you suddenly steal the ball and charge full speed down the court for a basket, oxygen cannot be delivered to the cells fast enough and they are forced to rely on energy produced from glucose by anaerobic metabolism.

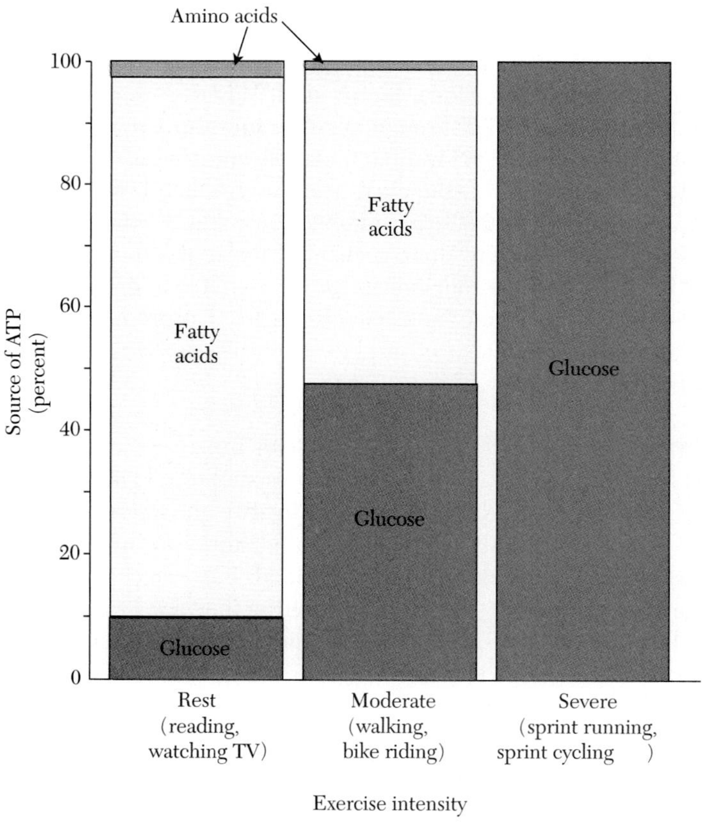

Figure 12.9

As exercise intensity increases, the proportion of energy supplied by carbohydrate increases. During exercise the total amount of energy expended is greater than at rest. (Adapted from Horton, E. S. Effects of low-energy diets on work performance. Am. J. Clin. Nutr. 35:1228–1233, 1982.)

Exercise Intensity During high-intensity exercise, the cardiorespiratory system cannot deliver oxygen to muscle cells fast enough to support aerobic metabolism. Without sufficient oxygen, glucose, either from the breakdown of glycogen or from that delivered by the blood, becomes the predominant fuel source (Figure 12.9). Under these conditions glucose provides about two thirds of energy needs, with the rest coming from fatty acids from the blood or stored in the muscle. When intensity reaches the VO_2 max, glucose is just about the only energy source. ATP production via anaerobic glycolysis is rapid, but it is not efficient and cannot sustain exercise for long periods. When high-intensity exercise can no longer be maintained, the individual is said to be experiencing **fatigue.** This occurs for two reasons: First, glucose stores are depleted, making fuel unavailable; and second, the by-products of anaerobic glycolysis—electrons and pyruvate—accumulate. When there is not sufficient oxygen to pick up the electrons, they are transferred to pyruvate, producing lactic acid. Excess lactic acid production changes the acidity of the muscle, which reduces the muscle's ability to contract and contributes to muscle fatigue. When exercise stops and oxygen is available again, lactic acid can be either carried away by the blood to other tissues to be broken down or metabolized aerobically in the muscle. After intense exercise, a mild cool-down, such as walking, may allow enough blood flow to the muscle to remove built-up lactic acid and prevent cramping.

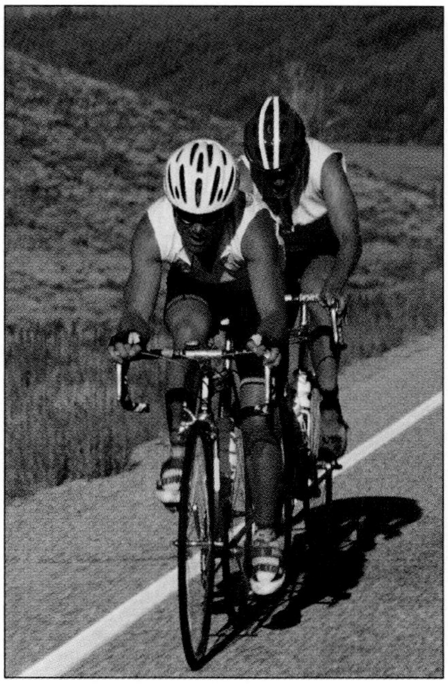

Figure 12.10
In moderate-intensity exercise of long duration, such as endurance cycling, fatty acids contribute the greatest proportion of energy. (Corbis)

Fatigue The inability to continue an activity at an optimal level.

Exercise Duration When the intensity of exercise is low, the duration of exercise becomes an important factor in determining what fuels are burned. When an individual begins an aerobic type of exercise, fuels present in the muscle—first ATP and creatine phosphate, and then glucose from muscle glycogen—are used for muscle contraction. Then glucose and fatty acids delivered by the blood provide an increasing proportion of the energy. As exercise progresses, the energy contribution of fatty acids from the breakdown of adipose stores continues to increase. For exercise lasting a few hours, more than half of the energy is supplied by fatty acids (Figure 12.10).[18] Even when exercise intensity is low, some glucose is used, eventually depleting glycogen stores and causing fatigue. When an athlete runs out of glycogen, he or she experiences a feeling of overwhelming fatigue that is sometimes referred to as "hitting the wall."

Long-term endurance exercise, such as Ironman triathlons and ultramarathons, where athletes are competing strenuously for many hours, also uses protein for fuel. Metabolically, exercise this strenuous for this duration is similar to starvation. Once glycogen stores are depleted, protein is broken down and the amino acids are used directly as an energy source or to make glucose in order to maintain blood glucose levels. The brain and nervous system have an absolute requirement for glucose; since glucose cannot be made from fatty acids, when carbohydrate stores are exhausted, amino acids from protein must be used to make glucose.

The Training of the Exerciser Training with repeated bouts of aerobic exercise causes physiological changes that increase the amount of oxygen that can be delivered to and used by the muscle cells. The heart becomes larger and stronger so that the stroke volume is increased. The number of capillary blood vessels in the muscles increases so that blood is delivered to muscles more efficiently. And the total blood volume and number of red blood cells expands, increasing the amount of hemoglobin so more oxygen can be transported to the cells. Training also causes changes at the cellular level that affect the ability of cells to use different types of fuel to produce ATP. There is an increase in the ability to store glycogen and there is an increase in the number and size of muscle-cell mitochondria (Figure 12.11). Because aerobic metabolism occurs in the mitochondria, this increases the cell's capacity to burn fatty acids to produce ATP. The use of fatty acids spares glycogen, which delays the onset of fatigue. Because trained athletes

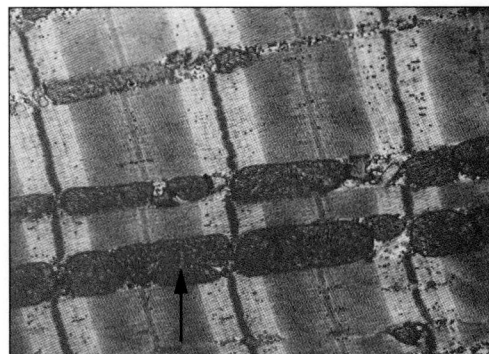

Figure 12.11
Mitochondria are the site of aerobic metabolism. In trained athletes, the number of mitochondria in muscle cells increases. (Don W. Fawcett/Visuals Unlimited)

store more glycogen and use it more slowly, they can sustain aerobic exercise for longer periods at higher intensities than can untrained individuals.

Living and working at high altitudes, where the atmosphere contains less oxygen, also causes adaptations that improve the capacity of the cardiorespiratory system to deliver oxygen. Therefore endurance athletes often train at high altitudes to enhance their aerobic capacity.

EXERCISING GOOD NUTRITION

Adequate nutrition is essential to performance whether you are a marathon runner or a mall walker. For every exerciser, diet must provide sufficient energy from the appropriate sources to fuel activity, protein to maintain muscle mass, micronutrients to allow utilization of the energy-containing nutrients, and water to transport nutrients and cool the body.

Energy Needs

Energy needs include those required for basal metabolic rate, activity, and the thermic effect of food. For a casual exerciser, the energy needed for activity may increase energy expenditure by a few hundred kcalories a day. For an endurance athlete, such as a marathon runner, the energy needed for training may increase expenditure by 2000 to 3000 kcalories per day. Some athletes require 6000 kcalories a day to maintain body weight.

Factors Affecting Energy Needed for Activity The amount of energy needed for an activity depends on the activity, the exerciser, and even the location. It also depends on the activity's intensity and duration and the frequency with which it is performed (see Table 12.2 and Appendix L). The more intense the activity, the more energy it requires. For example, riding a bicycle involves less work than running the same distance and therefore requires less energy. The more time spent exercising, the more energy it requires. Riding a bicycle for 10 minutes requires ten times the energy needed to ride for 1 minute. The body weight of the exerciser is another factor in determining energy needs. Moving a heavier body requires more energy than moving a lighter one. Therefore, it requires less energy for a 120-pound woman to walk for 5 minutes than it does for a 250-pound woman.

There are also some special considerations that affect the energy needs for activity. For example, although an obese woman would expend more energy walking a mile than a lighter counterpart, the obese woman would expend less energy when swimming because the buoyancy of her adipose tissue reduces the amount of work required to swim. If a lean individual and an obese individual were in the weightlessness of space, it would require no more energy for one to leap across the room than for the other. Also, special circumstances of the individual affect the amount of energy needed daily for activity. A paraplegic in a wheelchair may have lower energy needs because many of the major muscles in the body are always inactive. At the other extreme, a person with the form of cerebral palsy that causes uncontrolled muscle movements may have higher energy needs because the muscles never stop moving.

Desirable Body Weight and Composition Desirable body weight and composition for nonathletes can be estimated from body mass index or height-weight tables, or by measuring the percent body fat (see Chapter 7 or Appendix B). However, what is considered desirable body weight and composition for the general population may differ from what is viewed as optimal for some athletes. For example, the desirable body weight of a runner may be less than that of an average person, whereas that of a weight lifter may be greater. But both the runner

Table 12.2. *Energy Expended for Activity*

Activity	Energy (kcal/hr)						
Body Weight (kg)	**50**	**57**	**64**	**70**	**77**	**84**	**91**
(lb)	**110**	**125**	**140**	**155**	**170**	**185**	**200**
Aerobics (moderate)							
Male	455	480	506	531	556	582	607
Female	394	413	433	453	472	492	511
Biking (12 mph)							
Male	380	401	422	443	464	486	507
Female	329	345	361	378	394	410	427
Bowling (recreational)							
Male	121	128	135	142	148	155	162
Female	105	110	115	121	126	131	136
Dancing (recreational)							
Male	364	384	405	425	445	465	486
Female	315	331	346	362	378	393	409
Gardening (moderate)							
Male	303	320	337	354	371	388	405
Female	263	276	289	302	315	328	341
Golf (walking w/bag)							
Male	425	448	472	496	519	543	567
Female	368	386	404	422	441	459	477
Jumping rope (moderate)							
Male	595	628	661	694	727	760	793
Female	515	540	566	591	617	642	668
Running (10 min/mi)							
Male	619	653	688	722	757	791	826
Female	536	562	589	615	642	669	695
Sitting at ease							
Male	73	77	81	85	89	93	97
Female	63	66	69	72	76	79	82
Swimming (moderate)							
Male	364	384	405	425	445	465	486
Female	315	331	346	362	378	393	409
Walking (15 min/mi)							
Male	257	271	285	300	314	328	342
Female	222	233	244	255	266	277	288
Weight lifting							
Male	340	359	378	397	415	434	453
Female	294	309	323	338	352	367	382

Source: ESHA Research, Salem, Ore.

and the weight lifter are likely to have a lower percent body fat than sedentary individuals.

Athletes involved in activities where small, light bodies offer an advantage—for instance, ballet, gymnastics, and certain running events—may restrict energy intake to maintain a low body weight. While a slightly leaner physique may be beneficial, dieting to maintain an unrealistically low weight may threaten health and performance. An athlete who needs to lose weight should do so in advance of the competitive season to prevent the restricted diet from affecting performance. The general guidelines for healthy weight loss should be followed—reduce energy intake, increase activity, and change the behaviors that led to weight gain (see Chapter 7). To preserve lean body mass and enhance fat loss, weight loss should be at a rate of about 1/2 to 1 pound per week. This can be accomplished by reducing total energy intake by 200 to 500 kcalories per day and increasing exercise. If weight gain is desired, 200 to 500 extra kcalories should be consumed per day and weight gain should be accompanied by training to promote an increase in lean tissue.

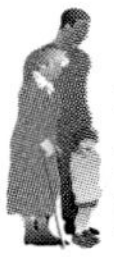

In adolescents, athletic activities combined with weight loss may affect the maturation process and increase the risks of developing anorexia or bulimia.[19] Female ballerinas and gymnasts who maintain extremely low levels of body fat often have delayed menses and delayed sexual maturation.[20] Sporadic diets that severely restrict fluid and energy intake are sometimes used by athletes in sports such as wrestling to fit into a specific weight class. Such dietary practices may be detrimental to health and performance (see discussion of fluid needs in the following section).[21]

Carbohydrate, Fat, and Protein Needs

The source of dietary energy is often as important as the amount of energy. In general, the diet of physically active individuals should contain the same proportion of carbohydrate, fat, and protein as is recommended to the general public—about 55 to 60% of total energy as carbohydrate, less than 30% of energy as fat, and about 12 to 17% of energy as protein.

Carbohydrate Most of the carbohydrate in the diet should be complex carbohydrates from whole grains and starchy vegetables, with some naturally occurring simple sugars from fruit and milk. These foods provide vitamins, minerals, phytochemicals, and fiber as well as energy. For athletes in training, adequate carbohydrate is necessary to rapidly replace muscle and liver glycogen stores depleted by daily exercise.

Fat Fat is an important source of energy for exercise, but excess dietary fat is unnecessary. Body stores of fat provide enough energy to support the needs of even the longest endurance events. The diet of physically active individuals should contain the same proportion of fat as is recommended to the general public—less than 30% of energy. Excess energy consumed as fat, carbohydrate, or protein can cause an increase in body fat.

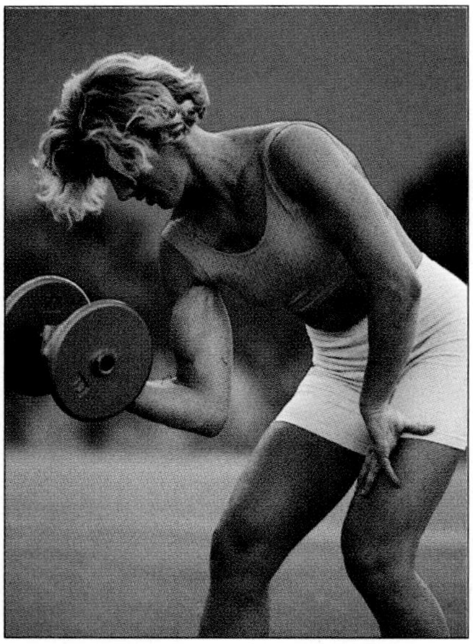

Figure 12.12
Increasing muscle size involves time and hard work. It is accomplished by increasing resistance exercise, not by simply increasing protein intake. (© Marc Romanelli/The Image Bank)

Protein Protein is essential to maintain muscle mass and strength. But eating extra protein does not produce bigger muscles. Muscle growth is stimulated by exercise, not by increasing protein intake (Figure 12.12). Supplements of synthetic anabolic steroids are often used by athletes to increase muscle mass; however, these are illegal and have dangerous side effects (see *Off the Shelf: The Anabolic Edge: From Steroids to Creatine*).

A diet that contains the 1989 RDA for protein (0.8 g/kg) provides adequate protein for most active individuals. Competitive athletes participating in endurance and strength sports may require more protein. In endurance events such as marathons, protein is used for energy and to maintain blood glucose so these athletes may benefit from 1.2 to 1.4 grams of protein per kilogram per day. Strength athletes who require amino acids to synthesize new muscle proteins may benefit from 1.4 to 1.8 grams per kilogram per day.[22] This amount, however, is not much more than the amount contained in the diets of typical American athletes. For example, a 85-kg man consuming 3000 kcalories, 18% of which is from protein, would be consuming 135 g, or 1.6 g of protein per kg body weight.

Protein Supplements Protein supplements are often marketed with the promise of enhancing muscle growth or improving performance. There are hundreds of protein powders and bars available. Although certain types of exercise do increase protein needs, the protein provided by expensive supplements will not meet an athlete's needs any better than the protein found in a balanced diet.

Amino Acid Supplements Amino acid supplements are also popular. Supplements of many single amino acids affect hormone levels and muscle physiology, but their effect on exercise performance is unclear. The amino acids ornithine and arginine are marketed with the promise that they will stimulate the release of growth hormone and, in turn, enhance the growth of muscles. Some studies have shown that large doses of arginine and ornithine can stimulate growth hormone release and may enhance the fat loss associated with strength training, but this result is not consistent.[23] Glutamine supplements also promise to increase the release of growth hormone as well as to increase muscle glycogen deposition. Although some studies have shown these effects, there is little research to support the use of glutamine for improving exercise performance. The amino acids leucine, isoleucine, and valine are the predominant amino acids used for fuel during exercise. Supplements of these are promoted to improve performance in endurance athletes. The results of studies examining these amino acids are conflicting, and the benefits associated with their use can also be obtained by consuming carbohydrate during exercise.[23]

Although some studies show benefits to athletes, in general amino acid supplements are not recommended. High doses of individual amino acids may interfere with the absorption of other amino acids from the diet (see Chapter 6). And, there have been several reports of illness caused by contaminants in the supplements. Like any dietary supplement, amino acid supplements should be taken with caution and the risks weighed against potential benefits.

Vitamin and Mineral Needs

Exercise increases energy needs and thus the need for vitamins and minerals involved in energy production. A balanced diet that meets energy needs generally provides these additional vitamins and minerals. However, this may not be true for exercisers consuming low-energy diets, such as individuals exercising to lose weight or athletes such as ballerinas or gymnasts who want to maintain very low body weights. To avoid deficiencies, these individuals must consume carefully planned diets or include a supplement in order to meet their vitamin and mineral needs. For some competitive athletes, particularly females, iron and calcium status are a concern.

Iron For most individuals, exercise does not increase iron needs. However, in athletes, particularly female athletes, a reduction in the amount of stored iron is common.[24] If this situation progresses to anemia, performance will be impaired.[25]

Poor iron status may be caused by an inadequate dietary iron intake, an increased demand for iron, increased iron losses, or a redistribution of iron due to exercise training. Dietary iron intake may be limited in athletes who are attempting to keep body weight low, or in those who consume a vegetarian diet and therefore do not eat meat—an excellent source of readily absorbable heme iron. Iron needs may be increased in athletes because exercise stimulates the production of red blood cells, so more iron is needed for hemoglobin synthesis. Iron is also needed for the synthesis of muscle myoglobin and the iron-containing proteins needed for ATP production in the mitochondria. Iron loss also may be increased by loss in sweat during exercise. Also, red blood cells may be broken by impact in events such as running (foot-strike hemolysis) or by the contraction of large muscles. However, this rarely causes anemia because the breaking of red blood cells stimulates the production of new ones.

Some athletes experience a condition known as sports anemia, which is a temporary decrease in hemoglobin concentration that occurs during exercise training. This is an adaptation to training that does not seem to impair delivery of oxygen to tissues. It occurs when blood volume expands to increase oxygen delivery, but the synthesis of red blood cells lags behind the increase in plasma volume.

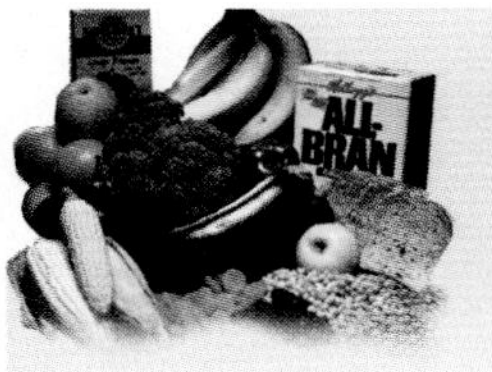

Off the Shelf

The Anabolic Edge: From Steroids to Creatine

For as long as there have been competitions, athletes have yearned for something—anything—that would give them the competitive edge. Everything from desiccated liver to bee pollen and shark cartilage has been tried as an ergogenic aid. The majority of these potential performance boosters have turned out to offer more of a psychological than a physiological edge. However, when athletes from Eastern European nations began to dominate international strength events, the athletic community became aware of the muscle-building effects of large doses of anabolic steroids. Finally an effective ergogenic aid had been found. Since then, however, anabolic steroids have been determined to be dangerous and their use is now illegal, so the search continues for the perfect performance booster.

Anabolic Steroids The term "anabolic steroid" refers to steroid hormones that accelerate protein synthesis and growth. The anabolic steroids used by athletes are synthetic versions of the human steroid hormone testosterone. Natural testosterone stimulates and maintains the male sexual organs and promotes the development of bones and muscles and the growth of skin and hair. The synthetic testosterone used by athletes has a greater effect on muscle development and bone, skin, and hair than it does on sexual organs. When synthetic testosterone is taken in conjunction with exercise and an adequate diet, muscle mass increases. However, these drugs also make the body think testosterone is being produced, and therefore they reduce the production of natural testosterone. Without natural testosterone, the sexual organs are not maintained; testes shrink and sperm production decreases. In adolescents, the use of synthetic testosterone causes bone growth to stop and height to be stunted. Anabolic steroid use may also cause oily skin and acne, water retention in the tissues, yellowing of the eyes and skin, coronary artery disease, liver disease, and sometimes death. Users may have psychological and behavioral side effects such as violent outbursts and depression, possibly leading to suicide. The dangers of steroid use are increased by the fact that they are illegal, so their manufacturing and distribution procedures are not regulated. Users can never be sure of the potency and purity of what they are taking.

Steroid Precursors Anabolic steroids are illegal, but their precursors are not. Compounds that can be converted into testosterone in the body can be purchased as dietary supplements. One of these, androstenedione, known as "Andro," is a precursor to the sex hormones testosterone and estrogen, and taking it is expected to cause an increase in levels of these hormones. Andro has been used for years by body builders, but it was launched to public prominence when Mark McGwire announced his use of it during the 1998 baseball season when he hit 70 home runs to break the single-season home-run record. This recent notoriety is projected to increase sales from $5 million to $100 million and has caused physicians, coaches, and athletes to revisit the safety issues associated with steroid use.[1]

As with any dietary supplement, the fact that Andro is available over-the-counter does not guarantee its safety. In fact, very little is known about either the safety or ergogenic effects of this supplement. Scientists do not know how much ingested or injected androstenedione is absorbed, where it acts, or how much is converted to testosterone. It is not known whether androstenedione will cause the testicular shrinkage, liver disease, and heart disease that anabolic steroids do. The purity of what is sold commercially is unknown, unregulated, and probably quite

Calcium In general, exercise—particularly weight-bearing exercise—increases bone density. This reduces the risk of osteoporosis. However, in female athletes with extremely low body weight and fat, calcium status can be at risk.

Female athletes who strive to reduce body weight and fat to improve performance, achieve an ideal body image, and meet goals set by coaches, trainers, or parents are at risk for eating disorders. The prevalence of eating disorders among female athletes is equal to or greater than in the general population.[26] Eating disorders can create a physiological condition similar to starvation and contribute to menstrual abnormalities. High levels of exercise are also hypothesized to affect the menstrual cycle by increasing energy demands or causing stress-related hormonal changes.[26] High levels of exercise combined with disordered eating can contribute to **amenorrhea**—the delayed onset or absence of menses in women. Amenorrhea in turn interferes with calcium status and consequently causes reductions in bone mass and bone mineral density. Amenorrhea results in low estrogen levels, which affects bone metabolism and reduces calcium absorption. Low estrogen levels combined with poor calcium intake, which is common in female athletes and females in general, leads to premature bone loss, failure to reach peak bone mass, and an increased risk of stress fractures. Neither adequate dietary calcium nor the increase in bone mass caused by weight-bearing exercise

Amenorrhea Delayed onset of menstruation or the absence of three or more consecutive menstrual cycles.

variable. Even its ability to improve athletic performance is not well documented. Although it can legally be purchased, its use is banned by the International Olympic Committee, the National Collegiate Athletic Association, and some but not all professional sports associations. Although the most well known, androstenedione is not the only steroid precursor available; others include androstenediol, DHEA, norandrostenediol, and norandrostenedione.

Creatine Creatine is another over-the-counter supplement that athletes are using for its anabolic effects. Creatine promises to produce steroidlike effects on muscle size and strength as well as to decrease fatigue and increase energy and performance.

Creatine is a chemical found in the body, primarily in muscle, where it is used to make creatine phosphate. Creatine phosphate replenishes ATP during short bursts of activity. When muscle activity begins, the small amount of ATP present in muscle is used rapidly. Muscle creatine phosphate then efficiently forms ATP to maintain levels until glycolysis can begin supplying ATP.

Creatine in muscle comes from that synthesized by the kidney, liver, pancreas, and other tissues as well as from that consumed in the diet.[2] Dietary creatine is found in muscle meats. The more creatine in the diet, the greater the muscle stores. Individuals who consume diets low in creatine, such as vegetarians, have lower body stores. Supplements of creatine monohydrate have been shown to increase levels of both creatine and creatine phosphate in muscle.[3] Once in the muscle, creatine levels remain elevated for several weeks after the supplement is stopped.

The benefits of creatine as an ergogenic aid have been well studied. Increasing muscle creatine and creatine phosphate has a number of advantages for athletes. It provides muscles with more quick energy for activity, delays fatigue, and allows creatine phosphate to be regenerated more quickly after exercise. And, it prevents the accumulation of lactic acid, which impairs performance.[2] These effects make creatine supplementation beneficial for repetitive short-term exhaustive anaerobic exercise such as sprinting and weight lifting, which require explosive bursts of energy. Creatine supplements have also been found to increase body mass mostly through lean tissue. This increase is believed to be due to an increase in protein synthesis as well as to fluid retention in the muscle.[3]

So, is creatine the magic pill that athletes have sought for generations? Is it an effective, safe, legal alternative to anabolic steroids? Research has shown it to be effective in the short term, but there are little data on whether chronic use further increases performance. Although a number of studies have suggested that it is safe, controlled toxicology studies are needed.[4] Finally, product purity is an issue. Since large doses of 5 to 30 grams (1 to 6 teaspoons) are needed to be effective, even a minor contaminant would be consumed in significant amounts. Whether beneficial or not, many athletes will choose to use creatine and other supplements in the hope that performance will be improved. The risks should be carefully weighed.

[1]Schnirring, L. Androstenedione et al.: nonprescription steroids. The Phys. Sport Med. 26:15–18, 1998.

[2]Maughan, R. J. Creatine supplementation and exercise performance. Int. J. Sport Nutr. 5:94–101, 1995.

[3]Greenhaff, P. L. Creatine and its application as an ergogenic aid. Int. J. Sport Nutr. 5:S100–S110, 1995.

[4]Toler, S. M. Creatine is an ergogen for anaerobic exercise. Nutr. Rev. 55:21–25, 1997.

can compensate for bone loss due to low estrogen levels. If menses resume, bone loss can at least be partially reversed, but whether these athletes are at greater risk of osteoporosis later in life is not known.[27]

The Importance of Water

Water is needed to regulate body temperature and to transport both oxygen and nutrients to the muscles and waste products away from muscles. Failure to consume adequate fluids to replace water lost through the lungs and in sweat can be critical to even the most casual exerciser.

Water and the Regulation of Body Temperature During exercise, heat production increases as exercise intensity increases. If heat cannot be lost from the body, body temperature rises and exercise performance as well as health may be jeopardized. The ability to dissipate the heat generated during exercise is affected by the hydration status of the exerciser as well as by environmental conditions. At rest in a temperate environment, an individual loses about 1.1 liters (about 4.5 cups) of water per day, or 50 ml per hour, from the skin and lungs. Exercise in a hot environment can increase this tenfold. Adequate fluids should be consumed

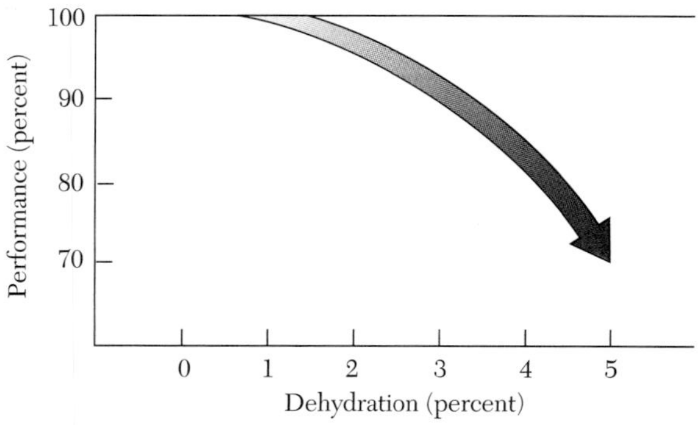

Figure 12.13
As dehydration increases, exercise performance declines. (Adapted from Saltin, B., and Castill, D. I. Fluid and electrolyte balance during prolonged exercise. In *Exercise, Nutrition, and Energy Metabolism*. Horton, E. S., and Tergung, R. I., eds. New York: Macmillan, 1988.)

before, during, and after exercise. Since thirst is not a reliable indicator of fluid needs, it is important for anyone exercising to schedule regular fluid breaks. Strenuous exercise should be avoided if the weather is too hot or too humid.

Consequences of Inadequate Hydration The water lost in sweat and evaporation from the lungs must be replaced. Inadequate body water leads to thermal distress which includes dehydration, heat cramps, heat exhaustion, and heat stroke. Dehydration occurs when water loss is great enough for blood volume to decrease, thereby reducing the ability to deliver oxygen and nutrients to exercising muscles. Even mild dehydration—a body water loss of 1% of body weight—can impair exercise performance (Figure 12.13). Heat cramps are involuntary cramps and spasms in the muscles involved in exercise. They occur when water and salt have been lost during extended exercise and are caused by an imbalance of the electrolytes sodium and potassium at the muscle cell membranes. Heat exhaustion occurs when fluid loss causes blood volume to decrease so much that it is not possible to both cool the skin and deliver oxygen to active muscles. It is characterized by a rapid weak pulse, low blood pressure, fainting, profuse sweating, and disorientation. Heat stroke, the most serious form of thermal distress, occurs when the temperature regulatory center of the brain fails. Heat stroke is characterized by elevated body temperature, hot dry skin, extreme confusion, and unconsciousness. It requires immediate medical attention.

Weight Loss Through Dehydration Athletes involved in sports with weight classes, such as wrestling and boxing, sometimes go to unhealthy extremes to keep body weight down so they can compete in lower weight classes (competing at the high end of a weight class is thought to give an advantage over smaller opponents).[21] Frequently, this rapid weight loss is accomplished by dehydration, through such practices as vigorous exercise, fluid restriction, wearing vapor-impermeable suits, and using hot environments such as saunas and steam rooms. More extreme measures include vomiting and the use of diuretics and laxatives. These practices can be dangerous and even fatal. They may reduce performance and can adversely affect heart and kidney function, temperature regulation, and electrolyte balance.[28]

Fluid Intake for Exercise Anyone exercising should consume extra fluids. Typically, however, exercising individuals ingest amounts of fluids that are equal to only about one to two thirds of the amount lost in sweat.[29]

How Much to Consume? To ensure adequate hydration, exercisers should drink about 2 cups of fluid 2 hours before exercise, and on warm days, they should consume an additional 1 to 2 cups about 30 to 60 minutes before exercising.[30] During exercise, whether casual or competitive, 3 to 6 ounces of fluid should be consumed every 10 to 15 minutes.

For endurance athletes, a good way to prevent dehydration is to consume enough fluid during exercise to minimize weight loss (Figure 12.14). And, immediately after exercise, each pound of weight lost should be replaced with 16 ounces (1 pound) of fluid (Table 12.3).

What to Consume? For most exercisers, water is the best fluid to drink.[30] Alcohol and beverages containing caffeine, such as colas, iced tea, and coffee, act as diuretics and therefore reduce body fluids rather than increase them.

Exercise lasting longer than 60 to 90 minutes may cause body carbohydrate stores to be depleted. For extended exercise, a beverage containing 4 to 8 grams of carbohydrate per 100 ml of fluid is therefore recommended. This is the amount of carbohydrate found in popular sports beverages such as Gatorade and Powerade (see *Off the Label: Sports Beverages and Bars: What Are You Really Getting?*). The carbohydrate in a beverage helps to maintain blood glucose levels, therefore providing a source of glucose for the muscle and delaying fatigue. As the amount of carbohydrate in the beverage increases, the rate at which the solution leaves the stomach decreases. Therefore, beverages containing larger amounts of carbohydrate, such as fruit juices and soft drinks, are not recommended unless they are diluted with an equal volume of water. Water and carbohydrate trapped in the stomach do not benefit the athlete.

Small amounts of minerals, including sodium and chloride, are lost in sweat, but for most activities, replacing electrolytes is not a primary concern because sweat consists mostly of water. The amounts of sodium and other minerals lost in sweat during exercise lasting even as long as 5 hours are not enough to affect health or performance and can easily be replaced by food eaten after the exercise has stopped. Only in extremely long events lasting longer than 8 hours, such as ultramarathons or Ironman triathalons, are there significant losses of sodium and other minerals in the sweat. If, during one of these endurance events, an athlete were to drink water without electrolytes, the water would dilute the sodium remaining in the blood. When the blood is diluted, it signals the brain to stop the thirst sensation and stimulates the production of urine by the kidneys, increasing water loss and resulting in dehydration. The consumption of fluids containing electrolytes will prevent blood from becoming too diluted.[31] It is recommended that these ultraendurance athletes include 0.5 to 0.7 gram of sodium per liter (1.2 to 1.8 g of sodium chloride per liter) in their rehydration drinks. Consuming salt alone in pill form is unnecessary and dangerous because the salt will draw water away from the tissues and may cause dehydration, nausea, and vomiting. Therefore, the common belief that salt pills are necessary to replace the sodium lost in sweat and prevent dehydration is a misconception.

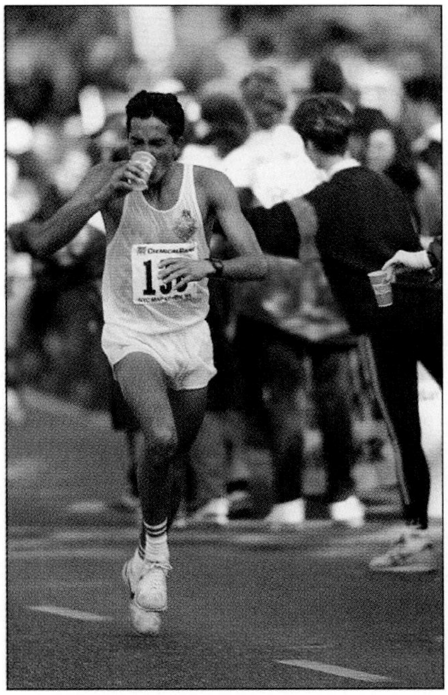

Figure 12.14
Fluids should be consumed before, during, and after exercise. (© John Kelly/The Image Bank)

Table 12.3 *Recommended Fluid Intake for Exercise*

Before Exercise
Begin exercise well hydrated by consuming fluids during the 2 hours before exercise.
Consume 14 to 20 ounces of fluid during the 30 minutes before exercise.

During Exercise
Consume 3 to 6 ounces of fluid every 15 minutes.
For exercise lasting less than 60 to 90 minutes, water is the best fluid.
For exercise lasting longer than 60 to 90 minutes, consuming a fluid containing about 6% carbohydrate may improve endurance.
For exercise lasting longer than 8 hours, a fluid containing carbohydrate and electrolytes may be beneficial.

After Exercise
Begin fluid replacement immediately after exercise.
Consume 16 ounces of fluid for each pound of weight lost.

Off the Label

Sports Beverages and Bars: What Are You Really Getting?

Exceed, Gatorade, Power Burst, Power Bar. . . . Beverages and bars claim to provide you with that extra boost that makes your workout more satisfying or your performance more competitive. They are marketed to people at all levels of activity, from strollers to professional athletes. Can they provide a convenient snack for your exercise program? Their benefits depend on what your individual needs are and when you want to consume them. Read labels carefully to be sure your ergogenic snack won't slow you down.

Sports Beverages Fluids before, during, and after exercise are important to prevent dehydration, and sports drinks claim to be the fluid you need for exercise. A glance at the label finds that sports drinks are really water, sugar, and salt. Most of what exercisers lose in sweat is water—so the best beverage to replace it is water. Because small amounts of minerals, including sodium, are also lost in sweat, many sports drinks are marketed with the promise of replacing these lost electrolytes. However, during everyday workouts and most athletic events only small amounts are lost in sweat, and these are easily replaced from foods eaten during the next meal. Although electrolyte replacement is unnecessary even for events lasting as long as a marathon, the amount of sodium in the typical sports drink is not harmful. And the sodium and other electrolytes in sports drinks may help increase the rate of fluid and glucose absorption from the gastrointestinal tract.[1]

The sugar in sports drinks is included to help maintain blood glucose. For moderate exercise such as a 20-minute jog, 40 minutes at the gym, or a brisk walk through the park, glucose-containing beverages offer no advantage over a water bottle filled at the drinking fountain. And they may be counterproductive if the goal of exercise is losing weight. A typical sports drink contains about 50 kcalories per cup, so drinking a 16-ounce bottle at the gym will replace about half of the 200 kcalories expended during your 40-minute ride on the stationary bicycle.

For exercise of longer duration (60 to 90 minutes), consuming glucose does help to maintain blood glucose and has been shown to increase endurance. To be effective, the drink should contain 4 to 8 grams of glucose in 100 ml (3 fluid ounces). The serving size for sports drinks is one cup, or about 240 ml, so the Nutrition Facts on your sports drink should list about 10 to 19 grams of total carbohydrate. Less than this may not enhance performance, and more may delay stomach emptying and cause abdominal cramps. The ingredient list shows you the source of the carbohydrate. Most provide glucose, but some beverages contain short chains of glucose molecules called glucose polymers. These leave the stomach more quickly than the same amount of glucose but have not been shown to offer any additional performance benefit.[2]

Other sports beverages use fructose instead of glucose, but studies have shown that there is no advantage over glucose in terms of stomach emptying or performance, and fructose is more likely to cause gastric distress. If fructose is tolerated, fruit juice diluted with an equal volume of water will provide the same amount of carbohydrate as a sports drink at about half the cost.

For most activities, sports drinks provide no performance or health advantages over plain water, but if a flavored beverage is consumed more readily than plain water, their use may provide the benefit of enhanced fluid intake.

Sports Bars Another type of "sports food" is the sports bar. There are many different types that vary in composition and in the promises they make. Some are high in carbohydrate and are advertised to optimize performance. Others are higher in protein and are advertised to build lean muscle, reduce body fat, increase strength, and speed recovery. All are marketed as a snack that can be eaten before, during, or after exercise.

If you are choosing a sports bar as a precompetition meal, read the label and choose one that provides about 300 kcalories—60 to 70% of kcalories as carbohydrate, 10 to 25% of kcalories as fat, and 10 to 20% of kcalories as protein. Use the total kcalories and grams of total carbohydrate, total fat, and protein to calculate the percent of energy from each (see figure). A bar that meets these recommendations can also be eaten during an activity to prevent hunger and maintain blood glucose. Bars that are lower in carbohydrate and higher in protein or fat may not significantly increase blood glucose and will take longer to digest, possibly causing stomach upset. Such a bar is fine for a snack during the day but is not the best choice immediately before or during exercise.

Although sports bars look and often taste like candy bars, comparing the labels will show that most are lower in fat than candy bars; provide more fiber; and contain vitamin C, vitamin E, calcium, iron, magnesium, copper, zinc, and a host of B vitamins. The percent Daily Value of many of these vitamins and minerals may not be included in the Nutrition Facts portion of the label, but the nutrients added will appear in the ingredient list. Whether sports bars are eaten before, during, or after an activity, they are just one part of the total diet and should not take the place of the whole grains, fresh vegetables and fruits, dairy products, and meats or meat substitutes that make up a healthy diet.

The greatest advantage of sports bars is convenience. They are pre-portioned,

FOOD AND DRINK FOR SPORT

For most of us, a trip to the gym requires no special nutritional planning beyond that needed to consume a balanced diet and plenty of water. For competitive athletes, however, foods eaten in preparation for competition may give or take away the extra seconds that can mean victory or defeat. Thus far, no magic pill that

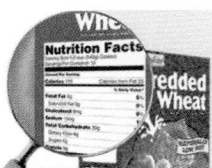

$$\% \text{ Kcalories from carbohydrate} = \frac{45 \text{ g} \times 4 \text{ kcal/g}}{230 \text{ kcal}} \times 100 = 78\%$$

$$\% \text{ Kcalories from fat} = \frac{2 \text{ g} \times 9 \text{ kcal/g}}{230 \text{ kcal}} \times 100 = 8\%$$

Nutrition Facts	Amount/Serving	% DV*	Amount/Serving	% DV*
Serving Size 1 bar (65g)	**Total Fat** 2g	3%	**Potassium** 145mg	4%
Calories 230	Saturated Fat 0.5g	3%	**Total Carb** 45g	15%
Calories from Fat 20	Polyunsat Fat 1.0g		Dietary Fiber 3g	12%
Calories from Sat Fat 5	Monounsat Fat 0.5g		Sugars 14g	
*Percent Daily Values (DV) are based on a 2,000 calorie diet.	**Cholesterol** 0mg	0%	Other Carb 28g	
	Sodium 90mg	4%	**Protein** 10g	

Vitamin A 0% • Vitamin C 100% • Calcium 30% • Iron 35% • Vitamin E 100%
Thiamin 100% • Riboflavin 100% • Niacin 100% • Vitamin B_6 100%
Folate 100% • Vitamin B_{12} 100% • Biotin 100% • Pantothenic Acid 100%
Phosphorus 35% • Magnesium 35% • Zinc 35% • Copper 35% • Chromium 20%

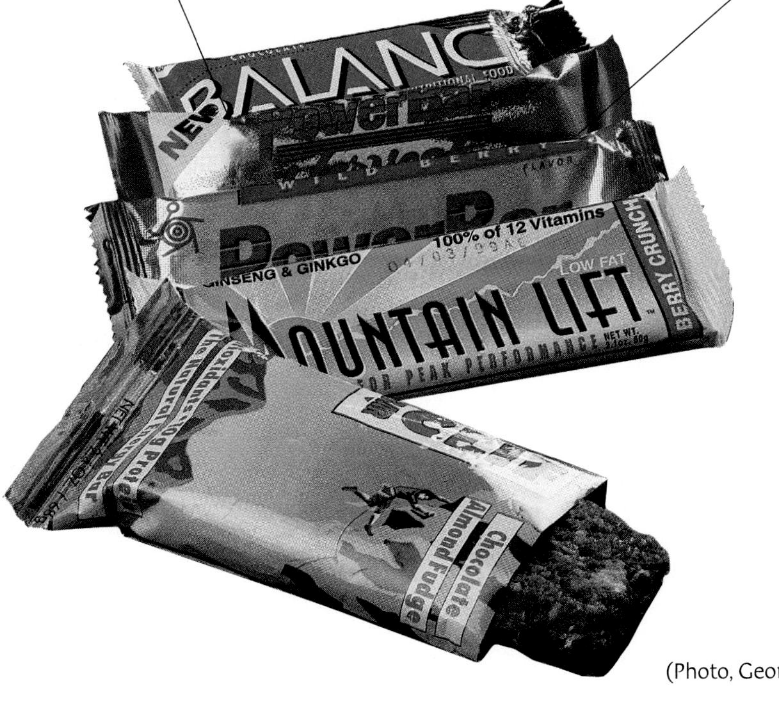

(Photo, George Semple)

ready to eat, and transportable. If having a compact, individually wrapped bar that will fit in a pocket or bicycle pack means the difference between consuming this food or no snack at all, they can be beneficial. They provide carbohydrate, protein, fat, and many micronutrients, but they don't provide fluid. If you choose to use these bars, eat them with plenty of water. Sports beverages and sports bars may also provide a psychological edge if the consumer believes they will enhance performance.

[1]Senay, L. C. Water and electrolytes during physical activity. In *Nutrition in Exercise and Sport,* 3rd ed. Wolinski, I., ed. Boca Raton, Fla.: CRC Press, 1998. 257–276.

[2]Puhl, S. M., and Buskirk, E. R. Nutrient beverages for exercise and sport. In *Nutrition in Exercise and Sport,* 3rd ed. Wolinski, I., ed. Boca Raton, Fla.: CRC Press, 1998. 277–314.

maximizes performance has been discovered, but there are a number of sound sports nutrition recommendations.

Glycogen Supercompensation: Maximizing Glycogen Stores

For the serious endurance athlete, larger glycogen stores allow exercise to continue for longer periods. One way to maximize glycogen stores before an event is to follow

Glycogen supercompensation or **carbohydrate loading** A regimen of diet and exercise training designed to maximize muscle glycogen stores before an athletic event.

a regimen of **glycogen supercompensation** or **carbohydrate loading.** This regimen involves depleting glycogen stores by exercising strenuously and then replenishing glycogen by consuming a high-carbohydrate diet for a few days before competition, during which time only light exercise is performed. This is more involved than consuming a large spaghetti dinner before running in a 10-kilometer fun run. Increasing glycogen stores requires a six-day regimen of diet and exercise. The current practice is to taper down exercise during the six days before competition while progressively increasing the carbohydrate content of the diet to about 550 grams, or 70% of energy, during the three days before competition.[32] Since consuming this much carbohydrate can be difficult, there are a number of high-carbohydrate beverages available which contain 20 to 25 grams of carbohydrate per 100 ml. These should not be confused with sports drinks designed to be consumed during competition, which contain only about 4 to 8 grams of carbohydrate per 100 ml. A glycogen supercompensation regimen will increase glycogen stores 20 to 40% above the level that would be achieved on a typical diet.[33]

Although carbohydrate loading is beneficial to endurance athletes, it will provide no benefit and even has some disadvantages for those exercising for periods less than 90 minutes For every gram of glycogen in the muscle, 3 grams of water are also deposited. This water will cause a 2- to 7-pound weight gain and may cause some muscle stiffness. As glycogen is used, the water is released. This can be an advantage when exercising in hot weather, but the extra weight is a disadvantage for those competing in events of short duration.

Meals for Competition

The goal of meals eaten before competition is to maximize glycogen stores and provide adequate hydration while minimizing any digestion, hunger, and gastric distress during the competition. The wrong precompetition meal can hinder performance more than the right one can enhance it. The goal for meals after competition is to replenish losses that occurred during the competition, including fluids and electrolytes lost during prolonged sweating.

The Precompetition Meal Meals before competition should ensure that liver glycogen stores are full. Muscle glycogen is depleted by exercise, but liver glycogen is used to supply blood glucose and is depleted even during rest if no food is ingested. A high-carbohydrate meal eaten 2 to 4 hours before the event will fill liver glycogen stores. The meal should be high in carbohydrate (60–70%), low in fat (10–25%), and moderate in protein (10–20%), and provide about 300 kcalories—for example, a cup of pasta with tomato sauce and a slice of bread, or a turkey sandwich and a cup of juice. High-fiber foods should be avoided to prevent feeling bloated during competition. Spicy foods that could cause heartburn, and large amounts of simple sugars that could cause diarrhea, should also be avoided unless the athlete is accustomed to eating these foods.

In addition to providing nutritional clout, a precompetition meal that includes "lucky" foods may impart an added psychological advantage. Some athletes find that in addition to a precompetition meal, a small high-carbohydrate snack or beverage consumed shortly before an event may enhance endurance.[33] Because foods affect people differently, athletes should test the effect of precompetition meals and snacks during training, not during competition.

Postcompetition Meals When exercise ends, the body must shift from the catabolic state of breaking down glycogen, triglycerides, and muscle proteins for fuel to the anabolic state of restoring muscle and liver glycogen, depositing lipids, and synthesizing muscle proteins. The first priority is to replace fluid losses. Appropriate postcompetition intake can replenish muscle and liver glycogen within 24 hours of the athletic event. This is critical to the ability to perform subsequent endurance activities. To maximize glycogen replacement, a high-carbohydrate meal or drink should be consumed as soon as possible after the event and again every 2 hours for 6 hours after the event. Ideally the meals should provide about 0.7 to 1.5 grams of carbohydrate per kg of body weight, which is about 50 to 100 grams of carbohydrate for a 70-kg person—the equivalent of two pancakes with syrup and a glass of fruit punch.[32] Approximately 600 grams of carbohydrate, or about 8 to 10 g per kg, should be consumed during the 24 hours after exercise. The consumption of fructose compared to glucose induces less muscle glycogen synthesis and more liver glycogen synthesis.

Ergogenic Aids: Do Supplements Enhance Athletic Performance?

Athletes use a variety of **ergogenic aids** to enhance their performance. Anything designed to enhance performance can be considered an ergogenic aid. For instance, the following are types of ergogenic aids: running shoes (mechanical aids); psychotherapy (psychological aid); increasing the number of red blood cells by having blood drawn and then readministered several days later, known as blood doping (physiological aid); and drugs to enhance red blood cell production (pharmacological aids). Many dietary supplements are also used as ergogenic aids.

Ergogenic aids Anything designed to increase work or improve performance.

The idea that specific foods might enhance athletic performance and confer athletic prowess is not new. In ancient Greece, the wrestler Milo of Croton was said to have subsisted on a daily diet of 20 pounds of bread, 20 pounds of meat, and 18 pints of wine.[34] Today, supplements ranging from carnitine and amino acids to bee pollen and ginseng are used with the hope that they will enhance performance. Although many of these supplements are expensive and most have not been shown to improve performance, athletes are vulnerable to their enticements.[35] When considering the use of an ergogenic supplement, an athlete should remember that, as dietary supplements, these products do not have to be proven safe or effective before they can be sold (see Chapter 9). Consumers should weigh health risks against potential benefits prior to using these products (see Figure 12.15 and Table 12.4).

Vitamin Supplements as Ergogenic Aids Many of the promises made about vitamin supplements are extrapolated from their biochemical functions. For example, thiamin, riboflavin, niacin, and pantothenic acid are all involved in muscle energy metabolism. Thiamin and pantothenic acid are needed for carbohydrate to enter the citric acid cycle for aerobic metabolism. Riboflavin and niacin are

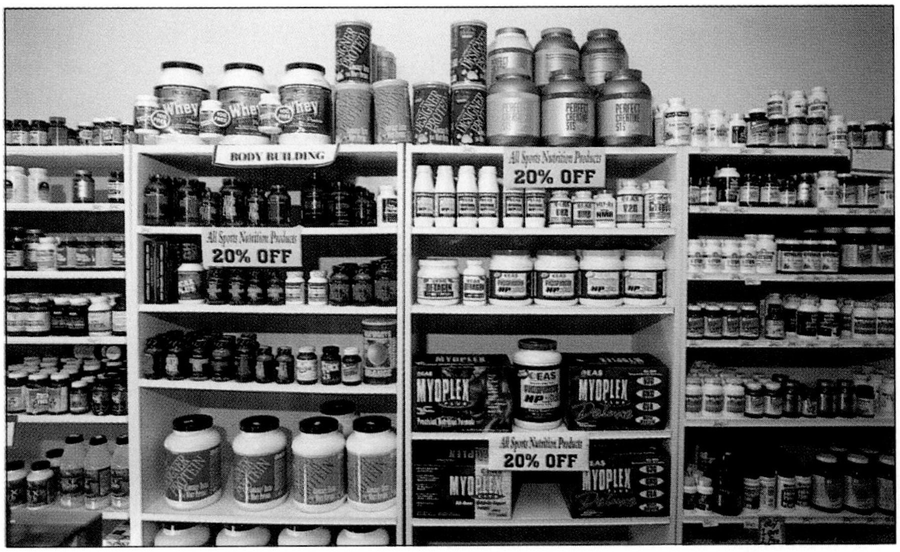

Figure 12.15
Many types of supplements are marketed to athletes as ergogenic aids. (George Semple)

Table 12.4 *Claims, Effectiveness, and Risks of Popular Ergogenic Aids*

Ergogenic Aid	Claim	Effectiveness	Risk
Androstenedione	Converted to testosterone, which increases muscle growth and strength.	No long-term human studies on safety or ergogenic effects.	May have risks similar to illegal steroids, such as stunted growth, acne, unwanted hair growth, premature baldness, increased blood cholesterol levels, and decreased sperm production.
Arginine and ornithine	Cause the release of growth hormone, which stimulates muscle development and decreases body fat.	Most studies show no increase in lean body mass with supplementation.	High levels of one amino acid may interfere with the absorption of others. Cause diarrhea at high doses.
Bee pollen	Causes faster recovery from training workouts, which enables a higher level of training.	No evidence that it improves training level or other parameters of performance.	Some individuals have allergic reactions.
Bicarbonate (sodium bicarbonate, baking soda)	Helps buffer lactic acid produced during exercise, thereby delaying fatigue.	Supplements increase blood pH and may enhance performance and strength in intense anaerobic activities but not in aerobic exercise.	Causes bloating, diarrhea, and high blood pH.
Branched chain amino acids (leucine, isoleucine, and valine)	Improve endurance and prevent fatigue.	Some studies show improvements in endurance and protection against muscle damage. Others showed no effect.	No toxicity reported.
Caffeine	Increases the release of fatty acids from adipose tissue, spares glycogen, and enhances endurance.	Research supports claims of increased endurance, but the effect depends on the individual.	Causes dehydration, nervousness, anxiety, insomnia, digestive discomfort, abnormal heartbeat, and memory impairment with amounts greater than 10 mg/kg.
Carnitine	Enhances the utilization of fatty acids and spares glycogen.	Most studies show no increase in fatty acid utilization or improvement in exercise performance.	L-carnitine form has little risk, but D,L-carnitine and D-carnitine forms can be toxic.
Chromium (chromium picolinate)	Increases lean body mass, decreases body fat, delays fatigue.	Chromium affects glucose utilization, protein synthesis, and lipid metabolism via its effect on insulin action, but supplements will not affect these processes unless a deficiency exists.	No toxicity reported in humans, but the chromium picolinate form has been shown to damage DNA in cells grown in the laboratory.

(continued)

needed to shuttle electrons to the electron transport chain so ATP can be formed. Other B vitamins are marketed for improving aerobic metabolism because of their roles in oxygen transport and delivery. For example, vitamin B_6 assists in the synthesis of hemoglobin and other proteins involved in oxygen transfer and utilization. Folic acid and vitamin B_{12} are both involved in the synthesis of red blood cells needed for oxygen transport. A deficiency of one or more of these would interfere with energy metabolism and impair athletic performance, but there is no evidence that consuming more than the recommended intake will enhance physical performance.

The claims that athletes should consume supplements of vitamin E, vitamin C, and beta-carotene focus on their antioxidant functions. Since exercise increases oxidative processes, it increases the production of free radicals. Free radicals can damage tissues and have been associated with fatigue during exercise.[17,36] It has been suggested that antioxidant supplements prevent free radical damage and delay fatigue. Vitamin E and vitamin C have been the most extensively studied. Vitamin E is particularly important in maintaining muscle function by protecting muscle cell membranes from free radical damage. Vitamin C acts as a free radical scavenger in aqueous solutions, such as the intracellular fluid and blood. Supplementation with mixtures of antioxidants has been shown to prevent free radical damage but has not been demonstrated conclusively to enhance perfor-

Table 12.4 *(continued)*

Ergogenic Aid	Claim	Effectiveness	Risk
Creatine (creatine monohydrate)	Increases energy production and speeds recovery after high-intensity exercise.	Creatine phosphate is rapidly converted into ATP for muscle contraction. Creatine supplements increase muscle creatine and creatine phosphate synthesis after exercise, and enhance strength, performance, and recovery from high-intensity exercise.	Causes stomach pain.
DHEA (dehydro-epiandosterone)	Converted into testosterone and estrogen inside the body and promises to build muscles, burn fat, and delay chronic diseases associated with aging.	No proven benefits.	May cause acne, oily skin, facial hair, voice deepening, hair loss, mood changes, liver damage; and stimulates existing cancers.
Glutamine	Prevents lactic acid accumulation; enhances muscle protein synthesis and growth hormone release; removes ammonia and increases muscle glycogen recovery; prevents decline in immune function with overtraining.	Some evidence exists for an increase in growth hormone release and an increase in bicarbonate to neutralize lactic acid.	No evidence of toxicity shown.
Ginseng	Spares glycogen, increases fatty acid oxidation, reduces fatigue.	No human research to support these claims.	Causes nervousness, confusion, and depression.
HMB (β-hydroxy β-methyl butyrate)	Increases ability to build muscle and burn fat in response to exercise.	Some studies support an increase in lean body mass and strength.	No toxicity in animals, but little information in humans.
Medium-chain triglycerides	Provide energy to body builders without promoting fat deposition; reduce muscle protein breakdown during prolonged exercise.	Provide energy and must be metabolized before they can be stored as body fat. They increase endurance and fatty acid oxidation in mice, but there is no evidence of a benefit in humans.	None known.
Vanadium (vanadyl sulfate)	Aids insulin action; allows more rapid and intense muscle pumping for body builders.	No evidence to support a benefit for body builders.	Reduces insulin production.

mance.[23,37] Although there is little risk associated with supplements of these nutrients, a diet with plenty of fruits and vegetables will ensure adequate intakes of vitamin E, vitamin C, and beta-carotene, as well as provide other dietary antioxidants.

Mineral Supplements as Ergogenic Aids Some of the minerals advertised as endurance enhancers include chromium, vanadium, selenium, zinc, and iron.

Chromium supplements, as chromium picolinate, claim to increase lean body mass and decrease body fat. Chromium is needed for insulin action and insulin promotes protein synthesis. Therefore, adequate chromium status is likely to be important for lean tissue synthesis. The picolinate form is believed to be absorbed better than other forms of chromium. Research has demonstrated an increase in muscle mass and decrease in body fat with supplemental chromium in pigs, but human trials have not consistently demonstrated an effect of supplemental chromium picolinate on body composition or body weight.[38] No adverse effects of chromium supplementation have been reported in humans,[39] but the picolinate form has been shown to cause DNA damage in cells in culture.[40] Although human studies using the standard supplemental dose of chromium picolinate have not detected an increase in DNA damage, more work is needed to completely rule out any risk.[41]

Vanadium, usually as vanadyl sulfate, is another mineral marketed for its ability to assist the action of insulin. Vanadium supplements promise to increase lean body mass, but there is no evidence that they have an anabolic effect, and toxicity is a concern.[23] Selenium is marketed for its antioxidant properties and zinc for its role in protein synthesis and tissue repair, but neither of these supplements have been found to improve athletic performance in individuals with adequate mineral status. Iron is also marketed as an ergogenic mineral because it is needed for hemoglobin synthesis. If an iron deficiency exists, as it frequently does in female athletes, supplements can be of benefit.

Other Ergogenic Aids Substances that are not nutrients are also marketed as ergogenic aids. Creatine, bicarbonate, and caffeine are non-nutrients which can have an ergogenic effect for some types of activity. Creatine supplements replenish creatine phosphate for quick energy and may increase muscle mass. They have been reported to improve performance in short-term intense exercise such as sprint cycling and running, but do not enhance performance in long-term endurance activities such as marathons (see *Off the Shelf: The Anabolic Edge: From Steroids to Creatine*).[42] Many other supplements that are sold to enhance performance, such as bee pollen, wheat germ oil, brewer's yeast, ginseng, royal jelly, DNA, and RNA, have not been found to be ergogenic.

Bicarbonate Bicarbonate ions act as buffers in the body. Bicarbonate supplements have been hypothesized to neutralize the lactic acid produced by anaerobic exercise and thus delay fatigue and allow improved performance. Taking bicarbonate before exercise has been found to improve performance and delay exhaustion in sports such as sprint cycling, which involve intense exercise for only 1 to 7 minutes, but it is of no benefit for lower-intensity aerobic exercise.[23]

Caffeine Some athletes may try to enhance endurance by consuming caffeine before an event. Caffeine has been shown to enhance performance during prolonged moderate-intensity endurance exercise and short-term intense exercise.[43] This is hypothesized to occur because caffeine enhances the release of fatty acids, and when fatty acids are used as a fuel source, glycogen is spared, delaying the onset of fatigue. The effect may vary, depending on the type of activity and the athlete. Athletes who are unaccustomed to caffeine respond better than those who routinely consume it. In some athletes caffeine may impair performance by increasing water loss in the urine or by causing gastrointestinal upset. Regardless of its effectiveness, athletes should know that excess caffeine is illegal. The International Olympic Committee prohibits athletes from competing when urine caffeine levels are 12 μg per ml or greater. For urine caffeine to reach this level, an individual would need to drink 6 to 8 cups of coffee within about a 2-hour period. Caffeine is also found in pill form in products such as NoDoz, which contains about 100 mg of caffeine per tablet—about the same amount as that in a cup of coffee (Table 12.5).

Other Supplements Bee pollen is a mixture of the pollen of flowering plants, plant nectar, and bee saliva. It contains no extraordinary factors and has not been shown to have any performance-enhancing effects. In addition, ingesting or inhaling bee pollen can be hazardous to individuals allergic to various plant pollens.[44] Brewer's yeast is a source of B vitamins and some minerals, but has not been demonstrated to have any ergogenic properties. Likewise, there is no evidence to support claims that wheat germ oil will aid endurance. As an oil, it is high in fat, but it is no better as an energy source than any other fat. Royal jelly is a substance produced by worker bees to feed to the queen bee. While it helps the queen bee

Table 12.5 ***The Caffeine Content of Commonly Consumed Foods and Medications***

Food or Medication	Amount	Caffeine (mg)
Coffee, regular	1 cup (240 ml)	139
Coffee, decaffeinated	1 cup	3
Tea, brewed	1 cup	45
Pepsi	12 oz (1 can)	37
Diet Pepsi	12 oz (1 can)	50
Mountain Dew	12 oz (1 can)	54
Hot chocolate	1 cup	7
Brownie	1	14
Chocolate bar	1 oz	15
NoDoz	1 tablet	100
Excedrin	1 tablet	65
Empirin, Anacin	1 tablet	32

grow to twice the size of worker bees and to live 40 times longer, royal jelly does not appear to enhance athletic capacity in humans. Ginseng is promoted to be ergogenic by increasing endurance. There are many different varieties of ginseng and thus far there is not sufficient evidence to support a role of ginseng in prolonging endurance in humans.[45] Although ginseng has been used for thousands of years with little toxicity, overdoses can cause insomnia, irritability, dizziness, and depression.[23] Finally, DNA and RNA are marketed to aid in tissue regeneration. In the body they carry genetic information and are needed to synthesize proteins, but DNA and RNA are not required in the diet, and supplements do not help replace damaged cells (see *Critical Thinking: Evaluating Ergogenic Aids*).

Critical Thinking

Evaluating Ergogenic Aids

Hector is on the college track team. He would like to improve his performance and decides to experiment with some ergogenic aids. Based on the advertisements in sports magazines, he selects bicarbonate to improve his sprint times and chromium to increase his lean body mass. But before he begins taking these he wants to explore their risks and benefits.

The ads and articles about these supplements make the following claims:

Bicarbonate will help neutralize the acidic lactic acid produced by muscles during anaerobic exercise and therefore improve performance in short-term exhaustive exercise.

Chromium will increase lean body tissue and enhance fat loss.

Do the claims made for these products make sense?

Bicarbonate is a buffer found naturally in the body that helps keep acidity in the normal range. So the claim that more might help buffer lactic acid is logical, assuming the bicarbonate from the supplement reaches the muscle cells where the lactic acid is produced.

Chromium is a mineral that is needed for insulin to perform its functions. Insulin is needed for many essential roles, including getting glucose into cells, turning on protein synthesis, and stimulating the synthesis of fat. The claim that it will increase lean tissue makes some sense metabolically, but Hector is not sure why taking chromium would enhance only the protein-building aspect of insulin's function.

Is there evidence that these supplements work?

The advertisements show photographs of sprinters and body builders and quote their testimonials on the effectiveness of these products. Hector is not convinced by this type of anecdotal evidence so he makes a trip to the library to explore the scientific literature.

What type of study should Hector look at?

Hector reviews Chapter 1 of his nutrition book to remind himself about what makes a good scientific study. He then looks for articles in well-respected peer-reviewed journals in the field of nutrition and sports, such as the *International Journal of Sport Nutrition,* and *Medicine and Science in Sports and Exercise.* He then focuses on papers that studied athletes involved in the types of activities he performs.

Do these supplements live up to their promoters' promises?

Hector finds several articles on bicarbonate and chromium. The studies of bicarbonate involve exhaustive exercise lasting 1 to 7 minutes and demonstrate enhanced performance in sprinters taking bicarbonate when compared to sprinters taking a placebo. For chromium, the studies are contradictory. One shows an increase in the amount of weight gained and a decrease in body fat in college weight trainers while another study found no significant effects.

What are the risks of taking bicarbonate and chromium?

Bicarbonate is sold as sodium bicarbonate, so it is high in sodium. Since it is not an essential nutrient, it is difficult to find information on toxicity. One article that Hector read used a dose of 0.3 gram per kilogram of body weight 2 to 3 hours before an event. At this dose some subjects experienced nausea, bloating, intestinal cramping, and diarrhea. Large intakes of water were recommended to prevent diarrhea.

Chromium is an essential mineral. Although the muscle-building effects of chromium are still questionable, the doses in supplements are about 200 μg per day—the upper end of the 1989 ESADDI for chromium. Although this amount of chromium does not pose a risk of toxicity, one study found that the picolinate form of chromium caused DNA damage in cells grown in the laboratory. He decides that he will wait for more research to be done before he takes chromium picolinate as an ergogenic aid. Because he eats a balanced diet and takes a multivitamin and mineral supplement that contains chromium, he concludes that he is getting adequate chromium. He is still unsure whether bicarbonate will offer more benefits than risks.

What would you recommend Hector do?

Answer:

APPLICATIONS

These exercises are designed to help you apply your critical thinking skills to your own lifestyle choices. They can be calculated using information in this text and its appendices.

1. Keep a log of your activity for one day.
   a. Note the number of hours you spend in (1) sleep, (2) very light activity, (3) light activity, (4) moderate activity, and (5) heavy activity (see Chapter 7).
   b. What is your RMR per hour? (Use Table 7.2 or Appendix B.)
   c. What are your energy needs for activity? (Use Table 7.3, Table 12.3, or Appendix L.)
   d. If you replaced very light activity with a 1-hour jog, what would your new energy expenditure be?
   e. Make a list of foods that you could add to your diet to balance the added expenditure of the jog.
2. Taking into consideration your typical weekly schedule of activities and events, design a reasonable exercise program for yourself using the Activity Pyramid. Include the types of activities, the times during the week you will be involved in each activity, and the length of time you will engage in each activity. Choose activities you enjoy and schedule them for reasonable lengths of time and at reasonable frequencies.
   a. What everyday changes have you made that will increase the energy expended in day-to-day activities?
   b. Which activities are aerobic, which improve flexibility, and which are for strength training?
   c. Can each of these activities be performed year-round? Suggest alternative activities and locations for inclement weather.
3. Do a risk-benefit analysis of an ergogenic aid (a quick way to do this is to use the Internet to collect information). List the risks and benefits and then write a conclusion as to why you would or would not take this substance.

Summary

1. Fitness, which is the ability to perform routine physical activity without undue fatigue, involves cardiorespiratory endurance, muscle strength and endurance, flexibility, and desirable body composition.
2. Regular exercise improves fitness in individuals of all ages and can reduce the risk of chronic diseases such as obesity, heart disease, diabetes, and osteoporosis. Exercise can also delay some of the changes in body composition and metabolism that occur with age.
3. A well-designed fitness program involves aerobic exercise, stretching, and strength training, and is carried out in a safe environment. There are numerous recommendations for how much exercise is enough; most agree that a minimum of 30 minutes of moderate activity should be performed on most

days of the week. One way to create a more active lifestyle is to choose enjoyable activities and follow the recommendations of the Activity Pyramid.

4. Activity is fueled by ATP generated from carbohydrate, fat, and protein. When oxygen is limited, anaerobic glycolysis produces ATP from carbohydrate. When oxygen is plentiful, aerobic metabolism generates ATP. Aerobic metabolism is more efficient than anaerobic glycolysis and can utilize carbohydrate, fatty acids, and amino acids as energy sources.
5. The availability of oxygen and the proportion of carbohydrate and fat used as fuel for a given activity depend on the intensity and duration of the activity and the training of the exerciser. For short-term, high-intensity activity, ATP is generated primarily from the anaerobic metabolism of glucose from muscle glycogen stores. For lower-intensity exercise of longer duration, aerobic metabolism predominates, and glucose and free fatty acids delivered to the tissues by the blood become important fuel sources. The proportion of energy generated from fatty acids increases with the duration of low-intensity exercise. Protein becomes an important source of energy only when exercise continues for many hours.
6. The daily diet of an active individual should provide sufficient energy to fuel activity. In general, it should contain about 55 to 60% of total energy as carbohydrate from whole grains, fruits, vegetables, and milk to ensure that glycogen stores are replenished after daily exercise; less than 30% of energy as fat; and about 12 to 17% of energy as protein.
7. Fluid intake before, during, and after exercise must replace water lost in sweat and from evaporation through the lungs. Water intake during activity must be sufficient to ensure that the body can be cooled and that nutrients and oxygen can be delivered to body tissues. If water intake is inadequate, exercise performance will decrease and thermal distress may occur. Plain water is the best fluid to consume for most exercise. During exercise lasting longer than 60 to 90 minutes, athletes might benefit from fluids containing glucose. Electrolyte replacement is only necessary during ultraendurance activities lasting more than 8 hours.
8. Sufficient micronutrients are needed to generate ATP from macronutrients and to transport oxygen and wastes to and from the cells. Some athletes are at risk for deficiencies of iron and calcium.
9. Competitive endurance athletes may utilize glycogen supercompensation regimens to maximize glycogen stores before an event.
10. Meals eaten before competition should provide about 300 kcalories; should be high in carbohydrate, low in fat, moderate in protein, and low in fiber; and should satisfy the psychological needs of the athlete. Postcompetition meals should replace lost fluids and electrolytes and begin restoring muscle and liver glycogen.
11. Many types of ergogenic aids are marketed to improve athletic performance. Some are beneficial for certain types of activity, but many offer little or no benefit. An individual risk-benefit analysis should be used to determine if a supplement is appropriate for you.

Review Questions

1. List the health benefits of fitness.
2. What is aerobic exercise?
3. What is strength training?
4. How does aerobic exercise affect resting heart rate?
5. How much exercise is enough?
6. What is maximal oxygen consumption and how is it affected by aerobic exercise?
7. What fuels are used to produce ATP in anaerobic metabolism?
8. Which is more efficient, aerobic or anaerobic metabolism?
9. What factors affect the availability of oxygen and the type of fuel used during exercise?
10. What fuels are used in exercise of long duration such as marathon running?
11. What are the recommendations for fluid intake before, during, and after exercise?
12. How does exercise affect protein needs?
13. What is glycogen supercompensation or carbohydrate loading?
14. Can ergogenic aids enhance exercise performance? How? Are they safe?

Nutrition Web Links

To further explore areas related to the material in this chapter, go to the *Nutrition: Science and Applications* Web site at ***www.Wiley.com/college/Smolin*** and *click on* **Student Companion Site** for chapter-by-chapter links. Some Web sites related to the information in Chapter 12 include:

Organizations that provide exercise recommendations such as the American Heart Association and the American Council on Exercise.

Organizations that provide information on exercise for specific groups such as the Fitness Partners Connection Jumpsite (for children) and the American Diabetes Association (for individuals with diabetes).

Locations that provide information on exercise and ergogenic aids such as Idea: The Fitness Source and the Physical Activity and Health Network.

References

1. Abernathy, R. P., and Black, D. R. Healthy body weights: an alternative perspective. Am. J. Clin. Nutr. 63(suppl):448S–451S, 1996.
2. U.S. Department of Health and Human Services, Centers for Disease Control and Disease Prevention, and the President's Council on Physical Fitness and Sports. *Physical Activity and Health: A Report of the Surgeon General* (Executive Summary), 1996.
3. Zelasko, C. J. Exercise for weight loss: what are the facts? J. Am. Diet. Assoc. 95:1414–1417, 1995.
4. American College of Sports Medicine. *ACSM's Guidelines for Exercise Testing and Prescription*, 5th ed. Baltimore: Williams & Wilkins, 1995.
5. NIH Consensus Development Panel on Physical Activity and Cardiovascular Health. J.A.M.A. 276:241–246, 1996.
6. American College of Sports Medicine. American College of Sports Medicine position stand: exercise and physical activity for older adults. Med. Sci. Sports Exerc. 30:992–1008, 1998.
7. Ivy, J. L. Role of exercise training in the prevention and treatment of insulin resistance and noninsulin dependent diabetes mellitus. Sports Med. 24:321–336, 1997.
8. Gammon, M. D., John, E. M., and Britton, J. A. Recreational and occupational physical activities and risk of breast cancer. J. Natl. Cancer Inst. 90:100–117, 1998.
9. Colditz, G. A., Cannuscio, C. C., and Frazier, A. L. Physical activity and reduced risk of colon cancer: implications for prevention. Cancer Causes Control 8:649–667, 1997.
10. Healthy People 2010. Online at http://web.health gov/healthypeople/2010Draft/
11. Jones, D. A., Ainsworth, B. E., Croft, J. B., et al. Moderate leisure-time physical activity: who is meeting the public health recommendations? A national cross-sectional study. Arch. Fam. Med. 7:285–289, 1998.
12. Exploring the Activity Pyramid, Institute for Research and Education. Healthsystem Minnesota. Online at http://www.hsmnet.com/HSM/BHC/IRE/HEC/EXPLORE.HTM
13. American Dietetic Association. Timely statement of the American Dietetic Association: nutrition guidance for child athletes in organized sports. J. Am. Diet. Assoc. 96:610–611, 1996.
14. Corbin, C. B., and Pangrazi, R. P. The new physical activity for children: a statement of guidelines. Council on Physical Education for Children, 1998. Online at http://www.aahperd.org/naspe/PressRelease.htm
15. Andersen, R. E., Crespo, C. J., Bartlett, S. J., et al. Relationship of physical activity and television watching with body weight and level of fatness among children: results from the Third National Health and Nutrition Examination Survey. J.A.M.A. 279:938–942, 1998.
16. American Academy of Pediatrics, Committee on Communications. Children, adolescents, and television. Pediatrics 96:786–790, 1995.
17. Kanter, M. M., and Williams, M. H. Antioxidants, carnitine, and choline as putative ergogenic aids. Int. J. Sport Nutr. 5:S120–S131, 1995.
18. Ratzin Jackson, C. G. Overview of human energy transfer and nutrition. In *Nutrition in Exercise and Sport*, 3rd ed. Wolinski, I., ed. Boca Raton, Fla.: CRC Press, 1998. 159–177.
19. Beals, K. A., and Manore, M. M. Nutritional status of female athletes with subclinical eating disorders. J. Am. Diet. Assoc. 98:419–425, 1998.
20. Arena, B., Maffulli, N., Maffulli, F., and Morleo, M. A. Reproductive hormones and menstrual changes with exercise in female athletes. Sports Med. 19:278–287, 1995.
21. Oppliger, R. A., Case, H. S., Horswill, C. A., et al. American College of Sports Medicine position statement: weight-loss in wrestlers. Med. Sci. Sports Exerc. 28:ix–xii, 1996.
22. Paul, G. L., Gautsch, T. A., and Layman, D. K. Amino acid and protein metabolism during exercise and recovery. In *Nutrition in Exercise and Sport*, 3rd ed. Wolinski, I., ed. Boca Raton, Fla.: CRC Press, 1998. 125–158.
23. Bucci, L. R. Dietary supplements as ergogenic aids. In *Nutrition in Exercise and Sport*, 3rd ed. Wolinski, I., ed. Boca Raton, Fla.: CRC Press, 1998. 315–368.
24. Smith, J. A. Exercise training and red blood cell turnover. Sports Med. 19:9–31, 1995.
25. Clarkson, P. M., and Haymes, E. M. Exercise and mineral status of athletes: calcium, magnesium, phosphorus and iron, Med. Sci. Sports Exerc. 27:831–843, 1995.
26. Otis, C. L., Drinkwater, B. L., Johnson, M., et al. American College of Sports Medicine position stand on the female athlete triad. Med. Sci. Sports Exerc. 29:i–ix, 1997.
27. Bennell, K. L., Malcolm, S. A., Wark, J. D., and Brukner, P. D. Skeletal effects of menstrual disturbances in athletes. Scand. J. Med. Sci. Sports 7:261–273, 1997.
28. Remick, D., Chancellor, K., Pederson, J., et al. Hyperthermia and dehydration-related deaths associated with intentional rapid weight loss in three collegiate wrestlers—North Carolina, Wisconsin, and Michigan, November–December, 1997. MMWR 47(06):105–108, 1998. Online at www.cdc.gov/epo/mmwr/mmwr_wk.html
29. Senay, L. C. Water and electrolytes during physical activity. In *Nutrition in Exercise and Sport*, 3rd ed. Wolinski, I., ed. Boca Raton, Fla.: CRC Press, 1998. 257–276.
30. American College of Sports Medicine. Position stand on exercise and fluid replacement. Med. Sci. Sports. Exerc. 28:i-vii, 1996.
31. Luetkemeir, M. J., Coles, M. G., and Askew, E. W. Dietary sodium and plasma volume levels with exercise. Sports Med. 23:279–286, 1997.
32. Wilkinson, J. G., and Liebman, M. Carbohydrate metabolism in sport and exercise. In *Nutrition in Exercise and Sport,* 3rd ed. Wolinski, I., ed. Boca Raton, Fla.: CRC Press, 1998. 63–99.
33. Coyle, E. F. Substrate utilization during exercise in active people. Am. J. Clin. Nutr. 61(suppl):968S–979S, 1995.
34. Harris, H. A. Nutrition and physical performance: the diet of Greek athletes. Proc. Nutr. Soc. 25:87–90, 1966.
35. Butterfield, G. Ergogenic aids: evaluating sport nutrition products. Int. J. Sport Nutr. 6:191–197, 1996.
36. Dekkers, J. C., van Doornen, L. J. P., and Kemper, H. C. G. The role of antioxidant vitamins and enzymes in the prevention of exercise-induced muscle damage. Sports Med. 21:213–238, 1996.
37. Kanter, M. M. Nutritional antioxidants and physical activity. In *Nutrition in Exercise and Sport*, 3rd ed. Wolinski, I., ed. Boca Raton, Fla.: CRC Press, 1998. 245–255.
38. Anderson, R. A. Effects of chromium on body composition and weight. Nutr. Rev. 56:266–270, 1998.
39. Hathcock, J. N. Vitamins and minerals: efficacy and safety. Am. J. Clin. Nutr. 66:427–437, 1997.
40. Stearns, D. M., Wise, J. P., Patierno, S. R., and Wetterhahn, K. E. Chromium (III) picolinate produces damage in Chinese hamster ovary cells. FASEB J. 9:1643–1648, 1995.
41. Kato, I., Vogelman, J. H., Dilman, V., et al. Effect of supplementation with chromium picolinate on antibody titers to 5-hydroxymethyl uracil. Eur. J. Epidemiol. 14:621–626, 1998.
42. Greenhaff, P. L. Creatine and its application as an ergogenic aid. Int. J. Sport Nutr. 5(suppl):S100–S110, 1995.
43. Spriet, L. L. Caffeine and performance. Int. J. Sport Nutr. 5(suppl): 84S–99S, 1995.
44. Bauer, L., Kohlich, A., Hirschwehr, R., et al. Food allergy: pollen or bee products? J. Allergy Clin. Immunol. 97:65–73, 1996.
45. Engels, H. J., and Wirth, J. C. No ergogenic effects of ginseng (Panax ginseng C. A. Meyers) during graded maximal aerobic exercise. J. Am. Diet. Assoc. 97:1110–1115, 1997.

Chapter 13

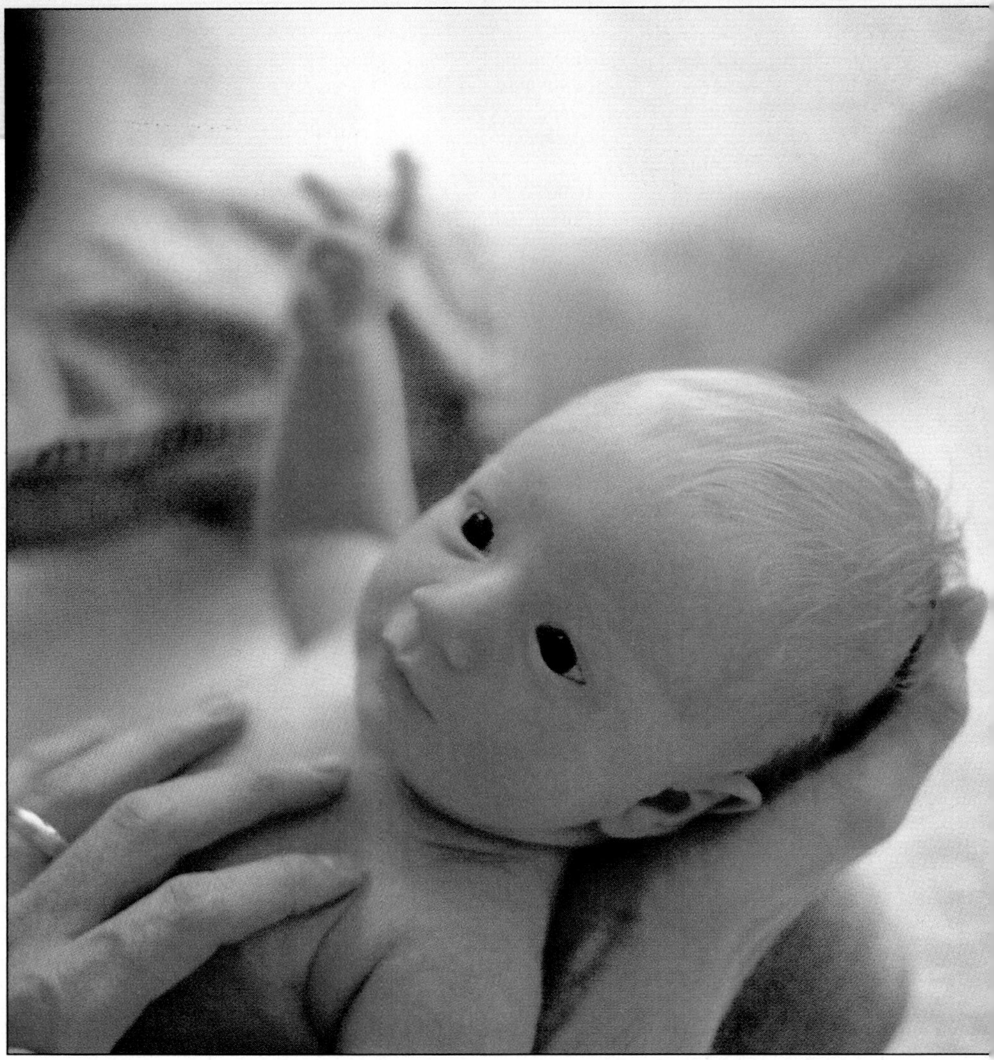

(© *Jeff Titcomb/Tony Stone Images*)

Chapter Outline

In the Beginning: Nutrition for Mothers and Infants

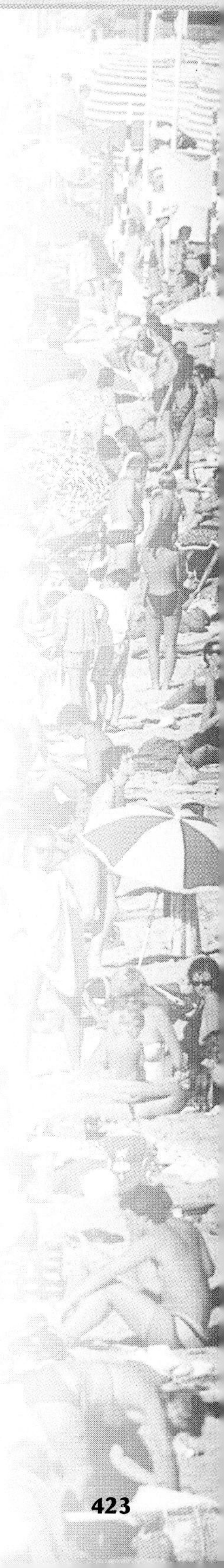

Chapter Concepts

1. A woman's nutrient intake during pregnancy must meet her needs and those of the fetus.
2. In order to support pregnancy and prepare for lactation, a pregnant woman's body undergoes many changes, including the development of a placenta and an amniotic sac, an increase in blood volume, enlargement of the breasts and uterus, and the accumulation of body fat.
3. Energy, protein, water, vitamin, and mineral needs increase during pregnancy.
4. Regardless of prepregnancy weight, adequate weight gain during pregnancy is essential to the health of the mother and unborn baby.
5. The age, health, and nutritional status of the mother and her use of drugs and alcohol during pregnancy can affect embryonic and fetal development.
6. Lactation increases the mother's nutrient needs. Her nutrient intake can affect the composition of the milk the baby consumes.
7. A newborn infant's energy and protein needs are higher per unit of body weight than at any other time of life.
8. Monitoring an infant's growth rate is the best measure of the adequacy of nutrient intake.
9. Breast feeding is the ideal way to nourish infants. Infant formula can also provide adequate nutrition.

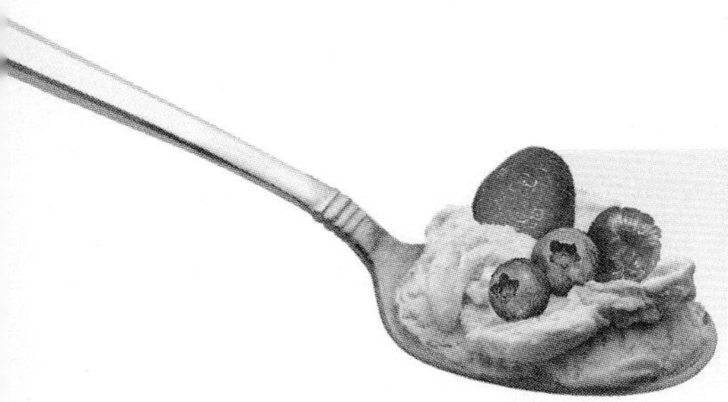

Just a Taste

Do pregnant women need vitamin and mineral supplements?

Should overweight women gain weight during pregnancy?

Is breast feeding the best option for all newborn infants and their mothers?

For a single cell to develop into a complete human being it must multiply and differentiate to form the specific shapes and specialized tissues of a human infant. This development requires a safe environment to which oxygen and nutrients are provided in the right amounts and at the right times and from which waste products are removed. The mother's uterus provides this environment and the nutrients and waste products are transported by her blood supply. Therefore, the mother's health and nutritional status are crucial to a successful pregnancy outcome. Even at the time of conception, the mother's nutritional status can affect the outcome of the pregnancy.

Most women pay special attention to their health and nutrition during pregnancy to help ensure the health of their babies. A woman must start her pregnancy in good nutritional health and, during pregnancy, her diet must be carefully planned to supply the nutrients needed to maintain her health, support the physiological changes in her body, and provide for the rapid growth and development of her unborn baby. A deficiency or excess of nutrients, as well as the use of alcohol, drugs, and cigarettes, may cause birth defects, premature births, and low birth weights. Although good nutrition cannot always prevent these problems, adequate nutrition and consistent prenatal care can reduce the number of babies born disabled, too soon, or too small.

After delivery, the newborn must continue to receive adequate nutrition. Breast-fed infants depend on nutrients from the mother to meet their needs. Lactation has high nutrient demands, and the composition of breast milk can be affected by maternal intake, so a nursing woman's diet must be selected carefully. Formula-fed infants rely on the nutrients in infant formulas to meet their needs.

THE PHYSIOLOGY OF PREGNANCY

Pregnancy, from **conception** to birth, usually lasts 40 weeks, or about nine months in humans. During pregnancy, a single cell grows and develops into an infant that is ready for life outside the womb. Many physiological changes take place in the mother to support her developing offspring and prepare her for **lactation.**

Conception The union of sperm and egg (ovum) that results in pregnancy.

Lactation Milk production and secretion.

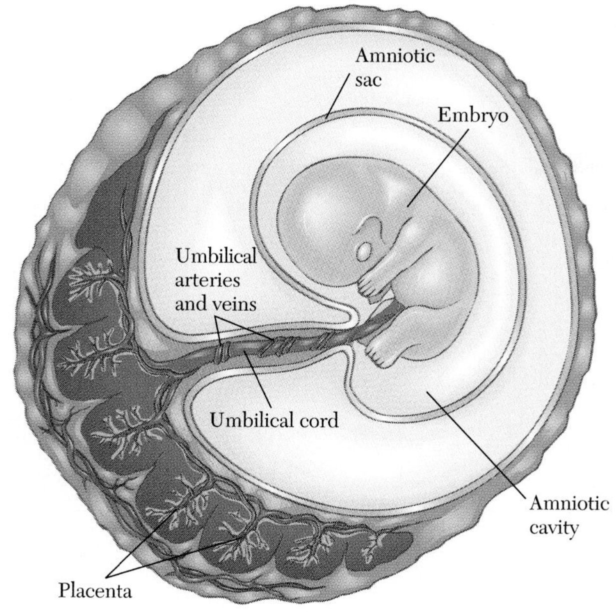

Figure 13.1
During pregnancy, the amniotic sac protects the fetus and the placenta allows nutrients and wastes to be transferred between mother and baby.

Prenatal Growth and Development

Reproduction requires the **fertilization** of an egg, or ovum, from the mother by a sperm from the father. Fertilization, which occurs in the **fallopian tube** or **oviduct,** produces a single-celled **zygote.** The zygote travels down the mother's fallopian tube into the uterus. Along the way the zygote divides many times to form a ball of smaller cells. In the uterus it attaches to the uterine lining in a process known as **implantation.** Once implantation has occurred, two new organs, the **amniotic sac** and **placenta,** form to protect and nourish the developing offspring (Figure 13.1). The amniotic sac is a fluid-filled membrane that surrounds the unborn baby and protects it from the bumps and bruises of the outside world. The placenta provides a network of blood vessels that allow nutrients and oxygen to be transferred from mother to baby and waste products to be transferred from the baby to the mother's blood for elimination. It is formed when the implanted ball of cells develops branchlike projections that grow into the lining of the uterus, allowing blood vessels that supply the developing baby to lie in close proximity to maternal blood. The placenta also secretes hormones necessary to maintain pregnancy.

As these structures develop, the ball of cells continues to grow. The cells differentiate to form the multitude of specialized cell types that make up the body, and arrange themselves in the proper shapes and locations to form body organs and structures. About two weeks after fertilization, the developing offspring is known as an **embryo.** The embryonic stage of development lasts until the eighth week after fertilization, when rudimentary organ systems have been formed. The embryo at this point is approximately 3 cm long (a little more than an inch) and has a beating heart. All major external and internal structures have been formed. Beginning at the ninth week of development and continuing until birth, the developing offspring is known as a **fetus** (Figure 13.2). During the fetal period of development, structures that appeared during the embryonic period continue to grow and mature. Anything that interferes with development can result in birth defects. If the defect is severe, it may result in a **spontaneous abortion** or **miscarriage.**

The fetal period usually ends after 40 weeks of **gestation** with the birth of an infant weighing about 3 to 4 kilograms (6.6 to 8.8 lb).[1] Infants who are born on time but have failed to grow well in the uterus are said to be **small-for-gestational-age.** Those born before 37 weeks of gestation are said to be **preterm** or **premature.**

Fertilization The union of sperm and egg (ovum).

Fallopian tubes or **oviducts** Narrow ducts leading from the ovaries to the uterus

Zygote The cell produced by the union of sperm and ovum during fertilization.

Implantation The process by which the developing ball of cells embeds in the uterine lining.

Amniotic sac A membrane surrounding the fetus that contains the amniotic fluid.

Placenta An organ produced from both maternal and embryonic tissues. It secretes hormones, transfers nutrients and oxygen from the mother's blood to the fetus, and removes wastes.

Embryo The developing human from two to eight weeks after fertilization. All organ systems are formed during this time.

Fetus The developing human from the ninth week to birth. Growth and refinement of structures occur during this time.

Spontaneous abortion or **miscarriage** Interruption of pregnancy prior to the seventh month.

Gestation The time between conception and birth, which lasts about nine months (or about 40 weeks) in humans.

Small-for-gestational-age An infant born at term weighing less than 2.5 kg (5.5 lb).

Preterm or **premature** An infant born before 37 weeks of gestation.

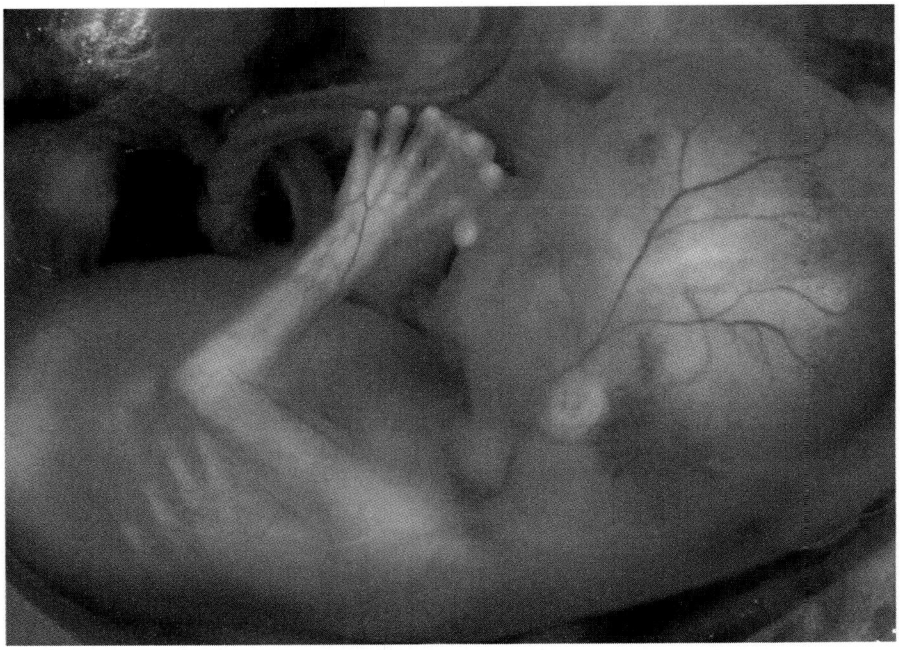

Figure 13.2
At 16 weeks the fetus is about 16 cm (6.4 inches) long. (Custom Medical Stock Photo)

Low birth weight A birthweight less than 2.5 kg (5.5 lb).

Very low birth weight A birthweight less than 1.5 kg (3.3 lb).

Whether born too soon or just too small, **low birth weight** infants (those weighing less than 2.5 kg [5.5 lb] at birth) and **very low birth weight** infants (those weighing less than 1.5 kg [3.3 lb]), are at increased risk for illness and early death.[2] They often require special care and a special diet in order to successfully continue to grow and develop. Survival improves with increasing gestational age and birth weight. Today, with advances in medical and nutritional care, infants born as early as 25 weeks of gestation and those weighing as little as 1 kg (2.2 lb) can survive.

Changes in the Mother

A woman's body undergoes many changes during pregnancy to develop and maintain the systems necessary to support the growing fetus. Her blood volume increases by 50%, and her heart, lungs, and kidneys work harder to deliver nutrients and oxygen and remove wastes. The placenta develops, and the hormones produced by it orchestrate other changes: They promote uterine growth; they relax muscles and ligaments to accommodate the growing fetus and allow for childbirth; they promote breast development; and they increase fat deposition to provide the energy stores that will be needed during late pregnancy and lactation. These changes all result in weight gain and can affect the type and level of physical activity that is safe. In some cases they can also cause uncomfortable or dangerous side effects that can occur and abate at different times during the pregnancy or continue throughout the pregnancy.

Weight Gain During Pregnancy Adequate weight gain during pregnancy is essential to the health of mother and fetus. Typically the weight of the infant at birth is only about 25% of the total pregnancy weight gain, that of the placenta is about 5%, and that of the amniotic fluid about 6%. Changes in maternal tissues account for most of the weight gained during pregnancy. This includes increases in the size of the uterus and breasts, in the volume of blood and extracellular fluid, and in fat stores (Figure 13.3).

Trimester A term used to describe each third, or three-month period, of a pregnancy.

The recommended weight gain during pregnancy is 25 to 35 pounds (11 to 15 kg) for healthy, normal weight women—those with a body mass index of 18.5 to 24.9 kg/m^2. The rate of weight gain is as important as the total weight gain. Little gain is expected in the first three months, or **trimester,** of pregnancy—usually

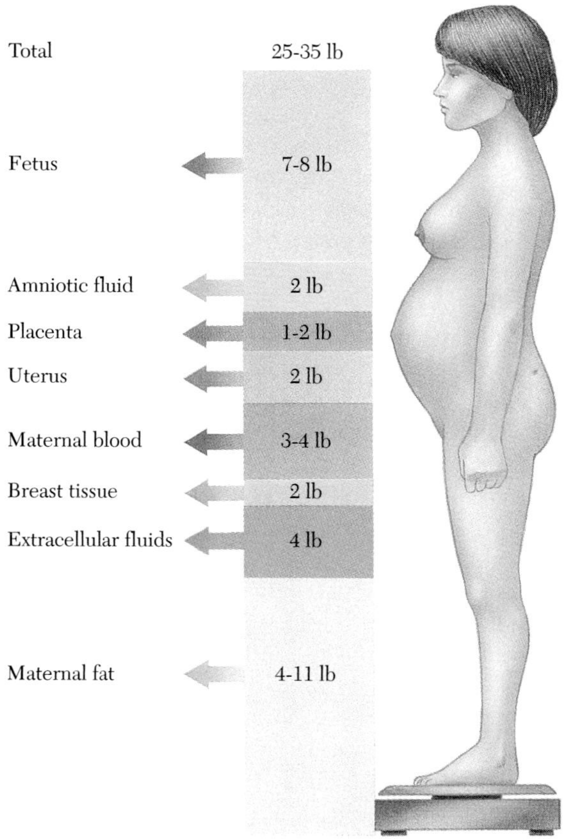

Figure 13.3

The weight gained by the mother during pregnancy includes increases in the weight of her tissues as well as the weight of the fetus, placenta, and the amniotic fluid.

about 2 to 4 pounds (0.9 to 1.8 kg). In the second and third trimesters, when the fetus grows from less than a pound to 6 to 8 pounds, the recommended maternal weight gain is about 1 pound (0.45 kg) per week. Women who are underweight or overweight at conception should also gain weight at a slow, steady rate (Figure 13.4). Weight gains of up to 40 pounds (18 kg) are recommended for women who begin pregnancy underweight. Overweight women should gain less, only about 15 to 25 pounds (6.8 to 11.4 kg) over the course of pregnancy.

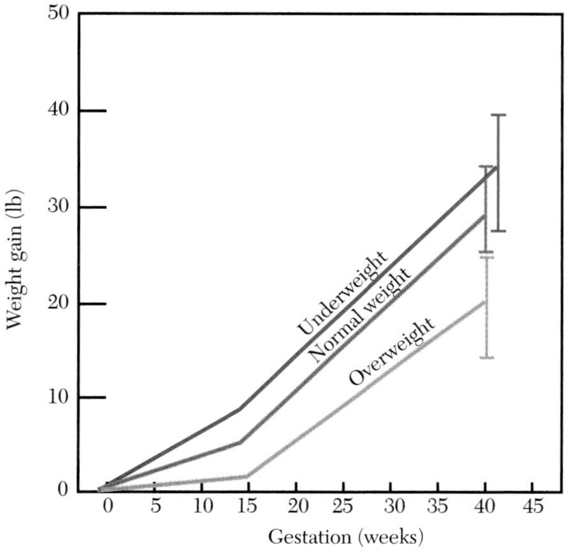

Figure 13.4

The same pattern of weight gain is recommended for women who are normal weight, underweight, or overweight at the start of pregnancy, but the recommendations for total weight gain are different. (Adapted from Committee on Nutritional Status During Pregnancy and Lactation. *Nutrition During Pregnancy*. Washington, D.C.: National Academy Press, 1990.)

Cesarean section The surgical removal of the fetus from the uterus.

Large-for-gestational-age An infant weighing greater than 4 kg (8.8 lb) at birth.

Gaining too much or too little weight as well as being underweight or overweight can affect the health of both mother and child.[1] Being underweight by 10% or more at the onset of pregnancy or gaining too little weight during pregnancy increases the risk of producing a low birth weight baby. Excess weight, whether present before conception or gained during pregnancy, can also compromise the outcome of the pregnancy. The mother's risks for high blood pressure, gestational diabetes, difficult delivery, and **cesarean section** are increased by excess weight, as is the risk of having a **large-for-gestational-age** baby. Dieting during pregnancy is not advised even for obese women. If possible, excess weight should be lost before the pregnancy begins or, alternatively, after the child is born and weaned. In either case the weight loss should be gradual and accomplished by increasing activity and consuming a low-energy, nutrient-dense diet.

Some women are concerned that weight gained during pregnancy will be permanent, but most lose all but about 2 pounds within a year of delivery.[3] Approximately 10 pounds are lost at birth from the weight of the baby, amniotic fluid, and placenta. In the week after delivery, another 5 pounds of fluid are typically lost. Once this initial fluid and tissue weight is lost, further weight loss requires that energy intake be less than energy output. After the mother has recovered from delivery, a balanced low-energy diet combined with moderate exercise will promote weight loss and the return of muscle tone. As discussed later in this chapter, breast feeding may help to promote weight loss.

Physical Activity During Pregnancy For healthy, well-nourished women, carefully chosen moderate exercise is recommended during pregnancy. Physical activity during pregnancy improves overall fitness, reduces stress, prevents excess weight gain, prevents low back pain, improves digestion, reduces constipation, prevents gestational diabetes, improves mood and body image, and speeds recovery from childbirth. Too much exercise that is too intense has the potential to harm the fetus by reducing the amount of oxygen and nutrients it receives or by increasing body temperature. Therefore, guidelines have been developed to minimize the risks and maximize the benefits of exercise during pregnancy (Table 13.1). However, all pregnant women should check with their physicians before engaging in any exercise program.

Women who were physically active before their pregnancy can continue their exercise programs, but women who begin an exercise program after becoming

Table 13.1 *Guidelines for Physical Activity During Pregnancy*

Obtain medical permission before beginning an exercise program.
If inactive before pregnancy, increase activity very gradually.
Regular exercise (at least three times per week) is preferable to intermittent activity.
Stop exercising when fatigued and do not exercise to exhaustion.
Choose non-weight-bearing activities such as swimming that have minimal risk of falls or abdominal injury.
Avoid strenuous exertion during the first trimester; at other times, strenuous exercise should not be continued for more than 15 minutes.
After the first trimester avoid exercise that is performed lying on one's back.
Avoid exercising in hot or humid environments.
Drink plenty of liquids before, during, and after exercise.
Prepregnancy exercise routines should be resumed gradually after the birth of the child.

Modified from Dewey, K. G., and McCrory, M. A. Effects of dieting and physical activity on pregnancy and lactation. Am. J. Clin. Nutr. 59 (suppl):446S–453S, 1994; and American College of Obstetricians and Gynecologists. *Exercise During Pregnancy and the Postpartum Period (Technical Bulletin #189)*. Washington, D.C.: ACOG, 1994.

pregnant should start slowly, with low-intensity, low-impact activities such as walking.[4] During pregnancy, the risk of injury is greater because women weigh more and carry that weight in the front of their bodies where it can interfere with balance and place stress on the bones, joints, and muscles. Activities that have a risk of abdominal trauma, falls, or joint stress, such as contact and racquet sports, should be avoided.[5] Exercise in the water is recommended because the body's buoyancy in water compensates for the changes in weight distribution (Figure 13.5).[6] To ensure adequate delivery of oxygen and nutrients to the fetus, intense exercise should be limited during pregnancy. To prevent overheating, plenty of fluids should be consumed and exercise should be carried out in a well-ventilated environment. Outdoor exercise in hot, humid weather should also be avoided. Women who exercise during pregnancy need to consume enough energy to meet the added demands of exercise and pregnancy.

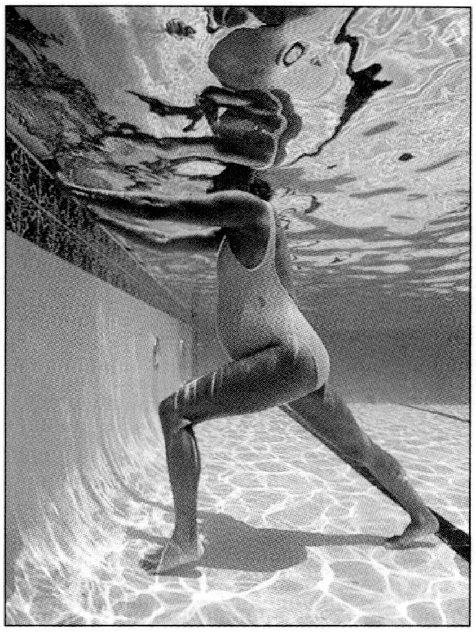

Figure 13.5
During pregnancy, exercising in the water can reduce stress on joints and help keep the body cool. (© Tracy Frankel/The Image Bank)

Digestive Discomforts of Pregnancy Hormonal changes during pregnancy affect the digestive tract and may cause discomfort for the mother. Most of these problems are minor, but in some cases they may endanger the mother and the fetus.

Morning sickness is a syndrome of nausea and vomiting that occurs during pregnancy. The term "morning sickness" is somewhat of a misnomer because symptoms can occur anytime during the day or night. It is thought to be related to the hormonal changes of pregnancy and may be alleviated to some extent by eating small frequent snacks of dry starchy foods, such as plain crackers or bread. In most cases symptoms decrease significantly after the first trimester, but in some cases the symptoms last for the entire pregnancy and, in severe cases, may require intravenous nutrition to assure that needs are met.

Morning sickness Nausea and vomiting that affects many women during the first few months of pregnancy and in some women can continue throughout the pregnancy.

Heartburn, a burning sensation caused by stomach acid leaking up into the esophagus, is another common digestive complaint during pregnancy because the hormones produced to relax the muscles of the uterus also relax the muscles of the gastrointestinal tract. This involuntary relaxation of the lower esophageal sphincter allows the acidic stomach contents to back up into the esophagus, causing irritation. The problem gets more severe as pregnancy progresses because the growing baby crowds the stomach. The fuller the stomach, the more likely that its contents will back up into the esophagus. Therefore, heartburn can be reduced by consuming many small meals throughout the day rather than a few large meals. Because high-fat foods, such as fried foods, rich sauces, and desserts, leave the stomach slowly, a lowfat diet of grains, fruits, vegetables, plain meats, and lowfat dairy products is less likely to cause heartburn. Because a reclining position makes it easier for acidic juices to flow into the esophagus, remaining upright after eating also reduces heartburn. Avoiding substances that are known to cause heartburn, such as caffeine and peppermint, can also be helpful.

Constipation is a frequent complaint during pregnancy. The pregnancy-related hormones that cause muscles to relax also decrease intestinal motility and slow transit time. Constipation becomes more of a problem late in pregnancy when the weight of the uterus puts pressure on the gastrointestinal tract. Maintaining a moderate level of physical activity and consuming at least one-half gallon of water and other fluids per day, as well as high-fiber foods such as whole grains, vegetables, and fruits, are recommended to prevent constipation. Hemorrhoids are also more common during pregnancy, as a result of both constipation and physiological changes in blood flow.

Complications of Pregnancy

Occasionally, the physiological changes that occur during pregnancy can lead to complications that affect blood glucose levels and fluid balance and threaten the health of both mother and baby.

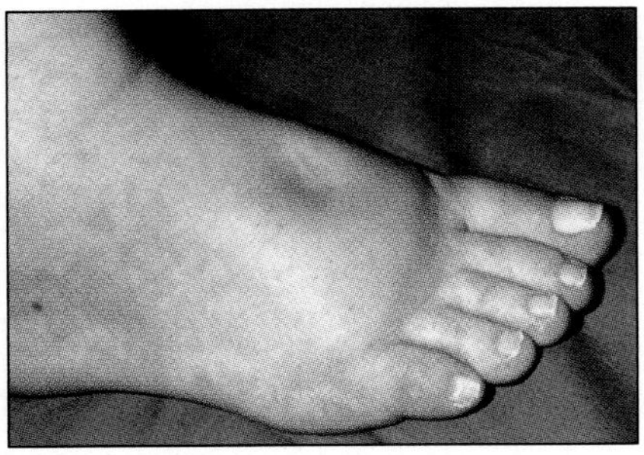

Figure 13.6
Edema of feet and ankles occurs when extracellular fluid accumulates in the tissues and is a common complication of pregnancy. Elevating the feet will help reduce swelling. (© Dr. P. Marazzi/Science Photo Library/Photo Researchers, Inc.)

Gestational diabetes A consistently elevated blood glucose level that develops during pregnancy and returns to normal after delivery.

Edema Swelling due to the buildup of extracellular fluid in the tissues.

Pregnancy-induced hypertension A spectrum of conditions involving elevated blood pressure during pregnancy. **Preeclampsia** is characterized by an increase in body weight, elevated blood pressure, protein in the urine, and edema. It can progress to **eclampsia,** which can be life threatening to mother and fetus.

Gestational Diabetes Consistently elevated blood glucose levels during pregnancy is known as **gestational diabetes.** It occurs in 2 to 6% of all pregnancies and is most common in obese women.[7] This form of diabetes usually disappears when the pregnancy is completed, although the mother remains at higher risk for developing type 2 diabetes (see Chapter 4).

High levels of glucose in the mother's blood can adversely affect the fetus. Glucose in the mother's blood passes freely across the placenta, so high maternal blood sugar provides extra energy to the fetus. This extra energy can produce a baby who is large for gestational age and consequently at increased risk of complications. As with other types of diabetes, the treatment of gestational diabetes involves consuming a carefully planned diet that is eaten at consistent intervals throughout the day, moderate daily exercise, and close monitoring by a physician.

Edema The hormonal changes of pregnancy cause blood volume to expand to nourish the fetus, but this expansion may also cause the accumulation of extracellular fluid in the tissues, known as **edema.** Edema is characterized by swelling, particularly in the feet and ankles (Figure 13.6). Restriction of dietary sodium below the amount recommended for the general population is not recommended, nor is fluid restriction. Edema can be uncomfortable but does not increase medical risks unless it is accompanied by a rise in blood pressure.

Pregnancy-Induced Hypertension Another complication of pregnancy is **pregnancy-induced hypertension,** which is a spectrum of conditions involving a rise in blood pressure. **Preeclampsia** is a form of pregnancy-induced hypertension that causes an increase in blood pressure, edema, and protein in the urine.[8] Its onset may be signaled by the gain of several pounds within a few days. It can progress to a more severe form, **eclampsia,** which is life threatening. Pregnancy-induced hypertension is most common in mothers under 20 or over 35 years of age, those in low-income groups, and those who are underweight. The cause is not known, but research suggests that low calcium intake may be involved. Calcium supplements during pregnancy have been shown in some trials to reduce the risk of pregnancy-induced hypertension, but this finding is not consistent.[9,10] Treatment includes bed rest and careful medical attention. Dietary sodium intake should be moderate, but sodium restriction is not a cure. The condition usually resolves after delivery.

The Nutritional Needs of Pregnancy

Nutrition is important before pregnancy to support conception and maximize the likelihood of a healthy pregnancy. During pregnancy maternal intake must provide all the nutrients needed to provide for the growth and development of the fetus while continuing to meet the mother's needs. Because the increased need for energy is proportionately smaller than the increased need for protein, vitamins, and minerals, a well-balanced, nutrient-dense diet is required.

The Importance of Nutrition Before Pregnancy

A woman's nutritional status before she becomes pregnant may affect her ability to conceive and successfully complete a pregnancy. For example, starvation diets, anorexia nervosa, and excessive athletic activity, such as marathon running, can interfere with ovulation and therefore make conception less likely. Obesity can alter hormone levels and decrease fertility. Deficiencies or excesses of nutrients can also affect pregnancy outcome. For instance, a deficiency of folate or an excess of vitamin A early in pregnancy can cause birth defects.[11]

Nutritional status can be affected by some birth control methods, and these can therefore have an impact on a subsequent pregnancy. For example, oral contraceptives are associated with reduced blood levels of vitamin B_{12}.[12] If conception occurs soon after oral contraceptive use stops, these levels will not have time to return to normal before pregnancy begins. The use of drugs—whether over-the-counter, prescribed, or illicit—can also affect both fertility and pregnancy outcome. A woman who is considering pregnancy should discuss her plans with her physician in order to determine the risks associated with any medication she is taking.

Energy and Macronutrient Needs During Pregnancy

A typical pregnancy requires a total of about 55,000 additional kcalories.[1] Although this number may seem staggering, it amounts to only about an extra sandwich and glass of milk, or about 300 kcalories, per day during the second and third trimesters of the pregnancy (Figure 13.7). During the first trimester the additional energy required is small, and the 1989 RDA is not increased. The macronutrient composition of the diet during pregnancy should be about the same as that recommended for the general population—55 to 60% of energy coming from carbohydrate and 30% or less from fat. If carbohydrate intake is less than 100 grams per day, ketosis may occur. Prolonged ketosis may be harmful to the fetus, even though some ketone production occurs normally after an overnight fast, and the fetus can metabolize ketones.[13]

Protein Needs Protein needs are also increased during pregnancy (see Figure 13.7). Protein is needed for the structure of all new cells in both the mother and the fetus. An increase of 10 grams of protein per day above the 1989 RDA for nonpregnant women is recommended throughout pregnancy to provide for the increase in maternal blood volume; the development of the placenta, breasts,

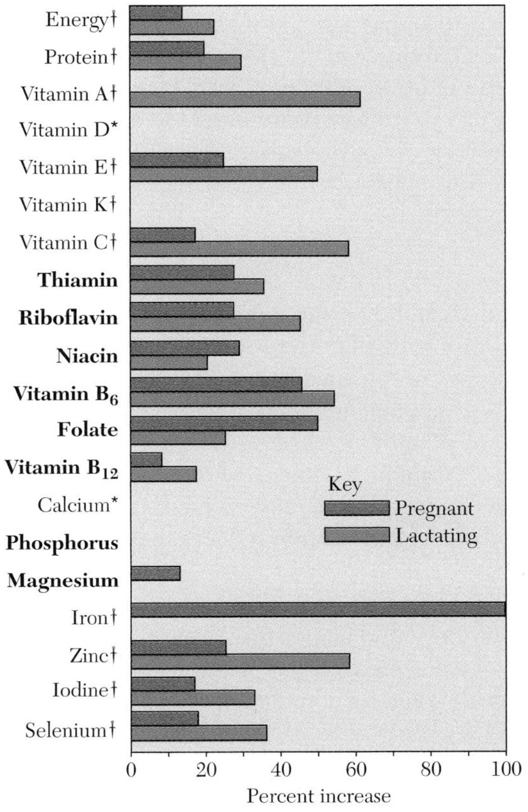

Figure 13.7
The percentage increase in recommended nutrient intakes for a 25-year-old woman during pregnancy and lactation. Nutrients in bold have Dietary Reference Intake RDAs values; nutrients followed by an asterisk have AIs, and those followed by a single dagger have 1989 RDAs.

uterus, and uterine muscles; and the development and growth of all fetal structures. For a woman weighing 136 pounds (62 kg), this increases protein needs to about 60 grams per day. Most nonpregnant women already consume this amount or more.

Fluid Needs The need for water is increased during pregnancy because of the increase in blood volume, the production of amniotic fluid, and the needs of the fetus. This requires the consumption of only an extra 30 ml per day. Adequate fluid consumption, about 2 liters per day, throughout pregnancy is important in preventing constipation.

Micronutrient Needs During Pregnancy

The need for many vitamins and minerals is increased during pregnancy. Due to growth in maternal and fetal tissues as well as increased energy utilization, the requirements for the B vitamins, such as thiamin, niacin, and riboflavin, increase. To meet the needs for increased protein synthesis in fetal and maternal tissues, the requirements for vitamin B_6 and zinc increase. The needs for micronutrients involved in the growth and development of bone and connective tissue and the synthesis of new cells are also greater (see Figure 13.7).

Micronutrient Needs for the Development of Bone and Connective Tissue Healthy bones require calcium for mineralization, vitamin D for calcium absorption and utilization, and vitamin C for connective tissue formation.

Calcium The fetus retains about 30 grams of calcium over the course of gestation. Most of the calcium is deposited in the last trimester when the fetal skeleton is growing most rapidly and the teeth are forming. The increased need for calcium does not increase maternal bone resorption and studies have found no correlation between the number of pregnancies a woman has had and the density of her bones. There is an increase in the absorption of calcium from the diet during pregnancy,[14] which may be due in part to an increase in estrogen and an increase in the concentration of active vitamin D in the blood.[15] Therefore, the AI for calcium for pregnant women age 19 and older—1000 mg a day—is not increased above nonpregnant needs.[14] This AI can be met by consuming 3 to 4 servings of milk or other dairy products daily. Women who are lactose intolerant may be able to meet their calcium needs with yogurt, cheese, reduced-lactose milk, and calcium-rich vegetables such as collard greens.

Vitamin D Adequate vitamin D is essential to ensure efficient calcium absorption, but the recommended intake for vitamin D is not increased above nonpregnant levels. When pregnant women receive regular exposure to sunlight, vitamin D supplements are unnecessary. If exposure to sunlight is limited and sufficient vitamin D is not consumed in the diet, supplements should be considered. Most prenatal supplements provide 10 μg of vitamin D, which is twice the AI but well below the UL of pregnancy of 50 μg.[14] Inadequate vitamin D may be a particular problem in African American women because their calcium intake is often low due to lactose intolerance and their darker pigmentation reduces the synthesis of vitamin D in the skin.

Vitamin C Vitamin C is important for bone and connective tissue formation because it is needed for the synthesis of collagen. Collagen is the major protein in connective tissue which gives structure to skin, tendons, and the protein matrix of bones. The 1989 RDA for vitamin C is increased to 70 mg per day during pregnancy. The requirement for vitamin C can easily be met with foods such as citrus fruit, and supplements are generally not necessary.

Micronutrient Needs for Increased Cell Division To form new fetal and maternal cells, the needs for folate, vitamin B_{12}, zinc, and iron are increased.

Folate Folate is needed for the synthesis of DNA and thus for cell division. During pregnancy, cells multiply to form the placenta, expand maternal blood, and allow for fetal growth. Adequate folate intake is crucial even before conception because rapid cell division occurs in the first days and weeks of pregnancy.

Folate is believed to be essential for proper formation of the **neural tube,** which is the portion of the embryo that develops into the brain and spinal cord. During development, neural tissue forms a groove; the groove closes when the sides fold together to form a tube (Figure 13.8). This neural tube closure occurs between 21 and 28 days of development. If it does not occur normally the infant will be born with a neural tube defect, such as spina bifida, a defect in which the neural tube does not close completely (see Chapter 8). The mechanism whereby folate reduces neural tube defects is unknown. It has been hypothesized that folate might overcome a deficit in the production of DNA or protein at a critical time in neural tube closure, or that it selectively increases the spontaneous abortion rate of affected fetuses.[16]

Neural tube A portion of the embryo that develops into the brain and spinal cord.

Because the neural tube closes so early in development, often before a woman even knows she is pregnant, the DRIs recommended that women capable of becoming pregnant consume 400 μg daily of synthetic folic acid from fortified foods, supplements, or a combination of the two, in addition to consuming a varied diet rich in natural sources of folate (see Chapter 8, *Critical Thinking: Four Hundred of Fortified Folate*).

Adequate folate continues to be important even after the neural tube closes. If folate is inadequate during pregnancy, megaloblastic anemia—the type of anemia in which blood cells do not mature properly—may result (see Chapter 8). Thus, to maintain red blood cell folate levels in pregnant women, the RDA for folate is set at 600 μg of dietary folate equivalents per day. Natural sources of folate include orange juice, legumes, leafy green vegetables, and organ meats. Fortified sources include breads, cereals, and other grain products. Folic acid supplements can also be used to meet this goal. Most prenatal supplements contain 400 μg of folic acid.

Vitamin B₁₂ Vitamin B_{12} is essential for the regeneration of active forms of folate, so a deficiency of vitamin B_{12} can also result in megaloblastic anemia. Vitamin B_{12} is transferred from the mother to the fetus during pregnancy. Based on the amount transferred and the increased efficiency of B_{12} absorption that occurs during pregnancy, the RDA for pregnancy is set at 2.6 μg per day.[17] This amount is easily met by a diet containing animal products. Deficiency has been observed in infants of vegan mothers. Vegans must consume foods fortified with vitamin B_{12} or take vitamin B_{12} supplements to meet their needs.

Zinc Zinc is involved in the synthesis and function of DNA and RNA and the synthesis of proteins. It is therefore extremely important for growth and development. The 1989 RDA is increased from 12 mg per day for nonpregnant women to 15 mg per day during pregnancy. Zinc deficiency during pregnancy is associated with an increased risk of fetal malformations and low birth weight.[18] Because zinc absorption is inhibited by high iron intakes, iron supplements may compromise zinc status if the diet is low in zinc.

Iron Iron deficiency anemia is common during pregnancy. It has been associated with an increased risk of low birth weight and preterm delivery.[19] Because low iron stores are so common among women of childbearing age, many women start pregnancy with diminished iron stores and quickly become deficient. This occurs despite the fact that iron absorption is increased during pregnancy and iron losses are decreased due to the cessation of menstruation.

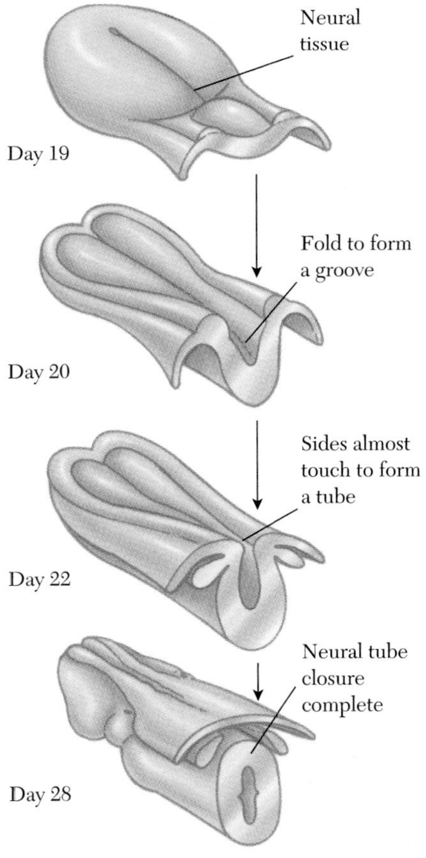

Figure 13.8
During embryonic development, a flat plate of neural tissue forms a groove and then the edges fold up and join to form the neural tube which will become the brain and spinal cord.

Iron needs are high during pregnancy to provide for the synthesis of hemoglobin and other iron-containing proteins in both maternal and fetal tissues. The fetus draws iron from the mother to ensure adequate fetal hemoglobin production, mostly during the last trimester. Babies born prematurely may not have had time to accumulate sufficient iron, but babies born at term usually have adequate iron stores even if the mother is deficient.

The 1989 RDA for iron during pregnancy is double that for nonpregnant women. It takes an exceptionally well-planned diet to meet iron needs during pregnancy. Red meats, leafy green vegetables, and fortified cereals are good sources of iron. Foods that enhance iron absorption, such as citrus fruit or meat, should also be included in the diet. Iron supplements are often recommended during the second and third trimesters (see *Critical Thinking: Nutrient Needs for a Successful Pregnancy*).

Meeting Nutrient Needs During Pregnancy

The energy and protein needs of pregnancy can be easily met by following the Food Guide Pyramid recommendations for pregnant women (Figure 13.9). The additional servings recommended from the Bread, Cereal, Rice, & Pasta Group and the Vegetable Group provide energy, protein, micronutrients, and fiber, particularly if whole grains are chosen. The extra serving of milk that is recommended provides energy, protein, calcium, vitamin D, and riboflavin. The

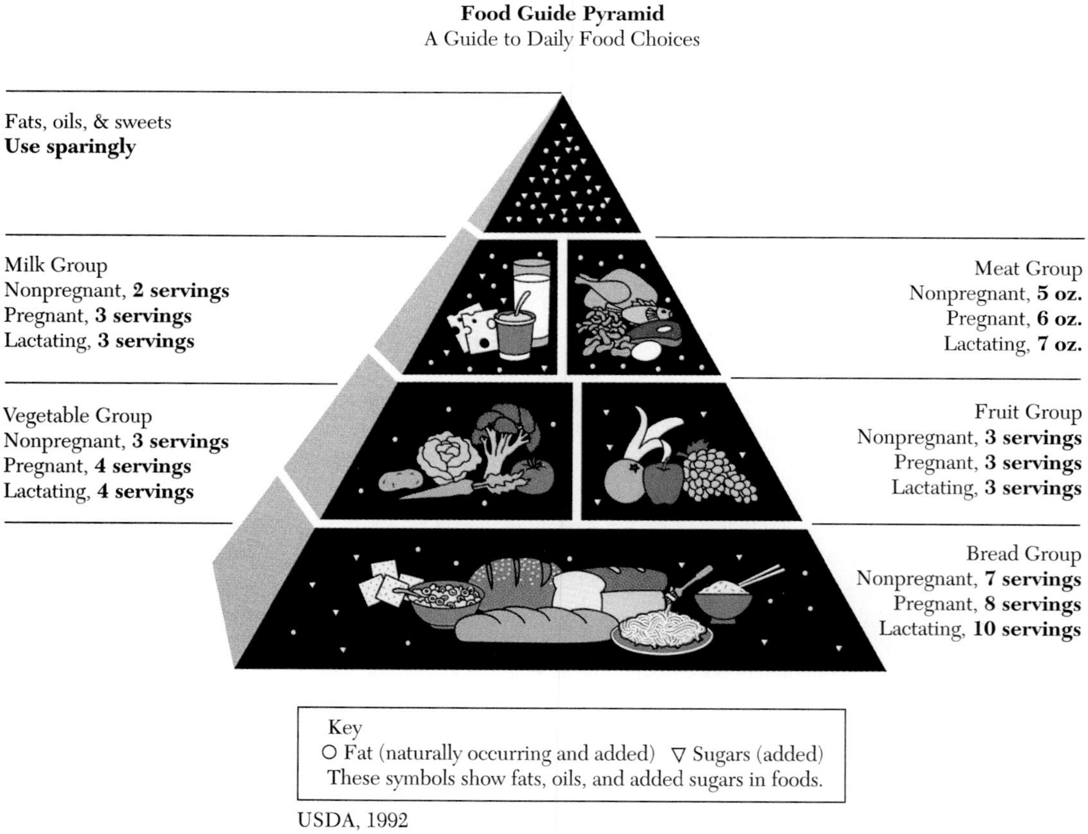

Figure 13.9

The recommendations of the Food Guide Pyramid can be applied during pregnancy and lactation. Shown here are the recommended servings for a 25-year-old woman before pregnancy and during pregnancy and lactation. (U.S. Department of Agriculture, Home and Garden Bulletin No. 252, 1992.)

additional one ounce of meat provides energy, protein, vitamin B_6, vitamin B_{12}, iron, and zinc. These recommendations can be met by adding a snack such as a roast beef sandwich and a glass of milk.

Food Cravings and Aversions Most women change their diets during pregnancy. Some changes are made in an effort to improve nutrition to ensure a healthy infant, but other changes are based on cravings, aversions, or cultural or family traditions. Foods that are commonly craved include sweets and dairy products. Common aversions include coffee and other caffeinated drinks, highly seasoned foods, or fried foods.[20] It has been suggested that hormonal or physiological changes during pregnancy—in particular, changes in taste and smell—may be the cause of such cravings and aversions.

An unusual type of food craving that is more common in pregnancy is **pica.** This is an abnormal craving for and ingestion of nonfood substances having little or no nutritional value. Commonly consumed substances include clay, laundry starch, ice and freezer frost, baking soda, cornstarch, and ashes.[21] Pica is more common in African American than Caucasian women, in rural than urban women, and in women with a family history of the practice.

Pica An abnormal craving for and ingestion of unusual food and nonfood substances.

Pica during pregnancy is potentially dangerous. The consumption of large amounts of nonfood substances may cause micronutrient deficiencies by reducing the intake of nutrient-dense foods and by reducing nutrient absorption from food. The substances consumed could also cause intestinal obstruction or perforation and may contain toxins or parasites. In addition, consumption of large amounts of starch provides kcalories and may cause excess weight gain.[20]

Anemia and pregnancy-induced hypertension are more common in mothers who practice pica, but it is not clear if pica is a result of these conditions or a cause. In newborns, anemia and low birth weight are often related to pica in the mother. Because of the association of these conditions with micronutrient intake, it was once thought that pica was an attempt to meet micronutrient needs. It is now believed that pica may be more related to cultural factors than the need for micronutrients.

Are Vitamin and Mineral Supplements Necessary? Meeting the increased micronutrient needs of pregnancy requires a very carefully planned nutrient-dense diet. Supplements that are generally recommended include folic acid before and during pregnancy, and iron during the second and third trimesters.[1] A multivitamin and mineral supplement may also be necessary in those whose food choices are limited, such as vegetarians, or in those whose needs are very high, such as pregnant teenagers. A healthy diet is essential to satisfy all of the requirements of pregnancy; even when a prenatal supplement is taken, a woman's diet must be carefully planned[1] (see *Off the Shelf: Prenatal Supplements*).

CRITICAL THINKING

Nutrient Needs for a Successful Pregnancy

Chevon is four months pregnant. From the start—before she tried to conceive—she has been careful about her nutritional health. She took care to consume plenty of both fortified grain products to obtain enough folic acid and foods that are naturally high in folate. Now that she is entering her second trimester, her doctor is concerned about her intake of iron and other nutrients and has prescribed a prenatal supplement. Chevon follows his advice and takes the supplement, but she evaluates her diet to see if she can meet the nutrient needs of pregnancy without supplements. She records her intake for a typical day:

Food	Food Guide Pyramid Group
Breakfast	
1 cup corn flakes	1 grain
with 1 cup reduced-fat milk	1 milk
3/4 cup orange juice	1 fruit
1 cup decaffeinated coffee	
with sugar and cream	fats, oils, and sweets
Lunch	
Tuna sandwich	
3 oz tuna	1 meat
2 tsp mayonnaise	fats, oils, and sweets
2 slices white bread	2 grain
20 french fries	2 vegetable
1 can orange soda	fats, oils, and sweets
3 chocolate chip cookies	1 grain
1 apple	1 fruit
Dinner	
3 oz chicken leg	1 meat
1/2 cup peas	1 vegetable
1 piece corn bread	2 grain
1 tsp margarine	fats, oils, and sweets
1 cup lettuce and tomato salad	1 vegetable
1 Tbsp dressing	fats, oils and sweets
1 cup reduced-fat milk	1 milk

Her current diet meets the recommendations of the Food Guide Pyramid for a nonpregnant woman, but during her second and third trimester she will require about 300 extra kcalories per day. To obtain this extra energy she should add a serving of vegetables, a serving of milk, an ounce of meat, and a serving of grain products.

What nutrients are provided by these additions?

An added serving of whole grains will add iron, zinc, and B vitamins. The extra serving of vegetables will add folate, fiber, and vitamin C or A. The extra serving of dairy products will add protein, riboflavin, vitamin D, and calcium. Even though the recommendation for calcium intake is not increased during pregnancy, most young women do not meet calcium needs, and three servings from this group provide about 1000 mg, the AI for young adults. The extra from the meat group adds protein, and if it is from red meat, it provides an excellent source of absorbable iron and zinc as well as vitamins B_{12} and B_6.

Chevon is overweight. Should she still add these foods to her diet?

Answer:

How could her original diet be improved to increase nutrient density?

Answer:

After she has added foods to increase her energy intake and improved her choices to increase nutrient density, Chevon enters her diet into a diet analysis program to see if it will meet all of her needs.

Can this diet meet the iron needs of pregnancy without supplements?

Answer:

Nutrition and the Risks of Pregnancy

Most of the four million women who give birth every year in the United States are healthy during pregnancy and produce healthy babies. However, childbearing is not without risks. In the United States, about 7 out of every 100,000 women die as a result of childbirth. Eleven percent of babies are born too soon, 7% are low birth weight, and 7.6 out of each 1000 born alive die within the first year of life.[22] The reasons for poor pregnancy outcome vary. Some women are at increased risk because of their age; others have limited access to health care before and during pregnancy, lack a supportive home environment, or lack the money and facilities to purchase, prepare, and consume nutritious foods. Others are at risk because they smoke, drink alcohol, or use illicit drugs.

Maternal Health Status

The health of the mother affects the outcome of pregnancy. As discussed earlier, being underweight or overweight as well as gaining too much or too little can negatively affect the health of both mother and child. Maternal age and reproductive history can also have an impact on nutritional status, maternal health, and pregnancy outcome.

Maternal Age: The Pregnant Teenager Teenage pregnancy is a major public health problem. One in every five babies is born to a teenager, and more than 10% of these mothers are age 15 or younger.[23] Pregnant teenagers face economic, social, and medical problems as well as nutritional problems.

Pregnancy places a nutritional strain on a woman's body at any age, but this stress is compounded when the mother herself is still growing. Adolescent girls continue to grow and mature physically for about four to seven years after menstruation begins. Therefore, the risk of pregnancy is greater during this time than it is in women who have stopped growing. To better assess the nutritional status and nutritional goals of the pregnant teenager, the Dietary Reference Intakes include an age category within pregnancy that focuses on the needs of pregnant teens. For example, the RDA for magnesium in pregnant girls age 18 or younger is greater than it is in either pregnant women 19 or older or in nonpregnant girls 18 or under.

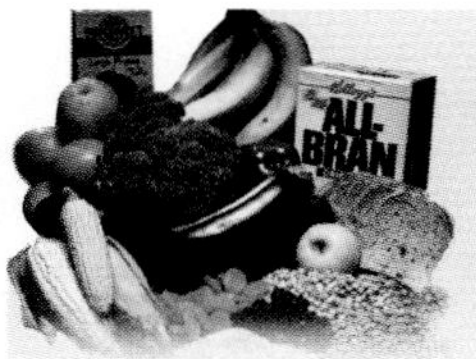

Off the Shelf

Prenatal Supplements

Most pregnant women leave their first prenatal doctor's visit with a prescription for a prenatal vitamin and mineral supplement. Yet public health agencies only recommend routine supplementation of iron and folate.[1,2] The supplements prescribed by physicians contain iron and folate, but they also contain about 15 other vitamins and minerals. Should women take these supplements?

There is nothing wrong with taking a multivitamin and mineral supplement during pregnancy as long as the recommended dosage is not exceeded. The concern of public health agencies is that individuals taking supplements may ignore other components of their diet, thinking that the supplement will meet all their needs. Even when a prenatal supplement is taken, a woman's diet must be carefully planned to satisfy all of the requirements of pregnancy.

Prenatal vitamin and mineral supplements supply many nutrients at levels that meet or slightly exceed the recommended intake for pregnancy, but some are present in amounts that do not meet the needs of pregnancy, and others are missing altogether. For example, the tablet shown in the table contains only 200 mg of calcium, which is only 20% of the AI for a pregnant woman age 19 or older.[3] The reason it does not contain more is that the tablet would have to be very large to provide the recommendation of 1000 mg. To meet her needs a pregnant woman would need to consume this tablet plus the amount of calcium in about three glasses of milk. For similar reasons, the tablet doesn't meet the recommendation for magnesium. Even if all the calcium and magnesium needed for pregnancy could be packed into a little pill, it still would not provide an adequate diet. Prenatal supplements do not contain the protein needed for tissue synthesis or the complex carbohydrates needed for energy. They lack fiber, which helps prevent constipation, and they do not contain fluid for expanding tissues and blood volume and maintaining normal bowel function. They are also lacking in food components such as the phytochemicals that are supplied by a diet rich in whole grains, fruits, and vegetables.

Prenatal supplements are not absolutely necessary to meet the nutrient needs of pregnancy, but a very carefully planned diet is necessary to provide all the nutrients needed to produce a healthy baby. If a prenatal supplement is taken, it must be part of a healthy diet.

Nutrients Commonly Contained in a Prenatal Supplement

Nutrient	Amount per Tablet	Recommendations for Pregnancy
Vitamin A (μg RE)	800	800†
Vitamin D (ergocalciferol) (μg)	10	5°
Vitamin E (mg α-TE)	11–15	10†
Vitamin C (mg)	80–120	70†
Folic acid (μg DFE)	400–1000	**600**
Thiamin (mg)	1.5	**1.4**
Riboflavin (mg)	1.6–3.0	**1.4**
Niacin (mg)	17–20	**18**
Vitamin B_6 (mg)	2.6–10	**1.9**
Vitamin B_{12} (μg)	2.5–12	**2.6**
Biotin (μg)	30	30°
Pantothenic acid (mg)	7	6°
Calcium (mg)	200	1000°
Iron (mg)	60–65	30†
Magnesium (mg)	100	**350**
Copper (mg)	2–3	1.5–3‡
Zinc (mg)	25	15†

Values given are for a pregnant woman 19 to 30 years of age during her third trimester.
Values in bold represent Dietary Reference Intake RDA values.
°Adequate Intake (AI).
†1989 RDAs.
‡ESADDI.

[1]Committee on Nutritional Status During Pregnancy and Lactation, National Academy of Science. *Nutrition During Pregnancy.* Washington, D.C.: National Academy Press, 1990.

[2]Institute of Medicine, Food and Nutrition Board. *Dietary Reference Intakes for Thiamin, Riboflavin, Niacin, Vitamin B-6, Folate, Vitamin B-12, Pantothenic Acid, Biotin, and Choline.* Washington, D.C.: National Academy Press, 1998.

[3]Institute of Medicine, Food and Nutrition Board. *Dietary Reference Intakes for Calcium, Phosphorus, Magnesium, Vitamin D, and Fluoride.* Washington, D.C.: National Academy Press, 1997.

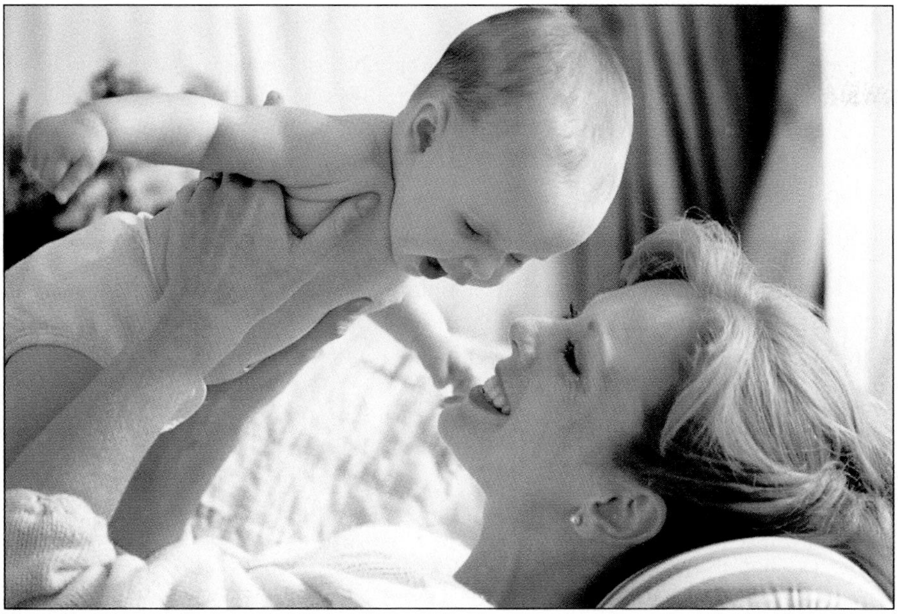

Figure 13.10
Prenatal care with careful medical monitoring can help older women have healthy pregnancies and produce healthy babies. (© Dennis O'Clair/Tony Stone Images)

Consuming a diet that meets the needs for a teenage mother's growth as well as the needs of pregnancy can be difficult. For example, pregnant teens typically consume a diet that contains less calcium, iron, zinc, magnesium, vitamin D, folate, and vitamin B_6 than is recommended. Teenagers are at greater risk of pregnancy-induced hypertension and are more likely to deliver preterm and low birth weight babies than are more mature women.[24] Socioeconomic and demographic factors also contribute to poor pregnancy outcomes in teenage girls. The pregnant teenager needs early medical intervention and nutritional counseling to produce a healthy baby.[23]

Maternal Age: The Older Mom Many women in ther 30s and 40s are having babies (Figure 13.10). The nutritional requirements for older mothers during pregnancy are no different than for women in their 20s, but pregnancy after the age of 35 does carry additional risks because older pregnant women are more likely to start pregnancy with medical conditions such as cardiovascular disease, kidney disorders, obesity, and diabetes.[25] During pregnancy, they also are more likely to develop gestational diabetes, pregnancy-induced hypertension, and other complications.[26] There is a higher incidence of low birth weight deliveries and of chromosomal abnormalities, especially **Down syndrome.** Today, careful medical monitoring throughout pregnancy is reducing the risks to older mothers and their babies.

Down syndrome A disorder caused by extra genetic material that results in distinctive facial characteristics, mental retardation, and other abnormalities.

Reproductive History Reproductive history is important for predicting pregnancy risk. Frequent pregnancies, with little time between, increase the risk for malnutrition because the mother may not have replenished nutrient stores depleted in the first pregnancy when she becomes pregnant again. A short interval between pregnancies also increases the risk of preterm and low birth weight infants. Women with a history of poor pregnancy outcomes are also at increased risk. For example, a women who has had a number of miscarriages is more likely to have another, and a woman who has had one child with a birth defect has an increased risk for defects in subsequent children.

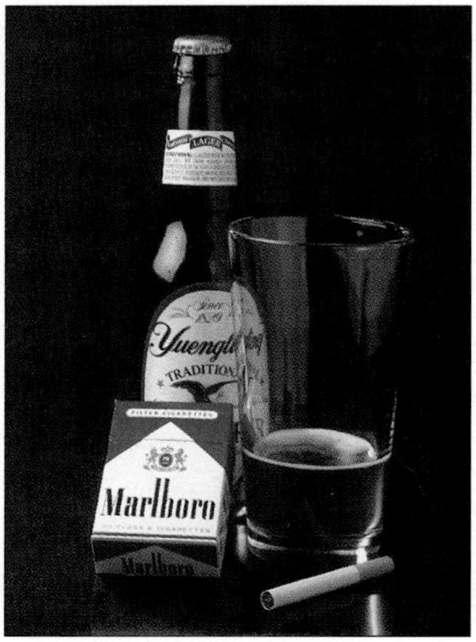

Figure 13.11
Women who smoke, drink alcohol, or use illicit drugs during pregnancy put their babies at risk. (George Semple)

Socioeconomic Factors

One of the greatest risk factors for poor pregnancy outcome is low income level. Poverty limits access to food and health care. Low-income women have a higher incidence of low birth weight and preterm infants. Race also affects pregnancy outcome. Poor African American women are more likely than poor white women to have very low birth weight infants.[20] In addition to poverty and race, inadequate health care, poor health practices, and lack of education are all related to poor pregnancy outcome.[27]

Ideally, prenatal care should start before conception. Low-income women, however, are unlikely to receive any care until late in pregnancy. One federally funded program that addresses the nutritional needs of pregnant women is the Special Supplemental Nutrition Program for Women, Infants, and Children (WIC). WIC has been shown to reduce health-care costs by providing preventative care to low-income pregnant women through nutrition education and food vouchers.[28] This program provides services to pregnant women, to nonlactating women for 6 months after birth, to lactating women for 12 months after birth, and to infants and children up to 5 years of age, but it does not address the need for good nutrition for women planning a pregnancy.

Substances That Affect Pregnancy Outcome

Many substances can affect the health of the embryo and fetus during pregnancy. Some of these are environmental toxins, some are consumed in the diet, and others are the result of maternal behaviors such as smoking and drug use (Figure 13.11).

Teratogen A substance that can cause birth defects.

Critical periods Times during growth and development when an organism is more susceptible to harm from poor nutrition or other environmental factors.

The Embryo and Fetus Are Particularly Vulnerable The rapidly dividing cells of the embryo and fetus are sensitive to many substances that might normally be a part of a woman's daily routine. Any chemical, biological, or physical agent that causes birth defects is called a **teratogen.** The placenta prevents some teratogens from passing from the mother's blood to the embryonic or fetal blood, but it cannot prevent the passage of all hazardous substances.

The developing embryo and fetus are particularly vulnerable to assault because both cell division and differentiation occur rapidly early in development. Times during development when teratogens are particularly damaging are called **critical periods** of development. Anything that interferes with development during a critical period causes irreversible damage. Critical periods correspond to times when cells are dividing, differentiating, and moving to form structures and organs. Because each organ system develops at a different rate and time, the period when a nutritional, chemical, or other insult occurs determines which organ system is primarily affected. Because the majority of cell differentiation occurs during the embryonic period, this is the time when exposure to teratogens can do the most damage, but vital body organs can still be affected during the fetal period (Figure 13.12). Severe damage to an embryo or fetus usually results in a spontaneous abortion.

Nutrients as Teratogens Deficiencies or excesses of some nutrients can have teratogenic effects. As discussed previously, inadequate folate intake may affect neural tube development. Excess vitamin D can cause mental retardation. Too much vitamin A is of particular concern because the risk of kidney problems and central nervous system abnormalities in the offspring increases even when maternal intake is not extremely high. Consumption by the mother of supplements containing 3000 μg RE or more of performed vitamin A, about four times the 1989 RDA, causes a fivefold increase in the risk of birth defects.[29] Supplements consumed during pregnancy should therefore contain beta-carotene, which is not teratogenic.

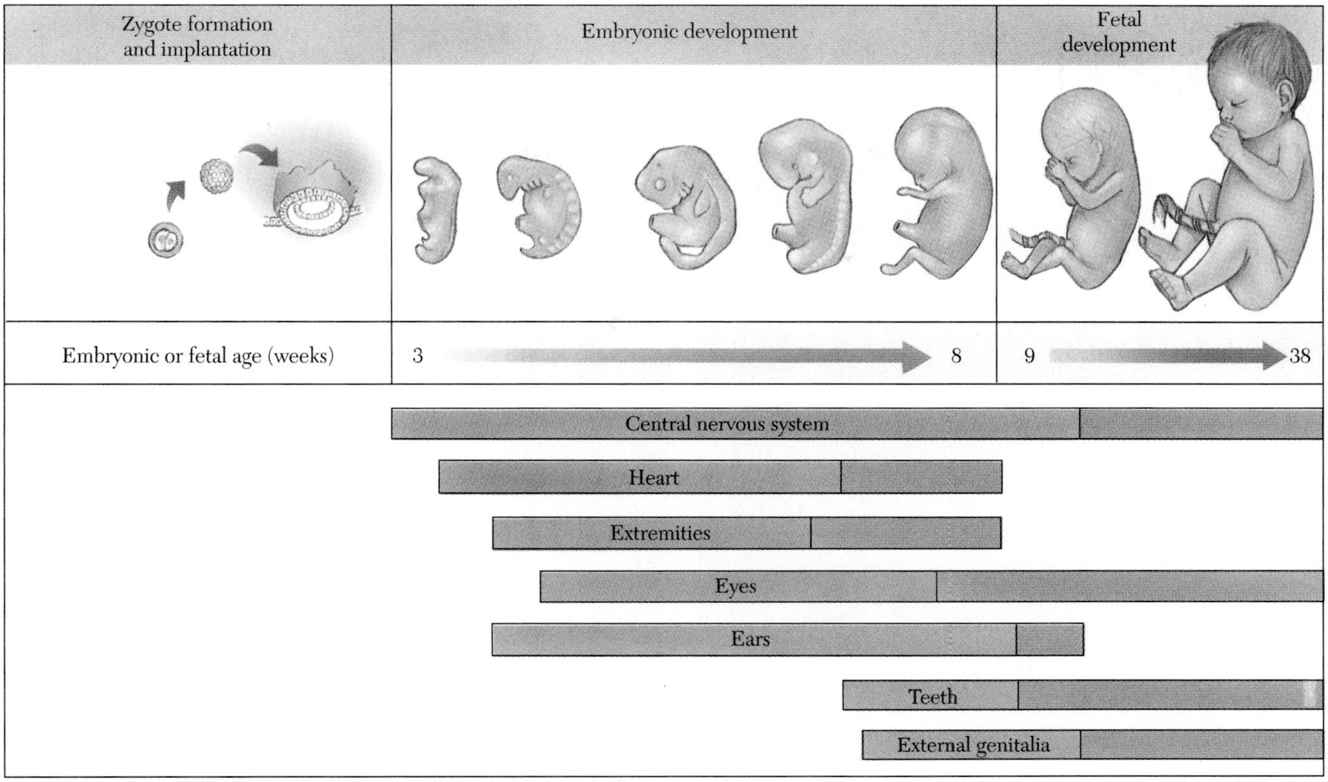

Figure 13.12

Critical periods of development are different for different body systems. The orange bars indicate when injury to the fetus from teratogens is likely to be the greatest. The purple bars indicate when damage may be less severe. (Adapted from Moore, K., and Persaud, T. *The Developing Human,* 5th ed. Philadelphia: W. B. Saunders Company, 1993.)

Alcohol Alcohol is a teratogen that impairs fetal growth and development. It is a toxin that reduces blood flow to the placenta thereby decreasing the delivery of oxygen and nutrients to the fetus. The use of alcohol can also impair maternal nutritional status, further increasing the risk to the embryo or fetus. Alcohol can cause learning and developmental disabilities and behavioral abnormalities referred to as **alcohol-related birth defects** or **fetal alcohol effects.** Alcohol-related birth defects are the leading cause of preventable birth defects and mental retardation.[30] They occur in 1 out of every 1000 live births in the United States and in 43 of every 1000 babies born to heavy drinkers. They are more common in babies born to minority women and in women of lower socioeconomic status.[31]

Alcohol-related birth defects or **fetal alcohol effects** A spectrum of abnormalities such as learning and developmental disabilities and behavioral abnormalities in a child due to maternal alcohol consumption during pregnancy.

Fetal alcohol syndrome A characteristic group of physical and mental abnormalities in an infant resulting from maternal alcohol consumption during pregnancy.

More severe alcohol-related damage during pregnancy is called **fetal alcohol syndrome.**[30] Fetal alcohol syndrome is a pattern of facial deformities, growth retardation, and permanent brain damage that causes problems throughout the child's lifetime. The most notable physical effects of fetal alcohol syndrome are visible in the head and face: The head circumference is small, the cheekbones are poorly developed, the nose is short with a low nasal bridge between the eyes, the area under the nose is flat, and the upper lip is thin (Figure 13.13a). Growth retardation either during gestation or after birth is common. Newborns with the syndrome may be shaky and irritable, with poor muscle tone and alcohol withdrawal symptoms. Other problems include heart and urinary tract defects, impaired vision and hearing, and delayed language development. Mental retardation is the most common and most serious effect.

Adolescents and adults diagnosed with fetal alcohol syndrome are plagued by debilitating behavioral problems, such as poor concentration and poor socialization and communication skills. These problems interfere with their ability to hold

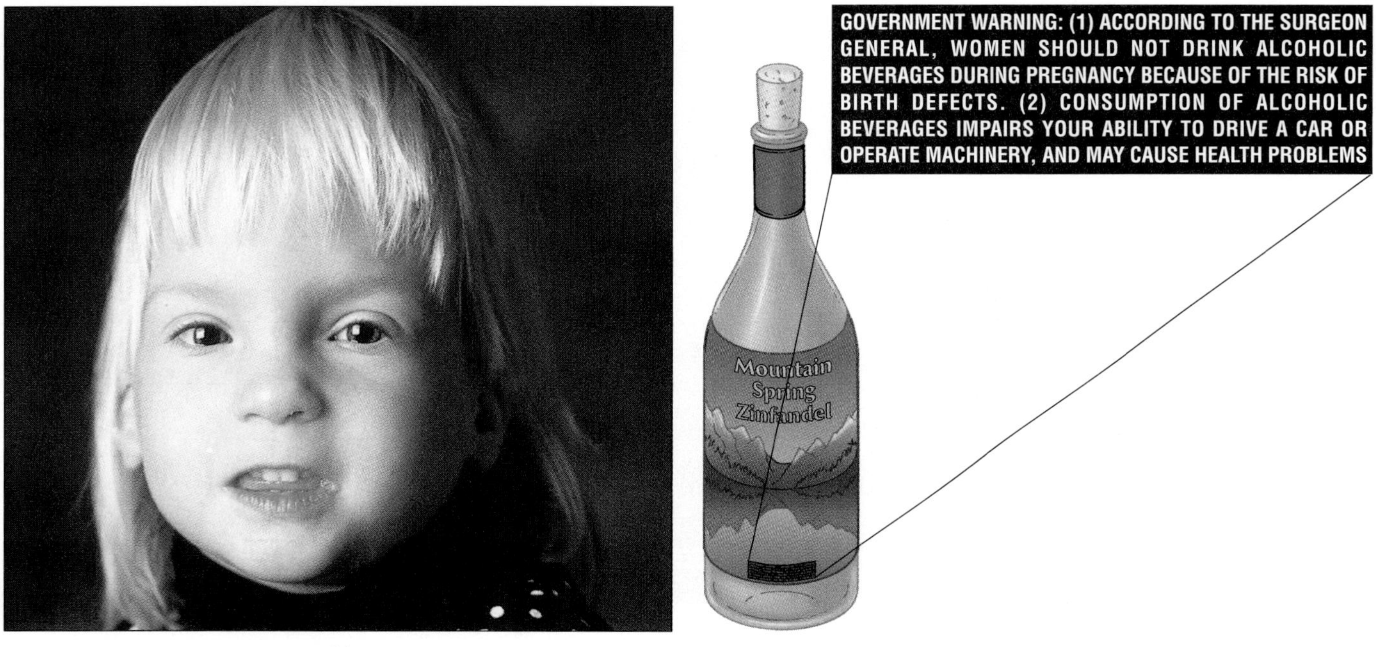
GOVERNMENT WARNING: (1) ACCORDING TO THE SURGEON GENERAL, WOMEN SHOULD NOT DRINK ALCOHOLIC BEVERAGES DURING PREGNANCY BECAUSE OF THE RISK OF BIRTH DEFECTS. (2) CONSUMPTION OF ALCOHOLIC BEVERAGES IMPAIRS YOUR ABILITY TO DRIVE A CAR OR OPERATE MACHINERY, AND MAY CAUSE HEALTH PROBLEMS
Mountain Spring Zinfandel

(a) (b)

Figure 13.13
(a) Children with fetal alcohol syndrome have common facial characteristics, including a low nasal bridge, a short nose, distinct eyelids, and a thin upper lip. (b) Alcoholic beverage packages include a warning against alcohol consumption during pregnancy. (*a,* © George Steinmetz)

jobs and live independently. Because alcohol consumption in each trimester has been associated with abnormalities, and because there is no level of alcohol consumption that is known to be safe during pregnancy, complete abstinence from alcohol during pregnancy is recommended, and warning labels to this effect appear on containers of beer, wine, and hard liquor (see Figure 13.13b).

Sudden infant death syndrome (SIDS) or **crib death** The unexplained death of an infant, usually during sleep.

Cigarettes It is estimated that 14.6% of pregnant women smoke cigarettes. Exposure to cigarette smoke affects the baby before birth and throughout life.[32] Compounds in tobacco smoke bind to hemoglobin and reduce oxygen delivery to fetal tissues. In addition, the nicotine absorbed from cigarette smoke constricts arteries and limits blood flow, reducing both oxygen and nutrient delivery to the fetus. Low birth weight babies are common among smokers; it is estimated that 20% of all such births could be prevented if women stopped smoking while pregnant. The risks of miscarriage, stillbirth, and premature birth are also increased in mothers who smoke.[33] The risk of **sudden infant death syndrome (SIDS, or crib death)** and respiratory problems are increased in children exposed to cigarette smoke both in the uterus and after birth.[34] The effects of maternal smoking follow children throughout life. Children whose mothers smoked while pregnant may have impaired intellectual development and a greater risk of developing lung disease in their youth.[35]

Caffeine Caffeine is a natural component of coffee, tea, and chocolate and is added to some soft drinks and medications. Caffeine has not been found to be a teratogen in humans, but consumption of more than 300 mg of caffeine per day by the mother during pregnancy has been associated with small reductions in birth weight and an increase in the risk for spontaneous abortion.[36] A typical cup of American coffee contains about 85 mg of caffeine, so this amount would be equivalent to about 4 to 5 cups of coffee per day. Table 12.5 lists the caffeine content of some commonly consumed foods, beverages, and medications.

Illicit Drug Abuse Substance abuse during pregnancy is a national health issue. Exposure to cocaine, opiates, or amphetamines has been shown to affect infant behavior and impact learning and attention span during childhood.[37]

Cocaine abuse during pregnancy has increased dramatically in the last decade. The health-care cost of treating cocaine-addicted infants is estimated at more than $500 million annually.[38] Cocaine increases the risk of complications to the mother and creates problems for the infant before, during, and after delivery. Cocaine use during pregnancy is associated with a high rate of miscarriages, intrauterine growth retardation, premature labor and delivery, low birth weight infants, birth defects, and sudden infant death syndrome.[39] This drug easily crosses the placenta and causes damage by constricting blood vessels, thereby reducing the flow of oxygen and nutrients to the rapidly dividing fetal cells.[40] At birth, cocaine-exposed babies are small and overly excitable. They have a small head circumference, which is associated with lower IQ scores. Cocaine also affects brain chemistry by altering the action of neurotransmitters. This may cause the impulsiveness and moodiness characteristic of some cocaine-exposed children. Some of these babies also have physical deformities, and most suffer from behavioral problems severe enough to sabotage their education and social development.

Marijuana also crosses the placenta and enters fetal blood. Thus far, results of studies on the effect of marijuana use on pregnancy outcome have been conflicting—some show no negative effects while others show that these infants are shaky and easily startled.[41]

LACTATION

The nutrient requirements of pregnancy include those needed to prepare for lactation. After childbirth, the breast-feeding mother's nutrient intake must support milk production and can influence the nutrient composition of her milk.

The Physiology of Lactation

During pregnancy, changes occur in the breasts to prepare for milk production, and body fat is deposited to ensure that energy is available for lactation. After birth, the suckling of the infant causes the release of the pituitary hormone prolactin, which stimulates milk production. The more the infant suckles, the more milk is produced. Once produced, the milk must move from storage lobules in the breast to the nipple, a process known as **let-down** (Figure 13.14). The let-down of milk is caused by oxytocin, another hormone produced by the pituitary gland. Oxytocin release is also stimulated by the suckling of the infant, but as nursing becomes more automatic, oxytocin release and the let-down of milk may occur in response to the sight or sound of an infant. It also can be inhibited by nervous tension, fatigue, or embarrassment—which can often occur in places such as the United States, where public breast feeding is sometimes frowned upon. The let-down response is essential for successful breast feeding and makes suckling easier for the child. If let-down is slow, the child can become frustrated and difficult to feed.

Let-down A hormonal reflex triggered by the infant's suckling that causes milk to be released from the milk ducts and flow to the nipple.

Maternal Nutrient Needs During Lactation

The need for energy and many nutrients is even greater during lactation than during pregnancy. This is because the mother is still providing for all of the nutrient needs of the infant, who is growing faster and is more active than the fetus. The newborn also has greater energy and nutrient needs for processes such as body temperature regulation and digestion that were partially or completely managed by the mother when the fetus was still in the womb.

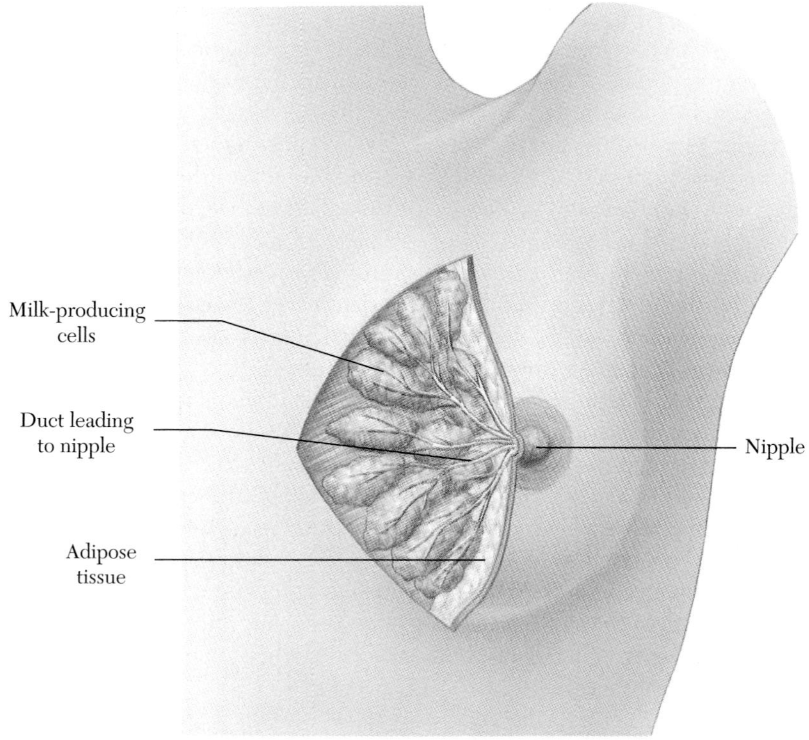

Figure 13.14
During lactation, milk travels from the milk-producing cell through the ducts that lead to the nipple.

Energy and Macronutrient Needs During Lactation During the first six months of lactation, approximately 600 to 900 ml, or 2.5 to 3.75 cups, of milk is produced daily. The amount is increased or decreased depending on the amount that the infant consumes.

Energy Needs During Lactation Producing a cup (240 ml) of breast milk requires about 225 kcalories. The milk itself contains approximately 175 kcalories, and the additional 50 kcalories are needed to synthesize the components of the milk. Providing an infant with 750 ml of milk would require approximately 700 kcalories from the mother. It is estimated that fat stored during pregnancy will provide 200 to 300 kcalories per day during the first three months of lactation. The remainder must be supplied by the diet. Therefore, an increase of about 500 kcalories per day over nonpregnant needs is recommended during early lactation (see Figure 13.7).

Many women are concerned about losing weight after pregnancy. It is normal to lose weight during the first six months after delivery. Some studies report that breast feeding does not affect the amount of weight lost,[42] whereas others suggest it does so initially[43] or if breast feeding continues for at least six months.[44] Beginning one month after birth, most lactating women lose 0.5 to 1 kilogram (1 to 2 lb) per month for six months. Some women will lose more and others may maintain or even gain weight regardless of whether or not they breast feed. Rapid weight loss is not recommended during lactation because it can decrease milk production; regular exercise may speed weight loss and does not impair milk production.[45]

Protein Needs During Lactation The protein needed to produce milk increases maternal protein needs; therefore, the 1989 RDA recommends an increase in protein intake of about 15 to 20 grams per day above nonpregnant needs.

Water Needs During Lactation To avoid dehydration and ensure adequate milk production, fluid intake should be increased by about 1 liter per day. This can be done by consuming an extra glass of milk, juice, or water at every meal and whenever the infant nurses. When fluid intake is low, the mother's urine will become more concentrated to conserve water for milk production.

Micronutrient Needs During Lactation The recommended intakes for several vitamins and minerals are increased during lactation to meet the metabolic needs of synthesizing milk and to replace the nutrients secreted in the milk itself (see Figure 13.7). Maternal intake of some vitamins can affect milk composition. This is particularly true of vitamins C, B_6, B_{12}, A, and D. When maternal intake is low, the amounts in milk are decreased. The recommended intakes of vitamin B_6, B_{12}, other B vitamins, and vitamin A are increased above nonlactating levels.

For other nutrients, including calcium and folate, levels in the milk are maintained at the expense of maternal stores. Much of the calcium secreted in human milk comes from an increase in maternal bone resorption. However, the AI for calcium is not increased above nonlactating levels because the loss of calcium from maternal bones is not prevented by increases in dietary calcium. Calcium supplements during lactation also do not affect the concentration of calcium in the milk or maternal bone mineral changes.[46] Although lactation is associated with maternal bone loss, the calcium lost is replaced after weaning.[47] Folate needs are increased above nonpregnant levels to account for the amount needed to replace folate secreted in milk plus the amount needed by nonlactating women to maintain folate status.[17] Iron needs are not increased during lactation because little iron is lost in milk, and, in most women, losses are decreased because menstruation is absent.

Meeting Maternal Nutrient Needs During Lactation Meeting the needs of lactation requires a varied nutrient-dense diet that follows the Food Guide Pyramid recommendations for lactating women (see Figure 13.9). The need for calcium can be met by consuming 3 servings of dairy products, and additional nutrients and energy are obtained from extra servings of vegetables and grains and a larger serving of meat or meat substitutes. Most lactating women can meet all their needs without supplements.

NUTRITION FOR THE INFANT

When a child is born and the umbilical cord is cut, he or she suddenly becomes actively involved in obtaining nutrients rather than being passively fed through the placenta (Figure 13.15). Nutrient needs are high to support growth, development, and activity. Suckling from either the breast or bottle must satisfy all nutrient needs.

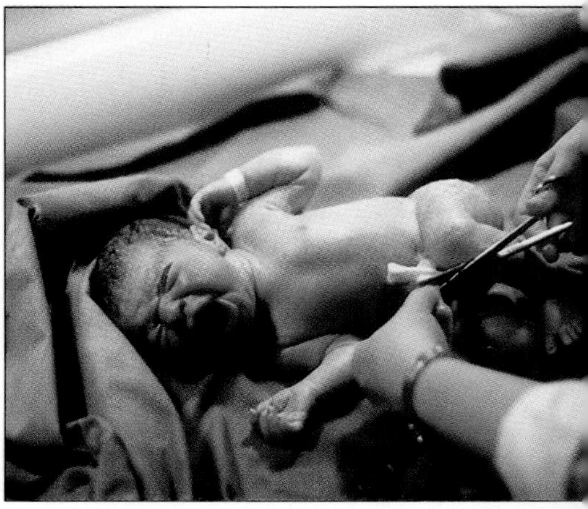

Figure 13.15
At birth the umbilical cord is cut and the child must obtain nutrients orally. (© Jerry Cooke/Photo Researchers, Inc.)

Nutrient Needs of the Newborn

During the first few months of life, growth is more rapid than at any other time of life. Many of the infant's organ systems and metabolic processes are still developing. Since infants' digestive abilities are limited and they have no teeth, a special type of diet is required.

Energy and Macronutrient Needs Energy requirements per unit of body weight are about three times greater in newborns than in adults. The 1989 RDAs for infants 0 to 6 months of age and 6 to 12 months of age are 108 and 98 kcalories per kilogram of body weight respectively, whereas adults require only 30 to 40 kcalories per kilogram.

Fat About 40 to 50% of the energy in an infant's diet should come from fat, with 3% from essential fatty acids. Breast milk and formulas contain approximately 50% of energy as fat. This high energy density allows the infant's small stomach to hold enough food to meet energy needs. A sufficient supply of the long chain polyunsaturated fatty acids docosahexaenoic acid (an omega-3 fatty acid) and arachidonic acid (an omega-6 fatty acid) are important for nervous system development. These fatty acids are constituents of cell membranes and are incorporated into the retina of the eye and brain tissue. Infants can synthesize docosahexaenoic acid and arachidonic acid from their precursors, alpha-linolenic acid and linoleic acid respectively, but the rate of conversion is not great enough to meet the need for optimal retinal and brain formation.[48] The need for these fatty acids is even greater in preterm infants. Development of the retina and brain continue to require dietary sources of these two fatty acids for about two years after birth.

Carbohydrate Carbohydrate is a major contributor to energy intake in the infant. The source of carbohydrate in breast-fed infants and most bottle-fed infants is lactose. About 39% of the energy in breast milk is from lactose. As the infant grows and solid foods are introduced into the diet, the percentage of kcalories from carbohydrate in the diet increases and the percent from fat decreases.

Protein As with energy, the infant's protein requirement per unit of body weight is very high compared with the adult requirement: The 1989 RDA is 2.2 grams per kilogram from birth to six months of age, compared with 0.8 gram per kilogram for an adult. The ideal protein source for newborns is human milk. Infant formulas are designed to mimic this amino acid pattern. The more closely the protein resembles that in human milk, the better it meets needs. A diet too high in protein may lead to dehydration because the excretion of metabolic wastes produced when excess protein is consumed increases water loss.

Water The fluid requirements of infants are also very high compared with those of adults. Infant kidneys are poorly developed and unable to reabsorb much of the water that is filtered out of the blood. Therefore, infants lose proportionately more water in their urine than adults. Infants also lose proportionately more water through evaporation than do adults because they have a large surface area compared with their total body weight. These factors, in addition to the fact that infants cannot tell us they are thirsty, puts them at risk for dehydration. They rely on their caregivers to provide them with enough fluid. It is recommended that infants consume 150 ml of water per kilogram of body weight. Usually the amount of water in breast milk or formula is enough to meet needs. Hot weather, fever, diarrhea, and vomiting increase water loss, and therefore require that additional water be given.

In the developing world, diarrhea is the most common cause of infant death, and in the United States it kills one child each day. The cause of the diarrhea is usually a bacterial or viral infection; the cause of death is dehydration. The fluid intake of infants with diarrhea should be monitored carefully, and a pediatrician should be contacted. Mixtures of sugar, water, and electrolytes are available to replace these lost fluids.

Micronutrients There are several vitamins and minerals that may be limited in the unsupplemented infant diet. Iron is the nutrient most commonly deficient in infants who are consuming adequate energy and protein. Iron deficiency is usually not a problem during the first four to six months of life because infants have iron stores at birth. In addition, the iron in human milk, though not particularly abundant, is very well absorbed, and iron-fortified infant formulas are available. After four to six months, the diets of breast-fed infants should contain other sources of iron, such as iron-fortified rice cereal.

Newborns are also potentially at risk for vitamin D deficiency. Breast milk is relatively low in vitamin D, so breast-fed infants who do not receive adequate exposure to sunlight, such as those living in cold climates, may not obtain adequate vitamin D. An AI of 5 μg of vitamin D has been set for infants 0 to 12 months of age. This may be provided as a supplement for breast-fed infants. Infant formulas contain 10 μg of vitamin D per liter of formula. To synthesize adequate vitamin D, about 15 minutes per day of sun exposure, with only the face exposed, is needed for light-skinned babies; a longer time is required for darker-skinned babies.

Vitamin K, important in blood clotting, is another nutrient for which newborns are at risk of deficiency. Little of this vitamin crosses the placenta from mother to fetus, and because the gut is sterile at birth, no microbial vitamin K synthesis occurs. Breast milk is also low in vitamin K, so breast-fed infants are at risk of hemorrhage due to vitamin K deficiency. Today, most newborns receive a vitamin K injection at birth to prevent the possibility of hemorrhage. This provides them with enough vitamin K to last until their intestines are colonized with the bacteria that synthesize it.

Fluoride is important in the development of teeth, even before they erupt. Breast milk is low in fluoride and formula manufacturers use unfluoridated water in preparing liquid formula. Therefore, breast-fed infants, infants fed premixed formula, and those fed formula mixed with low-fluoride water are often supplemented beginning at six months of age. In areas where the drinking water is fluoridated, infants fed formula reconstituted with tap water should not be given fluoride supplements.

Vitamin B_{12} may be deficient in the breast milk of vegan mothers. Therefore, infants of vegan mothers should be supplemented with vitamin B_{12}. Although vitamin B_{12} is not known to be toxic, iron, vitamin D, vitamin K, and fluoride are toxic at high doses. Nutrient supplements should be given to infants only when recommended by a pediatrician and only in the amounts prescribed.

How Much Is Enough: Assessing Infant Growth

Although nutrient needs for infants are fairly well defined, it is difficult to calculate an infant's actual nutrient intake. The best indicator of adequate nourishment is normal growth. Most healthy infants follow standard patterns of growth, so an infant's growth can be monitored by comparing length, weight, and head circumference to standard growth charts (Figure 13.16). (Charts for infants 0 to 36 months of age and children 2 to 18 years of age are included in Appendix B.) These charts plot typical growth patterns of infants and children in the United States. With them, an infant's pattern of growth can be monitored and compared with other infants of the same age. The resulting ranking, or percentile, indicates where the infant's growth falls in relation to population standards. For example, if a newborn boy is at the 20th percentile for weight, it means that 19% of newborn boys weigh less and 80% weigh more. Children usually continue at the same percentiles as they grow. For instance, a child who is at the 50th percentile for height and 25th percentile for weight should continue to follow approximately these height and weight curves. A dramatic deviation from the pattern could indicate overnutrition or undernutrition.

Whether an infant is 6 pounds or 8 pounds at birth, the rate of growth should be approximately the same—rapid initially and slowing slightly as the infant approaches one year of age. A rule of thumb is that an infant's birth weight should double by four months and triple by one year of age. In the first year of life, most infants increase their length by 50%. Breast-fed and bottle-fed infants have similar growth for the first three to four months, but then bottle-fed infants grow at a faster rate. Small infants and premature infants often follow a pattern parallel to but below the growth curve for a period of time and then experience catch-up growth that brings them onto the growth curve in a place compatible with their

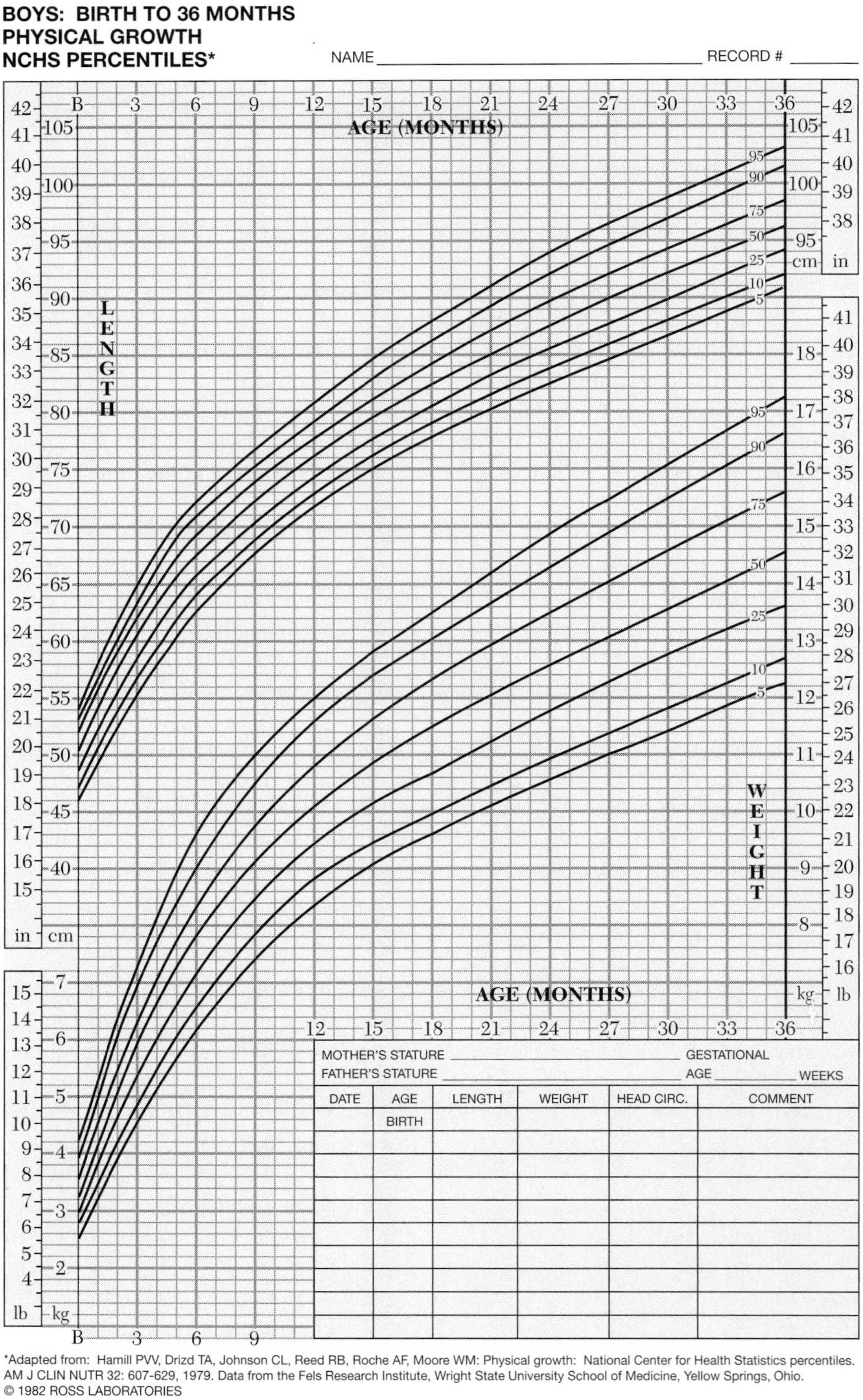

Figure 13.16
Growth charts, such as this one for boys from birth to 36 months of age, demonstrate typical patterns of growth. (© 1982 Ross Laboratories)

genetic growth potential. Slight fluctuations in growth rate are normal, but a consistent pattern of not following the growth curve or a sudden change in growth pattern is cause for concern.

A rapid increase in weight without an increase in height may be an indicator that the infant is being overfed. Growth that is slower than the predicted pattern indicates **failure to thrive.** This is a catch-all term for any type of growth failure in a young child. The cause may be a congenital condition, the presence of disease, poor nutrition, neglect, abuse, or psychosocial problems. Whatever the

Failure to thrive The inability of a child's growth to keep up with normal growth curves.

cause, the treatment is usually an individualized plan that includes adequate nutrition and careful monitoring by physicians, dietitians, and other health-care professionals. Just as there are critical periods in fetal life, there are critical periods for growth and development during infancy. For example, the brain is growing rapidly at birth, and undernutrition at this time can permanently affect brain development.

Feeding the Newborn

Newborns have small stomachs, can consume only liquids, and have high nutrient requirements. They should be fed on demand throughout the day and night, about eight times daily. The ideal food for the newborn is breast milk, but infant formula can also meet a newborn's needs. Solid food should not be introduced into the diet until the child is at least four to six months of age. Introducing solid food before four months is not recommended because the infant's feeding abilities and gastrointestinal tract are not mature enough to handle foods other than breast milk or formula.

Meeting Nutrient Needs With Breast Feeding Breast milk is the ideal food for the new baby. It is designed specifically for the human newborn, it requires no special preparation, and the amount available varies with demand. Thus, breast feeding is the preferred form of infant nutrition and is usually the recommended choice for feeding the newborn of a healthy, well-nourished mother.[49] Public health programs promote breast feeding, and as a result, the percent of infants who are breast fed has increased from 20% in 1970 to 59.4% in 1995. Breast feeding is most common among college-educated women over the age of 30, but the greatest increases in breast-feeding incidence have occurred among groups that historically have not had high rates, such as African Americans, women with low incomes, those less educated, those employed full-time, those less than 25 years of age, and women participating in the WIC program.[50]

Advantages to Mother and Child Breast feeding has nutritional, immunological, physiological, and psychological benefits for both mother and child.[49] Breast milk provides protection against infection early in life by passing immune factors from the mother to the infant. Breast-fed babies have fewer allergies, ear infections, respiratory illness, and urinary tract infections than formula-fed babies, and have fewer problems with constipation and diarrhea. There is also evidence that breast feeding protects against sudden infant death syndrome, diabetes, and chronic digestive diseases.[51] The strong suckling required by breast feeding aids in the development of facial muscles, which help in speech development and the correct formation of teeth. Breast-fed babies are also less likely to be overfed, because the amount of milk consumed cannot be monitored visually. In bottle feeding, it is often tempting to encourage the baby to finish the entire bottle whether or not he is hungry. For the mother, breast feeding has the advantage of providing a readily available and inexpensive source of nourishment for her infant. Breast feeding has been estimated to save more than $400 per child in food purchases during the first year. It requires no preparation or bottles and nipples that must be washed. It is more ecological because it doesn't require energy for manufacture or generate waste from discarded packaging. Physiologically, breast feeding causes contractions that help the mother's uterus return to size more quickly and may promote weight loss in some women, especially when continued for more than six months.[52] Women who breast feed have a lower risk of developing osteoporosis and breast and ovarian cancer.[51] Lactation also inhibits ovulation, lengthening the time between pregnancies; however, it does not reliably prevent ovulation and so cannot be effectively used for birth control. Oral contraceptives can be used immediately postpartum, but those containing only progestin are

Table 13.2 *Risks and Benefits of Breast and Bottle Feeding*

Risk/Benefit	Breast Feeding	Bottle Feeding
Nutrients	Ideal food for human babies. Composition changes as they eat and grow.	Modeled after human milk, but certain components cannot be duplicated. Composition does not change with time. Must be prepared carefully to supply the correct nutrient mix and ratio of nutrients to fluid.
Amount	Underfeeding can be a problem in newborns if the mother is not well versed in breast feeding and the signs of dehydration in the infant.	Overfeeding is a risk because of the desire of caregivers to have the baby empty the bottle.
Immunity	Immune factors are transferred from mother to infant.	There are no immune factors in formula.
Allergies	Allergies to breast milk are very rare and the risk of food allergies is reduced.	There are a variety of choices if the infant is allergic to one type of formula.
Risk from mother	Certain contaminants such as environmental pollutants, medications, illicit drugs, and disease-causing organisms such as HIV can pass from mother to baby.	None.
Environmental contamination	Breast milk is sterile, but pumped milk can become contaminated if stored improperly.	Bacterial contamination is a risk if formula is prepared under unsanitary conditions or stored improperly.
Ease for caregivers	No equipment to wash, always available, but may require more time from the mother.	Requires more preparation and washing, but other family members can share responsibility for feeding.
Ease for baby	Suckling is harder for the baby but aids in development of teeth and facial muscles needed for speech. Pumped breast milk can be easily consumed by weak or sick infants.	Easier for baby, which is especially important for weak or sick infants.
Benefit to mother	Promotes uterine contractions which help the uterus return to prepregnancy size. May promote loss of weight and body fat if continued for more than six months. May reduce risk of breast cancer.	May allow more sleep.
Cost	Cheaper, but the mother must be well nourished.	More expensive than nursing and includes cost of formula as well as equipment and energy used in preparation.

preferable because they do not affect milk volume or composition. Oral contraceptives containing estrogen may decrease milk volume.[53] Psychologically, breast feeding can be a relaxing, emotionally enjoyable interaction for both mother and infant (Table 13.2).

How Long Should Breast Feeding Continue? Physiologically, lactation can continue as long as suckling is maintained. Breast feeding alone is sufficient to support optimal growth for about six months, and the American Academy of Pediatrics recommends breast milk along with supplemental feeding of solids for the first year of life—and longer—as mutually desired by mother and child.[51] As part of its Integrated Management of Childhood Illness Program, the World Health Organization recommends that infants in developing nations be breast fed for two years.[54] After 12 months the baby no longer needs breast milk to meet nutrient needs. As the infant obtains more and more of its energy from solid foods, milk production decreases due to reduced demand by the infant. However, breast feeding beyond 12 months continues to provide nutrition, comfort, and an emotional bond between mother and child. The length of time a woman breast feeds is up to her and her baby. In most cultures it is acceptable to breast feed for two to three years, but in the United States, because of social pressures and convenience issues, few women continue for more than six months.

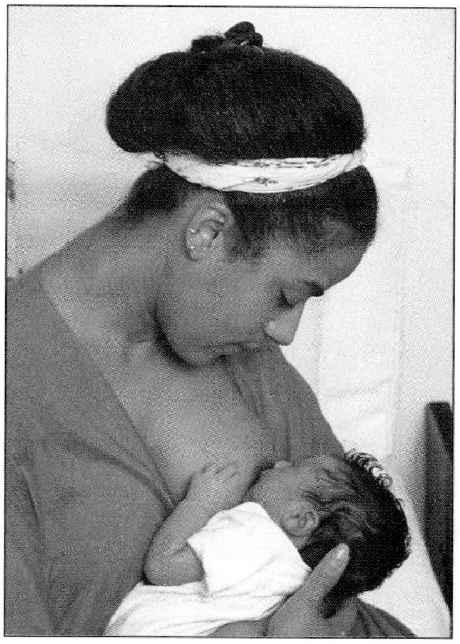

Figure 13.17
By the time the infant is a week old, mother and child have usually adjusted to breast feeding. (© Erika Stone/Photo Researchers, Inc.)

How Much Is Enough? A strong, healthy baby will be able to suckle shortly after birth. Within a week, milk production and breast feeding are usually fully established (Figure 13.17). Infants should be fed on demand every 1.5 to 3 hours. A feeding should last approximately 8 to 12 minutes at each breast. Although it is difficult to measure the amount of milk an infant takes from the breast, a well-fed newborn should urinate enough to soak six to eight diapers a day and gain about 1/3 to 1/2 pound per week.

Practical Aspects of Breast Feeding Breast feeding does not always come naturally to mother or infant and can require practice and patience. Effective suckling by the infant and relaxation of the mother are essential to successful breast feeding. Some foods and other substances in the mother's diet, such as garlic or spicy foods, contain chemicals or flavors that pass into breast milk and cause adverse reactions in some babies. These reactions seem to be individual to the mother and child. As long as a food does not affect the infant's response to feeding, it can be included in the mother's diet. Caffeine in the mother's diet can make the infant jittery and excitable, so large amounts should be avoided while breast feeding. Alcohol, which is harmful for infants, passes into breast milk. It is most concentrated an hour to an hour and a half after consumption and is cleared from the milk at about the same rate it disappears from the bloodstream. Therefore, occasional limited alcohol consumption while breast feeding is probably not harmful if intake is timed to minimize the amount present in milk when the infant is fed.

Breast feeding does not mean that a mother must be available for every feeding. Milk may be pumped from the breast and stored for later feedings. A working mother can nurse her baby in the morning and evening and provide formula or pumped breast milk to be fed from a bottle while she is away from home. If prescription drugs are taken by the mother for only a short time, a breast pump may be used to maintain milk production and the milk discarded, until the medication is no longer needed (Figure 13.18). Since pumped milk is exposed to pumps and bottles, care must be taken to avoid bacterial contamination. If pumped milk is not immediately fed to the baby, it should be refrigerated. It can be kept refrigerated for 24 to 48 hours, but if it will not be used within that period, it should be frozen in a clean container. Warming breast milk in a microwave is not recommended, because this destroys some of its immune properties and it may result in dangerously hot portions of the milk. The best way to warm milk is by running warm water over the bottle.

Colostrum The first milk, which is secreted in late pregnancy and up to a week after birth. It is rich in protein and immune factors.

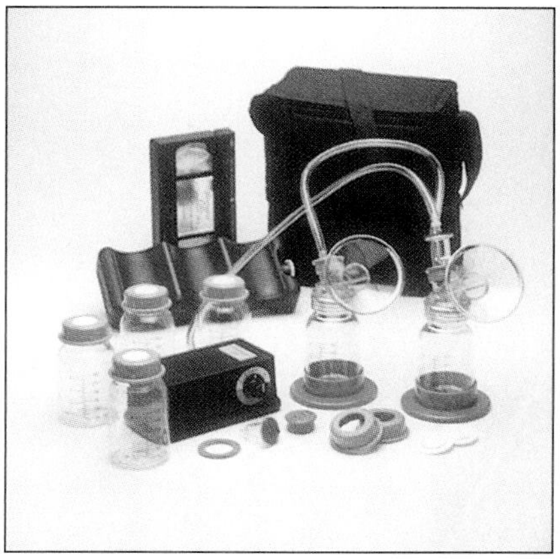

Figure 13.18
Breast pumps can be used to pump milk for bottle feedings. This relieves the mother from responsibility for all feedings. (Bailey Medical Engineering)

Composition of Human Milk The nutrient composition of breast milk is specifically designed for the human infant and changes as the infant develops. The first fluid that is produced by the breast after delivery is called **colostrum.** Not actually milk, colostrum is a yellowish fluid that is higher in water, protein, immune factors, minerals, and some vitamins than milk. It is produced for up to a week after delivery. While colostrum is produced, it may seem that the newborn is not receiving enough to eat; however, supplemental bottle feedings are not necessary. The nutrients in colostrum meet infant needs until actual milk production begins. During the first few months of life, the immune factors provided first by colostrum, and later by mature milk, compensate for the infant's immature immune system. Colostrum also has beneficial effects on the gastrointestinal tract, acting as a laxative that helps the baby excrete the thick, mucousy stool produced during life in the womb.

The composition of mature human milk changes over time, meeting the nutrient needs of the child for up to the first year of life. Mature human milk contains about 175 kcalories per cup (240 ml) and is a good source of protein, fat, magnesium, and calcium. When compared with cow's milk, it is very different in both appearance and composition. Human milk looks thin and watery and has less protein and minerals than cow's milk. Lactalbumin, the predominant protein in human milk, forms a soft, easily digested curd in the infant's stomach. The amino acids methionine and phenylalanine, which are difficult for the infant to metabolize, are present in lower amounts in human milk proteins than in cow's milk proteins. Human milk is also a good source of taurine, an amino acid needed for bile salt formation and eye and brain function.

The fat in human milk is more easily digested than that in cow's milk. Human milk is higher in cholesterol and the essential fatty acid linoleic acid. It is also higher in the long chain polyunsaturated fatty acids arachidonic acid and docohexaenoic acid, which are essential for normal brain development, eyesight, and growth.[55] The fat content of breast milk changes throughout a feeding, gradually increasing during the nursing session. Thus, for the baby to attain satiety and obtain adequate energy, it is important for nursing to continue long enough for the infant to obtain the higher-fat milk.

Lactose is the primary carbohydrate in human milk. It is digested slowly, so it stimulates the growth of acid-producing bacteria. It also promotes the absorption of calcium and other minerals and provides a source of galactose for nervous system development.

Human milk is low in iron, but the iron present is easily absorbed. About 50% of the iron in human milk is absorbed, compared with only 2 to 30% from many other foods.

Human milk also contains a number of other substances that protect the infant from disease. Antibody proteins and immune system cells pass from the mother into her milk to provide the infant immune protection. A number of enzymes and other proteins prevent the growth of harmful microorganisms. Several carbohydrates have been identified that protect against disease-causing organisms, including viruses that cause diarrhea.[56] One substance favors the growth of the beneficial bacterium *Lactobacillus bifidus* in the infant's colon, which inhibits the growth of disease-causing organisms (see *Critical Thinking: How to Nourish a New Baby*).

Meeting Nutrient Needs With Bottle Feeding A hundred years ago a baby who could not be breast fed had little chance of survival. Today infants who cannot breast feed can still thrive. When breast feeding is not the choice, there are many commercially available infant formulas modeled after the nutrient content of breast milk. Unmodified cow's milk should never be fed to infants; its higher protein and mineral content taxes the kidneys and predisposes the infant to dehydration. Young infants may also become anemic if fed cow's milk because it contains little absorbable iron and can lead to iron loss by causing small amounts of gastrointestinal bleeding.

When Is Bottle Feeding Best? Despite efforts to increase the number of women who breast feed, the infant formula business is booming. Many women prefer not to breast feed at all, and many breast feed for only a short time. Sometimes this is a lifestyle choice, but there are situations when breast feeding is not the best choice for health reasons. Bottle feeding is easier for the infant; less strength is needed to consume the same nutrients. An infant who is small or weak may not have the strength to receive adequate nutrition from breast feeding. In this case, formula, which provides almost the same nutrients as breast milk, can be used, or pumped breast milk can be offered to the infant in a bottle.

In some cases bottle feeding is the best choice because it reduces the transmission of drugs and disease via breast milk. Hepatitis and HIV infection, which causes AIDS, can be transmitted to the infant in breast milk, but common illnesses such as colds, flu, and skin infections should not interfere with breast feeding.[57] In the United States, women who are infected with HIV are advised not to breast feed, but in developing nations, the risks of malnutrition associated with not breast feeding outweigh the risk of passing this infection on to the infant. Women who are taking medications should check with their physician as to whether it is safe to breast feed. Because alcohol and drugs such as cocaine and marijuana can be passed to the baby in breast milk, alcoholic and drug-addicted mothers are counseled not to breast feed. Nicotine from cigarette smoke is also rapidly transferred from maternal blood to milk, and heavy smoking may decrease the supply of milk.[58] Also, secondhand exposure to smoke may be damaging to the infant's lungs and may increase the risk of sudden infant death syndrome.[34]

How Much Is Enough? As with breast-fed infants, formula-fed infants should be fed on demand every few hours. Newborns have small stomachs, so at each feeding they may consume only a few ounces of formula. As the infant grows, the amount consumed at each feeding will increase to 4 to 8 ounces. Caregivers should respond to cues from the infant that hunger is satisfied, even if a bottle of formula is not finished. Encouraging infants to finish every bottle can result in overfeeding and excess weight gain. As with breast-fed infants, adequate intake can be judged from the amount of urine produced and the amount of weight gained.

Practical Aspects of Bottle Feeding Infant formula must be prepared carefully in order to avoid mixing errors and contamination. If the proper measurements are not used in preparing formula, the child can receive an excess or deficiency of nutrients and an improper ratio of nutrients to fluids. If the water and all the equipment used in preparing formula are not clean or if the prepared formula is left unrefrigerated, food-borne illness may result. Because sanitation is often a problem in developing nations, infections that lead to diarrhea and dehydration occur more commonly in formula-fed than in breast-fed infants. Commercially prepared formulas are sterile and powdered formulas contain no harmful microorganisms. To avoid introducing harmful microorganisms, the water used to mix powdered formula should be boiled for one to two minutes and allowed to cool before mixing.[59] Hands should be washed before preparing formula, and bottles and nipples should be washed in a dishwasher or placed in a pan of boiling water for 5 minutes. Formula should be prepared immediately before a feeding, and any excess should be discarded. Opened cans of ready-to-feed and liquid concentrate formula should be covered and refrigerated and used within the time indicated on the can. Formula may be fed either warm or cold, but the temperature should be consistent.

The position of the child is important during feeding. The infant's head should be higher than the stomach, and the bottle should be tilted so that there is no air in the nipple (Figure 13.19). If the hole in the nipple is too large, the infant may feel full before receiving adequate nutrition. If the hole is too small, the infant may tire before nutrient needs are met. Just as breast-fed infants alternate breasts, bottle-fed infants should be held alternately between the left and right arms to promote equal development of the head and neck muscles.

Infants should never be put to bed with a bottle of formula. At night, while the child sleeps, the flow of saliva is decreased and the sugary formula liquid is allowed to remain in contact with the teeth for many hours. This causes the rapid

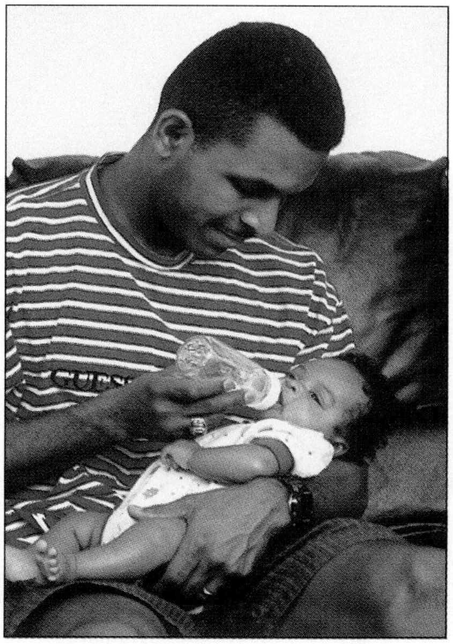

Figure 13.19
During bottle feeding, the position of the baby and the bottle are both important. (© Erika Stone/Photo Researchers, Inc.)

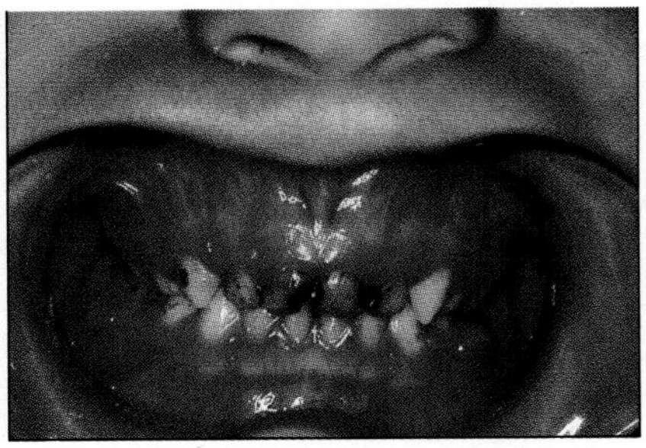

Figure 13.20
Nursing bottle syndrome causes rapid decay of the upper front teeth. (K. L. Boyd, D.D.S./Custom Medical Stock Photo)

Nursing bottle syndrome Extreme tooth decay in the upper teeth resulting from putting a child to bed with a bottle containing milk or other sweetened liquids.

and serious decay of the upper teeth referred to as **nursing bottle syndrome.** Usually, the lower teeth are protected by the tongue and are unaffected (Figure 13.20).

Formula Choices The modern era of infant formulas began with the development of artificial milk made from skimmed cow's milk to which homogenized animal and vegetable fats were added to approximate the fatty acid composition of human milk. Over the past 30 to 40 years, very few problems have resulted from inadequate or imbalanced formulas. In the 1950s, a few cases of vitamin A deficiency were seen in infants receiving formula made from defatted soy flour, and skin lesions have been seen in infants fed formulas low in linoleic acid. In 1978, a company accidentally left chloride out of two of its formulas, and infants fed these developed symptoms that included poor muscle control, delayed speech development, and slowed growth. Infant formulas can never duplicate the living cells, active hormones, enzymes, and immune system molecules in human milk, but formulas today try to replicate human milk as closely as possible in order to match the growth, nutrient absorption, and other parameters obtained with breast feeding. Formula is available in ready-to-feed, liquid concentrate, or powdered forms (see *Off the Shelf: Choosing an Infant Formula*).

Special Formulas for Special Needs There are a number of conditions, such as allergies, prematurity, and genetic abnormalities, that alter the dietary needs of newborns. To meet these unusual needs, special formulas are available. Milk allergy is an example of a relatively rare nutrition-related problem that can be life-threatening but is easily treated with a modified diet. There are over 25 proteins in milk that can be the cause of a milk allergy. Many, but not all, are inactivated by scalding the milk. For infants who cannot tolerate human or cow's milk, soy protein formulas are available. And for those who cannot tolerate soy protein, formulas made from predigested proteins, called protein hydrolysates, are an option.

Premature infants have special needs because they do not have fully developed organ systems or metabolic pathways. If they are too small or weak to nurse or take a bottle, pumped breast milk or formula can be fed through a tube. Some nutrients that are produced in the bodies of full-term infants are essential in the diets of premature infants. For example, preterm infants are less able to synthesize the amino acids tyrosine and cysteine and the fatty acid docosahexaenoic acid. These and other substances, such as taurine and carnitine, are needed in higher amounts by premature babies. The energy, protein, and micronutrient requirements of preterm infants are also higher due to their rapid growth and development. Preterm infant formulas are available to meet the needs of premature babies.

Genetic abnormalities that prevent the normal metabolism of specific nutrients may alter dietary needs. For instance, infants with the genetic disease phenylketonuria (PKU) lack an enzyme needed to metabolize the amino acid phenylalanine (see Chapter 6). If a child with PKU is fed breast milk or a formula that contains phenylalanine, the by-products of phenylalanine metabolism accumulate and can cause brain damage. This can be prevented by feeding infants with PKU a special formula that provides only enough phenylalanine to meet the need for protein synthesis. Because this special diet must be started as soon as possible, infants born in the United States and Canada are tested for PKU at birth.

Colic Inconsolable crying that is believed to be due to pain from gas buildup in the gastrointestinal tract or immaturity of the central nervous system.

A relatively common but not life-threatening problem in infants is **colic.** Colic involves daily periods of inconsolable crying that cannot be stopped by holding, feeding, or changing the infant. Colic usually begins at a few weeks of age and continues through the first two to three months. It occurs in both breast- and bottle-fed infants. Although its cause is unknown, it is hypothesized that colic is related to intestinal gas caused by milk intolerance, improper feeding practices, or immaturity of the central nervous system.

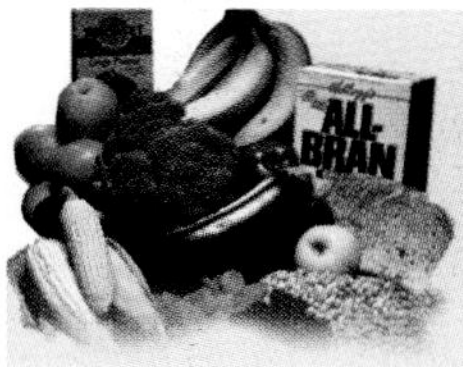

Off the Shelf

Choosing an Infant Formula

Which infant formula is best? Infants are often formula-fed from birth, and most are formula-fed after a few months of breast feeding. Selecting an infant formula can be confusing. Is cow's milk formula better than a soy-based formula? Is one safer or more nutritious than the other? Is a less expensive formula likely to be missing certain nutrients? Is premixed formula better than powdered?

Although cow's milk should never be fed to young infants, most formula is made from cow's milk. If cow's milk formula is not well tolerated by an infant, hydrolyzed cow's milk formula and soy-based formula are available. Cow's milk hydrolysates are usually recommended over soy formula because they provide higher quality protein and the calcium they contain is better absorbed. Soy-based formulas are necessary for infants who cannot tolerate the protein in cow's milk and for those who are lactose intolerant, because soy formula contains sucrose or corn syrup instead of lactose.

The safety of commercially prepared infant formulas is regulated by the FDA, which specifies the minimum, and in some cases maximum, amounts of nutrients that can be present in formulas according to recommendations by the American Academy of Pediatrics Committee on Nutrition.[1] These recommendations for the amounts of nutrients in infant formulas are based on the composition of human milk from a healthy mother. Strict quality control regulations require that each batch of formula be tested for stability and analyzed to ensure it contains the appropriate amounts of required nutrients. Each container must be coded to identify the batch.

Formulas are marketed in three basic forms: ready-to-feed, liquid concentrates, and powdered. Ready-to-feed formulas require no preparation and are available in sizes ranging from 4-ounce bottles to 32-ounce containers. Liquid concentrates are prepared for use by mixing equal amounts of the concentrate and water. Powdered formulas are prepared by mixing 1 tablespoon of powder for every 2 ounces of water. When properly prepared, all of these provide the needed nutrients in an appropriate concentration. Problems arise when formulas are mixed incorrectly or when the water used to prepare them is contaminated. Incorrect mixing can result from a lack of understanding, poor measuring techniques, the addition of extra water to make the formula last longer, or the belief that a more concentrated formula will make the baby grow better. Even correctly mixed formula is a health hazard if the water used to mix it contains contaminants such as lead or disease-causing microorganisms. Water for formula should come from a safe source and be boiled before use.

Since the composition and safety of infant formulas is regulated, the major considerations when choosing one are cost, ease of transport, and convenience of preparation. Ready-to-feed formulas are easiest to use but may cost more and are heavier and bulkier to carry home from the store. Liquid concentrates are a good compromise because they provide more formula for less weight and are easy to mix. Powders are the least expensive and the easiest to transport home in a grocery bag but require more measuring and mixing. Since all of these products are nutritionally comparable, the choice depends on the needs of the caregivers.

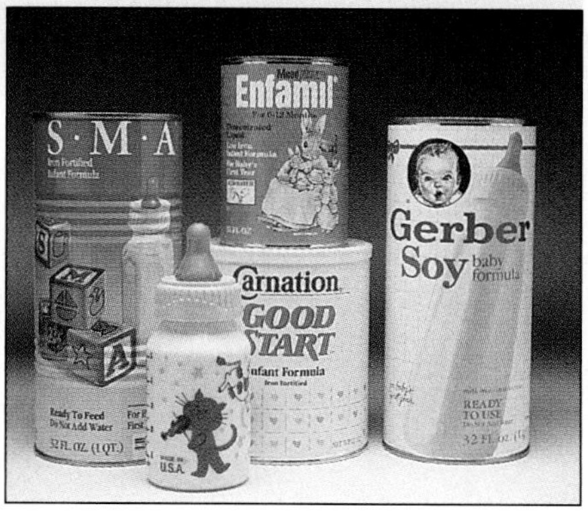

(Charles D. Winters)

[1]Stehlin, I. B. Infant formula: second best but good enough. FDA Consumer, 29:17–20, June 1996.

CRITICAL THINKING

How to Nourish a New Baby

Chevon had her baby last week. He is a healthy 7-pound, 19-inch-long boy, named Henry. Her grandmother has come to stay for a while to help with the baby. Chevon is breast feeding, but Grandma occasionally feeds Henry a bottle with pumped breast milk or formula. After three weeks the baby still wakes up at night to eat. Grandma says to give him a bottle of formula mixed with cereal before bed to help him sleep through the night.

Will this help?

There is no evidence that babies who consume cereal in their bottles sleep better. Henry is still too young to need any food other than breast milk or formula and may have difficulty digesting the cereal.

When Henry is six weeks old, Chevon must return to work. She would like to continue breast feeding even though Henry will be home with Grandma while she is at work across town.

What options does she have?

Even if she works full-time, she will still be able to nurse at home in the morning and evening. If there is a refrigerator in the lunch room at work, she can pump milk once or twice during the day and refrigerate the pumped milk to be fed to Henry the following day while she is at work. This will allow him to consume breast milk and will ensure that her milk production remains adequate. The refrigerated milk should be used within 24 to 48 hours. If no refrigerator is available, Chevon could try nursing mornings and nights and have Grandma feed him formula during the day.

Grandma says that Henry is so big that he can't possibly meet his needs from breast milk or formula alone. She wants to add solid food or mix a more concentrated formula to increase his energy intake. Chevon knows that an underdiluted formula will result in the wrong ratio of fluids to nutrients and can cause problems in the infant's organs and digestive tract.

Why should Grandma wait until Henry is four to six months old before feeding him solid food?

Answer:

APPLICATIONS

These exercises are designed to help you apply your critical thinking skills to your own nutrition choices. Many are best performed using a diet analysis software program. If you do not have access to a computer program, the exercises can be hand-calculated using the information in this text and its appendices.

1. Assume that one day of the food record you kept in Chapter 2 is the record of a 25-year-old pregnant woman.
   a. Does this diet meet her energy and protein needs? If not, what foods would you add to the diet to meet the needs of pregnancy?
   b. Does this diet meet the iron and calcium needs of a 25-year-old pregnant woman? List three foods that are good sources of each.
   c. Does this diet meet the folate needs of a 25-year-old pregnant woman? What foods could you add to a diet that is low in folate to meet needs without supplements? What foods in this diet are fortified with folic acid?
2. For each of the following nutrients, describe any differences between the needs of nonpregnant, pregnant, and lactating women. Explain why the requirements for pregnancy and lac-

tation do or do not differ from those for the nonpregnant state.
   a. Energy
   b. Protein
   c. Calcium
   d. Iron
   e. Folate
3. Use the Internet to find out about the WIC program in your area.
   a. Would it be easy for you to use this program if you were a pregnant or lactating woman or had a young child?
   b. What income levels does it serve?

Summary

1. Pregnancy begins with the fertilization of an egg by a sperm, producing a zygote. About three weeks after fertilization, the embryonic period of development begins. The embryo grows and the cells differentiate and move to form the organs and structures of the body. At nine weeks, the fetal period of development begins. It continues until birth, about 40 weeks after fertilization.
2. During pregnancy, maternal physiology changes to support the pregnancy and prepare for lactation. The amniotic sac and the placenta develop; maternal blood volume increases; the uterus and supporting muscles expand; body fat is deposited; the heart, lungs, and kidneys work harder; the breasts enlarge; and total body weight increases.
3. Recommended weight gain during pregnancy is 25 to 35 pounds for normal-weight women. If too little weight is gained, the infant may be small at birth and at increased risk for illness and death. Too much weight gain can place both mother and baby at risk, but weight loss should never be attempted during pregnancy. Normal-weight, underweight, and overweight mothers should gain weight at a steady rate during pregnancy.
4. During healthy pregnancies, a carefully planned program of moderate-intensity exercise can be beneficial and safe.
5. The hormones that direct changes in maternal physiology and the growth and development of the fetus sometimes cause unwanted side effects. Digestive system discomforts that are common in pregnancy include morning sickness, heartburn, constipation, and hemorrhoids. Changes in glucose utilization can cause gestational diabetes. An elevation in blood pressure, called pregnancy-induced hypertension, can cause edema, weight gain, and proteinuria (preeclampsia), and in severe cases can be life threatening (eclampsia).
6. Nutritional status is important before, during, and after pregnancy. Poor nutrition before pregnancy can decrease fertility or lead to a poor pregnancy outcome. During pregnancy the requirements for energy, protein, water, vitamins, and minerals increase. The B vitamins are needed to support increased energy and protein metabolism; calcium, vitamin D, and vitamin C are needed for bone and connective tissue growth; protein, folate, vitamin B_{12}, and zinc are needed for cell replication; and iron is needed for red blood cell synthesis.
7. Because the embryo and fetus are rapidly developing and growing, they are susceptible to damage from poor nutrition and physical, chemical, or other environmental teratogens.
8. Factors that increase the risks of pregnancy include a maternal age that is under 20 or over 35 years; a short interval between pregnancies; a history of poor reproductive outcomes; poverty; and behaviors such as smoking, alcohol use, and illicit drug use.
9. During lactation the need for energy, protein, fluid, and many vitamins and minerals is even greater than during pregnancy.
10. Newborns grow more rapidly and require more energy and protein per kilogram of body weight than at any other time in life. Fat and fluid needs are also proportionately higher than in adults. A diet that meets energy, protein, and fat needs may not necessarily meet the need for iron, fluoride, and vitamins D and K.
11. Breast milk is the ideal food for new babies. It is designed specifically for the human newborn, is always available, requires no special equipment, mixing, or sterilization, and provides immune protection. If breast feeding is not chosen, there are many infant formulas on the market that are patterned after human milk and provide adequate nutrition to the baby.
12. Infant formulas are the best option when the mother is ill or is taking prescription or illicit drugs, or when the infant has special nutritional needs. The major disadvantages of bottle feeding are the potential for bacterial contamination, overfeeding, and the possibility of errors in mixing formula.

Review Questions

1. List three physiological changes that occur in the mother's body during pregnancy.
2. How do the requirements for energy and protein change during pregnancy?
3. Why does the mother's recommended intake for iron double during pregnancy?
4. How much weight should a woman gain during pregnancy?
5. How do the recommendations for weight gain differ for overweight and underweight women?
6. What kind of exercise is safe during pregnancy?
7. Are vegetarian diets safe for pregnant women? Why or why not?
8. How does alcohol consumed by a woman during pregnancy affect the child?
9. How does maternal age affect nutrient requirements during pregnancy?
10. How do maternal energy and protein requirements change during lactation?
11. What are the advantages of breast feeding?
12. When is bottle feeding a better choice?

Nutrition Web Links

To further explore areas related to the material in this chapter, go to the *Nutrition: Science and Applications* Web site at ***www.Wiley.com/college/Smolin*** and *click on* **Student Companion Site** for chapter-by-chapter links. Some Web sites that provide additional information on topics discussed in Chapter 13 include:

Sites that provide information on pregnancy and health such as the New York Online Access to Health (NOAH) and the International Food Information Council.

Sites that provide information on normal development and the prevention of birth defects such as the March of Dimes.

Organizations that provide information on lactation and breast feeding such as the La Leche League.

References

1. Committee on Nutritional Status During Pregnancy and Lactation, National Academy of Sciences. *Nutrition During Pregnancy*. Washington, D.C.: National Academy Press, 1990.
2. Bryson, S. R., Theriot, L., Ryan, N. J., et al. Primary follow-up care in a multidisciplinary setting enhances catch-up growth of very-low-birth-weight infants. J. Am. Diet. Assoc. 97:386–390, 1997.
3. Smith, D. E., Lewis, J. L., Caveny, L. L., et al. Longitudinal changes in adiposity associated with pregnancy: the CARDIA study. J.A.M.A. 271:147–151, 1994.
4. American College of Sports Medicine. *ACSM's Guidelines for Exercise Testing and Prescription*, 5th ed. Baltimore: Williams & Wilkins, 1995.
5. Wang, T. W., and Apgar, B. S. Exercise during pregnancy. Am. Fam. Physician 57:1846–1852, 1998.
6. Katz, V. L. Water exercise in pregnancy. Semin. Perinatol. 20:285–291, 1996.
7. Sullivan, B. A., Henderson, S. T., and Davis, J. M. Gestational diabetes. J. Am. Pharm. Assoc. (Wash) 38:364–371, 1998.
8. Perloff, D. Hypertension and pregnancy-related hypertension. Cardiol. Clin. 16:79–110, 1998.
9. Bucher, H. C., Guyatt, G. H., Cook, R. J., et al. Effect of calcium supplementation on pregnancy-induced hypertension and preeclampsia: a meta-analysis of randomized trials. J.A.M.A. 275:1113–1117, 1996.
10. Levine, R. J., Hauth, J. C., Curet, L. B., et al. Trial of calcium to prevent preeclampsia. N. Engl. J. Med. 10:69–76, 1997.
11. Worthington-Roberts, B. The role of maternal nutrition in the prevention of birth defects. J. Am. Diet. Assoc. 97:S184–S185, 1997.
12. Green, T. J., Houghton, L. A., Donovan, U., et al. Oral contraceptives did not affect biochemical folate indexes and homocysteine concentrations in adolescent females. J. Am. Diet. Assoc. 98:49–54, 1998.
13. Mitchell, G. A., Kassovska-Bratinova, S., Boukaftane, Y., et al. Medical aspects of ketone body metabolism. Clin. Invest. Med. 18:193–216, 1995.
14. Food and Nutrition Board, Institute of Medicine. *Dietary Reference Intakes for Calcium, Phosphorus, Magnesium, Vitamin D, and Fluoride.* Washington, D.C.: National Academy Press, 1997.
15. Cross, N. A., Hillman, L. S., Allen, S. H., et al. Calcium homeostasis and bone metabolism during pregnancy, lactation, and postweaning: a longitudinal study. Am. J. Clin. Nutr. 61:514–523, 1995.
16. Hook, E. B., and Czeizel, A. E. Can terathanasia explain the protective effect of folic-acid supplementation on birth defects? Lancet 350:513–515, 1997.
17. Food and Nutrition Board, Institute of Medicine. *Dietary Reference Intakes for Thiamin, Riboflavin, Niacin, Vitamin B-6, Folate, Vitamin B-12, Pantothenic Acid, Biotin, and Choline.* Washington, D.C.: National Academy Press, 1998.
18. Goldenberg, R. L., Tamura, T., Neggers, Y., et al. The effect of zinc supplementation on pregnancy outcome. J.A.M.A. 274: 463–468, 1995.
19. Lops, V. R., Harte, L. P., and Dixon, L. R. Anemia in pregnancy. Am. Fam. Physican 5:1189–1197, 1995.
20. Mitchell, M. K. *Nutrition Across the Life Span*. Philadelphia: W. B. Saunders, 1997.
21. Rainville, A. J. Pica practices of pregnant women are associated with lower maternal hemoglobin level at delivery. J. Am. Diet. Assoc. 98:293–296, 1998.
22. Healthy People 2010. Online at http://web.health.gov/healthypeople2010/2010Draft
23. American Dietetic Association. Position of the American Dietetic Association: nutrition care for pregnant adolescents. J. Am. Diet. Assoc. 94:449–450, 1994.
24. Fraser, A. M., Brockert, J. E., and Ward, R. H. Association of young maternal age with adverse reproductive outcomes. N. Engl. J. Med. 332:1113–1117, 1995.
25. Prysak, M., and Kisly, A. Age greater than thirty-four years is an independent pregnancy risk factor in nulliparous women. J. Perinatol. 17:296–300, 1997.
26. Bianco, A., Stone, J., Lynch, L., et al. Pregnancy outcome at age 40 and older. Obstet. Gynecol. 87:917–922, 1996.
27. Stout, E. Prenatal care for low-income women and the health belief model: a new beginning. J. Community Health Nurs. 14:169–180, 1997.
28. Owen, A. L., and Owen, G. M. Twenty years of WIC: a review of some effects of the program. J. Am. Diet. Assoc. 97:777–782, 1997.
29. Rothman, K. J., Moore, L. L., Singer, M. R., et al. Teratogenicity of high vitamin A intake. N. Engl. J. Med. 333:1369–1373, 1995.
30. Appelbaum, M. G. Fetal alcohol syndrome: the nurse practitioner's perspective. Nurse Pract. 2:27–33, 1996.
31. Abel, E. L. An update on incidence of FAS: FAS is not an equal opportunity birth defect. Neurotoxicol. Teratol. 17:437–443, 1995.
32. Kendrick, J. S., and Merritt, R. K. Women and smoking: an update for the 1990s. Am. J. Obstet. Gynecol. 175:528–535, 1996.
33. DiFranza, J. R., and Lew, R. A. Effect of maternal smoking on pregnancy complications and sudden infant death syndrome. J. Fam. Pract. 40:385–394, 1995.
34. Klonoff-Cohen, H. S., Edelstein, S. L., Lefkowitz, E. S., et al. The effect of passive smoking and tobacco exposure through breast milk on sudden infant death syndrome. J.A.M.A. 273:795–798, 1995.
35. Chomitz, V. R., Cheung, L. W., and Leiberman, E. The role of lifestyle in preventing low birth weight. Future Child 5:121–135, 1995.
36. Hinds, T. S., West, W., Knight, E. M., and Hartland, B. F. The effect of caffeine on pregnancy outcome variables. Nutr. Rev. 54:203–207, 1996.
37. Wagner, C. L., Katikaneni, L. D., Cox, T. H., and Ryan, R. M. The impact of prenatal drug exposure on the neonate. Obstet. Gynecol. Clin. North Am. 25:169–194, 1998.
38. Rizk, B., Atterbury, J. L., and Groome, L. J. Reproductive risks of cocaine. Hum. Reprod. Update 2:43–55, 1996.

39. Fox, C. H. Cocaine use in pregnancy. J. Am. Board Fam. Pract. 7:225–228, 1994.
40. Plessinger, M. A., and Woods, J. R. Jr. Maternal, placental, and fetal pathophysiology of cocaine exposure during pregnancy. Clin. Obstet. Gynecol. 36:267–278, 1994.
41. Lee, M. J. Marijuana and tobacco use in pregnancy. Obstet. Gynecol. Clin. North Am. 25:65–83, 1998.
42. Potter, S., Hannum, S., McFarlin, B., et al. Does infant feeding method influence maternal postpartum weight loss? J. Am. Diet. Assoc. 91:441–446, 1991.
43. Kramer, E. M., Stunkard, A. J., Marshall, K. A., et al. Breast feeding reduces maternal lower body fat. J. Am. Diet. Assoc. 93:429–433, 1993.
44. Dewey, K. G., Heinig, M. J., and Nommsen, L. A. Maternal weight-loss patterns during prolonged lactation. Am. J. Clin. Nutr. 58:162–166, 1993.
45. Dewey, K. G. Effects of maternal caloric restriction and exercise during lactation. J. Nutr. 128:386S–389S, 1998.
46. Prentice, A. Calcium requirements of breast-feeding mothers. Nutr. Rev. 56:124–130, 1998.
47. Krebs, N. F., Reidinger, C. J., Robertson, A. D., and Brenner, M. Bone mineral density changes during lactation: maternal dietary and biochemical correlates. Am. J. Clin. Nutr. 65:1738–1746, 1997.
48. Bendich, A., and Brock, P. E. Rationale for the inclusion of long chain polyunsaturated fatty acids and for concomitant increase in vitamin E in infant formulas. Int. J. Vitam. Nutr. Res. 67:213–231, 1997.
49. American Dietetic Association. Position paper on promotion of breast-feeding. J. Am. Diet. Assoc. 97:662–666, 1997.
50. Ryan, A. S. The resurgence of breast-feeding in the United States. Pediatrics 99:596, 1997.
51. American Academy of Pediatrics, Working Group on Breast-Feeding. Breast-feeding and the use of human milk. Pediatrics 100:1035–1039, 1997.
52. Janney, C. A., Zhang, D., and Sowers, M. F. Lactation and weight retention. Am. J. Clin. Nutr. 66:1116–1124, 1997.
53. Kelsey, J. J. Hormonal contraception and lactation. J. Hum. Lact. 12:315–318, 1996.
54. WHO Fact Sheet No. 178: Reducing mortality from major childhood killer diseases. September 1997. Online at http://www.who.ch/inf/fs/fact178.html
55. Jensen, C. L., Prager, T. C., Fraley, J. K., et al. Effect of dietary linoleic/alpha-linolenic acid ratio on growth and visual function of term infants. J. Pediatr. 131:200–209, 1997.
56. Newburg, D. S., Peterson, J. A., Ruis-Palacios, G. M., et al. Role of human-milk lactadherin in protection against symptomatic rotavirus infection. Lancet 351:1160–1164, 1998.
57. Williams, R. D. Breast-feeding best bet for babies. FDA Consumer 28:19–23, October 1995.
58. Golding, J. Unnatural constituents of breast milk—medication, lifestyle, pollutants, viruses. Early Hum. Dev. 29 (suppl):S29–S43, 1997.
59. Stehlin, I. B. Infant formula: second best but good enough. FDA Consumer 29:17–20, June 1996.

Chapter 14

Chapter Outline

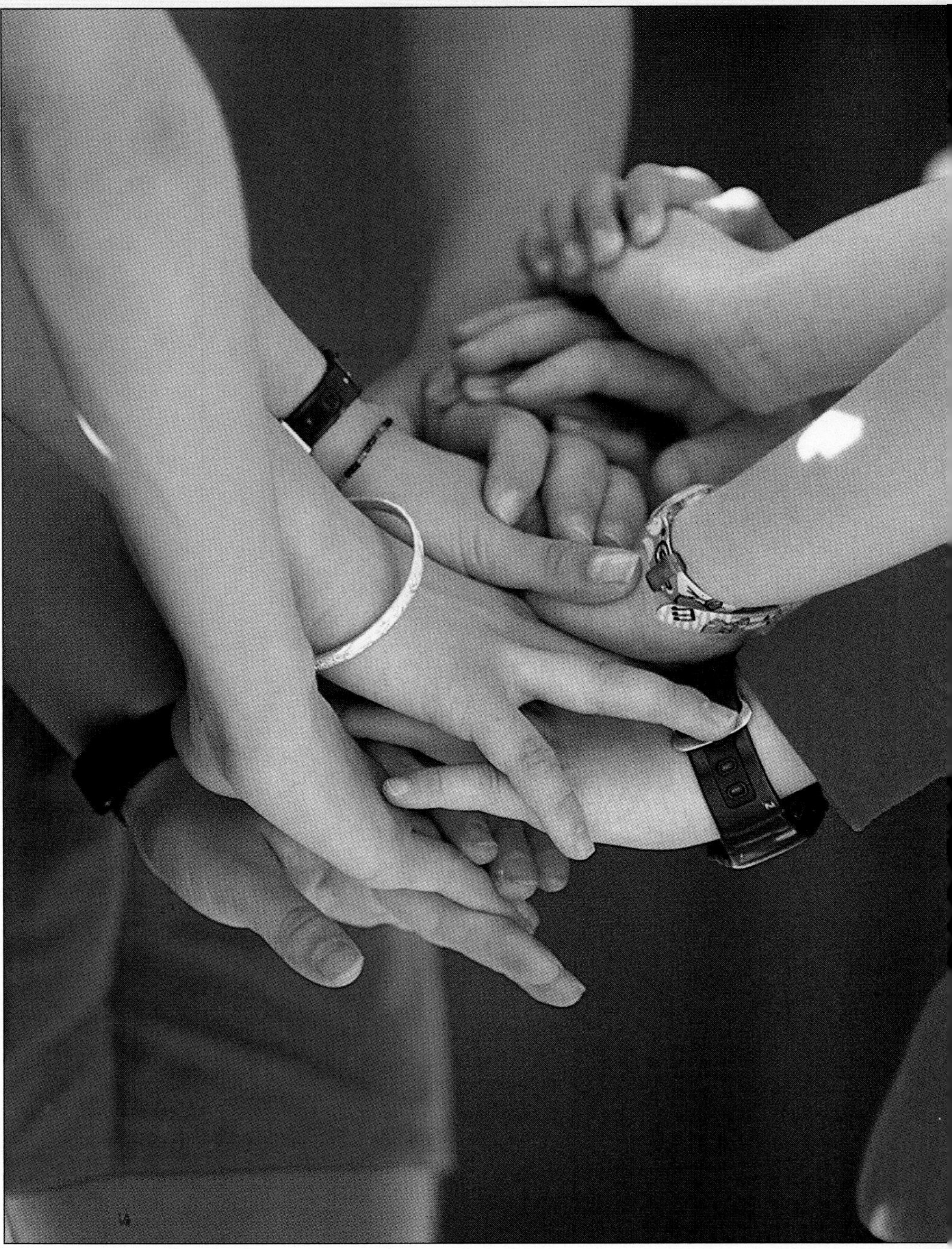

(© Caroline Wood/Tony Stone Images)

The Growing Years: Infancy to Adolescence

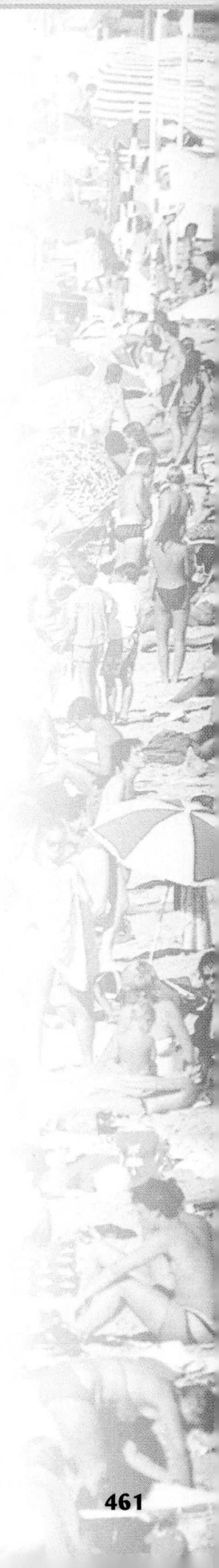

Chapter Concepts

1. The eating patterns learned in childhood can affect health over the course of a lifetime. Caregivers play a crucial role in helping children develop healthy eating habits.
2. Normal growth is the best indication of adequate nutrient intake in children and teens.
3. Nutrient intake throughout life can affect the risk of chronic disease. Children's diets, like those of adults, should be high in whole grains, fruits, and vegetables.
4. After four to six months of age, semisolid and solid foods can gradually be introduced into the infant's diet.
5. Nutrient intakes for children must meet the needs for growth and development as well as for maintenance and activity.
6. Meeting the nutrient needs of children and adolescents can be challenging as they exercise their personal preferences and are influenced more by their environment and their peers.
7. The physiological changes that occur during sexual maturation cause differences in the nutrient requirements of males and females.
8. Alcohol consumption can affect nutritional status, judgment, and health.

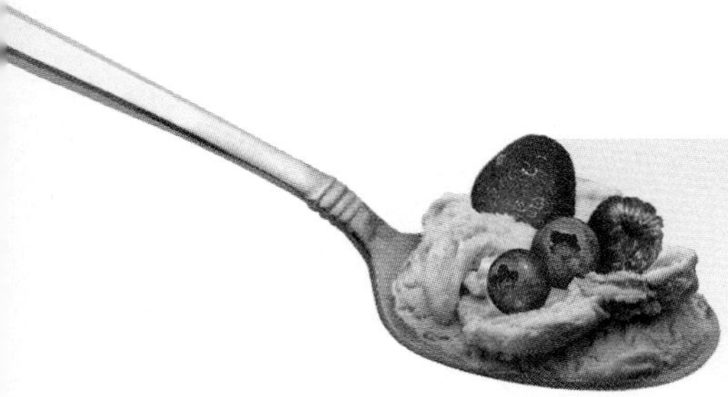

Just a Taste

Do parents' eating habits affect those of their children?

Are high blood cholesterol and high blood pressure concerns in children?

Can fast food and sweetened cereals be part of a healthy diet?

Nutrient intake during childhood helps shape the adult that the child will become. Thus, in the words of William Wordsworth, "the child is father of the man." Nutrition can affect health and the ability to achieve maximum growth potential as well as the propensity for developing chronic disease later in life. Eating habits developed during childhood and adolescence may last a lifetime.

Many physical changes occur between infancy and adulthood. During this period of rapid growth from birth to about 18 years of age, the diet must supply the nutrients needed for growth and development as well as for maintenance and activity. Many factors other than nutrient needs determine which foods a child consumes. From the start, which foods are offered is a major determinant of what is consumed, but individual taste always plays a role in food choices. As the child grows, influences from the outside world increase. When a child is enrolled in day-care or preschool programs, parents may no longer be in control of—or even aware of—what the child is eating. When the child is in school, carefully packed lunches may be discarded or traded for more appealing foods. During adolescence, physiological changes dictate nutritional needs but peer pressure may dictate food choices.

Starting Right: Healthy Eating for Life

Good nutrition early in life is key to health in later years. What children eat depends on what they have learned to eat as well as their personal preferences. A well-balanced eating pattern allows children to meet their nutrient needs for growth and development and to prevent or delay the onset of the chronic diseases that plague American adults.

Teaching Nutritious Eating Habits

The development of nutritious eating habits starts with caregivers offering a balanced and varied diet adequate in energy and essential nutrients and appropriate to the child's developmental needs. In addition, caregivers must provide a positive, supportive, and trusting eating environment. The caregiver is responsible for deciding what foods should be offered to the child, when they should be offered, and where they should be eaten. The child must then decide whether to eat, what foods to eat, and how much to consume.

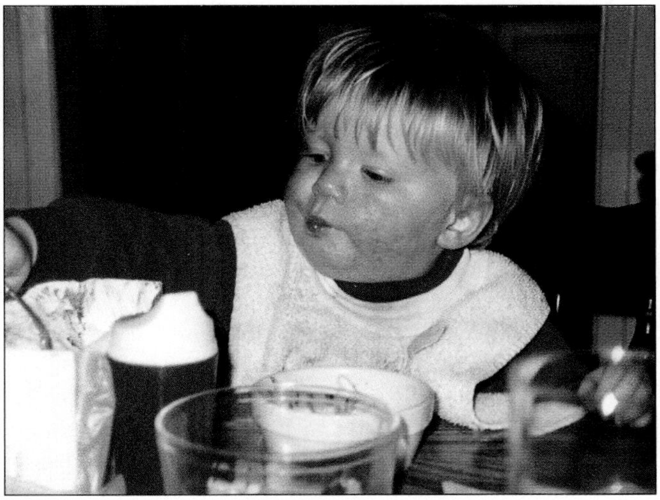

Figure 14.1
Caregivers should offer a variety of healthy food choices and allow children to select what they will eat and how much. (Mary Grosvenor)

Providing Nutritious Food Because children learn by imitation, caregivers should demonstrate healthy eating habits. If role models eat a diet high in fat and low in fruits and vegetables, children will follow suit. Parents and caregivers should choose the foods they want children to grow up eating. When children enter day care, preschool, or school, teachers, staff, and friends also influence their eating behavior.

What and When to Offer? Meals for children should be planned according to the groups and serving recommendations of the Food Guide Pyramid. Food choices should be developmentally appropriate. For example, finger foods can be offered when children have the coordination to put food in their mouths. Foods that pose a potential choking hazard should be avoided. Caregivers should also know how to administer the Heimlich maneuver in the event that food or another object does become lodged in the throat (see Chapter 3). The texture of foods should also be appropriate. Vegetables served to young children should be cooked until soft for easy chewing. Food should not be too hot or too spicy. As children grow, choices should change to meet their developmental abilities.

No matter how erratic children's food intake may be, caregivers should offer a variety of appropriate healthy food choices at each meal and let their children select what and how much they will eat (Figure 14.1). To increase the likelihood that a new food will be accepted, it should be introduced at the beginning of a meal when the child is hungry. If a new food becomes associated with a bad experience, such as burning the mouth, the child will be unlikely to try it again.

Young children have small stomachs and high energy needs, so frequent meals and snacks are necessary. A meal or snack should be offered every 2 to 3 hours and, because children thrive on routines and feel secure in knowing what to expect, a consistent pattern should be maintained from day to day.

Breakfast: Nutrition for Learning Does it really matter at what time during the day nutrients are consumed? Breakfast is often lost in the shuffle of getting a family up and off to work or school. Children and teens who are not particularly hungry first thing in the morning will gladly go off with an empty stomach. Whether the child is in preschool or high school, this may be detrimental to both total nutrient intake and school performance. An evaluation of the contribution of breakfast to daily nutrient intake found that children who eat breakfast consume more energy and are more likely to meet the recommended intakes for vitamins and minerals than children who skip breakfast.[1] Studies have also found that skipping breakfast can interfere with learning ability.[1] Children who eat breakfast perform better on achievement tests and have fewer behavior problems in school. In a study of children in the Philadelphia and Baltimore schools, breakfast eaters had better math grades, less hyperactivity, less absence and tardiness, and better psychosocial behaviors than nonbreakfast eaters.[2]

A good breakfast should meet a quarter to a third of the day's nutrient needs. For example, toast, a bowl of oatmeal with milk and raisins, and a glass of orange juice provides about 450 kcalories as well as B vitamins; vitamins C, A, and D; and calcium and iron. Though not every child will eat this good breakfast, even children who do not like breakfast may be willing to consume a slice of toast with peanut butter or a bowl of interestingly shaped colored cereal. Despite the high-sugar low-fiber content of breakfast cereals marketed to children, they have few other nutritional strikes against them. Even the most sugary cereal has some redeeming features. For example, while 40% of the energy in Cap'n Crunch is from simple sugars, it is still low in fat and provides 20% or more of the Daily Value for thiamin, riboflavin, niacin, vitamin B_6, folate, vitamin B_{12}, pantothenic acid, and iron. When 1/2 cup of reduced-fat milk is added to the cereal, it also provides 15% of the Daily Value for calcium. Children who eat ready-to-eat cereals, sugared or not, have a higher overall intake of vitamins and minerals than children who do not.[1] Although a bowl of oatmeal is preferable to a breakfast of Cookie Crisp, sugared cereals can make an important contribution to children's diets.

Children who cannot or will not eat breakfast before they leave the house can take a snack to be eaten on the way to school or during recess if they get hungry before lunch. Fruit, yogurt, a bag of dry cereal, or half a sandwich is certainly a better alternative than a candy bar from a vending machine. Having breakfast at school is also an option. The National School Breakfast Program is available in about half the nation's schools and serves more than seven million children. Children participating in the National School Breakfast Program have higher achievement test scores than eligible nonparticipants.[2] The breakfasts served must provide at least 25% of the 1989 RDA for certain nutrients and furnish at least 1 serving of milk; 1 serving of fruit, juice, or vegetables; and either 2 servings of bread, 2 servings of meat, or 1 serving of each. Meals are provided free or at a reduced cost for families who meet income guidelines.

A Positive Eating Environment Teaching sound eating habits also involves providing a positive eating environment. Companionship, conversation, and a pleasant location contribute to a positive atmosphere. Children eat better with company—caregivers should sit with children and eat what they eat (Figure 14.2).[3] Children need time to finish eating. Slow eaters are unlikely to finish eating if they are abandoned by siblings who run off to play and adults who leave to do dishes.

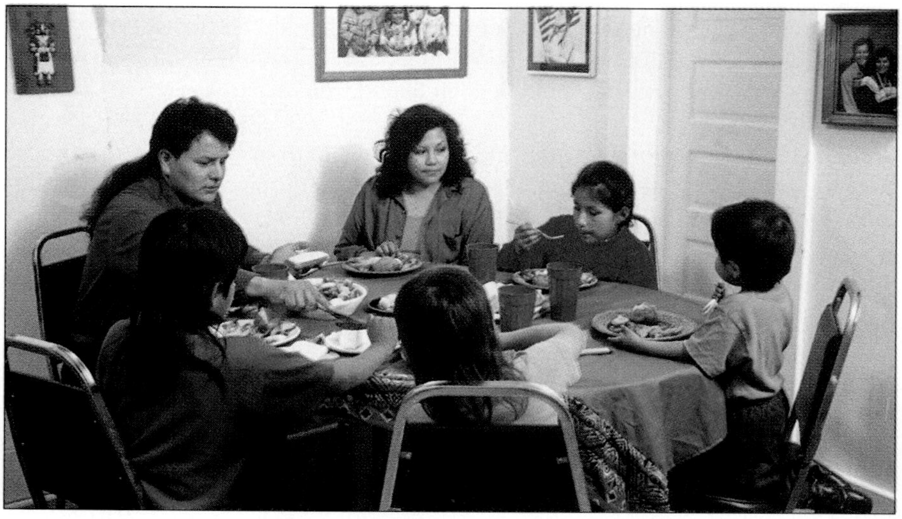

Figure 14.2
Companionship and conversation at meals helps create a positive eating environment. (© Lawrence Migdale/Photo Researchers, Inc.)

To make mealtime a nutritious, educational, and enjoyable experience, it should not be a battle zone.[3] Threats and bribes are counterproductive and can create a problem where none had previously existed. Food is not a reward or a punishment: It is simply nutrition. If caregivers follow these guidelines, it is then up to the child to decide whether to eat at all, what to choose from the offered foods, and how much to eat.

Providing for Optimal Growth and Development

The diets of children and adolescents must meet their needs for growth and development. Normal growth is the best indicator of adequate nourishment.

Growth Patterns Most children and adolescents follow standard patterns of growth. A child's growth can be monitored by comparing it to these patterns using growth charts (Appendix B). The rate of growth is slower in childhood than in infancy. In the second year of life, children generally grow about 5 inches; in the third year, 4 inches; and thereafter, about 2 to 3 inches per year. During adolescence, there is a period of growth that is almost as rapid as that of infancy.

Although growth patterns are predictable, growth occurs in spurts and plateaus. During a growth spurt, children's or adolescents' appetites may seem insatiable, while between spurts they may seem to eat nothing. If the pattern of growth suddenly changes, the child should be evaluated by a physician to determine if there is a physiological reason for the sudden change. Once medical causes have been ruled out, energy intake and activity should be assessed to determine which has changed and why.

Too Little Growth The maximum size that an individual will attain is affected by both genetic and environmental and lifestyle factors. For example, Asian children are usually smaller than African American and Caucasian children. Likewise, a child whose parents are 5 feet tall may not have the genetic potential to be 6 feet tall. Whatever the genetic potential may be, however, adequate nutrition is essential for a child to reach that potential. If a child is not growing, undernutrition is one possible reason. Poor nutrition in childhood causes growth retardation and interferes with normal brain development.

A child who is not consuming sufficient energy will first show a drop in weight, and if the deficiency continues, growth in height will slow or stop. Just as there are critical periods in prenatal development, there are critical periods in childhood when malnutrition can cause lasting damage. Growth and development can occur only when the proper hormonal signals are available; thus nutrient deficiencies at critical times can prevent cells from dividing, and adequate nutrition later on may not be able to compensate. Malnutrition in early childhood causes poorer IQ scores and cognitive function, behavioral problems, and poorer achievement when these children reach school age; and the disadvantages last at least until adolescence.[4]

Eating Disorders Typically, eating disorders are thought of as a problem affecting teens and young women; however, such disorders are becoming more and more common in younger children. Eating disorders are usually not diagnosed until adolescence, but the excessive concern about weight and body image that characterizes these conditions may begin as early as the preschool years. These abnormal concerns can lead to battles over food and eating and to excessive finickiness, resulting in poor growth and abnormal development.

Reducing the Risks of Chronic Disease

The diets of children and adolescents can affect their health and longevity. Nutrient deficiencies can affect growth and nutritional excesses can result in childhood obesity and an increased risk for chronic disease later in life. Most children and

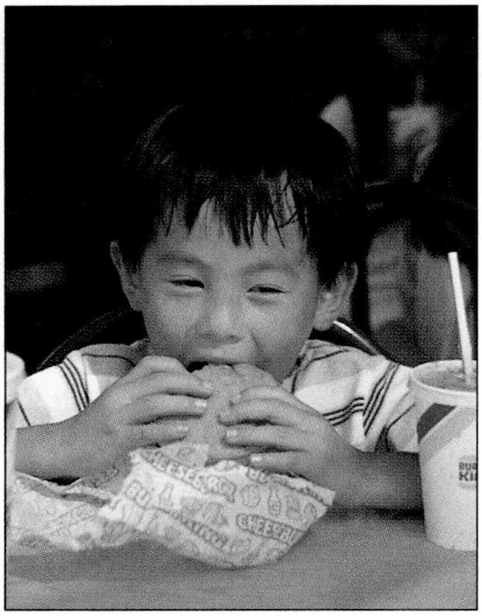

Figure 14.3
Many children in the United States consume a diet that is high in fat and low in fruits and vegetables. (© Arthur R. Hill/Visuals Unlimited)

adolescents in the United States consume more fat, saturated fat, and sodium than is recommended. They consume a dietary pattern that is low in fruits and vegetables and high in sweet and salty processed foods (Figure 14.3).

Obesity Obesity is a major problem in children in the United States.[5] A child is considered obese when weight for height, or BMI, falls at or above the 95th percentile.

Both heredity and environment and lifestyle play a role in childhood obesity. Obese parents are more likely to have obese offspring not only because they pass on a genetic tendency to be overweight but because their children may learn poor eating and exercise habits. If sound nutrition and exercise habits are developed early and are followed throughout life, obesity can be avoided despite a genetic predisposition.

As with adult obesity, childhood obesity increases the risks of chronic disease. Obese children may have high blood cholesterol and glucose levels and elevated blood pressure. These risk factors may increase the chances that they will develop heart disease, hypertension, and diabetes. In addition to its health impact, obesity's psychosocial impact is great for children. Obese children in the United States are less well accepted by their peers than normal-weight children and are frequently ridiculed and teased. They often have a poor self-image and low self-esteem.

Children with a BMI greater than or equal to the 95th percentile, and those with a BMI greater than or equal to the 85th percentile who have complications related to obesity, should undergo evaluation and possible treatment.[6] In addition, any sudden increase in the pattern of weight gain is a cause for concern (Figure 14.4). The goal of treatment should be healthy eating and increased activity. Whether weight maintenance or weight loss is recommended depends on the child's age, degree of overweight, and the presence of medical complications.[6] In many cases, slowing weight gain will be sufficient. The goal of this treatment is to allow the child to grow into his or her current weight. As long as the rate of weight gain is slowed, a child at the 95th percentile for weight at age 7 can be at the 90th percentile by age 9 and at the 75th percentile by age 11. This requires that the child's behavior be modified to reduce energy intake and increase activity. Changes should be gradual and stepwise, and involve the entire family. If weight control at home is not effective, professional help may be needed (see *Critical Thinking: At Risk for Malnutrition*).

Changing Behavior As with adults, weight gain in children is related to patterns of eating and exercise. Any permanent change in weight requires a permanent change in lifestyle. Changing eating patterns to provide balanced meals moderate in energy and increasing activity is key to developing and maintaining a healthy weight. Because children, like adults, may overeat for comfort, self-reward, or out of boredom, parent involvement in helping the child find other sources of gratification can be vital.

Reducing Intake Modifying a child's food consumption patterns can be difficult. Denying food may promote further overeating by making the child feel that there will not be enough to satisfy hunger. The child may then overeat whenever there is a chance. Thus, energy intake restrictions should be relatively mild, allowing adequate nutrition to continue growth in height with little weight gain. Healthy, lowfat foods such as whole grains, fruits and vegetables, lean meats, and reduced-fat dairy products should be offered at meals and for snacks.

Increasing Activity Promoting increased activity may be even more important than diet in treating childhood obesity. Although energy intake among American children overall is not increasing, they are getting heavier, suggesting that a major contributor to the increase in body weight is lack of physical activity.[7] Watching

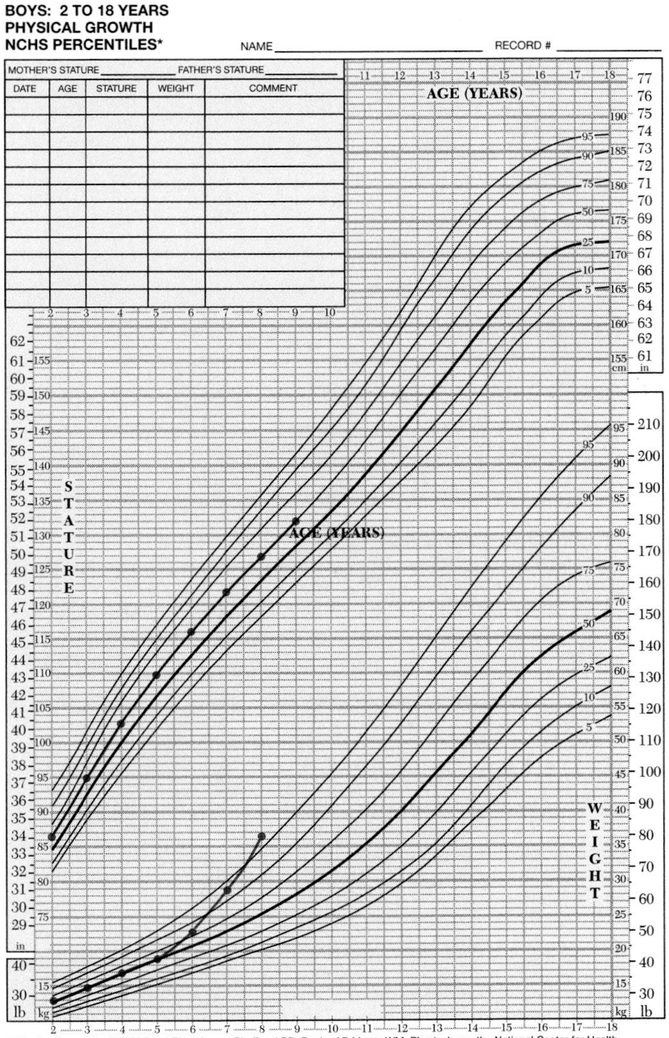

*Adapted from: Hamill PVV, Drizd TA, Johnson CL, Reed RB, Roche AF, Moore WM. Physical growth: National Center for Health Statistics percentiles. AM J CLIN NUTR 32: 607-629, 1979 Data from the National Center for Health Statistics (NCHS) Hyattsville, Maryland.

Figure 14.4

Plotting children's growth on growth charts is helpful in monitoring their pattern of growth.

television, playing video games, and surfing the Web have replaced neighborhood games of tag and soccer for many children.

Overweight children are less likely to be physically active than lean children. They may be embarrassed by their bodies and shy away from participating in group activities. For example, an overweight, inactive child might not join the swim team because she is too self-conscious to appear in a bathing suit. Inexperience in sports may also put obese children at a low skill level.

Increases in physical activity need to be gradual in order to make exercise a positive experience. A good way to start is to encourage activities such as games, walks after dinner, bike rides, hikes, swimming, and volleyball that can be enjoyed by the whole family. This sends a positive message to "be more active" rather than a negative message of "do not eat so much." An exercise program is most effective if the activities are enjoyable and not doled out as punishment. Again, involvement of the whole family is key. Parents who are active, play with their children, watch their children compete or play, or take children to physical activity or sports events have more active children.[8]

Activity Guidelines Whether or not a child is obese, he or she should be physically active. Most children are naturally active, and extended periods of inactivity are not normal for healthy children. The National Association for Sports and Physical Education recommends that preadolescent children be physically active

Fitness Pyramid for Kids

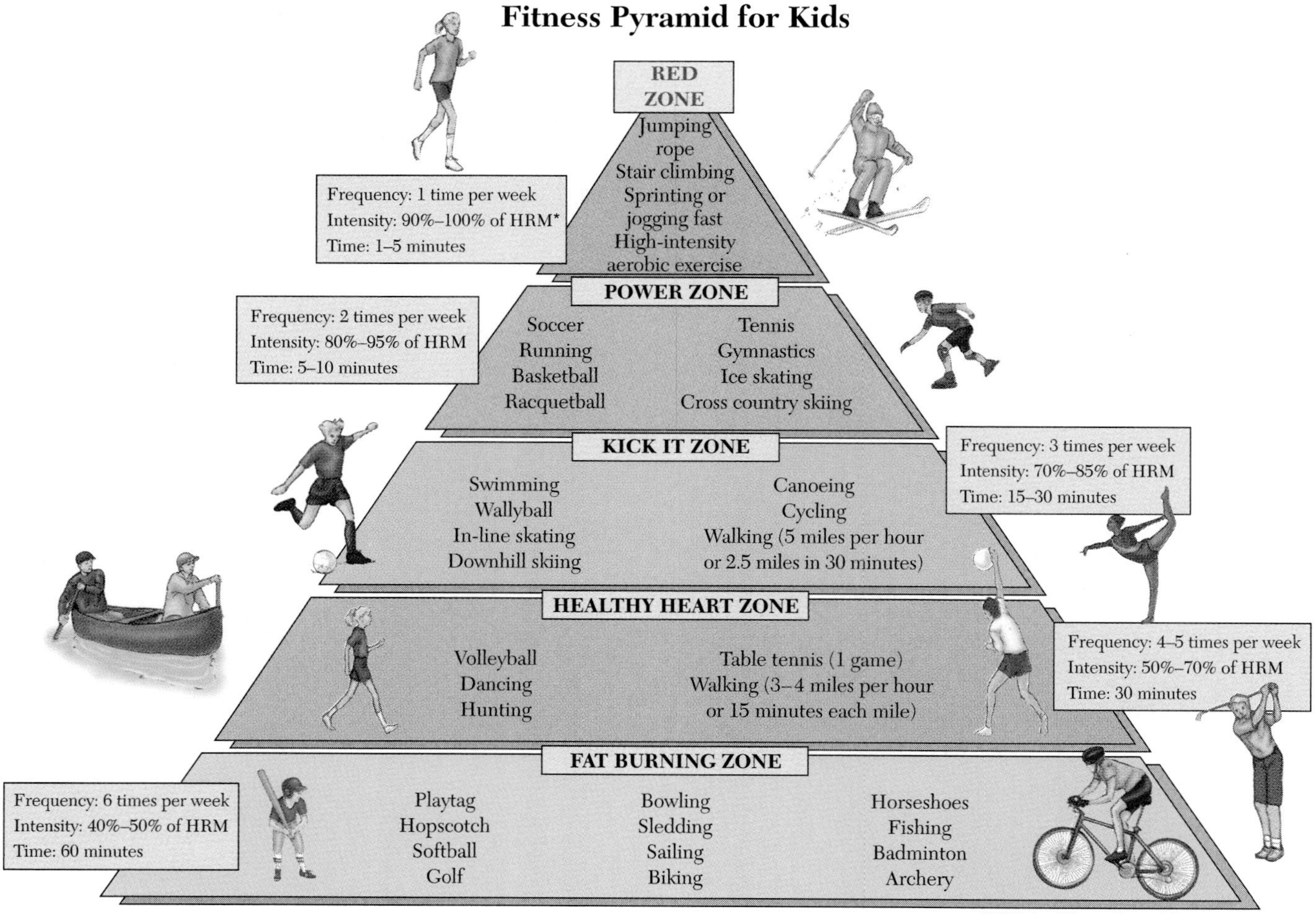

(Adapted from: American Dietetic Association. Position of the American Dietetic Association: Dietary guidance for healthy children aged 2 to 11 years. J. Am. Diet. Assoc. 99: 93–101, 1999.)

Figure 14.5
Children should enjoy participating in a variety of activities of varying intensity.

for at least an hour and up to several hours per day.[9] Children have short attention spans, so their activities should be intermittent. Periods of moderate to vigorous activity lasting 10 to 15 minutes or more each day should be interspersed with periods of rest and recovery. Preadolescent children should be exposed to a variety of different types of activities that are of various levels of intensity (Figure 14.5). Learning to enjoy sports and exercise in childhood will set the stage for an active lifestyle in adulthood.

Blood Cholesterol and Heart Disease Children in the United States and Canada currently consume about 34% of their energy from fat, with 13% from saturated fat.[10] This exceeds the amounts recommended for a healthy diet. As in adults, diets high in fat lead to elevated blood cholesterol levels in children. The recommended level for blood cholesterol in children aged 2 to 18 is less than 170 mg per 100 ml. In the United States, many children have blood cholesterol levels higher than this.[11] Elevated blood cholesterol levels during childhood and adolescence are associated with higher blood cholesterol and higher mortality rates from cardiovascular disease in adulthood.[12]

The American Academy of Pediatrics recommends blood cholesterol monitoring for high-risk children and teenagers. This includes those with parents or grandparents who developed heart disease before age 55, and those whose parents have cholesterol levels over 240 mg per 100 ml. To reduce the risk of developing high blood cholesterol levels and, subsequently, heart disease, the fat content of children's diets should gradually be reduced beginning at the age of two years. By the age of about five, the diet should contain no more than 30% of energy from fat—the same as is recommended for adults.[13]

Hypertension High blood pressure may also be a concern early in life. Those who have blood pressure at the high end of normal as youngsters are more likely to develop high blood pressure as adults.[14] Blood pressure can be affected by the amount of body fat, activity level, and sodium intake, as well as by the total pattern of dietary intake, so attention should be paid to these nutritional and lifestyle factors in children. This is particularly important if there is a family history of hypertension.

Critical Thinking

At Risk for Malnutrition

Bobby is eight years old and has a history of iron deficiency anemia. His parents have recently become concerned because all he wants to do is lie around and watch TV, and he is gaining weight. Previously he played active, imaginative games with his toys, enjoyed playing basketball with his friends, and was eager to go on hikes with the family. Since Bobby's parents are both overweight, they are concerned that he will also have a weight problem, so they take him to see their pediatrician.

The nurse weighs and measures Bobby and draws a blood sample to check for iron deficiency anemia. She compares Bobby's weight for height to last year's measurements. Last year he was at the 50th percentile and he is now almost at the 75th.

The pediatrician reports that Bobby is anemic again and prescribes an iron supplement. She refers Bobby and his parents to a dietitian for dietary counseling on weight management as well as iron intake. The dietitian reviews Bobby's diet and exercise patterns. She learns that Bobby has been watching TV or playing video games for about 6 hours a day. Below are the results of a food frequency questionnaire that she recorded:

		Frequency	
Food		**Servings/Day**	**Servings/Week**
Milk and dairy products:	Regular fat	6	
	Reduced fat		
	Fat free		
Meat and eggs:	Red meat		1
	Chicken		2
	Fish		1
	Eggs		
Grains and cereals:	Whole grains	2	
	Refined grains	2	
Fruit and juices:	Citrus	1	
	Other	2	
Vegetables:	Dark green leafy		
	Other	1	
Added fats:		3	
Snack foods:	Chips, etc.	1	
	Candy	1	

What nutrients are likely to be excessive or deficient in this dietary pattern?

Bobby's high intake of regular dairy products provides a good source of calcium but adds a lot of fat and saturated fat to his diet. His low intake of meats means that heme iron is low in the diet, and the lack of leafy green vegetables means his intake of nonheme iron from vegetables is low. His low intake of vegetables and whole grains means his fiber intake is low, and some vitamins and minerals may be low in the diet. The candy and chips add energy, fat, sugar, and/or salt with few other nutrients.

Why might excessive consumption of dairy products contribute to Bobby's anemia?

Dairy products are an important source of protein, vitamins, and minerals, particularly calcium, but they are a poor source of iron. In addition, the high calcium they provide decreases absorption of iron consumed at the same meal.

Suggest some dietary changes that would increase Bobby's iron intake and absorption.

Answer:

How can Bobby reduce the energy and fat content of his diet?

Because Bobby is well past the age when he needs a high-fat diet for growth and development and his weight is increasing more rapidly than his height, the dietitian recommends that he switch to lowfat milk and dairy products. The dietitian also suggests that the family make some changes in the types of food they have around the house so Bobby can have more low-kcalorie, nutrient-dense choices such as fruits and vegetables to snack on. The dietitian encourages the family to bake, broil, or grill their meat, trimming off excess fat. She also recommends the family work together to increase the amount of exercise they get.

Suggest some activities you enjoyed as a child that would help Bobby to increase his activity level.

Answer:

Nourishing the Infant: Introducing Solid Food

Solid and semisolid foods can be gradually introduced into the infant's diet starting between the fourth and sixth months of life when the infant's feeding abilities and gastrointestinal tract are mature enough to handle foods other than breast milk or formula. Since the young infant takes milk by a licking motion of the tongue called suckling, which strokes or milks the liquid from the nipple, solid food placed in the mouth at an early age is usually pushed out as the tongue thrusts forward. By four to six months of age the early reflex to bring the tongue to the front of the mouth to suckle has diminished, and the tongue is held farther back in the mouth, allowing solid food to be accepted without being expelled. By this age, the infant also can hold the head up steadily and is able to sit, either with or without support. Internally, the digestive tract has developed. Enzymes are present for starch digestion. The kidneys are more mature and better able to concentrate urine. With all of these changes, the child is ready to begin a new approach to eating.

Meeting the Infant's Nutrient Needs

Until one year of age, most nutritional needs are still met by breast milk or formula. Even though some suggest that the addition of infant cereal to the bottle during the first few months will help the infant sleep through the night, studies have shown that there is no difference in sleeping patterns based on such feeding practices.

First Foods The most commonly recommended food to be fed first to a child with a spoon is iron-fortified infant rice cereal mixed with formula or breast milk. Rice cereal is the recommended first food because it is easily digested and rarely causes allergic reactions. After rice has been successfully included in the diet, other grains can be introduced, with wheat cereal given last because it is most likely to cause an allergic reaction. To monitor for food allergies, it is important to introduce new foods one at a time. Each new food should be offered for a few days without the addition of any other new foods. If an allergic reaction occurs, it is most likely due to the newly introduced food. Foods that cause symptoms such as rashes, digestive upsets, or respiratory problems should be discontinued before any other new foods are added. After cereals are introduced, puréed vegetables or fruits can be tried; some suggest that vegetables be offered before fruits so that the child will learn to enjoy food that is not sweet before being introduced to sweet foods. Once teeth have erupted, foods with more texture can be added. For the 6- to 12-month-old child, small pieces of soft or ground fruits, vegetables, and meats are appropriate (Table 14.1).

Developmentally Appropriate Choices As the child becomes familiar with more variety, food choices should be made from each of the food groups in the Food Guide Pyramid. At one year of age, whole cow's milk should be offered and continued until two years of age. Reduced-fat and lowfat milk should not be used until after the age of two years; children younger than two need a high-fat diet to fuel their rapid growth and development. To avoid choking, foods that can easily lodge in the throat, such as carrots, grapes, and hot dogs, should not be offered to infants or toddlers.

As children become more independent, they will want to feed themselves. Although this is not always a neat and clean process, it is important for development (Figure 14.6). By the age of eight or nine months, infants can hold a bottle and self-feed finger food such as crackers. By ten months, most infants can drink from a cup, so water and fruit juices can be offered. Juice should not be served in a bottle because it may contribute to nursing bottle syndrome. Excess quantities

Table 14.1 *Typical Meal Patterns for Infants*

Food	Serving Size	Servings per Day 4–6 Months	6–8 Months	9–12 Months
		(tongue able to stay in back of mouth and not push food out)	(can easily move hand to mouth)	(can use a cup and easily consume finger foods)
Formula or breast milk*	8 oz	4	4	4
Dry infant cereal	2 Tbsp	2	4	4
Vegetables	2–3 Tbsp	—	2	3
Fruits	2 Tbsp	—	2	4
Fruit juice	4 oz	—	—	1 (by cup)
Meats (or egg yolk)	1 Tbsp	—	2–4 (strained)	4–6 (chopped)
Finger foods		—	1†	4‡

*Includes that added to cereal.
†Dry toast, teething biscuits.
‡Table foods except "choking" foods (foods in shapes and sizes that are likely to cause choking, such as large pieces of meat, whole grapes, or hot dogs or carrots cut in circular slices).

of apple and pear juice should be avoided; they contain sorbitol, a poorly absorbed sugar alcohol, that can cause diarrhea. Added sugars should be offered in moderation to ensure a nutrient-dense diet. Honey and corn syrup should not be served to children less than a year old because these foods may contain spores of *Clostridium botulinum,* the bacterium that causes botulism poisoning (see Chapter 16). Older children and adults are not at risk from botulism spores because the environment in a mature gastrointestinal tract prevents the bacterium from growing.

Allergen A foreign substance, usually a protein, that stimulates an immune response.

Nutrition-Related Problems in Infants

As the diet expands, the possibility of nutrition-related problems increases. The problems seen most commonly with first foods are food allergies and intolerances.

Food Allergies True allergic reactions to food, or food allergies, are relatively rare, occurring in about 1.4% of young children.[15] They occur when an **allergen** consumed in the diet is absorbed from the intestine, enters the lymph and/or bloodstream, and causes a reaction involving the immune system. Most food allergens are incompletely digested proteins that squeeze through gaps between the intestinal cells. Foods that commonly cause allergies include wheat, peanuts, eggs, milk, nuts, seafood, soy products, and some meats. Exposure to an allergen for the first time causes the immune system to produce antibodies to that allergen. When the allergen is encountered again by eating the same food, allergy symptoms such as vomiting, diarrhea, asthma, hives, eczema, runny nose and swelling of tissues, hay fever, and general cramps and aches may result as the immune system battles the allergen. The symptoms may occur almost immediately or take up to 24 hours to appear, and can vary from mild to severe and life threatening.

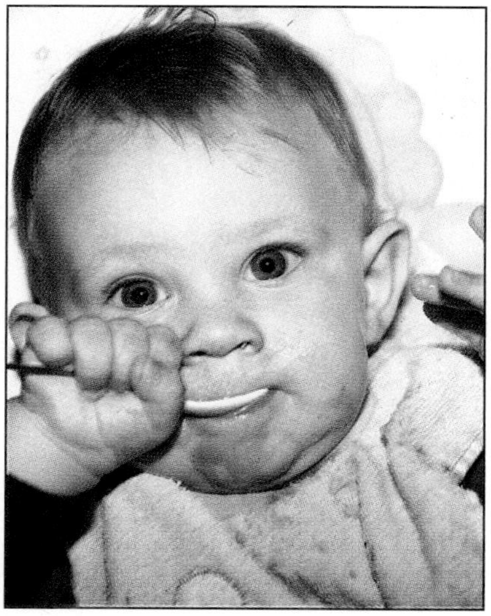

Figure 14.6
Self-feeding is important in infant development but is not a tidy process. (Gregory Smolin)

Age Groups at Risk Food allergies are common in infants because their digestive tracts are not fully mature. After about three months of age, the risk of developing food allergies is reduced because incompletely digested proteins are less likely to be absorbed. Many children who develop food allergies before the age of three will outgrow them. For example, of children allergic to eggs at one year of age, only 4% were still allergic by age five.[15] An offending food may be reintroduced under a doctor's supervision every six months after the age of one year to see if tolerance to it has increased. An allergy to peanuts is an exception. Because this allergy can be serious and even deadly, once it is identified, peanuts should not be reintroduced into the diet (see *Off the Shelf: Peanut Allergy*). Allergies that appear after three years are more likely to be a problem for life. If certain foods must be avoided in the diet, care must be taken to ensure that nutrient needs are met without these foods.

Diagnosis Food allergies can be diagnosed by several laboratory methods. Such tests may rule out a food and can identify foods that are likely to cause problems, but they cannot determine the source of the problem with 100% reliability. However, the cause of a food allergy can be confirmed by using an **elimination diet.** This diet involves removing all foods suspected of causing an allergic reaction from the diet. When a diet that causes no symptoms has been established, it is followed for two to four weeks. After that, foods suspected of causing mild reactions are reintroduced one at a time in small amounts under a doctor's supervision. If no reaction to the food occurs, then increasing amounts are introduced until a normal portion is offered. If there is still no reaction, then the food can be ruled out as an allergen.

Elimination diet A program that eliminates potential allergy-causing foods from an individual's diet and then systematically adds them back to identify any foods that cause an allergic reaction.

Prevention and Treatment Preventing food allergies is not always possible. Breast feeding can reduce the risk of food allergies and is recommended for infants from families with a history of allergies. Infants who are breast fed are less likely to be exposed to foreign proteins that cause food allergies. In addition, their gut matures earlier and they are protected by antibodies and other components of human milk.[15] The benefits of breast feeding are increased if the mother avoids eating common allergy-causing foods such as peanuts, eggs, fish, and dairy products during lactation. To decrease the chances of allergies when solid foods are introduced, wheat, eggs, and fish should not be introduced until the child is 12 months of age, and peanuts should not be given until 36 months.[15]

The best way to manage a food allergy is to avoid consuming the offending food. The information on food labels can be helpful (see Chapter 6, *Off the Label: Identifying Protein Sources*).

Food Intolerances Adverse reactions to foods are also caused by **food intolerances.** Food intolerances do not involve antibody production by the immune system. Rather, they are caused by foods that are difficult or impossible to digest. Food intolerances can be caused by chemical components in foods, by toxins that occur naturally in foods, by substances added to foods during processing or preparation, or simply by large amounts of foods, such as onions or prunes, that cause local GI irritation.[15] Lactose intolerance is an example of a food intolerance caused by a reduced ability to digest milk sugar. It is not an allergy to milk proteins.

Food intolerance An adverse reaction to a food that does not involve the immune system.

Nourishing Toddlers and Young Children

Nourishing a growing child is not always an easy task. Nutrient intake must meet the needs for maintenance and activity as well as growth. Foods offered must be appropriate for children's physical development as well as suit their developing tastes. Whether children are toddlers (ages one to three), or in early childhood (ages four through eight), they are becoming independent eaters. Suiting their tastes as well as meeting their needs can be a challenge to caregivers.

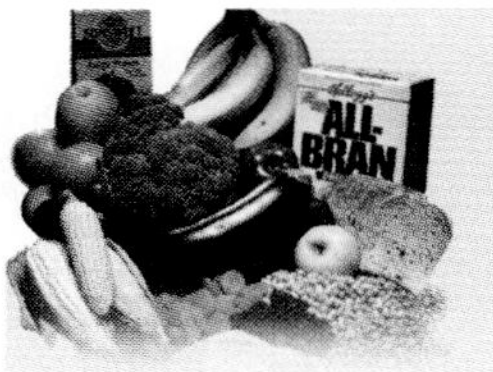

Off the Shelf

Peanut Allergy

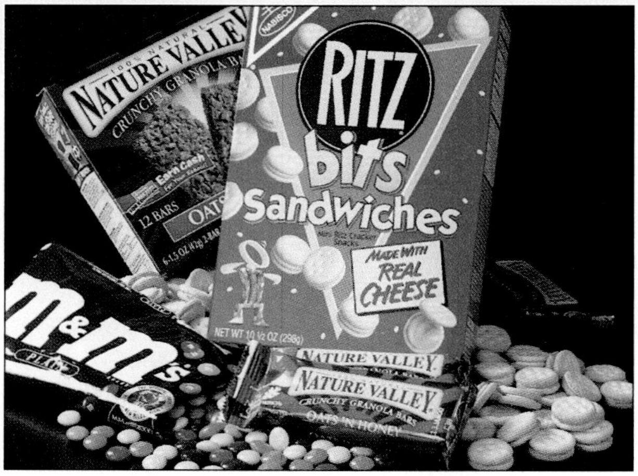

Parents of children with allergies must read labels carefully. These products all contain peanut products or indicate that they may have inadvertently become contaminated with peanuts during manufacture. (George Semple)

Peanut-free schools. Peanut-free airline seats. Why all the attention to peanuts? People with lactose intolerance or allergies to seafood do not force these items from their neighbor's plates, so is it a violation of civil rights to force a school to eliminate peanuts from the menu for the few children who have this allergy? Should we give up our bag of peanuts on the airplane because one passenger might be allergic to them? The answers to these questions are in the hands of the courts, but the rationale behind them is easily explained.

An allergy to peanuts is one of the most common food allergies. It is rarely outgrown, and reactions occur from exposure to minuscule doses, which can often be fatal. Amounts of peanut protein as low as 100 μg can cause a reaction, whereas for other food allergies, up to a thousandfold more—50–100 mg of an allergen—must be eaten before a reaction occurs.[1] And individuals who are allergic to peanuts may be at risk even if the peanuts do not find their way into their mouths. A survey found that 66% of allergic individuals develop symptoms simply from contact with peanuts.[2] Some even experience reactions when peanut allergen is merely inhaled. The typical reaction to peanuts varies but often includes difficulty breathing, skin reactions such as flushing and hives, and a drop in blood pressure. When an allergic individual has a reaction that includes respiratory symptoms, it must be treated immediately with an epinephrine injection and the person should be taken to a hospital emergency room for further treatment.

Because reactions occur with such low levels of peanut exposure, individuals with peanut allergy must avoid all contact with peanuts. This, however, may not be easy, especially for children. Peanut butter sandwiches are a staple of many children's diets, and a peanut butter–smeared finger or shirt could cause a reaction in an allergic friend. If the same knife that spread peanut butter is dipped into the jelly jar, the allergic child who is served only jelly crackers may suffer a peanut reaction.

Shopping for safe foods for someone with peanut allergy is challenging. Individuals with peanut allergy or their caregivers need to rely on food labels to identify safe and unsafe choices. Peanuts, peanut butter, and peanut butter candy are obvious foods to avoid. Others are not so obvious; some foods, such as cookies and crackers, contain peanut flour and peanut oil. Crude peanut oil (less refined) was found to cause an allergic reaction in 10% of allergic subjects, whereas refined peanut oil did not cause a reaction in any of those studied.[3] Food labels, however, do not indicate which type of oil is used in a product.

Even foods manufactured in the same location as peanut-containing foods can pose a risk. For instance, cheese "sandwich" crackers seem like a safe snack, but a thorough reading of the ingredient list reveals the last ingredient on the list to be peanuts. This is because the cheese crackers were manufactured in the same processing facility as peanut butter sandwich crackers, so the label reflects the possibility of cross-contamination. Other products may list "peanut fragments" or state either that the product "may contain peanuts" or that it was manufactured in a facility that processes peanuts. This information protects both the company from legal action and the allergic individual from inadvertently consuming peanut-containing products.

So should your school be peanut free? Serving peanut-free foods is challenging even for a mother trying to keep her own child safe, but it is nearly impossible for school cafeteria workers to be aware of all the ingredients in the food they serve. Even if allergic children bring all their own food from home, they are not necessarily safe if peanuts are being eaten all around them. So, will prohibition of peanuts prevent allergic reactions? Does it violate the rights of children who like peanut butter and jelly sandwiches? While this may be decided in the courts, awareness of the problem may protect an allergic child.

[1]Hourihane, J. O., Kilburn, S. A., Nordlee, J. A., et al. An evaluation of the sensitivity of subjects with peanut allergy to very low doses of peanut protein: a randomized, double-blind, placebo-controlled food challenge study. J. Allergy Clin. Immunol. 100:596–600, 1997.

[2]Hourihane, J. O., Kilburn, S. A., Dean, P., and Warner, J. O. Clinical characteristics of peanut allergy. Clin. Exp. Allergy 27:634–639, 1997.

[3]Hourihane, J. O., Bedwani, S. J., Dean, T. P., and Warner, J. O. Randomized double blind crossover challenge study of allergenicity of peanut oils in subjects allergic to peanuts. BMJ 314:1084–1088, 1997.

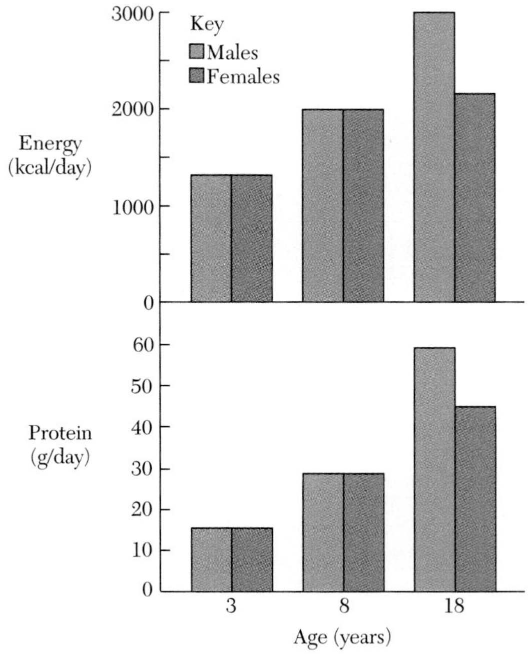

Figure 14.7
The total need for both energy and protein increases with age. The needs of males and females do not differ until adolescence.

Children's Nutrient Needs

As children grow, their nutrient requirements per unit of body weight decrease, but total needs increase because they gain weight and become more active. While a one-year-old will be standing and toddling, a two-year-old will be running, jumping, and climbing. Activity level in preschoolers is highly variable: Some children are relatively inactive, while others never slow down. Recommended intakes are not different for boys and girls until about nine years of age, at which time sexual maturation causes differences in nutrient needs between the sexes. The 1989 RDAs include three age groups: one through three, four through six, and seven through ten. The Dietary Reference Intakes have reduced this to two categories—toddlers (ages one through three), and early childhood (ages four through eight)—and include children nine and older with the adolescent group.

Energy and Macronutrient Needs Children need energy and protein for growth as well as for maintenance. Although growth and metabolic rate slow as children mature, the total need for energy and protein increases because body size increases. The average two-year-old needs about 1300 kcalories and 16 grams of protein per day. By age eight, that child will need about 2000 kcalories and 28 grams of protein per day (Figure 14.7).

Fluid requirements increase in proportion to energy requirements. By one year of age, a child's kidneys have matured and the fluid lost through evaporation has decreased, so fluid requirements are similar to those of adults: 1 ml of fluid per kcalorie of energy consumed.

Recommendations for Fat Intake From birth until the age of two, the requirement for dietary fat is greater than that of adults—about 40 to 50% of energy. This relatively high-fat diet is necessary for the development of the nervous system and to provide enough energy in a small volume of food to meet the needs for growth. After the age of two, the fat in children's diets should be gradually reduced to no more than 30% of energy from fat, the same as for adults[13] (Figure 14.8). Although a diet restricted to 30% fat can support normal growth and development in children, care should be taken to ensure that children's energy and nutrient needs are met while limiting fat intake[16] (see *Off the Label: Labeling Food for Young Children*).

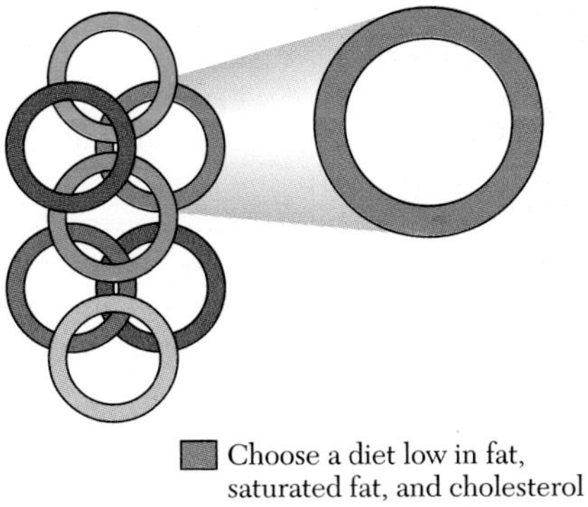

Choose a diet low in fat, saturated fat, and cholesterol

Figure 14.8
The Dietary Guidelines recommend a low-fat diet for everyone over the age of five years. (USDA, DHHS, 1995)

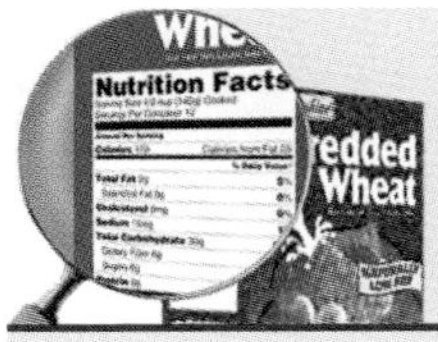

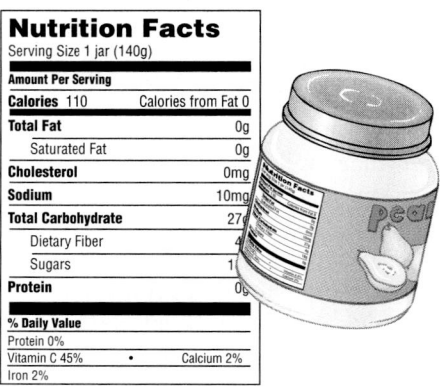

Off the Label

Labeling Food for Young Children

Children have different nutrient needs than adults. Therefore, the labels on foods designed for young children are regulated by different labeling rules.

Most of the population is concerned about excess dietary fat and cholesterol, but children under age two need a diet high in fat. Infancy and early childhood is a period of rapid growth and development, and dietary fat serves as an energy source, a carrier of fat-soluble vitamins, and a source of essential fatty acids. Thus, foods intended for children under two are not permitted to list the amount of saturated fat, polyunsaturated fat, monounsaturated fat, cholesterol, kcalories from fat, and kcalories from saturated fat on the label out of concern that caregivers might restrict fats in the diets of young children.[1] Labels for foods for children under two are also not allowed to carry most of the claims about a food's nutrient content, such as whether it is lowfat and low-cholesterol, and they cannot carry the FDA-approved health claims about the relationship between a nutrient or food and a health concern.[1]

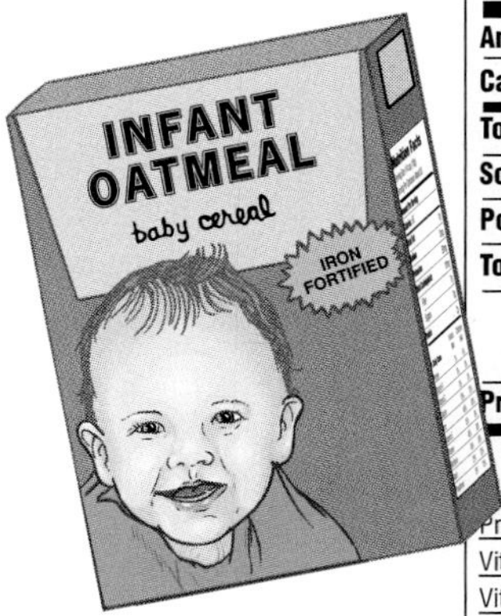

Nutrition Facts
Serving Size 1/4 cup (15g)
Serving Per Container About 30

Amount Per Serving	
Calories 60	
Total Fat	1g
Sodium	0mg
Potassium	50mg
Total Carbohydrate	10mg
Fiber	1g
Sugars	0g
Protein	2g

Daily Value	Infants **0-1**	Children **1-4**
Protein	7%	6%
Vitamin A	0%	0%
Vitamin C	0%	0%
Calcium	15%	10%
Iron	45%	60%
Vitamin E	15%	8%
Thiamin	45%	30%
Riboflavin	45%	30%
Niacin	25%	20%
Phosphorus	15%	10%

Nutrition label for foods for children under age two.

The Dietary Guidelines recommend that, after the age of two, the amount of fat in the diet be gradually reduced until it contains no more than 30% fat by about age five. Therefore, labels on foods designed for two- to four-year-olds must include information on the amount of cholesterol and saturated fat per serving and can voluntarily provide information on the number of kcalories from fat and saturated fat and the amount of polyunsaturated and monounsaturated fat per serving. The serving sizes listed are based on servings appropriate for small children.

Another difference between standard food labels and those for foods designed for children under age four is the absence of percent Daily Values for certain nutrients such as total fat, saturated fat, cholesterol, total carbohydrate, fiber, and sodium.[1] Daily Values for these nutrients have not been established for children under four; for this age group, the FDA has set Daily Values only for vitamins, minerals, and protein. Labels include the percent Daily Values for these nutrients when they are present in significant amounts.

A few nutrient and health claims are allowed on young children's foods. These include claims that describe the percentage of vitamins or minerals in a food as they apply to the Daily Values for children under age two, such as, "provides 50% of the Daily Value for vitamin C." Also, for children under two, the descriptors "unsweetened" and "unsalted" are allowed. "No sugar added" and "sugar free" are approved only for use on dietary supplements for children.

The labels of foods intended for young children provide information needed to make wise food selections, but many of the foods consumed by young children do not have special labels because they are also adult foods. When selecting these foods, keep in mind that the needs of young children, especially for fat, are different than the needs of adults.

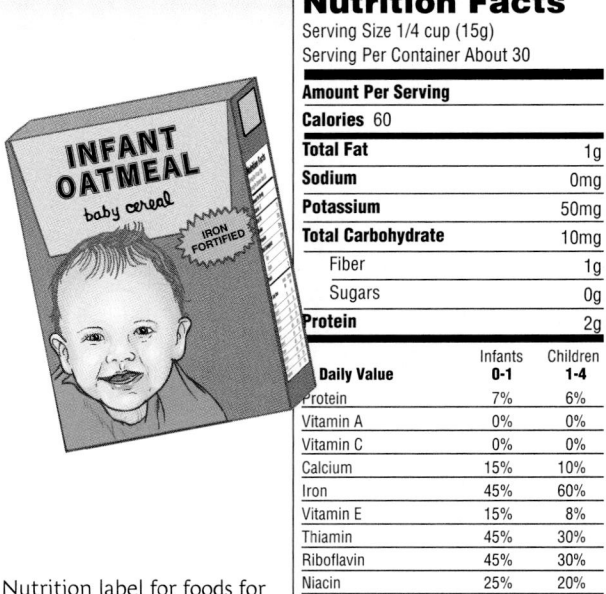

Nutrition Facts
Serving Size 1 jar (140g)

Amount Per Serving	
Calories 110	Calories from Fat 0
Total Fat	0g
Saturated Fat	0g
Cholesterol	0mg
Sodium	10mg
Total Carbohydrate	27
Dietary Fiber	4
Sugars	1
Protein	0g

% Daily Value
Protein 0%
Vitamin C 45% • Calcium 2%
Iron 2%

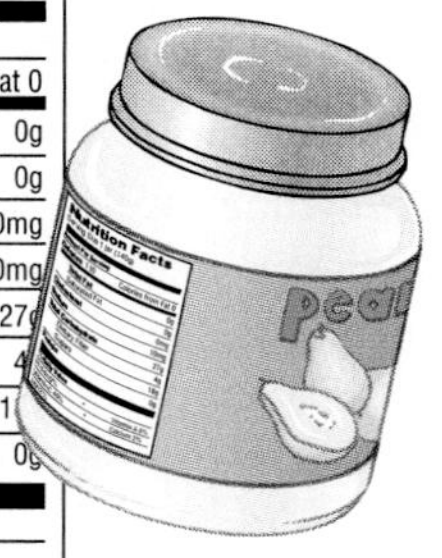

Nutrition label for foods for children ages two to four.

[1]Kurtzweil, P. Labeling rules for young children's foods. FDA Consumer 29:14–18, March 1995.

Carbohydrate and Fiber Recommendations Carbohydrate recommendations for children over about age two are the same as those for adults: 55 to 60% of energy. Specific fiber recommendations have not been made for children, but as a rule of thumb, the number of grams of fiber a child consumes should equal age in years plus 5 grams. For example, a five-year-old should consume 10 grams of fiber per day (5 + 5 = 10 grams).[17] Fiber supplements are not recommended for children, since high intakes can limit the amount of food and, consequently, the nutrients that a small child can consume. As in the adult diet, most of the carbohydrate in a child's diet should be complex carbohydrates. Foods high in added sugars, such as cookies, candy, and soda, should be limited because they are low in nutrient density and promote tooth decay.

Micronutrient Needs As children grow, so do their vitamin and mineral requirements. Surveys indicate that the diets of children in the United States are likely to be deficient in vitamin A, vitamin C, vitamin E, calcium, iron, and zinc.[18] The low intakes of vitamins A and C are most likely due to low intakes of fruits and vegetables.

Calcium Adequate calcium intake during childhood is essential for achieving maximum peak bone mass, which is important in preventing osteoporosis later in life (see Chapter 10). The AI for calcium for toddlers is 500 mg per day and for young children is 800 mg per day. Despite the importance of calcium for establishing peak bone mass, calcium intake in school-age American children is declining,[19] primarily due to a decrease in the consumption of dairy products, such as milk, yogurt, and cheese, which are the best sources of calcium. Children who cannot or do not consume dairy products should meet their calcium needs with fortified foods and calcium-rich vegetables.

Iron Iron deficiency anemia is one of the most prevalent forms of malnutrition in children. Although iron intake by American children has increased over the last 20 years, iron deficiency is still a public health problem.[20] Iron deficiency can affect learning ability, intellectual performance, stamina, and mood.[21] Iron deficiency anemia can also lower the child's resistance to illness and slow recovery time. Good sources of iron that are acceptable to small children include fortified grains and breakfast cereals, raisins, eggs, and lean meats. If anemia is diagnosed, iron supplements are usually prescribed until iron stores are repleted.

High doses of iron are toxic, so supplements should be kept out of the reach of children. Iron-containing supplements are the leading cause of poisoning deaths among children under six years of age.[22] To help protect children, products containing iron include a warning about the hazards to children of ingesting large amounts of iron. Products containing 30 mg or more per dose are packed in individual doses.[23] The time and effort required for a child to open these wrappers may reduce the chances of consuming enough to cause toxicity.

Do Children Need Vitamin and Mineral Supplements? As with adults, children who consume a well-selected, varied diet can meet all their vitamin and mineral requirements with food. Occasional skipped meals and unfinished dinners are a normal part of most children's eating behavior. However, children with particularly erratic eating habits, those on regimens to manage obesity, those with limited food availability, and those who consume a vegan diet may benefit from a multivitamin and mineral supplement that provides no more than 100% of the Daily Values. There are many children's supplements available, but they are rarely marketed for their nutrient content. Instead, the sales pitch focuses on their color, flavor, and shape. The choices are enticing—all look and taste like candy, and most children think they are candy. But supplements are not candy,

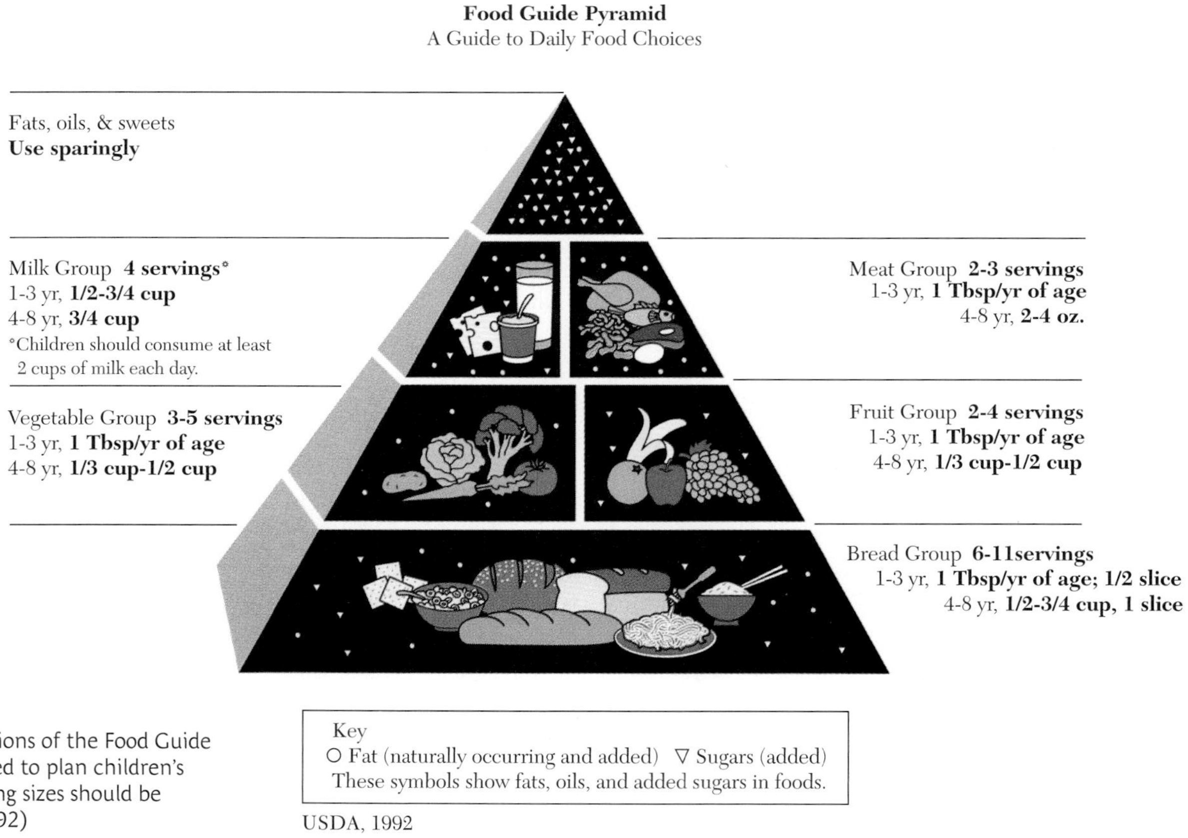

Figure 14.9
The recommendations of the Food Guide Pyramid can be used to plan children's diets, but the serving sizes should be smaller. (USDA, 1992)

and overdoses, particularly of iron-containing supplements, can be life threatening. If a children's supplement is offered, it should be monitored by caregivers and stored safely.

Meeting Children's Nutrient Needs

The physiological requirements for growth and development are important in dictating hunger and nutrient needs. However, food choices are affected by the child's stage of psychosocial development and the environment in which he or she lives and eats. Nourishing young children requires patience and creativity.

A Balanced Diet Children over the age of two, like adults, need a varied diet based on whole grains, vegetables, and fruits, adequate in milk and other high-protein foods, and moderate in fat and sodium. Snacks should be as nutritious as meals.

The recommendations of the Food Guide Pyramid can be used to plan children's diets by adjusting the serving sizes (Figure 14.9). For instance, an adult serving of milk would be 1 cup, whereas a serving for a two-year-old would be 4 ounces and for a five-year-old would be 6 ounces. Examples of meal patterns for a three-year-old and an eight-year-old are shown in Table 14.2. A version of the Food Guide Pyramid designed to be appealing for children two to six years of age has been developed by the U.S. Department of Agriculture (see Appendix J).

As previously mentioned, after the age of two, the fat content of the diet should be gradually reduced. Since much of the fat in young children's diets comes from milk and other dairy products, children two years of age and older should consume reduced-fat dairy products. Visible fat should be trimmed from meat, which should be broiled rather than fried; consumption of high-fat meats

Table 14.2 *A Typical Day's Food Intake for Three- and Eight-Year-Old Children*

Three-Year-Old Child			Eight-Year-Old Child		
Food	**Amount**	**Food Group**	**Food**	**Amount**	**Food Group**
Breakfast					
Corn flakes	3 Tbsp	1 grain	Corn flakes	3/4 cup	1 grain
Milk, 2%	1/2 cup	1 milk	Milk, 2%	3/4 cup	1 milk
Banana	3 Tbsp	1 fruit	Banana	half	1 fruit
Snack					
Peanut butter	1 Tbsp	1 meat			
Wheat crackers	3	1 grain			
Apple juice	1/2 cup	1 fruit			
Lunch					
Vegetable soup	1/4 cup	1 vegetable	Vegetable soup	1 cup	1 vegetable
Grilled tuna sandwich	half	1 grain, 1 meat	Grilled tuna sandwich	1	2 grain, 2 meat
Tomato	1/4	1 vegetable	Tomato	1/2	1 vegetable
Milk, 2%	1/2 cup	1 milk	Milk, 2%	3/4 cup	1 milk
Snack					
Hot cocoa	1/2 cup	1 milk	Hot cocoa	3/4 cup	1 milk
			Peanut butter and jelly sandwich	1	2 grain, 1 meat
Cookie	1	1 grain	Cookies	2	1 grain
Snack					
Pretzels	2	1 grain	Pretzels	4	1 grain
Orange juice	1/2 cup	2 fruit	Orange juice	1/2 cup	1 fruit
Dinner					
Rice	3 Tbsp	1 grain	Rice	3/4 cup	1 grain
Chicken	1 drumstick	1 meat	Chicken	2 drumsticks	1 meat
Broccoli	1 floret	1 vegetable	Broccoli	3 florets	1 vegetable
Milk, 2%	1/2 cup	1 milk	Milk, 2%	3/4 cup	1 milk
Ice cream	1/2 cup	1 milk	Ice cream	3/4 cup	1 milk

should be limited. However, the composition of the total diet should not be ignored when reducing fat intake. For instance, using reduced-fat hot dogs or lunch meats will reduce fat intake but will not increase the number of servings of fruits and vegetables in the diet (see *Off the Shelf: Snack Foods: Balancing Nutrition, Cost, and Convenience*).

Increased Variety Creativity may be necessary to convince a young child to consume a varied diet. Children often have periods known as food jags, when they will eat only certain foods and nothing else. For example, a child may refuse to eat anything other than peanut butter and jelly sandwiches for breakfast, lunch, and dinner. The general guideline is to continue to offer other foods along with those the child is focused on. It is the nutrient content of the total diet averaged over days or weeks that is important, so a few days of a food jag is unlikely to affect the child's overall nutritional health.

What children will not touch at one meal, they may eat the next day or the next week. Also, letting children participate in food preparation can increase interest in eating, and unusual shapes can make a disliked food an interesting one. Substituting appropriate nutritious choices for refused foods can increase the variety of the diet. If vegetables are refused, they can be added to soups and casseroles. Fruit can be served on cereals or in milkshakes. Cheese can be offered in recipes such as macaroni and cheese, cheese sauce, and pizza. Milk can be added to hot cereal, cream soups, puddings, and custards. And powdered milk can be used in baking. Meats can be added to spaghetti sauce, stews, casseroles, burritos, or pizza.

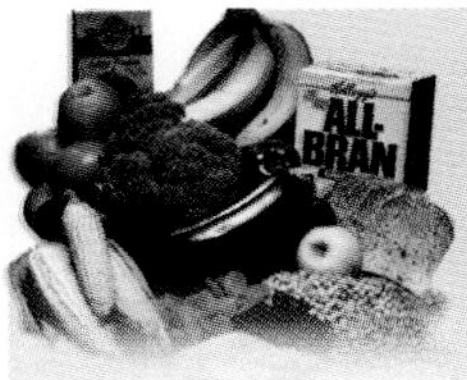

Off the Shelf

Snack Foods: Balancing Nutrition, Cost, and Convenience

Snacks are an important part of a child's diet. However, finding healthy snacks that fit your lifestyle and your pocketbook is not always easy. Advertising, glitzy packaging, and cartoon shapes often make packaged convenience snacks irresistible to children. Label statements such as "Made with skim milk" or "Made with real fruit" make them appear nutritious to parents. Convenient packaging tempts parents because it makes these products easy to send in school lunches or carry to soccer games. However, careful reading of food labels often reveals that the snack is not as healthy as the banner on the label implies. The benefits of convenience must be balanced against the cost and nutrient composition.

Labels boasting of skim milk, real fruit, or whole grains are often drawing attention away from the fat and sugar in the products. Pudding advertised to be "made with 70% skim milk" may be 70% skim milk by weight, but a look at the ingredient list reveals that the rest is mostly sugar and oil. Fruit snacks are another treat that a parent might serve as a healthy alternative to candy. After all, they are "made with real fruit." These snacks, however, contain so little fruit or juice that they don't even satisfy 2% of the Daily Value for any vitamin or mineral unless it is specifically added. Fruit or fruit juice may appear before sugar on the ingredient list, but ingredients are listed in order of weight. Fruit or juice contributes more weight because of its high water content, but it contributes far less energy than the added sugar.

Some granola or cereal bars also masquerade as a healthy snack when in many ways they resemble candy. They have an advantage over candy bars because of the oats they contain, but many contain more chocolate than oats. Granola bars often contain up to 50% of their energy as fat. Ingredients such as marshmallows and caramel, contained in many granola bar snacks, sound more like the ingredients in a candy bar than those in a healthy snack. Even granola bars that do not contain chocolate, caramel, or marshmallows are often higher in fat than a healthy snack should be.

Convenience snack foods can be part of a healthy diet. Pudding made at home with skim milk is less expensive and lower in fat, but prepackaged puddings are still a good source of calcium and are available in lowfat versions. Fresh fruit is a better choice than fruit snacks. It is higher in fiber and phytochemicals, cheaper, and just as easy to pack and transport as fruit snacks. But, an uneaten piece of fruit contributes no nutrients, and if the alternative is candy, at least many fruit snacks are fortified with vitamins A, C, and E.

The specific nutrients provided by a cereal bar depend on which you choose. Many are low in fat, provide some fiber and fruit, and are fortified with vitamins and minerals. They are high in sugar, but no more so than sugared breakfast cereal. However, if cost is an issue, a sandwich bag of dry cereal is just as convenient and costs about \$.05 per serving compared to about \$.50 for an individually packaged bar.

Convenience snacks are appealing to kids, easy to transport, and can contribute energy and nutrients to the diet. Although some are high in fat and sugar, they can be part of a healthy diet if they do not take the place of whole grains, fresh fruits and vegetables, and lowfat dairy products.

Nutrition-Related Problems in Children

In addition to nutrient deficiencies, a number of other problems related to food and nutrient intake can develop during childhood.

Dental Caries Diets high in sugary snacks promote tooth decay. Decay occurs when there is prolonged contact between sugar and bacteria on the surface of the teeth. Because the primary teeth guide the growth of the permanent teeth, maintaining healthy primary teeth is just as important as preserving permanent ones. Preventing tooth decay involves limiting carbohydrate snacks, especially those that stick to teeth; brushing teeth frequently to remove sticky sweets; and consuming adequate fluoride (Figure 14.10; see also Chapters 3, 4, and 11). Children three years of age and over should be seen by a dentist regularly.

Hyperactivity Hyperactivity is a problem in 5 to 10% of school-age children, occurring more frequently in boys than in girls. This syndrome involves extreme physical activity, excitability, impulsiveness, distractibility, short attention span, and a low tolerance for frustration. Hyperactive children have more difficulty learning but usually are of normal or above-average intelligence. Hyperactivity is now considered part of a larger syndrome known as **attention deficit hyperactive disorder.**

Attention deficit hyperactive disorder A condition in children that is characterized by a short attention span and a high level of activity, excitability, and distractibility.

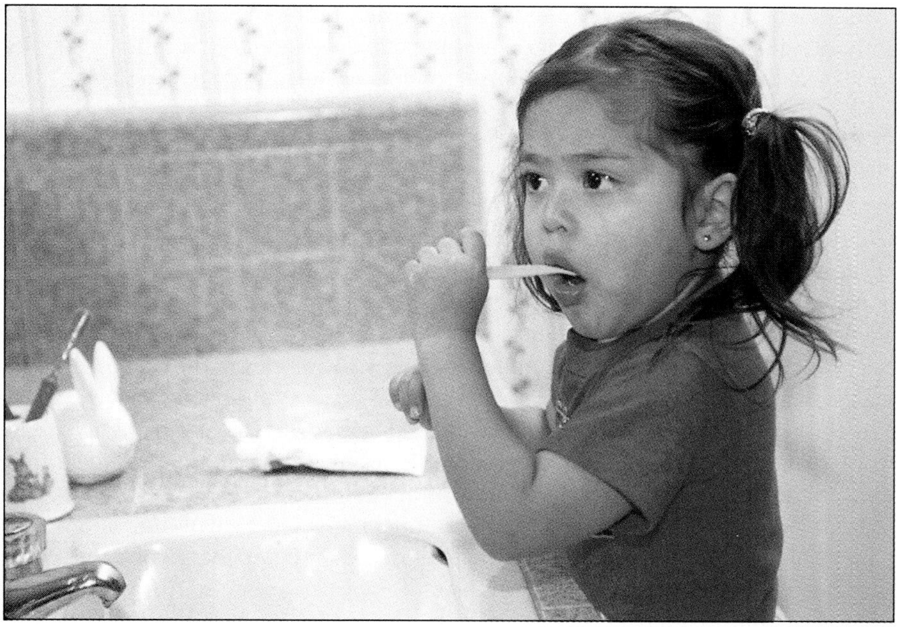

Figure 14.10
Frequent supervised toothbrushing by children can help prevent dental caries. (© David Young-Wolff/PhotoEdit)

One popular misconception is that hyperactivity is caused by a high sugar intake, but research on sugar intake and behavior has failed to support the hypothesis that sugar contributes to this behavior.[24] Hyperactive behavior that is observed after sugar consumption is likely the result of other circumstances in that child's life. For example, the excitement of a birthday party rather than the cake is most likely the cause of hyperactive behavior. Other situations that might cause hyperactivity include lack of sleep, overstimulation, the desire for more attention, or lack of physical activity.

Specific foods and food additives have also been implicated as a cause of hyperactivity. Numerous studies have been done to test the hypothesis that food sensitivities cause hyperactivity, but the results have been inconsistent.[25] Some children with this disorder seem to improve when particular foods or additives are eliminated, while others do not. Hyperactivity should be diagnosed and treated by a physician, using behavioral and dietary modification, special educational techniques, counseling, and in some cases medication.

Another possible cause of hyperactive behavior in children is caffeine. Caffeine is a stimulant that can cause sleeplessness, restlessness, and irregular heartbeats. Beverages, food, and medicines containing caffeine are often a part of children's diets (see Table 12.5 for the caffeine content of food, beverages, and medications). For example, caffeinated beverages such as Coke and Mountain Dew are often included in children's fast-food meals. A 12-ounce cola contains about 40 to 50 mg of caffeine. Because of children's small size, the same amount of caffeine in a child has a greater effect than it does in an adult.

Lead Toxicity Lead is an environmental contaminant that can be toxic, especially in children under six. Children are particularly susceptible because they absorb lead much more efficiently than do adults. It is estimated that children may absorb as much as 30 to 75% of ingested lead, whereas adults absorb only about 11%.[26] Once absorbed from the gastrointestinal tract, lead circulates in the bloodstream and then accumulates in the bones and, to a lesser extent, the brain, teeth, and kidneys. Lead disrupts the functioning of neurotransmitters and thus interferes with the functioning of the nervous system. Higher levels of lead can contribute to iron deficiency anemia, changes in kidney function, nervous system changes, and even seizures, coma, and death.[27] In young children, lead poisoning can cause learning disabilities and behavior problems. High lead levels in the bones of young boys have been linked to attention problems, aggressive behavior, and delinquency.[28] In adults, lead poisoning can damage the reproductive organs and cause high blood pressure.[29] During pregnancy, lead toxicity can damage the fetal nervous system.

Lead is found naturally in the earth's crust, but over the years industrial activities have redistributed it in the environment. Lead is now found in soil contaminated with lead paint dust; it also enters drinking water from old corroded lead plumbing, lead solder on copper pipes, or brass faucets. It is present in polluted air, and its presence in leaded glass and in glazes used on imported and antique pottery can contaminate food and beverages. Because of the risks of lead toxicity from environmental contamination, lead is no longer used in house paint, gasoline, or solder. As a result, the number of children with elevated blood lead levels has decreased by 85% over the last 20 years.[26] Despite these gains, nearly a million children under six years of age have blood lead levels that are high enough to cause damage.[30] For a number of reasons, the problem is greatest among children living in poverty. Older housing in both rural and urban settings is more likely to contain lead paint, and chipped paint is often consumed by children as they explore their environments. The old plumbing in these houses may contaminate the water with lead. In addition, children living in poverty are more likely to be malnourished, and malnutrition increases lead absorption because lead is better absorbed from an empty stomach and when other minerals such as calcium, zinc, and iron are deficient. An inverse relationship has been found between blood lead levels and dietary iron intake indicating that adequate iron intake prevents lead absorption and can help protect against lead toxicity.[27]

Children should have their blood lead levels tested.[26] The effects of lead poisoning are permanent, but if high levels are detected early, the lead can be removed with medical treatment. The best way to prevent lead poisoning is to learn how to avoid lead exposure (Table 14.3).

Table 14.3 *What You Can Do to Reduce Lead Exposure*

Reducing exposure from lead paint: If you live in a house built before 1978, it may contain lead paint or lead paint may have been sanded or scrapped off at some time.

- Wash floors and other surfaces weekly with warm water and detergent.
- Wipe soil off shoes before entering the house.
- Cover exposed soil in the yard with grass or mulch.

Reducing exposure from tap water: If your home has old plumbing, lead may be leaching into your tap water. More leaches into hot water than cold, and water that has been standing in the pipes has more lead.

- Use cold water for drinking and cooking.
- Allow water to run for 30 seconds before use.

Reducing exposure from food containers: Pottery glazes and lead crystal contain lead. The FDA limits the amount of lead allowed in ceramic foodware, but the lead content of pottery designed for ornamental use is not regulated.

- Look for engraved warnings such as "Not for Food Use—May Poison Food" and "For Decorative Purposes Only" to identify pottery that should not be used to serve food.
- Do not store acidic foods such as fruit juices or tomato juice in ceramic containers.
- Limit the use of antique or collectable housewares for food or beverages to special occasions.
- Use your lead crystal stemware to drink from, but do not store anything in lead crystal.
- Pregnant women should not routinely use lead crystal glasses.
- Infants should not be fed from lead crystal baby bottles.

For additional information: Contact the Centers for Disease Control and Prevention at 1-888-232-6789; the Environmental Protection Agency's Safe Drinking Water Hotline at 1-800-426-4791; the Consumer Product Safety Commission at 1-800-638-CPSC; the National Lead Information Center at 1-800-LEAD-FYI; or access Web sites for these agencies and organizations through links to this text's Web site.

Influences From the Outside World

Forty years ago mothers had a greater impact on children's food choices because they were home to offer three meals a day. Today, 60% of women with young children work outside the home,[7] fewer children live in homes with two parents, and many more have experienced divorce. The increase in working mothers and single-parent households means children consume an increasing number of meals away from home—in day-care facilities, schools, and restaurant/fast-food establishments. Because of modern lifestyles, children make many of their own food choices. They can prepare their own meals in the microwave and have a greater influence on food selection at the grocery store. Their food choices are influenced by their home life, time spent away from home, and what they see on television.

Fast Food Isn't All Bad Children generally love fast food, and there is nothing wrong with an occasional fast-food meal. But, these meals are typically lacking in milk, fruits, and vegetables. They are high in kcalories and fat and low in calcium, fiber, and vitamins A and C. To fit fast food into a healthy diet, more nutrient-dense fast-food choices need to be made and other meals and snacks throughout the day need to supply the missing nutrients. Many fast-food franchises now offer vegetables, salads, and milk. And some of the old standbys are not bad choices. A plain, single-patty hamburger provides a lot less fat and energy than one with two patties and a high-fat sauce. A chicken sandwich can be a lowfat choice if it is grilled or barbecued, not breaded and fried (see Appendix A). French fries are high in fat, but if they are combined with lowfat foods throughout the day, they can still be part of a healthy diet. A fast-food meal is only one part of the total diet. If the missing milk, fruits, and vegetables are consumed at other times during the day, the total diet can still be a healthy one.

Meals at Day Care or School As the number of single-parent families and families with both parents in the workforce has increased, so has the number of very young children that attend day care. Day-care providers therefore play a significant role in teaching children good eating habits. This does not mean the parent cannot be involved. In some day-care centers, meals are sent from home, and when meals or snacks are provided by the day-care center, parents can recommend favorite foods and foods to be avoided.

Whether it is a day care for toddlers, a preschool, or a public school, providing nutritious meals away from home is not always easy. A lunch taken to day care or school should contain foods that do not require refrigeration (even if a refrigerator is available, the child is likely to forget to put the lunch in it). Packing a lunch does not guarantee that it will be eaten, so caregivers should make sure the child likes what is sent; even the most carefully planned lunch is not nutritious if it is not eaten.

For children who buy their lunch at school, the National School Lunch Program provides low-cost meals designed to meet nutrient needs and promote healthy diets. The goals of this program are to improve the dietary intake and nutritional health of America's children, and to promote nutrition education by teaching children to make appropriate food choices.[31] Each lunch meal must provide one third of the 1989 RDA for protein, vitamin A, vitamin C, iron, calcium, and energy and meet the Dietary Guidelines recommendations of no more than 30% of energy from fat and 10% from saturated fat. Within these guidelines, each school or school district can decide which foods to serve and how they are prepared. In addition to lunches, federal guidelines regulate foods sold in snack bars and vending machines that compete with school lunch programs. These must provide at least 5% of the RDA for one or more of the following: protein, vitamin A, vitamin C, niacin, riboflavin, calcium, and iron. An analysis of the foods students choose to eat from the meal offered found that students who participated in the school lunch program consumed one third of the RDA for energy, protein,

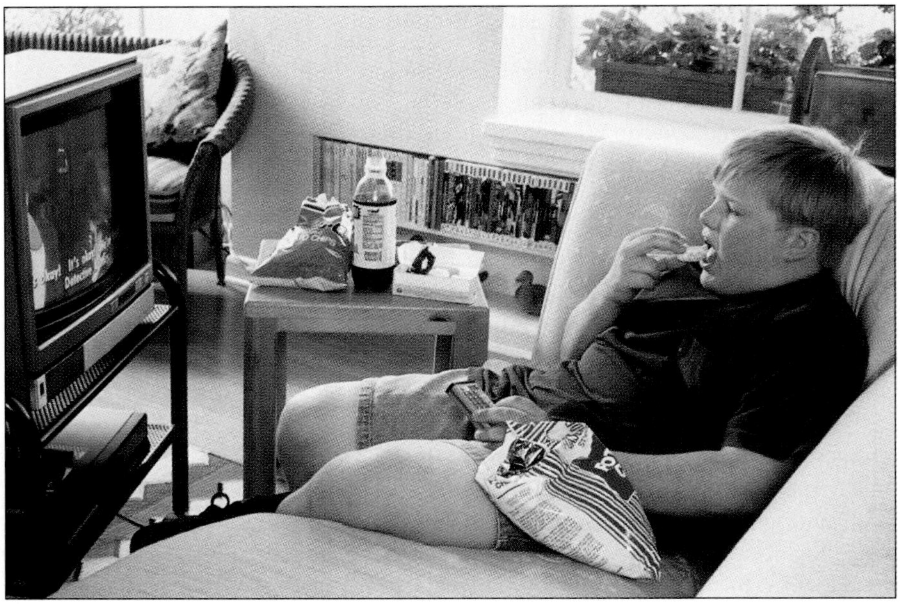

Figure 14.11
Television watching influences activity level, snacking behavior, and the kinds of foods children choose. (© Donna Day/Tony Stone Images)

vitamin A, vitamin C, vitamin B_6, calcium, iron, and zinc and drank twice as much milk as students not participating in school lunch programs. However, they consumed more fat than is recommended: 37% of the kcalories they consumed at lunch came from fat. Those who purchased meals from vending machines consumed fewer vitamins and minerals and an even greater percentage of kcalories from fat.[17]

Television Reduces Activity and Influences Food Choices Television viewing is another lifestyle factor that influences children's nutrition and health. Children today spend more time watching television than they do in school.[32] Television affects nutritional status in a number of ways: It introduces children to foods they might otherwise not be exposed to, it promotes snacking, and it reduces physical activity (Figure 14.11).

Through advertising, television has a strong influence on the foods selected by young children. A review of commercials broadcast during children's programming found that over 60% were for food products—primarily sweetened breakfast cereals; sweets such as candy, cookies, doughnuts, and other desserts; snacks; and beverages—that are high in sugar, fat, or salt.[33] Television also promotes snacking behavior.[33] Although snacks are an important part of a growing child's diet, many children snack on sweet and salty foods that are low in nutrient density while watching TV.

Perhaps the most important nutritional influence of television is that it reduces activity. Hours spent watching television are hours when physical activity is at a minimum. One study showed that children who watch four or more hours of TV per day had greater body fat and greater BMI than those who watch fewer than two hours a day.[34] In addition to television, children and adolescents today replace time spent at more physically demanding activities with time spent playing computer and video games.

ADOLESCENCE: TRANSITION TO ADULTHOOD

Once a child has reached about 9 to 12 years of age, the physical changes associated with sexual maturation begin to occur. The maturation process creates differences between the nutrient requirements of males and females. As with children, the nutrient intake of adolescents is also affected by psychosocial development and the environment in which they live. The DRIs begin recommendations for adolescent intake at age nine because the hormonal changes that mark the beginning of adolescence occur by this age in some girls, particularly in African Americans. The DRIs divide recommended intakes for adolescence into ages 9 through 13 and ages 14 through 18.[35] The 1989 RDAs begin recommendations for adolescence at age 11 and include recommendations for ages 11 through 14 and 15 through 18.

The Changing Body: Sexual Maturation

During adolescence, organ systems develop and grow, body composition changes, and the growth rates and nutritional requirements of boys and girls diverge. This period of rapid change, which ends in sexual maturation, is called **puberty.** Growth and development is more rapid in the early teens than at any time except for the first two years after birth. During adolescence, boys and girls grow about 11 inches and gain about 40% of their eventual skeletal mass.[36] From ages 10 to 17, girls gain about 53 pounds and boys about 70 pounds. During adolescence, there is an 18- to 24-month period of peak growth velocity, called the **adolescent growth spurt.** In girls, the growth spurt occurs between the ages of 10 and 13. In boys, it occurs between ages 12 and 15 (Figure 14.12).

Puberty A period in life characterized by rapid growth and physical changes that ends in the attainment of sexual maturity.

Adolescent growth spurt An 18- to 24-month period of peak growth velocity that begins at about ages 10 to 13 in girls and 12 to 15 in boys.

The hormonal changes that occur with sexual development orchestrate the type of growth that occurs and the change in body composition that results. During the growth spurt, boys tend to grow taller and heavier than girls and do so at a faster rate. Boys gain fat but also add so much lean mass as muscle and bone that their percentage of body fat actually decreases (Figure 14.13). In girls, **menarche,** the onset of menstruation, is typically followed by a deceleration in growth rate and an increase in fat deposition. By age 20, females have about twice as much adipose tissue as males and only about two thirds as much lean tissue. These physiologic changes affect nutrient needs. Because there is a large individual variation in the age at which these growth changes occur, the stage of maturation is often a better indicator of nutritional requirements than actual chronological age.

Menarche The onset of menstruation, which occurs normally between the ages of 10 and 15.

Nutrition during childhood and adolescence can affect sexual development. Nutritional deficiencies can cause poor growth and delayed sexual maturation. Taller, heavier children usually enter puberty sooner than shorter, lighter ones.[37]

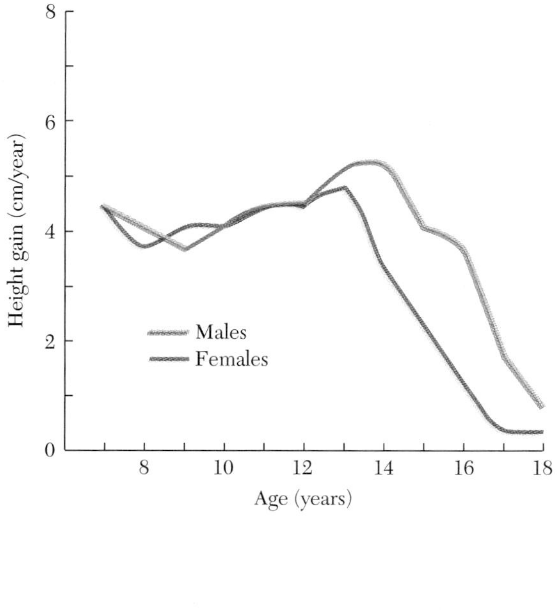

Figure 14.12
Peak growth occurs earlier in girls than in boys.

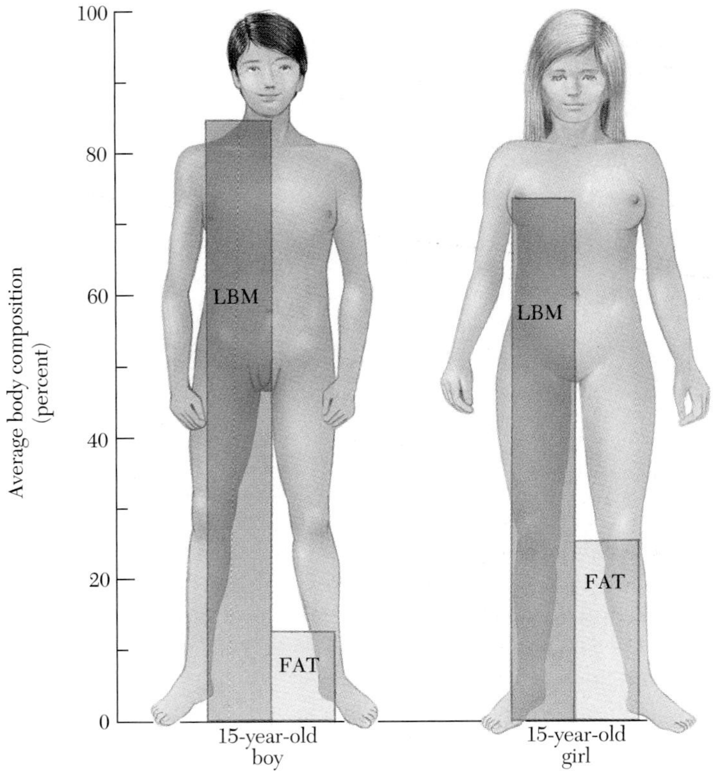

Figure 14.13
After puberty, males have a higher percentage of lean body mass and less body fat than females. (Adapted from Forbes, G. B. Body composition. In *Present Knowledge in Nutrition*, 6th ed. Brown, M. L., ed. Washington, D.C.: International Life Sciences Institute—Nutrition Foundation, 1990.)

Adolescent Nutrient Needs

Recommendations for nutrient intake in adolescents are based on the needs for growth and development; total nutrient needs are greater at this time than during any other time of life. The best indicators of adequate intake are satiety and growth that follows the curve of the growth charts.

Energy and Macronutrients Energy requirements for boys begin to exceed those for girls as they develop more muscle and a greater body size. Adolescent girls need 38 to 46 kcalories per kilogram of body weight, and boys' requirements range from 40 to 55 kcalories per kilogram (see Figure 14.7). Protein requirements for both groups reach the adult recommendation of 0.8 gram per kilogram by about age 19, but since boys are generally heavier, they require more total protein than girls. These higher requirements for males continue throughout life. Adolescents should follow the Dietary Guidelines by consuming a diet containing about 55 to 60% carbohydrate and no more than 30% of kcalories from fat.

Micronutrients The requirements for many vitamins and minerals are higher for adolescents than adults. Because data are often not available for this age group, the recommended intakes are often extrapolated from adult values.

Vitamins The need for B vitamins involved in energy metabolism is much higher in adolescence than in childhood because of high energy intake. Riboflavin is frequently low in teen diets, especially in those of girls, possibly due to low milk intake. Vitamin B_6 is needed for protein synthesis; therefore, need is increased during the rapid growth of adolescence. Folate and vitamin B_{12} needs are increased because of the high rate of cell division for tissue growth. Vitamin B_{12} intake is typically adequate, but folate is a vitamin at risk for deficiency in the adolescent population.[38] The need for vitamin D increases with skeletal growth. The AI for vitamin D is set at 5 μg per day, but in active teens who engage in outdoor activities, much of the requirement is met by synthesis. Additional amounts of vitamins A, C, and E are needed to preserve the structure and function of the newly synthesized cells. These vitamins are generally adequate in the teen diet.

Iron Iron deficiency anemia is common in adolescence. Iron is needed to synthesize hemoglobin for the expansion of blood volume and myoglobin for the increase in muscle mass. Because blood volume expands at a faster rate in boys than in girls, boys require more iron for tissue synthesis than girls. However, the iron loss due to menstruation makes total needs greater in young women, yet their intake is typically less than the recommended amount.[38] The 1989 RDA for adolescents is set at 12 mg for boys and 15 mg for girls. Good sources of iron acceptable to teens include fortified grains and breakfast cereals and lean red meats.

Calcium Bone contains 99% of the calcium in the body. The adolescent growth spurt increases both the length and the mass of bones; therefore, to form healthy bone, adequate calcium is essential. Calcium retention varies with growth rate, with the fastest-growing adolescents retaining the most calcium. The AI for calcium during adolescence is 1300 mg per day for both sexes. Although bone mass may continue to increase until age 30, about 45% of the bone present in the adult is laid down during adolescence. Calcium intake is typically low for adolescent boys and girls.[38] This may compromise the level of peak bone mass achieved, increasing the risk of developing osteoporosis later in life.

Foods common in the teen diet that are good sources of calcium include milk, yogurt and frozen yogurt, ice cream, and cheese added to hamburgers, nachos, and pizza. Although milk and cheese are the biggest source of calcium in teen diets, they can be high in saturated fat, so adolescents should be encouraged to consume reduced-fat dairy products and vegetable sources of calcium. Adolescent girls are likely to skimp on drinking milk, favoring low-kcalorie soft drinks. This may put them in double jeopardy, since diet soda does not supply calcium and some varieties are high in caffeine which increases calcium excretion and a form of phosphorus that increases calcium losses (Figure 14.14).[39]

Zinc Zinc is important in protein synthesis. During adolescence, the increase in protein synthesis required for the growth of skeletal muscle and the development of organs increases the need for zinc. A long-term deficiency results in growth retardation and altered sexual development. Although severe zinc deficiency is rare in developed countries, even mild deficiency can cause poor growth, affect appetite and taste, impair immune response, and interfere with vitamin A metabolism. Since adolescents are growing rapidly and maturing sexually, adequate zinc is essential for, but not typically consumed by, this age group.[38] Good sources include meats and whole grains.

Meeting Adolescent Nutrient Needs

Skipped meals and meals away from home are common among adolescents. No matter when foods are consumed throughout the day, an adolescent's diet should follow the recommendations of the Food Guide Pyramid—choosing at the high end of the range of serving recommendations. For example, a diet containing 3000 or more kcalories should contain 11 servings of grains. This may seem a staggering number, but it is not when spread over the course of a day. A large bowl of cereal and two slices of toast for breakfast is 4 servings; two tacos for lunch and crackers after school is 4 more servings; and a dinner of spaghetti and garlic bread can add another 3 or 4 servings. The diet should also provide 5 to 9 servings of fruits and vegetables. Unfortunately, fruits and vegetables are the food groups most likely to be lacking in the American diet: In a nationwide survey, only 29.3% of students had eaten 5 or more servings of fruits and vegetables on the preceding day.[40] French fries, which are high in fat and salt, are the most frequently consumed vegetable. And many people never consume fruit. Sources of

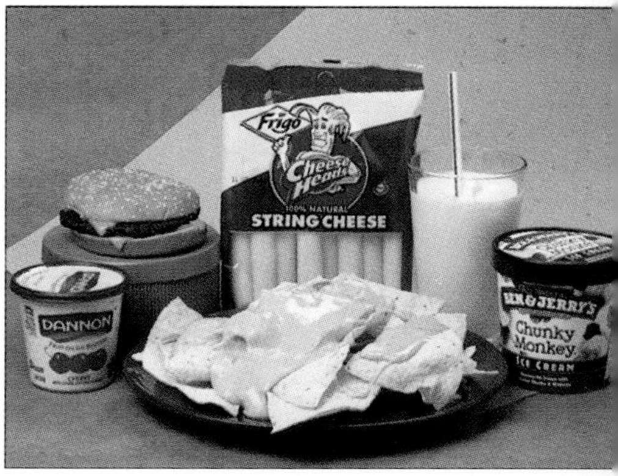

Figure 14.14
These foods provide good sources of calcium and are common choices for teens. (George Semple)

fruits and vegetables acceptable to teens include fruit juice, salads, and tomato sauce and vegetables on pizza and spaghetti.

Since the teen diet, especially that of teenage boys, is typically high in fat, saturated fat, cholesterol, and sodium,[41] meals offered at home should be low in fat and sodium. Teens are no longer fed by their parents, but healthy choices, such as reduced-fat milk and dairy products, vegetables, and fruits, should be available at home (see *Critical Thinking: Meeting Teen Needs*).

CRITICAL THINKING

Meeting Teen Needs

Jenny is a busy 16-year-old high school junior. Until recently she hadn't paid much attention to her diet because she ate all her meals at home or at school. Now she has a part-time job and frequently eats dinner and snacks on her own. She notices that she has gained a few pounds and decides that she should change her diet.

Jenny's Original Diet			Jenny's New Diet		
Food	Energy (kcal)	Fat (g)	Food	Energy (kcal)	Fat (g)
Breakfast					
Corn flakes	97	0	Bagel	187	1
Lowfat milk	120	5			
Orange juice	112	0			
Toast	140	2.2			
Margarine	68	7.6			
Lunch					
Hamburger	260	10	Frozen yogurt	288	13
Apple	81	0.5			
Lowfat milk	120	5			
Corn chips	153	9.5			
Snack					
Slice of pizza	200	5	Double burger	576	32
Cola	185	0	French fries	315	16
			Vanilla shake	503	14
Dinner					
Ham and cheese sandwich	350	15	Candy bar	300	21
Potato chips	150	10	Potato chips	150	10
Cola	185	0			
Total	**2221**	**69.8**		**2319**	**107**

How has Jenny's intake changed?

Although she eats less food, Jenny's new diet is actually higher in energy and fat, and lower in micronutrients. Her original diet provided 2221 kcalories, 28% of which was from fat, and met her micronutrient needs. Her new diet has more energy, contains 39% fat, and does not supply the RDA or AI for vitamin A, folate, vitamin C, vitamin E, calcium, magnesium, zinc, or iron.

How could she modify her original diet to reduce her energy intake, provide the essential nutrients she needs, and still fit her busy schedule?

Answer:

A Changing World: Influences on Adolescent Nutrition

The world of an adolescent changes from day to day, and nutrition is generally not a major concern. Marked psychosocial changes occur at this time. Teens are searching for their own identities and at the same time are afraid of some of the physical and social consequences of maturation. Social activities, peer pressure, and convenience are more important determinants of food intake and eating habits than is health. There is no sense of urgency about consuming a diet to reduce the risk of developing chronic disease. Nutrition concerns focus instead on environmental issues, appearance, weight loss or gain for appearance or athletic performance, or simply a full stomach. Factors outside the home, such as the use of drugs and alcohol, and other lifestyle choices that may have an impact on nutrition have more and more influence on what foods teens choose.

Environmental Concerns Many teens today are turning to vegetarian eating. According to one survey, 37% of teens said they try to avoid red meat,[42] and on any given day, 15% of college students choose vegetarian meals.[43] Some do it for health reasons or to lose weight, but most give up meat because they are concerned about animals and the environment. But vegetarian diets can have an impact on the nutritional health of adolescents. Meatless diets can be low in iron and zinc, and vegan diets, which contain no animal products, may put teens at risk of vitamin B_{12} deficiency and inadequate calcium intake. In addition, vegetarian diets are not necessarily low in fat, particularly if high-fat dairy products are chosen. A slice of cheese pizza and a can of cola provides calcium but is high in fat and low in iron. However, when chosen carefully, a vegetarian diet can be low in fat, saturated fat, and cholesterol and high in complex carbohydrate, fiber, and micronutrients. For example, a vegetarian lunch of a pita sandwich with hummus (chickpeas), tomatoes, and spinach, along with some dried fruit and a glass of reduced-fat milk, is low in fat and contains good sources of calcium and plant sources of iron.

Appearance and Body Image There is probably no other time in life when appearance is of more concern than during adolescence. The hormonal changes of puberty often cause acne, and many teens are unhappy with their bodies. Many girls want to lose weight even if they are not overweight. Many boys, on the other hand, want to gain weight to achieve a muscular, strong appearance.

Acne Acne, which is common in adolescence, is triggered by the hormonal changes that occur with the onset of puberty. At one time, acne was believed to be related to diet, and long lists of foods to avoid were doled out to teens with acne. Since then, restrictions on the intake of foods such as chocolate, french fries, and soft drinks have been found to have no effect on the severity of acne. Anxiety, lack of sleep, and hormonal fluctuations of the menstrual cycle are more likely to cause acne flare-ups than specific foods, but a well-balanced diet will ensure that the skin has all the nutrients needed to maintain its integrity. Medications are also available to treat acne. A prescription medication which is a derivative of vitamin A, called 13-cis-retinoic acid (Accutane), can be taken orally

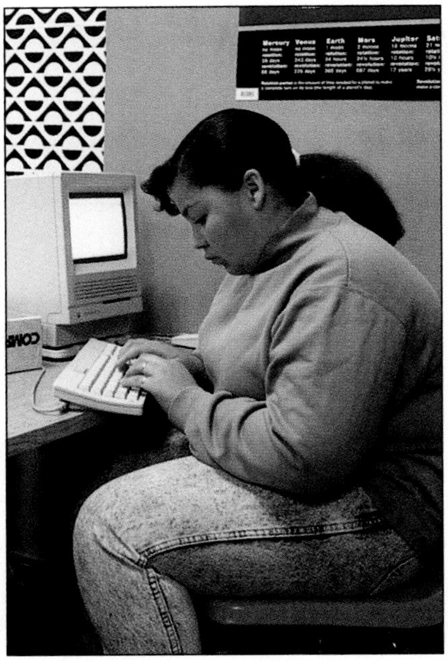

Figure 14.15
The prevalence of obesity is increasing among teens in the United States. (© Lawrence Migdale/Photo Researchers, Inc.)

to treat a severe form of acne called cystic acne. Another prescription vitamin A derivative, called Retin-A, is used topically to treat acne. In addition to reducing acne, Retin-A tightens the skin and decreases wrinkles, making it a popular drug with older adults. Neither Accutane nor Retin-A should be used during pregnancy. Although these drugs are derivatives of vitamin A, vitamin A supplements cannot be substituted as a treatment for acne. In addition, large doses of vitamin A are toxic.

Obesity Because of the importance of physical appearance during adolescence, being overweight can be particularly devastating. Obese adolescents may be discriminated against by adults as well as by their peers. This can lead to feelings of rejection, social isolation, and low self-esteem. The isolation of obese adolescents from teen society results in boredom, depression, inactivity, and withdrawal—all of which can cause an increase in eating and a decrease in energy output, worsening the problem (Figure 14.15).

Adolescent weight-loss diets should be carefully planned to supply essential nutrients for growth without excess energy. Meals should be low in fat and high in whole grains, vegetables, and fruits. Breakfast and lunch should not be skipped because this may actually increase energy intake by increasing the amount of food consumed later in the day. Behavior modification and increased physical activity are essential components of a weight-management program for adolescents. When planning meals and overall weight-management strategy, the social as well as physiological needs of the teen should be considered. Weight-management methods should not lead to isolation from peers. Planning ahead can help manage the eating that occurs at social events. For example, a teenage girl attempting to manage a weight problem might plan for a pizza party by deciding what she will eat earlier in the day and how many slices of pizza she will eat at the party. This plan may also allow for some extra kcalories on that day. Even if she eats more than she planned at the party, she should continue her low-energy eating plan the next day.

Eating Disorders Eating disorders are more common in adolescence than at any other time in life. The pressure of taking on the responsibilities of adulthood, combined with pressure from peers and society to be thin, may contribute to this high incidence. Many individuals with eating disorders feel ineffectual in their lives and may be using food to achieve some measure of self-control. Bulimia nervosa is an eating disorder characterized by a pattern of binge eating followed by inappropriate compensatory behavior, such as purging with self-induced vomiting or laxative abuse, or by other behaviors to eliminate the extra energy, such as dieting or exercise. When total food intake is extremely restricted and weight loss becomes severe, anorexia nervosa results. This eating disorder may cause so much weight loss that it can be fatal. Females are particularly at risk, but eating disorders also occur in males (see Chapter 7). Disordered eating is often hidden by other eating patterns. For example, vegetarian adolescent females were twice as likely as nonvegetarians to report frequent dieting, four times as likely to report intentional vomiting, and eight times more likely to purge using laxatives.[44]

The Impact of Athletics The desire to perform well in sports can motivate certain eating behaviors. Despite all the benefits of exercise, the nutrition misinformation that is common in school athletics can lead to serious health problems. Excessive use of dietary supplements, the use of anabolic steroids, inappropriate training diets, and fad diets can all cause problems (see Chapter 12).

Teen athletes may require more water, energy, protein, carbohydrate, and micronutrients than their less active peers, but supplements are rarely needed to meet these needs. Fluid should be consumed before, during, and after exercise to prevent dehydration. If the extra energy needs of teen athletes are met with whole grains, fresh fruits and vegetables, and dairy products, their protein, carbohydrate, and micronutrient needs will easily be met. An exception is iron, which may need to be supplemented, particularly in female athletes. The combination of poor iron intake, iron losses from menstruation and sweat, and increased needs for building new lean tissue puts many female athletes at risk for iron deficiency anemia (see Chapter 12).[45]

Some of the most dangerous practices associated with adolescent sports are those that attempt to control body weight. Some sports such as football demand that the athlete be large and heavy. Common supplements used to help high school athletes "bulk up" include anabolic steroids, androstenedione, and creatine. Anabolic steroids are illegal, and although they do increase muscle mass, the risks far outweigh the benefits (see Chapter 12, *Off the Shelf: The Anabolic Edge: From Steroids to Creatine*). Androstenedione is a testosterone precursor that is legally sold as a dietary supplement, but the long-term health effects of this supplement have not yet been determined. Creatine, if used correctly, is also associated with an increase in muscle mass, although some of this increase may be water. Creatine improves exercise performance in sports requiring short bursts of activity and has not been associated with serious side effects.[46] Despite the rising popularity of supplements, the best and safest way for young athletes to increase muscle mass is the hard way: Lift weights and eat more.

Female athletes involved in sports that require lean, light bodies, such as gymnastics and ballet, are likely to abuse weight-loss diets. Sexual maturation, which causes an increase in body fat and changes in weight distribution, can be disturbing to young women involved in such sports. This combination of athletic activities and weight loss may affect maturation and increase the risk of developing an eating disorder.[47]

Weight loss is also a concern for adolescents participating in sports such as wrestling that require athletes to fit into a specific weight class on the day of the event. In these athletes, dangerous methods of quick weight loss—such as severe energy intake restriction, water deprivation, vomiting, and diuretic and laxative abuse—are common practice. Low-energy diets can interfere with normal growth and may be too limited in variety to meet these athletes' needs for vitamins and minerals. Even more of a danger is the practice of restricting water intake and encouraging sweat loss to decrease body weight. This may achieve the temporary weight loss necessary to put the athlete in a lower weight class, but dehydration is dangerous and can impair athletic performance.[48]

Sexual Maturity As discussed earlier, sexual maturity in girls affects nutrition because it increases body fat, decreases energy needs, and increases iron needs. The use of oral contraceptives and pregnancy during adolescence can also affect nutritional status.

Oral Contraceptive Use Oral contraceptives may contain either estrogen or progesterone or a combination of the two. These hormones may be prescribed to adolescent girls for a number of reasons and can affect nutrition because they affect nutrient metabolism. Oral contraceptives may cause a rise in fasting blood sugar and a tendency toward abnormal glucose tolerance in those with a family history of diabetes. They may also cause changes in body composition, including weight gain due to water retention and an increase in lean body mass. Oral contraceptives may reduce the need for iron by reducing menstrual flow and increasing iron absorption. Blood levels of vitamin B_{12} have been found to be low in oral contraceptive users,[49] although it is not known whether these changes in blood levels reflect an increased need for this nutrient.

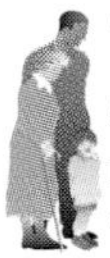

Teenage Pregnancy Because adolescent girls continue to grow and mature for several years after menstruation starts, the pregnant teenager must meet her own nutrient needs for growth and development as well as the needs of pregnancy. This puts the pregnant adolescent at nutritional risk. In order for the mother and fetus to remain healthy, special attention must be paid to all aspects of prenatal care, including nutrient intake (see Chapter 13). Due to the special nutrient needs of this group, the DRIs have included a life-stage group for pregnant girls age 18 or younger. For many nutrients, the recommended intake follows either the needs of adolescence or the needs of pregnancy, but for some, like magnesium, the needs of pregnant teens exceeds the needs of either nonpregnant teens or pregnant women age 19 or older.

Alcohol Use Although it is illegal to sell alcohol to individuals under a certain age (18 to 21 in most states), alcoholic beverages are commonly available at teen social gatherings, and the peer pressure to consume them is strong. Alcohol provides energy—7 kcalories per gram. It is also a drug that has short-term effects that occur soon after ingestion and long-term health consequences that are associated with overuse.

What Are the Immediate Effects of Alcohol Consumption? Alcohol is a small molecule that is rapidly and almost completely absorbed in the upper gastrointestinal tract. Some is absorbed directly from the stomach, so the effects of alcohol consumption are almost immediate, especially if it is consumed on an empty stomach. If there is food in the stomach when alcohol is consumed, less will be absorbed there because less is in contact with the stomach wall. Food also slows stomach emptying and therefore decreases the rate at which alcohol is absorbed in the small intestine. Some alcohol is metabolized by alcohol dehydrogenase in the stomach. Women tend to have less of this stomach enzyme, which may be one reason women become intoxicated after consuming less alcohol than men.

Absorbed alcohol is metabolized in the liver. It is broken down by liver alcohol dehydrogenase to form acetaldehyde, which is then further degraded to form acetyl-CoA. As the molecule is broken down, electrons are released and picked up by NAD, the coenzyme form of niacin. The amount of NAD available to accept electrons from glycolysis and the citric acid cycle is reduced. This inhibits acetyl-CoA from entering the citric acid cycle to produce ATP, so much of the acetyl-CoA generated is used to synthesize fatty acids (Figure 14.16).

The liver can break down about 0.5 oz of alcohol per hour, depending on body size, amount of previous drinking, food intake, and general health. When alcohol intake exceeds the ability of the liver to break it down, the excess circulates in the bloodstream until the liver enzymes can metabolize it. At the kidney, alcohol acts as a diuretic, increasing fluid excretion. Therefore, excessive alcohol intake can cause dehydration. At the brain, alcohol acts as a depressant. First it affects reasoning; if drinking continues, the vision and speech centers of the brain are affected. Next, large-muscle control becomes impaired, causing lack of coordination. Finally, the individual loses consciousness. If drinking were to continue, the anesthetic effects would suppress breathing and heart rate. It is possible for

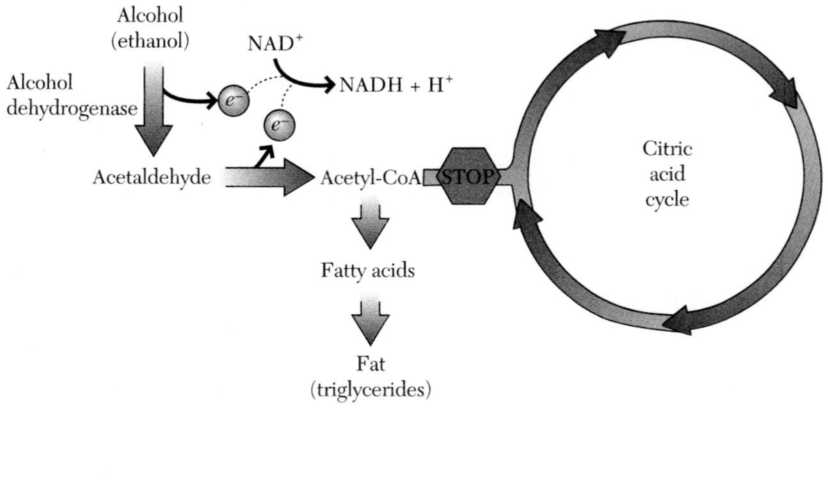

Figure 14.16
The breakdown of alcohol depletes the supply of NAD. This prevents acetyl-CoA from entering the citric acid cycle and diverts it for fat synthesis.

an individual to drink fast enough for alcohol levels to continue to rise after he or she has lost consciousness, resulting in death. This can occur with binge drinking, defined as frequently downing five or more drinks at a time. Binge drinking is a problem on college campuses that causes about 50 deaths and hundreds of cases of alcohol poisoning annually. About 43% of college students are binge drinkers and 21% are frequent binge drinkers; this behavior is most common among members of fraternities and sororities.[50]

Some alcohol is eliminated by the lungs. The amount lost through the lungs is predictable and reliable enough to be used to estimate blood alcohol level from a measure of breath alcohol. This is the basis of the Breathalyzer tests administered by the police to determine if an individual is driving under the influence of alcohol. The effects of alcohol on the central nervous system are what make driving while under the influence of alcohol so dangerous. Alcohol affects reaction time, eye-hand coordination, accuracy, and balance. Not only does alcohol impair one's ability to operate a motor vehicle, but it also impairs one's judgment in the decision to drive.

What Happens With Chronic Alcohol Use? One risk associated with regular alcohol consumption is the possibility of addiction. Alcohol addiction, like any other drug addiction, is a physiological problem that needs treatment. Alcoholism is believed to have a genetic component that makes some people more likely to become addicted, but environment also plays a significant role. Thus, someone with a genetic predisposition toward alcoholism whose peers do not consume alcohol is much less likely to become addicted. In general, the risk of developing chronic alcohol-related diseases is reduced if fewer than two drinks a day are consumed (assumes one drink contains about 0.5 ounce of alcohol, which can be obtained in 5 ounces of wine, 12 ounces of beer, or 1.5 ounces of distilled liquor).

Long-term excessive alcohol consumption has serious health implications. Alcohol either directly or indirectly affects every organ in the body and increases the risk of malnutrition and many chronic diseases. Alcohol contributes energy but few other nutrients and replaces more nutrient-dense energy sources in the diet. Alcohol damages the lining of the small intestine, decreasing the absorption of several B vitamins and vitamin C. Thiamin deficiency is a particular concern with chronic alcohol consumption. Alcohol can also alter the storage, metabolism, and excretion of other vitamins and some minerals.

The most significant physiological effects of chronic alcohol consumption occur in the liver. Alcoholic liver disease progresses in a number of phases. The first phase is **fatty liver,** a condition that occurs when alcohol consumption increases the synthesis and deposition of fat in the liver. The second phase, **alcoholic hepatitis,** is an inflammation of the liver. Both of these conditions are reversible if alcohol consumption is stopped and good nutritional and health practices are followed. If alcohol consumption continues, **cirrhosis** may develop. This is an irreversible condition in which fibrous deposits scar the liver and interfere with its function. Since the liver is the primary site of many metabolic reactions, cirrhosis is often fatal (Figure 14.17). In addition to causing liver disease, heavy drinking is associated with hypertension, heart disease, and stroke.

Fatty liver The accumulation of fat in the liver.

Alcoholic hepatitis Inflammation of the liver caused by alcohol consumption.

Cirrhosis Chronic liver disease characterized by the loss of functioning liver cells and the accumulation of fibrous connective tissue.

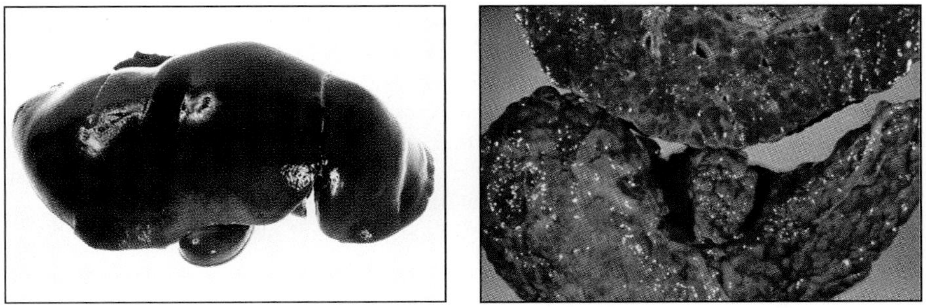

Figure 14.17
Chronic alcohol consumption can cause permanent liver damage. A normal liver is shown on the left, and a cirrhotic liver is shown on the right. (*Left,* Custom Medical Stock Photo; *right,* Phil Birn/Custom Medical Stock Photo)

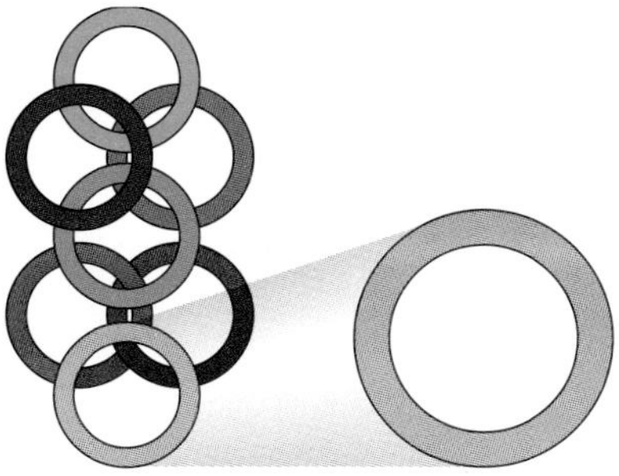

If you drink alcoholic beverages, do so in moderation

Figure 14.18
The Dietary Guidelines for Americans recommend that alcohol be consumed in moderation. (USDA, DHHS, 1995)

Safe Drinking Although moderate alcohol consumption is associated with a reduction in the risk of heart disease in some individuals, there are certain groups who should not drink, such as children, women who are pregnant or trying to conceive, alcoholics, individuals who plan to drive or engage in another activity that requires attention or skill, and individuals using prescription or over-the-counter medication[13] (see Chapter 15, *Off the Shelf: Alcohol: A Risk-Benefit Analysis*). Excess alcohol consumption, whether occasional or chronic, is hazardous to health. Individuals who do drink should not drink in excess (Figure 14.18). When alcohol is consumed, it should be consumed slowly with meals. Alcohol absorption is slowed when it is consumed with high-protein or high-carbohydrate foods. Also, the alcohol in an alcoholic punch is absorbed faster if mixed with a carbonated beverage than with a noncarbonated fruit juice base. It usually takes an hour to metabolize the alcohol in one drink (0.5 oz), so no more than one drink should be consumed every 1.5 hours. Sipping, not gulping, allows the liver time to break down what has already been consumed. Alternating nonalcoholic and alcoholic drinks will also slow down the rate of alcohol intake and prevent dehydration.

Unfortunately, once alcohol has been consumed, the rate at which it is metabolized and eliminated from the body cannot be accelerated. Cold showers, brisk walks, and black coffee may wake you up, but they will not sober you up.

APPLICATIONS

These exercises are designed to help you apply your critical thinking skills to your own nutrition choices. Many are best performed using a diet analysis software program. If you do not have access to a computer program, these exercises can be hand-calculated using the information in this text and its appendices.

1. Assume you had a Big Mac, fries, and a 16-ounce cola for lunch.
   a. How many servings from each food group of the Food Guide Pyramid does this represent?
   b. List the numbers of additional servings from each food group that you would need to satisfy the daily recommendations of the Food Guide Pyramid.
   c. Select foods from each group to complete your intake for the day.
   d. Do the foods you selected meet the selection recommendations of the Food Guide Pyramid and your energy needs?
2. The table gives height and weight measurements recorded for a girl from age six to age nine.
   a. Plot these values on the growth chart in Appendix B.
   b. What recommendations would you have about her weight?

Age	Height (in.)	Weight (lb)
6	45	44
7	48	53
8	50	77
9	52	97

3. Use the Internet or a diet analysis computer program to look up the nutrient composition of your favorite fast-food meal. What is the percent of kcalories from carbohydrate and fat in the meal?

Summary

1. Good nutrition in childhood sets the stage for nutrition and health in the adult years. The diet must meet the needs for growth and development as well as reduce the risk of chronic disease later in life. Growth that follows standard patterns indicates adequate nutrition. Obese children are likely to become obese adults and children with elevated blood pressure and blood cholesterol are more likely to have hypertension and heart disease as adults.
2. Introducing solid foods between four and six months of age adds iron and other nutrients to the diet and aids in muscle development. Newly introduced foods should be appropriate to the child's stage of development and offered one at a time to monitor for food allergies.
3. Food allergies are caused by the absorption of allergens, most of which are proteins. Food allergies involve the immune system and are more common in infancy because the infant's immature gastrointestinal tract is likely to absorb whole proteins. Specific foods that cause allergies can be identified

by an elimination diet. Unlike food allergies, food intolerances do not involve the immune system.

4. Children like to have control over what they eat. In order to meet nutrient needs and develop nutritious habits, a variety of healthy foods should be offered at meals and snacks throughout the day.
5. Energy and protein needs per kilogram of body weight decrease as children grow, but total needs increase because of the increase in total body weight and activity level. Beginning at two years of age, fat intake should be decreased gradually to 30% or less of energy. Dietary carbohydrates should come primarily from whole grains, vegetables, fruits, and milk.
6. Low dietary intakes of vitamin A, vitamin C, calcium, iron, and zinc put some American children at risk of deficiencies. Meals away from home at school or fast-food restaurants are common and impact overall nutrient intake.
7. During adolescence, accelerated growth and sexual maturation have an impact on nutrient requirements. Body composition and the nutritional requirements of boys and girls diverge. Males gain more lean body tissue, while females have a greater increase in body fat.
8. During the adolescent growth spurt, total energy and protein requirements are higher than at any other time of life. Young men require more protein and energy than young women.
9. In adolescence, vitamin requirements increase to meet the needs of rapid growth. The minerals calcium, iron, and zinc are likely to be low in the adolescent diet. Iron deficiency anemia is common, especially in girls as they begin losing iron through menstruation.
10. The food intake of adolescents may be determined more by social activities, peer pressure, and participation in athletics than by nutrient needs. Since meals are frequently missed, healthy snacks should be included in the diet.
11. Psychosocial changes occurring during the adolescent years make physical appearance of great concern. Obesity can be psychologically and socially devastating. Eating disorders are more common in adolescence than at any other time. Adolescent athletes are susceptible to nutrition misinformation, and they may try dangerous practices such as using anabolic steroids to increase muscle mass or fad diets and fluid restriction to lose weight.
12. During the teen years, pregnancy, the use of oral contraceptives, and the consumption of alcohol may affect nutritional status.
13. Alcohol has short-term effects on the central nervous system, including the impairment of reasoning, judgment, and coordination, and eventually the loss of consciousness. Chronic alcohol use damages the liver and can cause malnutrition by decreasing nutrient intake and absorption and interfering with nutrient utilization.

Review Questions

1. How does nutrient intake during childhood affect health later in life?
2. What is the best way to determine if a child is eating enough?
3. What impact does parents' weight have on a child's weight?
4. When should solid and semisolid foods be introduced into an infant's diet?
5. How should new foods be introduced to monitor for the development of food allergies?
6. What factors influence the maximum height a child will reach?
7. How do the recommendations for fat intake change when a child reaches the age of two years?
8. Why is anemia a problem in young children? In teenage girls?
9. Why are snacks an important part of children's diets?
10. Why is breakfast important?
11. What nutritional problems can be signaled by sudden changes in weight patterns?
12. How can fast foods be incorporated into a healthy diet?
13. What is the adolescent growth spurt? How does it affect nutrient requirements?
14. Describe two physiological differences between males and females after puberty that affect their nutrient needs.
15. Why are teenagers particularly susceptible to eating disorders?
16. How can alcohol consumption affect nutritional status?

Nutrition Web Links

To further explore areas related to the material in this chapter, go to the *Nutrition: Science and Applications* Web site at ***www.Wiley.com/college/Smolin*** and *click on* **Student Companion Site** for chapter-by-chapter links. Some Web sites related to the information in Chapter 14 include:

Organizations that provide nutrition recommendations for children such as the American Academy of Pediatrics and the Nemours Foundation.

Locations that provide information on weight management for children such as the Weight-Control Information Network and the American Heart Association.

Organizations that provide information on food allergies such as the American Dietetic Association and the Food Allergy Network.

References

1. Nicklas, T. A., O'Neil, C. E., and Berenson, G. S. Nutrient contribution of breakfast, secular trends, and the role of ready-to-eat cereals: a review of the data form the Bogalusa Heart Study. Am. J. Clin. Nutr. 67:757S–763S, 1998.
2. Kennedy, E., and David, C. USDA School Breakfast Program. Am. J. Clin. Nutr. 67:798S–803S, 1998.
3. Nahikian-Nelms, M. Influential factors of caregivers' behaviors at mealtime: a study of 24 child care providers. J. Am. Diet. Assoc. 97:505–509, 1997.
4. Grantham-McGregor, S. A review of studies of the effect of severe malnutrition on mental development. J. Nutr. 125:2233S–2238S, 1995.
5. Evers, C. Empower children to develop healthful eating habits. J. Am. Diet. Assoc. 97(suppl):S116, 1997.
6. Barlow, S. E., and Dietz, W. H. Obesity evaluation and treatment: Expert Committee recommendations. The Maternal and Child Health Bureau, Health Resources and Services Administration and the Department of Health and Human Services. Pediatrics 102:E29, 1998.
7. Kennedy, E., and Goldberg, J. What are American children eating? Implications for public policy. Nutr. Rev. 53:111–126, 1995.
8. Nutrition and Health Promotion Program, International Life Sciences Institute. A survey of parents and children about physical activity patterns. September–October 1996. Key findings online at http://www.ilsi.org/nhppress.html#2
9. National Association for Sports and Physical Activity. Physical activity guidelines for preadolescent children. 1998. Online at http://www.aahperd.org/naspe/PressRelease.htm
10. McDowell, M. A., Briefel, R. R., Alaimo, K., et al. Energy and macronutrient intakes of persons 2 months and over in the United States. *Third National Health and Nutrition Examination Survey, Phase I, 1988–1991.* Advance data from Vital and Health Statistics: No. 255. Hyattsville, Md.: NCHS, 1994.
11. Ernst, N., and Obarzanek, E. Child health and nutrition: obesity and high blood cholesterol. Prev. Med. 23:427–436, 1994.
12. Berenson, G. S., Wattigney, W. A., Srinivasan, S. R., and Radhakrishnamurthy, B. Rationale to study the early natural history of heart disease: the Bogalusa Heart Study. Am. J. Med. Sci. 310(suppl):22S–28S, 1995.
13. U.S. Department of Agriculture, U.S. Department of Health and Human Services. *Nutrition and Your Health: Dietary Guidelines for Americans*, 4th ed. Home and Garden Bulletin No. 232. Hyattsville, Md.: U.S. Government Printing Office, 1995.
14. Bao, W., Threefoot, S. A., Srinivasan, S. R., and Berenson, G. S. Essential hypertension predicted by tracking of elevated blood pressure from childhood to adulthood: the Bogalusa Heart Study. Am. J. Hypertens. 8:657–661, 1995.
15. Chandra, R. K. Food hypersensitivities and allergic disease: a selective review. Am. J. Clin. Nutr. 66(suppl):526S–529S, 1997.
16. Kleinman, R. E., Finberg, L. F., Klish, W. J., and Lauer, R. N. Dietary guidelines for children: U.S. recommendations. J. Nutr. 126:1028S–1030S, 1996.
17. American Dietetic Association. Position of the American Dietetic Association: child and adolescent food and nutrition programs. J. Am. Diet. Assoc. 96:913–917, 1996.
18. Zive, M. M., Taras, H. L., Broyles, S. L., et al. Vitamin and mineral intakes of Anglo-American and Mexican-American preschoolers. J. Am. Diet. Assoc. 95:329–335, 1995.
19. Tippett, K. S., Mickle, S. J., Goldman, J. D., et al. Food and nutrient intake by individuals in the United States, 1 day 1989–1991. Nationwide Food Surveys Report No. 91–92, 1995.
20. Centers for Disease Control and Prevention. Recommendations to prevent and control iron deficiency in the United States. MMWR Morb. Mortal. Wkly. Rep. 47:1–29, 1998. Online at www.cdc.gov/epo/mmwr/mmwr_rr.html
21. Pollitt, E. Iron deficiency and educational deficiency. Nutr. Rev. 55:133–141, 1997
22. Hingley, A. T. Preventing childhood poisoning. FDA Consumer 30:7–11, March 1996.
23. U.S. Food and Drug Administration. Iron-containing supplements and drugs: label warning statements and unit-dose packaging requirements. Federal Register, January 1997.
24. Wolraich, M. L., Wilson, D. B., and White, J. W. The effect of sugar on behavior or cognition in children: a meta analysis. J.A.M.A. 274: 1617–1618, 1995.
25. Breakey, J. The role of diet and behavior in childhood. J. Paediatr. Child Health 33:190–194, 1997.
26. Farley, D. Dangers of lead still linger. FDA Consumer 32:16–21, January/February, 1998.
27. Hammad, T. A., Sexton, M., and Langenberg, P. Relationship between blood lead and dietary iron intake in preschool children. Annals Epidemiol. 6:30–33, 1996.
28. Needleman, H. L., Reiss, J. A., Tobin, M. J., et al. Bone lead levels and delinquent behavior J.A.M.A. 275:363–369, 1996.
29. Fackelmann, K. Hypertension's lead connection: does low-level exposure to lead cause high blood pressure? Sci. News 149:382–383, 1996.
30. Update: blood lead levels—United States, 1991–1994. MMWR, Morb. Mortal. Wkly. Rep. 46:141–146, 1997.
31. U.S. Department of Agriculture. Nutrition Program Facts: National School Lunch Program: Qs and As on the National School Lunch Program. Online at http://www.usda.gov/fcs/cnp/school%7e2.htm
32. Gortmaker, S. I., Must, A., Sobol, and A. M. Television viewing as a cause for increasing obesity among children in the United States. Arch. Pediatr. Adolesc. Med. 150:356–360, 1996.
33. Sylvester, G. P., Achterberg, C., and Williams, J. Children's television and nutrition: friends or foes? Nutrition Today 30:6–15, February 1995.
34. Andersen, R. E., Crespo, C. J., Bartlett, S. J., et al. Relationship of physical activity and television watching with body weight and level of fatness among children: results from the third National Health and Nutrition Examination Survey. J.A.M.A. 279:938–942, 1998.
35. Institute of Medicine, Food and Nutrition Board. *Dietary Reference Intakes for Calcium, Phosphorus, Magnesium, Vitamin D, and Fluoride.* Washington, D.C.: National Academy Press, 1997.
36. Mitchell, M. K. *Nutrition Across the Life Span*, Philadelphia: W. B. Saunders, 1997.
37. Slyper, A. H. Childhood obesity, adipose tissue distribution and the pediatric practitioner. Pediatrics 102:e4, 1998.
38. USDA Agriculture Research Service. 1997 Results from USDA's 1994–1996 CSFII and 1994–1996 Diet and Health Knowledge Survey. ARS Food Surveys Research Group. Online at http://www.bare.usda.gov/bhnrc/foodsurvey/home.htm
39. Calvo, M. S., and Park, Y. K. Changing phosphorus content of the U.S. diet: potential for adverse effect on bone. J. Nutr. 126:1168S–1180S, 1996.
40. Centers for Disease Control and Prevention. Youth risk behavior surveillance, United States, 1997. CDC Surveillance Summaries, August 14, 1998. MMWR Morb. Mortal. Wkly. Rep. 47:1–89, 1998. Online at http://www.cdc.gov/epo/mmwr/mmwr_ss.html
41. U.S. Department of Agriculture, Human Nutrition Information Service. Food and nutrient intakes by individuals in the United States, 1 day, 1989. Nationwide Food Consumption Survey 1987088. NFCS Report No. 87-I-1, 1993.
42. Kaufman, L., Springen, K., Rogers, A., and Gordon, J. Children of the corn. Newsweek: 60–62, August 28, 1995.
43. Curcio, B. A. For college students, bulgur beats burgers. Eating Well: 21, September/October 1995.
44. Neumark-Sztainer, D., Story, M., Resnick, M. D., and Blum, R. W. Adolescent vegetarianism: a behavioral profile of a school-based population in Minnesota. Arch. Pediatr. Adolesc. Med. 151:833–838, 1997.

45. American Dietetic Association. Timely statement of the American Dietetic Association: nutrition guidance for adolescent athletes in organized sports. J. Am. Diet. Assoc. 96:611–612, 1996.
46. Greenhaff, P. L. Creatine and its application as an ergogenic aid. Int. J. Sport Nutr. 5:S100–110, 1995.
47. Beals, K. A., and Manore, M. M. Nutritional status of female athletes with subclinical eating disorders. J. Am. Diet. Assoc. 98:419–425, 1998.
48. Bazzarre, T. L. Nutrition and strength. In *Nutrition in Exercise and Sport*, 3rd ed. Wolinski, I., ed. Boca Raton, Fla.: CRC Press, 1998, 369–419.
49. Green,T. J., Houghton, L. A., Donovan,U., et al. Oral contraceptives did not affect biochemical folate indexes and homocysteine concentrations in adolescent females. J. Am. Diet. Assoc. 98:49–54, 1998.
50. Wechsler H., Dowdall, G. W., Maenner, G., et al. Changes in binge drinking and related problems among American college students between 1993 and 1997. Results of the Harvard School of Public Health College Alcohol Study. J. Am. Coll. Health 47:57–68, 1998.

Chapter

15

Chapter Outline

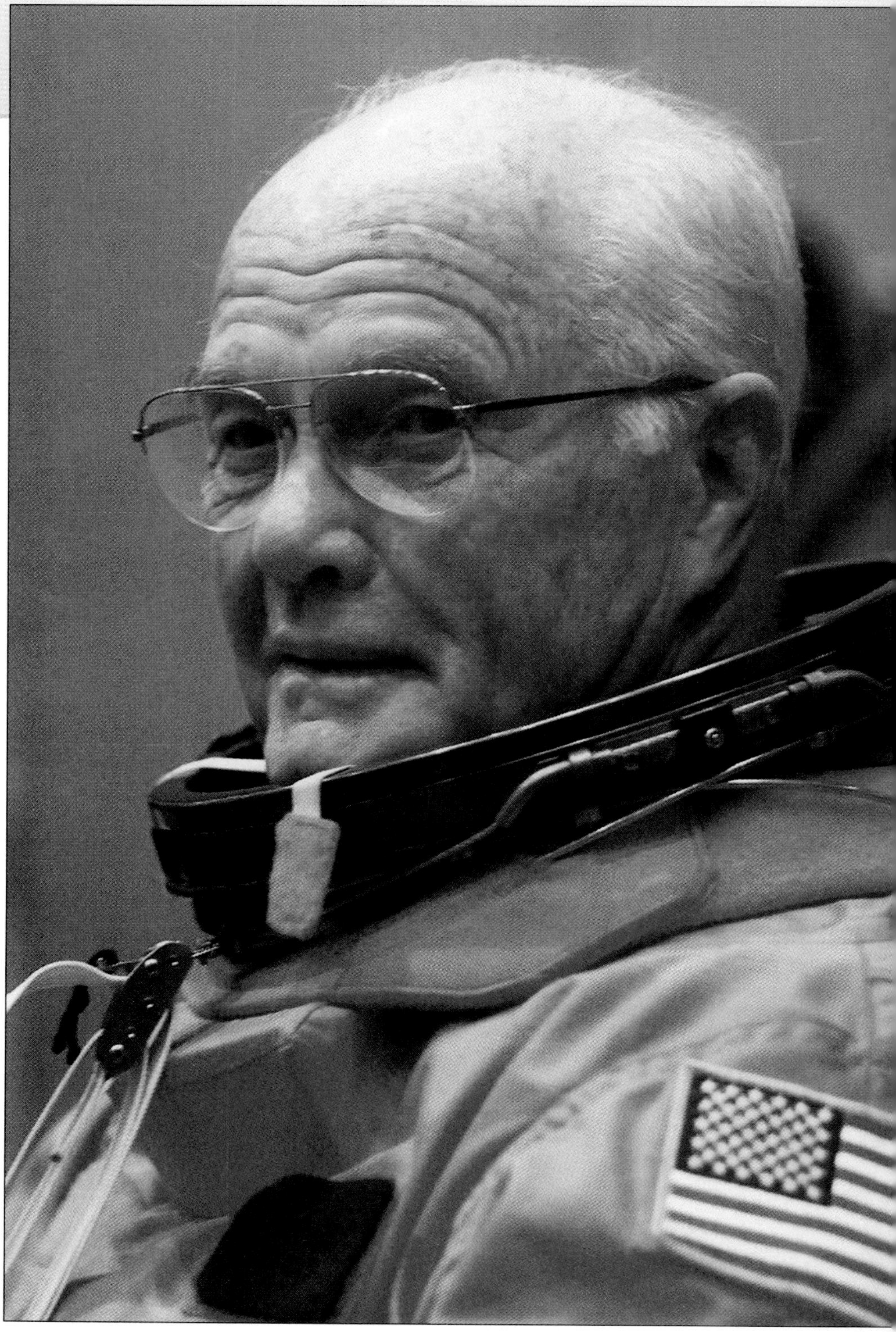

(© AP Photo)

Nutrition and Aging: The Adult Years

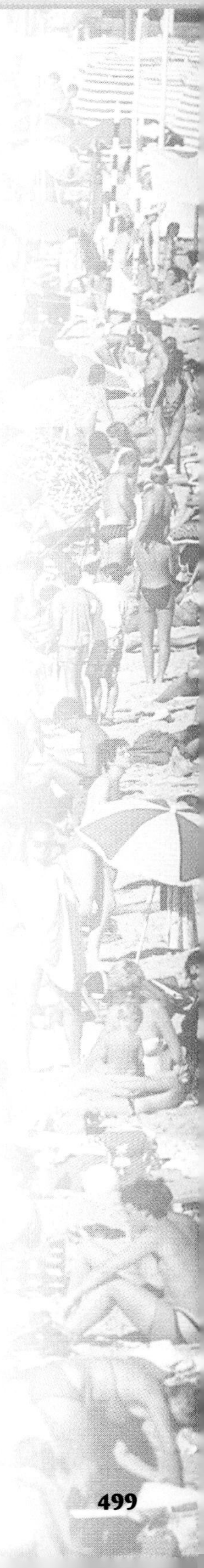

Chapter Concepts

1. Aging is the accumulation of changes that occur over a lifetime, resulting in an increasing susceptibility to malnutrition, disease, and death.
2. With advances in medicine and technology, Americans on average are living longer than ever before; now the goal is to increase the number of healthy years.
3. The risk of malnutrition increases with age because of physiological, medical, social, and economic changes that affect the ability to obtain, prepare, and consume an adequate diet.
4. With aging come physiological changes in sensory abilities, digestion and metabolism, hormonal balance, immune function, and body composition that affect nutritional status.
5. Aging increases the likelihood of disease and disability. These conditions may impair mobility, reduce mental capacity, and increase the use of medications—each of which can increase the risk of malnutrition.
6. Social and economic changes that occur with increasing age can also affect access to food and the risk of malnutrition.
7. A healthy lifestyle, including exercise and a nutritious diet, can prevent or postpone some of the degenerative changes that occur with aging.
8. Older adults need to consume nutrient-dense diets because their energy needs are decreased but their nutrient needs remain the same.
9. Meeting the nutritional needs of older adults requires consideration of their social, economic, and medical needs.

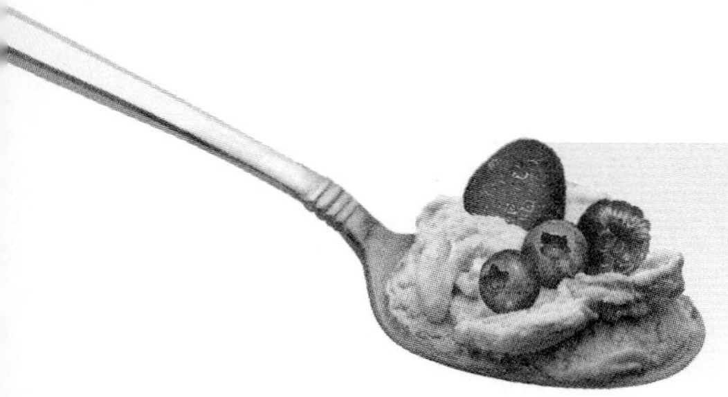

Just a Taste

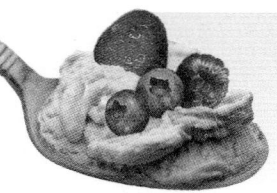

Can consuming a healthy diet delay the changes that occur with aging?

Is malnutrition inevitable in the elderly?

Can antioxidant supplements slow aging?

We are all getting older in a society obsessed with youth. Youth symbolizes beauty, fitness, and health. Aging is symbolized by gray hair, wrinkled skin, weak bodies, and forgetful minds. Are these unavoidable changes that occur with age, or can the diet and lifestyle choices we make slow or prevent these changes?

When trying to stop the physiological clock, nutrition is not always the first place people turn. They cover gray hair with dyes and washes and soften and fade wrinkles with creams, cleansers, and plastic surgery. These methods result only in cosmetic changes that help people look younger. They do not help maintain vitality at a youthful level. On the other hand, a healthy lifestyle may not remove the crow's feet, but it can affect the health and vitality of one's later years.

The discovery of areas of the world where inhabitants supposedly lived to a very old age generated hope that certain foods could extend life. Although the elderly in these regions are now believed to be no older than individuals throughout the rest of the world, they do remain healthier.[1] They are not overweight, hypertension is rare, and the incidence of both heart disease and osteoporosis is low. No one food has been determined to be common among these people, but there are a number of lifestyle similarities: All are societies in which people are physically active, consume largely vegetarian diets, and provide strong psychosocial support for the elderly. This suggests that although life is not extended by changes in lifestyle, the physiological changes, nutritional problems, and chronic illness common in old age can be postponed by a healthy diet and lifestyle.

Postponing the changes of aging is an important public health goal for the new millennium. Currently over 34 million Americans are over 65 years of age. It is estimated that this number will double to about 70 million by the year 2030. Because the incidence of disease and disability increases with increasing age, this older population accounts for a large part of the public health budget. Thus, keeping older adults healthy is beneficial not only for those individuals but for the national health-care system as well.[2]

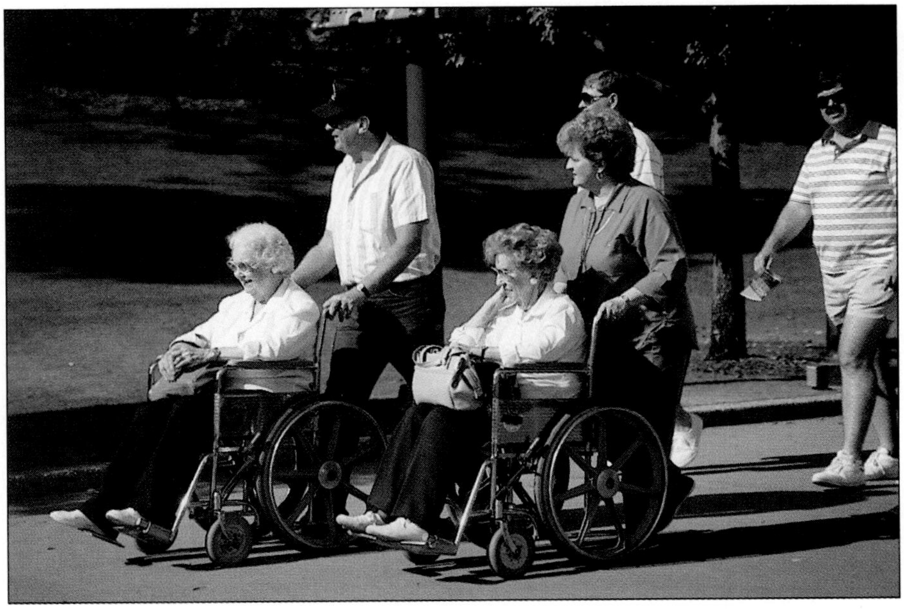

Figure 15.1
The diversity of health condition and physical ability among the elderly is greater than in other age groups. (© Dee Read/Visuals Unlimited)

What Is Aging?

Biologically, aging is not something that begins at age 55, 65, or 75; it is a process that begins with conception and continues throughout life (Figure 15.1). It can be defined as the inevitable accumulation of changes with time that are associated with and responsible for an ever-increasing susceptibility to disease and death. As organisms become older, the number of cells decreases and the function of the remaining cells declines. As tissues and organs lose cells, the ability of the organism to perform the physiological functions necessary to maintain homeostasis decreases; disease becomes increasingly common and the risk of malnutrition increases. Although universal to all living things, aging is a process we don't fully understand. How long we live and how long we remain healthy are affected by our genetic makeup and the environment and lifestyle in which we spend our years.

Who Is Old?

We are all aging. But when do we become "old"? Often the definition of "old" depends on who is defining the term. To a 5-year-old, anyone over age 15 seems old, but to a healthy 80-year-old, "old" may mean 90. Also, chronological age is not always the best indicator of health. A person who is chronologically 75 may have the vigor and health of someone only 55, or vice versa. There are 70-year-olds riding bicycles and others in wheelchairs; some are healthy, independent, and active, while others are chronically ill, dependent, and at high risk for malnutrition.

Although there is great diversity among the elderly, for the purposes of discussion in this chapter we will define older adults as those individuals 65 years of age and older; individuals 55 to 64 years of age are "approaching old age," the "young old" are those aged 65 to 74, "old" individuals are those aged 75 to 84, and the "oldest old" are those 85 years of age and older.[3]

What Causes Aging?

There are two major hypotheses to explain why aging occurs. One favors the idea of a genetic clock and argues that the cell death associated with aging is a genetically programmed event. The other views the events of aging as the result of cellular wear and tear. The actual cause of the cell death associated with aging is probably some combination of both of these, and the rate at which cell death occurs and at which aging proceeds is determined by the interplay among genetics, environment, and lifestyle.

Programmed Cell Death One hypothesis about aging proposes that cell death is triggered when genes that disrupt cell function are activated.[4] This causes the selective, orderly death of individual cells or groups of cells and is referred to as **programmed cell death.** This hypothesis is supported by the fact that cells grown in the laboratory divide only a certain number of times before they die. Cells from older individuals will divide fewer times than those from younger individuals, and those from longer-lived species will divide more times than those from shorter-lived species. If cells in an organism stop reproducing and continue to die, the total number of cells will decline, resulting in a loss of organ function.

Programmed cell death The death of cells at specific predictable times.

Wear and Tear Another hypothesis suggests that aging is the result of an accumulation of cellular damage. This wear and tear may result from errors in DNA synthesis, increases in glucose levels, or free radicals. Free radicals are reactive chemical substances that are generated from both normal metabolic processes and exposure to environmental factors. They cause oxidative damage to proteins, lipids, carbohydrates, and DNA, and may also indirectly harm cells by producing toxic products. For example, age spots—brown spots that appear on the skin with age—are caused by the oxidation of lipids, which produces a pigment called lipofuscin, or age pigment. The damage done to cells by free radicals is associated with aging and has been implicated in the development of a number of chronic diseases common among the aging, including cardiovascular disease and cancer.

Genetics, Environment, and Lifestyle The rate at which the changes associated with aging accumulate depends on genetics, environment, and lifestyle. Genes determine the efficiency with which cells are maintained and repaired. Individuals with less cellular repair capacity will lose cells and consequently age more quickly. Likewise, genes determine susceptibility to age-related diseases such as cardiovascular disease and cancer. However, individuals who inherit a low capacity to repair cellular damage may live long lives if they live in an environment with few factors that damage cells and if they eat well and exercise regularly. In contrast, individuals with exceptional cellular repair ability may accumulate cell damage rapidly if they smoke cigarettes, consume a diet high in fat and low in antioxidant nutrients, and live sedentary lives. No matter what individuals' genes predict about how long they will live, their actual **longevity** is also affected by lifestyle factors and the extent to which they are able avoid accidents and disease (see *Critical Thinking: Can Your Diet Keep You Young?*).

Longevity The duration of an individual's life.

How Long Can We Expect to Live?

The maximum age to which any human can live—the **life span**—is about 100 to 120 years. Most individuals do not live that long. **Life expectancy,** the average length of time that a person can be expected to live, varies between and within populations. It is affected by genetics, lifestyle, and environmental factors. In the United States in 1900, life expectancy was 50 years, but today, with advances in technology and improved nutrition and health care, the average is over 75 years.[5] African Americans have a life expectancy of 69.3 years; whites, 76.3 years; and Hispanics, 79.1 years.[6] Women in the United States on average live longer than men; white women live to be 79.6 years versus 72.9 years for men. African American women live an average of 73.8 years compared to 64.4 years for African American men.[6]

Life span The maximum age to which members of a species can live.

Life expectancy The average length of life for a population of individuals.

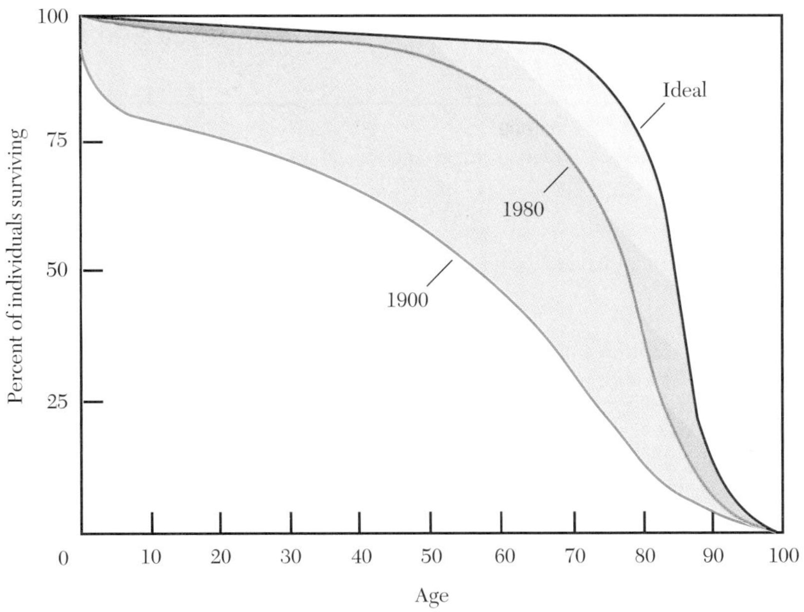

Figure 15.2
This graph illustrates the effect of compression of morbidity on survival in a population. The decline in deaths from infectious diseases between 1900 and 1980 allowed more people to survive into adulthood. Delaying the onset of chronic diseases will allow more people to remain healthy and survive into their seventies and eighties. (Adapted from Fries, J. F. Aging, natural death, and the compression of morbidity. N. Engl. J. Med. 303:130–135, 1980.)

How Long Can We Expect to Be Healthy?

Even though average life expectancy in the United States has increased to over 75 years, the average healthy life span is only about 64 years. The last 11 years of life are often restricted by disease and disability, which become more and more common with advancing age.[7] The goal of successful aging is to increase not only life expectancy but the number of years of healthy life that an individual can expect. This is achieved by slowing the changes that accumulate over time and postponing the diseases of aging long enough to approach or reach the limits of life span before any symptoms appear. This is referred to as **compression of morbidity.** When applied to the population as a whole, this term means that people are healthier and living longer (Figure 15.2); applied to the individual, it means staying healthy until the limits of life span are reached.

Compression of morbidity The postponement of the onset of chronic disease such that disability occupies a smaller and smaller proportion of the life span.

Maintaining and improving the health and well-being of older individuals has been called one of the greatest social challenges of the next century.[8] Currently 13% of the population of the United States is over 65 years of age; early in the next century, one out of every five people will be over 65 (Figure 15.3). The fastest-growing segment of the population in industrialized nations is the oldest

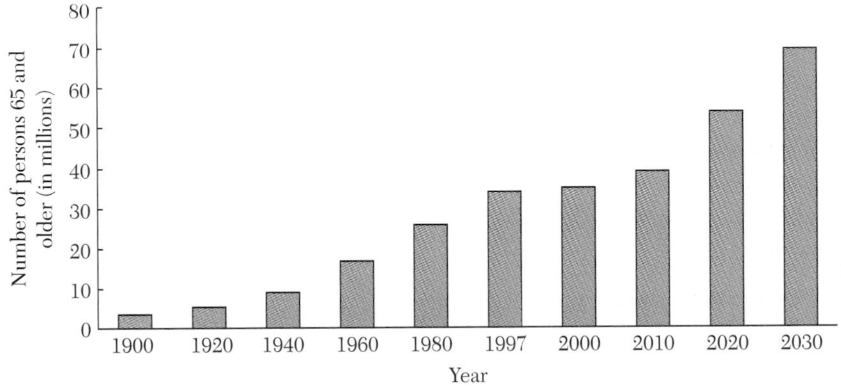

Figure 15.3
The number of people in the population who are age 65 or older has been increasing over the last century. By early in the next century it is projected that there will be almost 70 million people in the United States who are 65 or older. (Based on data from the U.S. Bureau of the Census. From the Administration on Aging. Information can be found online at http://www.aoa.dhhs.gov/aoa/stats/profile/default.htm #table1)

Table 15.1 *Factors That Increase the Risk of Malnutrition Among the Elderly*

Reduced food intake due to:
- Decreased appetite due to lack of exercise, depression, or social isolation
- Changes in taste, smell, and vision
- Dental problems
- Limitations in mobility
- Medications that restrict meal times or affect appetite
- Lack of money to buy food
- Lack of nutrition knowledge

Reduced nutrient absorption and utilization due to:
- Gastrointestinal changes
- Medications that affect absorption
- Diseases such as diabetes, kidney disease, alcoholism, and gastrointestinal disease

Increased requirements due to:
- Illness with fever or infection
- Injury or surgery

Increased losses due to:
- Medications that increase excretion of nutrients
- Diseases such as gastrointestinal and kidney disease

old—individuals over the age of 85.[9] Increasing the number of healthy years enjoyed by older adults is a major public health goal of Healthy People 2010.[7] Compression of morbidity benefits not only aging individuals but also the family members who must find the time and resources to care for them and the public health programs that attempt to meet their needs.

Malnutrition and Aging

Aging increases the risk of malnutrition. Although the aging process itself is usually not a cause of malnutrition in healthy active adults, nutritional health can be compromised by conditions that become increasingly common with advancing age[10] (see Table 15.1). Any circumstance, whether physical, psychological, emotional, social, or economic, that interferes with the availability of or the ability to acquire desirable foods in socially acceptable ways can lead to **food insecurity,** and, subsequently, malnutrition. It is estimated that from 2.5 to 4.9 million older Americans experience food insecurity in any given six-month period.[11] Yet this situation is often not recognized by health-care professionals or other caregivers.[12]

Food insecurity An inability to acquire appropriate foods in a socially acceptable way.

To address concerns over the nutritional health of the elderly, the federal Nutrition Screening Initiative was developed to promote screening for and intervention in nutrition-related problems in older adults.[13] This program recommends methods for increasing the awareness of nutritional problems in the elderly by involving practitioners and community organizations as well as relatives, friends, and others caring for the elderly in evaluating the nutritional status of the aging population. This program developed the DETERMINE checklist (see Table 15.2) based on an acronym for the physiological, medical, and socioeconomic situations that increase the risk of malnutrition among the elderly. The elderly themselves, family members, and caregivers can use this tool to identify when malnutrition is a potential problem.

Nutrition and the Aging Process

The physiological changes that occur with age can affect nutritional status. These changes also increase the frequency of disease and the need to take medications,

Table 15.2 *DETERMINE: A Checklist of the Warning Signs of Malnutrition*

Disease	Any disease, illness, or condition that causes changes in eating can predispose one to malnutrition. Memory loss and depression can also interfere with nutrition if they affect food intake.
Eating poorly	Eating either too little or too much can lead to poor health.
Tooth loss/mouth pain	A healthy mouth, teeth, and gums are needed to eat.
Economic hardship	Having to or choosing to spend less than $25–$30 per person per week on food interferes with nutrition.
Reduced social support	Being with people on a daily basis has a positive effect on morale, well-being, and eating.
Multiple medicines	The more medicines one takes, the greater the chances of side effects such as weakness, drowsiness, diarrhea, changes in taste and appetite, nausea, and constipation.
Involuntary weight loss/gain	Unintentionally losing or gaining weight is a warning sign that should not be ignored. Being overweight or underweight also increases the risk of malnutrition.
Needs assistance in self-care	Difficulty walking, shopping, and cooking increases the risk of malnutrition.
Elder above age 80	The risks of frailty and health problems increase with increasing age.

both of which can affect nutritional status. Likewise, there are social and economic changes that are common in aging and that increase the risk of food insecurity and, consequently, malnutrition (Figure 15.4).

Physiological Changes of Aging

It is difficult to determine which of the changes that occur with aging are inevitable consequences of the aging process and which are the effect of disease states. But whatever the cause, with aging there is a reduction in **reserve capacity**—the extent to which an organ or organ system can continue to function normally despite a decrease in the number and function of cells. In young adults, the reserve capacity of organs is four to ten times that required to sustain life. As a

Reserve capacity The amount of functional capacity that an organ has above and beyond what is needed to sustain life.

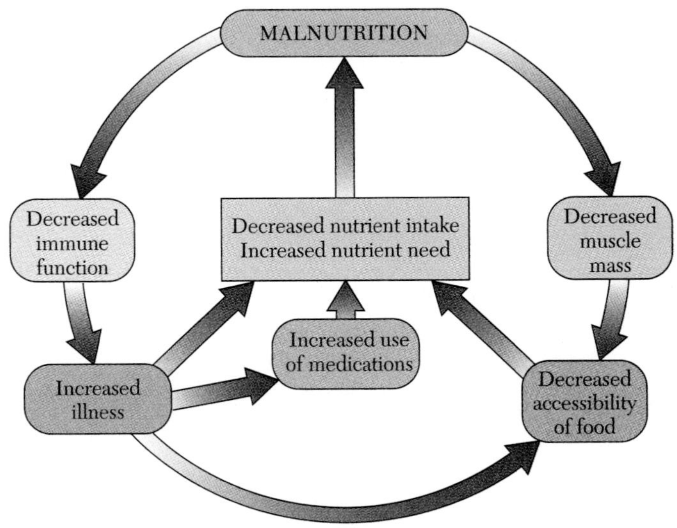

Figure 15.4
The causes and consequences of malnutrition are linked.

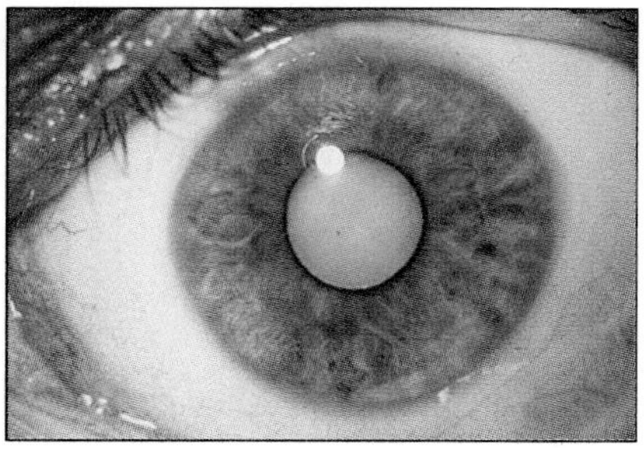

Figure 15.5
Cataracts cause the lens of the eye to become cloudy and impair vision. (© Science VU/Visuals Unlimited)

person grows older and reserve capacity becomes smaller, the effects of aging become evident in all body systems.[14] These changes can affect nutritional status by affecting the appeal of food, digestion and absorption, nutritional requirements, and the ability to obtain food.

Sensory Changes Beginning around age 60, there is a progressive decline in the ability to taste and smell which becomes more severe in persons over 70. The decline of these senses can contribute to impaired nutritional status by decreasing the appeal and enjoyment of food.[15] Some studies suggest that the decline in taste acuity is due to a reduction in the number of taste buds on the tongue; others suggest that it is the result of changes in sensitivity to specific flavors such as salty and sweet.[16] The sense of smell is important because odors provide important clues to food acceptability before food enters the mouth. Once in the mouth some molecules reach the nasal cavity where their odor is detected. It is the blending of the odor message from the nasal cavity and the taste message from the tongue that provides the overall food flavor. When the sense of smell is diminished, food is not as flavorful. Changes in taste and smell have been related to a greater intake of sweet foods among older adults.[16]

Macular degeneration Degeneration of a portion of the retina that results in a loss of visual detail and blindness.

Cataracts A disease of the eye that results in cloudy spots on the lens (and sometimes the cornea), which obscure vision.

Vision also typically declines with age, making shopping for and preparation of food difficult. **Macular degeneration** is the most common cause of blindness in older Americans. The macula is a small area of the retina of the eye that distinguishes fine detail. With age, oxidative damage reduces the number of viable cells in the macula. As the macula degenerates, visual acuity declines, ultimately resulting in blindness. **Cataracts** are another common reason for declining sight. Of people who live to age 85, half will have cataracts that impair vision (Figure 15.5). Oxidative damage is believed to cause both macular degeneration and cataracts. Therefore, a diet high in foods containing antioxidant nutrients might slow or prevent these eye disorders.[17]

Periodontal disease A degeneration of the area surrounding the teeth, specifically the gum and supporting bone.

Gastrointestinal Changes Aging causes changes in the gastrointestinal tract and its accessory organs that may alter the palatability as well as the digestion of food and the absorption of nutrients. One change is a decrease in the secretion of saliva into the mouth. Saliva mixes with food to allow it to be tasted and to provide lubrication for easy swallowing. A decrease in saliva causes dryness which decreases the taste of food and makes swallowing difficult. Saliva is also an important defense against tooth decay because it helps wash material away from the teeth and contains substances that kill bacteria. Thus a dry mouth increases the likelihood of tooth decay and **periodontal disease.** Loss of teeth and improperly fitting dentures also limit food choices and can contribute to poor nutrition in the elderly.

Atrophic gastritis An inflammation of the stomach lining that causes a reduction in stomach acid and allows bacterial overgrowth.

Aging may delay stomach emptying and cause changes in gastric secretions. Delayed stomach emptying can reduce hunger and, therefore, nutrient intake.[16] Reduced gastric secretions can affect the absorption of some nutrients. It is estimated that 10 to 30% of American adults over age 50 and 40% of those into their 80s have **atrophic gastritis,** an inflammation of the stomach lining accompanied by a decrease in the secretion of stomach acid.[18,19] Reduced stomach acid secretion allows microbial overgrowth in the stomach and small intestine.[18,20] Increased populations of microbes in the gut compete for absorption of vitamin B_{12}. In addition, when stomach acid is reduced, the enzymes that release vitamin B_{12} from food do not function properly and vitamin B_{12} in food cannot be absorbed.

With age there is also a reduction in digestive enzymes from the pancreas and small intestine, but there is enough reserve capacity that digestion and absorption are rarely significantly impaired. In the colon there are functional changes, including decreased motility and elasticity, weakened abdominal and pelvic muscles, and decreased sensory perception, that can lead to constipation. Low fiber and fluid intakes and lack of activity also contribute to constipation. Although constipation occurs in about the same frequency in all age groups,[21] it is

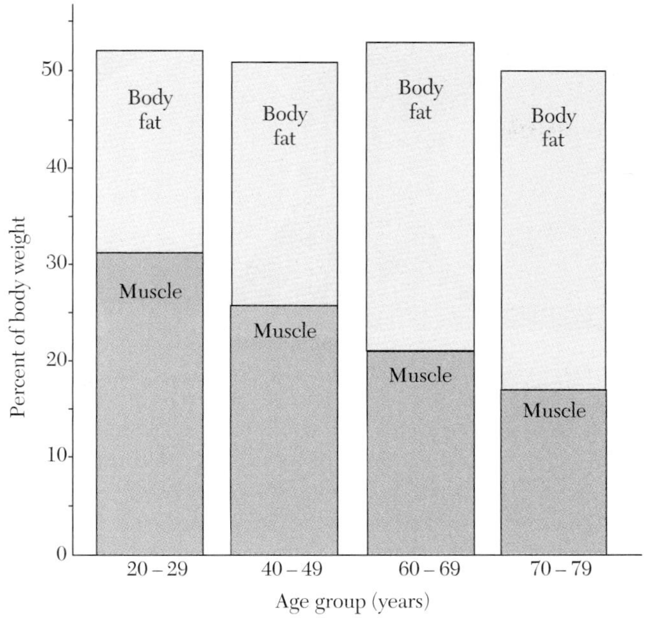

Figure 15.6
In most individuals, the proportion of muscle mass decreases and body fat increases with age. (Adapted from Cohen, S. H., et al. Compartmental body composition based on the body nitrogen, potassium, and calcium. Am. J. Physiol. 239:192–200, 1980.)

estimated that 20 to 30% of individuals over age 65 are dependent on laxatives.[22] Maintaining regular exercise and consuming adequate fluid and fiber are safer ways to prevent constipation.

Age-related changes in other organs may affect nutrient metabolism. Most absorbed nutrients travel from the intestine to the liver for metabolism or storage. The liver has a greater regenerative capacity than most organs, but with age, there is a decrease in liver size and blood flow and an increase in fat accumulation, which eventually decrease the liver's ability to metabolize nutrients and break down drugs and alcohol. With age, the pancreas may become less responsive to blood glucose levels, and the body cells may become more resistant to insulin, resulting in diabetes. Changes in the heart and blood vessels reduce blood flow to the kidneys, making waste removal less efficient. The kidneys themselves become smaller and their ability to filter blood and to excrete the products of protein breakdown declines.[23] In some individuals blood urea levels may increase if protein intake is too high. The kidney's ability to concentrate urine also decreases with age, as does the sensation of thirst, increasing the risk of dehydration.[23]

Changes in Body Composition and Weight Aging is accompanied by an increase in body fat and a decrease in lean tissue, including a loss in muscle mass and strength and a loss of bone (Figure 15.6).[24] Increases in body fat increase the risk of chronic disease but the risks associated with excess body fat are lower for older adults than for younger ones.[25] The decline in muscle size and strength affects both the skeletal muscles needed to move the body and the heart and respiratory muscles needed to deliver oxygen to the tissues. Therefore, both strength and endurance are decreased, making the tasks of day-to-day life more difficult. The changes in muscle strength contribute not only to physical frailty, which is characterized by general weakness, impaired mobility and balance, and poor endurance, but also to the risk of falls and fractures. Loss of bone mass also increases the risk of fractures. In the oldest old, loss of muscle strength becomes the limiting factor determining whether they can continue to live independently. Some of the reduction in muscle strength and mass is due to changes in hormone levels and in muscle protein synthesis, but a lack of exercise is also an important contributor (Figure 15.7).[26] Regular exercise can help maintain muscle mass, bone strength, and cardiorespiratory function and can increase energy needs.[27]

Figure 15.7
Magnetic resonance image of a thigh cross section from a 25-year-old man (left) and a 65-year-old man (right). The thighs are of similar size, but the thigh from the older man has a greater amount of fat (shown in white) around and through the muscle, indicating significant muscle loss. (S. A. Jubrias and K. E. Conley, University of Washington Medical Center)

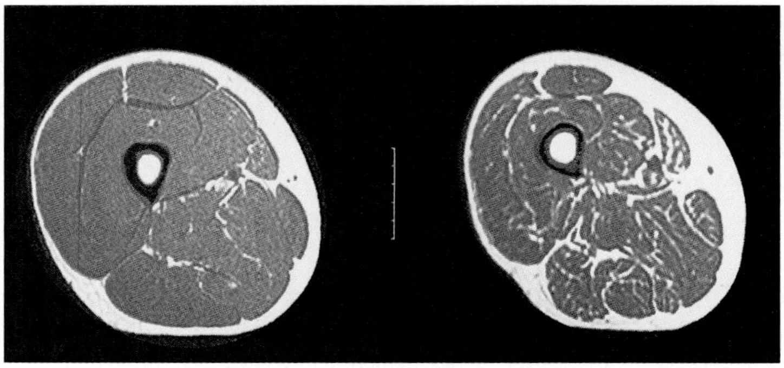

Stable body weight is a sign of good health. Extreme thinness or unintentional weight loss is a health risk, especially among older adults.[28] Although laboratory studies in animals have found that a diet deficient in energy can slow aging and extend life span,[29] this effect has not been demonstrated in humans.

Hormonal Changes Declining levels of some hormones are hypothesized to play a role in the aging process. Hormonal changes related to age can affect the ability to regulate blood glucose levels, body water, and body temperature and can cause changes in body composition. One of the most common hormone-related changes that occur with aging is elevated blood glucose. This is due to both a decrease in the amount of insulin released by the pancreas and a decrease in insulin sensitivity at the tissues. This decreased insulin sensitivity is related to poor diet, inactivity, increased abdominal fat mass, and decreased lean mass. About 40% of individuals between the ages of 65 and 74 and 50% of those over 80 have diabetes, and about half of these cases are undiagnosed.[24] Another common hormonal change that occurs with age is a decline in levels of thyroid hormones. Changes in insulin sensitivity and thyroid function are generally treated by administering hormones.

Many of the other hormonal changes, including decreases in growth hormone, DHEA (dehydroepiandosterone), melatonin, estrogen, and testosterone, are considered part of the normal physiology of aging. Some of these hormonal changes are partially responsible for the changes in body composition discussed above.

Growth hormone stimulates growth and protein synthesis; its levels gradually decline with age in both men and women and may be responsible for some of the decrease in lean body mass. When given to elderly people, injections of growth hormone increased muscle mass, skin thickness, and bone mineral content and decreased fat mass. However, growth hormone replacement did not increase muscle strength.[24] In addition, these injections are not without risk. They have caused such side effects as worsening diabetes, fluid retention, and joint pain. The long-term effects of growth hormone administration on the growth of tumors is unknown.

DHEA is a precursor to sex hormones such as testosterone, estrogen, and progesterone. Even though low levels of this hormone are not known to be the cause of age-associated disorders, DHEA supplements are available over-the-counter and promise to strengthen bones, muscles, and the immune system, and to prevent diabetes, obesity, heart disease, and cancer. Although some of these effects have been demonstrated when DHEA is administered to animals, beneficial effects of DHEA supplementation in humans have not been clearly established.[30] In addition, it is not clear whether the increases in sex hormones that may occur with DHEA administration create a risk of developing ovarian, prostate, or other types of cancer.[24]

Melatonin, a hormone that is secreted by the pineal gland, also declines with age. It is involved in regulating the body's cycles of sleep and wakefulness. The decline in melatonin is hypothesized to influence aging by affecting body rhythms and triggering genetically programmed aging at a cellular level.[31] Melatonin is also an antioxidant and may enhance immune function.[32] It is available as a dietary supplement, but its effect on aging in humans has not been determined.

The most striking and rapidly occurring age-related hormonal change is **menopause.** Menopause normally occurs in women around the age of 50. During menopause, the cyclical release of the female hormones estrogen and progesterone slows and eventually stops, causing ovulation and menstruation to cease. The period of decline in estrogen is accompanied by changes in mood, skin, and body composition (an increase in body fat and a decrease in muscle mass). The hormonal changes also have a powerful impact on the disease risks and nutritional status of older women. Reduction in estrogen decreases the risk of breast cancer but increases the risk of heart disease to a level more similar to that in men. Reduced estrogen also increases the risk of osteoporosis by increasing the rate of bone breakdown, and decreasing calcium absorption from the intestine. Menopause is also associated with a higher incidence of mental impairment. These effects can be treated with hormone replacement therapy; restoring estrogen to the levels found in younger women prevents changes in body composition and delays heart disease, loss of bone mass, and loss of mental function. However, this therapy may increase the risk of breast cancer.

Menopause Physiological changes that mark the end of a woman's capacity to bear children.

Menopause does not occur in men, but with age men do experience a gradual decrease in testosterone levels which may contribute to the decrease in muscle mass and strength.

Changes in Immune Function The ability of the immune system to fight disease declines with age.[33] As it does, the incidence of infections, cancers, and autoimmune diseases increases, and the effectiveness of immunizations declines. Some of the decrease in immune function may be due to nutritional deficiencies.[33,34] In turn, the increases in infections and chronic disease that occur can affect nutritional status.

The immune response depends on the ability of cells to divide rapidly and secrete immune factors, so nutrients that are involved in cell division and metabolism can influence the immune response. Antioxidants may influence immunity by preventing the free radical damage that accelerates aging and decreases the immune response. Supplements of beta-carotene and several micronutrients, including zinc, vitamin E, and vitamin B_6, have been shown to improve immune response in both healthy and diseased elderly.[33,35,36] Even supplements containing levels of vitamins and minerals near the RDA have been shown to significantly enhance parameters of immune function and decrease rates of infection.[37] Micronutrient supplementation may enhance immunity by correcting an underlying deficiency or by stimulating immunity in the absence of an underlying deficiency. Supplements may improve immune response in healthy elderly and prevent infections, but since high doses of some nutrients, including zinc, copper, and iron, depress immune function, supplements should be taken with care.

Medical Consequences of Aging

With age there is an increase in the incidence of both infectious and chronic diseases. Periodontal disease, atrophic gastritis, macular degeneration, and cataracts have already been discussed. These conditions and others impair the ability to maintain nutritional status by affecting nutritional requirements, mobility, and mental functioning. The increased incidence of disease increases the need for medications, some of which may further increase the risk of malnutrition.

Increased Frequency of Disease Both acute and chronic illness can cause food insecurity. Most older adults have at least one chronic medical condition.[2] The incidence of cardiovascular disease, diabetes, osteoporosis, hypertension, cancer,

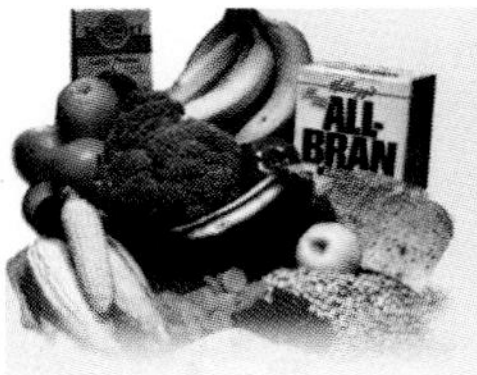

Off the Shelf

Arthritis Remedies

Osteoarthritis causes painful joints. It affects approximately 12% of the U.S. population and the incidence increases with advancing age.[1] It occurs when the connective tissue that keeps the bones in joints from rubbing together degenerates over time. A successful treatment should be able to control pain and slow or reverse the progression of the disease. Traditionally, arthritis has been treated with nonsteroidal anti-inflammatory drugs such as aspirin and ibuprofen and with pain relievers such as acetaminophen. These reduce pain and inflammation but do not repair the tissue. They also have side effects if taken over long periods of time. Over the years, many alternative treatments—ranging from copper bracelets to special diets and dietary supplements—have been promoted, but none have been successful.[2] Recently, however, the availability of glucosamine sulfate and chondroitin sulfate supplements has offered a new alternative for arthritis sufferers.

Glucosamine sulfate and chondroitin sulfate are not essential nutrients. They are molecules found in cartilage, the type of connective tissue that cushions our joints. Evidence is accumulating that supplements of these two substances reduce arthritis pain. It is hypothesized that they may also stop cartilage degeneration and, in some cases, stimulate the repair of damaged joint cartilage.

Glucosamine sulfate is a building block essential for the synthesis of large molecules called proteoglycans that are a structural component of cartilage. Limited data in human trials suggest that glucosamine sulfate, whether taken orally or by injection, may produce a gradual reduction in joint pain and tenderness, may increase the range of motion in the joint, and may increase the speed at which subjects can walk.[3] One hypothesis as to why glucosamine sulfate supplements benefit arthritis sufferers is that they provide the raw materials needed to synthesize proteoglycans. Another hypothesis is that these supplements increase the production of hyaluronic acid, a molecule that is responsible for the lubricating and shock-absorbing properties of the fluid that is present in joint spaces and within cartilage. Hyaluronic acid also has anti-inflammatory and pain-relieving properties. Previous studies have shown that the concentration of hyaluronic acid is reduced in individuals with arthritis; injections of hyaluronic acid have also been used to treat arthritis in animals.[4]

Chondroitin sulfate is also a precursor of the proteoglycans in cartilage and is hypothesized to be beneficial in treating arthritis because it provides building blocks for these important structural molecules. In randomized trials, patients treated with 800 to 1200 mg of chondroitin sulfate per day experienced a reduction in pain and an increase in mobility compared to control groups taking a placebo.[5–7] In addition, there was evidence suggesting that the amount of cartilage had increased in the group taking glucosamine sulfate supplements.[7]

Thus far, the only accepted dietary treatment for arthritis is to follow a balanced healthy diet and, for overweight arthritics, to lose weight. A controlled program of exercise can help improve conditioning and muscle tone, protect joints, and decrease disability. However, the benefits of chondroitin and glucosamine sulfates make them a promising treatment for an age-old disease. So far no adverse effects have been reported, but studies of chondroitin and glucosamine sulfates have been limited in the number of subjects used and the length of time the supplements were administered, so further research is needed to conclusively demonstrate both safety and effectiveness.

[1]Barclay, T. S., Tsourounis, C., and McCart, C. M. Glucosamine. Ann. Pharmacother. 32:574–579, 1998.

[2]Martin, R. H. The role of nutrition and diet in rheumatoid arthritis. Proc. Nutr. Soc. 57:231–234, 1998.

[3]daCamara, C. C., and Dowless, G. V. Glucosamine sulfate for osteoarthritis. Ann. Pharmacother. 32:580–587, 1998.

[4]McCarty, M. F. Enhanced synovail production of hyaluronic acid may explain the rapid clinical response to high-dose glucosamine in osteoarthritis. Med. Hypotheses 50:507–510, 1998.

[5]Bourgeois, P., Chales, G., Dehais, J., et al. Efficacy and tolerability of chondroitin sulfate 1200 mg per day vs. chondroitin sulfate 3 × 400 mg per day vs. placebo. Osteoarthritis Cartilage 6(suppl A):25–30, 1998.

[6]Bucsi, L., and Poor, G. Efficacy and tolerability of oral chondroitin sulfate as a symptomatic slow-acting drug for osteoarthritis (SYSADOA) in the treatment of knee osteoarthritis. Osteoarthritis Cartilage 6(suppl A):31–36,1998.

[7]Uebelhart, D., Thonar, E. J., Delmas, P. D., et al. Effects of oral chondroitin sulfate on the progression of knee osteoarthritis: a pilot study. Osteoarthritis Cartilage 6(suppl A):39–46, 1998.

---

arthritis, and Alzheimer's disease all increase with age. Kidney disease, cancer, and alcoholism can change nutrient needs and decrease the appeal of food. Other disease conditions also decrease mobility, making it difficult to acquire and prepare food. Some affect mental function, which further decreases independence. In addition, the reduction in reserve capacity and decline in immune function make infectious diseases more frequent and more serious in the elderly. Acute conditions such as infections, hip fracture, and surgery can increase nutrient requirements.

Conditions That Decrease Mobility More than half of the older population suffers from some form of physical disability and the incidence increases with age. Over 4.4 million older adults have difficulty carrying out the activities of daily life, including shopping, eating, and getting around the house.[2] These limitations affect the ability to maintain good nutritional health. A number of disease conditions can decrease mobility in the elderly. Arthritis, a condition that causes pain upon movement, is the most common cause of disability in older individuals. Osteoarthritis, the form of arthritis most common in the elderly, is characterized by abnormalities in the joint surfaces and is most likely the result of a lifetime of wear and tear (see *Off the Shelf: Arthritis Remedies*). Osteoporosis and its associated fractures can also affect mobility. Some of the decrease in mobility that is due to disease and normal aging can be prevented by a healthy diet and lifestyle.

Conditions That Affect Mental Status Altered mental status can affect nutrition. Although many individuals maintain adequate nervous system function into old age, the incidence of dementia increases with age. **Dementia** refers to an impairment in memory, thinking, and/or judgment that is severe enough to cause personality changes and affect daily activities and relationships with others. Causes of dementia include multiple strokes, alcoholism, and Alzheimer's disease. Vitamin B_{12} status may also affect mental function in the elderly. With aging there is a decrease in blood vitamin B_{12} levels and a rise in metabolites indicative of poor B_{12} status. In most cases, vitamin B_{12} supplements do not improve neurological function; however, in some elderly patients with mild dementia and low blood levels of vitamin B_{12}, supplementation improved mental function.[38]

Dementia A deterioration of mental state resulting in impaired memory, thinking, and/or judgment.

Over half of the cases of dementia in the elderly are due to **Alzheimer's disease,** a progressive, incurable loss of mental function. The brains of patients with Alzheimer's disease are characterized by the accumulation of an abnormal protein and a loss of certain types of nerve cells.[39] Its cause is currently unknown, but there does appear to be a genetic component in some cases. Many ineffective nutritional cures have been marketed for Alzheimer's disease. Supplements of choline and lecithin have been promoted to increase levels of the neurotransmitter acetylcholine, which is deficient in Alzheimer's patients. Antioxidant supplements have been suggested to prevent free radical damage. And when high aluminum levels were discovered in the brains of Alzheimer's patients, many people tried to reduce exposure by restricting the use of aluminum cookware and aluminum-containing deodorants. To date, neither nutritional supplements nor aluminum restriction has proved helpful in treating or preventing Alzheimer's disease.

Alzheimer's disease A disease that results in the relentless and irreversible loss of mental function.

Increased Use of Prescription and Over-the-Counter Drugs Because health problems increase with increasing age, older adults are likely to take medications. Almost half of older Americans take multiple medications daily.[40] The use of prescription and over-the-counter medications can affect nutritional status and contribute to malnutrition. The more medications taken, the greater the chance of side effects such as increased or decreased appetite, changes in taste, constipation, weakness, drowsiness, diarrhea, and nausea. Although these medications are necessary and provide beneficial effects, illness related to incorrect doses or inappropriate combinations of medications is a significant health problem in the elderly, accounting for 5 to 23% of all hospitalizations (Figure 15.8). Medications commonly used by older individuals include aspirin, antacids, laxatives, diuretics, anticoagulants (blood thinners), anticonvulsives, heart medications, and pain medications. Both the effects of drugs on nutritional status and the effects of nutritional status on the effectiveness of the drugs must be considered.

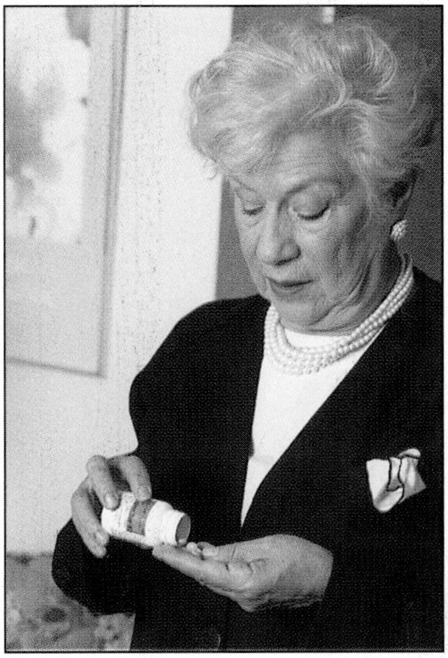

Figure 15.8
Many older adults take one or more medications every day. (© Michael Newman/ PhotoEdit)

The Effect of Drugs on Nutritional Status Drugs can affect nutrition by altering appetite, nutrient absorption, metabolism, or excretion (Table 15.3). These effects occur with both prescription and over-the-counter medications. In many situations, drugs do not significantly alter overall nutritional status, but they can have a significant impact on individuals who must take medications for extended

Table 15.3 *Commonly Used Drugs That May Cause Nutritional Deficiencies*

Drug Group	Drug	Potential Deficiency
Antacids	Sodium bicarbonate	Folate, phosphorus, calcium, copper
	Aluminum hydroxide	Phosphorus
Anticonvulsants	Phenytoin, phenobarbital, primidone	Vitamins D and K
	Valproic acid	Carnitine
Antibiotics	Tetracycline	Calcium
	Gentamicin	Potassium, magnesium
Antibacterial agents	Neomycin	Fat, nitrogen
	Boric acid	Riboflavin
	Trimethoprim	Folate
	Isoniazid	Vitamins B_6, D, and niacin
Anti-inflammatory agents	Sulfasalazine	Folate
	Prednisone	Calcium
	Aspirin	Vitamin C, folate, iron
Anticancer drugs	Colchine	Fat, vitamin B_{12}
	Methotrexate	Folate, calcium
Anticoagulant drugs	Warfarin	Vitamin K
Antihypertensive drugs	Hydralazine	Vitamin B_6
Diuretics	Thiazides	Potassium
	Furosemide	Potassium, calcium, magnesium
Hypocholesterolemic agents	Cholestyramine	Fat, fat-soluble vitamins, iron, folate, vitamin B_{12}
Laxatives	Mineral oil	Fat-soluble vitamins
	Phenolphthalein	Potassium, calcium
	Senna	Fat, calcium, vitamin B_6, folate, vitamin C
Tranquilizers	Chlorpromazine	Riboflavin

Adapted from Roe, D. A. *Diet and Drug Interactions*, New York: Van Nostrand Reinhold, 1989.

periods, who take multiple medications, or who already have marginal nutritional status.

Some medications directly affect the gastrointestinal tract. More than 250 drugs, including blood pressure medications, antidepressants, decongestants, and the pain reliever ibuprofen (found in Advil, Motrin, and Nuprin), can cause mouth dryness, which can decrease interest in eating by interfering with taste, chewing, and swallowing. Aspirin is a stomach irritant and can cause small amounts of painless bleeding in the gastrointestinal tract, resulting in iron loss. Digoxin, which is a heart stimulant, can cause gastrointestinal upset, loss of appetite, and nausea. Narcotic pain medications such as codeine can lead to constipation, nausea, and vomiting.

Other drugs can decrease nutrient absorption. Cholestyramine (Questran), which is used to reduce blood cholesterol, can decrease the absorption of fat-soluble vitamins, vitamin B_{12}, iron, and folate. Antacids that contain aluminum or magnesium hydroxide (Rolaids or Maalox) combine with phosphorus in the gut to form compounds that cannot be absorbed; chronic use can result in loss of phosphorus from bone and possibly accelerate osteoporosis. Repeated use of stimulant laxatives can deplete calcium and potassium. Mineral oil laxatives prevent the absorption of fat-soluble vitamins. If it is not possible to prevent constipation by consuming a diet high in fiber and fluid, bulk-forming laxatives are a safer choice.

The metabolism of drugs can also affect nutritional status. For example, anticonvulsive drugs taken by people prone to epileptic seizures increase the liver's capacity to metabolize and eliminate vitamin D, therefore increasing the need for vitamin D.

Some drugs affect nutrient excretion. Diuretics, which are used to treat hypertension and edema, cause water loss, but some types (thiazides) also increase the excretion of potassium. People taking thiazide diuretics are advised to include several good sources of potassium in their diet each day or are prescribed supplements.

The Effect of Food and Nutritional Status on the Utilization of Drugs Food components can either enhance or retard the absorption and metabolism of drugs. Some drugs, such as the pain medication Darvon, are absorbed better or faster if taken with food. Other drugs, such as aspirin and ibuprofen, should be taken with food because they are irritating to the gastrointestinal tract. Since food can delay how quickly drugs leave the stomach, some are best taken with just water. Other drugs interact with specific foods. For instance, the antibiotic tetracycline should not be taken with milk because it binds with calcium, making both unavailable.

Nutritional status can also affect drug metabolism. If nutritional status is poor, the body's ability to detoxify drugs may be altered. For example, in a malnourished individual, theophylline, used to treat asthma, is metabolized slowly, resulting in high blood levels of the drug, which can cause loss of appetite, nausea, and vomiting.

Specific nutrients can also affect the metabolism of drugs. High-protein diets enhance drug metabolism in general, and low-protein diets slow it. Vitamin K hinders the action of anticoagulants, taken to reduce the risk of blood clots. On the other hand, omega-3 fatty acids, such as those in fish oils, inhibit blood clotting and may intensify the effect of an anticoagulant drug and cause bleeding. It is safe to eat fish while taking anticoagulant drugs; however, the use of fish oil supplements is not recommended. Drugs can also interact with each other. For example, alcohol affects the metabolism of over a hundred medications. Drug interactions can exaggerate or, in some cases, diminish the effect of a medication. Mixing certain drugs can be fatal. Individuals taking any medication should consult their doctor, pharmacist, or dietitian regarding how the drug could affect the action of other drugs they may be taking, how the drug could affect their nutrition, and how their nutrition could affect the action of the drug.

Alcohol Use Alcohol consumption increases the risk of malnutrition in the elderly. Alcohol is high in kcalories and provides few other nutrients. Too much damages the brain, heart, liver, and other organs. It impairs judgment and balance and it therefore increases the frequency of falls and makes it harder to remember to eat and take medications correctly. Alcohol consumption should be limited to no more than one drink per day for women and two per day for men[40] (see *Off the Shelf: Alcohol: A Risk-Benefit Analysis*).

Social and Economic Impact of Aging

In addition to physiological and medical changes, there are a variety of social and economic changes that often accompany aging. These factors are all interrelated and affect nutritional status by decreasing the motivation to eat and the ability to acquire and enjoy food.

Economics About 3.4 million elderly persons live below the poverty level.[2] The highest rates of poverty occur among the oldest of the old, minorities, women, persons living alone, and those with disabilities. Many older individuals, regardless of income level, must live on a fixed income as they retire from their jobs,

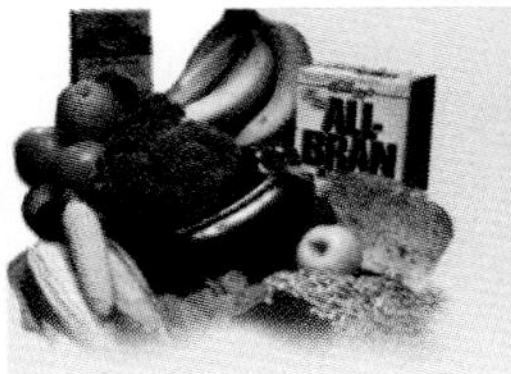

Off the Shelf

Alcohol: A Risk-Benefit Analysis

Almost every human culture since the dawn of civilization has produced and consumed some type of alcoholic beverage. The debate about whether the consumption of small amounts of alcohol is beneficial to health is almost as old. In Sumerian clay tablets dating back to 2100 B.C., physicians are shown to have prescribed beer, and doctors in ancient Egypt included beer or wine in many prescriptions. Today some people do not drink alcohol for religious, cultural, personal, or medical reasons. Others consume it in excess and suffer health and social consequences that affect their well-being and that of their families. Between these two extremes are the moderate drinkers who are unsure how to define "moderate" and unclear whether drinking alcoholic beverages is a risk or benefit.

For some, the risks far outweigh any benefits. For example, children should not consume alcohol. They are more sensitive than adults to alcohol's toxic effects, so it does not take much alcohol to cause drunkenness and poisoning leading to seizures, coma, and death.[1] Women who are pregnant or trying to conceive should not drink at all because it is not known what level of alcohol consumption is safe for the fetus. Individuals who plan to drive or engage in other activities that require attention or skill should not drink because alcohol impairs judgment, coordination, and reflexes. Finally, because alcohol is a drug that interacts with numerous medications, individuals using prescription or over-the-counter drugs should avoid its use.[2]

For everyone, the risks of *excess* alcohol consumption outweigh the benefits. The abuse of alcohol contributes to domestic violence and leads to more than 100,000 deaths per year, including 20,000 from traffic accidents. The incidence of alcohol poisoning, especially among college students who binge drink, is on the rise. Many college campuses are now prohibiting the consumption of alcohol and designing safe-drinking campaigns for their students. Alcoholics are ten times more likely to develop liver, pancreatic, and stomach cancer, and they have an increased risk of cirrhosis, peptic ulcers, and certain types of stroke.

The risks versus the benefits of *moderate* alcohol consumption are less clear. There is concern that recommending moderate drinking may lead to excessive drinking and addiction in susceptible individuals. Moderate alcohol consumption may also increase the risk of obesity.[3] Alcohol suppresses lipid oxidation, and in drinkers, fat is preferentially deposited in the abdominal region. This excess abdominal fat increases the risk of high blood pressure, heart disease, and diabetes. Alcoholic beverages may also contain chemical contaminants. Lead contamination can occur from older wine bottles that may be sealed with lead foil and liqueurs stored in leaded crystal. Urethane, which is a carcinogen in animals, is found in distilled liquors such as bourbon because it is a by-product of the distillation process.[4]

Moderate alcohol consumption also has benefits. Socially, alcohol can be relaxing, producing a euphoria that can enhance social interactions. Moderate alcohol can stimulate appetite and improve mood. And there is strong evidence that moderate alcohol consumption can decrease the risk of heart disease by increasing the concentration of HDL cholesterol. Certain alcoholic beverages, such as red wine, contain compounds such as phenols and other phytochemicals that may contribute to the reduction in heart disease risk. Wine consumption in particular is common in cultures with lower risks of heart disease. For example, the Mediterranean diet which has been associated with a reduced risk of heart disease includes daily consumption of wine in moderation, and one answer to the French paradox—the fact that the French eat a diet that is as high or higher in fat than Americans do but suffer from far less heart disease—is believed to be the glass of wine they drink with meals.

If you do choose to consume alcohol, consumption should be moderate—about 1 to 2 drinks per day (one drink equals approximately 5 ounces of wine, 12 ounces of beer, or 1.5 ounces of distilled liquor). Alcohol should be consumed slowly. It usually takes an hour to metabolize the alcohol in one drink, so no more than one drink should be consumed every one and a half hours. The best time to consume alcohol is with meals; alcohol absorption is slowed when it is consumed with high-protein or high-carbohydrate foods. Consuming alcohol with meals may also enhance its protective effects on the cardiovascular system. Like aspirin, alcohol prevents blood clotting, so it may counteract the tendency of a large meal to promote blood clotting and reduce the risk of an immediate heart attack. Also, the effect of alcohol on HDL is believed to be greater when the liver is processing nutrients in a meal.

Whether the benefits of alcohol consumption outweigh the risks, drinking is a personal decision that must take into account medical and social considerations.

[1] Hingley, A. T. Preventing childhood poisoning. FDA Consumer 30:7–11, March 1996.

[2] U.S. Department of Agriculture, U.S. Department of Health and Human Services. *Nutrition and Your Health: Dietary Guidelines for Americans*, 4th ed. Home and Garden Bulletin No. 232. Hyattsville, Md.: U.S. Government Printing Office, 1995.

[3] Suter, P. M., Häsler, E., and Vetter, W. Effects of alcohol on energy metabolism and body weight regulation: is alcohol a risk factor for obesity? Nutr. Rev. 55:157–171, 1997.

[4] Segal, M. Too many drinks spiked with urethanes. FDA Consumer 32:5–8, April 1998.

making it difficult to afford health care, especially medications, and a healthy diet. Food is often the most flexible expense in one's budget, so limiting the types and amounts of foods consumed may be the only option available for older adults trying to meet expenses. Substandard housing and inadequate food preparation facilities can make the situation worse because food cannot easily be prepared and eaten at home.

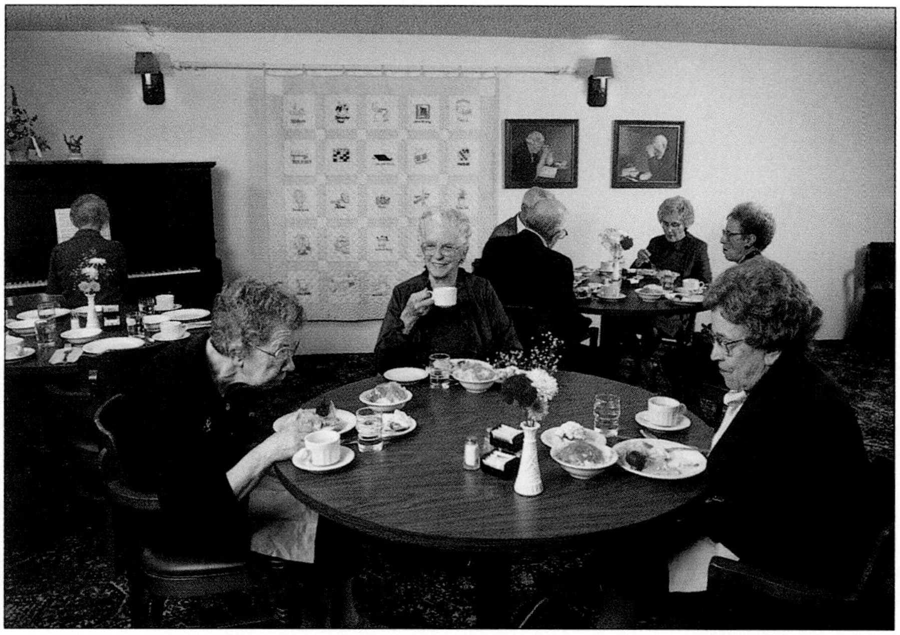

Figure 15.9
Social interaction may make eating more appealing. (© Blair Seitz/Photo Researchers, Inc.)

Dependent Living Most older individuals continue to live in a family setting: 66% of adults over 65 years of age live at home. However, this number decreases with age: Only 46% of individuals over 85 still live at home.[2]

Although many older adults continue to live independently in their own homes, the physical and psychological decline associated with aging causes some to eventually require assistance in living (Figure 15.9). Poor eyesight and other physical restrictions can limit the ability to drive a car. Without help, many older adults may be unable to get to markets and food programs, restricting the types of food available to them. While a social support system consisting of family members, friends, and other caregivers can help many people stay at home, others may require assisted-living facilities, where they have their own apartments but can obtain assistance around the clock. For some, however, the degenerative changes of age require a nursing home to provide the appropriate care.

Malnutrition can be a problem among older adults no matter where they live. Even older individuals living independently have been reported to have reduced intakes of energy and protein.[12] Those in nursing homes are at increased risk for malnutrition because they are more likely to have medical conditions that increase nutrient needs or that interfere with food intake or nutrient absorption, and because they are dependent on others to provide for their care.[41] In addition, 50% of institutionalized elderly suffer from some form of disorientation or confusion which further increases the likelihood of decreased nutrient intake. Even when adequate meals are provided, nursing-home residents frequently do not consume all of the food served, increasing the likelihood of fluid and energy deficits.[42] Whether an older adult resides in an assisted-living setting or in a nursing home, care must be taken to assess the needs of the individual and to provide appetizing meals that meet these needs.

Depression Social, psychological, and physical factors all contribute to depression in the elderly.[43] Retirement and the death or relocation of friends and family can cause social isolation which contributes to depression. Physical disability causes loss of independence. The inability to engage in normal daily activities, visit with friends and family easily, and provide for personal needs contributes to depression. Depression can make meals less appetizing and decrease the quantity and quality of foods consumed, thereby increasing the risk of malnutrition.

Critical Thinking

Can Your Diet Keep You Young?

Marilyn and Bob are a relatively healthy retired couple in their sixties. They have never paid much attention to their diet or lifestyle, but now that they are older, they decide they should get more exercise, increase their intake of antioxidant nutrients and omega-3 fatty acids, reduce their intake of fat, and take the antiaging hormone DHEA. To meet these goals they decide to begin a regular exercise program; take supplements of antioxidants, fish oil, and DHEA; and cut their meat intake to 3 ounces a week. Before beginning their program they check with their physician.

Are their plans safe?

The physician reviews their medical histories and current medication use. Bob is taking Questran for high blood cholesterol. Marilyn is taking Coumadin, an anticoagulant, because of problems with blood clots. The physician agrees that a moderate exercise program would be a good idea. She recommends that they slowly begin a program that includes some resistance exercise to preserve muscle mass as well as aerobic activity to improve cardiorespiratory health. She teaches them to monitor their pulse to keep exercise intensity at a level that does not raise their heart rates to more than 60 to 90% of maximum. She agrees that reducing dietary fat would be healthy, but she recommends that they get some counseling from a dietitian about how to modify their diet. Considering the medication Marilyn is taking, the physician tells her not to take fish oil supplements.

Why would fish oil supplements be dangerous for Marilyn?

Answer:

The antioxidant supplement that Bob and Marilyn are planning to take contains the following nutrients:

Vitamin C	1 gram
Beta-carotene	25,000 IU = 4167 μg RE
Vitamin E	400 IU = 400 mg α-TE
Selenium	125 μg

Should they take the antioxidant supplement?

There is evidence that high intakes of the antioxidants vitamin C, vitamin E, and beta-carotene improve immune function and prevent some of the chronic diseases associated with aging. Selenium supplements have been shown to decrease the risk of certain types of cancer. These antioxidants in the amounts present in this supplement pose little risk, but there are other substances—such as the nutrients zinc and vitamin B_6 that have also been shown to improve immune function, and phytochemicals that help prevent chronic disease—that are not included in this supplement. A better choice would be a diet high in fruits, vegetables, and grains, which are good sources of antioxidant nutrients and phytochemicals. If Marilyn and Bob want to take a supplement, a multiple vitamin and mineral supplement might be a better idea.

Is the supplement DHEA likely to offer any benefits or risks?

DHEA is a hormone that has been found to decline steadily with age. Although animal studies have shown some beneficial effects of DHEA supplementation, there is little evidence that it provides any long-term preventative or therapeutic benefits associated with aging in humans. In addition, it is still not clear whether supplements of DHEA pose a risk. In the body, DHEA can be converted to estrogen or testosterone—hormones that may affect the growth of tumors.

Is it safe for them to reduce their meat intake to 3 ounces a week?

Answer:

Nutrition for Older Adults

As stated earlier older adults are a diverse group, which makes defining and meeting nutrient needs challenging. The incidence of diseases that affect nutritional status is increased, and social and economic factors, such as a fixed income and social isolation, affect appetite and food availability. To meet the nutritional needs of the elderly, their individual medical, psychological, social, and economic circumstances must be considered (see *Critical Thinking: Dietary Modifications to Meet the Needs of the Elderly*).

Can Nutrition Keep Us Young?

What is the role of nutrition in aging? Is nutrition the key to immortality? Good nutrition may not keep us young but it can prevent malnutrition and delay the onset of chronic diseases.

Malnutrition causes a spiraling decline in physical and emotional well-being that contributes to illness and death. But malnutrition is not an inevitable consequence of aging. If the medical, social, and economic barriers to obtaining good nutrition can be overcome, good nutritional status can be maintained throughout life.

The diseases that are the major causes of disability in older adults—cardiovascular disease, hypertension, diabetes, cancer, and osteoporosis—are all nutrition-related. Exercise and a lifetime of healthy eating will not necessarily prevent these diseases, but they may slow the changes that accumulate over time, postponing the onset of disease symptoms. As discussed in Chapters 5 and 12, the risk of developing cardiovascular disease can be decreased by exercise and a diet low in total fat and saturated fat and high in whole grains, fruits, and vegetables. As discussed in Chapters 4 and 7, the risks and complications of diabetes are reduced by maintaining a healthy weight and regular exercise. As discussed in Chapter 10, hypertension may be reduced by consuming a diet moderate in sodium and high in fruits, vegetables, and lowfat dairy products. Osteoporosis may be prevented by adequate calcium intake and exercise throughout life. And, as discussed throughout this text, the likelihood of developing certain types of cancer can be reduced by consuming a diet low in fat and high in whole grains, vegetables, and fruits.

Nutrient Needs of Older Adults

General dietary recommendations are difficult to establish for older adults. For instance, the requirements of a wheelchair-bound 70-year-old are different from those of a more active individual. Dietary recommendations are developed to meet the needs of the majority of healthy individuals in a population, but "healthy" is difficult to define in such a diverse group. The 1989 RDAs divide adulthood into three age categories but the DRIs have expanded this to four: young adulthood, ages 19 through 30; middle age, 31 through 50 years; adulthood, ages 51 through 70; and older adults, those over 70 years of age. This recognizes the possible higher nutrient intake needs of younger adults, the decline with age in the need for nutrients involved in energy metabolism, and the variability in the functional capacity of older adults.

Energy and Macronutrient Needs Energy needs are typically reduced in the elderly. This occurs for several reasons. Energy requirements are the sum of the needs for basal metabolic rate (BMR), physical activity, and the thermic effect of food. A change in any one of these alters total energy needs. BMR is influenced by lean body mass, and because lean body mass usually decreases with age, there is a reduction in this component of energy expenditure in the elderly.[44] Physical activity also tends to decline with age. This causes a decrease in the activity component of energy expenditure and contributes to the reduction in lean body mass and BMR. The energy needed for the thermic effect of food does not change as adults age.[45]

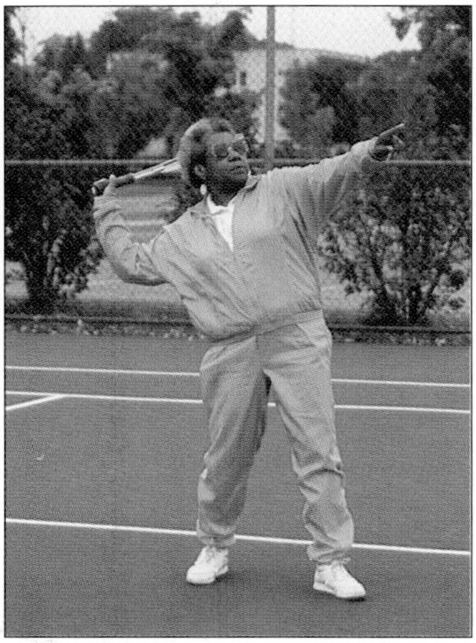

Figure 15.10
Exercise increases energy needs and helps to maintain lean body mass. (© CLEO/PhotoEdit)

The 1989 RDA recommends a reduction of 600 kcalories in men 51 and older and 300 kcalories in women 51 and older compared to younger age groups. Some of the decrease in energy requirement can be prevented by exercise, which increases energy output and helps prevent the loss of lean body mass (Figure 15.10).[44] Increasing energy needs through exercise also allows an increase in food intake without weight gain so micronutrient needs are more easily met.

Protein Needs Unlike energy requirements, the need for protein does not decline with age. Therefore, an adequate diet for older adults must be somewhat higher in protein relative to energy intake. Although the 1989 RDA for older adults is no different than that for younger adults, actual need depends on the individual. In some, the protein requirement may be less than the 1989 RDA because there is less lean body mass to maintain, whereas in others it may be greater than the 1989 RDA because protein absorption or utilization is reduced.

Water Needs The recommended water intake for older adults is the same as that for younger adults; however, changes in the homeostatic mechanisms that regulate water balance may make meeting these needs more challenging. With age there is a reduction in the sense of thirst, which can decrease fluid intake.[42] Changes in mobility may limit access to water even in the presence of thirst. In addition, the kidneys are no longer as efficient at conserving water, so water loss increases. Water loss may also increase in individuals with diabetes or diseases that cause vomiting or diarrhea. Depression, which decreases water intake, and medications that increase water loss such as laxatives and diuretics also increase the risk of dehydration in the elderly. Inadequate fluid intake also increases problems with constipation.

Micronutrient Needs The recommended intake for many of the micronutrients is not changed for older adults; however, the risk of micronutrient deficiencies increases in this age group due to deficient intakes as well as changes in digestion, absorption, and metabolism.

B Vitamins As mentioned earlier, with aging there is a decrease in blood vitamin B_{12} levels and a rise in metabolites indicative of poor B_{12} status. Low dietary intakes, especially among the poor, may contribute to this problem, but poor absorption of food-bound B_{12} is an important factor.[18] To prevent vitamin B_{12} deficiency in older adults, individuals over the age of 50 should meet their RDA for vitamin B_{12} by consuming fortified foods such as fortified breakfast cereals or soy-based products, or by taking a supplement containing vitamin B_{12}.[18] The B_{12} in fortified foods and supplements is not bound to proteins, so it is absorbed even when stomach acid is low.

The aging process does not appear to interfere with folate absorption or utilization, so the RDA is the same for all adult age groups.[18] The RDA for vitamin B_6 is greater in individuals age 51 and older than for younger adults, and in these older age groups the RDA for men is higher than for women. This is because higher dietary intakes are needed to maintain the same biochemical indicators of adequacy.

Vitamin D and Calcium Because vitamin D is necessary for calcium absorption, a deficiency may contribute to osteoporosis. Intakes of this vitamin are often low in the elderly population, usually due to limited consumption of dairy products. And, exposure to sunlight, which is necessary for the formation of provitamin D in the skin, is often limited in the elderly because they spend less time outdoors or tend to wear clothing that covers or shades their skin when they go out. Vitamin D deficiency is also a concern because the capacity to synthesize provitamin D in the skin and to form active vitamin D in the kidney decreases with age. Using bone loss as an indicator of adequacy, the AI for men and women aged 51 to 70 has been doubled from that of younger age groups to a value of 10 μg per day. For individuals over age 70, this is further increased to 15 μg per day.

Calcium status is a problem in the elderly because intakes are low and intestinal absorption decreases with age. The current AI for adults over age 51 is 1200 mg, greater than the AI of 1000 mg set for younger adults.[46] Although the decrease in estrogen that occurs at menopause causes bone loss, it cannot be prevented by increasing calcium intake, so the AIs for men and women are not different.

Antioxidant Nutrients: Do They Slow Aging? The hypothesis that aging is caused by oxidative damage has led to the popular conclusion that high dietary intakes of antioxidants will retard the aging process. In reality, antioxidant nutrients will not keep you young, but adequate intakes may reduce the incidence of disease. Dietary antioxidants, including vitamin E, vitamin C, and beta-carotene, have been found to improve immune function and may therefore help protect the body from infectious disease.[33,36] And there is evidence that antioxidant intake is correlated with a reduced incidence of various chronic diseases. Beta-carotene in foods and

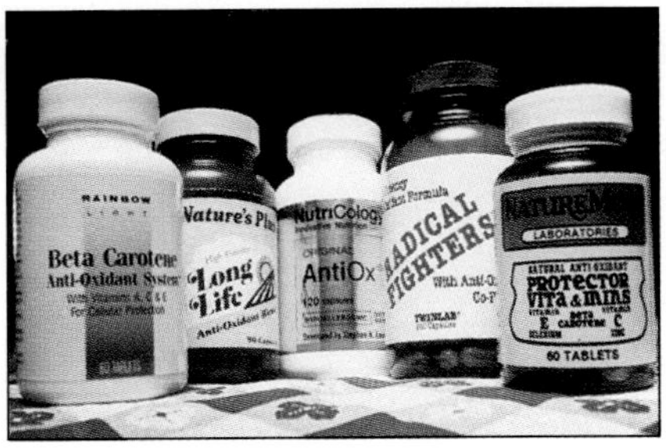

Figure 15.11
Supplements are often consumed to increase antioxidant intake. (Charles D. Winters)

supplements protects against cardiovascular disease,[47] and intakes of vitamin E greater than 100 IU per day or 70 mg α-TE per day have been associated with a reduced risk of heart disease.[48,49] Diets high in these nutrients are also associated with a reduced incidence of certain types of cancer. Nutritional status of vitamin C, vitamin E, and beta-carotene may be related to the risk of cataracts in healthy elderly.[17,50] The evidence that antioxidants in supplement form will have these effects is not as strong as the evidence supporting a diet plentiful in foods high in these nutrients (Figure 15.11). When these nutrients are obtained from foods, they bring with them phytochemicals, some of which offer additional antioxidant protection and some of which protect us from chronic disease in other ways.

Dietary Supplements: Are They Necessary? There are many supplements marketed to the elderly. Many of these have not been shown to be beneficial and could be toxic; others may provide some benefit. Coenzyme Q, a synthetic version of a compound in the electron transport chain, is purported to slow aging by enhancing the immune system. However, it does not boost immune function and may be dangerous for people with poor circulation. Lecithin is promoted to lower cholesterol and to treat Alzheimer's, but there is no proof that it does either. RNA is claimed to rejuvenate old cells, improve memory, and prevent wrinkling, but there are no controlled studies to support any of these claims. Superoxide dismutase (SOD), an enzyme that protects against oxidative damage, is promoted to slow aging and treat Alzheimer's. However, even if higher tissue levels of SOD provided extra antioxidant protection, SOD is a protein that is broken down to amino acids in the GI tract, so oral supplements will not increase blood or tissue levels of this enzyme.

Although supplements are not necessary to meet micronutrient needs, older adults may benefit from supplementing some nutrients. Because it can be difficult to consume 1200 mg of calcium from food without exceeding energy needs, a calcium supplement may be necessary to meet needs particularly for elderly women. Because the absorption of vitamin B_{12} decreases with age, supplemental vitamin B_{12} from pills or fortified foods is recommended for older adults. Nutrient supplements that have been shown to improve immune function include zinc and vitamin B_6. Antioxidants such as vitamin C, vitamin E, and beta-carotene may also improve the immune response and protect against chronic disease.[51] Supplements, however, should not take the place of a balanced, nutrient-dense diet high in grains, fruits, and vegetables. These foods also contain phytochemicals and other substances that may protect against disease (see Chapter 9). As with other age groups, the elderly should be cautious to avoid overdoses, and the resulting toxicities, when selecting supplements. A multivitamin and mineral supplement containing no more than 100% of the Daily Value is the safest way to supplement the diet.[51]

Meeting the Nutrient Needs of Older Adults

An understanding of the diversity in the elderly population as well as the factors that help maintain vitality and independence is key to meeting the nutrient needs of this segment of the population. In some cases, this involves providing education about nutrient requirements, economics, and food preparation; in other cases, assistance with shopping or meal preparation may be beneficial.

Nutritional Guidelines A well-planned diet for older adults should follow the recommendations of the Food Guide Pyramid at the low end of the range of servings. Most of the nutritional recommendations that have been made for the general public also apply to elderly individuals. The Dietary Guidelines are designed for everyone over about five years of age. The National Cholesterol Education Program, designed to reduce the risk of heart disease in the population, suggests that its guidelines be followed by older as well as younger adults. However, this program also cautions that, in the elderly, a very restrictive diet could lead to nutrient deficiencies.[52] Because of the decreased energy requirements of older adults, a nutrient-dense diet must be consumed to meet micronutrient needs.

Appropriate Choices Low intakes of fruits, vegetables, and dairy products is common among the elderly. Limited transportation for shopping, living and eating alone, and changes in the ability to chew and digest foods all contribute to this problem. If frequent shopping is difficult, dried, canned, or frozen fruits and vegetables are a good alternative to fresh ones. Fresh produce spoils easily, so it should be purchased in small quantities and stored in a visible location so it will be eaten shortly after purchase. If chewing and swallowing fresh produce is a problem, these items can be added to soups, stews, and casseroles. To increase dairy product consumption, cheese or yogurt can be eaten by those who do not drink milk. Fruit can be mixed with yogurt or pudding to increase both dairy and fruit consumption.

Flexible Meal Patterns Older individuals may have small appetites. For many, consuming frequent small meals and snacks throughout the day rather than three large meals can increase overall intake. Keeping easy-to-fix foods such as fruit, yogurt, cheese and crackers, milk and cereal, canned soups, and medical nutritional products, such as Ensure or Sustacal, on hand can make getting enough food easier. Older adults with dementia may sometimes forget to eat, so setting a timer can provide a reminder to eat.

Overcoming Limitations to Meet Nutrient Needs There are many reasons why older individuals may not consume diets that meet their nutrient needs. In order to increase nutrient intake, nutrient-dense meals need to be available, appetizing, and easy to prepare and consume.

Overcoming Economic Limitations Being able to afford a healthy diet is a problem for many older individuals. Thus, education about low-cost nutritious food choices can help reduce food costs. Low-cost choices that are high in protein include eggs, beans, turkey, chicken, and some types of fish. Also, cooking and eating at home costs less than eating out. Family and friends can help by giving food gifts, dropping off a weekly bag of groceries, and bringing a meal or food with each visit. Help with shopping can allow the purchase of large amounts of nonperishable foods, such as rice, at a lower cost. Reduced-cost food and meals at senior centers, food stamps, food banks, soup kitchens, and commodity foods are available to people on limited incomes.

Overcoming Social Limitations Another problem that contributes to poor nutrient intake is loneliness. Living, cooking, and eating alone can decrease interest in food. Preparing food for only one person can be frustrating and may contribute to poor intake. This can be a problem not only for the elderly but for anyone who typically eats alone. It is important for people of all ages to keep socially active and share and cook meals with others as often as possible.

Even when eating alone, single people can eat convenient, nutritious, delicious foods. Buying single servings of food is an option, although it can be expensive. To avoid spoilage of perishable items, grocers can be asked to break up packages of meat, eggs, fruits, and vegetables so small amounts can be purchased. Cooking larger portions and freezing foods in meal-size batches can be helpful not only with cost but also to relieve the boredom of eating the same leftovers several days in a row. Creativity and flexibility in what defines a meal can also help. An easy single meal can be prepared by topping a potato with cooked vegetables and cheese, or with leftover chili or spaghetti sauce (Figure 15.12). Yogurt or a bowl of cereal with fruit and milk is also a nutritious dinner option.

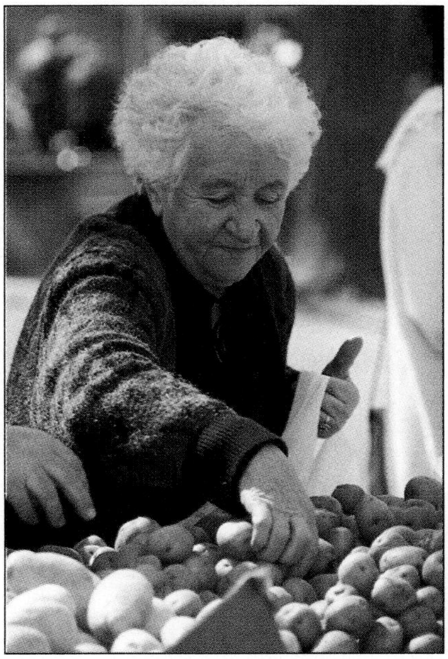

Figure 15.12
Selecting acceptable foods that are nutritious and easy to prepare is important in meeting the needs of the elderly. (© Tony Freeman/PhotoEdit)

Off the Label

Using Food Labels to Follow Special Diets

It is estimated that 85% of elderly individuals have nutrition-related diseases.[1] The treatment of many of these ailments includes restricting or increasing specific nutrients. Food choices may be limited by these special diets, but often individuals are not provided with adequate instruction about how to follow such diets. Understanding the basis for special dietary recommendations and how to use the information on food labels can enhance the food choices of individuals consuming special diets.[2]

One of the most important pieces of information for people with dietary limitations is the nutrient composition of a food. For many nutrients, this information is included in the Nutrition Facts section of the food label. For example, a diabetic who is counting carbohydrates can find the carbohydrate content on the label of almost any packaged food. Individuals with diverticular disease or constipation who are monitoring their fiber intake can use food labels to determine a food's fiber content. Those with kidney disease can use food labels to monitor their protein intake.

There are a number of disease conditions that require altering the micronutrient content of the diet. Food labels can also be helpful for some of these. For example, restricting sodium intake can be important for individuals with hypertension or those with kidney disease. The total amount of sodium in milligrams is listed on all packaged food. However, not all micronutrients are listed on all food labels. For example, individuals taking certain types of hypertension medications may need to monitor potassium intake, but inclusion of potassium information on food labels is voluntary. Individuals with osteoporosis or kidney disease may need to increase their intake of calcium and vitamin D. Good food sources of calcium can be identified because calcium is listed as a percent of the Daily Value on food labels. To determine the milligram amount of calcium in a product, these percentages can be multiplied by the DRI for calcium, which is 1000 mg (see Table 9.2). Information about vitamin D is not required on food labels, but foods that are a good source of vitamin D may include the percent Daily Value voluntarily, and can carry descriptors such as "high in vitamin D," "a good source of vitamin D," or "fortified with vitamin D."

While food labels are a readily available source of information, they must be used carefully. Individuals following a special diet must understand that the Daily Values are goals for a healthy population and may not be appropriate for their special needs. Those consuming special diets must also be aware that the serving sizes on food labels may not be the same as those prescribed in their diets. For example, a typical serving of cooked fish may be 3 ounces, but someone on a protein-restricted diet may be allowed only a 1-ounce serving.

A thorough knowledge of one's dietary prescription and a working knowledge of food labels can enhance one's ability to comply with dietary restrictions and meet nutrient needs while consuming a varied diet.

[1]White, J. V., Ham, R. J., Lipschitz, D. A., et al. Consensus of the Nutrition Screening Initiative: risk factors and indicators of poor nutritional status in older Americans. J. Am. Diet. Assoc. 91: 783–787, 1991.

[2]Kurtzweil, P. The new food label: better information for special diets. FDA Consumer 29: 19–25, January/February, 1995.

Overcoming Physical Limitations Difficulty in cooking due to limited mobility can also reduce food intake. Precooked foods, frozen dinners, or salad bar items, as well as instant foods such as cereals, rice and noodle dishes, and soups that just require adding water, can provide a meal with almost no preparation. Medical nutritional products can also be used to supplement intake. Frozen meals and canned foods are helpful too. Microwave ovens are easy to use, if the individual is instructed in their use, and can cook foods quickly. Food can also be ordered by phone if it is affordable. Eating out at senior centers or low-cost restaurants or sharing shopping and cooking chores with a friend can reduce cooking demand and increase social interaction. Home health services can help with cooking and eating, and most senior centers, health departments, or social service agencies offer meals, rides, and in-home care.

Overcoming Medical Limitations Medical conditions and the use of medications often affect food choices. Meals need to be appealing and easy to prepare and consume, as well as compatible with medical conditions. For instance, an individual with dental problems may not be able to chew fresh fruits and vegetables. Therefore, a texture modification is required. Fully cooked, canned, or soft fruit and fruit juices can be substituted for hard-to-chew fruits, and cooked vegetables can replace raw ones. Eggs and stewed meats can provide easy-to-chew protein sources. To overcome changes in the sense of taste and smell, spicy or acidic foods may be limited or emphasized, depending on individual tastes.

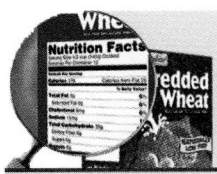

Medical conditions often require special diets. These diets may contribute to malnutrition if they restrict favorite foods and if individuals prescribed the diet are not provided with enough information about how to substitute foods that will give them adequate energy, nutrients, and eating pleasure. Education about what foods are appropriate and how to read food labels can help identify products that fit within dietary restrictions (see *Off the Label: Using Food Labels to Follow Special Diets*).

The use of prescription or over-the-counter medications to treat medical conditions can also affect eating habits. Physicians, pharmacists, and dietitians can provide information about possible effects on food intake. Purchasing all prescription medications from the same pharmacy will ensure that the pharmacist is aware of all medications taken and can advise of possible interactions. Health-care providers also need to be informed about all nonprescription medications and vitamin, mineral, or other dietary supplements used and whether or not medications are taken according to the prescription instructions.

Nutrition Programs for the Elderly The federal Older Americans Act provides nutrition services to older individuals who are in economic need, particularly low-income minorities. Programs that provide nutritious meals in communal settings promote social interaction and can improve nutrient intake. The Congregate and Home-Delivered Nutrition Programs established by the Older Americans Act provide congregate meals at locations such as senior centers, community centers, schools, and churches. For those who are unable to attend congregate meals, home-delivered meals are available.

Although such programs are a first step in meeting nutritional needs, currently most provide only one meal a day for five days a week. Each meal served must provide at least a third of the 1989 RDA.[53] In practice, participants in these elder nutrition programs are receiving 40 to 50% of their daily needs from the meal consumed.[54] Studies have shown that individuals who receive these meals have a better-quality diet and fewer hospitalizations than those who do not.[55] These and other programs addressing the nutritional needs of older adults are described in Table 15.4 (page 525).

CRITICAL THINKING

Dietary Modifications to Meet the Needs of the Elderly

Shirley is 70 years old. She lives alone in the city. Recently, she had most of her teeth extracted because of periodontal disease. Her new dentures are uncomfortable so she has difficulty chewing, and as a result she has eaten only cottage cheese and milk for the past week. Her granddaughter, Anna, begins to worry about Shirley's nutrition.

First, Anna takes her grandmother back to the dentist to see if he can improve the comfort of her dentures. Then she consults a dietitian to learn ways she can help her grandmother eat a nutritious diet. A review of Shirley's medical history finds that she is basically healthy except for her dental problems and being underweight. The dietitian asks Shirley to recall the diet she ate before her teeth were extracted. Anna also points out that the groceries that Shirley buys must be carried home on the bus.

Original Diet		Modified Diet	
Food	**Amount**	**Food**	**Amount**
Breakfast			
~~Bran flakes~~	3/4 cup	Oatmeal	1/2 cup
Lowfat milk	1 cup	Lowfat milk	1 cup
Coffee	1 cup	Coffee	1 cup
Lowfat milk	1 Tbsp	Lowfat milk	1 Tbsp
Sugar	2 tsp	Sugar	2 tsp
Snack			
—	—	Orange juice	1 cup
		Banana bread	1 slice
Lunch			
Gefilte fish	1 oz	Gefilte fish	1 oz
Chicken soup	1 cup	Chicken soup	1 cup
~~Matzoh~~	1	Whole wheat bread	2 slices
~~Apple~~	1 small	Apple juice	1 cup
Dinner			
Lowfat milk	1 cup	Lowfat milk	1 cup
~~Instant rice~~	1 cup	Stew with	
Beef	3 oz	Beef	3 oz
		Potatoes	1 medium
Peas	1 cup	Peas and carrots	1/2 cup
		Gravy	1/2 cup
Snack			
—	—	Banana bread	1 slice
Total energy (kcal)	**1035**		**1720**

Even before her dental problems, Shirley's diet was low in energy, vitamins, and minerals. The dietitian suggests a diet that includes foods that are not only easy to prepare and carry home on the bus but that are also easy to chew. She suggests that Anna take Shirley shopping once a month for the heavy, bulky items like paper goods, laundry soap, rice, cereal, and canned foods. Shirley will be able to handle the smaller, more perishable items when she takes the bus to the store. The dietitian also suggests that Shirley add some snacks to her diet, and recommends meals like stew, which can be made in advance and frozen in individual servings, in order to decrease the amount of time Shirley spends cooking each day. These changes will increase the energy and nutrient content of her diet.

How would Shirley benefit from participating in a congregate meal program at the local senior center?

Answer:

Table 15.4 *National Programs Promoting Better Nutrition Among Older Americans*

Older Americans Act Title III Congregate and Home-Delivered Nutrition Programs

Serves at least one meal five days a week to persons 60 years and older. Meals are served at home or in churches, schools, senior centers, or other facilities.

Older Americans Act Title VI Congregate and Home-Delivered Nutrition Programs

Provides home-delivered and congregate meals to Native American organizations.

Older Americans Act Title III Health Promotion and Disease Prevention Program

Provides health-promotion and disease-prevention services in areas where there are large numbers of economically needy older adults.

Nutrition Screening Initiative

Promotes nutritional screening and more attention to nutrition in all health-care and social-service settings that provide for older adults.

Food Stamp Program

Provides food stamps to low-income individuals including the elderly. These can be used instead of cash to purchase food.

Nutrition Program for the Elderly

Provides grants, cash, and commodity foods to states and tribes to supplement congregate and home-delivered meal programs.

Commodity Supplemental Food Program—Elderly

Provides food, nutrition education, and health-service referrals to individuals with low incomes, including the elderly.

Adult Day Care in the Child and Adult Care Food Program

Provides cash reimbursements and food commodities to community day-care centers that serve meals and snacks to children and elderly with special needs.

Food Distribution Program on Indian Reservations

Distributes commodity foods to low-income persons including the elderly living on or near Indian reservations.

APPLICATIONS

These exercises are designed to help you apply your critical thinking skills to your own nutrition choices. Many are best performed using a diet analysis software program. If you do not have access to a computer program, the exercises can be hand-calculated using the information in this text and its appendices.

1. Use one day of the food record you kept in Chapter 2 and compare it with the RDA for energy for a person who is 70 years old. Modify your food choices to meet the recommendations of the Food Guide Pyramid while not exceeding what your energy needs would be at age 70.
2. Many elderly people have conditions that require dietary modifications. How might you modify your food choices to accommodate a
   a. low-sodium diet?
   b. restriction of protein to 0.6 gram per kilogram of body weight?
   c. loss of smell and taste?
   d. dry mouth and poorly fitting dentures?
3. Using the Internet, assess what kind of nutrition information is available to individuals planning for the care of their elderly parents or relatives.
   a. What types of services are available?
   b. What are the costs?

Summary

1. Aging is the accumulation of changes over time that results in an ever-increasing susceptibility to disease and death. A combination of genetic, environmental, and lifestyle factors determines how long we live and how long we remain healthy.
2. As a population, we are living longer but not necessarily healthier lives. Compression of morbidity, that is increasing the number of healthy years, is an important public health goal. The elderly are the fastest-growing segment of the American population.
3. Life span is a characteristic of a species. The average age to which people in a population live, or life expectancy, is a characteristic of a population. An individual's longevity is affected by genetic background, diet, and lifestyle.
4. The risk of malnutrition increases with age due to the physical, psychological, social, and economic changes that accompany aging.
5. As the body ages, reserve capacity decreases, causing organ function to decline. There are changes in vision and the sense of smell, affecting the ability to eat as well as the appeal of food; changes in digestion and absorption, decreasing the intake and absorption of nutrients; changes in metabolism, affecting nutrient utilization; changes in hormonal patterns, affecting body function; and changes in mobility and mental capacity, limiting the ability to acquire, prepare, and consume food.
6. The incidence of disease increases with increasing age. Both infectious and chronic diseases affect nutrient requirements and the ability to consume a nutritious diet. The medications used to treat disease also affect nutrition, especially when the medications are taken over long periods of time and when multiple medications are taken simultaneously.
7. The social and economic changes that occur with aging, such as loneliness due to retirement and the death of family and friends, can affect nutrient intake.
8. A healthy diet and lifestyle cannot stop aging but can postpone the onset of many of the changes and diseases that are common in older adults.
9. Dietary guidelines for the elderly are not different from those for younger adults. However, since energy needs are decreased but the need for protein, fluid, and most micronutrients is not, meals for the elderly must be nutrient-dense. In addition, individual medical, psychological, social, and economic circumstances must be considered. In some cases, assistance with shopping and meal preparation may be needed.
10. The federal Older Americans Act includes programs that provide older adults with low-cost or free meals in their homes or in a social setting. Although these programs are helpful, they do not ensure adequate nutrition for all elderly.

Review Questions

1. How long can each of us expect to live?
2. What is meant by compression of morbidity?
3. What factors determine at what age the consequences of aging become apparent?
4. Why are older adults at risk for malnutrition?
5. List three physiological changes that occur with aging.
6. List three ways in which medication use and nutrition interact.
7. What social and economic factors increase nutritional risk among the elderly?
8. What causes the energy needs of older adults to be reduced?
9. Why is it so important that elderly individuals consume a nutrient-dense diet?
10. How do recommendations such as the RDAs and the Dietary Guidelines for Americans apply to individuals over the age of 65 years?

Nutrition Web Links

To further explore areas related to the material in this chapter, go to the *Nutrition: Science and Applications* Web site at ***www.Wiley.com/college/Smolin*** and *click on* **Student Companion Site** for chapter-by-chapter links. Some Web sites related to the information in Chapter 15 include:

Organizations that provide resources for elderly persons and their families such as the Administration on Aging and National Institute on Aging.

Organizations that provide information about diseases that become more common with advancing age such as the Arthritis Foundation and the National Eye Institute.

Locations that provide information on local programs that provide services to the elderly such as Meals on Wheels.

References

1. Mazess, R. B., and Forman, S. H. Longevity and age exaggeration in Vilcabamba, Ecuador. J. Gerontol. 34:94–98, 1979.
2. U.S. Department of Health and Human Services, Administration on Aging. Profile of Older Americans. 1998. Online at http://www.aoa.dhhs.gov/aoa/stats/profile/default.htm
3. American Dietetic Association: Position of the American Dietetic Association: nutrition, aging, and the continuum of care. J. Am. Diet. Assoc. 96:1048–1052, 1996.
4. Kirkwood, T. B. L. Comparative life spans of species: why do species have the life spans they do? Am. J. Clin. Nutr. 55(suppl):1191S–1195S, 1992.
5. Shoaf, L. R., and Bishirjina, K. O. Standards of practice for gerontological nutritionists: a mandate for action. J. Am. Diet. Assoc. 95:1433–1438, 1995.
6. Bernard, M. A., Lampley-Dallas, V., and Smith, L. Common health problems among minority elders. J. Am. Diet. Assoc. 97:771–776, 1997.
7. Healthy People 2010. *National Health Promotion and Disease Prevention Objectives.* Washington, D.C.: U.S. Department of Health and Human Services, 1998. Online at http://web.health.gov/healthypeople
8. Hodes, R. J., Cahan, V., and Pruzan, N. The National Institute of Aging at its twentieth anniversary: achievements and promise of research on aging. J. Am. Geriatr. Soc. 44:204–206, 1996.
9. U.S. Department of Health and Human Services, Administration on Aging. 1997 Census Estimates of the Older Population. Online at http://www.aoa.dhhs.gov/aoa/stats/97pop/popx5.htm
10. Blumberg, J. Nutritional needs of seniors. J. Am. Coll. Nutr. 16:517–523, 1997.
11. Wellman, N. S., Weddle, D. O., Brain, C. T., and Kranz, S. Elder insecurities: poverty, hunger, and malnutrition. J. Am. Diet. Assoc. 97:S120–S122, 1997.
12. Coulston, A. M., Craig, L., and Coble Voss, A. Meals on wheels applicants are a population at risk for poor nutritional status. J. Am. Diet. Assoc. 96:570–573, 1996.
13. American Academy of Family Physicians. Nutrition Screening Initiative. Online at http://www.aafp.org/nsi/index.html
14. Young, A. Ageing and physiological functions. Philos. Trans. R. Soc. Lond. B. Biol. Sci. 352:1837–1843, 1997.
15. Duffy, V. B., Backstrand, J. R., and Ferris, A. M. Olfactory dysfunction and related nutritional risk in free-living elderly women. J. Am. Diet. Assoc. 95:879–884, 1995.
16. Morley, J. E. Anorexia of aging: physiologic and pathologic. Am. J. Clin. Nutr. 66:760–773, 1997.
17. Christen, W. G. Antioxidant vitamins and age-related eye disease. Proc. Assoc. Am. Physicians 111:16–21, 1999.
18. Institute of Medicine, Food and Nutrition Board. *Dietary Reference Intakes for Thiamin, Riboflavin, Niacin, Vitamin B6, Folate, Vitamin B12, Pantothenic Acid, Biotin, and Choline.* Washington, D.C.: National Academy Press, 1998.
19. Russell, R. M. New views on the RDAs for older adults. J. Am. Diet. Assoc. 97:515–518, 1997.
20. van Asselt, D. Z., van den Broek, W. J., Lamers, C. B., et al. Free and protein-bound cobalamin absorption in healthy middle-aged and older subjects. J. Am. Geriatr. Soc. 44:949–953, 1996.
21. Harari, D., Gurwitz, J. H., Avorn, J., et al. Bowel habits in relation to age and gender: findings from the National Health Interview Survey and clinical implications. Arch. Intern. Med. 156:315–320, 1996.
22. Brucker, M. C., and Faucher, M. A. Pharmacologic management of common gastrointestinal health problems in women. J. Nurse-Midwifery 42:145–162, May/June 1997.
23. Lubran, M. M. Renal function in the elderly. Ann. Clin. Lab. Sci. 25:122–133, 1995.
24. Lamberts, S. W. J., van den Beld, A. W., and van der Lely, A-J. The endocrinology of aging. Science 278:419–424, 1998.
25. Stevens, J., Cai, J., Pamuk, E. R., et al. The effect of age on the association between body-mass index and mortality. N. Engl. J. Med. 338: 1–7, 1998.
26. Proctor, D. N., Balagopal, P., and Nair, K. S. Age-related sarcopenia in humans is associated with reduced synthetic rates of specific muscle proteins. J. Nutr. 128:351S–355S, 1998.
27. Evans, W. J., and Cyr-Campbell, D. Nutrition, exercise and healthy aging. J. Am. Diet. Assoc. 97:632–638, 1997.
28. Wallace, J. I., and Schwartz, R. S. Involuntary weight loss in elderly outpatients: recognition, etiologies and treatment. Clin. Geriatr. Med. 13:717–735, 1997.
29. Masoro, E. J. Possible mechanisms underlying the antiaging actions of caloric restriction. Toxicol. Pathol. 24:738–741, 1996.
30. Bastianetto, S., and Quirion, R. Any facts behind the DHEA hype? Trends Pharmacol. Sci. 18:447–449, 1997.
31. Rieter, R. J. The pineal gland and melatonin in relation to aging: a summary of the theories and the data. Exp. Gerontol. 30:199–212, 1995.
32. Maestroni, G. J. P-helper-2 lymphocytes as a peripheral target of melatonin. J. Pineal Res. 18:84–89, 1995.
33. Lesourd, B. M., Mazari, L., and Ferry, M. The role of nutrition in immunity in the aged. Nutr. Rev. 56 (II):S113–S125, 1998.
34. Lesourd, B. Protein undernutrition as the major cause of decreased immune function in the elderly: clinical and functional implications. Nutr. Rev. 53:S86–S94, 1995.
35. Meydani, S. N., Meydani, M., Blumberg, J. B., et al. Vitamin E supplementation and in vivo immune responses in healthy elderly subjects. J.A.M.A. 277:1380–1386, 1997.
36. Meydani, S. N., Wu, D., Santos, M. S., et al. Antioxidants and immune response in aged persons: overview of the present evidence. Am. J. Clin. Nutr. 62(suppl):1426S–1476S, 1995.
37. Bogden, J. D. Studies on micronutrient supplements and immunity in older people. Nutr. Rev. 53:S59–S65, 1995.
38. Stabler, S. P., Lindenbaum, J., and Allen, R. H. Vitamin B12 deficiency in the elderly: current dilemmas. Am. J. Clin. Nutr. 66:741–749, 1997.
39. Vogel, G. Tau protein mutations confirmed as neuron killers. Science 280:1524–1525, 1998.
40. American Academy of Family Physicians. The Nutrition Checklist. Online at http:www.aafp.org/nsi
41. American Dietetic Association: Position of the American Dietetic Association: liberalized diets for older adults in long-term care. J. Am. Diet. Assoc. 98:201–204, 1998.
42. Chidester, J. C., and Spangler, A. A. Fluid intake in the institutionalized elderly. J. Am. Diet. Assoc. 97:23–28, 1997.
43. Cui, X. J., and Vaillant, G. E. Antecedents and consequences of negative life events in adulthood: a longitudinal study. Am. J. Psychiatry 153:21–26, 1996.
44. Evans, W. J., and Cyr-Campbell, D. Nutrition, exercise and healthy aging. J. Am. Diet. Assoc. 97:632–638, 1997.
45. Young, V. R. Energy requirements in the elderly. Nutr. Rev. 50:95–101, 1992.
46. Institute of Medicine, Food and Nutrition Board. *Dietary Reference Intakes: Calcium, Phosphorus, Magnesium, Vitamin D, and Fluoride.* Washington, D.C.: National Academy Press, 1997.
47. Kohlmeier, L., and Hastings, S. B. Epidemiologic evidence of a role of carotenoids in cardiovascular disease prevention. Am. J. Clin Nutr. 62(suppl):1370S–1376S, 1995.
48. Rimm, E. B., Stampfer, M. J., Ascherio, A., et al. Vitamin E consumption and the risk of heart disease in men. N. Engl. J. Med. 328:1450–1456, 1993.

49. Stampfer, M. J., Hennekens, C. H., Manson, J. E., et al. Vitamin E consumption and the risk of heart disease in women. N. Engl. J. Med. 328:1487–1489, 1993.
50. Taylor, A., Jacques, P. F., and Epstein, E. M. Relations among aging, antioxidant status and cataract. Am. J. Clin. Nutr. 62(suppl):1439S–1447S, 1995.
51. Diplock, A. T. Safety of antioxidant vitamins and beta-carotene. Am. J. Clin. Nutr. 62(suppl):1510S–1516S, 1995.
52. The Expert Panel. Summary of the Second Report of the National Cholesterol Education Program Expert Panel on Detection, Evaluation and Treatment of High Blood Cholesterol in Adults. J.A.M.A. 269:3015–3023, 1993.
53. Fogler-Levitt, E., Lau, D., Csima, A., et al. Utilization of home-delivered meals by recipients 75 years of age or older. J. Am. Diet. Assoc. 95:552–557, 1995.
54. U.S. Department of Health and Human Services, Administration on Aging. Elderly Nutrition Program. Online at http://www.aoa.gov/nutrition/default.htm
55. Roe, D. A. Development and current status of home-delivered meals programs in the United States: are the right elderly served? Nutr. Rev. 52:29–33, 1994.

V

Nutrition in Today's World

Chapter 16
How Safe Is Our Food Supply?

Chapter 17
The Global View: Feeding the World

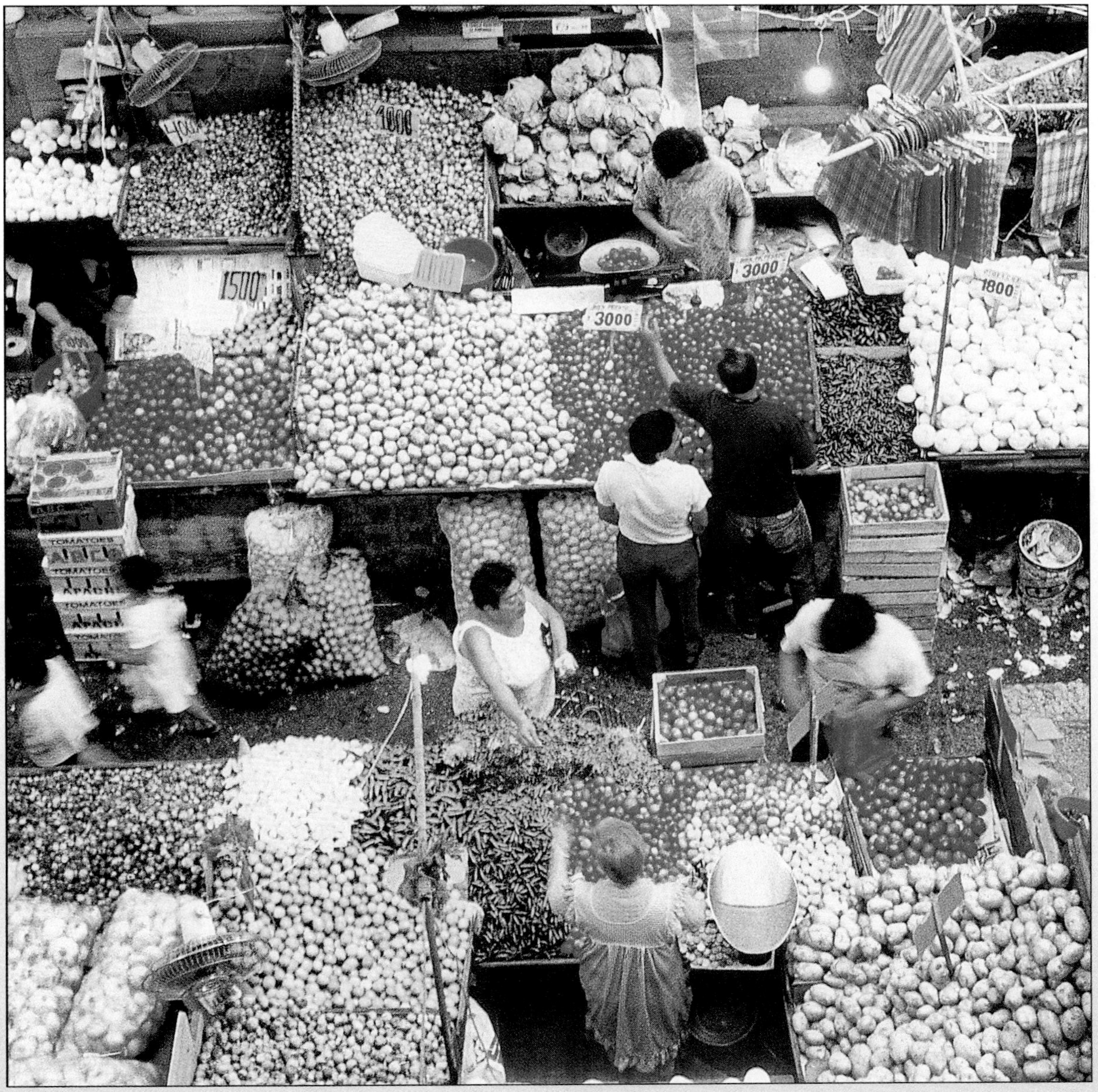

Chapter 16

Chapter Outline

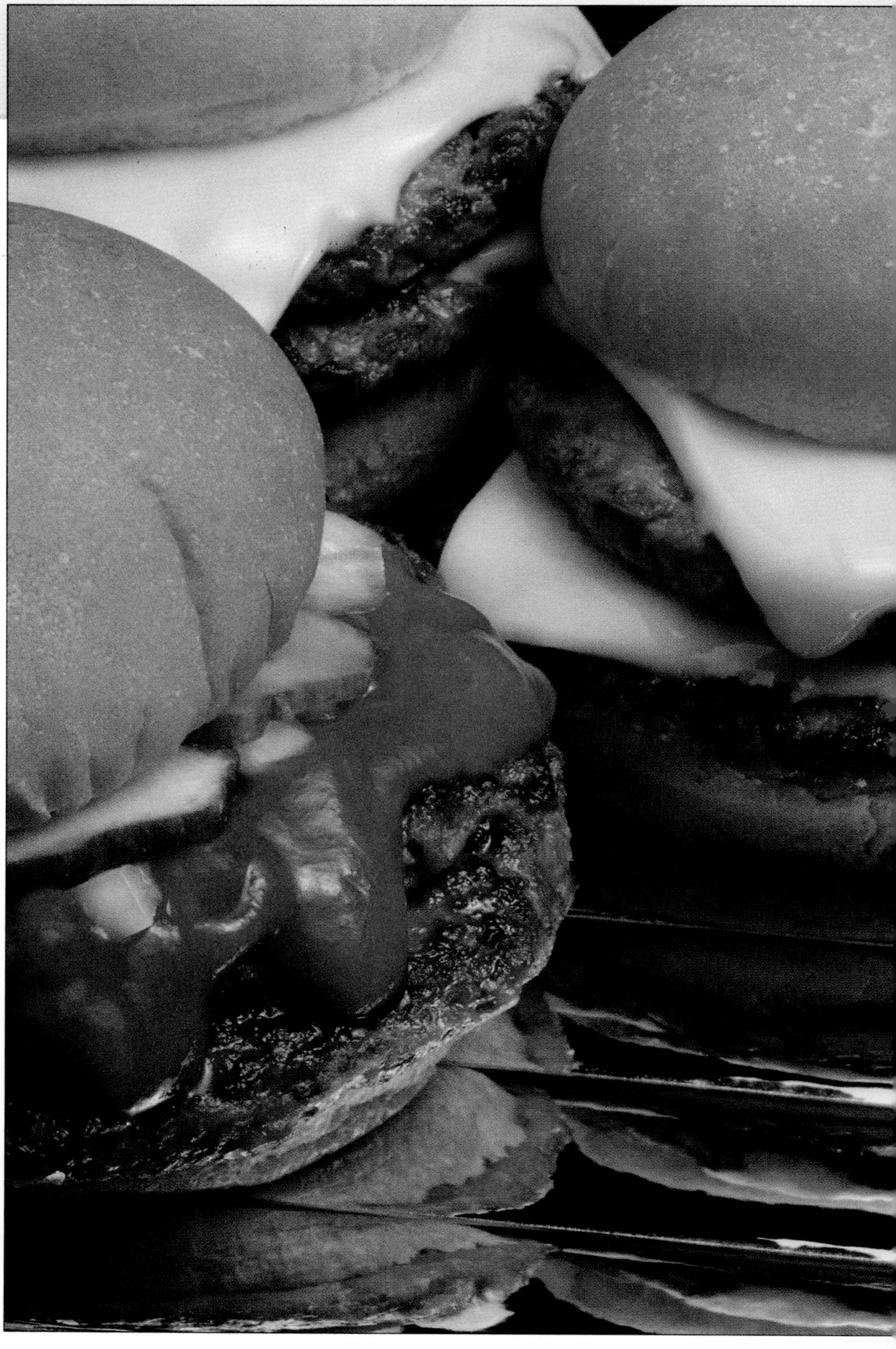

(Corbis)

How Safe Is Our Food Supply?

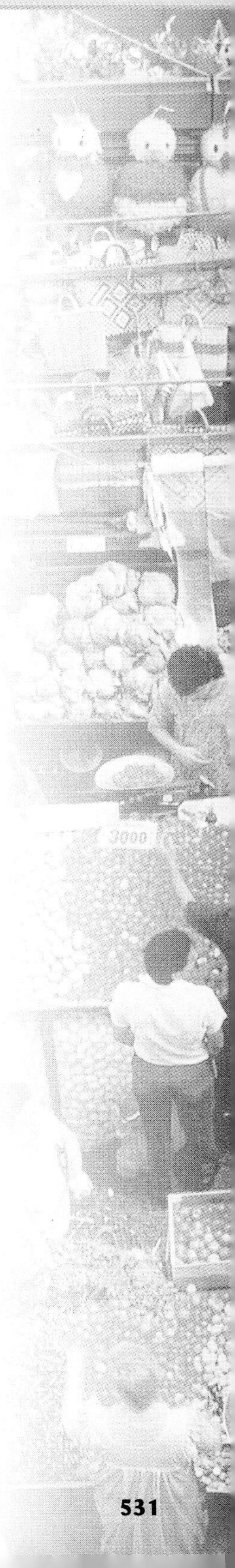

Chapter Concepts

1. Microbial contamination is the number one cause of food-borne illness in the United States. Chemical contamination can also affect the safety of the food supply.
2. Food-borne illness results when food contains a large enough amount of a contaminant to cause harm to the individual consuming it.
3. Public health concern about the safety of the food supply has led to the initiation of programs to prevent food contamination, improve monitoring of the food supply, and enhance communication systems for tracking food-related illness.
4. Bacteria, viruses, molds, and parasites all contaminate food and have the potential to cause food-borne illness.
5. Care in choosing, preparing, cooking, handling, and storing food can reduce the risk of consuming contaminants.
6. Chemicals used in agriculture and industry can contaminate the environment and make their way into the food supply.
7. Direct food additives are used to protect foods from microbial contamination, enhance nutrient content, increase shelf life, aid in processing, and increase the appeal of food products.
8. Packaging and processing can improve the safety of the food supply but may also pose risks.
9. Newer food technologies include irradiation, which uses x-rays, gamma rays, or high-energy electrons to preserve foods, and biotechnology, which creates new foods and products by manipulating DNA.

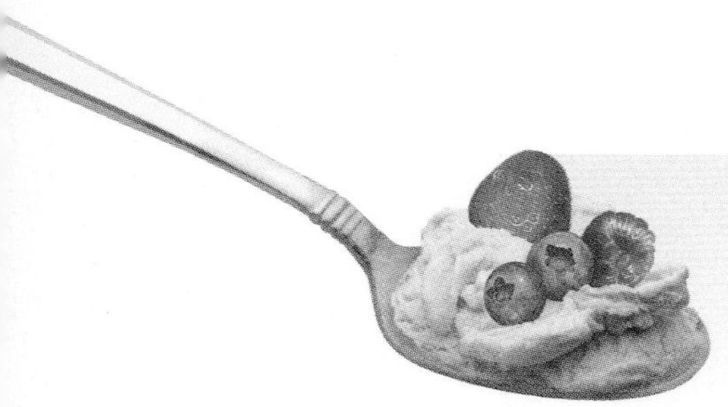

Just a Taste

Is it safe to eat hamburgers cooked medium rare?

Can you tell if your food is contaminated with bacteria?

Do food additives make the food supply safer?

The American food supply is the most carefully monitored in the world; nonetheless, *Salmonella* bacteria contaminate chicken sold in the United States, pesticide residues are found on our fruit, and industrial waste has polluted some of our waterways. Headlines announce *E. coli* in meat and apple juice; *Salmonella* in eggs, on vegetables, and in cereal; *Cyclospora* on fruit; *Cryptosporidium* in drinking water; and hepatitis A in frozen strawberries. In 1997, 25 million pounds of hamburger suspected of harboring a disease-causing strain of *E. coli*—*E. coli* O157:H7—were voluntarily recalled by the food distributor. Although the American food supply may in fact be the safest in the world, it is not risk free or beyond improvement. As many as 9,000 people in the United States, mostly children and the elderly, die each year of food-related illness and millions more become ill.[1]

If given a choice, most people would elect to consume food that contains no harmful substances. However, it is nearly impossible to choose a diet that is free of all potential hazards. Food has always carried the risks of bacterial contamination and naturally occurring toxins. In the modern world, changes in agricultural technology, trade patterns, food processing, and dietary habits have increased the risks associated with bacterial contamination and introduced new risks. Pesticides used to increase crop yields in South America contaminate fruits and vegetables shipped to New York, materials in food packaging may be leaching into the foods they are designed to protect, and additives used to preserve food may cause allergies and intolerances. Regulatory agencies, food manufacturers, and retailers as well as consumers must work together to maximize the safety of the food supply.

Weighing the Risks and Benefits

People need to eat to stay alive. However, an unsafe food supply can cause illness and even death. The risks of consuming a contaminated food must be weighed against the benefits that food provides. Risk-benefit analyses are done by regulatory agencies when they evaluate the safety and sanitation of food processing methods and food service establishments. Consumers must also consider the risks and benefits when they choose which foods to buy, which to eat, and how to handle, store, and cook these foods (Figure 16.1).

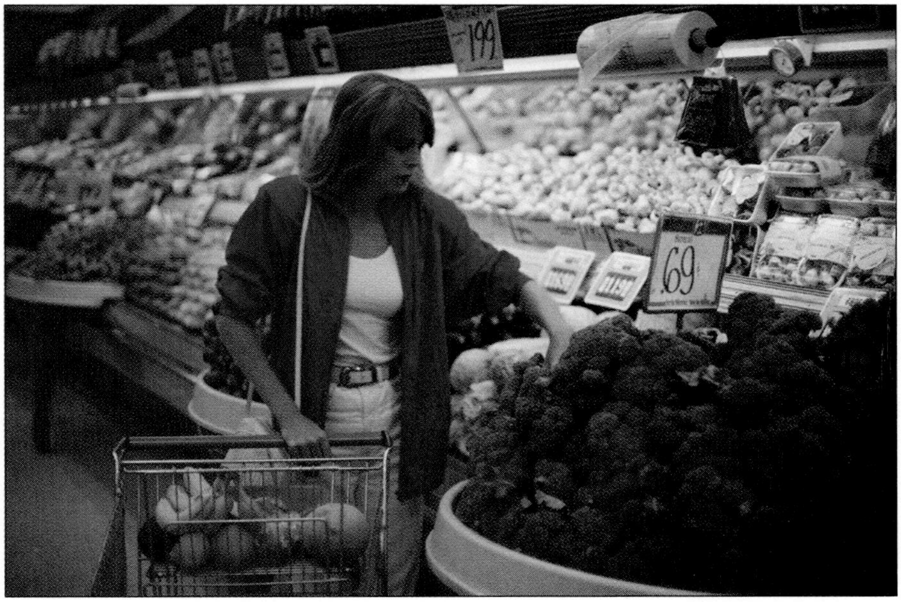

Figure 16.1
Choosing safe, nutritious foods is one way that consumers help control the safety of the foods they eat. (© 1999 PhotoDisc, Inc.)

The Risks of Food-Borne Illness

Most of the **food-borne illness** in the United States is caused by the contamination of food with **pathogens,** microorganisms or microbes that can cause disease. **Toxins** produced by these microorganisms, as well as those present in the environment and those used in the processing and packaging of food, can also contaminate food and increase risk to the consumer. However, the presence of contaminants in a food does not always mean that the food is hazardous.

Food-borne illness An illness caused by consumption of food containing a toxin or disease-causing microorganism.

Pathogen An organism capable of causing disease.

Toxins Substances that can cause harm at some level of exposure.

Where Does Food Get Contaminated? Many foods are contaminated where they are grown or produced. *Salmonella enteritidis* may enter eggs directly from the hen, and *E. coli* from the intestinal tract of a single cow may spread contamination to thousands of pounds of hamburger during processing. Fish and seafood may be contaminated by agricultural runoff, sewage, and other toxins in our waterways. Molds grow on grains during unusually wet or dry growing seasons. Milk, eggs, seafood, meat, and poultry can be contaminated by the misuse of veterinary drugs and poor production or harvesting practices. Food can also be contaminated during processing or storage, at retail facilities, and even at home. Most of these sources of contamination, can be controlled by careful sanitation and food handling. Regardless of the original source of contamination, most of the cases of food-borne illness are caused by foods prepared at home.[2]

When Do Contaminants Make Us Sick? The potential of a substance to cause harm depends on how potent it is, the amount or dose that is consumed, how frequently it is consumed, and who consumes it. Some contaminants in food cause harm even when minute amounts are consumed, and almost any substance can be toxic if a large enough amount is consumed. Many substances have a **threshold effect;** that is, they are harmless up to a certain dose or threshold, after which negative effects increase with increasing intake. Body size, nutritional status, and how a substance is metabolized by the body can affect toxicity. Small doses are more dangerous in children and small adults because the amount of toxin per unit of body weight is greater. Poor nutritional or health status may decrease the body's natural ability to detoxify harmful substances. The way that a substance is stored or excreted also determines its potential for harm. Substances that are stored in the body are more likely to be toxic because they accumulate over time. They are deposited in bone, adipose tissue, the liver, or other organs until toxicity

Threshold effect A reaction that occurs at a certain level of ingestion and increases as the dose increases. Below that level there is no reaction.

symptoms occur. For instance, vitamin A is stored in the liver and can be toxic if excess amounts are consumed over a long period. Substances that are easily excreted when consumed in excess, such as vitamin C, are less likely to cause toxicity. The interaction of toxins with one another and with other dietary factors also affects toxicity. For example, mercury, which is extremely toxic, is not absorbed well if the diet is high in selenium, and the absorption of lead is decreased by the presence of iron and calcium in the diet.

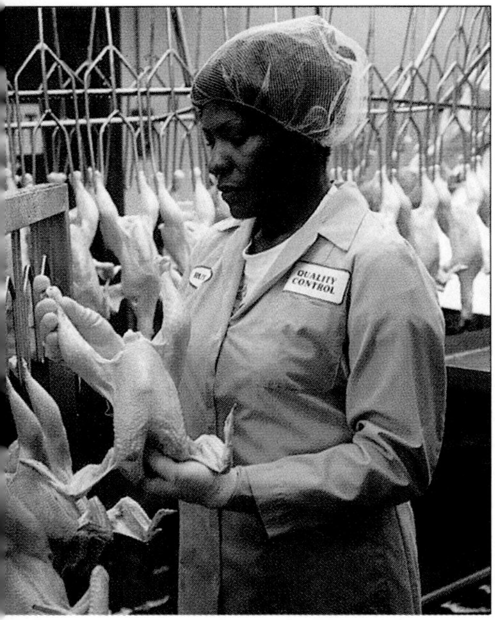

Figure 16.2
Traditional methods of protecting the food supply rely on spot-checks by food safety inspectors. (© Don Smetzer/Tony Stone Worldwide-Click/Chicago Ltd.)

Safeguarding Our Food Supply

Concern about the safety of our food supply is not new. In the early 1900s, a novel by Upton Sinclair, *The Jungle*, caused a public outcry by its description of Chicago's meatpacking industry. Repulsive conditions in the rat-infested processing plants, where spoiled meat was processed alongside fresh, were revealed. This led to the passage of the nation's first food regulations, and since then the government has been involved in safeguarding the food supply.

Traditional methods for protecting the food supply have involved setting standards for food safety and conducting spot-checks of manufacturing conditions and products (Figure 16.2). These spot-checks often rely on visual inspection to detect contamination. Inspecting all food-processing establishments is a daunting task and contamination is easily missed using this method. Recently, media coverage of large outbreaks of food-borne illnesses has heightened concern about food safety and encouraged regulatory agencies and food manufacturers to establish a better system for safeguarding the food supply. These concerns have been addressed at the federal level in the National Food Safety Initiative, which targets all aspects of food safety from the farm to the table. This program promotes the implementation of a system called **Hazard Analysis Critical Control Point (HACCP)** to improve food safety. HACCP is designed to prevent food contamination rather than catch it after it occurs.

Hazard Analysis Critical Control Point (HACCP) A food safety system that focuses on identifying and preventing hazards that could cause food-borne illness.

National Food Safety Initiative The National Food Safety Initiative was conceived to reduce the incidence of food-borne illness by improving food safety practices and policies throughout the United States. The focus is on reducing the risk of microbial food-borne illness because microorganisms are the most common cause of food-borne illness. However, the initiative also recognizes that chemical contaminants can cause food-borne illness.[3]

The Food Safety Initiative includes programs to enhance food safety and monitoring; to promote an increase in research into methods for more rapid detection of food-borne pathogens; to improve intergovernmental tracking of and response to food-borne outbreaks; and to educate food service personnel as well as consumers.[1]

In response to the Food Safety Initiative, a national computer network linking public health laboratories is in place.[4] This enables epidemiologists to quickly respond to serious and widespread food contamination problems. With this system, the distinctive DNA fingerprint of a pathogenic strain of a microorganism can be tracked. For example, if outbreaks of food-borne illness in Ohio and Minnesota are both caused by the same strain of an organism, epidemiologists know that the outbreaks were caused by the same food source. They can focus their search for the source of contamination on foods distributed to both locations. To confirm the source, the DNA fingerprint isolated from the organisms found in victims can be matched to the DNA fingerprint from a contaminated food source.

HACCP The HACCP approach to food safety is based on identifying points in the handling of food, called **critical control points,** where chemical, physical, or microbial contamination can occur.[1] Once these points have been identified, a plan is devised to prevent, control, or eliminate the contamination before the food reaches the consumer. This requires establishing standardized procedures for

Critical control points Possible points in food production, manufacturing, and transportation at which contamination could occur or be prevented.

monitoring control points, taking corrective actions when the control or prevention isn't effective, and establishing record-keeping procedures to verify the system is working consistently. Each manufacturer or processor is required to set up its own HACCP plan based on the system used in the industry.

The HACCP system allows companies to anticipate where contamination will occur and to design plans to prevent the food hazard from reaching the consumer. For example, contamination with *Salmonella* has been identified as a risk in the production of shelled frozen eggs. To produce this product, eggs are removed from their shells; mixed together in large vats; heated, in a process called **pasteurization,** to kill *Salmonella* and other microbial contaminants; packaged; and then frozen (Figure 16.3). The critical control point for preventing contaminated eggs from getting to consumers is the pasteurization process. To monitor the effectiveness of pasteurization in the frozen egg industry, bacterial tests are performed. Once the eggs are pasteurized, samples are removed to test for *Salmonella.* The eggs are held refrigerated or frozen until the results of the bacterial tests have been obtained. If the eggs are *Salmonella*-free, they are released to the market. If they contain *Salmonella*, the batch of eggs cannot be sold and pasteurization conditions are adjusted to ensure that *Salmonella* is killed in the next batch. Extensive record keeping enables the manufacturer to trace which eggs were pasteurized when, for how long, and at what temperature, and when and where they were shipped in the event of an outbreak of food-borne illness.

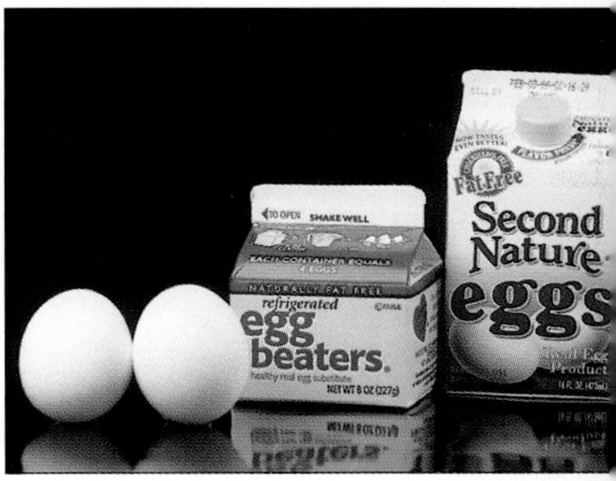

Figure 16.3
Salmonella contamination is a concern in the production of frozen eggs. (George Semple)

Pasteurization The process of heating food products to kill disease-causing organisms.

Although the focus in this example is microbial, HACCP also identifies other food hazards such as chemicals, toxins, and physical objects such as broken glass and rodent hair. Currently HACCP is required in the seafood industry and is being implemented in other areas of food production, such as the processing of meat, poultry, and fruit and vegetable juices. The advantage of this system over standard inspections by the FDA is that the plan is preventative rather than punitive, oversight is easier, and the responsibility for food safety is placed on the manufacturer, not the regulatory agencies.

Monitoring Foods From Farm to Table The safety of the food supply is monitored by agencies at the international, federal, state, and local levels. International cooperation on food inspection and regulatory standards helps to ensure the safety of imported foods. Approximately 40 different nations are now partners with the United States in ensuring food safety through agreements that regulate a variety of food products. The Food and Drug Administration (FDA), the Food Safety and Inspection Service (FSIS) of the U.S. Department of Agriculture (USDA), the Environmental Protection Agency (EPA), the Centers for Disease Control and Prevention (CDC), the Department of Commerce's National Oceanic and Atmospheric Administration, and other federal agencies all monitor segments of the food supply (see Table 16.1). These agencies set standards and establish regulations for the safe and sanitary handling of food and water as well as the use of additives and packaging techniques. They also set standards for both the nutrition information and the safe-handling information on food labels. They inspect food processing and storage facilities, monitor both domestic and imported foods for contamination, and investigate outbreaks of food-borne illness. These agencies work together to ensure a safe food supply from the farm to the table.

On the Farm Food on the farm is regulated primarily by state and federal agencies. The EPA approves pesticides and establishes acceptable levels of pesticide use. The FDA oversees the use of drugs and feed in milk- and food-producing animals. The Animal and Plant Health Inspection Service (APHIS) works to control disease in animals. Federal agencies also monitor the environmental impact of production, harvesting, and waste elimination procedures that could contaminate groundwater or grazing land.

Table 16.1 *Agencies Responsible for Food Safety*

Agency	Responsibility
FDA (Food and Drug Administration)	Ensures the safety and wholesomeness of all foods sold across state lines with the exception of red meat (beef, veal, pork, and lamb), poultry, and egg products; inspects food-processing plants and imported foods; sets standards for food composition; oversees use of drugs and feed in food-producing animals; and enforces regulations for food labeling, food and color additives, and food sanitation.
FSIS (Food Safety and Inspection Service) at the USDA (U.S. Department of Agriculture)	Enforces standards for the wholesomeness and quality of red meat, poultry, and egg products.
EPA (Environmental Protection Agency)	Regulates pesticide levels and must approve all pesticides before they can be sold in the United States; establishes water quality standards.
National Marine Fishery Service at the Department of Commerce	Oversees the management of fisheries and fish harvesting. Operates a voluntary program of inspection and grading of fish products.
Animal and Plant Health Inspection Service (APHIS)	Helps control disease in food-producing animals.
CDC (Centers for Disease Control and Prevention)	Monitors and investigates the incidence and causes of food-borne diseases.
ATF (Bureau of Alcohol, Tobacco, and Firearms)	Enforces laws regulating the production, distribution, and labeling of alcoholic beverages.

Food Processing The FDA regulates the processing of foods other than meat, poultry, and egg products (except shelled eggs). The processing of meat, poultry, and egg products is regulated by the FSIS of the USDA. State and local governments can also inspect food-processing plants.

Food Transported Interstate and From Foreign Countries Foods that are produced in the United States and transported across state lines are subject to federal and state regulations. Meat, poultry, and most egg products imported from other countries are overseen by the FSIS, and the FDA oversees all other imported foods. If a food is suspect, it can be tested for contamination and entry into the country denied.

Restaurants, Supermarkets, and Institutional Food Food in these institutions is regulated by state and local health authorities. The FDA provides guidelines to state and local governments for regulating dairy products and food sold at restaurants. States then have the primary responsibility for milk safety and the inspection of restaurants, retail food stores, dairies, grain mills, and other food-related establishments within their borders (Figure 16.4). As a result, regulations vary from state to state. The FDA publishes the **Food Code,** which provides recommendations for safeguarding public health when food is offered to the consumer. National standards for drinking water are set by the EPA but enforced by local public water authorities. The FDA establishes comparable standards for bottled water (see Chapter 10, *Off the Shelf: Is Bottled Water Better?*).

Food Code A set of recommendations published by the FDA for the handling and service of food sold in restaurants and other establishments that serve food.

In the Home Consumers must also be actively involved in preventing food-borne illness. Individuals must decide what foods they will consume and evaluate the risks involved. A food that has been manufactured, packaged, and

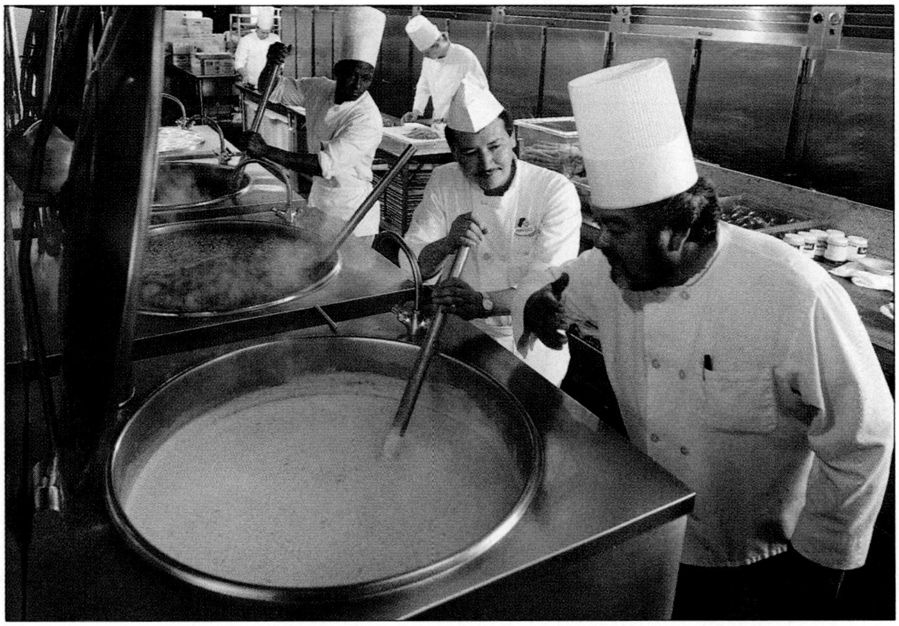

Figure 16.4
State and local governments are responsible for regulating the safety of food sold at restaurants. (Art Montes de Oca/FPG International)

transported with the greatest care can still cause food-borne illness if it is not carefully handled at home. For example, foods such as eggs, chicken, or hamburger when undercooked can cause microbial food-borne illness. Consumers can help prevent this by following safe food-handling, cooking, and storage practices. Consumers can also protect themselves and others by reporting incidents involving unsanitary, unsafe, deceptive, or mislabeled food to the appropriate agencies (Table 16.2).

Pathogens and Parasites in Food

Food-borne illness can be caused by consuming food contaminated with bacteria, viruses, molds, or parasites or by consuming foods contaminated with toxins produced by these organisms (Table 16.3). It is estimated that about 9000 deaths and as many as 81 million cases of food-borne illness occur in the United States each year.[5] Food-borne illness is usually suspected only when a large number of people who consumed the same food develop the same symptoms shortly after eating. In most cases, the symptoms of a microbial food-borne illness include abdominal pain, nausea, diarrhea, and vomiting. These relatively mild symptoms are often mistaken for the flu. Food-borne illness can also cause symptoms other than those involving the gastrointestinal tract. It can cause spontaneous abortion; hemolytic uremia syndrome, which can lead to kidney failure and death; and long-lasting conditions like arthritis and Guillain-Barré syndrome, which is the most common cause of acute paralysis in adults and children. Young children, pregnant women, elderly persons, and individuals with compromised immune systems, such as AIDS and cancer patients, are most susceptible to severe reactions.[1] Avoiding microbial food-borne illness requires a knowledge of how contamination occurs and how to handle, store, and prepare food safely.

Bacteria

Bacteria are ubiquitous in our environment. They are present in the soil, on our skin, on most surfaces in our homes, and in the food we eat. Most of the bacteria in our environment are harmless. Pathogenic bacteria cause disease either by

Table 16.2 *How to Report an Incident Involving Unsanitary, Unsafe, Deceptive, or Mislabeled Food*

First, get all the facts. Have you used the product as intended and according to the manufacturer's instructions? Check to be sure the item is not being used past its expiration date. Once these steps have been taken, immediately report the item or incident to the appropriate agency. Do not wait.

Then report the incident to the appropriate agency:

- **Problems relating to any food except meat and poultry,** including adverse reactions, should be reported to the FDA Food and Seafood Information line (1-800-332-4010). If it is an emergency requiring immediate action, such as a case of food-borne illness, call the FDA's emergency number (1-301-443-1240). For a problem not requiring immediate attention, the FDA district office consumer complaint coordinator for your geographic area can be contacted.[1]
- **Issues relating to meat and poultry** should be reported first to your state's department of agriculture and then to the USDA hotline (1-800-535-4555).
- **Restaurant food and sanitation** problems can be reported directly to local or state health departments.
- **Issues related to alcoholic beverages** should be reported to the Department of the Treasury's Bureau of Alcohol, Tobacco, and Firearms.
- **Accidental poisonings** should be reported to state or local poison control centers or hospitals before calling the Centers for Disease Control and Prevention.
- **Pesticide, air, and water pollution** should be reported first to your state's environmental protection department and then to the EPA.
- **Products purchased at the grocery store** should be returned to the store. Grocery stores are concerned with the safety of the foods they sell, and they will take the responsibility of tracking down and correcting the problem as well as refunding your money or replacing the product with one that is safe.
- **Hazardous household products** are the responsibility of the state department of consumer protection and, federally, the Consumer Product Safety Commission (http://www.cpsc.gov/).
- **False advertising** should be reported first to your state's department of consumer protection and then to the Federal Trade Commission.
- **Unsolicited products in the mail** should be reported to the U.S. Postal Service.

[1]How to report adverse reactions and other problems with products regulated by FDA. FDA Backgrounder, April 29, 1998. Online at http://www.fda.gov/opacom/backgrounders/problem.html

growing in the gastrointestinal tract or by producing toxins. Bacterial pathogens are responsible for most outbreaks of food-borne illness.[2]

Pathogenic bacteria frequently contaminate food before it is purchased. Food may also be infected by **cross-contamination.** This occurs when a contaminated food or anything that has touched it comes in contact with an uninfected food, resulting in transfer of bacteria. If the contaminated food is not properly handled, the bacteria will multiply. The more bacteria a food contains when it is consumed, the more likely it is to cause a food-borne illness. Most bacteria grow and reproduce in the temperature range between 41°F and 140°F. Storing food at temperatures below 40°F will slow or stop most bacterial growth. And because high temperatures kill most bacteria, cooking food to above 140°F can destroy the bacteria that have contaminated a food (Figure 16.5).

Cross-contamination The transfer of contaminants from one food to another.

Bacterial Food-Borne Infection **Food-borne infection** is caused when a food containing pathogenic bacteria is ingested and the bacteria grow in the gastrointestinal tract. Subsequently, these bacteria may also grow in other tissues or produce toxins within the body. Usually a large number of bacteria must be consumed to cause illness. Some common causes of bacterial infections include *Salmonella, Campylobacter jejuni, Listeria monocytogenes*, and *Vibrio vulnificus*. The most frequent sources of food-borne illness and the symptoms associated with them are included in Table 16.3.

Food-borne infection Illness produced by the ingestion of food containing microorganisms that can multiply inside the body and produce injurious effects.

Table 16.3 *Which Bug Has You Down?*

Microbe	Sources	Symptoms	Onset	Duration
Bacteria				
Salmonella	Fecal contamination, raw or undercooked eggs and meat, especially poultry	Nausea, abdominal pain, diarrhea, headache, fever	6–48 hrs	1–2 days
Campylobacter jejuni	Unpasteurized milk, undercooked meat and poultry	Fever, headache, diarrhea, abdominal pain	2–5 days	1–2 wks
Listeria monocytogenes	Raw milk products, raw and undercooked poultry and meats, raw and smoked fish, produce	Fever, headache, stiff neck, chills, nausea, vomiting	Days to weeks	6 wks
Vibrio vulnificus	Raw seafood from contaminated water	Cramps, abdominal pain, weakness, watery diarrhea, fever, chills	15–24 hrs	2–4 days
Staphylococcus aureus	Human contamination from coughs and sneezes, eggs, meat, potato and macaroni salads	Severe nausea, vomiting, diarrhea	2–8 hrs	24–48 hrs
Escherichia coli O157:H7	Fecal contamination, undercooked ground beef	Abdominal pain, bloody diarrhea, kidney failure	5–48 hrs	3 days to 2 wks or longer
Clostridium perfringens	Fecal contamination, deep-dish casseroles	Fever, nausea, diarrhea, abdominal pain	8–22 hrs	6–24 hrs
Clostridium botulinum	Canned foods, deep casseroles, honey	Lassitude, weakness, vertigo, dizziness, respiratory failure, paralysis	18–36 hrs	10 days or longer (must administer antitoxin)
Shigella	Fecal contamination of water or foods, especially salads such as chicken, tuna, shrimp, and potato salad	Diarrhea, abdominal pain, fever, vomiting	12–50 hrs	5–6 days
Yersinia enterocolitica	Pork, dairy products, and produce	Diarrhea, vomiting, fever, abdominal pain; often mistaken for appendicitis	24–48 hrs	Weeks
Viruses				
Norwalk virus	Fecal contamination of seafood	Diarrhea, nausea, vomiting	1–2 days	2–6 days
Hepatitis A virus	Human fecal contamination of food or water, raw shellfish	Jaundice, liver inflammation, fatigue, fever, nausea, anorexia, abdominal discomfort	10–50 days	1–2 wks to several months
Parasites				
Giardia lamblia	Fecal contamination of water and uncooked foods	Diarrhea, abdominal pain, gas, anorexia, nausea, vomiting	5–25 days	1–2 wks but may become chronic
Cryptosporidium parvum	Fecal contamination of food or water	Severe watery diarrhea	Hours	2–4 days but sometimes weeks
Trichinella spiralis	Undercooked pork, game meat	Muscle weakness, flu symptoms	Weeks	Months
Anisakis simplex	Raw fish	Severe abdominal pain	1 hr to 2 wks	3 wks
Toxoplasma gondii	Meat, primarily pork	Toxoplasmosis (can cause central nervous system disorders, flu-like symptoms, and birth defects in women exposed during pregnancy)	10–23 days	May become chronic carrier

Source: U.S. Food and Drug Administration, Center for Food Safety and Nutrition. Foodborne Pathogenic Microorganisms and Natural Toxins Handbook: The "Bad Bug Book." Online at http://vm.cfsan.fda.gov/~mow/intro.html

Estimates of the number of people infected with *Salmonella* each year in the United States range from 800,000 to 4 million. Most of these people just experience diarrhea, but sometimes more serious infections can be fatal. *Salmonella* is found in animal and human feces and infects food through contaminated water or improper handling. *Salmonella* outbreaks have been caused by contaminated meat, meat products, dairy products, seafood, fresh vegetables, and cereal, but

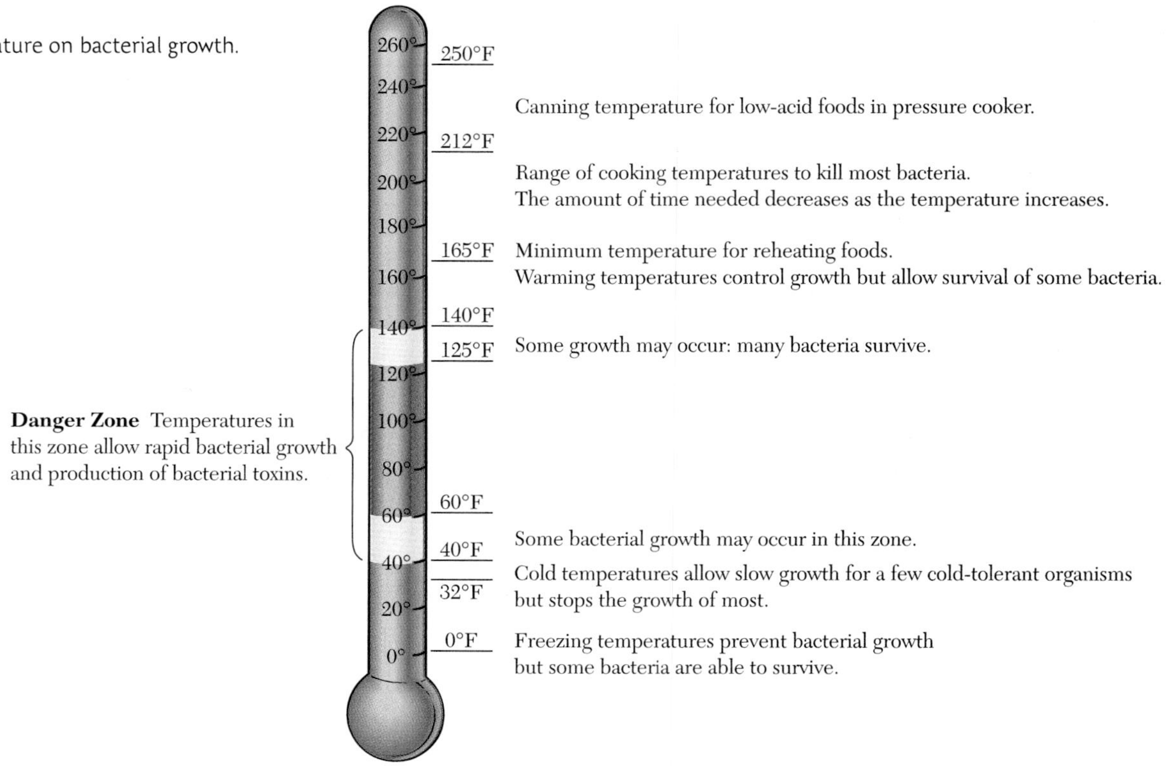
260°
240°
220°
200°
180°
160°
140°
120°
100°
80°
60°
40°
20°
0°
250°F
212°F
165°F
140°F
125°F
60°F
40°F
32°F
0°F
Canning temperature for low-acid foods in pressure cooker.
Range of cooking temperatures to kill most bacteria.
The amount of time needed decreases as the temperature increases.
Minimum temperature for reheating foods.
Warming temperatures control growth but allow survival of some bacteria.
Some growth may occur: many bacteria survive.
Danger Zone Temperatures in this zone allow rapid bacterial growth and production of bacterial toxins.
Some bacterial growth may occur in this zone.
Cold temperatures allow slow growth for a few cold-tolerant organisms but stops the growth of most.
Freezing temperatures prevent bacterial growth but some bacteria are able to survive.

Figure 16.5
The effect of temperature on bacterial growth.

poultry and eggs are the most common food sources. Poultry products are often contaminated because poultry farms house large numbers of chickens in close proximity allowing one infected chicken to infect thousands of others. A new way to reduce infection is to spray chicks with beneficial bacteria (Figure 16.6). The FDA has approved the use of a spray that includes of 29 types of living, nontoxic bacteria that are present in the normal gut of adult chickens.[6] The chicks ingest the bacteria when they preen their feathers and the bacteria colonize the digestive tract, leaving no room for pathogens. The spray prevents chicks from being infected with *Salmonella, Listeria,* and *E. coli* O157:H7.

Even if food contaminated with *Salmonella* is brought into the kitchen, careful handling and cooking of the food can prevent the organisms from causing illness. Washing food can remove some of the bacteria, and washing hands, cutting boards, and utensils can prevent cross-contamination. If a contaminated food is stored in the refrigerator, the multiplication of the *Salmonella* will be slowed. If a contaminated food is left at room temperature, the *Salmonella* will multiply rapidly, and when the food is ingested, large numbers of bacteria will be ingested with it. *Salmonella* is killed by heat—so foods likely to be contaminated, such as poultry and eggs, should be cooked thoroughly.

Two species of *Campylobacter, Campylobacter jejuni* and *Campylobacter coli*, also cause food-borne infection. *Campylobacter* is the most frequent cause of acute infectious diarrhea in developed countries.[3] Common sources are undercooked chicken, unpasteurized milk, and untreated water. This organism grows slowly in the cold and is killed by heat, so, as with *Salmonella*, thorough cooking and careful storage help prevent infection.

Another cause of bacterial infection is *Listeria monocytogenes*. Although most cases of *Listeria* infection result in flu-like symptoms, in high-risk groups such as pregnant women, children, the elderly, and the ill, it can cause meningitis and serious blood infections. *Listeria* frequently contaminates dairy products, but it is destroyed by pasteurization, so avoiding raw milk products will help prevent this source of infection. It is also found on produce and raw and undercooked

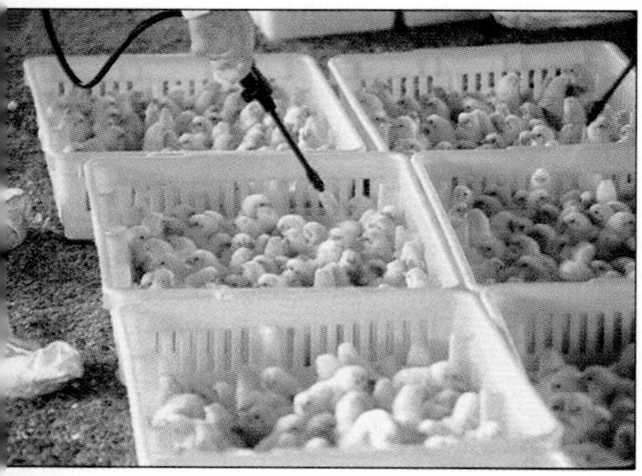

Figure 16.6
A shower of beneficial bacteria prevents chicks from being infected with bacteria that are pathogenic to humans. (Agricultural Research Service/USDA)

meat, poultry, and seafood. *Listeria* is a very resistant organism that survives at higher and lower temperatures than most bacteria; it can survive and grow at refrigerator temperatures.

Vibrio vulnificus infection usually causes gastrointestinal upset but can be deadly in vulnerable populations. The bacteria are most common in mollusks such as oysters, clams, and mussels harvested from the Gulf of Mexico in the summer when the water is most likely to be contaminated with human fecal matter. Foods that pose a risk include raw and undercooked seafood.

Bacterial Food-Borne Intoxication **Food-borne intoxication** is caused by consuming food containing toxins or microbes that produce toxins. The symptoms of food-borne intoxication are caused by the toxin, not the organism itself. Unlike food infections, which are usually caused by ingesting large numbers of bacteria, intoxication can be caused by only a few microorganisms that have produced a toxin. Although the bacteria are fairly easy to kill, some food toxins may be difficult to destroy.

Food-borne intoxication Illness caused by consuming a food containing a toxin or microbes that produce toxins.

Staphylococcus aureus is a common cause of microbial food-borne intoxication. These bacteria live in human nasal passages and can be transferred through coughing or sneezing when handling food. Foods that are common sources include cooked ham, salads, bakery products, and dairy products.

Escherichia coli (E. coli) is a bacterium that inhabits the gastrointestinal tracts of humans and other animals. Some strains of *E coli* are harmless but others cause both infection and intoxication. One strain of *E. coli*, found in water contaminated by human or animal feces, is the cause of "travelers' diarrhea." Another strain, *E. coli* O157:H7, causes abdominal pain, bloody diarrhea, and, in severe cases, kidney failure and even death.

Transmission of *E. coli* is a risk at day-care centers from cross-contamination if caregivers do not carefully wash their hands after diaper changes. *E. coli* comes in contact with food through fecal contamination of water or unsanitary handling of food. *E. coli* can multiply slowly even at refrigerator temperatures, but if a contaminated food is thoroughly cooked to 160°F, both the bacteria and the toxin are destroyed.

Hamburger contaminated with *E. coli* O157:H7 is a particular risk because the bacteria are mixed throughout the meat during grinding. The *E. coli* on the outside of the hamburger are quickly killed during cooking, but those in the interior survive if the hamburger is not cooked thoroughly. This strain was responsible for the deaths of several children who consumed undercooked, contaminated hamburgers from a fast-food chain in 1993. In 1996, unpasteurized apple juice contaminated with *E. coli* O157:H7 caused illness in 66 people and the death of one child.

The bacterium *Clostridium perfringens* may cause illness by both infection and intoxication. It is found in soil and in the intestines of animals and humans. It thrives in conditions with little oxygen (anaerobic conditions) and is difficult to kill because it forms heat-resistant **spores,** which are a stage of bacterial life that remains dormant until environmental conditions favor growth. *Clostridium perfringens* is often called "cafeteria germ" because foods stored in large containers have anaerobic centers that provide an excellent growth environment. Sources include improperly prepared roast beef, turkey, pork, chicken, and ground beef.

Spore A dormant state of some bacteria that is resistant to heat but can germinate and produce a new organism when environmental conditions are favorable.

Another strain of *Clostridium, Clostridium botulinum*, produces the deadliest bacterial food toxin. The bacteria survive in spore form for long periods and develop and multiply only in low-acid anaerobic conditions. Although the bacteria themselves are not harmful, a deadly toxin is produced as the spores begin to grow and develop. The toxin blocks nerve function, resulting in vomiting, abdominal pain, double vision, dizziness, and paralysis causing respiratory failure. If untreated, botulism poisoning is often fatal, but today modern detection methods and rapid administration of antitoxin have reduced mortality. Low-acid foods, such as potatoes or stew, that are held in anaerobic conditions provide optimal conditions for botulism spores to germinate. Canned foods, particularly improperly home-canned foods, can also be a source of botulism. Canned foods should be discarded if the can is bulging because this indicates the presence of gas produced by bacteria as they grow. Once formed, botulism toxin can be destroyed by boiling, but if the safety of a food is in question, it should be discarded; even a taste of botulism toxin can be deadly.

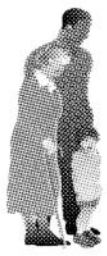

The most common form of botulism is infant botulism.[7] It occurs when ingested botulism spores germinate in the body, producing toxin and blocking nerve function. In healthy adults, conditions in the gastrointestinal tract prevent the spores from germinating, but in infants the spores can germinate. Botulism spores can contaminate honey, so it should never be fed to infants.

Viruses

Viruses Minute particles not visible under an ordinary microscope that depend on cells for their metabolic and reproductive needs.

We usually think of **viruses** as the cause of respiratory infections, but they can also cause water-borne and food-borne illnesses. Viruses are easily spread. They come in contact with food when it is contaminated with human or animal feces. To reproduce, viruses require living cells. Although the viruses that cause human disease cannot grow and reproduce in foods, they can contaminate foods and then infect the consumer.

Shellfish are notorious carriers of viral infections. Norwalk virus, found in water polluted with human or animal feces, causes most of the gastrointestinal illness that results from eating mollusks and other shellfish.[8] Because Norwalk virus is destroyed by cooking, uncooked foods such as raw shellfish and salads are the most common cause of food-borne illness from this virus.

Hepatitis A virus causes an inflammation of the liver. It is a highly contagious disorder that can be contracted from food contaminated by unsanitary handling or from eating raw or undercooked shellfish caught in sewage-contaminated waters. Hepatitis A can require a long recovery period and, in some cases, results in permanent liver damage. Individuals who have contracted the hepatitis A virus may remain carriers for years; it is also possible to carry the virus without having disease symptoms. Hepatitis in drinking water is destroyed by chlorination. Cooking destroys the virus in food, and good sanitation can prevent its spread (Figure 16.7).

Molds

Molds Multicellular fungi that form a filamentous branching growth.

Parasites Organisms that live at the expense of others without contributing to the survival of the host.

Many types of **molds** grow on foods such as bread, cheese, and fruit. If a food is moldy, it should be discarded, the area where it was stored should be cleaned, and neighboring foods should be checked to see if they have also become contaminated with mold.

Molds produce toxins that can lead to food intoxication. Mold toxins, such as aflatoxin, are among the most potent mutagens and carcinogens known. To safeguard the consumer, the FDA has set a maximum tolerable level of aflatoxin that may be present in foods. Another mold toxin that contaminates grain, particularly rye, is ergot. It causes hallucinations and is a natural source of the hallucinogenic drug LSD. Today, modern milling removes the part of the grain that harbors the mold, so the disease ergotism is rare. Other foods on which toxin-producing molds grow include corn, nuts, flour, whole grains, rice, legumes, and peanut butter. These should be discarded if moldy.

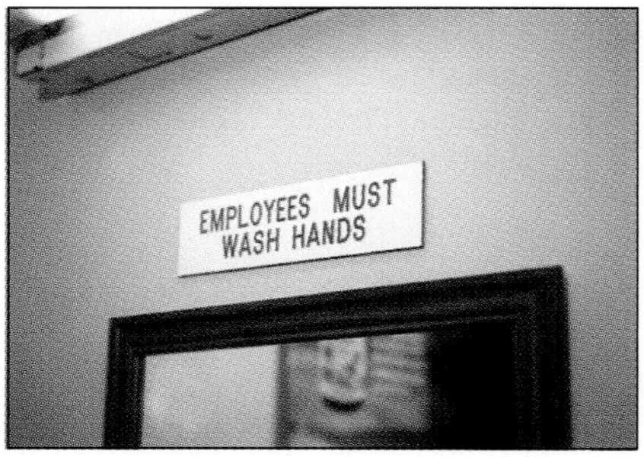

Figure 16.7
Good sanitation when preparing food is important for preventing food-borne illness. (George Semple)

Parasites

Many different types of **parasites** can enter the body through the diet. Some are single-celled animals while others are worms that can be seen with the naked eye. There are only a few that create problems in the food supply in North America. *Giardia lamblia* is a single-celled animal that can infect the gastrointestinal tract through water or food contaminated with human or animal feces. It is the most frequent cause of diarrhea not due to bacteria.[9] *Giardia* is sometimes contracted by hikers who drink untreated water from streams contaminated with animal feces, and it is becoming a problem from cross-contamination in day-care centers. Another single-celled animal is *Cryptosporidium parvum*. It causes watery diarrhea and is commonly spread by contaminated water, but cases have also been reported from unpasteurized apple juice and homemade chicken salad.[10,11]

Trichinella spiralis is a parasite found in raw and undercooked pork, pork products, and game meats, particularly bear. Once ingested, these small, wormlike organisms find their way to the muscles, where they grow, causing flu-like symptoms, muscle weakness, fever, and fluid retention. Trichinosis, the disease caused by *Trichinella* infection, can be prevented by thoroughly cooking meat to kill the parasite before it is ingested. The parasites are also destroyed by curing, smoking, canning, or freezing.

Fish are a common source of parasitic infections. Fish can carry the larvae (a wormlike stage of an organism's life cycle) of parasites such as roundworms, flatworms, flukes, and tapeworms. One such infection, Anisakis disease, is caused by the larval form of the small roundworm *Anisakis simplex*, or herring worm, found in raw fish.[9] Once consumed, these parasites invade the stomach and intestinal tract, causing severe abdominal pain. As the popularity of eating raw fish has increased, so has the incidence of parasitic infections from fish. The fresher the fish is when it is eviscerated, the less likely it is to cause this disease because the larvae move from the fish's stomach to its flesh only after the fish dies. Parasitic infections from fish can be avoided by consuming cooked fish or freezing fish for 72 hours before consumption. If raw fish is consumed, it should be very fresh (Figure 16.8).

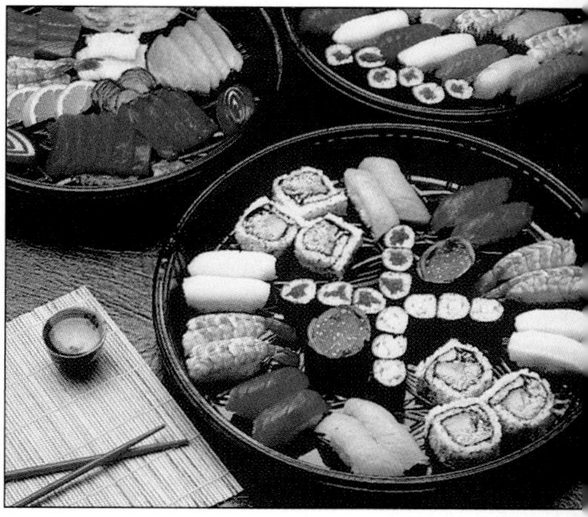

Figure 16.8
The incidence of parasitic infections has increased with the popularity of raw fish, such as this sushi. (R. Pleasant/FPG International)

Reducing the Risks: From Store to Table

Despite the variety of organisms that can cause food-borne illness, most cases can be avoided if food is handled properly. This requires safe practices by both manufacturers and consumers. Just as manufacturers are asked to identify critical control points in food handling where contamination can be prevented and monitored, consumers can take a similar approach in selecting, storing, preparing, and serving food and leftovers (see Table 16.4).

Table 16.4 *Tips for Handling Food Safely*

Choose wisely
Jars should be closed and seals unbroken. Cans should not be rusted, dented, or bulging. Check product expiration dates. Select frozen foods from below the frost line in the freezer.

Store foods properly
Fresh or frozen foods brought from the store should be refrigerated or frozen immediately. Food that has been in your refrigerator for longer than is safe should be discarded.

Wash
Hands, cooking utensils, and surfaces should be washed with warm soapy water before each food preparation step. This will prevent cross-contamination.

Cook thoroughly
Thorough cooking destroys most bacteria, toxins, viruses, and parasites.

Refrigerate promptly
Cooked food can be recontaminated, so it should be refrigerated as soon as possible after it is served.

Reheat thoroughly
Thorough reheating to 165°F will destroy microorganisms that have recontaminated cooked foods and toxins that have been produced.

When in doubt, throw it out.

Selecting Safe Foods The first critical control point in preventing food-borne illness is making safe selections at the store to reduce the contaminants that are brought into the home. Food should come from reputable vendors who are known to purchase their stocks with safety in mind. Foods should appear fresh; meat and fish should not be gray or brown. Frozen fish should be in sealed packages. Frozen foods should not contain frost or ice crystals, which may indicate that the product has been stored for a long time or that the food has been thawed and refrozen. Thawing allows food to reach temperatures at which bacteria may grow. Items stored low in the freezer are more likely to remain at a constant temperature.

Food packaging should be secure. Jars should be firmly closed, seals should not be broken, and cans should not be rusty, dented, or bulging. Most packaged products are dated as either "sell by" or "use by." A "sell by" date indicates when the grocery store should take the product off the shelf. A "use by" date indicates the date by which the product should be consumed. Outdated products should not be purchased and store managers should be notified if they are on the shelves. Although dates are helpful, they do not ensure food safety; one food may be safe and wholesome after the expiration date, while another, if it has not been handled properly, may be spoiled before it reaches its expiration date. Foods that are discolored or smell contaminated and those in damaged packages should not be purchased or consumed. Generally, grocery stores encourage customers to return damaged or tainted products.

Safe Food Storage Storage is another critical control point in the home. Proper storage both before and after cooking can reduce the risk of food-borne illness. Consumers need to pay attention to storage as soon as the food leaves the grocery store. Cold foods should be purchased last and refrigerated or frozen as quickly as possible. Cold foods should be kept cold, at 40°F or less, and hot foods should be kept hot, greater than 140°F. Refrigerator temperature should be set between 38° and 40°F and freezers at 0°F. Produce should be stored in the refrigerator. Fresh meat, poultry, and fish should be frozen immediately if it will not be used within a day or two. Processed meats such as hot dogs and bologna must also be kept refrigerated but can be kept longer than fresh meat.

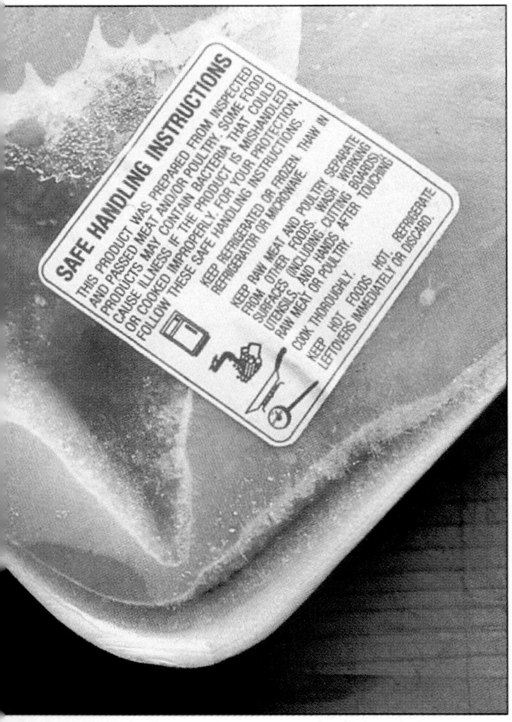

Figure 16.9
Meat carries labels offering safe handling guidelines. (Dennis Drenner)

Preparing and Serving Food Safely The next critical control point is preparation. Even when microorganisms come into the home, most food-borne illness can be prevented by proper kitchen precautions. A clean kitchen is essential for safe food preparation. Hands, countertops, cutting boards, and utensils should be washed with warm soapy water before each food preparation step. Food should be thawed in the refrigerator, in the microwave oven, or under running water—not at room temperature. Foods that are going to be cooked should not be prepared on the same surfaces as foods that are eaten raw. Uncooked foods such as meat and poultry may contain microbes that can contaminate any food that touches it or its juices. For example, if a chicken contaminated with *Salmonella* is cut up on a cutting board and the unwashed cutting board is then used to chop vegetables for a salad, the vegetables will become contaminated with *Salmonella*. When the chicken is cooked, the bacteria will be killed, but the contaminated vegetables are not cooked, so the bacteria can grow and cause food-borne illness. Cutting boards used to cut raw meat, poultry, or fish should be washed with soap and hot water and then sanitized with a mild bleach solution after each use.[12] Cross-contamination can also occur when uncooked foods containing live microbes come in contact with foods that have already been cooked. Therefore, cooked meat should never be returned to the same dish that held the raw meat, and sauces used to marinate uncooked foods should never be used as a sauce on cooked food. Meat packaging is labeled with safe handling guidelines (Figure 16.9).

Making sure that cooked food is thoroughly cooked is one of the most important control points in the home because heat will destroy most harmful microorganisms. A meat thermometer should be used because color is not a good indicator of safety. Red meat and fish should be cooked to an internal temperature of 160°F and poultry to 180°F. Shellfish should be cooked to an internal temperature of 145°C for 15 seconds. Eggs should not be eaten raw, since *Salmonella* can contaminate the inside of the shell; they should be boiled for 7 minutes, poached for 5 minutes, or fried for 3 minutes on a side. Thorough cooking may be a problem when using a microwave oven, because these appliances do not cook evenly and therefore bacteria may survive in cold pockets in the food.

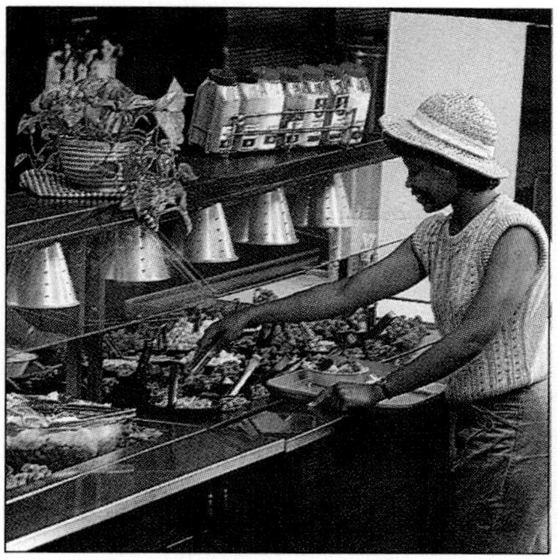

Figure 16.10
Clear plastic shields, or "sneeze guards," above salad bars prevent customers from contaminating food with microorganisms transmitted by coughs and sneezes.
(© Charles Gupton/Tony Stone Images)

Handling of Leftovers Cooked food can be recontaminated, so it must be refrigerated as soon as possible after serving and should not be left out to cool at room temperature. The best temperatures for bacterial growth are the temperatures at which food usually sets between service and storage. Large portions of food should be divided before refrigeration so they will cool quickly and not remain at bacterial growth temperatures for long periods in the refrigerator. When refrigerated leftovers are reheated, they should be heated thoroughly enough to destroy any bacteria that may have grown in them.

Food Safety Away From Home Safe food practices at home will not prevent food-borne illness when eating away from home. Although most of the food-borne illness in the United States is caused by food prepared in homes, an outbreak in a commercial or institutional establishment usually involves more people at a time and is more likely to be reported. Food in retail establishments has many opportunities to be contaminated because of the large volume of food that is handled and the large number of people involved in food preparation. Consumers should choose restaurants with food safety in mind. Restaurants should be clean, and cooked foods should be served hot. Cafeteria steam tables should be kept hot enough that the water is steaming. Cold foods such as salad bar items should be held refrigerated or on ice. The safest salad bar items, as well as the most nutritious, are fresh fruits and vegetables and dried fruits. However, recent incidents of food-borne illness from salad bar fruit have made even these suspect. For example, an outbreak of food-borne illness was caused by cantaloupe that was contaminated with *Salmonella* in the field and cut up before the outer skin was washed. The bacteria were carried onto the fruit, and, when it was left at room temperature, enough bacteria grew to cause illness.

Even when a restaurant uses extreme care in food preparation, customers can be a source of contamination. Because customers serve themselves at salad bars, cross-contamination from one customer to another is a risk. Salad and dessert bars in restaurants are usually equipped with "sneeze guards"—clear plastic shields placed above the food to prevent contamination from coughs and sneezes (Figure 16.10). Customers are also asked to use a clean plate if they go back for second helpings.

Picnics and other large events where food is served provide a prime opportunity for microbes to flourish because food is often left at room temperature or in the sun for hours before it is consumed. Foods that last well without refrigeration, such as fresh fruits and vegetables, breads, and crackers, should be selected for these occasions.

Any food that is transported should be kept cold. Lunches should be transported to and from work or school in a cooler or an insulated bag. They should be refrigerated upon arrival or kept cold with ice packs. Most foods that are brought home from work or school uneaten should be thrown out and not saved for another day (see *Critical Thinking: Are These Choices Safe?*).

CRITICAL THINKING

Are These Choices Safe?

Eleanor is in charge of organizing a potluck dinner. Because food at a potluck usually sets at room temperature for several hours and many people serve themselves from the same serving dishes, Eleanor is concerned about the potential for food-borne illness. She collects the following list of food items that her friends intend to bring:

Chicken salad	Cheese and crackers
Tamales	Cheesecake
Fruit salad	Cookies
Raw vegetables	Mushrooms stuffed with crab meat
Chips and onion dip	Lasagna

Do the foods on this list pose a risk of food-borne illness?

The more food is handled, the more likely it is to be contaminated. The chicken salad, tamales, mushrooms, and lasagna pose a risk because they are handled extensively in preparation. The lasagna and stuffed mushrooms are cooked, but when left at room temperature, the inside may stay warm enough to provide a good environment for microbial growth. The raw fruits and vegetables are safe if they are not contaminated during handling. The cookies, chips, and cheese and crackers are safe choices. The onion dip and cheesecake are probably safe during the party as long as they have been refrigerated beforehand.

How might raw vegetables and fruit salad become contaminated?

Answer:

What suggestions might Eleanor make that would decrease the chances of microbial contamination?

Foods such as cheese and crackers that are designed to be served at room temperature are safest, but a potluck without both hot and cold dishes is missing out on variety and taste. To prevent food from becoming contaminated before the potluck, safe kitchen food handling and preparation practices should be followed. Once at the potluck, hot dishes like the lasagna should be kept on a hot plate to ensure that they remain hot. Cold dishes like the fruit salad can be placed in a bowl of ice. Store-bought dips are a good choice because they can remain unopened until the party begins. Acidic dips such as tomato-based salsa are safe. Layer cakes and fruit pies keep better at room temperature than cheesecake.

After the party is over, what foods would you consider safe to keep as leftovers and what would you throw out?

Answer:

Chemical Toxins in Food

The safety of the food supply can be affected by compounds used in agricultural production and by industrial wastes that contaminate the environment. These chemical contaminants are taken up by plants and consumed by small animals. These plants and animals are then eaten by larger animals, which are in turn eaten by still larger animals, thus passing the contaminants up through the food chain to all levels of the food supply. Contaminants are found in the greatest concentration in foods of animal origin because animals are at the top of the food chain (Figure 16.11).

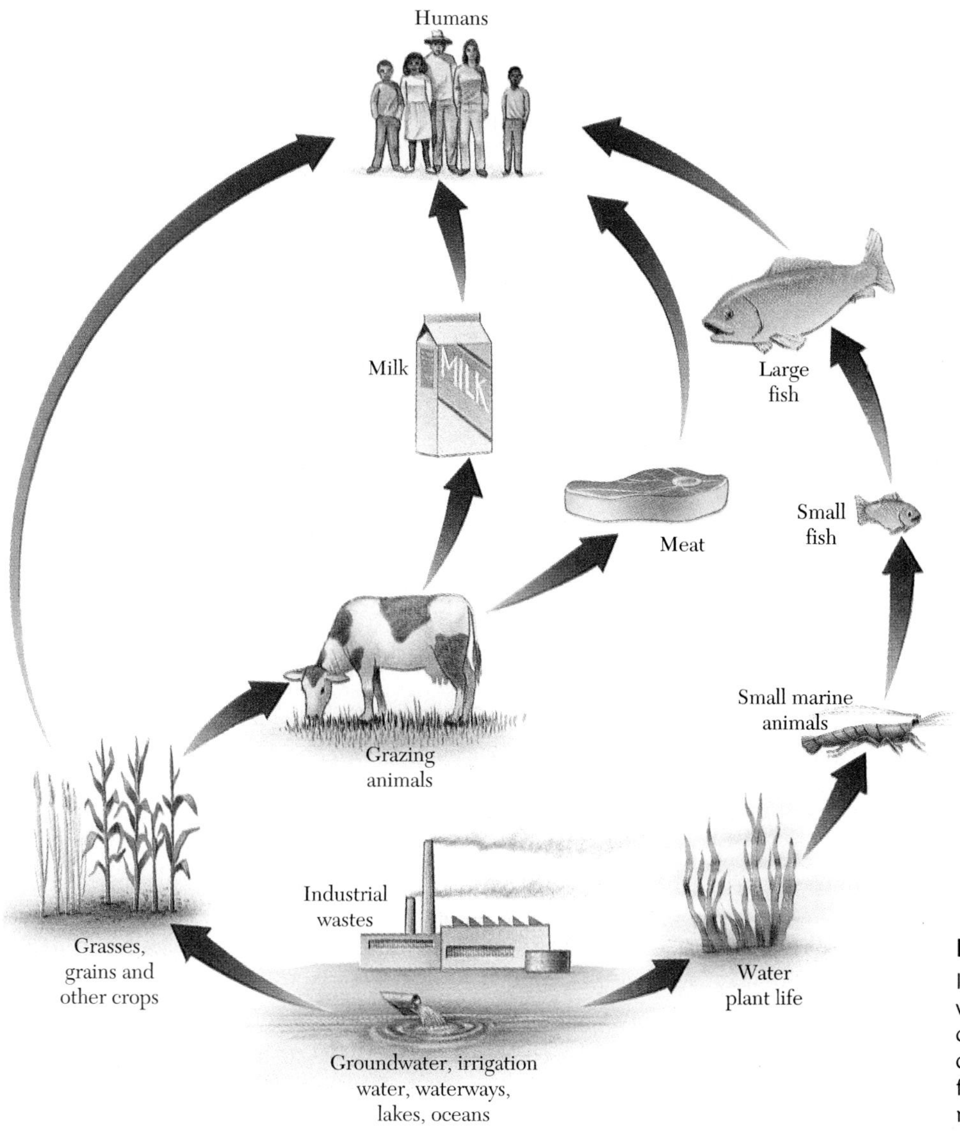

Figure 16.11
Industrial pollutants that contaminate the water supply become more and more concentrated as they are passed up the food chain. Large organisms like cattle and large fish may have high levels of these contaminants in their adipose tissue.

Risks and Benefits of Pesticides

Pesticides are used to prevent plant diseases and insect infestations. They are applied to crops growing in the fields as well as after harvesting to prevent spoilage and extend the shelf life of produce. Crops grown using pesticides generally produce higher yields and look more appealing because insect damage is limited. Some residues of these chemicals remain on the food when it arrives at our tables, and pesticides may travel from the fields where they are applied into water supplies, soil, and other parts of the environment. For instance, pesticides are found not only on treated produce but also in meat, poultry, fish, dairy products, and lard, as well as in groundwater.[13]

The potential risks of pesticides to consumers depend on the type and amount consumed as well as who consumes it. For example, a large volume of pesticide spilled on a farm worker could cause an acute toxic reaction such as a burn or skin rash. The small amounts of pesticides that remain in the food supply will cause no immediate reaction but could cause health problems if routinely consumed over a long period.

Regulating Pesticide Use The types of pesticides that can be used on food crops and the amounts of residues that can remain when foods reach consumers are regulated. New pesticides are now so carefully tested for safety that years may pass between the time they are developed and when they can be used. The EPA must approve and register pesticides that are used in food production and establish allowable limits, or **tolerances.** The FDA and USDA then monitor pesticide levels in foods. To establish tolerances for pesticides, the risk of toxicity is weighed against the benefit that the pesticide provides. The risks are based on the known incidence of toxicity and the predicted exposure that consumers will have to the toxin. Tolerance levels are then set at the minimum amount of the pesticide needed to be effective; these levels are often several hundred times lower than the level found to cause reactions in test animals.[14]

Tolerances The maximum amount of pesticide residues that may legally remain in food, set by the EPA.

In the past, tolerance levels were set based on weights and food consumption patterns of adults. However, pesticides may be more of a danger to children than adults. Children are smaller, so the same amount of pesticide provides a larger dose per unit of body weight. And, children often have less varied diets than adults. For example, a two-year-old who drinks nothing but apple juice for weeks at a time is consuming more than the predicted amount of pesticide residue. The 1996 Food Quality Protection Act requires the EPA to determine that a tolerance level of a pesticide is safe for children as well as adults.[15]

In general, the amounts of pesticides to which people are exposed through foods are small. According to the FDA's pesticide residue monitoring program, the levels of pesticides found in the American food supply are below tolerances. Less than 2% of the food samples studied had residues of pesticides that either exceeded tolerance levels or contained pesticides for which there is no legal tolerance, and the overall incidence was comparable for domestic and imported foods.[16] Because of country-to-country differences in crops, pests, growing conditions, and pesticide regulations, imported foods are more likely to contain pesticides that are not used in the United States and for which the EPA has not set tolerance levels. However, a report by the National Research Council in 1996 concluded that the majority of synthetic chemicals, including pesticides, in the diet are present at levels below which any significant adverse biological effect is likely and that they are unlikely to pose a cancer risk.[17] Although special-interest groups concerned with overuse of pesticides disagree with this conclusion,[18] the fact remains that repeated consumption of large doses of any one pesticide is unlikely because most people consume a variety of foods produced in many different locations.

Reducing Pesticide Risks New, more effective chemical pesticides are being developed, and the use of older, more toxic products is decreasing in the United States. One approach to the development of safer pesticides is **genetic engi-**

Genetic engineering A set of techniques used to manipulate DNA for the purpose of changing the characteristics of an organism or creating a new product.

neering. In 1991, the EPA approved the first genetically engineered pesticides. They are insect-killing proteins that are produced by bacteria. The bacteria containing the pesticides are killed and then sprayed on plants.

In addition to developing safer pesticides, production methods are being implemented to make low-pesticide and pesticide-free produce available to the consumer. One such system is called **integrated pest management (IPM).** IPM combines chemical and nonchemical methods of pest control and emphasizes the use of natural toxins and more effective pesticide application. Another system is organic farming, which does not use synthetic pesticides, herbicides, or fertilizers at all. These farming techniques reduce the exposure of farm workers to pesticides and decrease the quantity of pesticides introduced into the food supply and the environment.

Integrated pest management (IPM) A method of agricultural pest control that integrates nonchemical and chemical techniques.

Exploiting Natural Toxins Many toxins occur naturally in plants. They function as natural pesticides that offer protection from bacteria, molds, and insect pests. These naturally pest-resistant crops are advantageous in developing countries because they thrive without the use of expensive added pesticides. Plants high in natural pesticides are being produced through special breeding programs. The natural toxins in plants can also be isolated and applied to crops like synthetic pesticides.

As with all chemical toxins, natural toxins move through the food supply. For example, a cow that has foraged on toxic plants can pass the toxin into her milk and poison the consumer of the milk. Abraham Lincoln's mother died from drinking milk from a cow that had eaten poisonous snakeroot plants. The potential for toxicity, however, depends on the dose of toxin and the health of the consumer. Most natural toxins in the food supply are consumed in doses that pose little risk to the consumer. For instance, solanine, a neurotoxin found in the green layer under potato skins, is not toxic in amounts typically consumed. But consuming ten times the typical amount of potatoes could cause symptoms (see *Off the Shelf: Herbal Tea: Healthy or Hazardous?*).

Using Organic Techniques Organically grown foods are those produced without the use of synthetic pesticides or fertilizers. Consumer demand for organic produce increased sales from $78 million in 1980 to $3.5 billion in 1996.[19] Despite this increasing demand, organically produced foods are usually more expensive and available in less variety than conventionally grown foods. It is also often assumed that organic foods are healthier and safer than foods grown using other methods. However, organically grown foods are not superior in quality, taste, or nutrient content to conventionally grown foods. Organic methods reduce both the risk of pesticide ingestion by consumers and the contamination of the environment by chemicals used in traditional growing methods, but organically produced foods are not necessarily pesticide-free. Irrigation water, rain, or a variety of other sources can introduce traces of pesticides into organically grown foods. And use of untreated manure fertilizers can increase the risks of microbial food-borne illness.

To assure consumers that the organically produced products they buy meet consistent standards, the USDA is currently developing regulations governing the use of fertilizers, herbicides, insecticides, fungicides, preservatives, and other chemicals during the production and handling of organic foods.[20] These national standards will replace guidelines that vary from state to state. Farmers who follow USDA guidelines can certify and market their products as organic, and these products can bear the USDA seal on their labels and in marketing information (Figure 16.12).

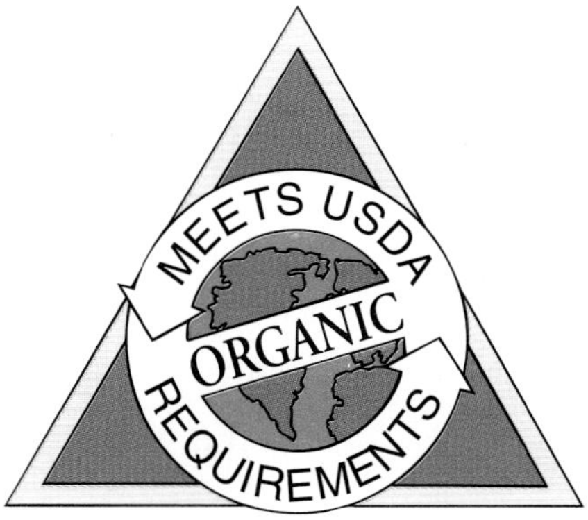

Figure 16.12
The USDA organic seal can appear on the label of agricultural products that meet USDA standards for the production and handling of organic foods.

Antibiotics and Hormones in Food

The use of antibiotics to increase weight gain in cattle and to increase egg production in poultry was once common. These drugs produced greater yields at a lower

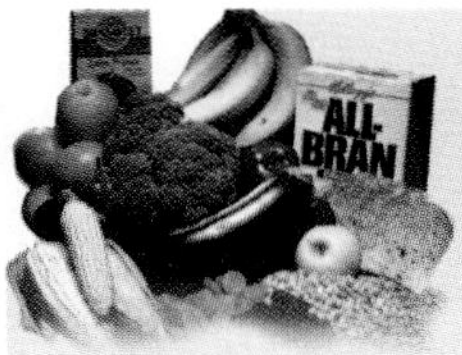

Off the Shelf

Herbal Tea: Healthy or Hazardous?

For thousands of years, herbs have been used medicinally, and today herbal teas are consumed for their aroma and flavor as well. While consuming herbal teas is thought to be a healthy alternative to caffeinated beverages, little is really known about the safety of some of the herbs.

Many of the herbal teas on the market have ingredient lists that look like a garden tour: lemon grass, rosehips, spearmint, raspberry leaves, chamomile flowers. Most of these and other ingredients used in commercially prepared teas have been used for centuries with relative safety. However, problems arise when people consume herbal teas in excessive amounts or concoct their own brews. For example, comfrey tea can cause liver disease. Comfrey roots and leaves contain chemicals that have been found to cause cancer in rats. Lobelia, also known as Indian tobacco, was used in the 19th century to treat asthma, but, when used in large amounts, it can cause vomiting, breathing problems, convulsions, coma, and death. Sassafras tea, which was once used as a stimulant, blood thinner, and reputed cure for rheumatism and syphilis, causes cancer in rats. Oil of sassafras and safrole from sassafras root bark were taken out of root beer over 30 years ago, and today sassafras bark is banned in all food products. There have been reports of illness caused by tea made from the leaves of foxglove plant, from which the heart drug digitalis is derived. Abnormal menstrual bleeding was reported in a woman consuming a homemade brew that included, among others, tonka beans, melilot, and woodruff. These contain coumarin, an anticoagulant. Herbal teas containing plant-derived laxatives such as senna, aloe, cascara, buckthorn, rhubarb root, and castor oil are marketed as "dieter's teas." Senna, cascara, and castor oil, found in over-the-counter laxatives, are regulated as drugs. When consumed in excessive amounts, plant-derived laxatives can cause stomach cramps, fainting, vomiting, diarrhea, and even death.[1]

Currently, the regulation of herbal teas depends on the types of claims made about their use. If an herbal tea makes a claim to prevent or cure a disease, the FDA regulates it as a drug, and it must be approved as safe and effective for its intended use. For example, products claiming to help with smoking cessation, weight loss, constipation, or sore throats are considered drugs. Herbal teas claiming less dramatic effects, such as calming, relaxing, and soothing, are classified as dietary supplements by the FDA and therefore regulated as foods rather than drugs or additives.

Concern about the effects of herbs has prompted the FDA to collect samples of herbal products to determine health hazards and assess unsubstantiated claims. In Canada, an advisory committee was established to review information about herbs and make recommendations. The result was a ban on 57 herbs and warning labels on five others that may cause problems during pregnancy. The herb industry itself has also initiated a program to evaluate 200 or so commercially available herbs that are currently not approved for use as food flavorings. Their evaluations include factors such as the use of the herb in other countries, chemical composition, pharmacological properties, reports of adverse reactions, and toxicity studies. Advice for tea drinkers is to stick to commercial varieties, to not steep teas too long, and to avoid consuming any one variety in excess.

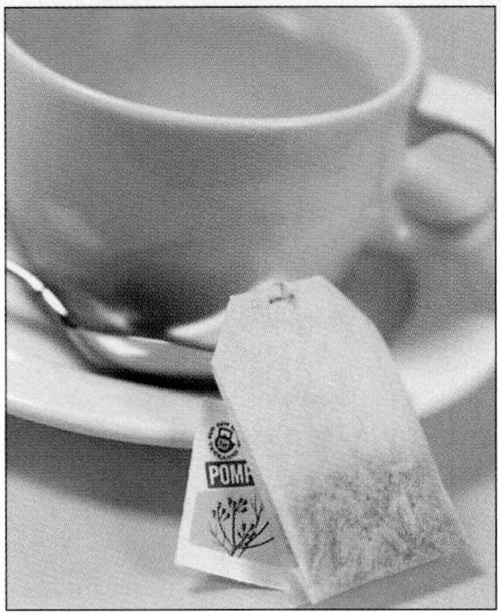

(© Index Stock Photography)

[1]Kurtzweil, P. Dieter's brews make tea time a dangerous affair. FDA Consumer, July/August 1997; updated December 1997. Online at http://www.fda.gov/fdac/features/1997/597_tea/html

cost. Today antibiotics are used primarily to treat illness in cattle and dairy cows. The FDA regulates which drugs can be used to treat animals used for food production. If a dairy cow has been treated with medication, the milk may not be sold until the treatment has been stopped and the drugs cleared from the milk. According to the USDA and the FDA, the majority of milk samples they test do not contain any drug residues, and those that do, contain amounts that are very low and not known to be harmful to humans.[21] The known benefits of drinking milk outweigh the potential risks.

Perhaps a more important concern raised in relation to antibiotic use in animals is the creation of antibiotic-resistant bacteria. When bacteria are exposed to an antibiotic, those that are resistant to that antibiotic survive and produce offspring that are also resistant to the antibiotic. If these resistant bacteria infect humans, the resulting illness cannot be treated with that antibiotic. Since nearly half

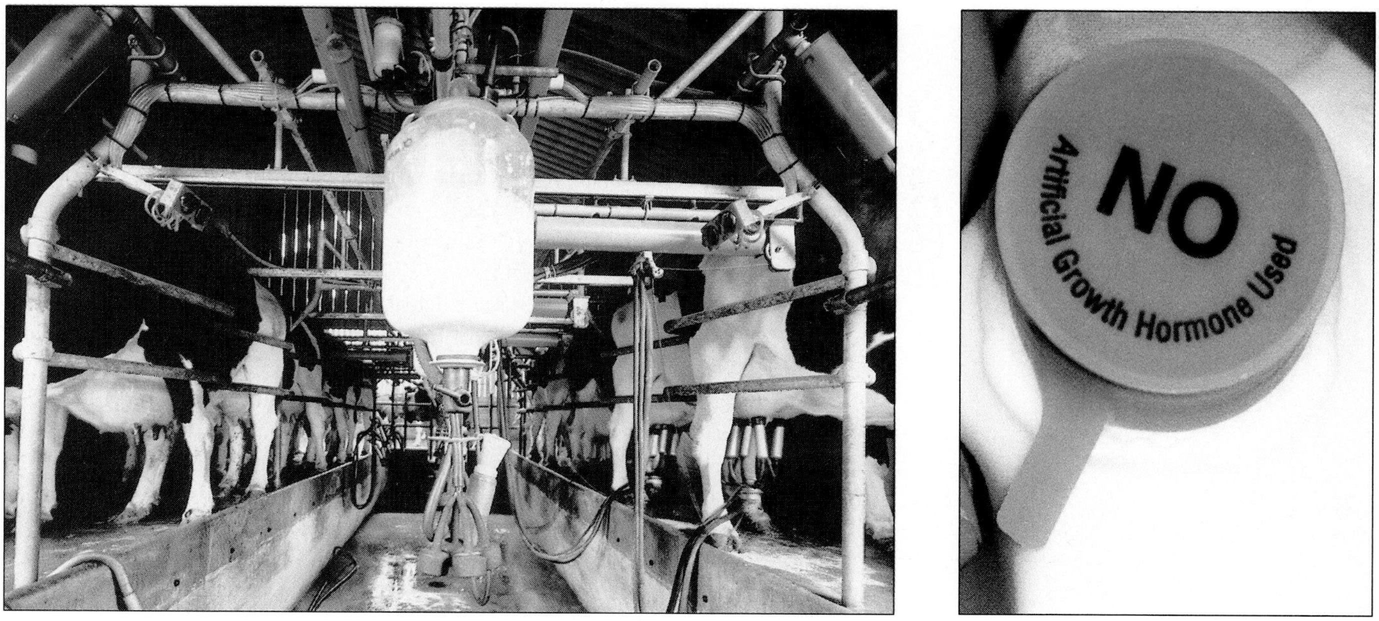

(a) (b)

Figure 16.13
(a) When administered to cattle, genetically engineered bovine somatotropin increases milk production. (b) Milk from cows treated with genetically engineered bovine somatotropin is indistinguishable from other milk, but dairies that do not use bovine somatotropin may choose to indicate this on the label. (*a,* Graeme Norways/Tony Stone Images; *b,* Lori Smolin)

the antibiotics produced in the United States are used to prevent disease in animals, this use is suspected of being a major contributor to the development of antibiotic-resistant strains of bacteria.[22]

A hormone that has created public concern is genetically engineered bovine somatotropin (bST) which is used to increase milk production in dairy cows (Figure 16.13a). Cows naturally produce somatotropin, a hormone that stimulates milk production. Genetically engineered bST is produced by bacteria and injected into cows to increase their milk production. Consumer groups contend that genetically engineered bST causes health problems for the cows and for humans who consume milk or meat from the cows.

An FDA review of the effect of bST concluded that it causes no serious long-term health effects in cows. The only concern is a possible increase in udder infections. Since these infections are often treated with antibiotics, there is concern that this could increase the antibiotic residues in the milk from cows treated with bST. Monitoring is currently in place to ensure that this does not occur. The FDA has concluded that milk and meat from bST-treated cows is not a health risk to consumers.[23] Cow's milk naturally contains bST, and it is not possible to detect a difference between milk from bST-treated and untreated cows. Pasteurization destroys 90% of bST, and digestion breaks down the rest. The milk from treated and untreated cows is identical, so the FDA does not require milk from bST-treated cows to be specially labeled. Companies may voluntarily label their products as long as the labeling is truthful and not misleading (Figure 16.13b).

Contamination From Industrial Wastes

Fish accumulate substances that are in the waters where they live and feed. This can cause a food hazard when the water is polluted. For example, **polychlorinated biphenyls (PCBs)** are a group of carcinogenic chemicals that were used extensively in the manufacture of electrical capacitors and transformers, plasticizers, waxes, and paper. In the past, PCBs in runoff from manufacturing plants

Polychlorinated biphenyls (PCBs) Carcinogenic industrial compounds that have found their way into the environment and, subsequently, the food supply. Repeated ingestion causes them to accumulate in biological tissues over time.

contaminated water, particularly near the Great Lakes. Although they are no longer produced, these compounds do not degrade, and they are still found in the environment and in fish. The fish accumulate PCBs in their adipose tissue; humans who consume large quantities of contaminated fish accumulate PCBs in their adipose tissue.

PCBs are a particular problem for mothers and infants. Prenatal exposure may cause learning deficits in children.[24,25] Because PCBs are secreted in breast milk, the American Academy of Pediatrics recommends that breast-feeding women in areas where high exposures of PCBs have occurred check with their local health department for recommendations on fish consumption. However, they have concluded that the benefits of breast-feeding outweigh the risks of low levels of PCBs.[26]

Other contaminants from manufacturing, such as chlordane (used to control termites), radioactive substances such as strontium-90, and toxic metals such as cadmium, lead, arsenic, and mercury have also found their way into fish and shellfish. Cadmium and lead can interfere with the absorption of other minerals, as well as have a direct toxic effect: Cadmium can cause kidney damage; lead can impair brain development. Arsenic is believed to contribute to cancer development, and mercury, which has been found in large fish, particularly swordfish and shark, damages nerve cells.[27] Large fish at the top of the food chain are more likely to contain high levels of industrial contaminants, but shellfish also accumulate contaminants because they feed by passing large volumes of water through their bodies (Figure 16.14).

Choosing Wisely to Reduce Risk

Even though individual consumers cannot detect chemicals in food, care in selection and preparation can reduce the amounts that are consumed. Pesticide consumption can be reduced by careful selection and preparation of plant and animal food products. Despite widespread fear of pesticides, the health risk of eliminating foods from the diet that may contain pesticide residues, such as fresh fruits and vegetables, is probably greater than that of the pesticide exposure.

Consumers should be aware that domestically grown produce is less likely to contain unapproved pesticides. And, locally grown produce is likely to contain fewer pesticides because many pesticides are not applied in the fields; rather, they are used to prevent spoilage and extend the shelf life of produce that is shipped. Foods produced organically or using IPM are also likely to contain fewer pesticide residues.

Pesticides can be removed or reduced on conventionally grown produce by peeling it or washing it with tap water and scrubbing with a brush if appropriate.[28] For leafy vegetables such as lettuce and cabbage, the outer leaves should be removed and discarded. Some produce, such as cucumbers, apples, eggplant, squash, and tomatoes, are coated with wax to maintain freshness by sealing in moisture. But wax also seals in pesticides and is often combined with fungicides to inhibit the growth of molds. Although federal law requires that stores have a sign on any bulk produce that has been waxed, this is rarely enforced. Much of the wax can be removed by rinsing produce in warm water and scrubbing it with a brush, but to eliminate all wax, the produce must be peeled. Although peeling fruits and vegetables eliminates some pesticides, it also eliminates fiber and some micronutrients.

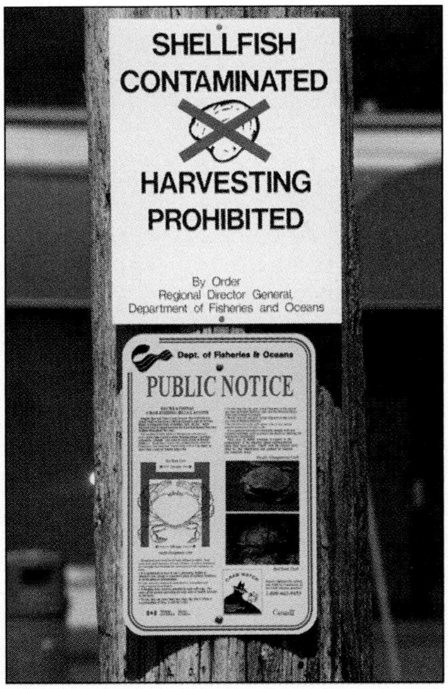
SHELLFISH
CONTAMINATED
HARVESTING
PROHIBITED
By Order
Regional Director General
Department of Fisheries and Oceans
Dept. of Fisheries & Oceans
PUBLIC NOTICE

Figure 16.14
It is unsafe to consume shellfish from contaminated waters. (Corbis/Paul A. Souders)

Fish and seafood can also be contaminated by chemical pesticides moving up the food chain. The risk of ingesting chemical pollutants from fish can be minimized by choosing wisely. Small fish are lower on the food chain and therefore will have lower levels of contaminants than larger fish. The safest fish are saltwater varieties caught well offshore, away from polluted waters. Freshwater fish and saltwater fish that live near shore or spend part of their life cycle in freshwater are more likely to contain contaminants. Migratory fish such as striped bass and bluefish are a problem because they may contain contaminants even when they are caught in clean water well offshore. Consuming a variety of fish rather than just one or two kinds can also reduce the risk of ingesting dangerous amounts of contaminants from fish. Most toxins concentrate in adipose tissue, so amounts can be reduced by trimming all fat from fish (and meat) before cooking or eating. Internal organs such as the green-colored "tomale" in lobster and the "mustard" in blue crabs should not be consumed because toxins such as PCBs and cadmium accumulate in these organs.

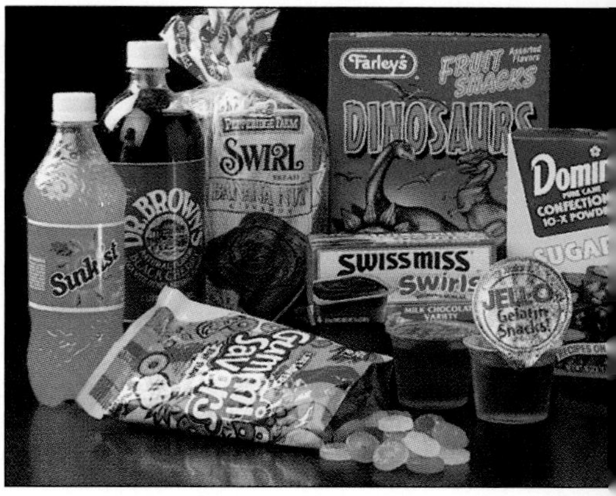

Figure 16.15
The additives in these foods prevent the bread from molding, the fruit snacks from hardening, and the powdered sugar from clumping; they also smooth the texture of the pudding and give color to soft drinks and candy. (George Semple)

Food Technology: A Risk-Benefit Analysis

Advances in food and agricultural technology have improved the safety and availability of foods. Such technology includes techniques to preserve food and develop new food products. While technology offers many benefits, it also creates risks.

Food and agricultural technology ensures that food is available even if the local growing season is not ideal. Without these modern processing, packaging, and storage techniques, we would be forced to rely on locally grown foods and to eat them soon after harvest or slaughter. While this has some appeal, it would limit the variety of foods in our diet, particularly during the winter months, and place us at risk for malnutrition if food production were interrupted by a natural or man-made disaster.

In the process of improving food availability and safety, food technology may intentionally add some substances to foods and other substances may contaminate food unintentionally. Substances added to preserve or enhance the appeal of food products are called **food additives** (Figure 16.15). By legal definition, a food additive is a substance that can reasonably be expected to become a component of a food during processing. This includes **direct food additives** that are intentionally added during the preparation, packaging, transport, and holding of food. It also includes **indirect food additives,** which are substances known to enter food, although unintentionally, during processing. Indirect food additives are regulated as food additives. All processing and packaging techniques as well as direct and indirect food additives are regulated to ensure that their risks do not outweigh their benefits. However, if foods or packaging materials are handled improperly, unexpected substances may accidentally enter food. These **accidental contaminants** are not regulated by the FDA.

Food additives Substances that can reasonably be expected to become a component of a food during processing. The foods that may contain them and the amounts that may be present are regulated by the FDA.

Direct food additives Substances intentionally added to foods. They are regulated by the FDA.

Indirect food additives Substances that are expected to unintentionally enter foods during manufacturing or from packaging. They are regulated by the FDA.

Accidental contaminants Substances not regulated by the FDA that unexpectedly enter the food supply.

Regulating What Gets Into Food

The nation's first food regulations were the Pure Food and Drug Act of 1906 and the Meat Inspection Act of 1906. The Pure Food and Drug Act stated that only additives that were proven to be safe and effective could be used in foods. In 1938, the federal Food, Drug, and Cosmetic Act provided exemptions and safe tolerance levels for additives that were necessary or unavoidable in production. This law established **standards of identity** for foods. These prescribed recipes define exactly the ingredients that can be contained in certain foods such as mayonnaise, jelly, and orange juice. These foods were originally exempt from listing the product's ingredients on the food label; however, today even foods with standards of identity must list ingredients.[29] The Food, Drug, and Cosmetic Act also gave the FDA the responsibility of testing food additives for safety. Because the FDA could not possibly test all additives, the 1958 Food Additives Amendment transferred the responsibility for testing from the FDA to the manufacturer.

Standards of identity Regulations that define the allowable ingredients, composition, and other characteristics of foods.

Testing Food Additives for Safety Since 1958 all new additives have had to be demonstrated to be safe before they could be added to food. Safety tests must be done using at least two animal species, usually rats and mice. These tests are used to determine the highest level of a substance at which no deleterious effects are observed. The highest amount of the substance that can be added to food is then set at 1/100 of this level.

When a manufacturer wants to use a new food additive, a petition must be submitted to the FDA. The petition describes the chemical composition of the additive, how it is manufactured, and how it is detected and measured in food. The manufacturer must prove that the additive will be effective for its intended purpose at the proposed levels, that it is safe for its intended use, and that its use is necessary.

Generally recognized as safe (GRAS) A group of chemical additives that are generally recognized as safe based on their longstanding presence in the food supply without obvious harmful effects.

The GRAS List When the 1958 Food Additives Amendment was passed, over 600 chemicals defined as food additives were already in common use. The amendment added a category of materials that were considered **generally recognized as safe (GRAS).** GRAS substances are exempt from the regulations applied to substances defined as food additives, color additives, or pesticides. If the safety of a substance on the GRAS list is questioned, the FDA must provide evidence that the substance is unsafe before it can be removed from the list. For example, the artificial sweetener cyclamate was removed from the GRAS list because it was found to cause cancer in laboratory animals. Substances on the GRAS list are subject to ongoing review.

Delaney Clause A clause added to the 1958 Food Additives Amendment of the Pure Food and Drug Act that prohibits the intentional addition to foods of any compound that has been shown to induce cancer in animals or humans at any dose.

The Delaney Clause The 1958 Food Additives Amendment also included the **Delaney Clause,** which was designed to protect the public from additives found to be carcinogenic. The Delaney Clause states that a substance that induces cancer in either an animal species or humans at any dosage, no matter how large, may not be added to food. Currently, support is growing to amend the Delaney Clause to allow the use of substances that are added at a level so low that they would not represent a significant health risk. Like other substances, carcinogens would then be evaluated using a risk-benefit analysis.

Direct Food Additives

Food additives enhance the quality of our food supply. Although some have been questioned as potential hazards, additives are used only if it is concluded that the benefits they offer outweigh any risk they might pose. Food additives are used to improve the nutritional quality of food, to preserve foods, to enhance flavor or improve taste, and to aid in processing or preparation. They may not be used to disguise inferior products or to deceive the consumer. They are also not permitted in foods where they significantly destroy nutrients or where the same effect can be achieved by sound manufacturing processes. For example, sulfites cannot be used on meats because they restore the red color, giving a false appearance of freshness, and they cannot be used in foods that are important sources of thiamin, such as enriched flour, because they destroy thiamin.

Additives to Maintain or Improve Nutritional Quality Many nutrients are added to foods. As discussed in Chapter 8, refined grains are enriched with iron and some of the B vitamins that are lost in processing. In other cases, food is fortified with nutrients typically lacking in the diet. For instance, grains are fortified with folic acid.

Preservatives Compounds that extend the shelf life of a product by retarding chemical, physical, or microbiological changes.

Additives to Maintain Product Quality Many different substances are added to foods to maintain their quality. **Preservatives** are added to food to prevent bacteria and molds from causing food spoilage, to extend shelf life, or to protect natural color and flavor. Sugar and salt are two of the oldest preservatives. They prevent microbial growth by decreasing the water availability in the product;

without adequate water, microbes cannot grow. For example, the high concentration of sugar in jams and jellies draws water away from the microbial cells and prevents them from growing.

Most preservatives have little documented risk. However, for some, the risks have been carefully weighed against the benefits. For example, nitrites and nitrates are used in cured meats such as ham and hot dogs to retard the growth of bacteria, particularly *Clostridium botulinum*, which causes deadly botulism poisoning. However, they also react with amino acids to form **nitrosamines** in the body. Nitrosamines are known to be carcinogenic in animals, but there is little evidence that they pose a serious risk in the amounts consumed in the human diet.[30] To minimize any risk of nitrosamines without increasing the risk of bacterial illness, the FDA has limited the amount of nitrites that can be added to food and has required the addition of antioxidants, which reduce nitrosamine formation, to foods containing nitrites. Consumers can reduce the risk of nitrites by limiting cured meat consumption to 3 to 4 ounces per week and maintaining adequate intakes of vitamins C and E.

Sulfites are another preservative that can be a health risk to consumers. The use of sulfites is restricted because some individuals are sulfite sensitive—in them, exposure may cause symptoms that range from stomachache and hives to severe asthmatic reactions.[31] Sulfite use is prohibited on foods intended to be eaten raw, but they may be used to prevent discoloration in dried fruits and fresh-cut potatoes, to control black spots in freshly caught shrimp, and to prevent discoloration, bacterial growth, and fermentation in wine (Figure 16.16).

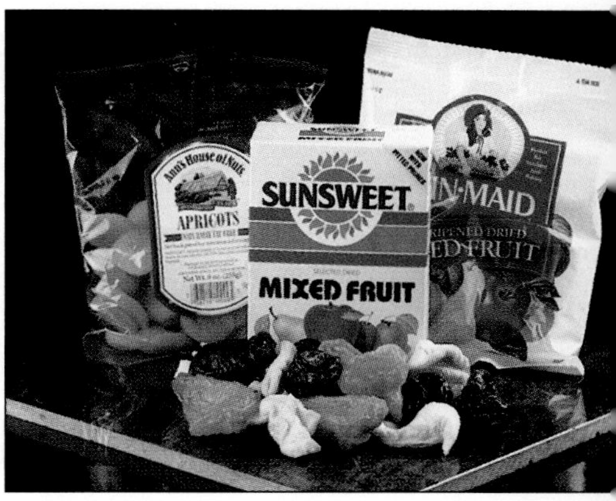

Figure 16.16
Sulfites are used in products such as dried fruit, but they can cause deadly reactions in sulfite-sensitive individuals. (George Semple)

Nitrosamines Carcinogenic compounds produced by reactions between nitrites and amino acids.

Additives That Aid in Processing or Preparation Many different types of additives are used in product processing and preparation. Emulsifiers improve the homogeneity, stability, and consistency of products such as ice cream. Stabilizers, thickeners, and texturizers, such as pectins and gums, are used to improve consistency or texture in pudding and to stabilize emulsions in foods such as salad dressing. Leavening agents are added to incorporate gas into breads and cakes, causing them to rise. Acids are added as flavor enhancers, preservatives, and antioxidants. Humectants, such as propylene glycol, cause moisture to be retained so products stay fresh. Anticaking agents prevent crystalline products such as powdered sugar from absorbing moisture and caking or lumping.

Additives to Affect Color and Flavor Additives are also used to enhance the flavor and color of foods. Flavor additives may supplement, magnify, or modify the original taste or aroma of a food. For example, both natural and artificial sweeteners are added to enhance the flavor of foods (see Chapter 4). Fat replacers such as Simplesse and Olestra increase the appeal of fat-free and lowfat foods by adding body, texture, and taste that simulates fat (see Chapter 5).

Colors can be used to make foods appear more appetizing; however, they cannot be used as deception to conceal inferiority. The FDA's list of permitted colors includes two categories: certified food colors and those exempt from certification. Certification means that each batch of the food color is tested to ensure safety, quality, consistency, and strength of color. Certified food colors are synthetic dyes derived primarily from petroleum and coal sources. About 10% of the food consumed in the United States contains certified food colors. Colors derived from plant, animal, and certain mineral sources are exempt from certification. Examples include beet juice, caramel, and paprika extract. The soft drink industry is the single largest user of color additives. Colors found to be potential hazards have been removed from the list of permissible additives.[32] However, the certified food color FD&C Yellow No. 5, which may cause itching and hives in hypersensitive individuals, was not considered a great enough risk to be removed from the food supply (see *Off the Label: Identifying Things Added to Your Food*).

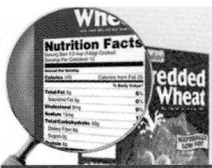

Off the Label

Identifying Things Added to Your Food

For many of us, the ingredients listed on food labels sound like a chemical soup. There is calcium propionate added to bread, disodium EDTA added to canned kidney beans, and BHA in potato chips. Are these chemical additives necessary in our food supply?

For most individuals, concerns about food additives are unfounded. Food additives are not approved by the FDA unless they are safe for most consumers. Understanding what these chemicals are used for can help make the ingredient list a source of information rather than a cause for concern. Food additives are used to make food safer; improve color, flavor, or texture; aid in processing; and enhance nutritional value. The table to the right provides some examples of food additives that might appear on food labels, the type of additive each is, and what it does in particular foods.

For individuals who are sensitive or allergic to certain additives, such as preservatives or colors, these lists provide essential information that can be lifesaving. Sulfites are preservatives used in many foods—for example, baked goods, canned vegetables, condiments, and maraschino cherries. Sulfites allowed in packaged foods include sulfur dioxide, sodium sulfite, sodium and potassium bisulfite, and sodium and potassium metabisulfite.[1] In sensitive individuals, they can cause deadly asthmatic reactions. Individuals sensitive to sulfites should read food labels to identify foods that contain them, and should be aware that foods served in restaurants could contain sulfites. For example, a potato dish served in a restaurant may be prepared using potatoes that were peeled and soaked in a sulfite solution before cooking.

Food colors can also cause reactions in sensitive individuals. For instance, the color additive FD&C Yellow No. 5, which is listed as tartrazine on medicine labels, may cause itching and hives in sensitive people. It is found in beverages, desserts, and processed vegetables. The ingredient list of the food label can be used to identify the presence of color additives. All foods that contain FDA-certified color additives must list them by name in the ingredient list. Colors that are exempt from certification, such as dehydrated beets and carotenoids, do not have to be specifically identified and may be listed on the label collectively as "artificial color."[2]

Reactions to food ingredients are relatively rare. The FDA estimates that 1 in 100 people are sulfite-sensitive and that sensitivity to FD&C Yellow No. 5 occurs in fewer than 1 in 10,000 people. The FDA monitors problems related to food additives using the Adverse Reaction Monitoring System (ARMS). Adverse reactions can be reported by contacting the FDA district office listed in your phone directory or by writing to:

ARMS
HFS-636
Food and Drug Administration
200 C Street, N.W.
Washington, DC 20204

[1]Papazian, R. Sulfites: safe for most, dangerous for some. FDA Consumer 30:11–14, December 1996. Online at http://www.fda.gov/fdac/featues/096 sulf.html

[2]U.S. Food and Drug Administration. Food Color Facts. January 1993. Online at http://vm.cfsan.fda.gov/~lrd/colorfac.html

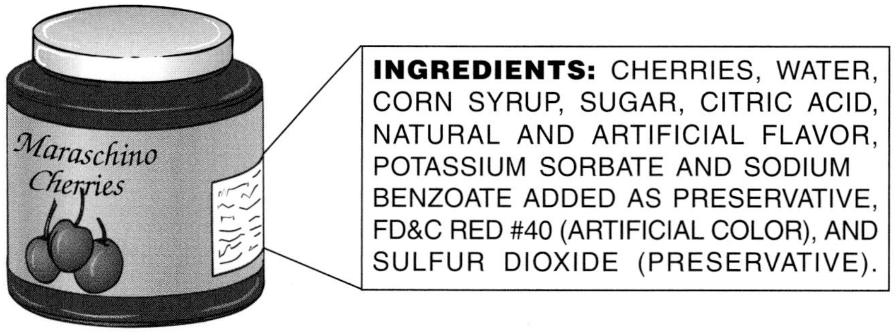

Maraschino Cherries
INGREDIENTS: CHERRIES, WATER, CORN SYRUP, SUGAR, CITRIC ACID, NATURAL AND ARTIFICIAL FLAVOR, POTASSIUM SORBATE AND SODIUM BENZOATE ADDED AS PRESERVATIVE, FD&C RED #40 (ARTIFICIAL COLOR), AND SULFUR DIOXIDE (PRESERVATIVE).

Processing and Packaging

Fermentation A process in which microorganisms metabolize components of a food and therefore change the composition, taste, and storage properties of the food.

For thousands of years, humans have been treating foods in order to protect them from spoilage by microorganisms. Most of the oldest methods of food preservation—including drying, smoking, **fermentation,** the addition of sugar or salt, and the use of heat or cold—are still used today.

Additive	Function	Example of Use
Acetic acid	Provides acidity	Gives tartness to dressings and sauces.
Ascorbic acid	Preservative, nutrient	Keeps fruit from darkening, inhibits rancidity in fatty foods, enhances nutritional value of beverages.
Baking soda (sodium bicarbonate)	Leavening agent	Generates gas so ensures baked goods rise.
Beet extract	Natural color	Gives deep red color to foods.
BHA	Preservative	Acts as an antioxidant to prevent rancidity of fats, oils, and dried meats; keeps baked goods fresh.
BHT	Preservative	Acts as an antioxidant to prevent rancidity in potato flakes, enriched rice, and shortenings.
Calcium silicate	Anticaking agent	Absorbs moisture to keep powdered foods like baking powder free-flowing
Carrageenan	Stabilizer, texturizer	Improves consistency and texture of chocolate milk, frozen desserts, puddings, and syrup.
Citric acid	Preservative, provides acidity	Provides acidity in beverages and dessert products.
FD&C colors	Color	Adds color to foods, drugs, and cosmetics.
Gelatin	Thickener	Provides texture to desserts, confectionery products, and canned meat products.
Glycerides (monoglycerides and diglycerides)	Emulsifier	Prevents ice cream from separating while melting, keeps oil in peanut butter from separating.
Glycerine (glycerol)	Humectant	Binds water to prevent moisture losses in flaked coconut, marshmallows, and toaster foods.
Guar gum	Thickener	Thickens liquids such as gravies and sauces.
Gum arabic	Stabilizer, emulsifier	Keeps butter mixed in buttered syrups and stabilizes flavors in dry-mix food products.
Lactic acid	Preservative	Controls molds in pickles, sauerkraut, cheese, buttermilk, and yogurt.
Lecithin	Emulsifier	Prevents separation of oil and vinegar in mayonnaise.
Magnesium stearate	Anticaking agent	Prevents clumping in flour.
Pectin	Thickener	Gels jams, jellies, and preserves.
Potassium sorbate	Preservative	Controls surface molds on cheese, syrups, margarine, and mayonnaise.
Propylene glycol	Humectant	Improves texture of foods by holding moisture.
Sodium benzoate	Preservative	Controls molds in syrup, margarine, soft drinks, and fruit products.
Sodium nitrite	Preservative	Prevents botulism growth in cured meats, fish, and poultry.
Sorbitol	Sweetener, humectant	Keeps fruit snacks and gummy candies soft.
Sulfites (sulfur dioxide, sodium sulfide, sodium and potassium bisulfite, and sodium and potassium metabisulfite)	Preservative	Acts as an antioxidant to prevent discoloration in fruits and vegetables like dried apples and dehydrated potatoes.
Tartaric acid	Increases acidity	Adds tartness to carbonated fruit-flavored drinks.

Using Temperature to Ensure Safety Cooking food is one of the oldest methods of ensuring food safety. It kills disease-causing organisms and destroys toxins. Cooling food with refrigeration or freezing also protects us by slowing or stopping microbial growth. Other preservation techniques that rely on temperature include canning, pasteurization, and sterilization. These techniques benefit us by providing appealing safe food, but they are not risk free, particularly if used incorrectly. If foods are not heated long enough or to a high enough temperature, or if they are not kept cold enough, there is a risk of food-borne illness.

Toxins Produced During Cooking Cooking can also generate food hazards such as mutagens and carcinogens. These are considered accidental contaminants, so they are not regulated by the FDA. The most familiar group of chemicals produced during cooking is the **polycyclic aromatic hydrocarbons (PAHs).** PAHs are formed when fat from beef, pork, lamb, poultry, or fish drips onto the flame of a grill. As early as 1775, PAH-containing soot was linked to cancer in chimney sweeps. Several of the PAHs found in food have been shown to cause cancer in laboratory animals. Eating grilled fatty meat every day is not recommended, but occasional grilling, particularly with lowfat meat, presents little risk.

Polycyclic aromatic hydrocarbons (PAHs) A class of mutagenic substances produced during cooking when there is incomplete combustion of organic materials—such as when fat drips on a grill.

Broiled foods, which are cooked with the heat source at the top, are low in PAHs. However, broiled and pan-fried meats contain another potential hazard—**heterocyclic amines (HAs),** such as benzopyrene, which are formed from the burning of amino acids and other substances in meats. Well-done meat and meat cooked using hotter temperatures contain greater amounts. The cooking temperatures recommended by the FDA are designed to prevent microbial food-borne illness and minimize the production of heterocyclic amines. The levels of heterocyclic amines can be reduced by precooking meat in the microwave and discarding the juice.

Heterocyclic amines (HAs) A class of mutagenic substances produced when there is incomplete combustion of amino acids during the cooking of meats—such as when meat is charred.

Using Packaging to Ensure Safety Some of the newer methods of food preservation rely on modern packaging. In one type of preservation, referred to as **aseptic processing,** sterilized foods are placed in sterilized packages using sterilized packaging equipment.[33] Aseptic processing is currently used to produce boxes of sterile milk and juices. These can remain free of microbial growth at room temperature for years.

Aseptic processing A method that places sterilized food in a sterilized package using a sterile process.

Consumer demand for fresh foods has led to a new generation of fresh refrigerated foods such as pasta, vegetables, fish, chicken, and beef. They are delicious, nutritious, and convenient, but are they safe? To make fresh refrigerated foods—for example, beef teriyaki—the raw ingredients are sealed in plastic pouches, the air is vacuumed out, and the pouch and its contents are partially precooked and immediately refrigerated. This type of processing eliminates the need for the extreme cold of freezing or the extreme heat of canning, so flavor and nutrients are better preserved. Unlike canned foods, fresh refrigerated products are not heated to sufficient temperatures to kill all bacteria, and unlike frozen foods, they are not kept at temperatures low enough to prevent all bacteria from growing. In some products, the oxygen in the package is replaced with a gas such as carbon dioxide or nitrogen, in which microbes are unlikely to grow.[34] This is called **modified atmosphere packaging (MAP).** These foods should be purchased only from reputable vendors, used by the expiration date printed on the package, refrigerated constantly until use, and heated according to the time and temperature on the package directions.

Modified atmosphere packaging (MAP) A type of food packaging in which the gases inside the package control or retard chemical, physical, and microbiological changes.

Contamination From Packaging Packaging can protect food from spoilage, but even the best packaging can introduce risk if it becomes a part of the food. A variety of substances leach into foods from plastics, paper, and even dishes. Substances that are known to contaminate foods are indirect food additives and the amounts and types are regulated by EPA tolerance levels and FDA inspections. However, these regulations apply only to the intended use of the product. When used improperly, packaging can migrate into food and become an accidental contaminant. For instance, some plastics migrate into food when heated in a microwave oven. Thus only packages designated for microwave cooking should be used.

Lead from pottery glazes, leaded crystal wine glasses and decanters, and lead solder in water pipes can also contaminate food and water. For information about lead contamination and kits that test the amount of lead leaching from ceramic ware, call your local FDA office or check the FDA Web site. In addition, most ceramic manufacturers in the United States maintain toll-free lines that can provide information about lead levels in their products (see Chapter 14).

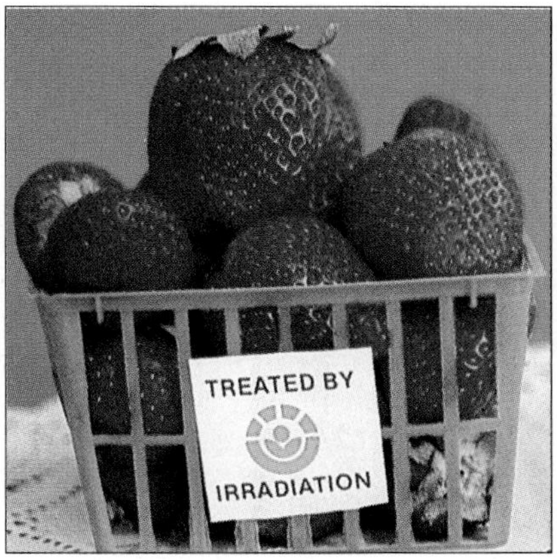

Figure 16.17
Foods that have been treated with irradiation can be identified by the radura symbol. (Courtesy of Nordion International, Inc.)

Irradiated Foods

Irradiation is a process that exposes food to a high dose of x-rays, gamma radiation, or high-energy electrons. It kills microorganisms and insects and slows vital processes such as the germination and ripening of fruits and vegetables. It may, therefore, be used in place of chemicals to reduce insect and microbial contamination and to slow ripening during food storage.[35] It is used in more than 40 countries to treat everything from frog legs to rice. It has been endorsed by the United Nations Food and Agriculture Organization, the World Health Organization, as well as the FDA.[36] It is one of the technologies singled out in the National Food Safety Initiative because of its potential for improving the safety of food and reducing the incidence of food-borne illness.

Irradiation A process of exposing foods to radiation to kill contaminating organisms and retard ripening and spoilage of fruits and vegetables.

Food irradiation is not a new technique; astronauts have eaten irradiated food since Apollo 17 went to the moon in 1972, but it is used relatively infrequently in the United States. Part of the reason for its underuse is lack of irradiation facilities, but public fear and suspicion of the technology also limits its use. The word "irradiation" fosters the belief that the food itself becomes radioactive. Opponents to food irradiation claim that it introduces carcinogens, depletes the nutritional value of food, and is used to allow the sale of previously contaminated foods. In fact, irradiated food is not radioactive and there is no evidence to support the claim that it causes cancer. FDA scientists have concluded that irradiation does not compromise nutritional quality or noticeably change food texture, taste, or appearance as long as it is properly applied to a suitable product.[35,37] Irradiation can decrease the amounts of certain nutrients; as much as 10% of vitamin A, thiamin, vitamin E, and vitamin K in a food can be destroyed. But this is similar to the losses that occur with canning or cold storage.[36]

The FDA has approved irradiation to destroy pathogens in red meat and poultry and contaminants in spices; prevent insect infestation in flour and spices; increase the shelf life of potatoes; eliminate *Trichinella* in pork; control insects in fruits, vegetables, and grains; and slow the ripening and spoilage of some produce. Irradiated foods must be labeled with the radura symbol (Figure 16.17) and the statement "treated with radiation" or "treated by irradiation." Products that contain irradiated spices or other irradiated ingredients do not need to display this symbol, and irradiation labeling requirements do not apply to restaurant food.[37] Because irradiation produces unique compounds in irradiated foods, it is treated as a food additive, and the level of radiation that may be used is regulated by the FDA and USDA. At the allowed levels of radiation, the amounts of these unique compounds produced are almost negligible and have not been found to be a risk to consumers. Irradiated foods may cost more because of the cost of adding an extra processing step, but in the future this may be offset by a longer shelf life[37] (Figure 16.18). Irradiation should be used to complement, not replace, proper food handling by producers, processors, and consumers.

Biotechnology

In addition to the technological advances that have created new methods of processing and packaging foods, technology has also produced new foods and products. Some of these are produced using traditional food chemistry and plant breeding procedures, but many are now being made using biotechnology.

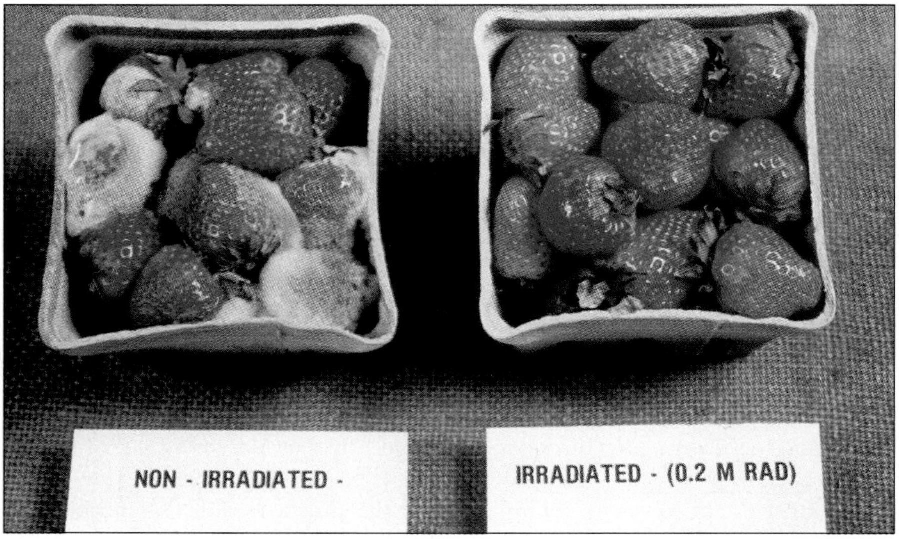

Figure 16.18
After two weeks in cold storage, the strawberries treated by irradiation remain free of mold (*right*), whereas the untreated strawberries picked at the same time are covered with mold (*left*). (Council for Agricultural Science and Technology)

Clones Copies that are identical to the original.

Biotechnology refers to the use of genetic modification or genetic engineering to alter the DNA of plants and animals to produce new traits or enhance desirable ones. The first step is to identify a stretch of DNA, or gene, for a given desirable trait, such as resistance to a particular disease. This gene could be in a plant, an animal, or a bacterial cell. The gene can be clipped out with specific DNA-cutting enzymes and then pasted into or recombined with the DNA of a virus or bacterium (Figure 16.19). The virus or bacterium containing the gene for the desired trait then reproduces. Each reproduction produces **clones,** or copies of the gene. Each of the clones can now produce the protein that is coded for by that gene. For example, insulin, used to treat diabetes, is produced by genetically engineered bacteria.

Bacteria or viruses containing recombined genes can also be used to produce plants or animals with specific characteristics. To do this, the gene of interest must be inserted into a target plant or animal cell. For example, a gene for disease resistance might be introduced into the cells of wheat plants, making the wheat disease resistant. One way genes are inserted is by allowing a virus containing the desired gene to infect the target cell, hence introducing the recombinant DNA.

The Benefits of Biotechnology The uses of biotechnology are as varied as the imagination. Crops being developed using biotechnology include fruits and vegetables that ripen more slowly so they will arrive at stores at their peak, virus-resistant vegetables, insect-resistant produce, vegetables with increased levels of amino acids, low-caffeine coffee, long-lasting raspberries, potatoes that absorb less fat when fried, and bananas that deliver a dose of hepatitis B vaccine.[38] Vegetable crops can be developed that do not need as much cooking when they are canned or that are more resistant to freezing.

Other advances in biotechnology that will impact on the quantity, quality, safety, and shelf life of foods include environmentally friendly pesticides and safer additives and preservatives. Genetically engineered enzymes are also used in food processing, and food colors and flavors are being produced from plant tissue grown in the laboratory. Improvements in the treatment, prevention, and diagnosis of animal disease as well as developments that improve animal growth and fertility all can enhance food production.

Does Biotechnology Carry Risks? As with any new process or product, consumers may be reluctant to use genetically engineered foods. The FDA has ruled that there is no reason for extra regulations on most foods produced by genetic engineering.[39] No premarket approval is required for the production of genetically engineered foods unless the food contains substances not commonly found

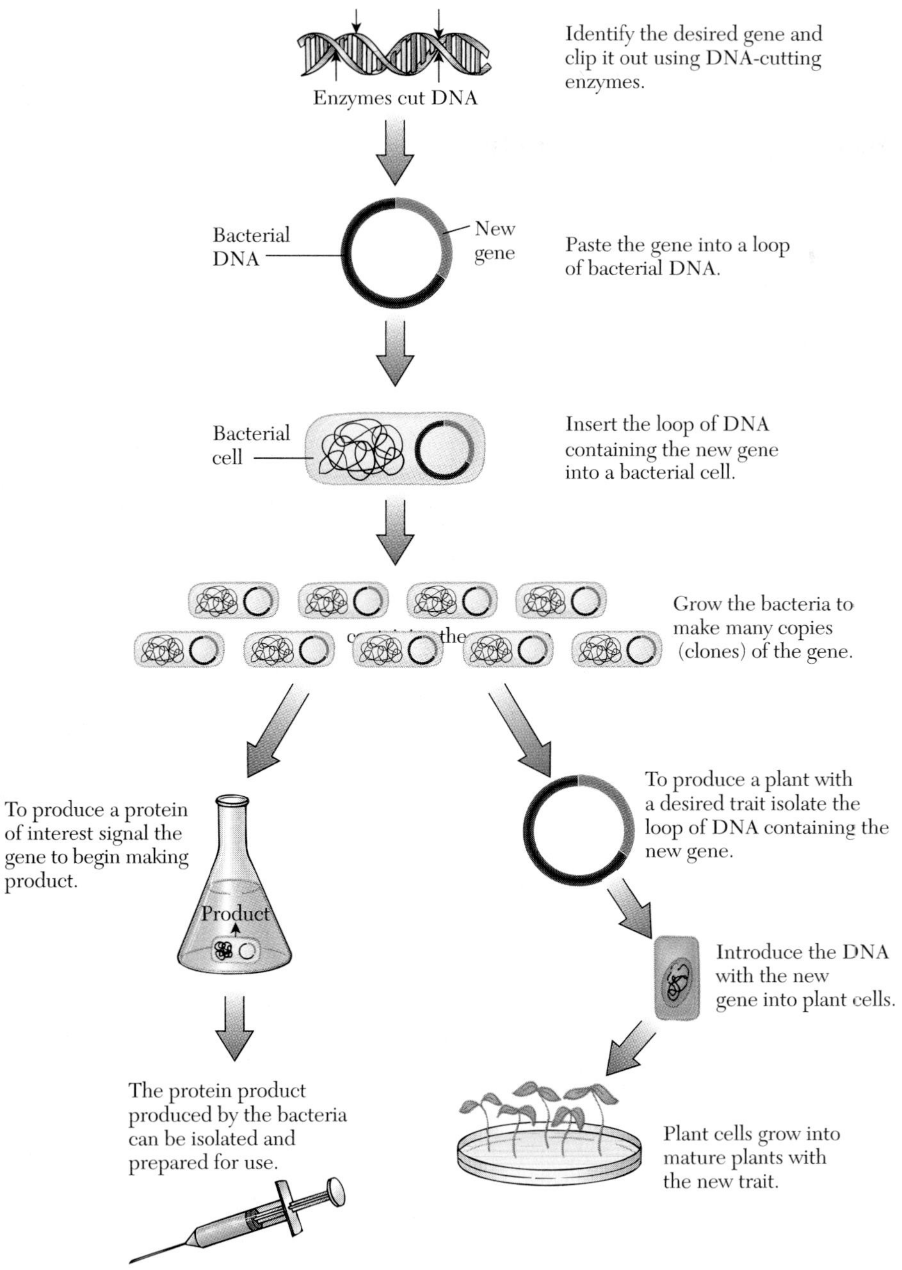
Enzymes cut DNA
Identify the desired gene and clip it out using DNA-cutting enzymes.
Bacterial DNA
New gene
Paste the gene into a loop of bacterial DNA.
Bacterial cell
Insert the loop of DNA containing the new gene into a bacterial cell.
Grow the bacteria to make many copies (clones) of the gene.
To produce a protein of interest signal the gene to begin making product.
Product
The protein product produced by the bacteria can be isolated and prepared for use.
To produce a plant with a desired trait isolate the loop of DNA containing the new gene.
Introduce the DNA with the new gene into plant cells.
Plant cells grow into mature plants with the new trait.

Figure 16.19
Genetic engineering involves inserting a gene for a desired trait into an organism to create a new strain of plant or animal or to produce large amounts of a desired gene product.

in foods or contains a substance that does not have a history of safe use in foods. To help assure the public that this approach is appropriate for genetically engineered foods, producers are required to notify the FDA before these products are marketed so the FDA is kept aware of all new developments.

Because genetically engineered foods are essentially no different from other foods, they do not need special labeling. Exceptions are foods into which a potential allergen has been introduced. For example, if DNA from fish or peanuts—foods that commonly cause allergic reactions—is introduced into tomatoes or corn, these foods would have to be labeled in order to alert allergic consumers. Labeling would also be required if the nutrient content of a food were significantly altered. For example, tomatoes are an excellent source of vitamin C. If a tomato were developed that had no vitamin C, it would have be labeled to disclose this information.

The standard concerns about safety and labeling have been addressed, but genetic engineering has introduced some new concerns. One relates more to the environment than to the consumer. If a trait introduced into a plant species could be passed on to one of its wild relatives, it might produce a plant that would become a fast-growing weed or that would be harmful to species that depend on it for food. If fish engineered to grow faster and produce more young entered the ecosystem, they might have an adaptive advantage over their wild relatives and would ultimately reduce diversity. Ethical and religious issues also need to be resolved. For example, can a tomato that contains some DNA from a fish be included in a vegan diet? Is corn that contains DNA from a pig appropriate for Jews and Muslims to eat? The FDA currently believes that the answer to these questions is yes, since plants and animals already share some of the same types of DNA, but this issue and others will continue to be debated.[40] Genetically engineered foods are one part of the solution to the challenge of producing more food of better quality and, in the case of the vaccine-bearing banana, may even protect children in developing nations from disease (see *Critical Thinking: Individual Risk-Benefit Analysis*).

CRITICAL THINKING

Individual Risk-Benefit Analysis

After reading a newspaper article about a child who died of food-borne illness contracted by eating an undercooked hamburger, Rex became concerned about the safety of the foods his family was eating. He thought more carefully about other food safety issues, such as eggs and poultry contaminated with *Salmonella*; pesticide residues on fruits and vegetables; and fish contaminated with industrial pollutants, bacteria, viruses, and parasites. He started to think it was too risky to eat at all but then decided to look at the foods his family eats and see if the benefits they provide are worth the risk.

In general his family eats a healthy diet and is rarely sick, but he knows that a few of the things they like carry risks. He enjoys his meat rare, his son is an athlete who drinks protein shakes containing raw eggs, his young daughter likes to lick the bowl where cookie dough containing raw eggs is mixed, and he and his wife enjoy eating sushi and raw oysters. He made the following list of foods and then recorded the risks and benefits of each:

Food	Risk	Benefit
Hamburger	Can be contaminated with pathogenic *E. coli*.	A good source of protein and iron in the diet.
Chicken	Is often contaminated with *Salmonella*.	An economical source of protein that is low in fat.
Eggs	Can contain *Salmonella* or *Campylobacter*.	An inexpensive source of protein.
Fish	Can be contaminated with environmental pollutants such as PCBs and toxic metals.	A lowfat source of high-quality protein. Consumption has been associated with a reduced risk of cardiovascular disease
Raw fish and shellfish	May be a source of bacterial, viral, and parasitic infections.	A lowfat source of high-quality protein and omega-3 fatty acids.
Fruits and vegetables	May contain pesticide residues.	An excellent source of fiber and vitamins in the diet. They also contain health-promoting phytochemicals.

After reviewing the risks and benefits of his family's diet, Rex realizes he can minimize the risk of eating hamburger and chicken by thoroughly cooking them, because *E. coli* and its toxins and *Salmonella* are destroyed by heat.

What other changes can he make to minimize the risks associated with his family's typical diet while including foods that are beneficial?

Answer:

APPLICATIONS

These exercises are designed to help you apply your critical thinking skills to your own nutrition choices.

1. Read the labels from food products in your cupboard or the store.
   a. List ten additives and the food product in which they are contained.
   b. Describe why each additive is used and what might happen in each case if the additive were not used in the product.
2. After 67 people became ill from consuming food at a company picnic, investigators determined that the tossed salad, the egg salad, and the turkey slices were all contaminated with *Salmonella*. Invent a scenario that would explain how all three became contaminated (the FDA Web page can be helpful here).
3. Use the Internet to go to the FDA/CFSAN Web site. Complete the exercise at this site called "Can Your Kitchen Pass the Food Safety Test?"
   a. What was your score?
   b. Based on how you answered these questions, what changes should you make in the way you store and handle foods in your kitchen?
   c. Based on how you answered these questions, are there foods that you will eliminate from your diet?

Summary

1. The safety of the food supply can be affected by biological as well as chemical contamination. The harm caused by contaminants in the food supply depends on the type of toxin, the dose, the length of time over which it is consumed, and the size and health status of the consumer.
2. The food supply is monitored for safety by food manufacturers and regulatory agencies at the international, federal, state, and local levels. In addition, consumers play an important role in limiting the risks of developing food-borne illness.
3. The use of HACCP (Hazard Analysis Critical Control Point) offers a method for preventing food contamination, monitoring food processing methods, and tracking contaminated foods to prevent food-borne illness.
4. The most common cause of food-borne illness is microbial contamination, which often produces acute gastrointestinal symptoms. Some bacteria cause food-borne infection because they are able to grow in the gastrointestinal tract when ingested. Others produce toxins in food or in the body and cause food-borne intoxication. Some may do both. Viruses that contaminate food can also cause food-borne illness, as can toxins produced by molds that grow on foods, and parasites consumed in contaminated water or food.
5. The risk of food-borne illness can be decreased by proper food selection, preparation, and storage. Consumers should choose the freshest meats and produce, select frozen foods that have been kept at constant temperatures, and avoid packages with broken seals or contents that appear spoiled. Once in the home, foods should be cooked thoroughly and leftovers stored properly. Kitchen surfaces, hands, and cooking utensils should be cleaned between preparation steps.
6. Contaminants such as pesticides applied to crops, drugs given to animals, and industrial wastes that leach into water may find their way into the food supply.
7. To decrease the potential risk of pesticides, safer ones are being developed and American farmers are reducing the amounts applied by using integrated pest management and organic methods.
8. Industrial pollutants such as PCBs, radioactive substances, and toxic metals have contaminated some waterways and the fish that live in them. As these contaminants move up the food chain their concentrations increase.
9. Consumers can reduce the amounts of pesticides and other environmental contaminants in food by careful selection and handling of produce; selection of lowfat saltwater varieties of fish caught well offshore in unpolluted waters; and trimming fat from meat, poultry, and fish before cooking.
10. Food additives include all substances that can reasonably be expected to find their way into a food during processing. This includes direct food additives, which are used to preserve or enhance the appeal of food, and indirect food additives, which are substances known to find their way into food during cooking, processing, and packaging. Direct and indirect food

additives are regulated by the FDA. Accidental contaminants that enter food when it is used or prepared incorrectly are not regulated by the FDA.

11. Processing and packaging techniques are used to prevent food spoilage. Cold temperatures slow or prevent microbial growth. High temperatures used in canning, pasteurization, sterilization, and cooking kill microorganisms. Packaging also preserves foods. Aseptic processing sterilizes the food and the package; modified atmosphere packaging reduces the oxygen available for microbial growth. However, cooking and packaging can also introduce hazards into foods.
12. Irradiation preserves food by exposing it to x-rays, gamma radiation, or high-energy electrons. It kills microorganisms, destroys insects, and slows the germination and ripening of fruits and vegetables.
13. New foods and products can be produced using biotechnology. These techniques alter the DNA of plants or animals to produce new varieties with desired traits, such as disease resistance, increased nutrient content, or delayed spoilage.

Review Questions

1. What is the major cause of food-borne illness in the United States today?
2. List three factors that affect the toxicity of a substance.
3. Explain what HACCP is and how it can prevent food contamination.
4. List three ways in which the federal government is involved in providing a safe food supply.
5. List three common bacterial food contaminants. What can be done to avoid the food-borne illnesses caused by them?
6. What temperature range allows the most rapid bacterial growth?
7. What is the difference between a food-borne infection and a food-borne intoxication?
8. How do pesticides applied to crops find their way into animal products?
9. List some ways in which food processing reduces food-borne illnesses.
10. What is the GRAS list?
11. List four reasons for using food additives.
12. What is food irradiation? Is it safe?
13. How does genetic engineering introduce new traits into plants or animals?

Nutrition Web Links

To further explore areas related to the material in this chapter, go to the *Nutrition: Science and Applications* Web site at ***www.Wiley.com/college/Smolin*** and *click on* **Student Companion Site** for chapter-by-chapter links. Some Web sites related to information in Chapter 16 include:

Sites that provide information on food safety such as the government's centralized Food Safety Web site.

Sites that provide information about environmental issues such as the Environmental Protection Agency and the USDA's National Organic Food Standards site.

Sites that provide information on biotechnology such as the Biotechnology Information Center.

References

1. Hingley, A. Food safety initiative calls on government, industry, consumers to stop food-related illness. FDA Consumer 31:8–11, September/October 1997.
2. Knabel, S. J. Institute of Food Technologists Scientific Status Summary: Foodborne illness: role of home food handling practices. Food Technol. 49:119–131, 1995.
3. U.S. Food and Drug Administration, Department of Agriculture, and Environmental Protection Agency. Food Safety From Farm to Table: A New Strategy for the 21st Century. February 21, 1997. Online at http://vm.cfsan.fda.gov/~dms/fs-draft.html
4. U.S. Department of Health and Human Services. National computer network in place to combat foodborne illness (press release). May 22, 1998. Online at http://www.cdc.gov/od/oc/media/pressrel/r980522.htm
5. National Academy of Sciences. *Ensuring Safe Food From Production to Consumption.* Washington, D.C.: National Academy Press, 1998.
6. Stephenson, J. Fighting flora with flora: FDA approves an anti-Salmonella spray for chickens. J.A.M.A. 279:1152, 1998.
7. Cerington, M. Clinical spectrum of botulism. Muscle Nerve 21:701–710, 1998.
8. Kohn, M. A., Farley, T. A., Ando, T., et al. An outbreak of Norwalk virus gastroenteritis associated with eating raw oysters: implications for maintaining safe oyster beds. J.A.M.A. 273:466–471, 1995.
9. U.S. Food and Drug Administration, Center for Food Safety and Nutrition. Foodborne Pathogenic Microoganisms and Natual Toxins Handbook: The "Bad Bug Book." Online at http://vm.cfsan.fda.gov/~mow/intro.html
10. Outbreaks of Escherichia coli O157:H7 infection and cryptosporidosis associated with drinking unpasteurized apple cider—Connecticut and New York, October 1996. MMWR Morb. Mortal. Wkly. Rep. 46:4–8, 1997.

11. Foodborne outbreak of diarrheal illness associated with Cryptosporidium parvum—Minnesota, 1995. MMWR Morb. Mortal. Wkly. Rep. 45:783–784, 1996.
12. Kurtzweil, P. Can your kitchen pass the food safety test? FDA Consumer 28:14–18, October 1994.
13. Kolpin, D. W., Barbash, J. E., and Gilliom, R. J. Occurrence of pesticides in shallow groundwater of the United States—initial results from the National Water-Quality Assessment Program. Environ. Sci. Technol. 32:558–566, 1998.
14. Foulke, J. E. FDA reports on pesticides in foods. FDA Consumer 27:29–32, June 1993.
15. Cooney, C. M. New pesticide law drops "zero-tolorance" standard, focuses on exposure to children. Environ. Sci. Technol. 30:380A, September 1996.
16. U.S. Food and Drug Administration. FDA Report: Pesticides in Our Food, 1998. Online at http://vm.cfsan.fda.gov/~dms/pes97.html
17. National Research Council, Committee on Comparative Toxicology of Naturally Occurring Carcinogens. Individual chemicals in the diet generally pose no risk to Americans, NRC concludes. Food Chem. News 37:32–33, February 19, 1996.
18. Acquavella, J., Burns, C., Flaherty, D., et al. A critique of the World Resource Institute's report "Pesticides and the Immune System: The Public Health Risks." Environ. Health Perspect. 106:51–54, 1998.
19. U.S. Department of Agriculture. Remarks of Secretary Glickman. Proposed Organic Standards. December 15, 1997. Online at http://www.usda.gov/news/releases/1997/12/0443
20. U.S. Department of Agriculture. Agricultural Marketing Program, National Organic Program. Online at http://www.ams.usda.gov/nop
21. Russell, L. Consumers face little danger from residues in meat and poultry. Food News 6:10–11, 1990.
22. Kaneene, J. B., and Miller, R. Problems associated with drug residues in beef from feeds and therapy. Rev. Sci. Tech. 16:694–708, 1997.
23. Ropp, K. L. New animal drug increases milk production. FDA Consumer 28:24–27, May 1994.
24. Clarkson, T. W. Environmental contaminants in the food chain. Am. J. Clin. Nutr. 61(suppl):682S–686S, 1995.
25. Jacobson, J. L., and Jacobson, S. W. Intellectual impairment in children exposed to polychlorinated biphenyls in utero. N. Engl. J. Med. 335:783–789, 1996.
26. American Academy of Pediatrics, Committee on Environmental Health. PCBs in breast milk. Pediatrics 84:122–123, 1994.
27. Foulke, J. E. Mercury in fish: cause for concern? FDA Consumer 28:5–8, September 1994.
28. Kurtzweil, P. Fruits and vegetables: eating your way to five a day. FDA Consumer 31:16–23, March 1997.
29. Segal, M. Ingredient labeling: what's in a food? FDA Consumer 27:14–18, April 1993.
30. Eichholzer, M., and Gutzwiller, F. Dietary nitrates, nitrites, and N-nitroso compounds and cancer risk: a review of the epidemiologic evidence. Nutr. Rev. 56:95–105, 1998.
31. Papazian, R. Sulfites: safe for most, dangerous for some. FDA Consumer 30:11–14, December 1996.
32. U.S. Food and Drug Administration. Food Color Facts. January 1993. Online at http://vm.cfsan.fda.gov/~lrd/colorfac.html
33. Gould, G. W. Methods of preservation and extension of shelf life. Int. J. Food Microbiol. 33: 51–64, 1996.
34. Marth, E. H. Scientific Status Summary: extended-shelf-life refrigerated foods: microbiological quality and safety. Food Technol. 52:57–62, 1998.
35. American Dietetic Association. Position of the American Dietetic Association: Irradiated Foods. J. Am. Diet. Assoc. 96:69–72, 1996.
36. Skerrett, P. J. Food irradiation: will it keep the doctor away? Technol. Rev. 100:28–36, November/December 1997.
37. Henkel, J. Irradiation: a safe measure for safer food. FDA Consumer 32:12–17, May/June 1998.
38. Henkel, J. Genetic engineering: fast forwarding to future foods. FDA Consumer 29:6–11, April 1995.
39. Genetically engineered foods: fears and facts. FDA Consumer 27:11–14, January/February 1993.
40. Kendall, P. Food biotechnology: boon or threat? J. Nutr. Educ. 29:112–115, 1997.

Chapter

17

Chapter Outline

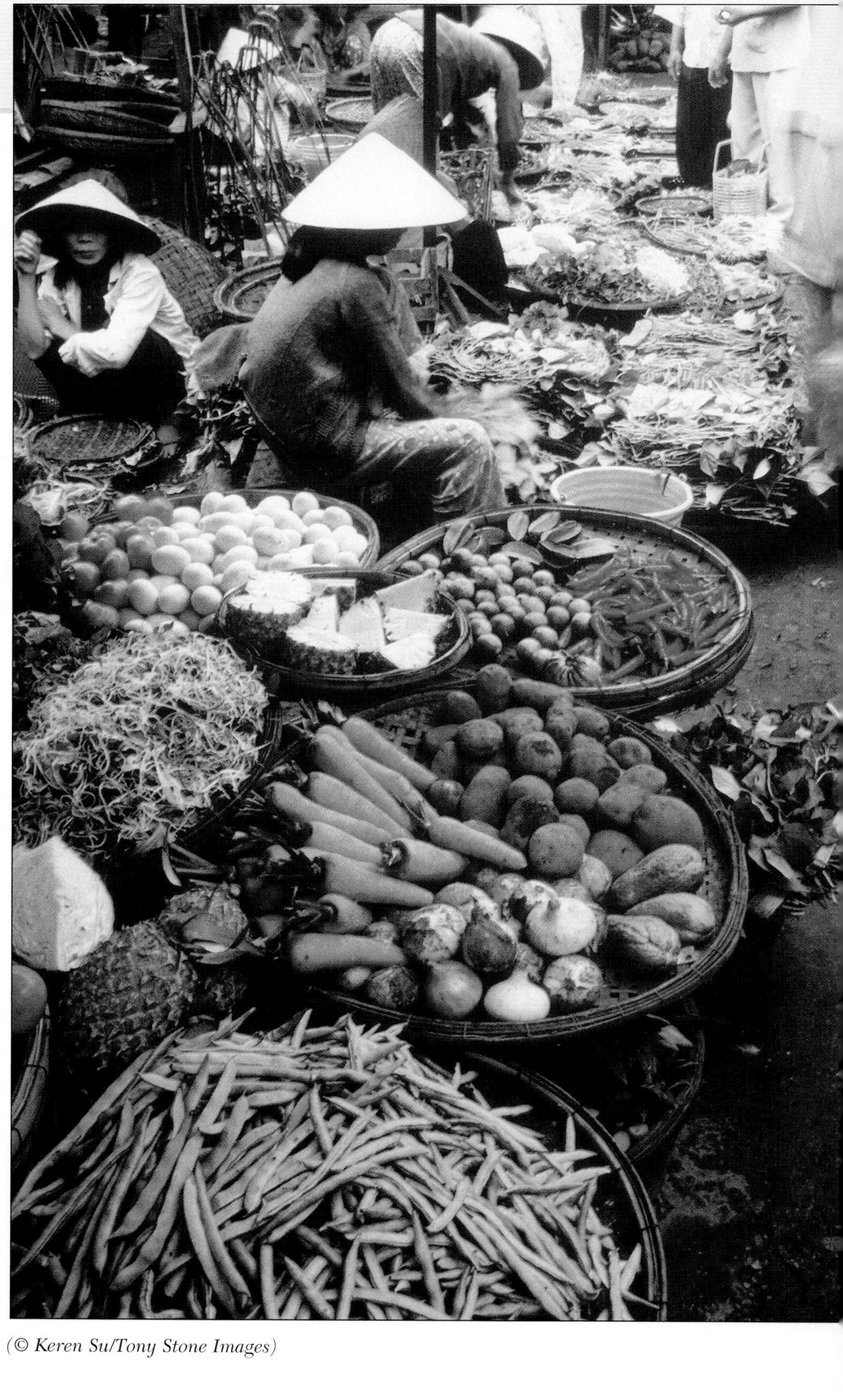

(© Keren Su/Tony Stone Images)

The Global View: Feeding the World

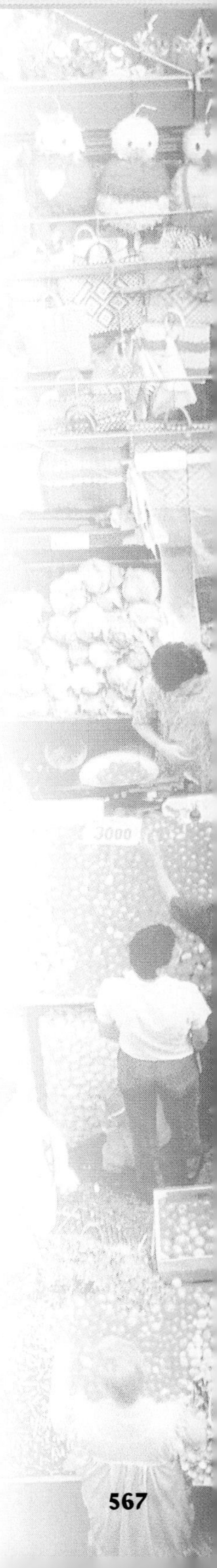

Chapter Concepts

1. The overnutrition that is prevalent in developed countries contrasts sharply with the undernutrition that is a problem in much of the developing world.
2. Undernutrition can result from a general lack of food or a diet that is deficient in one or more essential nutrients.
3. When food and nutrients are limited, a cycle of malnutrition produces poorly nourished infants who are at risk for infection, illness, and early death. Those who survive often grow to be unhealthy adults who are unable to reach their full potential.
4. A shortage of food can occur in entire populations or among subgroups of a given population. Food shortages are caused by natural and man-made disasters and by overpopulation, inequitable distribution of money and other resources, and agricultural practices that damage the environment, limiting food production.
5. Poor-quality diets and increased nutrient needs cause malnutrition even in populations with adequate food supplies.
6. Solutions to the problem of worldwide undernutrition include short-term programs to feed the hungry and long-term programs that balance population size with resources, foster economic self-sufficiency among households and nations, encourage the development of a nutritionally adequate food supply, and promote food production methods that preserve the environment for future use.
7. In the United States, the majority of the population is at risk for overnutrition, but poverty—particularly among women and children, the homeless, and the elderly—creates pockets of undernutrition.
8. Solutions to hunger at home involve providing access to affordable food, education, and medical care.
9. Overnutrition, with the resulting increase in the incidence of chronic disease, is a growing international problem.

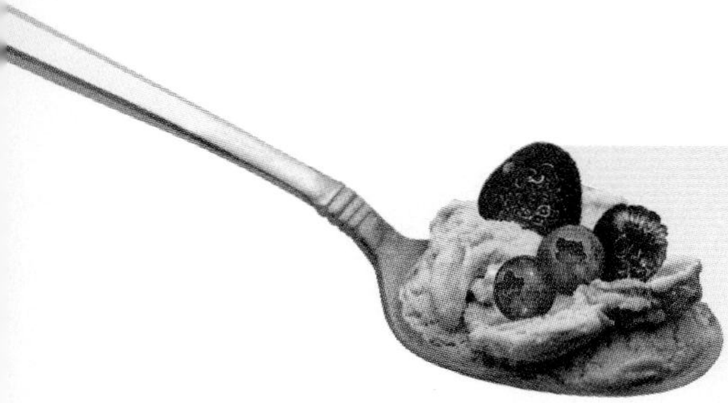

Just a Taste

Is there enough food to feed the world?

Is hunger a problem in the United States?

Can the food choices you make affect the environment?

In developed nations today, the majority of nutritional problems are related to overconsumption. Yet people around the world are starving. Undernutrition is the major form of malnutrition in developing nations, where 840 million people are chronically undernourished.[1,2] In addition, there are pockets of undernutrition in developed countries, including the United States.

Why does this dichotomy exist? Why are there two faces of malnutrition in the world? There are many reasons, but the underlying one is that the food produced in the world is not distributed equitably, so that in some places there is plenty and in others there is not enough. Overpopulation, inefficient land use, and inequitable distribution of land, wealth, and food cause populations and individuals within populations to be malnourished. Solving these problems involves controlling population growth, providing food, and changing agricultural, political, social, and economic systems.

Feeding the world involves every aspect of nutrition. It requires understanding nutrient needs and how to meet these needs. It involves the politics and economics of providing food. It involves technology to increase food production and environmental consciousness to maintain resources for future generations.

Undernutrition: A World Health Problem

Hunger is one of the first images that comes to mind when the topic of global nutrition is raised (Figure 17.1). Over time, hunger leads to undernutrition—a lack of energy or one or more nutrients. Undernutrition is the result of an insufficient diet or of a disease state that increases nutrient needs or interferes with the ability to consume and utilize nutrients. An insufficient diet either does not contain enough food or it contains the wrong combination of foods to meet nutrient needs. Solutions to the problem of undernutrition must first feed the hungry and then develop strategies to promote a balance between the population, the production of food, and the use of environmental resources.

Cycle of malnutrition A cycle in which malnutrition is perpetuated by an inability to meet nutrient needs at all life stages.

The Cycle of Malnutrition

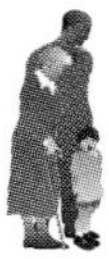

In populations where undernutrition is a chronic problem, a **cycle of malnutrition** prevents the development of a healthy productive population (Figure 17.2). The cycle of malnutrition begins when women consume a deficient diet during

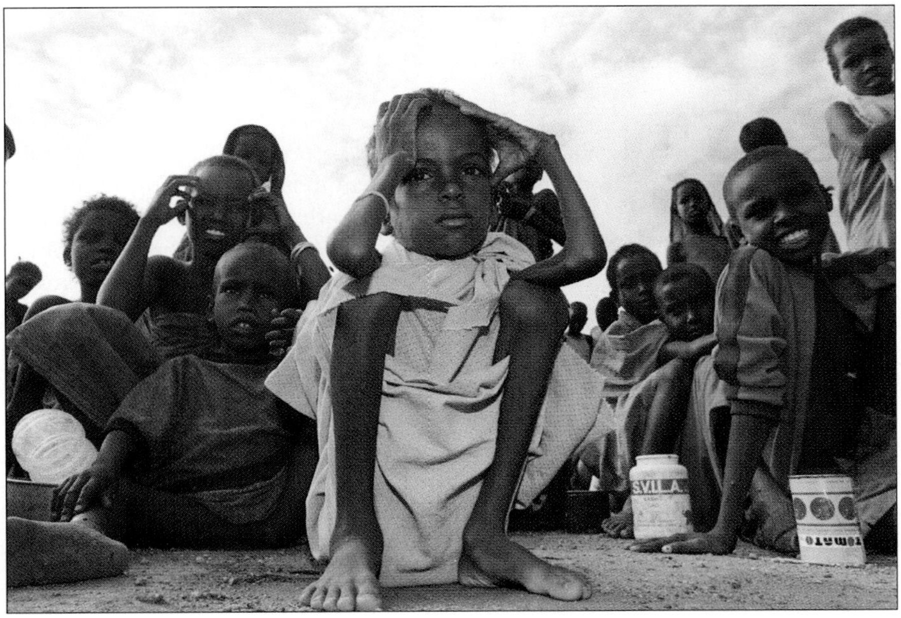

Figure 17.1
Undernutrition is more common in developing nations, especially among children because of their high nutrient needs. (Reuters/Bettmann)

pregnancy. These women are more likely to give birth to low birth weight infants who are susceptible to illness and early death. The children who do survive may be small and weakened physically and mentally. They grow into undernourished adults unable to contribute optimally to economic and social development. Thus, the women in this next generation also begin their pregnancies poorly nourished and are therefore likely to give birth to low birth weight infants. Interruption of this cycle of malnutrition at any point can benefit the individuals and the society. Healthy children can then grow into healthy adults who produce healthy offspring and can contribute fully to society.

Low Birth Weight and Infant Mortality Low birth weight infants—those weighing less than 2500 grams (about 5.5 pounds) at birth—are at greater risk of complications, illness, and early death. A higher number of low birth weight infants means a higher **infant mortality rate,** the number of deaths per 1000 live births in a population. The infant mortality rate and the number of low birth weight births are indicators of the health and nutritional status of a population. The average infant mortality rate worldwide is about 64 per 1000, but in developing nations the average rate is 120 per 1000, as compared to only 7 per 1000 in more developed countries.[3] Low birth weight infants who do survive require extra

Infant mortality rate The number of deaths during the first year of life per 1000 live births.

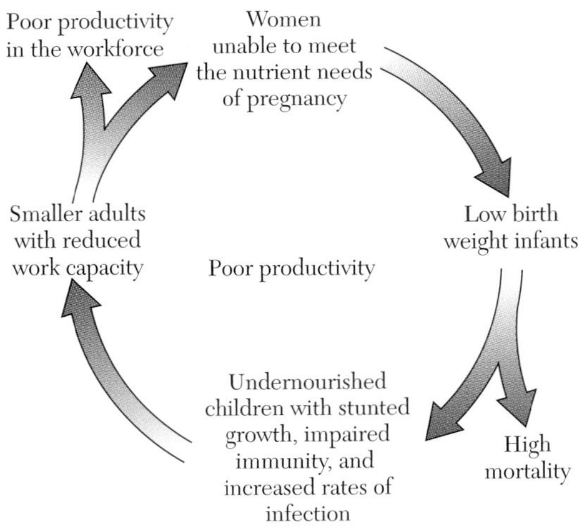

Figure 17.2
The cycle of malnutrition affects both the health and the productivity of a population.

nutrients, which are usually not available. Malnutrition in infancy and childhood has a profound effect on growth and development as well as susceptibility to infectious disease.

Stunting A decrease in linear growth rate, which is an indicator of the nutritional well-being in populations of children.

Stunting Malnourished children grow poorly. The prevalence of decreased linear growth, referred to as **stunting,** is used as an indicator of the well-being of populations of children.[4] The prevalence of stunting in developing countries varies dramatically, but in some places it is as high as 62%.[5] Deficiencies of energy, protein, iron, and zinc, as well as prolonged infections, have been implicated as causes of stunting. Stunting in childhood produces smaller adults who have a reduced work capacity. Stunted women are more likely to give birth to low birth weight babies.

Infectious Disease Undernourished children have depressed immune systems, which reduces their ability to resist infection. Of the 50 million deaths that occur worldwide each year, 80% are in developing countries, and half of mortality is due to infectious diseases and parasites.[3] Infections decrease appetite and increase energy requirements and nutrient losses—which further contribute to undernutrition. Undernourished children may die of infectious diseases that would not be life-threatening in well-nourished children. Even immunization programs, designed to reduce the incidence of infectious disease, may be ineffective because the immune systems of undernourished individuals cannot respond normally. Mortality is increased even among children with mild to moderate malnutrition.[6]

Food Shortage: A Cause of Undernutrition

Food shortage Insufficient food to feed a population.

Famine A widespread lack of access to food due to a disaster that causes a collapse in the food production and marketing systems.

While much of the world currently has an abundant supply of food, there are areas where the total amount of food available is insufficient to feed the population. These **food shortages** cause widespread protein-energy malnutrition in local populations. Shortages of food occur for many reasons. The most obvious example of a food shortage is **famine,** which is a widespread failure in the food supply due to a collapse in the food production and marketing systems. Famines can be brought on by nature and by humans. Drought, floods, earthquakes, and crop destruction by diseases or pests cause nature-induced famines (Figure 17.3).

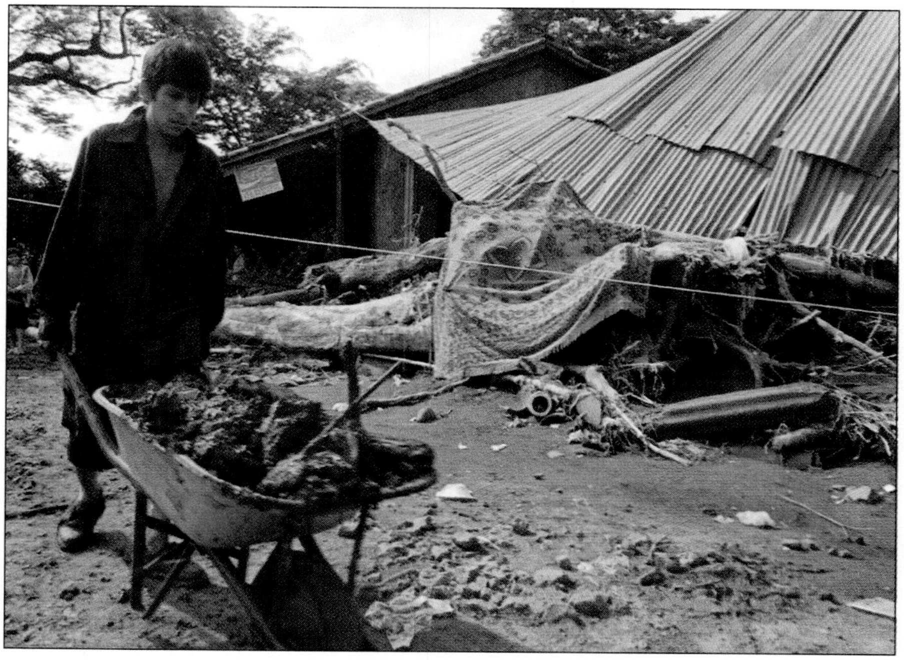

Figure 17.3
Natural disasters, such as hurricanes, destroy homes, farms, and infrastructure and can lead to famine. (© AP Photo/Luis Romero)

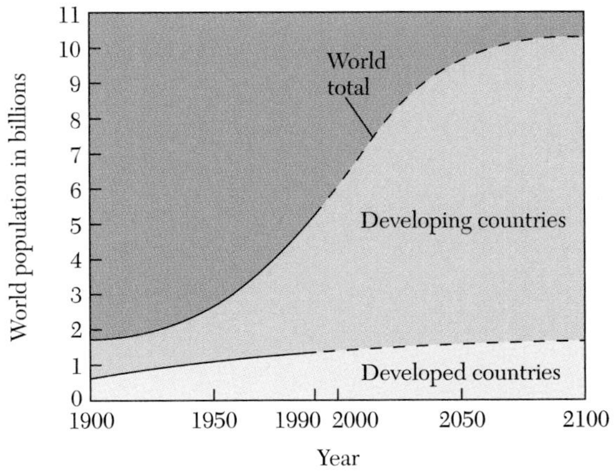

Figure 17.4
Since 1950, most of the increase in world population has occurred in developing countries, and this trend is expected to continue.

Wars and civil conflicts create man-made famines. Regions that produce barely enough food for survival under normal conditions are vulnerable to the disaster of famine. Populations living at this level do not have reserves of food, money, or livestock. This situation is analogous to a man standing in water up to his nostrils: If all is calm, he can breathe, but if there is a ripple, he will drown. When a ripple such as a natural or civil disaster occurs, it cuts the margin of survival and creates famine.

Food shortage due to famine is very visible because it causes many deaths in one area during a short period of time. More chronic food shortages occur when the food supply is insufficient to feed the population; when cultural practices limit food choices; when economic inequities result in lack of money, health care, and education for individuals or populations; and when environmental resources are misused, limiting the ability to continue to produce food. Any of these factors can result in food insecurity (the inability to obtain food for any reason) within a population.

Food Shortage: A Problem of Overpopulation Overpopulation exists when a region has more people than its natural resources can support. Some regions can support more people than others before food shortages occur. For example, a fertile river valley can produce more food per acre than can a desert environment. Even in fertile regions of the world, however, if the number of people increases too much, resources are overwhelmed and food shortages occur.

The human population is currently growing at a rate of more than 80 million persons per year, and most of this growth is occurring in developing countries (Figure 17.4). These countries cannot escape from poverty because their economy cannot keep pace with such fast population growth.[7] In addition, the growing populations reduce the amount of available agricultural land by using it for housing and industry. Efforts to produce enough food can damage the soil and deplete environmental resources, further reducing the capacity to produce food in the future. The problem of hunger today is due primarily to the unequal distribution of resources, but it is estimated that, worldwide, food production has begun to lag behind population growth.[8] If this trend continues there will soon be too little food in the world to feed the population (Figure 17.5).

Food Shortage: A Cultural Problem In some cultures, access to food may be limited for certain individuals within households. For example, women and girls may receive less food than men and boys because culturally they are viewed as less important. How much food is available to an individual within a household depends on gender, control of income, education, age, birth order, and genetic endowments.[9]

The cultural acceptability or unacceptability of foods also contributes to food shortages and malnutrition. If available foods are culturally unacceptable, a food

Figure 17.5
Worldwide food production has increased greatly since 1980, but because the world population has also grown, the amount of food available per person has changed little. (Data from FAO Production Yearbook, vol. 43, 1989.)

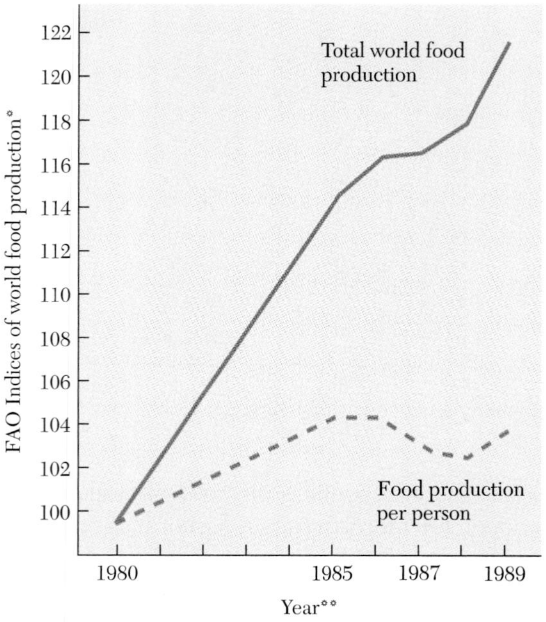

* Numbers show the relative level of food produced for each year in comparison with the base period 1979–81.

** Data not available for years 1981–1984.

shortage exists unless the population can be educated to use and accept the new food. For example, insects are eaten in some cultures and provide an excellent source of protein, but they are unacceptable to others. Another example is greens, which are often available locally but are underutilized because people have traditionally not eaten them and do not know how to prepare them.

Food Shortage: An Economic Problem About a quarter of the world's population lives in poverty, surviving on less than a dollar a day.[1] Poverty is at the root of the problem of undernutrition. The link between hunger and poverty is so strong that in most parts of the world their incidence is almost identical (Figure 17.6). Poverty can be viewed as the cause as well as the result of inadequate food production, distribution, and storage; of inappropriate utilization of resources; of unsanitary living conditions; and of lack of health care and education. Poverty and food insecurity occur in countries, in households, and among individuals when food and resources are not distributed equitably. And, food insecurity increases the risk of malnutrition.

Economic Policies On the national level, lack of money limits the ability to produce, transport, and distribute food. National economic priorities also contribute to food shortages in populations. Nations have traditionally grown **subsistence crops,** the crops they need to feed their people. However, colonialism and the development of modern trade practices has shifted the emphasis from producing food for local consumption to producing **cash crops,** which can be sold on the national and international market. This improves the cash flow of the country but uses local resources to produce crops for export and leaves the least fertile land to grow food for local consumption.

Subsistence crops Crops grown as food for the local population.

Cash crops Crops grown to be sold for monetary return rather than to be used for food locally.

Household and Individual Poverty At the household and individual level, poverty is an important cause of food insecurity and malnutrition. If money is scarce, food cannot be obtained and malnutrition increases. The poorest poor do not own land to grow food and do not have money to buy enough food or enough of the right

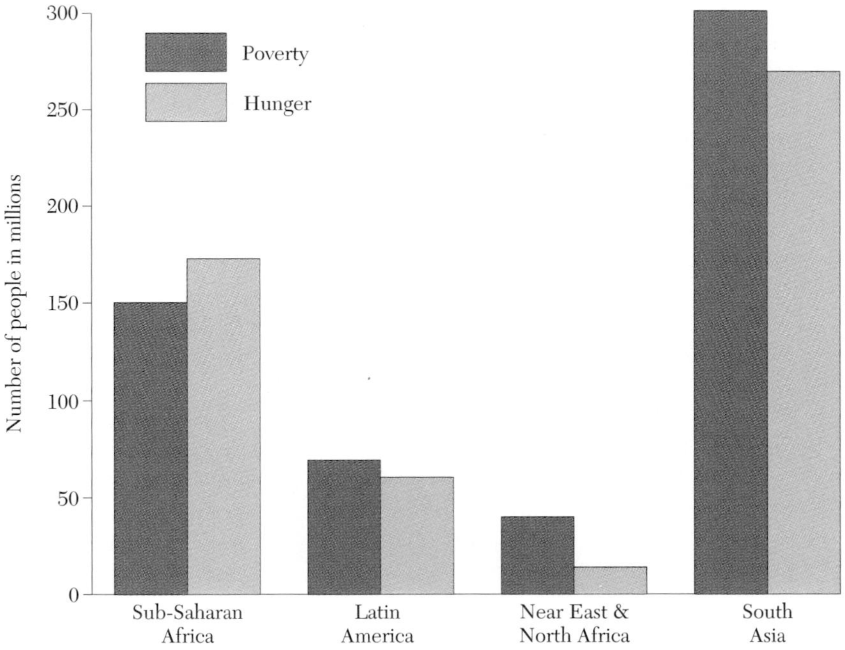

Figure 17.6
The incidences of hunger and poverty are almost identical in most parts of the world. (Adapted from Uvin, P. The state of world hunger. Nutr. Rev. 52:151–161, 1994.)

kinds of food to meet nutritional needs. They do not have access to transportation to get to markets and must walk long distances to buy food and collect firewood for cooking.

The poor also have less access to health care. Malnutrition increases the incidence of disease and disability, and, in turn, disease further increases malnutrition. Because health care is unavailable, diseases go untreated—which can increase nutrient needs and limit the ability to acquire food. Lack of health care also increases infant mortality and the incidence of low birth weight births. Lack of immunizations and treatment for infections and other illnesses results in an increased incidence and morbidity from infectious disease and a decrease in survival rates from chronic diseases such as cancer.

Lack of education and subsequent illiteracy go hand in hand with poverty, reducing opportunities to escape poverty and increasing the risk of undernutrition and disease.[10] Inadequate education leads to inadequate care for infants, children, and pregnant women. A lack of education about food preparation and storage can affect food safety and the health of the household—unsanitary food preparation increases the incidence of gastrointestinal diseases, which contribute to malnutrition (Figure 17.7).

Food Shortage: An Environmental Problem The land and resources available for food production are limited. Some resources, such as minerals and fossil fuels, are present in the earth in limited amounts and are nonrenewable—that is, once used they cannot be replaced in a reasonable amount of time. Technology will need to find substitutes for these resources. Other resources are **renewable** if they are not damaged and are used at a rate at which the earth can restore them. For example, if agricultural land is used wisely—crops rotated, erosion prevented, contamination limited—it can be reused almost endlessly. However, if this land is not used carefully, soil erosion, nutrient depletion, and accumulation of pollutants in soil and water may occur at a rate that exceeds the earth's ability to restore and repair these resources. As agricultural lands are depleted, forests are cut down to create more agricultural land. This contributes to soil erosion. Deforestation combined with air pollution contribute to global climate changes. Lack of water and pollution of existing water limit agricultural productivity, and overgrazing destroys rangelands. Whether animal products, agricultural crops, or fish or seafood are

Renewable resources Resources that are restored and replaced by natural processes and that can therefore be used forever.

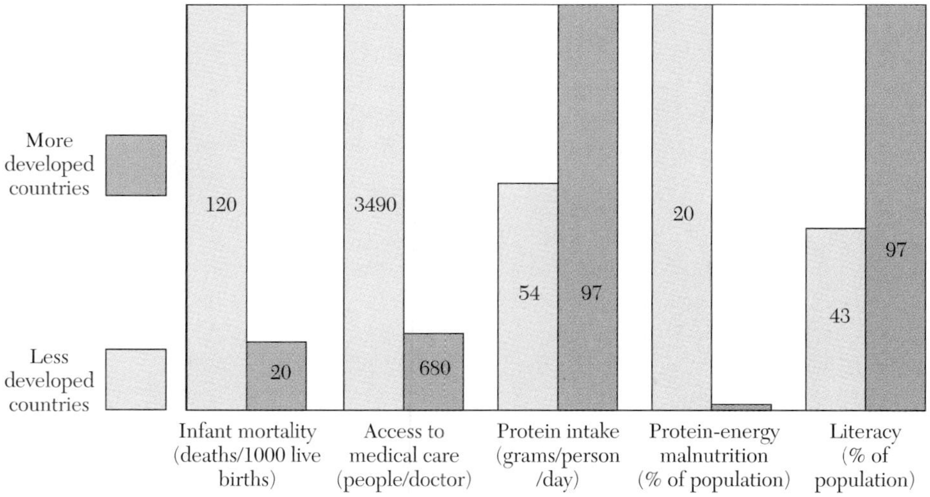

Figure 17.7
Populations in less developed countries have a higher infant mortality rate, less access to medical care, a lower protein intake, a greater incidence of protein-energy malnutrition, and a lower literacy rate. (Adapted from Olson, R. E. World food production and problems of human nutrition. Nutr. Today 24:15–21, 1989.)

being produced and distributed, the environmental cost could be high. To maintain adequate agricultural land and water resources, those available must be used in ways that will sustain them for continued use.

Environmental Cost of Meat Production Modern meat production is an example of the inefficient use of natural resources. Modern methods of raising cattle use grain, water, and fossil fuels, and create both air and water pollution. Cattle raised in the United States spend most of their lives eating grass from grazing lands; then, for about their last 100 days, the animals are kept in stockyards and fed grain to increase their body fat. A large proportion of the grain produced in the United States is used for this purpose. To produce this feed grain, fertilizers and pesticides are used, soil is eroded, and groundwater is contaminated. Much of the grain is grown on land that must be irrigated, so water supplies are depleted as well (about 87% of the fresh water in the world today is consumed by agriculture[11]). The animals themselves produce methane gas in their gastrointestinal tracts which enters the air and contributes to the greenhouse effect. And when animal sewage is stored in ponds and heaps, it decomposes anaerobically, producing more methane.

Environmental Cost of Agricultural Crops The environmental cost of producing plant-based foods is lower than that of animals products, but it may still be substantial. For example, growing a head of lettuce in California using pesticides and fertilizer and then trucking it in a refrigerated car to New York requires a great deal of energy. The price of our food may reflect some of these costs, but the cost of the damage to soil, groundwater, and farm workers caused by pesticides and fertilizers is not included. These and other social, medical, and ecological costs associated with modern agricultural practices are difficult to measure.

Overfishing and Water Pollution Throughout human history fish have been an important source of protein. However, increases in population have increased demand for fish to the point that the earth's oceans are being depleted. Because the ocean is open to fishermen from around the world, its use has been difficult to control. Many marine species have been harvested until their numbers are severely depleted. According to the United Nations Food and Agriculture Organization, 70% of the world's fish stocks are either fully exploited, overexploited, or depleted. Pollution also threatens the world's fishing grounds. Oil spills and deliberate dumping can occur offshore, and sewage, pesticides, organic pollutants, and sediments from erosion wash into coastal waters where most fish spend at least part of their lives. Heavy metals such as lead, cadmium, and mercury can enter the food chain and are toxic to fish and humans.

Diet Quality: A Cause of Undernutrition

Undernutrition can be caused by a poor-quality diet as well as by a shortage of food. The typical diet in developing countries is based on high-fiber grain products and has little variety. Adults who are able to consume a relatively large amount of this diet may be able to meet their nutrient needs. But those with increased needs or a limited capacity to consume these foods are at risk for nutrient deficiencies. Children, pregnant women, the elderly, and the ill may not be able to eat enough of this bulky grain diet to meet their needs. Deficiencies of protein, iron, iodine, and vitamin A are common because of poor-quality diets.

Protein-Energy Malnutrition Over 200 million children under the age of five suffer from deficiencies of protein and energy.[2] Protein and energy deficiencies usually occur together. However, in individuals with high protein needs—those who are growing, developing, or healing—protein deficiency can predominate (see Chapter 6). Kwashiorkor (a deficiency of protein but not energy) occurs as a result of the wrong combination of foods rather than of a general lack of food. It is common in children over 18 months of age when the main energy source is a bulky cereal grain low in high-quality protein. Children have small stomachs and are not able to consume enough of this diet to meet their protein needs (Figure 17.8). Other factors such as metabolic changes caused by infection may also play a role in the development of kwashiorkor.[12]

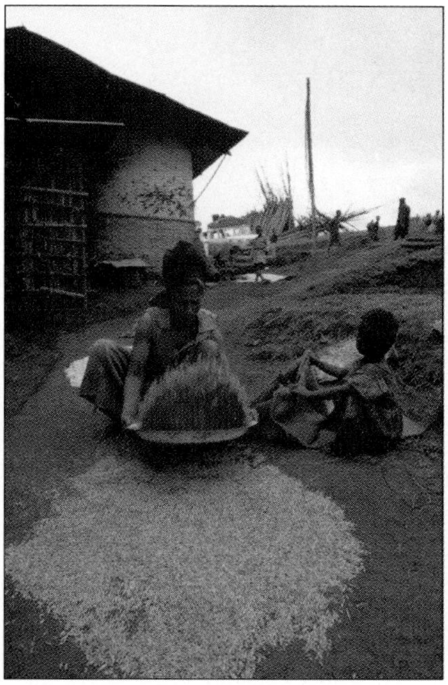

Figure 17.8
Because of their size, children are often unable to eat enough of a bulky grain diet to meet their nutrient needs. (Corbis/Jim Sugar Photography)

Micronutrient Deficiencies Micronutrient malnutrition affects about 2 billion people worldwide and impacts the mortality, morbidity, reproductive health, growth, and development of individuals and the economic productivity of societies.[13]

Iron Deficiency Iron deficiency anemia is the most common nutritional problem in both developed and developing nations, but the prevalence is almost fourfold higher in the developing world, where it affects 43% of all women and 34% of all men.[4] When the amount of iron available in the diet does not meet individual needs, it causes iron deficiency which can lead to anemia. It is estimated that worldwide over 2 billion people suffer from iron deficiency and more than half of them are anemic.[14] The prevalence of iron deficiency in poor countries is over 50% among infants, children under two years of age, and pregnant women.[15] The highest prevalence of iron deficiency anemia is in Southeast Asian countries, where almost 80% of pregnant woman are anemic.[4]

Iron deficiency can result from an increased need for iron, chronic loss of iron due to blood loss, or a diet with inadequate amounts of iron-containing foods or one that limits iron bioavailability. Nonheme iron from plant sources is the major dietary source of iron in many parts of the developing world where meat consumption is economically unfeasible. This dietary pattern increases the risk for iron deficiency because nonheme iron is poorly absorbed. Also, intestinal parasites, especially hookworm infections, cause gastrointestinal blood loss which leads to iron deficiency anemia.[4] The greater rates of both acute and chronic infections, such as malaria and schistosomiasis, in the developing world aggravate dietary iron deficiency.

Iron deficiency can have a major impact on the health and productivity of a population. Anemia during pregnancy increases the risk of maternal and fetal mortality, premature delivery, and low birth weight. Iron deficiency in infants and children can stunt growth and retard mental development, decrease resistance to infection, and increase morbidity due to disease.[16] In older children and adults it causes fatigue and decreased productivity (see Chapter 11).

Iodine Deficiency Diseases Iodine is a trace element that is an essential constituent of the thyroid hormones. It is estimated that 1.6 billion people live in areas considered to be at risk for iodine deficiency and that about 655 million, or 12% of the global population, have goiter.[4,17] Iodine deficiency occurs in regions with iodine-deficient soil that rely extensively on locally produced food. Areas of the world with the greatest percent of their population at risk of iodine deficiency disorders include the Eastern Mediterranean region and Africa. These disorders affect virtually all members of a community and worldwide are believed to be the greatest single cause of preventable brain damage and mental retardation.[18] Iodine deficiency during pregnancy increases the incidence of stillbirths, spontaneous abortions, and developmental abnormalities such as cretinism. Cretinism is characterized by irreversible mental and physical retardation. Iodine-deficient children have lower IQs and impaired school performance.[19] Iodine deficiency in children and adults causes goiter and is associated with apathy and decreased initiative and decision-making capabilities. Because soil iodine is low in regions where deficiency is common, the problem can be solved only by dietary diversification or interventions to add iodine to the diet.

Vitamin A Deficiency It is estimated that 250 million children worldwide suffer from vitamin A deficiency.[20,21] The incidence of clinical vitamin A deficiency in children is greatest in East and South Africa. Vitamin A deficiency causes blindness; depresses immune function, which increases the risk of infections; retards growth; and is often accompanied by anemia.

Vitamin A deficiency can be caused by a low intake of the vitamin in relation to need. Obtaining sufficient vitamin A is a particular problem during periods of rapid growth and development, such as infancy, early childhood, pregnancy, and lactation. Need is increased by frequent infections, such as those causing diarrhea, and illnesses such as measles.[4] Deficiencies of other nutrients, including fat, protein, and zinc, can contribute to vitamin A deficiency. Vitamin A cannot be absorbed without fat, so a diet very low in fat can cause a deficiency by preventing absorption. Protein and zinc are needed for the transport and metabolism of vitamin A, so deficiencies of either can make vitamin A unavailable to body tissues (see Chapter 9). Control of vitamin A deficiency is a major public health goal of the World Health Organization (WHO).

Food for All: Solutions to World Hunger

Solving the problem of world hunger is a daunting task. It involves controlling population growth, meeting the nutritional needs of a large and diverse population with culturally acceptable foods, increasing food production, and maintaining the global ecosystem. It requires international cooperation, commitment from national and local governments, and the involvement of local populations. The solutions involve economic policies, technical advancement, education, and legislative measures. They require input from politicians, nutrition scientists, economists, and the food industry.

Solutions: An International View In 1996, world leaders met at the World Food Summit in Rome to renew their commitment to the eradication of hunger and malnutrition around the world and achieve food security for all people.[22] The delegates at the summit adopted a Declaration on World Food Security and Plan of Action that encompasses commitments for national and international action. These include policies to prevent and meet transitory emergencies due to natural disasters and man-made emergencies, to eradicate poverty, to increase food production in a **sustainable** manner, to improve access to adequate food, and to develop trade policies that foster food security for all.[23] They defined food security as a condition in which "all people, at all times, have physical and economic access to sufficient, safe, and nutritious food to meet their dietary needs and food prefer-

Sustainable Refers to methods of using resources that prevent overuse of natural systems and allow the environment to be maintained indefinitely without a decline.

ences for an active and healthy life." This World Food Summit pledged to cut in half the number of hungry people in the world by the year 2015.

Government representatives at the World Food Summit focused on food security as a supply problem that could be solved by controlling population growth and increasing agricultural production. Nongovernmental organizations at the summit viewed food security as a demand problem that could be solved by more equitable food distribution, reduction in overconsumption in certain areas, and improving small sustainable agricultural food production by reducing the industrialization of farming. However the problem is viewed, programs and policies must first provide food and then establish sustainable programs to allow continuous production and distribution (see *Off the Shelf: Aquaculture: A Benefit in the Developed and the Developing World*).

Short-Term Solutions: Responding to Emergency Situations The first step toward solving the problem of undernutrition is to stop starvation. Although short-term food and medical aid do little to prevent future hunger, this type of relief is necessary for a population to survive an immediate crisis such as famine. The standard approach has been to bring food into the stricken area (Figure 17.9). These foods generally consist of agricultural surpluses from other countries and often are not well planned in terms of their nutrient content.[24] Famine relief efforts are frequently hindered by war, looting, and the lack of supporting infrastructure, such as roads, bridges, and airports, that is necessary to deliver food.

There are many international, national, and private organizations working toward the goal of relieving world hunger. The World Health Organization and the United Nations (UN) Food and Agriculture Organization (FAO) and World Food Bank provide food relief. The emphasis of the FAO is on the production, intake, and distribution of food. WHO targets community health centers and emphasizes the prevention of nutrition problems, such as micronutrient deficiencies. The World Bank finances projects such as supplementation and fortification to foster economic development. The United Nations Children's Fund (UNICEF), which relies on volunteer support, distributes food to all countries in need with a goal of assisting developing countries that occasionally suffer periods of starvation. The Red Cross, the UN Disaster Relief Organization, and the UN High Commissioner for Refugees concentrate on famine relief. The Peace Corps focuses more on fostering long-range development. More and more agencies are

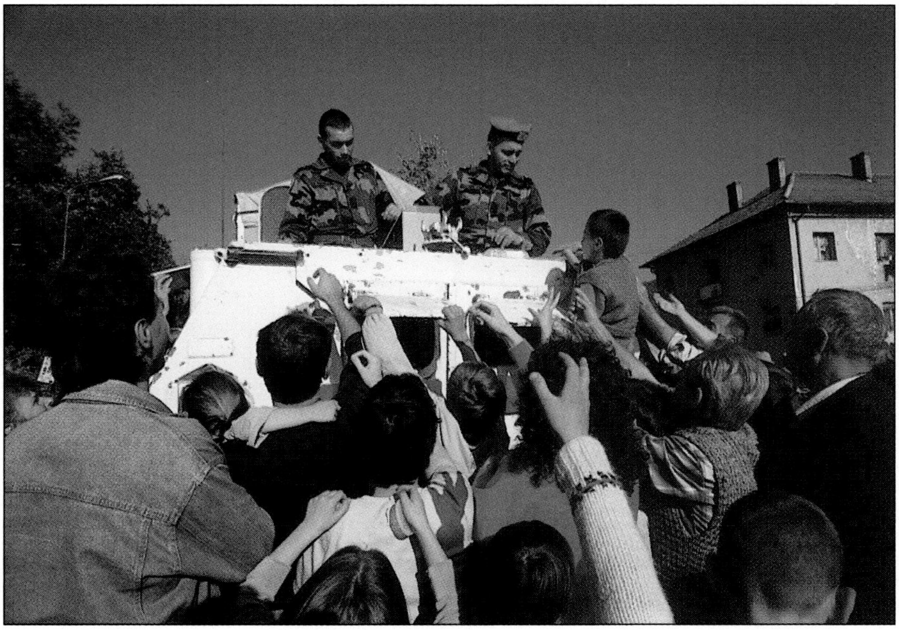

Figure 17.9
There are many international relief organizations that provide food to hungry people throughout the world. (© Wesley Bocxe/Photo Researchers, Inc.)

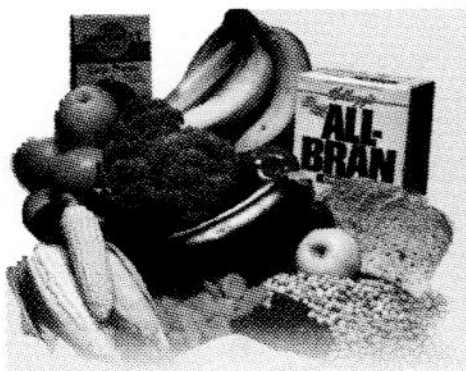

Off the Shelf

Aquaculture: A Benefit in the Developed and the Developing World

Feeding the world requires developing methods of producing food that minimize the use of resources. Keeping the world healthy means providing foods containing the right combination of nutrients to meet needs without increasing the risks of chronic disease. Aquaculture, the breeding of fish and other aquatic organisms, meets both of these needs.

Aquaculture, which is more like farming than fishing, is not a new technology. It was developed in China several thousand years ago, but its potential to produce large amounts of food has been recognized only recently. It produces much of the bass, rainbow trout, and catfish that are available on the commercial market and is a $5-billion-a-year business in the United States.[1] In developing countries it has the potential for providing both a high-protein addition to the local diet and an economically beneficial product for export. Fish may be raised in ponds or in floating cages in rivers, lakes, estuaries, or the open ocean. It is labor-intensive and so requires an inexpensive labor force, which is a resource available in developing nations.

Despite the advantages, setting up aquaculture is expensive, requires careful research to ensure that the fish can be adapted to domestication, and is not without food-safety risks and environmental costs. When raised in rivers, lakes, and oceans, farm-raised fish, like those in the wild, can be exposed to chemical pollution and human and animal wastes. In addition, the chemicals used to prevent health problems in the fish, including disinfectants to kill bacteria, herbicides to control plant growth in ponds, vaccines to prevent disease, and drugs to treat diseases and parasites, may remain in the flesh of the fish and move through the food chain. Despite these environmental risks, aquaculture can also be environmentally friendly. In some Asian countries, rural communities use fish ponds to recycle food waste. Marine algae grown using aquaculture can be used as a nonchemical treatment for wastewater. In wastewater treatment plants algae have been shown to reduce the amounts of bacteria, phosphorus, nitrogen, ammonia, and heavy metals in the water and increase its amino acid content.

Care must also be taken to ensure that marine animals produced by aquaculture are as healthful as those caught in the wild. Fish is a lowfat source of high-quality protein, and its consumption has been associated with a decreased incidence of heart disease.[2] Some of this effect is likely due to the omega-3 fatty acids in fish. When fish are domesticated, their diet is changed, causing changes in their fatty acid composition. The result may be fish that are not as healthful as those caught in the wild. Scientists monitor the fatty acid composition of fish produced by aquaculture to ensure that it remains a healthy food for humans.[3]

When managed efficiently, aquaculture has the potential to increase the productivity of existing resources by offering a product that will help decrease malnutrition in developing nations and that may reduce chronic disease in developed nations.

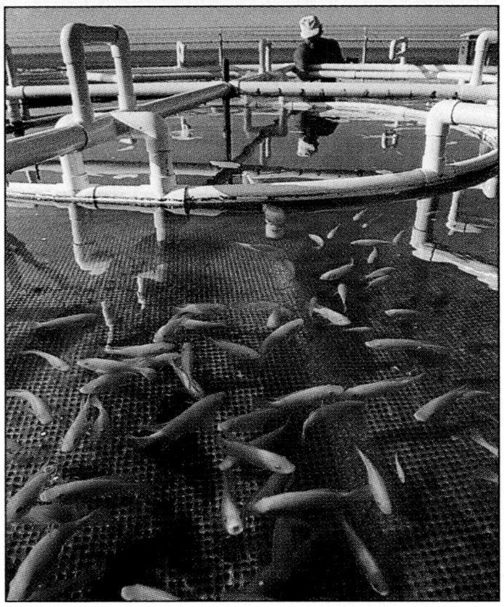

(Greg Vaughn/Tom Stack and Associates)

[1]Raven, P. H., Berg, L. R., and Johnson, G. B. *Environment*, 2nd ed. Philadelphia: Saunders College Publishing, 1998.

[2]Ascherio, A., Rimm, E. B., Stampfer, M. J., et al. Marine n-3 fatty acids, fish intake, and the risk of coronary disease among men. N. Engl. J. Med. 332:977–982, 1995.

[3]Craig, S. R., and Gatlin, D. M. Coconut oil and beef tallow, but not tricaprylin, can replace menhaden oil in the diet of red drum (*Sciaenops ocellatus*) without adversely affecting growth or fatty acid composition. J. Nutr. 125:3041–3048, 1995.

engaging in both development and relief. A few examples include the U.S. Agency for International Development, Oxfam, the Hunger Project, and Catholic Relief Services.

Long-Term Solutions: Increasing the Ratio of Food to People Short-term crises can be solved by international intervention, but long-term solutions need to be based on the cultural and economic needs of the local population. Local governments need to work to increase the ratio of food to people by controlling population growth and increasing food production.

Controlling Population The problem of world hunger can be solved only by bringing the population into line with the ability to produce food. One solution is to decrease the rate of population growth by controlling birthrates. Although the rate of population growth worldwide has slowed from more than 6 children per woman in 1950 to 3.3 in 1998, the world's population is still growing faster than the food supply.[7] More than 50% of developing countries currently have policies to reduce birthrates. To be successful, family-planning efforts must be acceptable to the population and compatible with their cultural and religious needs.

A number of approaches, such as provision of contraceptives, education, and economic incentives, have been used to decrease population growth. In Singapore, Thailand, Colombia, and Costa Rica, programs that provide contraceptive information, services, and supplies have been somewhat successful in slowing population growth. Population-control education is being integrated into the school curriculum, and in Mexico and Egypt popular television shows carry family-planning messages.

In addition to family-planning education, an increase in the general level of education has been shown to reduce population growth.[9] When the social and economic status of women is improved, birthrates decrease.[25] Women with more education tend to marry later and have fewer children. Education also increases the likelihood that women will have control over their fertility, provides knowledge to improve family health, decreases infant and child mortality rates, and offers options other than having numerous children. In Botswana, women with a secondary-level education have an average of 3.1 children. Those with only a primary-level education have 5.1 children, and women with no education have an average of 5.9 children.[25]

Changes in economic policies can also help reduce population growth. In many areas, children provide economic security.[25] They are needed to work the farms, support the elders, and otherwise contribute to the economic survival of the family. Thus people are resistant to family-planning messages because of high infant mortality rates—they choose to have many children to ensure that some will survive. They feel safe having fewer children only when they are financially secure and able to acquire the necessities of life. Programs that foster economic development and ensure access to food, shelter, and medical care have been shown to cause a decline in birthrates. For example, a reduction in birthrates occurred along with economic success in South Korea. Another approach is to offer incentives for families with fewer children. In China, stringent family-planning programs offer economic advantages to urban families with only one child and to rural families with no more than two, if the first is a girl.

Economic Solutions: Better Access to Food In order to provide long-term food security, populations must develop manageable systems for producing acceptable, sustainable sources of food. **Food self-sufficiency,** the country's capacity to feed its population, can help to prevent food shortages. To assure that the food produced can be acquired by all, economic solutions must also strive to eliminate poverty.

Food self-sufficiency The ability of an area to produce enough food to feed its population.

Trade Policies to Foster Food Self-Sufficiency. Trade policies often determine what crops will be grown on a nation's arable land. A decision to grow a cash crop instead of food for local consumption may mean that less food is available for the local diet. If, however, the cash from the crop is used to purchase nutritious foods from other countries, this decision may help alleviate undernutrition. Countries that have few natural resources must rely on international trade to distribute world resources more equitably. Trade can provide an economic advantage if food is imported and other products on which a good monetary return is obtained are exported. The newly industrialized countries of Asia such as Japan and Korea are examples of how an increase in food imports can decrease the number of hungry people (Figure 17.10). In general, the countries of the world are becoming

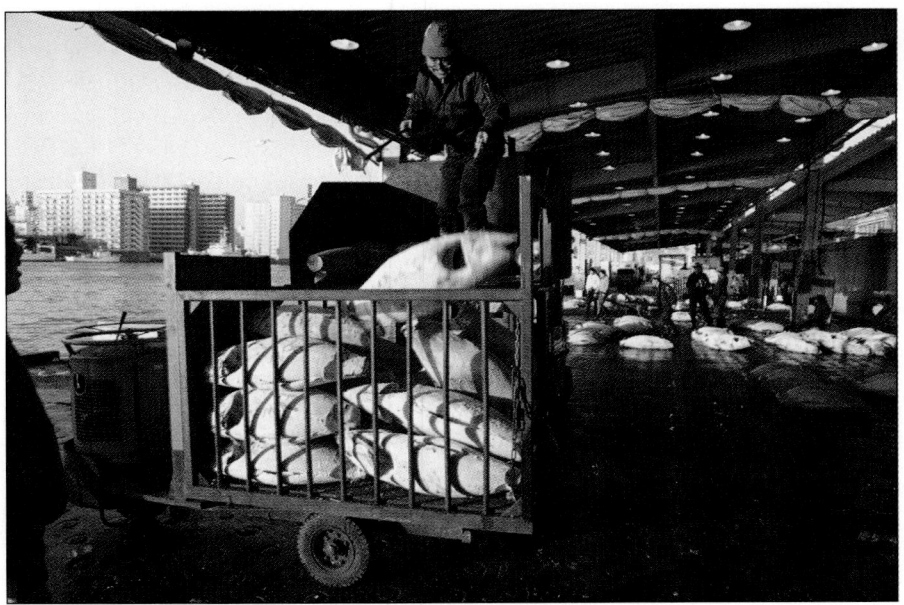

Figure 17.10
Many countries rely on imports to meet their local food needs. (© 1999 Photo Disc, Inc.)

more interdependent on food imports and on exports to pay for this food.[26] If this interdependence increases the availability of food for the world population, it is beneficial; but policies and practices in each nation must be developed to ensure that the population can be fed (see *Off the Label: Food Labels: An International Perspective*).

Alleviating Poverty. Although controlling population growth and ensuring adequate food production or importation are essential steps in eliminating world hunger, hunger will still exist as long as there is poverty. Even when food is plentiful in a region, the poor do not have access to enough of the right foods to maintain their nutritional health. Economic development that guarantees safe and sanitary housing, access to health care and education, and the resources to acquire enough food are essential to eliminate hunger. Poor, hungry people have little influence on government policies, but these policies can result in higher incomes, lower food prices, or feeding programs for the poor, all of which can improve food security.

Education: Increasing Food Availability and Safety Educational programs as well as technology may be necessary to make food available and safe. Providing food or technology does little if individuals do not know how to use it. For example, a new crop variety is not beneficial unless local farmers know how to grow it and the population accepts it as a food source and knows how to prepare it for consumption. For instance, white yams are used by some cultures but are a poor source of provitamin A. If the yellow yam, which is is rich in provitamin A, became an acceptable choice, the provitamin A content of the diet would increase. Food safety is also a concern when changing traditional dietary practices. For example, introducing papaya to the diet as a source of vitamin A will not improve nutritional status if it is washed in unsanitary water and causes dysentery among the people it is meant to nourish.

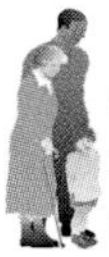

Education to encourage breast feeding can also improve nutritional status and health. Breast feeding reduces the risk of infectious diseases in infants. When infants are not breast fed, education about nutritious breast milk substitutes and safe preparation of formulas is essential. However, this information is often lacking among the poor.

Solutions for the Life of the Planet: Environmental Awareness Solutions to the problem of providing enough food must assure that natural resources are con-

Off the Label

Food Labels: An International Perspective

Importing foods from other countries can enhance the nutrient content and diversity of a nation's food supply. Foods imported to the United States must meet U.S. standards, including those for food labeling. Likewise, foods we export to other countries must meet the labeling guidelines from those nations. Over the last decade, an increase in the international trade of both raw agricultural commodities and processed foods has made food labeling an international issue.[1]

Food labels appear to be simply a source of nutrition information. So why are they an issue? The information on the label is actually of interest at the national, political, cultural, economic, and consumer levels.[2] Governments want labeling information to be compatible with their national nutrition and food-safety guidelines, such as regulations for food additives, standards for composition of common products, and limits or thresholds of ingredients. Businesses want labels to emphasize features that give the product a competitive advantage. Consumers want labels to tell them how foods fit into their diets. Achieving all of these goals among countries is a difficult task. Despite the high priority of setting international standards for trade, a standard food label is unlikely to be agreed upon.

Without standardized food labels, food for export must be specially labeled. This is expensive even when the labeling guidelines are not too different between countries. For example, if a Canadian food manufacturer wants to export cookies to the United States, it must relabel its product to meet all of the specifications of the U.S. Nutrition Labeling and Education Act. The amount of each nutrient must be adjusted to U.S. serving sizes, and the percent Daily Values must be added. For countries with no labeling guidelines, even getting the information about product composition may be costly.

Currently there are some minimum standards for international labeling of prepackaged foods. They are determined by the Codex Alimentarius Commission (Latin for "code concerned with nourishment") and state simply that "prepackaged foods should not be described or presented on any label or in any labeling material in a manner that is false, misleading, or deceptive or is likely to create an erroneous impression regarding its character in any respect." Guidelines also state that when a nutrition claim or representation is made on the label, the declaration of a standardized list of nutrients becomes mandatory. Canadian and European nutrition labeling systems are similar to Codex guidelines. Labeling regulations in the United States are not contradictory to these but are much more stringent.

Harmonization of food labels and requirements for composition, formulations, and allowable additives would permit manufacturers to produce and label foods for sale in any country. Without some standardization of labeling, the burden of specially labeling foods for export will limit what foods are sold in the United States and therefore limit consumer choices, corporate choices, and government choices.

[1]Potter, N. N., and Hotchkiss, J. H. *Food Science*, 5th ed. New York: Chapman & Hall, 1995.

[2]Food labeling: a Canadian and international perspective. Nutr. Rev. 53:103–105, 1995.

served to allow continued food production for future generations. This requires maintaining the earth's renewable resources while developing technologies to increase production. It may also require changes in consumption and production patterns. Promoting sustainable use of land and resources requires the support of consumers and government policy makers.

Maintaining Renewable Resources Renewable resources such as fertile agricultural land; grazing land; fish in lakes, rivers, and oceans; fresh water; and clean air can be used forever if they are not exploited. For instance, rotating the crops grown in a field prevents the depletion of specific nutrients in the soil, whereas growing the same crop year after year depletes the soil and increases the need for added fertilizers. Producing these fertilizers uses resources, and applying fertilizers increases water pollution. Pollution of the water reduces the amount available to irrigate the crops and nourish the population. Restoring water once it has become polluted takes long periods of time or expensive resources.

Sustainable Food Production Maintaining the world food supply for the long term requires development of policies that promote sustainable agriculture. Sustainable methods produce food while allowing the environment to restore itself so food can be produced indefinitely. This type of agriculture relies on ecological

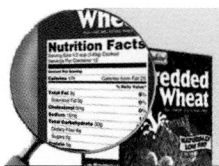

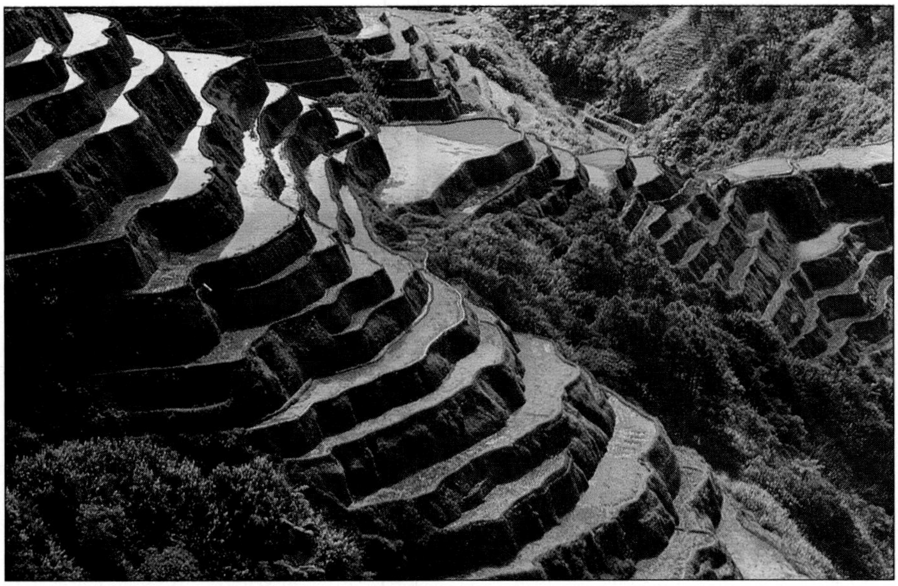

Figure 17.11
Terracing and contour-plowing help sustain the environment by preventing soil erosion. (David Cavagnaro)

principles, normal biological processes, and the use of chemicals that do not damage the environment.

Techniques of sustainable food production rely more on natural predator-prey relationships and disease-resistant crops than man-made pesticides. Chemical fertilizers are avoided or minimized by using integrated pest-management and fertilizing with animal manure. Crop rotation, plowing techniques, and terracing maintain soil fertility and prevent soil erosion (Figure 17.11). Other techniques include agroforestry, in which techniques from forestry and agriculture are used together to restore degraded areas; natural systems agriculture, which attempts to develop agricultural systems that include many types of plants and therefore function like natural ecosystems; and the technique of reducing fertilizer use by matching nutrient resources with the demands of the plant.[25,27] Policies are beginning to reflect environmental issues. For example, concern about pesticides in the environment has led government intervention in the pesticide market to focus on the development of natural means of pest control.[28]

Water and energy are conserved by relying more on labor-intensive agricultural methods which produce less food in the short term but will protect water and land resources in the long term. These methods are often more appropriate in developing nations than are high-technology methods, because these areas typically have large populations but little access to modern machinery such as tractors and pumps.

Technology to Improve Food Production New technologies are needed to increase food production without damaging the environment. Technological advances such as high-yielding crop varieties, irrigation, and mechanization have dramatically increased our ability to produce food. For example, corn yields in eastern Colorado have increased by 400 to 500% since 1940.[27] Technological development must interface with cultural needs and economic structures. For instance, tractors increase food production in the United States, but providing tractors to developing nations does no good if there is no gas to power them or mechanics or parts to repair them. In addition, technology needs to be evaluated for its impact on the environment in order to maintain high levels of production without further compromising natural resources.

Genetic engineering is one technology that is being implemented to increase food production while minimizing environmental damage. Genetic engineering is in reality just a more sophisticated approach to the traditional plant and animal breeding techniques that have been used for centuries. Using the traditional method, the best stocks are bred so that their traits will be passed on to the next generation. Productive crops are crossed with disease-resistant ones to produce hybrids containing the traits of both parents. Genetic engineering has the advantage of being faster, more precise, and more powerful. Traditional breeding may take 12 or more years to create a new strain, whereas genetic engineering can produce one in only about five years.[29] It is being used to produce plants and animals with new or more desirable traits. This technology can help meet the world's nutrient needs by creating safer pesticides, disease-resistant crops, foods with greater nutrient density, and products to increase the intake of deficient nutrients. To accomplish this, governments, industry, and academia need to cooperate and focus research efforts on the development of environmentally friendly technologies.[13]

Changing Production and Consumption Patterns The resources needed to support food production depend on the methods used. In developing countries, the resources used by a single person are small, but the numbers of people are so great that in many cases sufficient food cannot be produced without depleting and damaging soil, forests, and water supplies. In developed nations, the population is less dense but the resource demands made by each individual are far greater because of lifestyle and the production methods used. A single child born in a developed country like the United States causes a greater impact on the environment and resources than do dozens or more children born in developing nations.[25] For example, the resources used to feed a child in the United States include those needed to produce, package, ship, and prepare the variety of foods available in American grocery stores. A typical person in the United States draws 10 to 1000 times more resources daily than the average Chilean, Ghanaian, or Yemenite.[11] In both developed and developing nations natural resources are being depleted (see *Critical Thinking: What Can You Do?*).

Some consumers may believe that we should all become vegetarians to save the environment. This is not the answer because, in addition to their nutritional contribution to the diet, animals help to fully use available resources. Livestock can graze on land that is not suitable for crops, and they can eat plant materials such as cornstalks and corncobs that would otherwise go to waste (see Chapter 6, *Off the Shelf: Are Vegetarian Diets Better for Our Environment?*). A more effective option for consumers might be to reduce consumption of animal products and increase consumption of foods produced in ways that are less energy intensive and ecologically damaging.

Providing the Right Combination of Nutrients In addition to sufficient energy, the right mix of nutrients is necessary to ensure the nutritional health of the population. If the foods and crops that are grown or imported do not meet all nutrient needs, the quality of the diet will be poor and malnutrition will occur. If the right mix of foods is not available, either dietary patterns must be changed or nutrients must be added to the diet by fortifying foods or including dietary supplements. Strategies to reduce micronutrient deficiencies also include parasitic disease control. Consumers must also learn how to choose foods that provide the needed nutrients and how to handle them safely.

Nutrification **Nutrification** is the process of adding one or more nutrients to commonly consumed foods with the goal of adding to the nutrient intake of a population. Nutrification will not provide energy to a hungry population, but it can increase the protein quality of the diet and eliminate micronutrient deficiencies. Nutrification programs have been created by a combination of partnerships among industry, academia, and governments.[13] Industry and academia must provide the technology for adding the nutrient and governments must promote the consumption of the nutrified foods so that consumers will use them.

Nutrification The process of adding one or more nutrients to commonly consumed foods with the goal of adding to the nutrient intake of a group of people.

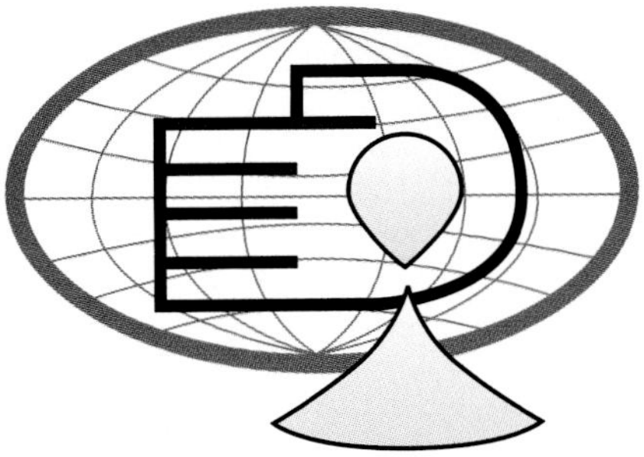

Figure 17.12
This global iodized salt logo can be recognized around the world as an indicator of iodized salt.

In order for nutrification to solve a nutritional problem in a population, it must be implemented wisely. Nutrification works if vulnerable groups consume centrally processed foods. The foods selected for nutrification should be among those consistently consumed by the majority of the population so that extensive promotion and re-education are not needed to encourage their consumption. The nutrient should be added uniformly and in a form that optimizes its utilization. Nutrification has been used successfully in preventing health problems in the United States: The fortification of cow's milk to increase vitamin D intake was a major factor in the elimination of infantile rickets (see Chapter 9), and the enrichment of grains with niacin helped eliminate pellagra. The most recent addition is the fortification of grains with folate to reduce neural tube defects in newborns (see Chapters 8 and 13). Nutrification has also been used successfully in developing countries. The addition of iodine to salt reduced iodine deficiency from 84% to almost zero in school children in Thailand (Figure 17.12). And fortification of sugar with iron has been found to improve iron status in Guatemalan communities.[30] In the Philippines, the fortification of margarine with vitamin A has improved the population's vitamin A status,[31] and the effectiveness of vitamin A–fortified sugar is being evaluated in Bolivia.[32] In Guatemala, where subclinical vitamin A deficiency is prominent, fortification of sugar has moved the country toward adequate vitamin A status.[4] Iron fortification of flour is being pursued in Latin America, the Caribbean, Central and South America, the Middle East, North Africa, and Central Asia. Iron fortification in Venezuela was shown to be effective at reducing the prevalence of anemia in school-age children.[33]

Supplementation Supplementation can also be used to reduce the prevalence of micronutrient malnutrition. Of countries where vitamin A deficiency is a public health problem, 78% have policies supporting regular vitamin A supplementation in children. Many have also adopted the World Health Organization recommendation to provide all breast-feeding women with a high-dose supplement of vitamin A within eight weeks of delivery. This improves maternal vitamin A status and raises the amount of vitamin A that is in breast milk and therefore passed to the infant.[34] Supplementation, along with regular deworming programs, is also used to reduce iron deficiency anemia. Many countries have adopted programs to supplement children older than six months with iron and pregnant women with iron and folate.

Education In order for any of these programs to work, consumers must use the foods that have been fortified or change their diets to include natural sources of nutrients that are deficient. Education to modify dietary patterns may promote the use of produce from home gardens. This education must include information about which foods are good nutrient sources so choices made when purchasing foods or growing vegetables at home can meet micronutrient needs.

CRITICAL THINKING

What Can You Do?

Keesha is concerned about the problems of hunger, malnutrition, and global ecology. Although she is a college student who cannot afford to make monetary contributions to relief organizations, she would like to contribute in other ways. She enjoys working with children, so she arranges to spend one afternoon a week helping with nutrition education programs for children. She also volunteers to spend one evening a week helping to prepare and serve food in a church soup kitchen near campus.

To be more ecological, Keesha buys a canvas bag to take to the grocery store. This will reduce the amount of waste she generates by eliminating the need for a new paper or plastic bag each time she shops. She asks her grocer to wrap the meat and chicken she buys in recyclable paper, and she begins recycling cans, bottles, and paper goods and tries to avoid purchasing products in nonrecyclable containers. This will reduce the amount of nonrecyclable, nonbiodegradable waste she generates.

What impact will the following changes Keesha makes have on the environment?

Action	Impact
Instead of driving her car the 2 miles from home to campus, she rides her bike, takes the bus, or carpools with a friend	This reduces the use of fossil fuels and reduces air pollution.
She contacts her local utility company to come and do an energy audit of her home and make energy-saving suggestions.	This will reduce energy usage in her home.
Instead of buying nonrecyclable juice boxes for her lunch, she brings juice in a thermos.	Answer:
She decides to begin composting the leftover vegetable scraps and other plant matter from her kitchen.	Answer:
When she can afford it, she chooses organically grown produce.	Answer:
She selects locally grown foods when possible.	Answer:

Suggest some other changes Keesha could make to decrease her impact on the environment.

Answer:

Food Insecurity at Home

In the United States, most of the nutritional problems are related to overnutrition. It is estimated that approximately half of adults in the United States are overweight.[35,36] Heart disease, hypertension, and cancer—all related to obesity—are the leading causes of death. While much of the population is concerned with consuming a diet to lower the risks for these chronic diseases, hungry families are standing in line at soup kitchens. Problems such as poverty and unemployment lead to food insecurity in a land of plenty (Figure 17.13). Government food and nutrition policy must be concerned with improving economic security as well as

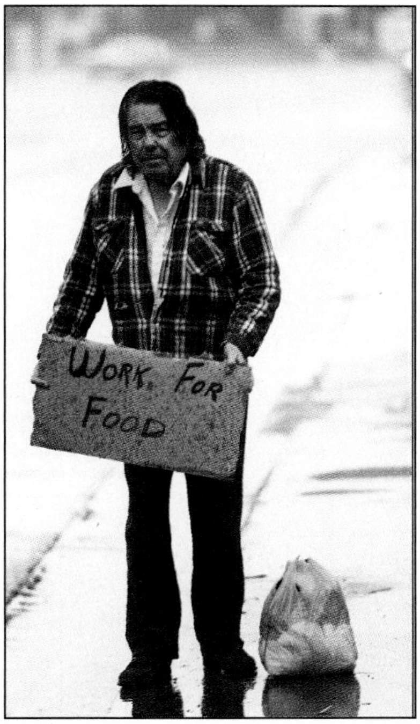

Figure 17.13
Hunger due to poverty, unemployment, and homelessness is an important problem in the United States today. (Ron Chapple/ FPG International Corporation)

providing food to the hungry and maintaining the food supply at an affordable level—at the same time policy must promote healthy diets to reduce diseases related to overconsumption.

Causes of Food Insecurity at Home

In the United States, general food shortage is not the cause of undernutrition, but food insecurity and hunger still occur. It is estimated that 10 million Americans, including 4 million children, do not get enough to eat.[37] Poverty is a major contributor, but disabilities and poor health also cause food insecurity by making it more difficult to acquire and prepare foods. Access to food is also compromised by lack of accessible grocery stores, lack of education about selecting an economical nutritious diet, and lack of access to health care. Within the population are subgroups, such as children, pregnant women, and the elderly, who are at particularly high risk for malnutrition due to food insecurity.

Economic Insecurity and Limited Access to Food Food security depends on economic security. About 13.8% of Americans live at or below the poverty level, and 20.8% of children live in households below the poverty level.[38] The poor have less money to spend on food and often have less access to affordable food. Lower profits have driven supermarkets out of the cities and into the suburbs. Because many low-income families do not own cars, they must shop at small, expensive corner stores or pay cab fares to take advantage of less expensive bulk items that are difficult to transport.

Lack of education, which is more common among the poor, also contributes to food insecurity. In the short term, lack of knowledge about how to stretch limited food budgets and select healthy diets contributes to malnutrition. Too little food may cause the diet to be deficient in energy or particular nutrients, but poor food choices also allow food insecurity to coexist with obesity. Lack of education about food safety can also increase the incidence of food-borne illness. In the long term, lack of education prevents people from getting well-paying jobs which allow them to escape from poverty.

Poverty is linked not only to undernutrition but also to diet-related chronic disease. For example, iron deficiency is more than twice as frequent in low-income children, and the incidence of heart disease, cancer, hypertension, and obesity increases with decreasing income.[38] As in developing nations, poverty is reflected in infant mortality rates. Average infant mortality in the United States population is about 7.6 per 1000 live births.[39] However, there are groups within the population that have infant mortality rates as high as those in impoverished nations. Among African Americans, the infant mortality rate is 14.2 per 1000 live births—almost twice that of the general population.[39] This difference mirrors the the higher poverty rate in this group.

Although poverty is associated with poor nutritional and health status, it cannot be assumed that everyone living in poverty is food insecure, or that those above the poverty line have plenty to eat. Illness, disability, a sudden decrease in income, or high living expenses can put anyone at risk for food insecurity. A recent Census survey showed that 7.8% of all U.S. households are food insecure. The highest prevalence is in inner city areas and the lowest is in the suburbs. Food insecurity occurs less often among white households than Hispanic and African American households. Households with children have the greatest frequency of hunger and food insecurity.

Vulnerable Populations Certain subgroups within the U.S. population are at increased risk of hunger and undernutrition. These include the homeless; women, infants, and children; the elderly; Native Americans and Alaska Natives; and migrant and seasonal workers. According to a 1997 survey by the hunger-relief organization Second Harvest, 62% of people who rely on emergency food assistance are women, 38% are children under age 18, and 16% are over 65.[40] Considering that children make up only 27% of the U.S. population and the elderly 13%, a disproportionate number of children and elderly are seeking food assistance.

The Homeless The poor must use most of their income to pay for shelter. It is estimated that people who live in poverty spend about 80% of their income on housing, which seriously reduces the chances that their families will be adequately fed.[41] The high cost of housing not only limits food budgets but also has created a growing problem of homelessness in the United States. It is estimated that over half a million Americans are homeless, and one of the major health problems of the homeless population is malnutrition.[42] The homeless are at high risk of food insecurity because they lack not only money but also cooking and food storage facilities. Without cooking facilities, they must rely on ready-to-eat foods. Without storage facilities, they cannot use less expensive staples such as rice and dried beans, which can be purchased in bulk.[43] Homeless individuals often rely on soup kitchens and shelters to obtain adequate food (Figure 17.14). A study of homeless preschool children found that several times each month the children did not have enough food to eat and that they rarely consumed the recommended amounts of grains, fruits, vegetables, or dairy products.[44]

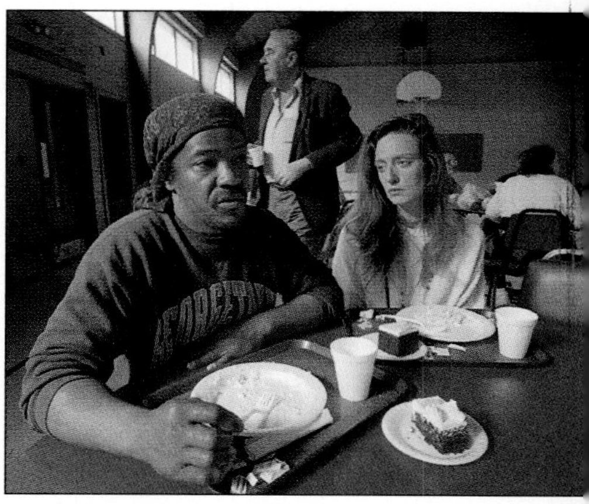

Figure 17.14
Soup kitchens and shelters provide meals to the homeless and others in need. (Paula A. Scully/AP Photo)

Women and Children Poverty has become a women's issue. More than 35% of households headed by women are below the poverty level. Significantly greater numbers of minority women live in poverty than ever before. Statistics show that 66% of African American women and 61% of Hispanic women live in poverty compared with 22% of white non-Hispanic women.[45] Nearly 40% of the American poor are children, especially Hispanic and African American children. Poverty places these women and children at risk of malnutrition, and their special nutritional needs magnify this risk. Because of their increased need for some nutrients, malnutrition may occur in pregnant women, infants, and children even when the rest of the household is adequately fed. For example, the amount of iron in the family diet may be enough to prevent anemia in all but a pregnant teenager.

Impact of Aging Due to diseases and disabilities, the elderly may be limited in their ability to purchase, prepare, and physically ingest food. This puts the elderly, especially the elderly poor, at risk for malnutrition. A recent survey found that 8 to 14% of older adults experience food insecurity at some point in a six-month period.[42] Greater nutritional risk among older adults is associated with more hospital admissions and hence greater health-care costs. The number of individuals over age 85 is expected to quadruple by the year 2050; as the number of elderly increases so will the number at risk of food insecurity. Thus providing food security for older adults both improves their quality of life and reduces health-care costs for the public health system (see Chapter 15).[42]

Native Americans and Alaska Natives Many Native Americans and Alaska Natives live in remote locations, which reduces access to food (Figure 17.15). The unemployment and poverty rates are high among these groups. Unemployment for the United States as a whole was 5.6% in 1995 but was 35% among Native Americans living on or adjacent to reservations; only 29% of those employed earned more than $9048 a year.[38]

Migrant and Seasonal Farm Workers Migrant workers have limited access to food because labor camps are in remote locations and transportation is limited. Low incomes and difficult working and living conditions limit their ability to purchase food and prepare adequate meals.

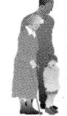

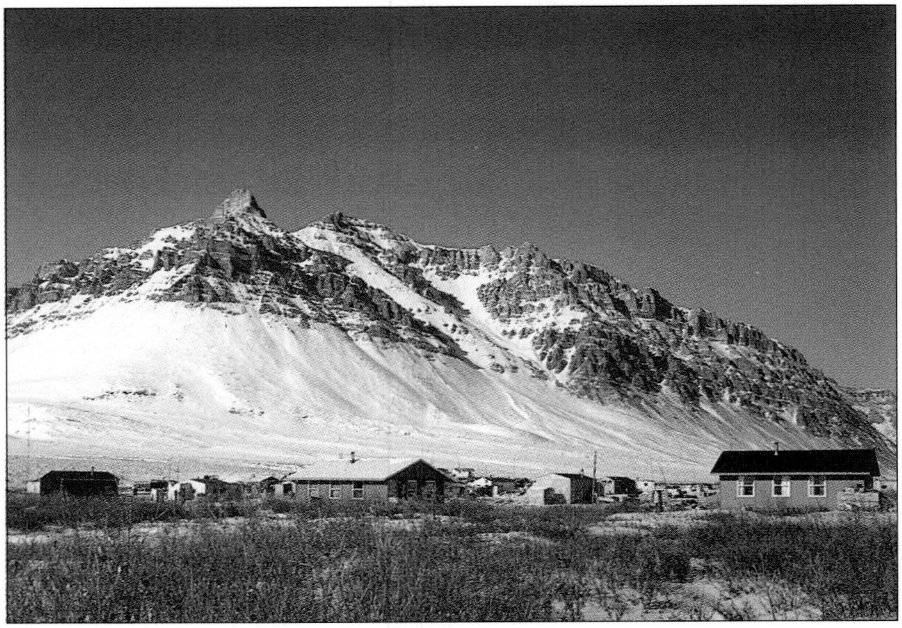

Figure 17.15
Living in remote locations limits access to food. (© McCutcheon/Visuals Unlimited)

Solutions to Food Insecurity at Home

Solving the problem of undernutrition in the United States requires alleviating poverty and providing access to an adequate nutritious food supply at a reasonable cost. Historically, many approaches have been attempted to meet this goal. Some have met with success and others have done little to increase access to a nutritious diet for all. Programs which provide access to affordable food and promote healthy eating have been referred to as a nutrition safety net for the American population.

A Historical Perspective Government response to hunger first occurred in the United States during the Great Depression with the distribution of farm surpluses by the Federal Supplies Relief Corporation.[46] Awareness of undernutrition in the United States was again aroused during World War II, when it was determined that 70% of the men rejected from the military draft had poor nutritional histories. At this time, the School Lunch Program (see Chapter 14) was initiated to improve the nutritional status of American youth and create the potential for a strong military.[42]

Between 1952 and 1960 the government showed little interest in the problems of hunger and malnutrition—an attitude that may have stemmed from the assumption that every citizen was well-fed in a land overflowing with food. In the 1960s, the Food Stamp Program and the Commodity Program were developed in response to the hunger witnessed by John F. Kennedy on his travels through the United States during his presidential campaign. At the same time, Martin Luther King Jr.'s Southern Christian Leadership Conference cited areas of hunger in cotton-growing states, where replacement of cotton by corn and soybeans had put many field hands out of work. Reports of hunger also began to appear from other parts of the country, such as Appalachia, northern Maine, Indian reservations in the Southwest, ghettos in large cities, and Native sections of Alaska. In 1967, teams of nutritionists and physicians were sent around the country to assess the problem of hunger. The resulting report indicated widespread malnutrition in every ethnic group in every part of the country, urban and rural. The report was brought to Congress and broadcast on prime-time television in the CBS documentary "Hunger in America." It was a rude awakening for the American public, and the awareness prompted interested organizations to coalesce into the National Council on Hunger and Malnutrition in the United States. The U.S. Senate formed the Senate Select Committee on Nutrition and Human Needs, and a White House Conference on Food, Nutrition, and Health was convened in 1969 to develop workable, implementable recommendations. There were 1800 such recommendations relating to poverty programs, diet, health, and consumer concerns. The Commodity Program was expanded, the Food Stamp Program was made permanent, the Special Supplemental Food Program for Women, Infants, and Children (WIC) was developed, child nutrition programs were expanded, and nutrition programs for the elderly were created[42] (Figure 17.16).

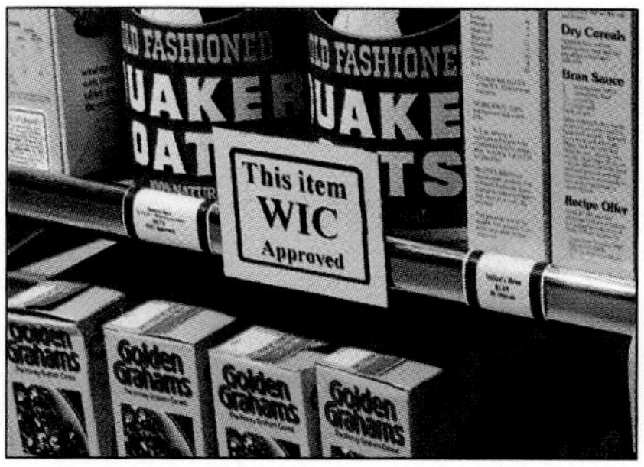

Figure 17.16
WIC supplies vouchers for foods that provide nutrients needed for healthy pregnancy and childhood. (© Tony Freeman/PhotoEdit)

In 1977, a follow-up survey to assess hunger in America found that although poverty had not changed, the number of hungry people had decreased. There had been a major improvement in the diets of poor people from 1965–66 to 1977. This change was attributed solely to federal food assistance programs. The reduction in hunger was a major social advance, but as times change, so do political agendas. Many of the attempted solutions of the 1960s and 1970s fell by the wayside in the 1980s and 1990s. However, a key group of programs still provide access to food and nutrition education to the poor and other at-risk groups. In addition, nutrition guidelines, such as the Dietary Guidelines and the Food Guide Pyramid, have been developed to promote the consumption of not only an adequate diet but one that will reduce the risks of chronic disease.

As we move into the 21st century, the structure of the nutrition safety net is being influenced by measures designed to reduce the number of welfare recipients in the United States. The federal Personal Responsibility and Work Opportunity Reconciliation Act of 1996 will not affect WIC or the School Breakfast and Lunch Program, but other components of the nutrition safety net will be changed drastically. For instance, the maximum food-stamp benefits that a family can receive will be reduced, and the length of time able-bodied adults can receive food stamps will be limited to 3 months out of every 36 unless the adult is working or engaged in a work-related program.[47] Only time will reveal the effects of these types of changes in federal assistance programs. If net household income is decreased by these changes, the number of individuals who are at risk for food insecurity at any given time may increase. If, on the other hand, these changes move people out of poverty, the result may be to promote long-term food and financial security.

Programs to Provide Access to Food In the United States the two major programs designed to make sure that all people have access to an adequate diet are the Food Stamp Program and the Emergency Food Assistance Program (see Table 17.1). The Food Stamp Program provides monthly benefits in the form of coupons or electronic transfers using a plastic card that can be used to purchase food, thereby supplementing the food budgets of low-income individuals and families. The Food Stamp Program served about 22.9 million people per month in 1997.[48] The Emergency Food Assistance Program distributes USDA food commodities to individuals for home use as well as to organized programs. Available commodities vary depending on market conditions. Products that are typically available include canned and dried fruits, canned vegetables, canned meats, peanut butter, and pasta products. This program provided states with about $80 million worth of USDA commodities in 1997.[48]

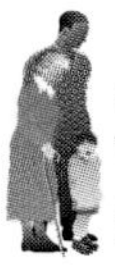

Because women, infants, children, the elderly, and the homeless are at highest risk of malnutrition, a number of programs target these particular groups. The WIC program (see Chapter 13) provides coupons to purchase nutrient-dense foods for pregnant women, lactating and non-breast-feeding postpartum women, and infants and children.[49] Preschool and school meal programs provide meals to children once they reach preschool age (Figure 17.17; see also Chapter 14). And the Nutrition Program for the Elderly helps prevent malnutrition in the elderly by providing nutritious meals in congregate settings and by home delivery (see Chapter 15).

Table 17.1 *Programs to Prevent Undernutrition in the United States*

Program	Target Population	Goals and Methods
Food Stamp Program	Low-income individuals	Increases access to food by providing coupons that can be used to purchase food at the grocery store.
Commodity Supplemental Food Program	Low-income pregnant women, breast-feeding and non-breast-feeding postpartum women, infants and children under six years of age, and the elderly	Provides food by distributing USDA commodity foods.
Special Supplemental Nutrition Program for Women, Infants, and Children (WIC)	Low-income pregnant women, breast-feeding, and non-breast-feeding postpartum women, and infants and children under five years of age	Increases access to the right mix of foods by providing coupons for purchasing foods that are good sources of those nutrients at risk of deficiency in these groups.
WIC Farmers Market Nutrition Program	WIC participants	Increases access to fresh produce by providing coupons to purchase produce at authorized local farmers' markets.
National School Breakfast Program	Low-income children	Provides free or low-cost breakfasts to improve the nutritional status of children.
National School Lunch Program	Low-income children	Provides free or low-cost lunches at school to improve the nutritional status of children.
Special Milk Program	Low-income children	Provides milk for children in schools, camps, and child-care institutions with no federally supported meal program.
Summer Food Service Program	Low-income children	Provides meals for children during the summer months.
Child and Adult Care Food Program	Children up to age 12 and handicapped adults	Provides cash reimbursements and food commodities to child-care programs and community adult day-care centers.
Head Start	Low-income preschool children and their families	Provides education, including nutrition education, to low-income children and their families.
Nutrition Program for the Elderly	Individuals age 60 or over and their spouses	Provides free congregate meals in churches, schools, senior centers, or other facilities, and home-delivers to the homebound.
Homeless Children Nutrition Program	Preschoolers living in shelters	Reimburses providers for meals served to homeless preschool children in shelters.
Emergency Food Assistance Program	Low-income people	Provides commodities to soup kitchens, food banks, and individuals for home use.
Healthy People 2010	U.S. population	Sets national health promotion objectives to improve the health of the U.S. population through health-care system and industry involvement, and individual actions.
Expanded Food and Nutrition Education Program (EFNEP)	Low-income families	Provides education in all aspects of food preparation and nutrition.
Nutrition Education and Training Program (NET)	Children, parents, teachers, and food service personnel	Provides a comprehensive, school-based nutrition education program.
Temporary Assistance for Needy Families (TANF)	Low-income households	Provides money to ensure housing, food, and clothing to low-income families. Exact requirements and provisions are determined by the states.

There are few specific programs that serve the homeless. In 1991 the Healthy Meals for Healthy Americans Act created the Homeless Children Nutrition Program to provide meals for homeless preschool-age children living in shelters. Most of the homeless rely on food banks, feeding centers, and other community resource agencies to provide food; however, this does not guarantee an adequate nutrient intake. Often meals at feeding centers are based more on the types of foods donated than the definition of an adequate diet. However, innovative approaches are being developed to feed homeless people. One approach is to provide kitchens and cooking facilities in shelters for the homeless. Inhabitants of such shelters have been found to have better nutritional status.[43]

Even with federal assistance programs, many individuals still rely on church, community, and charitable emergency food shelters to provide for their basic nu-

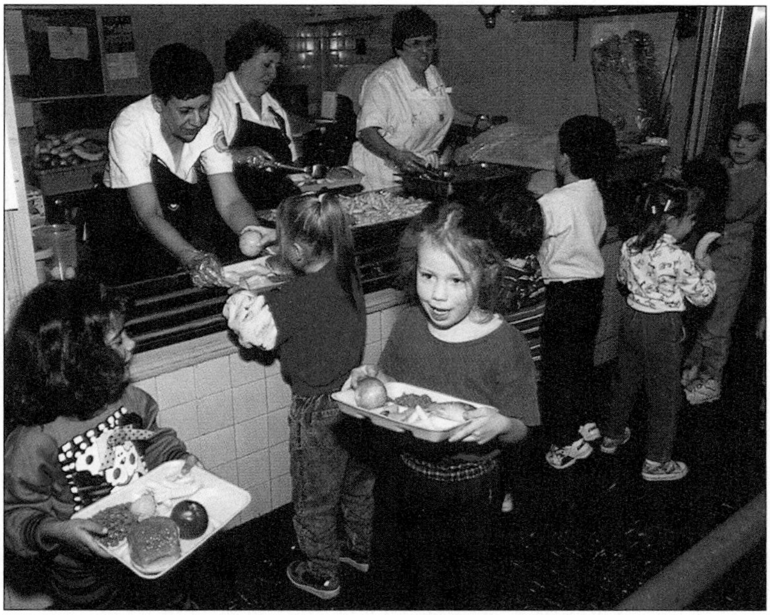

Figure 17.17
The School Lunch Program provides nutritious meals to school-age children.

tritional needs. Second Harvest, the nation's largest charitable hunger relief organization, provided food to 21 million people in 1997.[40]

Nutrition Education The link between nutrition education and diet quality is strong. People with more nutrition information and more awareness of the relationship between diet and health consume healthier diets.[50] Healthy diets not only improve current health by optimizing growth, productivity, and well-being, but are essential for preventing chronic diseases in the future. Increasing nutrition knowledge can reduce medical care costs and improve the quality of life. Education can help individuals with lower incomes stretch limited food dollars by making wise choices at the store and reducing food waste at home. Education can promote community gardens to increase the availability of seasonal vegetables. It can teach people how to prepare foods that become available through commodity distribution and food banks. It can teach safe food handling and food preparation methods. Knowing which foods to choose and how to handle them safely is as important in preventing malnutrition as having the money to buy enough food.

There are a number of government programs designed to provide nutrition education. One of the goals of Healthy People 2010 is to increase the nutrition education provided by schools as well as by work sites. The Expanded Food and Nutrition Education Program (EFNEP) provides education in all aspects of food preparation and nutrition to low-income families. The Family Nutrition Program provides funding to develop and provide nutrition education programs for people on food stamps. In addition, the Dietary Guidelines for Americans, the Food Guide Pyramid, and food labels educate the general public about making wise food choices.

Policies to Control Food Costs The price of food depends on the amount produced and the consumer demand, so controlling the supply of food is important in determining cost. If the supply is large, prices will be low, but if supply forces prices to drop too much, the profit to the farmer and food industry may be too low to justify harvesting the crop. Government policy has tried to prevent this by controlling agricultural production with programs like the Grain Reserve Program and the Price Support Program. The Grain Reserve Program draws surplus grain off the market when excess is produced or prices decline. This practice keeps grain prices more stable and saves food for times when the harvest is not as plentiful. The Price Support Program also protects farmers from the drop in prices that results from overproduction. While these programs protect farmers, moderate food prices, and limit what reaches the marketplace, they may not provide incentive for farmers to limit production when demand is low. Federal programs also have the potential to support sustainable agriculture by regulating the use of natural resources and agricultural chemicals.

Policies to Affect the Foods Produced Food policy can have an effect on what foods are produced and consumed by the population. For example, the grading of meat is based on the fat content, which is associated with flavor and tenderness. The greater the fat content, the higher the grade and the greater the cost. Beef labeled "prime" is higher in fat and cost than that labeled "choice" or "select." A change in grading policy could encourage the production of lower-fat meats.

An example of how policy can affect production is pricing in the dairy industry. For years the USDA milk pricing system favored the production of milk high in fat and protein. To respond to the health needs of the consumer, the USDA is now changing its policy—lowering the price it pays farmers for butterfat and increasing the price it pays for skim milk. The goal is to provide less of an incentive for farmers to produce milk with a high butterfat content. Thus changes in technology and policy affect what foods are produced and in turn consumed, which can then affect the nutritional health of the population (see *Critical Thinking: Cutting Food Costs*).

NUTRITION TRANSITION: THE GROWING PROBLEM OF OVERNUTRITION

Undernutrition is not the only world nutrition problem. Problems of overnutrition coexist with undernutrition in both industrialized and developing nations. Nutrition-related noncommunicable diseases such as cardiovascular disease, cancer, diabetes, and osteoporosis are newly appearing, rapidly rising, or already established in every country around the world,[51,52] and obesity levels in some developing countries are as high as those in the developed world.[53] This situation occurs because developing nations follow a pattern of transition toward the diet and lifestyle of developed countries. Traditional diets that are high in whole grains and vegetables are replaced by diets that are higher in meat, fat and saturated fat, and sugar. Along with these dietary transitions come changes in lifestyle that decrease activity. There is a shift toward less physically demanding occupations, an increase in the use of transportation to get to work or school, more labor-saving technology in the home, and more passive leisure time.[53]

Nutrition transition The shift in dietary pattern that occurs as incomes increase—from a diet high in complex carbohydrates and fiber to a more varied diet higher in fats, saturated fat, and sugar.

Some of the effects of this economic and **nutrition transition** are positive. Typically, the diet in developing countries is based on a limited number of foods—primarily starchy roots and coarse grains. As incomes increase, the diet becomes more varied. Meat, fish, milk, cheese, eggs, and fresh fruits and vegetables—sources of iron, vitamin A, and protein—can be incorporated into the diet.[54] These shifts in diet are accompanied both by increases in life expectancy and by decreases in the birthrate and in the incidence of infectious diseases and nutrient deficiencies. However, at the same time, rates of heart disease, cancer, diabetes, obesity, and childhood obesity increase.[54] The increased reliance on animal proteins as well as on refined and processed foods also increases the use of energy and natural resources, which may damage the environment and deplete nonrenewable resources.

A problem facing international development agencies is how to promote economic growth and at the same time prevent the undesirable effects of nutrition transition. To address these growing health concerns, individual countries have developed public health campaigns and policies (see Appendix G). In addition, an international campaign, the INTERHEALTH program, has been developed by the World Health Organization to work toward the prevention and control of chronic noncommunicable diseases.[52] Each country involved in INTERHEALTH must assess its nutritional behaviors and intakes, physical activity levels, blood pressure and blood cholesterol levels, as well as other risk factors for chronic diseases such as smoking, alcohol consumption, and obesity. The country must then implement strategies for reducing these risk factors, monitor trends in mortality, and evaluate the success of their programs. INTERHEALTH strategies must simultaneously address more than one disease and emphasize total community involvement, health promotion activities, behavioral interventions, and prevention and control activities.

INTERHEALTH programs and strategies focus on activities at every level of society.[52] At the macro level, the food supply and mass media are targets. For example, agricultural policy may be modified to encourage the production of milk that is lower in fat, or weekly radio programs may educate people about chronic disease topics. At the intermediate level, communities, work sites, schools, and health professions are targeted. This could involve risk-factor screening, nutrition education in the schools, and training and education of health professionals. Finally, at the micro level, the family and individual are targeted. This might include home visits to monitor and promote nutrition behavior changes and referral networks for high-risk individuals.

A component of the INTERHEALTH program, called the INTERHEALTH Nutrition Initiative, was developed to collect information about global population and nutrition trends and to evaluate programs related to food and nutrition. Nutrition goals for countries involved must emphasize the availability of a safe and adequate food supply, as well as the promotion of dietary practices to reduce chronic disease risk. For countries where chronic disease rates are low and infectious disease rates and undernutrition are high, programs directed toward feeding the population are emphasized. For countries with high chronic disease risks, nutrition recommendations similar to the Dietary Guidelines for Americans encourage maintenance of appropriate body weight; decreased consumption of total fat, saturated fat, cholesterol, and sodium; increased consumption of fiber-rich foods and complex carbohydrates; and moderate alcohol intake.[52]

CRITICAL THINKING

Cutting Food Costs

Cecelia works part-time at the local market and her husband is a house painter. Their combined income is about $15,000 per year. At this income level, she is just above the poverty line and so feels she should be able to feed her family without accepting federal assistance or charity. Despite this, by the end of the month the money is gone and she must go to a soup kitchen to get meals for her family.

According to the USDA Center for Nutrition Policy and Promotion's thrifty meal plan, it is possible for Cecelia to feed her family of four on $82.30 per week. The cost of her current meals for one day is given below.

Current Diet		Modified Diet	
Food	Cost per Serving (dollars)	Food	Cost per Serving (dollars)
Breakfast			
Frosted flakes	.20	Oatmeal	.05
Lowfat milk	.15	Lowfat milk	.15
Banana	.30	Banana	.30
Doughnut	.25	Toast	.12
Coffee with creamer and sugar	.10	Coffee with creamer and sugar	.10
Orange juice	.25	Orange juice	.25
Lunch			
Roast beef	1.00	Peanut butter	.05
with cheese and	.20	and jelly	.03
mayonnaise	.03	on wheat bread	.12
on wheat bread	.12		
Grapes	.35	Apple	.15
Potato chips (1-oz bag)	.30	Potato chips (from a large bag)	.15
Juice (box)	.35	Juice (from a large bottle)	.15
Cookies, 3 (brand-name)	.25	Cookies, 3 (store-brand)	.10
Dinner			
Pork chops	1.15	Spaghetti	
Potatoes au gratin	.25	with tomato and meat sauce	.80
Broccoli	.25		
Tossed salad	.05	Tossed salad	.05
Salad dressing (bottled)	.10	Oil and vinegar dressing (homemade)	.02
Dinner rolls	.24	Bread	.12
Lowfat milk	.15	Lowfat milk	.15
Ice cream sandwich	.35	Ice cream (from a large container)	.12
Total	**$6.39**		**$2.98**

At $82.30 a week, one day's meals for the entire family should cost $11.76. Currently, Cecelia's meals alone cost $6.39. To meet the recommendations of the thrifty meal plan, her meals should cost about $3.00. She needs to make some changes.

What changes could Cecelia make to reduce food costs without major changes in her meal pattern?

She could switch to a cooked cereal or a store brand of cereal. She could buy large containers instead of individual servings of yogurt, ice cream, juice, and potato chips.

Does her modified diet meet the recommendations of the Food Guide Pyramid?

Answer:

One of the problems with buying bulk items is they are hard to transport without a car. In addition, although they cost less per serving, the amount of money needed at the time of purchase is greater. Cecelia does not always have the money available to buy larger sizes such as a gallon of apple juice, so she must settle for a smaller size.

What other changes could Cecelia make to reduce food costs without requiring the purchase of bulk items?

Answer:

Applications

These exercises are designed to help you apply your critical thinking skills to your own nutrition choices.

1. Keep a record of how much money you spend on food in a day and use this to estimate your monthly food costs.
   a. Suggest specific changes in the foods you choose that will reduce your food costs.
   b. How do these changes affect the nutrient content of your diet?
   c. Modify your choices so that your food cost for the day is $3.00.
   d. Would this modified diet meet your nutrient needs? Which nutrients are deficient? Which are excessive?
2. World Food Day is October 16. List some ideas for campus-wide programs to increase awareness of global nutrition issues.
3. Use the Internet to locate Web sites for organizations such as Worldwatch or Bread for the World Institute. Research one area of the world where hunger and undernutrition are a major problem:
   a. What is the cause of undernutrition in this area?
   b. What solutions are in place or proposed to solve these problems?

Summary

1. Both insufficient amounts of food and a poor quality diet cause undernutrition—the predominant nutritional problem worldwide.
2. In poorly nourished populations, a cycle of malnutrition exists in which poorly nourished women give birth to low birth weight infants at risk of disease and early death. If these children survive, they grow into adults who are physically unable to fully contribute to society. Indicators of the nutritional status of a population are the infant mortality rate and the incidence of low birth weight and stunting.
3. Hunger and undernutrition occur when there is a shortage of food. Short-term food shortage, such as famine, may result from a natural or man-made disaster. Chronic food shortage occurs when overpopulation and limited natural resources create a situation in which there are more people than food. The inequitable distribution of food and resources caused by poverty creates food insecurity within a population even if there is enough total food.
4. Malnutrition also occurs when the quality of the diet is poor. High-risk groups such as pregnant women, children, the elderly, and the ill may not be able to meet their nutrient needs. Protein, iron, iodine, and vitamin A deficiencies are common worldwide.
5. Short-term solutions to undernutrition provide food through relief at the local, national, and international levels. Long-term solutions include control of population growth, economic and agricultural policies that promote self-sufficiency and alleviate poverty, improvements in the quality of the food supply, and the development of sustainable systems that will provide food without damaging the environment.
6. Technology can help solve the problems of world hunger by providing environmentally safe pesticides, disease-resistant crops, and foods with greater nutrient density.
7. Both undernutrition and overnutrition are problems in the United States. As in developing nations, undernutrition is associated with poverty, but food insecurity can also occur when income is adequate. The homeless, women, children, the elderly, and minority groups are most often food insecure.
8. Nutrition programs in the United States focus on maintaining a nutrition safety net which will provide access to affordable

food and promote healthy eating in the United States. Some programs designed to help feed the hungry address the general population, whereas others focus on specific high-risk groups. Most programs provide access to food and some provide nutrition education.

9. Problems of overnutrition coexist with undernutrition in both developed and developing nations. Policies and education must work to feed the population when hunger is prevalent, prevent the population from adopting dietary and lifestyle patterns that result in an increase in chronic disease, and reduce the incidence of chronic diseases where they are a problem.

Review Questions

1. What is the cycle of malnutrition?
2. How does overpopulation contribute to food shortage?
3. How does poverty contribute to world hunger?
4. How are economic growth and population growth related?
5. What segments of the world population are at greatest risk for undernutrition?
6. List three micronutrient deficiencies that are world health problems.
7. Why are environmental issues important in maintaining the world's food supply?
8. How does sustainable agriculture reduce environmental damage?
9. How can nutrification help eliminate malnutrition?
10. List four groups in the United States population that are at risk for undernutrition.
11. List three federal programs that address malnutrition in the United States.
12. Why is overnutrition a concern in all countries around the world?

Nutrition Web Links

To further explore areas related to the material in this chapter, go to the *Nutrition: Science and Applications* Web site at ***www.Wiley.com/college/Smolin*** and *click on* **Student Companion Site** for chapter-by-chapter links. Some Web sites related to the information in Chapter 17 include:

International organizations that provide information on food and nutrition such as the World Health Organization and the Food and Agriculture Organization of the United Nations.

Private organizations that provide information on world hunger and the environment such as the Worldwatch Institute and the World Hunger Program.

United States government agencies that support nutrition programs such as the Department of Health and Human Services.

References

1. Bread for the World Institute. Executive Summary: Hunger in a Global Economy: Hunger 1998. Online at http://www.bread.org/bfwi/esumm98.html
2. Table set thinly as Food Summit pledges to halve world hunger in 20 years. UN Chronicle, 33:24–28, 1996.
3. Bengoa, J. M. A half-century perspective on world nutrition and the international nutrition agencies. Nutr. Rev. 55:309–314, 1997.
4. United Nations, Administrative Committee on Coordination, Sub-Committee on Nutrition, *Third Report on the World Nutrition Situation*. Geneva: ACC/SCN, December 1997.
5. World Health Organization. *Global Database on Child Growth and Malnutrition*. Geneva: WHO, 1997.
6. Pelletier, D. L. The potentiating effects of malnutrition on child mortality: epidemiologic evidence and policy implications. Nutr. Rev. 52:409–415, 1994.
7. National Geographic Society. Millennium in maps: population. Supplement to *National Geographic Magazine*, October 1998.
8. International Food Policy and Research Institute (IFPRI). *A 2020 Vision for Food, Agriculture, and the Environment: The Vision, Challenge, and Recommended Action*. Washington, D.C.: IFPRI, 1995.
9. Beckman, D., Cohen, M. J., and Kennedy, E. Position of the American Dietetic Association: world hunger. J. Am. Diet. Assoc. 95:1160–1162, 1995.
10. Olson, R. E. World food production and problems of human nutrition. Nutr. Today 24:15–21, 1989.
11. Raloff, J. The human numbers crunch. Sci. News 149:396–397, June 22, 1996.
12. Torún, B., and Chew, F. Protein-energy malnutrition. In *Modern Nutrition in Health and Disease*, 9th ed. Shils, M. E., Olson, J. A., Shike, M., and Ross, A. C., eds. Baltimore: Williams & Wilkins, 1999, 963–988.
13. Darnton-Hill, I. Developing industrial-government-academic partnerships to address micronutrient malnutrition. Nutr. Rev. 55:76–81, 1997.
14. Freiri, W. B. Strategies of the Pan American Health Organization/World Health Organization for the control of iron deficiency in Latin America. Nutr. Rev. 55:183–188, 1997.
15. United Nations Children's Fund. The state of the world's children 1998: a UNICEF report. Malnutrition: causes, consequences, and solutions. Nutr. Rev. 56:115–123, 1998.
16. Pollitt, E. Functional significance of the covariance between protein energy malnutrition and iron deficiency anemia. J. Nutr. 125:2272S–2277S, 1995.
17. Ramalingaswami, V. New global perspectives on overcoming malnutrition. Am. J. Clin. Nutr. 61:259–263, 1995.
18. Delange, F. The disorders induced by iodine deficiency. Thyroid 4:107–128, 1994.
19. Hetzel, B. S., and Clugstrum, G. A. Iodine. In *Modern Nutrition in Health and Disease*, 9th ed. Shils, M. E., Olson, J. A., Shike, M., and Ross, A. C., eds. Baltimore: Williams & Wilkins, 1999, 253–264.

20. World Health Organization. Vitamin A—the good news. Donald McLaren highlights recent developments. Online at http://www.who.int/chd/pub/newslet/dialog/9/vitamin_a.htm
21. Ross, D. A. Vitamin A and public health. Proc. Nutr. Soc. 57:159–165, 1998.
22. UN Food and Agriculture Organization. World Food Summit briefing, United Nations, November 1996. Online at http://www.fao.org
23. UN Food and Agriculture Organization. Rome Declaration on World Food Security and World Food Summit Plan of Action, United Nations, November 13, 1996. Online at http://www.fao.org
24. Sloham, J. Emergency feeding programmes: still not delivering the goods. Br. J. Med. 305:596–597, 1992.
25. Raven, P. H., Berg, L. R., and Johnson, G. B. *Environment,* 2nd ed. Philadelphia: Saunders College Publishing, 1998, 185.
26. Uvin, P. The state of world hunger. Nutr. Rev. 52:151–161, 1994.
27. Matson, P. A., Parton, W. J., Power, A. G., and Swift, M. J. Agricultural intensification and ecosystem properties. Science 277:504–509, 1997.
28. Waibel, H. Government intervention in crop protection in developing countries. Ciba Found. Symp. 177:76–90, 1993.
29. Henkel, J. Genetic engineering fast forwarding to future foods. FDA Consumer 29:6–11, April 1995.
30. Viteri, F. E., Alvarez, E., Batres, R., et al. Fortification of sugar with iron sodium ethylenediaminotetraacetate (FeNaEDTA) improves iron status in semirural Guatemalan populations. Am. J. Clin. Nutr. 61:1153–1163, 1995.
31. Solon, F. S., Solon, M. S., Meshansho, H., et al. Evaluation of the effect of vitamin A–fortified margarine on the vitamin A status of preschool Filipino children. Eur. J. Clin. Nutr. 50:720–723, 1996.
32. Arraya, J. C., and Canelas, W. Assessment of vitamin A in fortified sugar—simplified. Abstract, 17th International Vitamin A Consultative Group Meeting, Guatemala City, 1996. Washington, D.C.: International Vitamin A Consultative Group, 1996.
33. Layrisse, M., Chaves, J. F., Mendez-Castellano, H., et al. Early response to the effect of iron fortification in the Venezuelan population. Am. J. Clin. Nutr. 64:903–907, 1996.
34. World Health Organization/United Nation's Children's Fund/International Vitamin A Consultative Group. *Vitamin A Supplements: A Guide to Their Use in the Treatment and Prevention of Vitamin A Deficiency and Xerophthalmia,* 2nd ed. Geneva: WHO, 1997.
35. National Institutes of Health; National Heart, Lung, and Blood Institute. Clinical Guidelines on the Identification, Evaluation, and Treatment of Overweight and Obesity in Adults. Executive Summary. June, 1998. Online at http://www.nhlbi.nih.gov/nhlbi/cardio/obes/prof/guidelines/ob_xsum.htm
36. Update: prevalence of overweight among children, adolescents, and adults—United States, 1988–1994. MMWR Morb. Mortal. Wkly. Rep. 46:198–202, March 7, 1998.
37. National Center for Health Statistics. Fact sheets: ten million Americans do not get enough to eat. Online at http://www.cdc.gov/nchswww/releases/98factsheets
38. U.S. Department of Agriculture, Foreign Agricultural Service. Discussion paper on domestic food security, February 13, 1998. Online at http://www.fas.usda.gov/icd/summit/discussi.html
39. U.S. Department of Health and Human Services, Centers for Disease Control and Prevention, National Center for Health Statistics. Online at http://www.cdc.gov/nchswww
40. Second Harvest. Hunger: the faces and facts: a profile of who is hungry. Online at http://www.secondharvest.org/websecha/d_ffla.htm
41. Mayer, J. Hunger and undernutrition in the United States. J. Nutr. 120:919–923, 1990.
42. American Dietetic Association. Position on domestic food and nutrition security. J. Am. Diet. Assoc. 98:337–342, 1998.
43. Wiecha, J. L., Dwyer, J. T., Jacques, P. F., and Rand, W. M. Nutritional and economic advantages for homeless families in shelters providing kitchen facilities and food. J. Am. Diet. Assoc. 93:777–783, 1993.
44. Taylor, M. L., and Oblinsky, S. A. Food consumption and eating behavior of homeless preschool children. J. Nutr. Ed. 26:20–25, 1994.
45. Chernoff, R. Baby boomers come of age: nutrition in the 21st century. J. Am. Diet. Assoc. 95:650–654, 1995.
46. Poppendieck, J. Hunger and public policy lessons from the Great Depression. J. Nutr. Ed. 24(Suppl):6S–10S, 1992.
47. Oliveira, V. Cost of food-assistance programs declined slightly in first half of 1996. Food Review 26-33, USDA Food and Consumer Service, September/December, 1996.
48. U.S. Department of Agriculture. Food, nutrition, and consumer service mission. Online at http://www.usda.gov/mission/fncs.htm
49. Owen, A. L., and Owen, G. M. Twenty years of WIC: a review of some effects of the program. J. Am. Diet. Assoc. 97:777–782, 1997.
50. U.S. Department of Agriculture Economic Research Service, USDA Center for Nutrition Policy and Promotion. USDA's healthy eating index and nutrition information. Online at http://www.econ.ag.gov/epubs/pdf/tb1866
51. Posner, B. M., Franz, M., Quatromoni, P., and the INTERHEALTH steering committee. Nutrition and the global risk for chronic diseases: the INTERHEALTH Nutrition Initiative. Nutr. Rev. 52:201–207, 1994.
52. Posner, B. M., Quatromoni, P. A., and Franz, M. Nutrition policies and interventions for chronic disease risk reduction in international settings: the INTERHEALTH Nutrition Initiative. Nutr. Rev. 52:179–187, 1994.
53. Popkin, B. M., and Doark, C. M. The obesity epidemic is a worldwide phenomenon. Nutr. Rev. 56:106–114, 1998.
54. Drewnowski, A., and Popkin, B. M. The nutrition transition: new trends in the global diet. Nutr. Rev. 55:31–43, 1997.

Appendices

Appendix A

Nutrient Composition of Foods

Key: Esha Code = computer code for Esha Software; Qty = quantity; Meas = measurement; Wgt = weight; Wtr = water; Cals = kcalories; Prot = protein; Carb = carbohydrate; Fib = fiber; SatF = saturated fat; MonoF = monounsaturated fat; PolyF = polyunsaturated fat; Choles = cholesterol; Calc = calcium; Phos = phosphorus; Sod = sodium; Pot = potassium; Zn = zinc; Magn = magnesium; VitA = vitamin A; VitE = vitamin E; VitC = vitamin C; Thia = thiamin; Ribo = riboflavin; Nia = niacin; B6 = vitamin B6; Fola = folate; B12 = vitamin B12.

Esha Code	Food Item	Qty	Meas	Wgt (g)	Wtr (g)	Cals	Prot (g)	Carb (g)	Fib (g)	Fat (g)	SatF (g)
90095	Ac'cent flavor enhancer	0.25	tsp	1	—	0	0	0	0	0	0
4639	Acorns, dried	1	oz.	28	1	144	2	15	1.2	9	1.2
26000	Allspice, ground	0.25	tsp	0	0	1	0	0	0.1	0	0
4567	Almond butter, honey+cinnamon	2	Tbs	31	1	188	5	8	1.2	16	1.6
4572	Almond butter, plain, salted	2	Tbs	31	0	198	5	7	1.2	18	1.8
4534	Almond butter, plain, unsalted	2	Tbs	32	0	203	5	7	1.2	19	1.8
15907	Almond chicken	0.5	cup	121	93	137	10	9	1.9	7	1
4657	Almond meal, partially defatted	1	oz.	28	2	116	11	8	1	5	0.5
4553	Almond paste, packed	2	Tbs	28	4	131	3	14	1.4	8	0.8
4500	Almond, dried, unblanched, whole	0.25	cup	36	2	209	7	7	3.9	18	1.8
4549	Almond, dry roasted, unsalted, whole	0.25	cup	34	1	203	6	8	4.7	18	1.7
4548	Almonds, blanched, slices	0.25	cup	26	1	154	5	5	1.8	14	1.3
4547	Almonds, blanched, whole	0.25	cup	36	2	212	7	7	2.4	19	1.8
4727	Almonds, blanched, whole	0.25	cup	36	2	222	8	7	4.8	18	—
4501	Almonds, dried, unblanched, chopped	0.25	cup	32	1	191	6	7	3.5	17	1.6
4503	Almonds, dried, unblanched, slivered	0.25	cup	34	1	199	7	7	3.7	18	1.7
4571	Almonds, dry roasted, salted	0.25	cup	34	1	203	6	8	4.7	18	1.7
4730	Almonds, dry roasted, whole	0.25	cup	34	1	206	7	7	3.7	18	1.5
4732	Almonds, natural, whole	0.25	cup	36	2	213	7	7	4.4	18	1.3
4640	Almonds, oil roasted, blanched	0.25	cup	36	1	218	7	6	4	20	1.9
4620	Almonds, oil roasted, salted	0.25	cup	39	1	243	8	6	4.4	23	2.2
4505	Almonds, oil roasted, unsalted	0.25	cup	39	1	243	8	6	4.4	23	2.2
4729	Almonds, oil roasted, whole	0.25	cup	39	1	244	9	5	3.7	23	1.7
4566	Almonds, whole, toasted	1	oz.	28	1	167	6	6	3.2	14	1.4
5377	Amaranth leaves, cooked, drained	0.5	cup	66	60	14	1	3	1.2	0	0
5375	Amaranth leaves, raw, chopped	0.5	cup	14	13	3	0	1	0.2	0	0
38070	Amaranth, grain	0.5	cup	98	10	365	14	64	14.8	6	1.6
5376	Amaranth, raw leaf	1	each	14	13	3	0	1	0.2	0	0
26106	Anise seed	1	tsp	2	0	8	0	1	0.3	0	0
26484	Annatto seed	1	oz.	28	3	102	4	19	10.2	1	—
49005	Apple brown betty	0.75	cup	155	96	264	4	46	3.8	8	4.2
23000	Apple butter	1	Tbs	17	10	30	0	7	0.3	0	0
49031	Apple crisp, recipe	1	cup	282	173	460	5	91	4.8	10	2.1
45549	Apple dumpling	1	each	190	62	670	7	84	2.9	35	8.6
3008	Apple juice, canned/bottled	1	cup	248	218	117	0	29	0.2	0	0

This table of food composition has been prepared for Saunders College Publishing and is copyrighted by ESHA Research in Salem, Oregon, developer and publisher of The Food Processor® and Genesis™ nutrition and labeling software systems. The table includes nutrient data for over 3900 foods, including brand-name items, ethnic foods, vegetarian products, nonfat and low-sodium alternatives, baby foods and formulas, and a large selection of common food items. The foods are presented alphabetically with corresponding units of measure. Over 1000 sources of scientific information are researched to provide the most accurate, reliable data available. Government sources of information are the base for all the data: the USDA Handbook series and its current supplemental data, as well as current data from both published and unpublished provisional data. Even with all the government data available, there are still missing values for some nutrients. Dashes in the table appear where there are no data available. Considerable effort has been made to report the most accurate data available and to eliminate missing values. Please be advised that the folate values in this table include the amount added in fortification for all non–brand-name items. Values for brand-name items may or may not include added folic acid. The authors welcome any suggestions or comments for future editions.

MonoF (g)	PolyF (g)	Choles (mg)	Calc (mg)	Phos (mg)	Sod (mg)	Pot (mg)	Zn (mg)	Iron (mg)	Magn (mg)	VitA (μg RE)	VitE (mg α-TE)	VitC (mg)	Thia (mg)	Ribo (mg)	Nia (mg)	B6 (mg)	Fola (μg)	B12 (μg)
0	0	0	0	—	160	—	—	0	—	0	—	0	—	—	—	—	—	0
5.6	1.7	0	15	29	0	201	0.2	0.3	23	0	—	0	0.04	0.04	0.7	0.2	33	0
0	0	0	3	1	0	5	0	0	1	0	0	0	0	0	0	0	0	0
10.6	3.4	0	84	162	3	234	0.9	1.1	94	0	5.63	0	0.04	0.19	0.9	0.02	20	0
12	3.9	0	84	163	141	237	1	1.2	95	0	6.34	0	0.04	0.19	0.9	0.02	20	0
12.3	4	0	86	167	4	243	1	1.2	97	0	6.5	0	0.04	0.2	0.9	0.02	21	0
2.6	2.9	18	40	119	307	275	0.8	1	30	38	1.32	5	0.04	0.1	4.3	0.21	16	0.12
3.4	1.1	0	120	259	2	397	0.8	2.4	82	0	3.8	0	0.09	0.48	1.8	0.03	16	0
5.1	1.7	0	49	74	3	90	0.4	0.5	37	0	5.79	0	0.02	0.12	0.4	0.01	21	0
12	3.9	0	94	185	4	260	1	1.3	105	0	8.52	0	0.08	0.28	1.2	0.04	21	0
11.6	3.7	0	97	189	4	266	1.7	1.3	105	0	1.91	0	0.04	0.21	1	0.03	22	0
9	2.9	0	65	140	3	197	0.8	1	75	0	5.33	0	0.04	0.18	0.8	0.03	10	0
12.4	4	0	90	193	4	272	1.2	1.3	104	0	7.36	0	0.06	0.24	1.2	0.04	14	0
—	—	0	94	192	0	221	1.2	1.4	109	—	7.5	—	0.05	0.23	1.1	0.04	14	0
11	3.6	0	86	169	4	238	0.9	1.2	96	0	7.8	0	0.07	0.25	1.1	0.04	19	0
11.4	3.7	0	90	176	4	247	1	1.2	100	0	8.1	0	0.07	0.26	1.1	0.04	20	0
11.6	3.7	0	97	189	269	266	1.7	1.3	105	0	1.91	0	0.04	0.21	1	0.03	22	0
11.5	3.2	0	111	—	1	243	—	—	—	—	7.62	—	0.02	0.49	0.8	—	15	0
11.2	4.1	0	—	—	—	—	—	—	—	—	8.09	—	0.07	0.32	1.1	0.04	16	0
13	4.2	0	69	205	4	246	0.5	1.9	103	0	1.95	0	0.03	0.1	1.4	0.03	22	0
14.7	4.8	0	92	215	306	268	1.9	1.5	119	0	2.18	0	0.05	0.39	1.4	0.03	25	0
14.7	4.8	0	92	215	4	268	1.9	1.5	119	0	2.18	0	0.05	0.39	1.4	0.03	25	0
13.1	5.4	0	120	196	0	232	1.2	1.5	101	—	8.6	—	0.04	0.43	1.4	—	12	0
9.4	3	0	80	156	3	219	1.4	1.4	86	0	4.54	0	0.04	0.17	0.8	0.02	18	0
0	0.1	0	138	48	14	423	0.6	1.5	36	183	0.33	27	0.01	0.09	0.4	0.12	38	0
0	0	0	30	7	3	87	0.1	0.3	8	42	0.11	6	0	0.02	0.1	0.03	12	0
1.4	2.8	0	149	444	20	357	3.1	7.4	259	0	1	4	0.08	0.2	1.3	0.22	48	0
0	0	0	30	7	3	86	0.1	0.3	8	41	0.11	6	0	0.02	0.1	0.03	12	0
0.2	0.1	0	14	10	0	32	0.1	0.8	4	1	0.02	0	0.01	0.01	0.1	0.01	0	0
—	—	—	51	—	4	—	—	9.2	—	2	—	1	—	—	—	—	—	0
2.3	0.9	17	70	49	295	147	0.4	1.9	16	61	0.42	0	0.22	0.13	1.9	0.07	7	0.02
0	0	0	2	2	1	16	0	0.1	1	2	0	0	0	0	0	0.01	0	0
4.3	3.3	0	79	70	513	274	0.5	2.1	20	87	—	6	0.24	0.2	2.2	0.12	14	0
15.2	9.2	0	14	75	607	129	0.5	3.1	16	10	3.2	2	0.39	0.3	3.5	0.05	11	0
0	0.1	0	17	17	7	295	0.1	0.9	7	0	0.02	2	0.05	0.04	0.2	0.07	0	0

A

Esha Code	Food Item	Qty	Meas	Wgt (g)	Wtr (g)	Cals	Prot (g)	Carb (g)	Fib (g)	Fat (g)	SatF (g)
3010	Apple juice, prepared from frozen	1	cup	239	210	112	0	28	0.2	0	0
3005	Apple rings, dried	10	each	64	20	156	1	42	5.6	0	0
3148	Apple slices, canned, sweetened	0.5	cup	102	84	68	0	17	1.7	0	0.1
3149	Apple slices, frozen, heated	0.5	cup	103	90	48	0	12	2	0	0.1
3009	Apple slices, peeled, cooked	0.5	cup	85	72	48	0	12	2.4	0	0.1
49015	Apple strudel	1	each	71	31	195	2	29	1.6	8	1.4
45550	Apple turnover	1	each	82	27	289	3	36	1.2	15	3.7
3308	Apple, baked, unsweetened	1	each	161	133	102	0	26	3.8	1	0.1
3145	Apple, dried, cooked w/o sugar	0.5	cup	128	108	73	0	20	2.6	0	0
3146	Apple, dried, cooked w/sugar	0.5	cup	140	110	116	0	29	2.7	0	0
3003	Apple, no peel	1	each	128	108	73	0	19	2.4	0	0.1
3004	Apple, peeled slices	0.5	cup	55	46	31	0	8	1	0	0
3000	Apple, w/peel	1	each	138	116	81	0	21	3.7	0	0.1
3002	Apple, w/peel, slices	0.5	cup	55	46	32	0	8	1.5	0	0
3147	Applesauce, canned, sweetened	0.5	cup	128	101	97	0	25	1.5	0	0
3006	Applesauce, unsweetened	0.5	cup	122	108	52	0	14	1.5	0	0
3332	Apricot halves w/skin, canned in water	3	each	84	78	23	1	5	1.3	0	0
3217	Apricot halves, dried, cooked	0.5	cup	125	94	106	2	27	4	0	0
3013	Apricot halves, dried, sulfured	10	each	35	11	83	1	22	3.2	0	0
3015	Apricot nectar, canned	1	cup	251	213	141	1	36	1.5	0	0
3218	Apricot nectar, canned, vitamin C added	1	cup	251	213	141	1	36	1.5	0	0
3157	Apricot, pitted, fresh	3	each	106	92	51	1	12	2.5	0	0
3011	Apricot, w/skin, canned in heavy syrup	0.5	cup	129	100	107	1	28	2.1	0	0
3153	Apricot, w/skin, canned in light syrup	0.5	cup	126	104	80	1	21	2	0	0
3151	Apricot, w/skin, canned w/juice	0.5	cup	124	107	60	1	15	2	0	0
3155	Apricots, frozen, sweetened	0.5	cup	121	89	119	1	30	2.7	0	0
3156	Apricots, halves, fresh	0.5	cup	78	67	37	1	9	1.9	0	0
3333	Apricots, peeled, canned in water	2	each	90	84	20	1	5	1	0	0
56335	Arby's Bac'n cheddar sandwich, deluxe	1	each	231	136	512	21	39	0.3	32	8.7
69055	Arby's Philly beef'n swiss sandwich	1	each	197	105	467	24	38	—	25	9.6
69045	Arby's Q sandwich	1	each	190	104	389	18	48	—	15	5.4
69046	Arby's chicken sandwich, grilled, deluxe	1	each	230	143	430	24	42	—	20	3.5
56337	Arby's roast beef sandwich, Junior	1	each	89	42	233	12	23	0.5	11	3.8
56336	Arby's roast beef sandwich, regular	1	each	155	72	383	22	35	1.1	18	6.9
69051	Arby's sandwich, light roast beef, deluxe	1	each	182	118	294	18	33	—	10	3.4
69052	Arby's sandwich, light roast chicken, deluxe	1	each	195	129	276	24	33	—	7	1.7
53256	Arby's sauce	0.5	oz.	14	10	15	0	3	—	0	0
69048	Arby's sub sandwich, Italian	1	each	297	174	671	34	47	—	39	12.8
69049	Arby's sub sandwich, roast beef	1	each	305	185	623	38	47	—	32	11.5
69050	Arby's sub sandwich, tuna	1	each	284	118	663	74	50	—	37	8.2
69044	Arby's sub sandwich, turkey	1	each	277	173	486	33	46	—	19	5.3
57015	Arby's, Cheddar fries	5	oz.	142	64	399	6	46	—	22	9
69056	Arby's, Steak'n cheddar sandwich	1	each	194	96	508	25	43	—	26	7.7
6432	Arby's, curly fries	3.5	oz.	99	31	337	4	43	—	18	7.4
69042	Arby's, roast chicken club sandwich	1	each	238	142	503	30	37	—	27	6.9
5191	Artichoke heart, marinated	6	oz.	170	138	168	4	13	7.5	14	2
5360	Artichoke heart, raw	0.5	cup	84	73	37	2	9	5	0	0
6493	Artichoke heart, raw	0.5	cup	84	73	37	2	9	5	0	0
5077	Artichoke, Jerusalem, raw, freshly harvested	0.5	cup	75	58	57	2	13	1.2	0	0
5192	Artichoke, frozen, cooked	9	oz.	240	208	108	7	22	11	1	0.3
5000	Artichoke, globe, cooked	1	each	120	101	60	4	13	6.5	0	0
6032	Arugula leaf, raw	5	each	10	9	2	0	0	0.2	0	0
6033	Arugula, chopped, raw	0.5	cup	10	9	2	0	0	0.2	0	0
5007	Asparagus spears, canned, drained	4	each	80	75	15	2	2	1.3	1	0.1
5245	Asparagus spears, canned, not drained, low sodium	4	each	80	75	12	1	2	0.8	0	0
5004	Asparagus spears, cooked, unsalted	4	each	60	55	14	2	3	1	0	0
5006	Asparagus spears, frozen, cooked	4	each	60	55	17	2	3	1	0	0.1
5842	Asparagus, canned w/liquid, low sodium	0.5	cup	122	115	18	2	3	1.2	0	0.1
5361	Asparagus, frozen, uncooked spears	4	each	58	53	14	2	2	1.1	0	0
5002	Asparagus, raw spears	4	each	58	54	13	1	3	1.2	0	0
42454	Aunt Anne's pretzel, original, soft	1	each	138	—	390	12	84	3	1	0
42456	Aunt Anne's pretzel, whole wheat, soft	1	each	140	—	390	13	82	8	2	0
3018	Avocado cubes	0.5	cup	75	56	121	1	6	3.8	12	1.8
3019	Avocado slices	1	piece	10	7	16	0	1	0.5	2	0.2
3210	Avocado, California	1	each	173	126	306	4	12	8.5	30	4.5

MonoF (g)	PolyF (g)	Choles (mg)	Calc (mg)	Phos (mg)	Sod (mg)	Pot (mg)	Zn (mg)	Iron (mg)	Magn (mg)	VitA (μg RE)	VitE (mg α-TE)	VitC (mg)	Thia (mg)	Ribo (mg)	Nia (mg)	B6 (mg)	Fola (μg)	B12 (μg)
0	0.1	0	14	17	17	301	0.1	0.6	12	0	0.02	1	0.01	0.04	0.1	0.08	1	0
0	0.1	0	9	24	56	288	0.1	0.9	10	0	0.35	2	0	0.1	0.6	0.08	0	0
0	0.1	0	4	5	3	69	0	0.2	2	5	0.01	0	0.01	0.01	0.1	0.04	0	0
0	0.1	0	5	8	3	78	0.1	0.2	3	2	0.21	0	0.01	0.01	0	0.03	1	0
0	0.1	0	4	7	1	79	0	0.1	3	3	0.01	0	0.01	0.01	0.1	0.04	1	0
2.3	3.8	4	11	23	191	106	0.1	0.3	6	6	2.19	1	0.03	0.02	0.2	0.03	10	0.16
6.6	4	0	6	32	262	56	0.2	1.3	7	4	1.38	1	0.17	0.13	1.5	0.02	5	0
0	0.2	0	12	12	0	179	0.1	0.3	9	7	1.02	8	0.02	0.02	0.1	0.08	3	0
0	0	0	4	12	26	134	0.1	0.4	5	3	0	1	0.01	0.02	0.2	0.06	0	0
0	0	0	4	11	27	137	0.1	0.4	4	3	0.34	1	0.01	0.02	0.2	0.07	0	0
0	0.1	0	5	9	0	145	0.1	0.1	4	5	0.1	5	0.02	0.01	0.1	0.06	1	0
0	0	0	2	4	0	62	0	0	2	2	0.04	2	0.01	0.01	0	0.02	0	0
0	0.1	0	10	10	0	159	0.1	0.2	7	7	0.44	8	0.02	0.02	0.1	0.07	4	0
0	0.1	0	4	4	0	63	0	0.1	3	3	0.18	3	0.01	0.01	0	0.03	2	0
0	0.1	0	5	9	4	78	0.1	0.4	4	1	0.01	2	0.02	0.04	0.2	0.03	1	0
0	0	0	4	9	2	92	0	0.1	4	4	0.01	1	0.02	0.03	0.2	0.03	1	0
0.1	0	0	7	11	3	161	0.1	0.3	6	108	0.75	3	0.02	0.02	0.3	0.04	1	0
0.1	0	0	20	51	4	611	0.3	2.1	21	295	0.62	2	0.01	0.04	1.2	0.14	0	0
0.1	0	0	16	41	4	482	0.3	1.6	16	253	0.52	1	0	0.05	1	0.06	4	0
0.1	0	0	18	23	8	286	0.2	1	13	331	0.2	2	0.02	0.04	0.7	0.06	3	0
0.1	0	0	18	23	8	286	0.2	1	13	331	0.23	137	0.02	0.04	0.7	0.06	3	0
0.2	0.1	0	15	20	1	314	0.3	0.6	8	277	0.94	11	0.03	0.04	0.6	0.06	9	0
0	0	0	12	16	5	181	0.1	0.4	9	159	1.15	4	0.03	0.03	0.5	0.07	2	0
0	0	0	14	16	5	175	0.1	0.5	10	167	1.13	3	0.02	0.02	0.4	0.07	2	0
0	0	0	15	25	5	205	0.1	0.4	12	210	1.1	6	0.02	0.02	0.4	0.07	2	0
0.1	0	0	12	23	5	277	0.1	1.1	11	203	1.08	11	0.02	0.05	1	0.07	2	0
0.1	0.1	0	11	15	1	229	0.2	0.4	6	202	0.69	8	0.02	0.03	0.5	0.04	7	0
0	0	0	7	14	10	139	0.1	0.5	8	163	0.8	2	0.02	0.02	0.4	0.05	2	0
12.7	10.1	38	110	—	1094	491	3	4.3	—	40	—	11	0.34	0.46	9.6	—	—	—
10.6	5.1	53	290	—	1144	409	3.8	4.1	—	—	—	19	0.28	0.46	8.8	—	—	—
6.3	3.5	29	70	—	1268	456	—	9.2	—	—	—	—	0.27	0.39	9.2	—	—	—
5.1	4.4	44	70	—	901	659	—	2.5	—	80	—	8	0.32	0.29	13.6	—	—	—
4.8	2.3	22	40	60	519	201	1.5	2.7	8	—	—	—	0.18	0.26	6.6	0.1	7	—
7.9	3.4	43	60	120	936	422	3.8	4.9	16	0	—	1	0.28	0.48	11	0.2	14	—
4.6	2	42	130	—	826	392	—	4.5	—	40	—	8	0.27	0.49	8.4	—	—	—
2.9	2.5	33	130	—	326	392	—	2.9	—	40	—	7	0.44	0.75	9.4	—	—	—
0.1	0.1	0	—	—	113	28	—	0.4	—	—	—	—	—	—	—	—	—	—
15.7	8.5	69	410	—	2062	565	—	4.3	—	100	—	11	0.92	0.49	8.2	—	—	—
13	6.8	73	410	—	1847	708	—	7.7	—	100	—	9	0.56	0.71	10.1	—	—	—
11.8	17	43	410	—	1847	708	—	7.7	—	100	—	9	0.56	0.71	14.2	—	—	—
6	7	51	400	—	2033	500	—	4.7	—	20	—	—	13.2	0.54	18.8	—	—	—
10	1.7	9	80	—	443	742	0.9	1.4	—	—	—	—	0.06	0.14	2	—	—	0
12	6.8	52	150	—	1166	321	3	6.1	—	—	—	1	0.42	0.63	9.8	—	—	—
7.6	1.5	0	20	—	167	724	0.6	1.4	—	0	—	—	0.06	0.07	2	—	—	0
9.8	10.4	46	180	—	1143	534	2.2	2.9	—	—	—	8	0.51	0.71	10.6	—	—	—
3	7.7	0	39	102	899	439	0.5	1.6	48	28	1.87	52	0.06	0.17	1.4	0.15	149	0
0	0.1	0	33	50	55	221	0.3	1.1	33	12	0.17	6	0.05	0.04	0.5	0.07	37	0
0	0.1	0	33	50	55	221	0.3	1.1	33	12	0.17	6	0.05	0.04	0.5	0.07	37	0
0	0	0	10	58	3	322	0.1	2.6	13	2	0.14	3	0.15	0.04	1	0.06	10	0
0	0.5	0	50	146	127	634	0.9	1.3	74	38	0.46	12	0.15	0.38	2.2	0.21	286	0
0	0.1	0	54	103	114	425	0.6	1.6	72	22	0.23	12	0.08	0.08	1.2	0.13	61	0
0	0	0	16	5	3	37	0	0.1	5	24	0.04	2	0	0.01	0	0.01	10	0
0	0	0	16	5	3	37	0	0.1	5	24	0.04	2	0	0.01	0	0.01	10	0
0	0.2	0	13	34	230	138	0.3	1.5	8	42	0.34	15	0.05	0.08	0.8	0.09	76	0
0	0.1	0	12	30	227	138	0.4	0.5	7	42	1.72	13	0.04	0.07	0.7	0.08	68	0
0	0.1	0	12	32	7	96	0.3	0.4	6	32	0.23	6	0.07	0.08	0.6	0.07	88	0
0	0.1	0	14	33	2	131	0.3	0.4	8	49	0.75	15	0.04	0.06	0.6	0.01	81	0
0	0.1	0	18	46	32	210	0.6	0.7	11	65	0.15	20	0.07	0.11	1	0.12	104	0
0	0.1	0	14	37	5	147	0.3	0.4	8	55	1.25	18	0.07	0.08	0.7	0.06	111	0
0	0.1	0	12	32	1	158	0.3	0.5	10	34	1.16	8	0.08	0.07	0.7	0.08	74	0
—	—	0	40	—	1100	—	—	2.7	—	0	—	—	—	—	—	—	—	—
—	—	0	40	—	1290	—	—	2.7	—	0	—	—	—	—	—	—	—	—
7.2	1.5	0	8	31	8	449	0.3	0.8	29	46	1.01	6	0.08	0.09	1.4	0.21	46	0
1	0.2	0	1	4	1	60	0	0.1	4	6	0.13	1	0.01	0.01	0.2	0.03	6	0
19.4	3.5	0	19	73	21	1096	0.7	2	71	106	2.32	14	0.19	0.21	3.3	0.48	113	0

A

Esha Code	Food Item	Qty	Meas	Wgt (g)	Wtr (g)	Cals	Prot (g)	Carb (g)	Fib (g)	Fat (g)	SatF (g)
3211	Avocado, California, mashed	0.5	cup	115	84	204	2	8	5.6	20	3
3212	Avocado, Florida	1	each	304	242	340	5	27	16.1	27	5.4
3213	Avocado, Florida, mashed	0.5	cup	115	92	129	2	10	6.1	10	2
3016	Avocado, average	1	each	201	149	324	4	15	10.1	31	4.9
60754	Baby Food, bananas, strained, Heinz	1	Tbs	16	12	16	0	4	0.3	0	0
60763	Baby Food, beef dinner supreme, stage 2, Beech-nut	1	each	128	106	147	2	9	1.1	10	—
60769	Baby Food, beef stew, toddler	1	Tbs	14	12	7	1	1	0.2	0	0.1
60765	Baby Food, carrots, stage 1, Beech-nut	1	oz.	28	26	12	0	2	1	0	0
60759	Baby Food, cereal, mixed, w/formula	1	Tbs	18	14	22	1	3	—	1	—
60761	Baby Food, cereal, rice w/fruit, Gerber	1	Tbs	14	12	11	0	3	0.1	0	—
60757	Baby Food, chicken w/broth, stage 1, jar, Beech-nut	1	each	71	59	70	8	0	0	3	—
60758	Baby Food, chicken-rice dinner, stage 2, Beech-nut	4	oz.	113	100	80	1	9	1	3	—
60755	Baby Food, peaches, strained, Heinz	1	Tbs	16	13	12	0	3	0.4	0	0
60762	Baby Food, pudding, cherry vanilla, Gerber	1	Tbs	14	12	10	0	2	0	0	—
60770	Baby Food, spaghetti w/meat sauce, toddler	1	Tbs	14	12	11	1	2	—	0	—
60766	Baby Food, sweet potatoes, stage 3, jar, Beech-nut	1	each	170	148	110	1	25	1	0	0
60756	Baby Food, tropical fruit medley, Gerber	1	Tbs	14	12	9	0	2	0	0	—
60764	Baby Food, turkey sticks, Gerber	1	each	10	8	13	1	0	0	1	0.3
60768	Baby Formulat, similac, liquid, 27cal/oz, Ross Labs	0.46	cup	114	95	100	3	10	—	5	—
12002	Bacon, Canadian style, grilled	2	piece	47	29	87	11	1	0	4	1.3
12000	Bacon, cooked, regular	3	piece	19	2	109	6	0	0	9	3.3
44061	Bagel chips	2	piece	28	1	119	2	21	2.2	3	0.5
42092	Bagel, 100% whole wheat	1	each	55	16	145	6	31	5.4	1	0.1
42100	Bagel, cinnamon raisin	1	each	71	23	195	7	39	1.6	1	0.2
42101	Bagel, cinnamon raisin, toasted	1	each	66	18	194	7	39	1.6	1	0.2
42041	Bagel, egg	1	each	71	23	197	8	38	1.6	1	0.3
42102	Bagel, egg, toasted	1	each	66	18	197	8	38	1.6	1	0.3
42103	Bagel, oat bran	1	each	71	23	181	8	38	2.6	1	0.1
42104	Bagel, oat bran, toasted	1	each	66	18	181	8	38	2.5	1	0.1
42000	Bagel, plain	1	each	68	22	187	7	36	1.6	1	0.2
42099	Bagel, plain, toasted	1	each	66	18	195	7	38	1.6	1	0.2
23119	Baking chips, butterscotch	0.5	cup	85	1	458	2	57	0	25	20.5
23120	Baking chips, peanut butter	0.5	cup	85	5	422	16	38	7.1	25	11.1
23121	Baking chips, white chocolate	0.5	cup	85	1	458	5	50	0	27	16.5
23180	Baking chocolate, bar, semi-sweet, Nestle	1	oz.	28	0	142	2	18	4	8	5.1
23179	Baking chocolate, bar, unsweetened, Nestle	1	oz.	28	0	162	4	9	6.1	14	4
28208	Baking chocolate, unsweetened, liquid, pkt	1	each	28	0	134	3	10	5.1	14	7.2
23178	Baking chocolate, unsweetened, premelted, ChocoBake	1	oz.	28	1	162	0	10	6.1	16	10.2
28059	Baking mix, reduced fat, Bisquick	1	cup	120	—	450	9	84	1.5	8	1.5
28004	Baking powder, double acting, Calumet	1	tsp	5	0	2	0	1	0	0	0
28005	Baking powder, double acting, Rumford	1	tsp	5	0	2	0	1	0	0	0
28006	Baking powder, low sodium	1	tsp	4	0	4	0	2	0.1	0	0
28003	Baking soda/sodium bicarbonate	1	tsp	5	0	0	0	0	0	0	0
45516	Baklava	1	piece	78	20	333	5	29	1.6	23	9.3
5403	Balsam pear, leaftips, cooked	0.5	cup	29	26	10	1	2	0.6	0	0
5405	Balsam pear, pods, cooked	0.5	cup	62	58	12	1	3	1.2	0	0
5401	Bamboo shoot, sliced, canned	0.5	cup	66	62	12	1	2	0.9	0	0.1
5230	Bamboo shoot, sliced, raw	0.5	cup	76	69	20	2	4	1.7	0	0.1
5249	Bamboo shoots, cooked slices	0.5	cup	60	58	7	1	1	0.6	0	0
5250	Bamboo shoots, cooked, whole	1	each	144	138	17	2	3	1.4	0	0.1
3020	Banana	1	each	114	85	105	1	27	2.7	1	0.2
3307	Banana chips, fried	0.5	cup	46	2	239	1	27	3.5	16	13.3
3325	Banana nectar	1	cup	250	202	177	1	46	1.4	0	0.2
3021	Banana slices	0.5	cup	75	56	69	1	18	1.8	0	0.1
2070	Banana split w/whipped cream	1	each	425	221	1076	15	120	1.2	66	37.9
23113	Banana, chocolate-covered, w/nuts	1	each	145	74	336	7	43	4.6	19	7
3023	Banana, dehydrated	0.5	cup	50	2	173	2	44	3.8	1	0.3
3306	Banana, ripe, fried	1	each	91	54	184	1	24	1.6	11	2.2
38003	Barley, pearled, cooked	0.5	cup	78	54	97	2	22	3	0	0.1
38002	Barley, pearled, dry	0.5	cup	100	10	352	10	78	15.6	1	0.2
38001	Barley, whole, cooked	0.5	cup	100	65	135	4	30	6.8	1	0.2
38000	Barley, whole, dry	0.5	cup	92	9	326	12	68	15.9	2	0.4
26001	Basil, dried	0.25	tsp	0	0	1	0	0	0.2	0	0
26046	Basil, fresh leaves	5	each	2	2	1	0	0	0.1	0	0
26045	Basil, fresh, chopped	1	Tbs	3	2	1	0	0	0.1	0	0

MonoF	PolyF	Choles	Calc	Phos	Sod	Pot	Zn	Iron	Magn	VitA	VitE	VitC	Thia	Ribo	Nia	B6	Fola	B12
(g)	(g)	(mg)	(mg)	(mg)	(mg)	(mg)	(mg)	(mg)	(mg)	(μg RE)	(mg α-TE)	(mg)	(mg)	(mg)	(mg)	(mg)	(μg)	(μg)
12.9	2.4	0	13	48	14	729	0.5	1.4	47	70	1.54	9	0.12	0.14	2.2	0.32	75	0
14.8	4.5	0	33	119	15	1483	1.3	1.6	103	185	2.37	24	0.33	0.37	5.8	0.85	162	0
5.6	1.7	0	13	45	6	561	0.5	0.6	39	70	0.9	9	0.12	0.14	2.2	0.32	61	0
19.3	3.9	0	22	82	20	1203	0.8	2	78	123	2.69	16	0.22	0.24	3.9	0.56	124	0
—	—	—	1	3	0	52	0	0.1	—	2	—	6	0	0.02	0.1	0.04	—	—
—	—	—	27	—	51	192	—	0.3	—	813	—	0	0.01	0.06	1	—	—	—
0.1	0	2	1	6	49	20	0.1	0.1	2	36	0.03	0	0	0.01	0.2	0.01	1	0.07
0	0	—	6	—	25	40	—	0	—	300	—	0	0	0	0.1	—	—	—
—	—	—	7	—	3	—	—	0.9	—	7	—	1	0.02	0.02	0.3	0.04	—	—
—	—	—	2	3	1	7	0.1	0.4	1	0	—	1	0.02	0.02	0.3	0.02	—	—
—	—	—	12	—	55	120	—	0.6	—	0	—	0	0.02	0.08	1.2	—	—	—
—	—	—	36	—	70	115	—	0.6	—	1260	—	0	0.02	0.03	0.6	—	—	—
—	—	—	1	1	0	34	0	0.1	—	16	—	10	0	0.01	0.2	0	—	—
—	—	—	1	1	1	6	—	0	0	0	—	0	0	0	0	0	—	—
—	—	—	3	6	51	23	0.1	0.1	2	12	—	1	0.01	0.01	0.2	0.01	5	0.03
0	0	—	12	—	15	360	—	0.3	—	855	—	0	0.03	0.04	0.5	—	—	—
—	—	—	1	0	1	6	—	0	1	2	—	2	0	0	0	0.01	—	—
—	—	9	10	13	43	12	0.2	0.1	1	0	—	0	0	0.02	0.2	0.01	—	—
—	—	—	90	70	34	132	0.8	0.2	7	90	2.01	9	0.1	0.15	1	0.06	15	0.25
1.9	0.4	27	5	139	727	183	0.8	0.4	10	0	0.12	0	0.39	0.09	3.2	0.21	2	0.37
4.5	1.1	16	2	64	303	92	0.6	0.3	5	0	0.1	0	0.13	0.05	1.4	0.05	1	0.33
0.8	1.4	0	4	58	168	67	0.4	0.6	16	0	0.19	0	0.05	0.05	0.6	0.08	23	0
0.1	0.3	0	16	159	270	190	1.3	1.8	59	0	0.49	0	0.17	0.14	2.8	0.18	40	0
0.1	0.5	0	14	71	229	105	0.8	2.7	20	6	0.11	0	0.27	0.2	2.2	0.04	64	0
0.1	0.5	0	13	55	228	108	0.5	2.7	15	5	0.12	0	0.22	0.18	2	0.04	51	0
0.3	0.5	17	9	60	359	48	0.5	2.8	18	23	0.1	0	0.38	0.17	2.4	0.06	62	0.11
0.3	0.5	17	9	59	358	48	0.5	2.8	18	21	0.07	0	0.3	0.15	2.2	0.06	11	0.11
0.2	0.3	0	9	78	360	82	0.6	2.2	22	0	0.1	0	0.24	0.24	2.1	0.03	58	0
0.2	0.3	0	9	117	360	145	1.5	2.2	41	0	0.17	0	0.19	0.22	1.9	0.13	23	0
0.1	0.5	0	50	65	363	69	0.6	2.4	20	0	0.03	0	0.37	0.21	3.1	0.04	60	0
0.1	0.5	0	53	68	379	72	0.6	2.5	20	0	0.02	0	0.31	0.2	2.9	0.03	50	0
1.9	0.4	0	29	27	76	159	0.1	0.1	4	0	1.91	0	0.07	0	0.1	0.01	1	0.08
8.2	4.5	0	94	264	213	429	1.7	1.4	94	2	2.55	0	0.04	0.17	7	0.19	82	0.05
7.7	0.9	18	169	150	76	243	0.6	0.2	10	3	1.91	0	0.05	0.24	0.6	0.05	14	0.52
—	—	0	0	—	0	109	—	0.7	—	0	—	0	0.02	0	0.2	—	—	—
5.2	0.7	0	0	—	0	239	—	0	—	0	—	0	0.03	0.04	0.4	—	—	—
2.6	3	0	15	96	3	331	1	1.2	75	0	1.71	0	0.01	0.08	0.6	0.02	5	0
—	—	0	0	—	0	—	—	1.5	—	0	—	0	0.04	0.04	0.4	—	—	—
—	—	0	120	—	1380	90	—	4.3	—	—	—	—	0.45	0.31	4.8	—	—	—
0	0	0	270	101	488	1	0	0.5	1	0	0	0	0	0	0	0	0	0
0	0	0	339	456	363	0	0	0.5	2	0	0	0	0	0	0	0	0	0
0	0	0	186	295	4	434	0	0.4	1	0	0	0	0	0	0	0	0	0
0	0	0	0	0	1258	0	0	0	0	0	0	0	0	0	0	0	0	0
8.5	3.8	36	34	88	291	139	0.5	1.7	34	124	1.99	1	0.17	0.13	1.3	0.05	9	0.02
0	0	0	12	22	4	175	0.1	0.3	27	50	0.14	16	0.04	0.08	0.3	0.22	25	0
0	0	0	6	22	4	198	0.5	0.2	10	7	0.43	20	0.03	0.03	0.2	0.02	32	0
0	0.1	0	5	16	5	52	0.4	0.2	3	1	0.25	1	0.02	0.02	0.1	0.09	2	0
0	0.1	0	10	44	3	402	0.8	0.4	2	2	0.76	3	0.11	0.05	0.5	0.18	5	0
0	0.1	0	7	12	2	320	0.3	0.1	2	0	0.4	0	0.01	0.03	0.2	0.06	1	0
0	0.1	0	17	29	6	768	0.7	0.3	4	0	0.96	0	0.03	0.07	0.4	0.14	3	0
0	0.1	0	7	23	1	451	0.2	0.4	33	9	0.31	10	0.05	0.11	0.6	0.66	22	0
0.9	0.3	0	8	26	3	247	0.3	0.6	35	4	2.48	3	0.04	0.01	0.3	0.12	6	0
0	0.1	0	8	18	5	347	0.2	0.3	27	7	0.24	8	0.04	0.09	0.5	0.5	17	0
0	0.1	0	4	15	1	297	0.1	0.2	22	6	0.2	7	0.03	0.08	0.4	0.43	14	0
18.8	5	209	468	477	354	779	2.7	1.5	89	545	0.49	2	0.15	0.9	0.5	0.17	19	1.41
7.5	3.2	0	28	153	7	596	1.8	1.4	93	8	1.92	9	0.1	0.19	3.3	0.63	42	0
0.1	0.2	0	11	37	2	746	0.3	0.6	54	16	0	4	0.09	0.12	1.4	0.22	7	0
4.8	3.4	0	10	23	120	366	0.2	0.3	30	142	1.89	6	0.04	0.1	0.5	0.53	10	0.01
0	0.2	0	9	42	2	73	0.6	1	17	1	0.04	0	0.06	0.05	1.6	0.09	13	0
0.1	0.6	0	29	221	9	280	2.1	2.5	79	2	0.13	0	0.19	0.11	4.6	0.26	23	0
0.1	0.6	0	13	115	1	115	0.8	1	22	0	0.6	0	0.08	0.03	1.4	0.09	8	0
0.3	1	0	30	243	11	416	2.6	3.3	122	2	0.55	0	0.59	0.26	4.2	0.29	18	0
0	0	0	8	2	0	13	0	0.2	2	4	0.01	0	0	0	0	0	1	0
0	0	0	4	2	0	12	0	0.1	2	10	—	0	0	0	0	0	2	0
0	0	0	4	2	0	12	0	0.1	2	10	—	0	0	0	0	0	2	0

A

Esha Code	Food Item	Qty	Meas	Wgt (g)	Wtr (g)	Cals	Prot (g)	Carb (g)	Fib (g)	Fat (g)	SatF (g)
26107	Bay leaf, crumbled	1	tsp	1	0	2	0	0	0.2	0	0
7084	Bean cake, Japanese style	1	each	32	7	130	2	16	0.9	7	1
7167	Bean paste, sweetened	1	oz.	28	13	60	2	14	1.5	0	0
5197	Bean sprouts, mung, canned, drained	0.5	cup	62	60	8	1	1	0.5	0	0
5021	Bean sprouts, mung, cooked, drained	0.5	cup	1	1	0	0	0	0	0	0
5020	Bean sprouts, mung, raw	0.5	cup	52	47	16	2	3	0.9	0	0
5246	Bean sprouts, mung, stir fried	0.5	cup	62	52	31	3	7	1.2	0	0
5240	Bean, Italian green, canned, drained, low sodium	0.5	cup	120	112	24	1	5	2.3	0	0
7031	Bean, winged/goabean, dry, cooked	0.5	cup	86	58	126	9	13	2.1	5	0.7
7000	Beans Garbanzo/Chickpeas, dry	0.25	cup	50	6	182	10	30	8.7	3	0.3
7035	Beans, Adzuki, canned, sweetened	0.5	cup	145	59	344	6	80	4.2	0	0
7034	Beans, Adzuki, cooked	0.5	cup	115	76	147	9	28	1	0	0
57054	Beans, B & M baked, fat free	0.5	cup	130	—	160	8	31	7	1	0
7001	Beans, Garbanzo/chickpea, cooked from dry	0.5	cup	82	49	134	7	22	6.2	2	0.2
5232	Beans, Italian green, canned, not drained, low sodi	0.5	cup	120	114	18	1	4	1.8	0	0
7022	Beans, Navy, dry, cooked	0.5	cup	91	58	129	8	24	5.8	1	0.1
7038	Beans, baked, canned, vegetarian	0.5	cup	127	92	118	6	26	6.4	1	0.1
7040	Beans, baked, canned, w/pork	0.5	cup	126	90	134	7	25	6.9	2	0.8
7037	Beans, baked, home prepared	0.5	cup	126	82	190	7	27	6.9	6	2.5
7085	Beans, baked, low sodium	0.5	cup	126	92	118	6	26	7	1	0.2
7042	Beans, black turtle soup, canned w/liquid	0.5	cup	120	91	109	7	20	8.3	0	0.1
7041	Beans, black turtle soup, cooked	0.5	cup	92	60	120	8	22	4.9	0	0.1
7012	Beans, black, dry, cooked, no added salt	0.5	cup	86	56	114	8	20	7.5	0	0.1
7027	Beans, broadbean/fava dry, cooked	0.5	cup	85	61	94	6	17	4.6	0	0.1
7055	Beans, broadbean/fava, canned w/liquid	0.5	cup	128	103	91	7	16	4.7	0	0
7043	Beans, cranberry, cooked	0.5	cup	88	57	120	8	22	8.8	0	0.1
7045	Beans, french, cooked	0.5	cup	86	57	111	6	21	8.1	1	0.1
7088	Beans, garbanzo/chickpeas, canned w/liquid	0.5	cup	120	84	143	6	27	5.3	1	0.1
7021	Beans, great northern, dry, cooked	0.5	cup	88	61	104	7	19	6.2	0	0.1
5016	Beans, green, Italian, canned, drained	0.5	cup	68	63	14	1	3	1.3	0	0
5017	Beans, green, Italian, canned, not drained	0.5	cup	120	114	18	1	4	1.8	0	0
5012	Beans, green, Italian, cooked	0.5	cup	62	56	22	1	5	2	0	0
5014	Beans, green, Italian, frozen, cooked, drained	0.5	cup	68	62	19	1	4	2	0	0
5010	Beans, green, Italian, raw	0.5	cup	55	50	17	1	4	1.9	0	0
5239	Beans, green, canned, drained, low sodium	0.5	cup	68	63	14	1	3	1.3	0	0
5231	Beans, green, canned, not drained, low sodium	0.5	cup	120	114	18	1	4	1.8	0	0
5571	Beans, green, seasoned, canned	0.5	cup	114	108	18	1	4	1.7	0	0.1
5015	Beans, green, snap/string, canned, drained	0.5	cup	68	63	14	1	3	1.3	0	0
5013	Beans, green, snap/string, frozen, cooked, drained	0.5	cup	68	62	19	1	4	2	0	0
5603	Beans, green, string, pickled	0.5	cup	68	61	19	1	4	1.1	0	0
5009	Beans, green/snap/string, raw	0.5	cup	55	50	17	1	4	1.9	0	0
5011	Beans, green/snap/string, raw, cooked	0.5	cup	62	56	22	1	5	2	0	0
7029	Beans, hyacinth, dry, cooked	0.5	cup	97	67	113	8	20	3.5	1	0.1
7046	Beans, kidney, California red, cooked	0.5	cup	88	59	109	8	20	8.2	0	0
7087	Beans, kidney, all, canned w/liquid	0.5	cup	128	100	104	7	19	4.5	0	0.1
7064	Beans, kidney, red, canned w/liquid, low sodium	0.5	cup	128	99	109	7	20	8.2	0	0.1
7135	Beans, kidney, red, canned, drained	0.5	cup	128	88	151	9	28	11.4	1	—
7047	Beans, kidney, red, cooked	0.5	cup	88	59	112	8	20	6.5	0	0.1
7049	Beans, kidney, royal red, cooked	0.5	cup	88	59	108	8	19	8.2	0	0
5527	Beans, lima, baby, canned, w/liquid, low sodium	0.5	cup	87	71	62	4	12	3.1	0	0.1
7009	Beans, lima, baby, dry	0.25	cup	48	6	159	10	30	9.8	0	0.1
7058	Beans, lima, baby, dry, cooked	0.5	cup	91	61	115	7	21	7	0	0.1
5019	Beans, lima, baby, frozen, cooked	0.5	cup	90	65	94	6	18	5.4	0	0.1
5193	Beans, lima, canned, drained	0.5	cup	85	57	82	5	16	3.7	0	0.1
5247	Beans, lima, fordhook, frozen, cooked	0.5	cup	85	62	85	5	16	4.9	0	0.1
5570	Beans, lima, immature, canned w/liquid	0.5	cup	124	101	88	5	16	4.5	0	0.1
5319	Beans, lima, immature, raw, cooked	0.5	cup	85	57	105	6	20	4.5	0	0.1
7011	Beans, lima, large, canned, not drained	0.5	cup	120	93	95	6	18	5.8	0	0
7010	Beans, lima, large, dry, cooked	0.5	cup	94	66	108	7	20	6.6	0	0.1
7059	Beans, mung, cooked, unsalted	0.5	cup	101	73	106	7	19	7.7	0	0.1
7061	Beans, mungo, cooked	0.5	cup	90	65	94	7	16	5.8	0	0
7050	Beans, pink, cooked	0.5	cup	84	51	125	8	23	4.4	0	0.1
7051	Beans, pinto, canned w/liquid	0.5	cup	120	93	103	6	18	5.5	1	0.2
7013	Beans, pinto, dry, cooked	0.5	cup	86	55	117	7	22	7.4	0	0.1
7007	Beans, red kidney, dry	0.25	cup	46	5	155	10	28	7	0	0.1

MonoF	PolyF	Choles	Calc	Phos	Sod	Pot	Zn	Iron	Magn	VitA	VitE	VitC	Thia	Ribo	Nia	B6	Fola	B12
(g)	(g)	(mg)	(mg)	(mg)	(mg)	(mg)	(mg)	(mg)	(mg)	(μg RE)	(mg α-TE)	(mg)	(mg)	(mg)	(mg)	(mg)	(μg)	(μg)
0	0	0	5	1	0	3	0	0.3	1	4	0.01	0	0	0	0	0.01	1	0
2.9	2.6	0	3	21	55	58	0.2	0.7	6	0	1.14	0	0.07	0.05	0.5	0.02	9	0
0	0	0	4	23	30	105	0.2	0.5	9	0	0.04	0	0.03	0.01	0.1	0.03	17	0
0	0	0	9	20	88	17	0.2	0.3	6	1	0.01	0	0.02	0.04	0.1	0.02	6	0
0	0	0	0	0	0	1	0	0	0	0	0	0	0	0	0	0	0	0
0	0	0	7	28	3	78	0.2	0.5	11	1	0	7	0.04	0.06	0.4	0.05	32	0
0	0	0	8	49	6	136	0.6	1.2	20	2	0.01	10	0.09	0.11	0.7	0.08	43	0
0	0.1	0	31	23	2	131	0.3	1.1	16	42	0.17	6	0.02	0.07	0.2	0.04	38	0
1.8	1.3	0	122	132	11	241	1.2	3.7	46	0	0.09	0	0.25	0.11	0.7	0.04	9	0
0.7	1.4	0	52	183	12	438	1.7	3.1	58	4	0.41	2	0.24	0.11	0.8	0.27	279	0
0	0	0	32	107	316	173	2.3	1.6	45	1	0.04	0	0.15	0.08	0.9	0.12	155	0
0	0	0	32	193	9	612	2	2.3	60	1	0.12	0	0.13	0.07	0.8	0.11	139	0
0	0.5	0	60	—	220	—	—	3.6	—	0	—	0	—	—	—	—	—	—
0.5	1	0	40	138	6	239	1.2	2.4	39	2	0.29	1	0.1	0.05	0.4	0.11	141	0
0	0.1	0	29	23	17	110	0.2	1.1	16	38	0.17	4	0.03	0.06	0.2	0.04	22	0
0	0.2	0	64	143	1	335	1	2.3	54	0	0.36	1	0.18	0.06	0.5	0.15	127	0
0	0.2	0	64	132	504	376	1.8	0.4	41	22	0.67	4	0.19	0.08	0.5	0.17	30	0
0.8	0.3	9	67	136	522	389	1.8	2.1	43	23	0.49	3	0.07	0.05	0.6	0.08	46	0
2.7	0.9	6	77	137	532	451	0.9	2.5	54	0	0.66	1	0.17	0.06	0.5	0.11	61	0
0.1	0.2	0	63	132	1	374	1.8	0.4	40	22	0.67	4	0.19	0.08	0.5	0.16	30	0
0	0.2	0	42	130	461	370	0.6	2.3	42	0	0.31	3	0.17	0.14	0.7	0.07	73	0
0	0.1	0	51	140	3	398	0.7	2.6	45	1	0.28	0	0.21	0.05	0.5	0.07	79	0
0	0.2	0	23	120	1	305	1	1.8	60	1	0.07	0	0.21	0.05	0.4	0.06	128	0
0.1	0.1	0	31	106	4	228	0.9	1.3	37	2	0.08	0	0.08	0.08	0.6	0.06	88	0
0.1	0.1	0	33	101	580	310	0.8	1.3	41	1	0.1	2	0.03	0.06	1.2	0.06	42	0
0	0.2	0	44	119	1	341	1	1.8	44	0	0.09	0	0.18	0.06	0.5	0.07	182	0
0	0.4	0	54	88	5	318	0.6	0.9	48	0	0.1	1	0.11	0.05	0.5	0.09	64	0
0.3	0.6	0	38	108	359	206	1.3	1.6	35	2	0.18	5	0.04	0.04	0.2	0.57	80	0
0	0.2	0	60	146	2	346	0.8	1.9	44	0	0.27	1	0.14	0.05	0.6	0.1	90	0
0	0	0	18	13	177	74	0.2	0.6	9	24	0.1	3	0.01	0.04	0.1	0.02	22	0
0	0.1	0	29	23	311	110	0.2	1.1	16	38	0.14	4	0.03	0.06	0.2	0.04	22	0
0	0.1	0	29	24	2	187	0.2	0.8	16	42	0.09	6	0.05	0.06	0.4	0.04	21	0
0	0.1	0	33	21	6	85	0.3	0.6	16	27	0.1	3	0.02	0.06	0.3	0.04	16	0
0	0	0	20	21	3	115	0.1	0.6	14	37	0.23	9	0.05	0.06	0.4	0.04	20	0
0	0	0	18	13	1	74	0.2	0.6	9	24	0.1	3	0.01	0.04	0.1	0.02	22	0
0	0.1	0	29	23	17	110	0.2	1.1	16	38	0.17	4	0.03	0.06	0.2	0.04	22	0
0	0.1	0	25	18	425	106	0.2	0.5	15	60	0.14	4	0.03	0.06	0.3	0.05	20	0
0	0	0	18	13	177	74	0.2	0.6	9	24	0.1	3	0.01	0.04	0.1	0.02	22	0
0	0.1	0	33	21	6	85	0.3	0.6	16	27	0.1	3	0.02	0.06	0.3	0.04	16	0
0	0	0	22	23	148	127	0.1	0.6	16	38	0.24	8	0.04	0.06	0.4	0.04	18	0
0	0	0	20	21	3	115	0.1	0.6	14	37	0.23	9	0.05	0.06	0.4	0.04	20	0
0	0.1	0	29	24	2	187	0.2	0.8	16	42	0.09	6	0.05	0.06	0.4	0.04	21	0
0.1	0.3	0	39	116	7	327	2.8	4.4	80	0	0.1	0	0.26	0.04	0.4	0.04	4	0
0	0	0	58	121	4	369	0.8	2.6	42	0	0.18	1	0.11	0.06	0.5	0.09	65	0
0	0.2	0	35	134	444	329	0.7	1.6	40	0	0.26	2	0.14	0.09	0.6	0.09	63	0
0	0.2	0	31	120	436	329	0.7	1.6	36	0	0.06	1	0.13	0.11	0.6	0.03	65	0
—	—	0	—	166	—	—	1	—	50	0	—	—	0.19	0.16	0.8	0.04	90	0
0	0.2	0	25	125	2	355	0.9	2.6	40	0	0.07	1	0.14	0.05	0.5	0.11	114	0
0	0.1	0	39	125	4	333	0.8	2.4	37	0	0.07	1	0.08	0.06	0.5	0.09	65	0
0	0.1	0	24	62	3	248	0.6	1.4	30	13	0.25	8	0.02	0.04	0.5	0.05	14	0
0	0.2	0	38	176	6	666	1.2	2.9	89	0	0.19	0	0.27	0.1	0.8	0.16	190	0
0	0.2	0	26	116	3	365	0.9	2.2	48	0	0.16	0	0.15	0.05	0.6	0.07	137	0
0	0.1	0	25	101	26	370	0.5	1.8	50	15	0.58	5	0.06	0.05	0.7	0.1	14	0
0	0.2	0	24	60	201	189	0.8	1.5	35	16	0.26	5	0.03	0.04	0.4	0.02	20	0
0	0.1	0	19	54	45	347	0.4	1.2	29	16	0.25	11	0.06	0.05	0.9	0.1	18	0
0	0.2	0	35	88	312	353	0.8	2	42	19	0.36	9	0.04	0.05	0.7	0.08	20	0
0	0.1	0	27	111	14	485	0.7	2.1	63	32	0.12	9	0.12	0.08	0.9	0.16	22	0
0	0.1	0	25	89	405	265	0.8	2.2	47	0	0.12	0	0.07	0.04	0.3	0.11	61	0
0	0.2	0	16	104	2	478	0.9	2.2	40	0	0.17	0	0.15	0.05	0.4	0.15	78	0
0.1	0.1	0	27	100	2	269	0.8	1.4	48	2	0.52	1	0.17	0.06	0.6	0.07	161	0
0	0.3	0	48	140	6	208	0.7	1.6	57	3	0.14	1	0.14	0.07	1.4	0.05	85	0
0	0.2	0	44	139	2	427	0.8	1.9	55	0	0.33	0	0.22	0.05	0.5	0.15	141	0
0.2	0.3	0	52	110	353	292	0.8	1.8	32	3	1.13	1	0.12	0.08	0.4	0.09	72	0
0.1	0.2	0	41	137	2	400	0.9	2.2	47	0	0.8	2	0.16	0.08	0.3	0.13	147	0
0	0.3	0	38	187	6	625	1.3	3.1	64	0	0.1	2	0.28	0.1	1	0.18	181	0

Esha Code	Food Item	Qty	Meas	Wgt (g)	Wtr (g)	Cals	Prot (g)	Carb (g)	Fib (g)	Fat (g)	SatF (g)
7008	Beans, red kidney, dry, cooked	0.5	cup	88	59	112	8	20	5.7	0	0.1
7082	Beans, red mexican, dry, cooked	0.5	cup	112	78	126	8	24	9	0	0.1
7024	Beans, refried/frijoles, canned	1	cup	253	192	238	14	39	13.4	3	1.2
7003	Beans, small white, dry, cooked	0.5	cup	90	57	127	8	23	9.3	1	0.1
7054	Beans, white, canned w/liquid	0.5	cup	131	92	153	10	29	6.3	0	0.1
7053	Beans, white, dry, cooked, unsalted	0.5	cup	90	57	125	9	23	5.7	0	0.1
7030	Beans, winged/goabean, dry, mature	0.5	cup	91	8	372	27	38	6.2	15	2.1
7033	Beans, yardlong, dry, cooked	0.5	cup	86	59	101	7	18	3.2	0	0.1
7032	Beans, yardlong, dry, mature	0.5	cup	84	7	290	20	52	9.2	1	0.3
5438	Beans, yellow snap, canned, low sodium	0.5	cup	68	63	14	1	3	0.9	0	0
5196	Beans, yellow wax, canned, drained	0.5	cup	68	63	14	1	3	0.9	0	0
5194	Beans, yellow wax, cooked, drained	0.5	cup	62	56	22	1	5	2.1	0	0
5195	Beans, yellow wax, frozen, cooked, drained	0.5	cup	68	62	19	1	4	2	0	0
7052	Beans, yellow, dry, cooked	0.5	cup	88	55	127	8	22	9.2	1	0.2
7036	Beans, yokan adzuki, confection, slices	3	piece	43	15	112	1	26	0.9	0	0
4642	Beechnuts, dried	1	oz.	28	2	163	2	10	1	14	1.6
56153	Beef & noodles, w/tomato sauce, Hamburger Helper	0.5	cup	124	93	140	15	10	1.4	4	1.4
56150	Beef (roast) hash	0.5	cup	95	65	158	11	10	1.1	8	2.5
10073	Beef cube steak, fried, lean	4	oz.	113	63	261	38	0	0	11	3.8
10051	Beef jerky	1	each	20	5	81	7	2	0.4	5	2.2
16234	Beef pot pie, Banquet	1	each	198	134	330	9	38	3	15	7
70734	Beef pot pie, Swanson	1	each	198	120	415	11	41	2	23	9
10077	Beef round steak, fried, lean	4	oz.	113	63	261	38	0	0	11	3.8
10078	Beef sirloin steak, fried, lean	4	oz.	113	63	261	38	0	0	11	3.8
11008	Beef stroganoff	0.5	cup	128	91	202	13	8	0.7	13	5.3
10021	Beef, London Broil, broiled, lean	1	piece	21	13	44	6	0	0	2	0.9
10021	Beef, London Broil, broiled, lean	3	oz.	85	52	176	23	0	0	9	3.7
10035	Beef, bacon, Sizzlean	2	piece	22	6	99	7	0	0	8	3.2
10057	Beef, bottom round, pot roast, braised, lean	3	oz.	85	49	178	27	0	0	7	2.4
10057	Beef, bottom round, pot roast, braised, lean	4	oz.	113	65	237	36	0	0	9	3.1
10036	Beef, brisket, corned, cooked, lean	1	piece	42	25	105	8	0	0	8	2.7
10036	Beef, brisket, corned, cooked, lean	3	oz.	85	51	213	16	0	0	16	5.4
10053	Beef, chuck, arm pot roast, braised, lean	3	oz.	85	49	184	28	0	0	7	2.6
10053	Beef, chuck, arm pot roast, braised, lean	4	oz.	113	66	245	37	0	0	9	3.4
10008	Beef, corned, canned	4	oz.	113	65	284	31	0	0	17	7
10081	Beef, cube steak, bread/flour fried, lean	4	oz.	113	54	313	30	12	0.7	15	4.5
10009	Beef, dried, cured 6	0.75	piece	28	16	47	8	0	0	1	0.5
10060	Beef, filet mignon steak, broiled, lean	4	oz.	113	68	239	32	0	0	11	4.2
10455	Beef, ground, baked, well done, extra lean	4	oz.	113	60	311	34	0	0	18	7.1
10722	Beef, ground, broiled, well done, extra lean	4	oz.	113	61	301	32	0	0	18	7
10032	Beef, ground, broiled, well done, lean	1	each	88	47	246	25	0	0	16	6.1
10724	Beef, ground, broiled, well done, lean	4	oz.	113	60	318	32	0	0	20	7.9
10463	Beef, ground, broiled, well done, regular	4	oz.	113	59	331	31	0	0	22	8.7
10030	Beef, ground, extra lean, broiled, well done	1	each	96	52	254	28	0	0	15	6
10461	Beef, ground, fried, well done, lean	4	oz.	113	61	314	31	0	0	20	7.9
10457	Beef, ground, fried, well, extra lean	4	oz.	113	61	298	32	0	0	18	7.1
10031	Beef, ground, patty, baked, well done, lean	1	each	88	45	257	26	0	0	16	6.3
10015	Beef, heart, simmered	4	oz.	113	73	198	33	0	0	6	1.9
10010	Beef, liver, fried	3	oz.	85	47	184	23	7	0	7	2.3
13000	Beef, lunchmeat, thin sliced	1	oz.	28	16	50	8	2	0	1	0.5
10052	Beef, meat stick, smoked	1	each	20	4	109	4	1	—	10	4.1
11018	Beef, meatloaf	1	piece	108	67	230	18	7	0.4	14	5
10028	Beef, porterhouse steak, choice, broiled, lean	1	each	170	102	366	44	0	0	20	6.9
10024	Beef, rib eye steak, broiled, lean	4	oz.	113	67	255	32	0	0	13	5.4
10056	Beef, rib steak, broiled, lean	4	oz.	113	66	251	32	0	0	13	5.1
10022	Beef, rib, whole, roasted, lean	1	piece	42	24	102	12	0	0	6	2.4
10022	Beef, rib, whole, roasted, lean	3	oz.	85	49	207	23	0	0	12	4.8
10002	Beef, rib, whole, roasted, lean & fat	3	oz.	85	39	320	19	0	0	26	10.7
10002	Beef, rib, whole, roasted, lean & fat	4	oz.	113	52	426	25	0	0	35	14.3
10004	Beef, roast, rump, braised, lean	3	oz.	85	50	167	27	0	0	6	2
10004	Beef, roast, rump, braised, lean	4	oz.	113	66	222	36	0	0	8	2.6
10003	Beef, roast, rump, braised, lean & fat	3	oz.	85	45	220	25	0	0	13	4.8
10003	Beef, roast, rump, braised, lean & fat	4	oz.	113	61	294	33	0	0	17	6.5
10069	Beef, round steak, fried, lean & fat	4	oz.	113	57	327	35	0	0	20	7.5
10058	Beef, round tip, sirloin roast, roasted, lean	4	oz.	113	74	210	32	0	0	8	2.7

MonoF	PolyF	Choles	Calc	Phos	Sod	Pot	Zn	Iron	Magn	VitA	VitE	VitC	Thia	Ribo	Nia	B6	Fola	B12
(g)	(g)	(mg)	(mg)	(mg)	(mg)	(mg)	(mg)	(mg)	(mg)	(μg RE)	(mg α-TE)	(mg)	(mg)	(mg)	(mg)	(mg)	(μg)	(μg)
0	0.2	0	25	126	2	357	0.9	2.6	40	0	0.19	1	0.14	0.05	0.5	0.11	115	0
0.1	0.2	0	42	139	240	369	0.9	1.9	48	0	0.08	2	0.13	0.07	0.4	0.12	94	0
1.4	0.4	20	89	218	756	676	3	4.2	84	0	0	15	0.07	0.04	0.8	0.36	28	0
0	0.2	0	65	151	2	414	1	2.5	61	0	0.36	0	0.21	0.05	0.2	0.11	123	0
0	0.2	0	96	119	7	595	1.5	3.9	67	0	0.24	0	0.13	0.05	0.1	0.1	86	0
0	0.1	0	81	102	5	505	1.2	3.3	57	0	0.2	0	0.11	0.04	0.1	0.08	73	0
5.5	3.9	0	400	410	35	889	4.1	12.2	163	0	0.26	0	0.94	0.41	2.8	0.16	41	0
0	0.2	0	36	155	4	269	0.9	2.3	84	2	0.24	0	0.18	0.06	0.5	0.08	125	0
0.1	0.5	0	115	467	14	966	2.9	7.2	282	4	0.24	1	0.74	0.2	1.8	0.31	549	0
0	0	0	18	13	1	74	0.2	0.6	9	7	0.2	3	0.01	0.04	0.1	0.02	22	0
0	0	0	18	13	169	74	0.2	0.6	9	7	0.2	3	0.01	0.04	0.1	0.02	22	0
0	0.1	0	29	24	2	187	0.2	0.8	16	5	0.18	6	0.05	0.06	0.4	0.04	21	0
0	0.1	0	33	21	6	85	0.3	0.6	16	7	0.1	3	0.02	0.06	0.3	0.04	16	0
0.1	0.4	0	55	161	4	286	0.9	2.2	65	0	0.44	2	0.16	0.09	0.6	0.11	71	0
0	0	0	12	17	36	19	0	0.5	8	0	0.02	0	0	0	0	0	4	0
6.2	5.7	0	0	0	11	288	0.1	0.7	0	0	—	4	0.09	0.1	0.2	0.19	32	0
1.7	0.3	47	13	144	343	390	2.4	2.1	28	50	0.8	6	0.13	0.16	2.9	0.32	10	1.39
2.9	1.7	29	10	103	427	294	2.5	1.2	18	0	0.62	4	0.08	0.1	1.9	0.25	8	0.91
4.6	1	110	9	317	345	555	6.1	3.9	38	0	0.16	0	0.14	0.34	5.6	0.63	13	4
2.2	0.2	10	4	81	438	118	1.6	1.1	10	0	0.1	0	0.03	0.03	0.3	0.04	26	0.2
—	—	25	20	—	1000	—	—	1.1	—	150	—	0	—	—	—	—	—	—
—	—	25	20	—	740	—	—	1.8	—	150	—	0	—	—	—	—	—	—
4.6	1	110	9	317	345	555	6.1	3.9	38	0	0.16	0	0.14	0.34	5.6	0.63	13	4
4.6	1	110	9	317	345	555	6.1	3.9	38	0	0.16	0	0.14	0.34	5.6	0.63	13	4
3.7	3.3	42	46	153	610	276	2.4	1.8	20	49	0.78	1	0.09	0.19	2.2	0.14	10	1.29
0.9	0.1	14	1	50	17	87	1	0.5	5	0	0.04	0	0.02	0.04	1.1	0.07	2	0.68
3.5	0.3	57	6	201	71	352	4.1	2.2	20	0	0.14	0	0.09	0.16	4.3	0.29	7	2.76
3.7	0.3	26	2	52	496	91	1.4	0.7	6	0	0.05	0	0.02	0.06	1.4	0.07	2	0.76
3	0.3	82	4	231	43	262	4.7	2.9	21	0	0.12	0	0.06	0.22	3.5	0.31	9	2.1
4.1	0.4	109	6	308	58	349	6.2	3.9	28	0	0.16	0	0.08	0.3	4.6	0.41	12	2.8
3.9	0.3	41	3	52	476	61	1.9	0.8	5	0	0.07	0	0.01	0.07	1.3	0.1	3	0.68
7.8	0.6	83	7	106	964	123	3.9	1.6	10	0	0.14	0	0.02	0.14	2.6	0.2	5	1.39
3	0.3	86	8	228	56	246	7.4	3.2	20	0	0.12	0	0.07	0.25	3.2	0.28	9	2.89
3.9	0.4	115	10	304	75	328	9.8	4.3	27	0	0.16	0	0.09	0.33	4.2	0.37	12	3.86
6.8	0.7	98	14	126	1140	154	4	2.4	16	0	0.17	0	0.02	0.17	2.8	0.15	10	1.84
5.5	3.7	86	36	260	386	438	5.7	4	35	3	0.55	0	0.17	0.34	4.4	0.44	14	3.23
0.5	0.1	12	2	49	986	126	1.5	1.3	9	0	0.04	0	0.02	0.06	1.6	0.1	3	0.76
4.3	0.4	95	8	270	71	475	6.3	4.1	34	0	0.16	0	0.15	0.34	4.4	0.5	8	2.91
7.9	0.7	121	10	184	73	330	7.9	3.4	25	0	0.2	0	0.06	0.35	6.1	0.33	12	2.11
7.8	0.7	112	10	215	93	418	7.3	3.1	28	0	0.2	0	0.08	0.36	6.6	0.36	12	2.9
6.8	0.6	89	11	160	78	307	5.5	2.2	21	0	0.18	0	0.05	0.21	5.2	0.26	10	2.39
8.8	0.7	115	14	206	101	396	7	2.8	27	0	0.23	0	0.07	0.27	6.8	0.34	12	3.08
9.7	0.8	115	14	217	105	371	6.6	3.1	25	0	0.26	0	0.04	0.24	7.3	0.34	11	3.72
6.6	0.6	95	9	182	79	354	6.2	2.7	24	0	0.17	0	0.07	0.31	5.6	0.31	11	2.46
8.8	0.7	108	12	205	99	386	6.7	2.8	26	0	0.22	0	0.07	0.27	6.2	0.36	11	2.93
7.9	0.7	105	9	210	92	408	7.1	3.1	27	0	0.2	0	0.08	0.34	6.2	0.35	11	2.63
7.1	0.6	87	11	144	62	252	5.7	2.3	18	0	0.18	0	0.06	0.21	4.8	0.23	11	1.99
1.4	1.6	219	7	284	71	264	3.6	8.5	28	0	0.82	2	0.16	1.75	4.6	0.24	2	16.2
1.4	1.4	410	9	392	90	309	4.6	5.3	20	9119	0.54	20	0.18	3.52	12.2	1.22	187	95.2
0.5	0.1	12	3	48	409	122	1.1	0.8	5	0	0.05	0	0.02	0.05	1.5	0.1	3	0.73
4.1	0.9	26	14	36	293	51	0.5	0.7	4	34	0.06	1	0.03	0.09	0.9	0.04	0	0.2
6	0.7	90	43	161	409	293	3.6	2	22	17	0.17	1	0.08	0.28	4	0.14	12	1.64
8.9	0.6	117	12	359	117	624	9	5.3	46	0	0.24	0	0.19	0.42	7.9	0.68	14	3.86
5.6	0.4	91	15	236	78	447	7.9	2.9	31	0	0.18	0	0.11	0.25	5.4	0.45	9	3.76
5.4	0.4	91	15	236	78	447	7.9	2.9	31	0	0.16	0	0.11	0.25	5.4	0.45	9	3.76
2.5	0.2	34	4	90	30	157	2.9	1.2	10	0	0.06	0	0.03	0.09	1.8	0.11	3	1.22
5	0.4	68	8	182	61	318	5.9	2.4	21	0	0.12	0	0.07	0.18	3.5	0.23	7	2.47
11.4	0.9	72	9	146	54	252	4.4	2	16	0	0.2	0	0.06	0.14	2.9	0.2	6	2.14
15.2	1.3	96	12	195	71	336	5.9	2.6	22	0	0.27	0	0.08	0.19	3.8	0.26	8	2.86
2.5	0.2	82	4	231	43	262	4.7	2.9	21	0	0.08	0	0.06	0.22	3.5	0.31	9	2.1
3.4	0.3	109	6	308	58	349	6.2	3.9	28	0	0.1	0	0.08	0.3	4.6	0.41	12	2.8
5.6	0.5	82	5	210	42	241	4.2	2.7	20	0	0.09	0	0.06	0.2	3.2	0.28	8	2.01
7.4	0.6	109	7	280	57	321	5.6	3.6	26	0	0.12	0	0.08	0.27	4.2	0.37	11	2.68
8.4	1.2	110	10	287	340	500	5.5	3.6	34	0	0.2	0	0.13	0.31	5.1	0.57	12	3.71
3.1	0.3	92	6	274	74	438	8	3.3	31	0	0.16	0	0.11	0.31	4.2	0.45	9	3.28

Esha Code	Food Item	Qty	Meas	Wgt (g)	Wtr (g)	Cals	Prot (g)	Carb (g)	Fib (g)	Fat (g)	SatF (g)
10014	Beef, round, bottom, braised, lean	1	piece	42	24	92	13	0	0	4	1.3
10014	Beef, round, bottom, braised, lean	3	oz.	85	48	187	27	0	0	8	2.7
10027	Beef, round, broiled, lean & fat	4	oz.	113	62	311	29	0	0	21	9.2
10016	Beef, round, pot roasted, lean & fat	1	piece	42	22	116	12	0	0	7	2.7
10016	Beef, round, pot roasted, lean & fat	3	oz.	85	44	234	24	0	0	14	5.4
10047	Beef, sandwich steak, Steak Ums	1	each	41	24	105	10	0	0	7	2.6
10026	Beef, short ribs, choice, braised, lean	2	each	102	51	301	31	0	0	18	7.9
10624	Beef, shortrib, braised, lean & fat	4	oz.	113	40	534	24	0	0	48	20.2
10005	Beef, sirloin steak, broiled, lean	1	each	156	96	315	47	0	0	12	4.8
10005	Beef, sirloin steak, broiled, lean	3	oz.	85	52	172	26	0	0	7	2.6
10064	Beef, sirloin strip steak, broiled, lean	4	oz.	113	68	235	32	0	0	11	4.1
10049	Beef, stew meat, cooked, lean & fat	4	oz.	113	57	345	32	0	0	23	9.2
10050	Beef, stew meat, cooked, lean only	0.5	cup	70	39	164	22	0	0	8	3
10007	Beef, t-bone steak, broiled, lean	1	each	184	113	377	49	0	0	19	6.6
10007	Beef, t-bone steak, broiled, lean	3	oz.	85	52	174	23	0	0	9	3.1
10006	Beef, t-bone steak, broiled, lean & fat	1	each	219	114	677	51	0	0	51	19.9
10006	Beef, t-bone steak, broiled, lean & fat	3	oz.	85	44	263	20	0	0	20	7.7
10061	Beef, tenderloin steak, broiled, lean	4	oz.	113	68	239	32	0	0	11	4.2
10059	Beef, top round steak, broiled, lean	4	oz.	113	70	204	36	0	0	6	1.9
10065	Beef, top sirloin steak, broiled, lean	4	oz.	113	70	221	34	0	0	8	3.2
10019	Beef, tripe, pickled	1	oz.	28	25	18	3	0	0	0	0.1
14008	Beefalo, roasted	4	oz.	113	70	213	35	0	0	7	3
22612	Beer, Lowenbrau Special	1	cup	237	—	105	1	10	—	0	0
22610	Beer, Lowenbrau dark, 12 fl oz	1	each	356	—	158	1	14	—	0	0
22627	Beer, Milwaukee's Best Ice	1	cup	237	—	90	1	5	—	0	0
22630	Beer, Red Dog	1	cup	237	—	98	0	9	—	0	0
22598	Beer, lager, bottled 355ml can	1	each	357	336	107	1	6	0.7	—	—
22512	Beer, light	1	cup	236	225	66	0	3	0	0	0
20276	Beer, non-alcoholic, Sharp's	1	cup	237	—	39	0	8	—	0	0
22500	Beer, regular, alcoholic	1	cup	237	219	97	1	9	0.5	0	0
13035	Beerwurst/beer salami	1	piece	23	12	76	3	0	0	7	3
5025	Beet greens, cooked, no added salt	0.5	cup	72	64	19	2	4	2.1	0	0
5605	Beets & onions, pickled	0.5	cup	84	72	42	1	10	1.2	0	0
5024	Beets, canned, drained	0.5	cup	85	77	26	1	6	1.4	0	0
5357	Beets, canned, w/liquid, low sodium	0.5	cup	123	113	34	1	8	1.5	0	0
5309	Beets, canned, w/liquid, regular	0.5	cup	123	113	34	1	8	1.5	0	0
5022	Beets, cooked, no added salt	0.5	cup	85	74	37	1	8	1.7	0	0
5310	Beets, pickled slices	0.5	cup	114	93	74	1	19	2.3	0	0
5573	Beets, raw slices	0.5	cup	68	60	29	1	6	1.9	0	0
5572	Beets, raw, whole	1	each	82	71	35	1	8	2.3	0	0
5538	Beets, w/Harvard sauce	0.5	cup	123	91	135	1	25	1.5	4	0.8
5023	Beets, whole, cooked, no added salt	2	each	100	87	44	2	10	2	0	0
5311	Beets, whole, pickled	1	each	50	41	32	0	8	1	0	0
45551	Berry turnover	1	each	78	25	277	3	36	1.4	14	3.4
42107	Biscuit dough, higher fat, chilled	1	oz.	28	10	90	2	12	0.4	4	1
42108	Biscuit dough, higher fat, chilled, baked	1	each	27	8	93	2	13	0.4	4	1
42110	Biscuit dough, lower fat, chilled, baked	1	each	21	6	63	2	12	0.4	1	0.3
42002	Biscuit mix, dry, prepared	1	each	28	8	95	2	14	0.5	3	0.8
42206	Biscuit, cheese	1	each	30	8	115	3	12	0.4	6	2.2
42001	Biscuit, homemade	1	each	28	8	101	2	13	0.4	5	1.2
42112	Biscuit, mixed grain, chilled, baked	1	each	41	11	125	3	23	1.1	3	0.7
42063	Biscuit, plain, fast food	1	each	74	20	276	4	34	1.4	13	8.7
42105	Biscuit, plain/buttermilk, baked	1	each	35	9	127	2	17	0.5	6	0.9
42205	Biscuit, whole wheat	1	each	63	17	201	6	29	4.8	8	2.2
14009	Bison, roasted	4	oz.	113	75	162	32	0	0	3	1
3024	Blackberries, fresh	0.5	cup	72	62	37	1	9	3.8	0	0
3028	Blackberries, frozen, unsweetened	0.5	cup	76	62	48	1	12	3.8	0	0
3027	Blackberry, canned w/heavy syrup	0.5	cup	128	96	118	2	30	4.4	0	0
5115	Blackeyed cowpeas, frozen, cooked	0.5	cup	85	56	112	7	20	5.4	1	0.1
5213	Blackeyed peas, cooked from raw, drained	0.5	cup	82	62	80	3	17	4.1	0	0.1
49018	Blintz, fruit-filled	1	each	70	44	124	4	17	0.4	5	1.4
3030	Blueberries, canned w/heavy syrup	0.5	cup	128	98	113	1	28	1.9	0	0
3029	Blueberries, fresh	0.5	cup	72	61	41	0	10	2	0	0
3231	Blueberries, frozen, sweetened, pkg	0.5	cup	115	89	93	0	25	2.4	0	0
3031	Blueberries, frozen, unsweetened	0.5	cup	78	67	40	0	9	2.1	0	0

MonoF	PolyF	Choles	Calc	Phos	Sod	Pot	Zn	Iron	Magn	VitA	VitE	VitC	Thia	Ribo	Nia	B6	Fola	B12
(g)	(g)	(mg)	(mg)	(mg)	(mg)	(mg)	(mg)	(mg)	(mg)	(μg RE)	(mg α-TE)	(mg)	(mg)	(mg)	(mg)	(mg)	(μg)	(μg)
1.7	0.2	40	2	114	21	129	2.3	1.4	10	0	0.08	0	0.03	0.11	1.7	0.15	5	1.04
3.5	0.3	82	4	231	43	262	4.7	2.9	21	0	0.15	0	0.06	0.22	3.5	0.31	9	2.1
10.5	0.9	95	8	239	68	415	4.7	2.7	27	0	0.29	0	0.1	0.23	4.2	0.5	10	3.12
3.1	0.3	40	3	103	21	118	2.1	1.3	9	0	0.08	0	0.03	0.1	1.6	0.14	4	0.99
6.2	0.5	82	5	208	42	240	4.2	2.6	19	0	0.16	0	0.06	0.2	3.2	0.28	8	2
3	0.2	33	3	66	29	128	2.2	1	9	0	0.07	0	0.02	0.11	1.9	0.11	4	0.82
8.1	0.6	95	11	240	59	319	8	3.4	22	0	0.14	0	0.07	0.21	3.3	0.29	7	3.53
21.4	1.7	107	14	184	57	254	5.5	2.6	17	0	0.33	0	0.06	0.17	2.8	0.25	6	2.97
5.3	0.5	139	17	381	103	629	10.2	5.2	50	0	0.22	0	0.2	0.45	6.7	0.7	16	4.45
2.9	0.3	76	9	207	56	343	5.5	2.9	27	0	0.12	0	0.11	0.25	3.6	0.38	8	2.42
4.3	0.4	86	9	247	77	449	5.9	2.8	31	0	0.16	0	0.1	0.23	6.1	0.48	9	2.27
10.1	0.8	113	12	248	333	285	8.5	3.5	23	0	0.2	0	0.08	0.27	3.3	0.32	8	2.78
3.4	0.3	71	7	172	208	193	6.1	2.5	16	0	0.1	0	0.06	0.19	2.2	0.21	5	1.83
8.3	0.6	109	11	396	131	696	9.8	5.8	52	0	0.26	0	0.2	0.46	8.5	0.72	15	4.18
3.8	0.3	50	5	183	60	321	4.5	2.7	24	0	0.12	0	0.09	0.21	3.9	0.33	7	1.93
22.3	1.8	147	18	403	140	703	9.8	5.9	50	0	0.46	0	0.2	0.46	8.6	0.72	15	4.66
8.7	0.7	57	7	156	54	273	3.8	2.3	20	0	0.18	0	0.08	0.18	3.4	0.28	6	1.81
4.3	0.4	95	8	270	71	475	6.3	4.1	34	0	0.16	0	0.15	0.34	4.4	0.5	8	2.91
2.2	0.2	95	7	279	69	501	6.3	3.3	35	0	0.16	0	0.14	0.31	6.8	0.64	14	2.81
3.5	0.3	101	12	277	75	457	7.4	3.8	36	0	0.16	0	0.15	0.33	4.8	0.51	11	3.23
0.1	0	19	36	24	13	5	0.5	0.5	2	0	0.03	0	0	0.04	0.5	0	0	0.26
3	0.2	66	27	284	93	521	7.3	3.5	0	0	0.2	10	0.03	0.12	5.6	0.45	20	2.89
0	0	0	—	—	5	—	—	—	—	—	—	—	—	—	—	—	—	0
0	0	0	—	—	7	—	—	—	—	—	—	—	—	—	—	—	—	0
0	0	0	—	—	3	—	—	—	—	—	—	—	—	—	—	—	—	0
0	0	0	—	—	3	—	—	—	—	—	—	—	—	—	—	—	—	0
—	—	0	14	—	14	121	0	—	—	—	—	0	—	0.07	—	0.07	14	0.5
0	0	0	12	28	7	42	0.1	0.1	12	0	0	0	0.02	0.07	0.9	0.08	10	0.02
0	0	0	—	—	2	—	—	—	—	—	—	—	—	—	—	—	—	0
0	0	0	12	28	12	59	0	0.1	14	0	0	0	0.01	0.06	1.1	0.12	14	0.05
3.2	0.3	14	2	22	236	40	0.6	0.3	3	0	0.04	0	0.02	0.03	0.8	0.04	1	0.45
0	0	0	82	30	174	654	0.4	1.4	49	367	0.22	18	0.08	0.21	0.4	0.1	10	0
0	0	0	8	21	209	211	0.2	0.5	27	1	0.22	3	0.02	0.01	0.2	0.02	27	0
0	0	0	13	14	165	126	0.2	1.6	14	1	0.26	3	0.01	0.03	0.1	0.05	26	0
0	0	0	16	20	26	175	0.3	0.8	20	4	0.37	3	0.01	0.05	0.2	0.07	36	0
0	0	0	16	20	310	162	0.3	0.8	20	4	0.35	3	0.01	0.05	0.2	0.07	36	0
0	0.1	0	14	32	66	259	0.3	0.7	20	3	0.26	3	0.02	0.03	0.3	0.06	68	0
0	0	0	12	19	301	169	0.3	0.5	17	1	0.15	3	0.01	0.06	0.3	0.06	30	0
0	0	0	11	27	53	221	0.2	0.5	16	3	0.2	3	0.02	0.03	0.2	0.05	74	0
0	0	0	13	33	64	265	0.3	0.7	19	3	0.24	4	0.02	0.03	0.3	0.06	89	0
1.7	1.2	0	12	30	287	288	0.2	0.7	36	53	0.87	5	0.03	0.02	0.2	0.03	45	0
0	0.1	0	16	38	77	305	0.4	0.8	23	4	0.3	4	0.03	0.04	0.3	0.07	80	0
0	0	0	6	8	132	74	0.1	0.2	8	0	0.06	1	0	0.02	0.1	0.02	13	0
6.1	3.7	0	6	32	230	54	0.2	1.3	8	2	1.51	3	0.18	0.13	1.5	0.02	6	0
2.1	0.5	0	5	100	314	41	0.1	0.7	4	0	0.51	0	0.11	0.06	0.9	0.01	16	0
2.2	0.5	0	5	104	325	42	0.1	0.7	4	0	0.49	0	0.09	0.06	0.8	0.01	12	0
0.6	0.2	0	4	98	305	39	0.1	0.6	4	0	0.14	0	0.09	0.05	0.7	0.01	14	0
1.2	1.2	1	52	133	271	53	0.2	0.6	7	7	0.11	0	0.1	0.1	0.9	0.02	2	0.06
2.4	1.2	6	80	70	197	42	0.3	0.7	6	17	0.43	0	0.1	0.1	0.8	0.01	3	0.04
2	1.2	1	67	47	165	34	0.2	0.8	5	7	0.37	0	0.1	0.09	0.8	0.01	17	0.02
1.4	0.4	0	8	158	319	217	0.3	1.3	14	0	0.57	0	0.15	0.09	1.5	0.02	4	0
3.4	0.5	5	90	260	584	87	0.3	1.6	9	24	0.44	0	0.27	0.18	1.6	0.03	6	0.1
2.4	2.2	0	17	151	368	78	0.2	1.2	6	0	1.03	0	0.15	0.1	1.2	0.02	21	0.05
3	1.9	4	120	177	468	200	1.2	1.5	56	9	0.98	0	0.14	0.12	2.2	0.13	13	0.06
1.1	0.3	93	9	237	65	409	4.2	3.9	30	0	0.16	0	0.11	0.31	4.2	0.45	9	3.24
0	0.2	0	23	15	0	141	0.2	0.4	14	12	0.51	15	0.02	0.03	0.3	0.04	24	0
0	0.2	0	22	23	1	106	0.2	0.6	17	8	0.54	2	0.02	0.04	0.9	0.05	26	0
0	0.1	0	27	18	4	127	0.2	0.8	22	28	0.91	4	0.04	0.05	0.4	0.05	34	0
0.1	0.2	0	20	104	4	319	1.2	1.8	42	7	0.33	2	0.22	0.05	0.6	0.08	120	0
0	0.1	0	106	42	3	345	0.8	0.9	43	65	0.18	2	0.08	0.12	1.2	0.05	105	0
1.8	1	50	33	56	151	75	0.3	0.8	6	78	0.69	1	0.05	0.13	0.3	0.04	8	0.2
0.1	0.2	0	6	13	4	51	0.1	0.4	5	8	1.28	1	0.04	0.07	0.1	0.05	2	0
0	0.1	0	4	7	4	64	0.1	0.1	4	7	0.72	9	0.04	0.04	0.3	0.03	5	0
0	0.1	0	7	8	1	69	0.1	0.4	2	5	0.82	1	0.02	0.06	0.3	0.07	8	0
0.1	0.2	0	6	9	1	42	0.1	0.1	4	6	0.78	2	0.02	0.03	0.4	0.05	5	0

Esha Code	Food Item	Qty	Meas	Wgt (g)	Wtr (g)	Cals	Prot (g)	Carb (g)	Fib (g)	Fat (g)	SatF (g)
13002	Bologna, beef	1	piece	23	13	72	3	0	0	7	2.8
13006	Bologna, beef & pork	1	piece	28	15	90	3	1	0	8	3
13032	Bologna, cured pork	1	piece	23	14	57	4	0	0	5	1.6
13007	Bologna, turkey	1	piece	28	18	56	4	0	0	4	1.4
3032	Boysenberries, canned w/heavy syrup	0.5	cup	128	98	113	1	28	3.3	0	0
3026	Boysenberries, fresh	0.5	cup	72	62	37	1	9	3.8	0	0
3034	Boysenberries, frozen, unsweetened	0.5	cup	66	57	33	1	8	2.6	0	0
13079	Bratwurst, cooked link	1	each	85	48	256	12	2	0	22	7.9
42004	Bread crumbs, dry, grated, plain	0.25	cup	25	2	99	3	18	0.6	1	0.3
42144	Bread crumbs, seasoned, dry, grated	0.25	cup	30	2	110	4	21	1.3	1	0.2
42009	Bread crumbs, soft	0.25	cup	11	4	30	1	6	0.2	1	0.2
42036	Bread stick, w/o salt coating, plain	10	each	100	6	412	12	68	3	10	1.4
42035	Bread stick, w/salt coating	1	each	35	2	134	4	26	0.8	1	0.2
42038	Bread stuffing, homemade	1	cup	203	132	341	8	45	4	15	3
42037	Bread stuffing, mix, prepared	1	cup	140	91	249	4	30	4.1	12	2.4
42467	Bread, 7-grain, Pepperidge Farm	1	piece	38	15	100	3	18	2	2	0
42171	Bread, Armenian	1	piece	20	7	55	2	10	0.6	1	0.1
42172	Bread, Armenian, toasted	1	piece	18	5	55	2	10	0.6	1	0.1
42052	Bread, Boston brown, canned	1	piece	45	21	88	2	20	2.1	1	0.1
42173	Bread, Cuban-Spanish-Portuguese	1	piece	20	6	58	2	11	0.5	1	0.1
42174	Bread, Cuban-Spanish-Portuguese, toasted	1	piece	18	3	61	2	12	0.6	1	0.1
42043	Bread, French	1	piece	35	12	96	3	18	1	1	0.2
42132	Bread, Hollywood, dark	1	piece	18	7	39	2	8	1.4	0	0.1
42133	Bread, Hollywood, dark, toasted	1	piece	16	6	39	2	8	—	0	0.1
42134	Bread, Hollywood, light	1	piece	18	7	41	2	8	0.9	0	0
42135	Bread, Hollywood, light, toasted	1	piece	16	6	40	2	8	—	0	0
42118	Bread, Indian fry, 5 inch diameter	1	piece	90	24	296	6	48	1.6	9	2.1
42046	Bread, Italian	1	piece	30	11	81	3	15	0.8	1	0.3
42120	Bread, Italian, toasted	1	piece	27	8	80	3	15	0.8	1	0.3
42189	Bread, Spanish coffee	1	each	85	21	292	7	49	1.6	7	1.1
42039	Bread, banana, homemade, w/margarine	1	piece	50	15	163	2	27	0.6	5	1.1
42113	Bread, banana, recipe, w/vegetable shortening, 1/18	1	piece	60	17	203	3	33	0.8	7	1.8
42191	Bread, barley	1	piece	26	10	69	2	13	1.2	1	0.3
42175	Bread, batter	1	piece	33	12	93	3	15	0.6	2	0.7
42194	Bread, buckwheat	1	piece	27	10	71	2	13	1	1	0.3
42195	Bread, buckwheat, toasted	1	piece	25	7	73	2	14	1	1	0.3
42086	Bread, cheese	1	piece	26	10	71	2	12	0.6	1	0.5
42088	Bread, cheese, toasted	1	piece	24	7	71	2	12	0.6	1	0.5
42176	Bread, corn & molasses	1	piece	32	12	86	2	15	0.6	2	0.6
42177	Bread, corn & molasses, toasted	1	piece	29	9	87	2	15	0.6	2	0.6
42042	Bread, cracked wheat	1	piece	25	9	65	2	12	1.4	1	0.2
42053	Bread, cracked wheat, toasted	1	piece	21	6	59	2	11	1.3	1	0.2
42203	Bread, crumpet biscuit	1	each	45	24	80	3	17	0.8	0	0.1
42204	Bread, crumpet biscuit, toasted	1	each	41	19	82	3	18	0.8	0	0.1
42484	Bread, dark pumpernickel, Pepperidge Farm	1	piece	32	12	80	3	15	1	1	0.5
42211	Bread, date nut	1	piece	56	12	217	3	30	0.8	10	2.2
42090	Bread, egg/challah	1	piece	23	8	66	2	11	0.5	1	0.4
42091	Bread, egg/challah, toasted	1	piece	21	6	66	2	11	0.5	1	0.3
42210	Bread, fruit, w/o nuts	1	piece	41	10	150	2	23	0.5	6	1.5
42209	Bread, hoecake, 1/8 pone	1	piece	61	29	136	3	25	3.6	3	0.7
42178	Bread, milk & honey	1	piece	28	10	74	2	15	0.6	1	0.2
42179	Bread, milk & honey, toasted	1	piece	29	9	84	2	17	0.6	1	0.2
42047	Bread, mixed grain	1	piece	25	9	62	2	12	1.6	1	0.2
42048	Bread, mixed grain, toasted	1	piece	23	7	63	3	12	1.5	1	0.2
42097	Bread, multigrain, low calorie, high fiber	1	piece	23	10	46	2	10	2.8	1	0
42098	Bread, multigrain, low calorie, high fiber, toasted	1	piece	21	8	47	2	10	2.8	1	0
42069	Bread, oat bran	1	piece	30	13	71	3	12	1.4	1	0.2
42076	Bread, oat bran, low calorie	1	piece	28	13	56	2	12	3.4	1	0.1
42077	Bread, oat bran, low calorie, toasted	1	piece	25	9	60	2	12	3.6	1	0.1
42121	Bread, oat bran, toasted	1	piece	27	10	70	3	12	1.3	1	0.2
42049	Bread, oatmeal	1	piece	25	9	67	2	12	1	1	0.2
42125	Bread, oatmeal, low calorie	1	piece	23	10	48	2	10	—	1	0.1
42126	Bread, oatmeal, low calorie, toasted	1	piece	19	6	48	2	10	—	1	0.1
42050	Bread, oatmeal, toasted	1	piece	23	7	67	2	12	1	1	0.2
42087	Bread, onion cheese	1	piece	26	10	71	2	12	0.6	1	0.5

MonoF	PolyF	Choles	Calc	Phos	Sod	Pot	Zn	Iron	Magn	VitA	VitE	VitC	Thia	Ribo	Nia	B6	Fola	B12
(g)	(g)	(mg)	(mg)	(mg)	(mg)	(mg)	(mg)	(mg)	(mg)	(μg RE)	(mg α-TE)	(mg)	(mg)	(mg)	(mg)	(mg)	(μg)	(μg)
3.2	0.3	13	3	20	226	36	0.5	0.4	3	0	0.04	0	0.01	0.02	0.6	0.04	1	0.33
3.8	0.7	16	3	26	289	51	0.6	0.4	3	0	0.06	0	0.05	0.04	0.7	0.05	1	0.38
2.2	0.5	14	3	32	272	65	0.5	0.2	3	0	0.06	0	0.12	0.04	0.9	0.06	1	0.21
1.4	1.2	28	24	37	249	56	0.5	0.4	4	0	0.15	0	0.02	0.05	1	0.06	2	0.08
0	0.1	0	23	13	4	115	0.2	0.6	14	5	0.91	8	0.03	0.04	0.3	0.05	44	0
0	0.2	0	23	15	0	141	0.2	0.4	14	12	0.51	15	0.02	0.03	0.3	0.04	24	0
0	0.1	0	18	18	1	92	0.1	0.6	11	5	0.3	2	0.04	0.02	0.5	0.04	42	0
10.4	2.3	51	37	127	473	180	2	1.1	13	0	0.21	1	0.43	0.16	2.7	0.18	2	0.81
0.6	0.3	0	57	37	216	55	0.3	1.5	12	0	0.14	0	0.19	0.11	1.7	0.02	27	0
0.3	0.2	0	30	40	795	81	0.3	1	11	1	0.04	0	0.05	0.05	0.8	0.04	33	0.01
0.2	0.1	0	9	11	57	12	0.1	0.3	2	0	0.02	0	0.04	0.03	0.4	0	4	0
3.6	3.6	0	22	121	657	124	0.9	4.3	32	0	1.48	0	0.59	0.55	5.3	0.07	122	0
0.4	0.3	1	10	35	586	32	0.2	1.5	7	0	0.04	0	0.23	0.18	2.2	0.01	4	0
6.5	4.3	0	130	100	936	266	0.6	3.3	30	140	2.44	3	0.34	0.29	3.2	0.11	34	0
5.3	3.6	0	45	59	760	104	0.4	1.5	17	113	1.96	0	0.19	0.15	2.1	0.06	141	0.01
0.5	0	0	0	—	180	—	—	0.7	—	0	—	0	0.12	0.07	1.2	—	—	—
0.1	0.3	0	16	15	117	15	0.2	0.6	5	0	0.05	0	0.08	0.05	0.7	0.01	5	0
0.1	0.3	0	16	15	116	15	0.2	0.6	5	0	0.04	0	0.06	0.05	0.7	0.01	4	0
0.1	0.3	0	32	50	284	143	0.2	0.9	28	5	0.25	0	0.01	0.05	0.5	0.04	5	0
0.2	0.2	0	9	17	116	18	0.1	0.6	4	0	0.02	0	0.08	0.05	0.7	0.01	6	0
0.2	0.2	0	9	18	121	19	0.1	0.6	4	0	0.01	0	0.07	0.05	0.7	0.01	6	0
0.4	0.2	0	26	37	213	40	0.3	0.9	9	0	0.1	0	0.18	0.12	1.7	0.02	33	0
0.1	0.2	0	139	29	92	36	0.3	0.6	12	0	0.02	0	0.08	0.07	0.7	0.02	5	0
0.1	0.2	0	137	29	91	36	0.3	0.6	12	0	0.02	0	0.06	0.06	0.6	0.02	4	0
0.1	0.2	0	130	15	124	34	0.2	0.6	7	0	0.04	0	0.08	0.06	0.7	0.01	4	0
0.1	0.1	0	128	14	123	34	0.2	0.6	7	0	0.03	0	0.06	0.05	0.7	0	3	0.01
3.6	2.3	0	210	141	626	67	0.4	3.2	14	0	0.7	0	0.39	0.27	3.3	0.02	67	0
0.2	0.4	0	23	31	175	33	0.3	0.9	8	0	0.11	0	0.14	0.09	1.3	0.01	28	0
0.2	0.4	0	23	31	173	33	0.3	0.9	8	0	0.05	0	0.11	0.08	1.2	0.01	6	0
4.8	0.8	32	12	81	12	82	0.5	2.6	14	15	1.08	0	0.34	0.31	3	0.05	34	0.06
2.2	1.6	22	10	29	151	67	0.2	0.7	7	60	0.9	1	0.09	0.1	0.7	0.08	16	0.05
3	1.8	26	11	34	119	79	0.2	0.8	8	14	0.84	1	0.1	0.12	0.9	0.09	7	0.05
0.3	0.3	1	10	31	96	39	0.3	0.7	8	2	0.06	0	0.09	0.08	1.1	0.02	9	0.01
0.9	0.5	14	20	41	127	50	0.2	0.9	7	9	0.25	0	0.12	0.13	1	0.03	13	0.05
0.4	0.3	1	11	38	100	57	0.3	0.8	18	2	0.12	0	0.1	0.08	1.2	0.04	10	0.01
0.4	0.3	1	11	40	103	59	0.3	0.8	19	2	0.12	0	0.1	0.08	1.2	0.04	11	0.01
0.4	0.3	2	38	32	144	30	0.2	0.7	7	4	0.02	0	0.12	0.09	1	0.01	9	0.01
0.4	0.3	1	38	32	145	30	0.2	0.7	6	4	0.02	0	0.1	0.09	1	0.01	7	0.01
0.7	0.4	2	27	35	261	100	0.2	0.9	16	6	0.17	0	0.11	0.11	1	0.05	11	0.03
0.7	0.4	2	27	35	263	101	0.2	0.9	16	6	0.17	0	0.11	0.11	1	0.06	11	0.03
0.5	0.2	0	11	38	135	44	0.3	0.7	13	0	0.15	0	0.09	0.06	0.9	0.08	15	0
0.4	0.2	0	10	35	123	40	0.3	0.6	12	0	0.13	0	0.07	0.05	0.8	0.06	6	0.01
0	0.2	0	50	72	324	37	0.2	0.4	7	0	0.02	0	0.08	0.01	0.4	0.02	4	0
0	0.2	0	51	74	332	38	0.2	0.5	7	0	0.02	0	0.08	0.01	0.4	0.02	4	0
0	0.5	0	20	—	230	—	—	1.1	—	0	—	0	0.12	0.07	1.2	—	—	—
3.8	3.5	28	47	54	140	100	0.3	1	15	14	0.88	1	0.12	0.12	0.9	0.12	9	0.05
0.5	0.3	12	21	24	113	26	0.2	0.7	4	5	0.14	0	0.1	0.1	1.1	0.02	24	0.02
0.6	0.2	12	21	25	113	26	0.2	0.7	4	5	0.18	0	0.08	0.09	1	0.01	19	0.02
2.5	1.5	22	34	32	109	62	0.2	0.7	7	11	0.61	1	0.08	0.09	0.7	0.08	5	0.04
1.2	1	0	69	94	245	94	0.6	1.1	41	0	0.27	0	0.1	0.06	1.1	0.09	6	0
0.1	0.2	1	10	29	53	35	0.2	0.9	5	2	0.08	0	0.12	0.1	1	0.02	13	0.01
0.1	0.3	1	12	33	60	40	0.2	1	6	2	0.1	0	0.11	0.12	1.2	0.03	13	0.01
0.4	0.2	0	23	44	122	51	0.3	0.9	13	0	0.16	0	0.1	0.09	1.1	0.08	20	0.02
0.4	0.2	0	23	44	122	51	0.3	0.9	13	0	0.15	0	0.08	0.08	1	0.08	16	0.02
0	0.1	2	18	57	117	40	0.5	0.6	20	0	0.04	0	0.1	0.07	0.9	0.03	14	0
0	0.1	2	18	58	118	40	0.5	0.6	20	0	0.04	0	0.08	0.07	0.9	0.03	12	0
0.5	0.5	0	20	42	122	44	0.3	0.9	10	0	0.19	0	0.15	0.1	1.4	0.02	24	0
0.2	0.5	0	16	39	98	29	0.3	0.9	15	0	0.13	0	0.1	0.06	1	0.03	18	0
0.2	0.5	0	17	36	105	30	0.3	0.9	14	0	0.13	0	0.08	0.05	1	0.02	14	0
0.5	0.5	0	19	31	121	33	0.3	0.9	9	0	0.12	0	0.12	0.09	1.3	0.01	19	0
0.4	0.4	0	16	32	150	36	0.3	0.7	9	0	0.15	0	0.1	0.06	0.8	0.02	16	0.01
0.2	0.3	0	26	23	89	28	0.2	0.5	6	0	0.09	0	0.08	0.06	0.7	0.01	13	0.02
0.2	0.3	0	26	27	88	35	0.2	0.5	6	0	0.08	0	0.06	0.06	0.6	0.01	5	0.03
0.4	0.4	0	17	32	150	35	0.3	0.7	9	0	0.09	0	0.08	0.05	0.7	0.02	12	0
0.4	0.3	2	38	32	144	30	0.2	0.7	7	4	0.02	0	0.12	0.09	1	0.01	9	0.01

Esha Code	Food Item	Qty	Meas	Wgt (g)	Wtr (g)	Cals	Prot (g)	Carb (g)	Fib (g)	Fat (g)	SatF (g)
42089	Bread, onion cheese, toasted	1	piece	24	7	71	2	12	0.6	1	0.5
42007	Bread, pita pocket, white	1	each	60	19	165	5	33	1.3	1	0.1
42080	Bread, pita pocket, whole wheat	1	each	45	14	120	4	25	3.3	1	0.2
42081	Bread, pita, 100% whole wheat, toasted	1	each	41	9	120	5	26	4.7	1	0.1
42180	Bread, potato	1	piece	26	10	69	2	13	0.6	1	0.2
42181	Bread, potato, toasted	1	piece	24	7	70	2	13	0.6	1	0.2
42122	Bread, protein	1	piece	19	8	47	2	8	0.6	0	0.1
42123	Bread, protein, toasted	1	piece	17	6	46	2	8	0.6	0	0.1
42006	Bread, pumpernickel	1	piece	32	12	80	3	15	2.1	1	0.1
42054	Bread, pumpernickel, toasted	1	piece	29	9	80	3	15	2.1	1	0.1
42051	Bread, raisin	1	piece	25	8	68	2	13	1.1	1	0.3
42055	Bread, raisin, toasted	1	piece	21	6	62	2	12	1	1	0.2
42200	Bread, rice	1	piece	25	9	79	2	10	0.6	4	0.4
42129	Bread, rice bran, low calorie	1	piece	27	11	66	2	12	1.3	1	0.2
42130	Bread, rice bran, toasted, low calorie	1	piece	25	9	66	2	12	1.3	1	0.2
42201	Bread, rice, toasted	1	piece	23	6	81	2	10	0.6	4	0.4
42005	Bread, rye	1	piece	25	9	65	2	12	1.4	1	0.2
42056	Bread, rye, light, toasted	1	piece	22	7	62	2	12	1.4	1	0.2
42127	Bread, rye, low calorie	1	piece	23	11	47	2	9	2.8	1	0.1
42128	Bread, rye, low calorie, toasted	1	piece	19	7	46	2	9	—	1	0.1
42045	Bread, sourdough	1	piece	25	9	68	2	13	0.8	1	0.2
42003	Bread, sourdough starter	1	Tbs	16	10	22	1	4	0.3	0	0
42075	Bread, sourdough, toasted	1	piece	23	7	68	2	13	0.8	1	0.2
42196	Bread, soy	1	piece	26	10	69	3	12	0.7	1	0.4
42197	Bread, soy, toasted	1	piece	24	7	71	3	12	0.7	1	0.4
42078	Bread, sprouted wheat	1	piece	26	10	68	2	12	1.4	1	0.2
42198	Bread, sunflower meal	1	piece	27	10	75	3	12	0.5	1	0.5
42199	Bread, sunflower meal, toasted	1	piece	25	7	76	3	12	0.5	1	0.5
42182	Bread, sweet potato	1	piece	25	8	72	2	12	0.6	2	0.3
42192	Bread, triticale	1	piece	25	9	63	2	12	1.6	1	0.2
42193	Bread, triticale, toasted	1	piece	23	7	64	2	12	1.7	1	0.2
42044	Bread, vienna	1	piece	25	9	68	2	13	0.8	1	0.2
42012	Bread, wheat	1	piece	28	10	74	3	13	1.2	1	0.3
42013	Bread, wheat berry	1	piece	26	10	68	2	12	1.1	1	0.2
42032	Bread, wheat berry, toasted	1	piece	24	8	68	2	12	1.3	1	0.2
42136	Bread, wheat bran	1	piece	36	14	89	3	17	1.4	1	0.3
42137	Bread, wheat bran, toasted	1	piece	33	10	90	3	17	1.4	1	0.3
42095	Bread, wheat, low calorie, thin sliced	1	piece	23	10	46	2	10	2.8	1	0.1
42096	Bread, wheat, low calorie, thin sliced, toasted	1	piece	21	7	50	2	11	2.8	1	0.1
42031	Bread, wheat, toasted	1	piece	25	8	70	2	13	1.3	1	0.2
42217	Bread, white, composite, firm & soft, toasted	1	piece	23	7	67	2	12	0.6	1	0.2
42216	Bread, white, compostite, firm & soft	1	piece	25	9	67	2	12	0.6	1	0.2
42011	Bread, white, firm	1	piece	33	12	91	3	17	0.7	1	0.4
42028	Bread, white, firm, toasted	1	piece	29	7	93	3	17	0.8	1	0.4
42084	Bread, white, low calorie, thin sliced	1	piece	20	9	41	2	9	1.9	0	0.1
42085	Bread, white, low calorie, thin sliced, toasted	1	piece	18	6	44	2	9	2	1	0.1
42138	Bread, white, recipe, w/2% milk	1	piece	42	15	120	3	21	0.8	2	0.5
42139	Bread, white, recipe, w/2% milk, toasted	1	piece	38	11	119	3	21	0.8	2	0.5
42140	Bread, white, recipe, w/nonfat dry milk	1	piece	44	15	121	3	24	0.9	1	0.2
42141	Bread, white, recipe, w/nonfat dry milk, toasted	1	piece	40	11	120	3	24	0.9	1	0.2
42008	Bread, white, soft	0.25	cup	8	3	20	1	4	0.2	0	0.1
42010	Bread, white, soft	1	piece	28	10	76	2	14	0.6	1	0.4
42030	Bread, white, soft, toasted	1	piece	24	6	75	2	14	0.6	1	0.3
42073	Bread, white, very low sodium	1	piece	26	10	69	2	13	0.6	1	0.2
42074	Bread, white, very low sodium, toasted	1	piece	24	7	70	2	13	0.6	1	0.2
42014	Bread, whole wheat	1	piece	35	13	86	3	16	2.4	1	0.3
42142	Bread, whole wheat, recipe	1	piece	23	8	64	2	12	1.4	1	0.2
42143	Bread, whole wheat, recipe, toasted	1	piece	42	11	128	4	24	2.8	2	0.4
42029	Bread, whole wheat, toasted	1	piece	29	9	80	3	15	2.2	1	0.3
3239	Breadfruit, raw	0.5	cup	110	78	113	1	30	5.4	0	0.1
23226	Breath Savers, spearmint breath mints	1	each	2	—	10	0	0	0	0	0
5678	Broccoflower, raw	0.5	cup	50	45	16	1	3	1.6	0	0
5679	Broccoflower, steamed	0.5	cup	78	70	25	2	5	2.5	0	0
5557	Broccoli floweret, raw	5	each	55	50	15	2	3	1.6	0	0
5028	Broccoli pieces, cooked, no added salt	0.5	cup	78	71	22	2	4	2.3	0	0

MonoF	PolyF	Choles	Calc	Phos	Sod	Pot	Zn	Iron	Magn	VitA	VitE	VitC	Thia	Ribo	Nia	B6	Fola	B12
(g)	(g)	(mg)	(mg)	(mg)	(mg)	(mg)	(mg)	(mg)	(mg)	(μg RE)	(mg α-TE)	(mg)	(mg)	(mg)	(mg)	(mg)	(μg)	(μg)
0.4	0.3	1	38	32	145	30	0.2	0.7	6	4	0.02	0	0.1	0.09	1	0.01	7	0.01
0.1	0.3	0	52	58	322	72	0.5	1.6	16	0	0.02	0	0.36	0.2	2.8	0.02	57	0
0.2	0.5	0	7	81	239	76	0.7	1.4	31	0	0.41	0	0.15	0.04	1.3	0.12	22	0
0.1	0.3	0	13	133	173	161	1.1	1.5	50	0	0.43	0	0.14	0.12	2.3	0.15	34	0
0.3	0.3	0	30	27	143	30	0.2	0.8	6	0	0.01	0	0.12	0.09	1	0.01	9	0
0.3	0.3	0	31	27	145	31	0.2	0.8	7	0	0.01	0	0.1	0.09	1	0.01	8	0
0	0.2	0	24	35	104	61	0.3	0.8	12	0	0.07	0	0.07	0.08	0.8	0.01	20	0
0	0.2	0	23	32	102	59	0.2	0.8	10	0	0.01	0	0.05	0.07	0.7	0.01	13	0
0.3	0.4	0	22	57	215	67	0.5	0.9	17	0	0.14	0	0.1	0.1	1	0.04	26	0
0.3	0.4	0	22	57	214	66	0.5	0.9	17	0	0.17	0	0.08	0.09	0.9	0.04	20	0
0.6	0.2	0	16	27	98	57	0.2	0.7	6	0	0.13	0	0.08	0.1	0.9	0.02	22	0
0.5	0.2	0	15	25	89	52	0.2	0.7	6	0	0.17	0	0.06	0.08	0.7	0.01	16	0
0.6	2.7	0	3	52	69	93	0.3	0.3	14	0	1.32	0	0.05	0.04	0.9	0.08	19	0
0.4	0.5	0	19	48	119	58	0.4	1	22	0	0.22	0	0.18	0.08	1.8	0.07	18	0
0.4	0.5	0	19	44	120	53	0.3	1	19	0	0.2	0	0.14	0.07	1.7	0.05	14	0
0.6	2.8	0	3	53	71	96	0.3	0.3	15	0	1.36	0	0.05	0.05	0.9	0.08	20	0
0.3	0.2	0	18	31	165	42	0.3	0.7	10	0	0.09	0	0.11	0.08	1	0.02	22	0
0.3	0.2	0	18	30	160	40	0.3	0.7	9	0	0.13	0	0.08	0.07	0.8	0.02	16	0
0.2	0.2	0	18	18	93	22	0.2	0.7	5	0	0.06	0	0.08	0.06	0.6	0.02	11	0.01
0.2	0.2	0	17	19	92	22	0.2	0.7	4	0	0.03	0	0.07	0.05	0.5	0.01	4	0.02
0.3	0.2	0	19	26	152	28	0.2	0.6	7	0	0.07	0	0.13	0.08	1.2	0.01	24	0
0	0	0	8	18	3	26	0.1	0.3	2	4	0.02	0	0.06	0.07	0.5	0.01	16	0.02
0.3	0.2	0	19	26	152	28	0.2	0.6	7	0	0.06	0	0.1	0.07	1.1	0.01	19	0
0.4	0.3	1	23	44	74	110	0.2	0.9	14	3	0.07	0	0.1	0.08	0.9	0.03	12	0.02
0.4	0.3	1	24	46	76	112	0.2	0.9	14	3	0.07	0	0.1	0.09	1	0.03	13	0.02
0.3	0.4	0	23	33	138	35	0.4	0.7	13	0	0.28	0	0.09	0.06	0.8	0.02	7	0
0.5	0.4	1	17	40	61	34	0.3	0.8	13	3	0.12	0	0.15	0.09	1.2	0.03	10	0.02
0.5	0.4	1	17	40	62	34	0.3	0.8	13	3	0.12	0	0.16	0.1	1.2	0.03	10	0.02
0.6	0.4	14	5	28	228	40	0.2	0.8	5	50	0.3	1	0.09	0.1	0.9	0.03	14	0.03
0.2	0.4	0	22	47	136	52	0.4	0.7	17	0	0.06	0	0.07	0.04	0.7	0.02	12	0
0.2	0.4	0	22	47	137	53	0.4	0.7	17	0	0.07	0	0.06	0.04	0.7	0.02	10	0
0.3	0.2	0	19	26	152	28	0.2	0.6	7	0	0.07	0	0.13	0.08	1.2	0.01	24	0
0.5	0.3	0	30	43	151	57	0.3	0.9	13	0	0.15	0	0.12	0.08	1.2	0.03	22	0
0.4	0.2	0	27	39	138	52	0.3	0.9	12	0	0.14	0	0.11	0.07	1.1	0.02	20	0
0.4	0.2	0	27	39	138	52	0.3	0.9	12	0	0.14	0	0.09	0.07	1	0.02	16	0
0.6	0.2	0	27	67	175	82	0.5	1.1	29	0	0.17	0	0.14	0.1	1.6	0.06	25	0
0.6	0.2	0	27	67	176	82	0.5	1.1	29	0	0.24	0	0.12	0.09	1.4	0.06	7	0
0.1	0.2	0	18	24	118	28	0.3	0.7	9	0	0.03	0	0.1	0.07	0.9	0.03	16	0
0.1	0.2	0	20	23	128	31	0.2	0.7	7	0	0.04	0	0.08	0.07	0.9	0.03	5	0.02
0.5	0.2	0	28	41	144	54	0.3	0.9	12	0	0.15	0	0.09	0.07	1	0.02	16	0
0.4	0.2	0	27	24	136	30	0.2	0.8	6	0	0.07	0	0.1	0.08	0.9	0.01	19	0
0.4	0.2	0	27	24	135	30	0.2	0.8	6	0	0.1	0	0.12	0.08	1	0.02	24	0.01
0.5	0.2	1	32	34	163	40	0.2	0.9	7	0	0.25	0	0.13	0.08	1.1	0.01	12	0
0.5	0.2	1	32	34	163	40	0.2	0.9	7	0	0.26	0	0.11	0.08	1.1	0.01	12	0
0.2	0.1	0	19	24	91	15	0.3	0.6	5	0	0.03	0	0.08	0.06	0.7	0.01	19	0.06
0.2	0.1	0	20	29	97	16	0.3	0.7	6	0	0.04	0	0.07	0.06	0.7	0.01	5	0.05
0.5	1.2	1	24	48	151	61	0.3	1.2	8	9	0.36	0	0.17	0.16	1.5	0.02	38	0.03
0.5	1.2	1	24	48	150	61	0.3	1.2	8	8	0.46	0	0.14	0.14	1.4	0.02	12	0.03
0.2	0.6	0	14	42	148	49	0.3	1.4	7	5	0.17	0	0.19	0.16	1.6	0.02	37	0.01
0.2	0.6	0	14	42	148	49	0.3	1.4	8	5	0.16	0	0.15	0.14	1.5	0.01	8	0.01
0.1	0.1	0	6	7	38	8	0	0.2	2	0	0.01	0	0.03	0.02	0.2	0	3	0
0.5	0.2	1	24	28	143	30	0.2	0.8	6	0	0.05	0	0.11	0.07	0.9	0.01	10	0
0.3	0.2	1	24	27	142	30	0.2	0.8	6	0	0.05	0	0.09	0.07	0.9	0.01	10	0
0.4	0.2	0	28	24	7	31	0.2	0.8	6	0	0.1	0	0.12	0.09	1	0.02	25	0.01
0.4	0.2	0	29	25	7	31	0.2	0.8	6	0	0.08	0	0.1	0.08	0.9	0.02	23	0
0.6	0.4	0	25	80	184	88	0.7	1.2	30	0	0.3	0	0.12	0.07	1.3	0.06	18	0
0.3	0.7	0	8	43	80	72	0.3	0.7	19	0	0.31	0	0.07	0.05	0.9	0.05	14	0
0.5	1.4	0	15	86	160	145	0.7	1.4	37	0	0.67	0	0.11	0.1	1.6	0.08	24	0
0.5	0.3	0	24	75	172	82	0.6	1.1	28	0	0.34	0	0.09	0.06	1.1	0.05	10	0
0	0.1	0	19	33	2	539	0.1	0.6	28	4	1.23	32	0.12	0.03	1	0.11	15	0
0	0	0	—	—	0	0	—	—	—	—	—	—	—	—	—	—	—	—
0	0.1	0	16	32	12	161	0.2	0	10	4	0.15	37	0.04	0.05	0.4	0.1	28	0
0	0.1	0	25	50	18	251	0.4	0.5	16	5	0.23	49	0.06	0.07	0.6	0.14	38	0
0	0.1	0	26	36	15	179	0.2	0.5	14	165	0.91	51	0.04	0.06	0.4	0.09	39	0
0	0.1	0	36	46	20	228	0.3	0.7	19	108	1.32	58	0.04	0.09	0.4	0.11	39	0

A

Esha Code	Food Item	Qty	Meas	Wgt (g)	Wtr (g)	Cals	Prot (g)	Carb (g)	Fib (g)	Fat (g)	SatF (g)
5030	Broccoli pieces, frozen, cooked, no added salt	0.5	cup	92	83	26	3	5	2.8	0	0
5026	Broccoli pieces, raw	0.5	cup	44	40	12	1	2	1.3	0	0
5653	Broccoli pieces, steamed	0.5	cup	62	56	17	2	3	1.9	0	0
5654	Broccoli pieces, stir fried	0.5	cup	78	71	22	2	4	2.3	0	0
5029	Broccoli spears, cooked, no added salt	1	each	180	163	50	5	9	5.2	1	0.1
5234	Broccoli spears, frozen, cooked	1	piece	30	27	8	1	2	0.9	0	0
5027	Broccoli spears, raw	1	each	151	137	42	4	8	4.5	1	0.1
6445	Broccoli, Chinese, Gai Lan	4	oz.	113	104	34	3	5	—	0	—
5513	Broccoli, batter-dipped, fried	0.5	cup	42	32	61	2	4	1	4	0.7
5456	Broccoli, cooked w/cheese sauce	0.5	cup	114	92	110	6	6	2	7	3.5
5558	Broccoli, stalk only, raw	0.5	cup	44	40	12	1	2	1.4	0	0
50305	Broth, beef, fat free, Health Valley	4	oz.	113	111	14	2	1	0	0	0
50193	Broth, chicken, dry, cube	1	each	5	0	10	1	1	0	0	0.1
50034	Broth, chicken, dry, prepared	0.5	cup	122	118	11	1	1	0	1	0.1
47030	Brownie, mix, low calorie, low sodium, prepared	1	each	22	3	84	1	16	0.8	2	1.1
47028	Brownie, mix, w/nuts, prepared	1	each	33	4	140	1	20	0.9	7	1.4
47323	Brownie, peanut butter fudge, Weight Watchers	1	each	35	8	110	2	21	3	2	0.5
47000	Brownie, w/nuts	1	each	25	3	101	1	16	0.5	4	1.1
47019	Brownie, w/walnuts, homemade	1	each	20	3	93	1	10	0.4	6	1.5
5034	Brussels sprouts, cooked, drained	4	each	84	73	33	2	7	2.2	0	0.1
5033	Brussels sprouts, cooked, drained, cup measure	0.5	cup	78	68	30	2	7	2	0	0.1
5035	Brussels sprouts, frozen, cooked	0.5	cup	78	67	33	3	6	3.2	0	0.1
5032	Brussels sprouts, raw	4	each	76	65	33	3	7	2.9	0	0
5031	Brussels sprouts, raw, cup measure	0.5	cup	44	38	19	1	4	1.7	0	0
38073	Buckwheat groats, roasted/cooked	0.5	cup	99	75	91	3	20	2.7	1	0.1
38072	Buckwheat, w/outside skin	0.5	cup	85	8	292	11	61	8.5	3	0.6
38028	Bulgur wheat, cooked	0.5	cup	91	71	76	3	17	4.1	0	0
42020	Bun, hamburger	1	each	45	15	129	4	23	1.2	2	0.5
42163	Bun, hamburger/hot dog, low calorie, extra fiber	1	each	43	20	84	4	18	2.7	1	0.1
42162	Bun, hamburger/hot dog, mixed grain	1	each	43	16	113	4	19	1.6	3	0.4
42021	Bun, hotdog/frankfurter	1	each	40	14	114	3	20	1.1	2	0.5
57002	Burger King, BK broiler, chicken sandwich	1	each	248	146	550	30	41	2	29	6
56354	Burger King, Whopper sandwich	1	each	270	157	640	27	45	3	39	11
56355	Burger King, Whopper sandwich, w/cheese	1	each	294	167	730	33	46	3	46	16
57001	Burger King, cheeseburger, double	1	each	213	104	609	42	28	1	36	17.2
56360	Burger King, chicken sandwich	1	each	229	104	710	26	54	2	43	9
56362	Burger King, fish fillet sandwich, Ocean Catch	1	each	255	130	700	26	56	3	41	6
57000	Burger King, whopper Jr. w/cheese	1	each	180	96	468	23	30	2	28	10.2
56999	Burger King, whopper junior sandwich	1	each	168	90	430	22	30	2	25	8.2
45591	Burrito, apple, small	1	each	155	55	484	5	73	—	20	9.6
56629	Burrito, bean & cheese	2	each	186	100	378	15	55	—	12	6.8
57283	Burrito, black bean, Life Choice	1	each	374	269	410	12	86	13	2	0
70756	Burrito, sausage, Great Starts	1	each	99	52	240	9	24	1	12	4
8133	Butter replacement, dry (Butter Buds)	1	Tbs	5	0	19	0	4	0	0	0
8160	Butter, lightly salted	1	Tbs	14	2	102	0	0	0	12	7.2
8000	Butter, regular, salted	1	Tbs	14	2	100	0	0	0	11	7.1
8001	Butter, regular, salted, pat	1	each	5	1	36	0	0	0	4	2.5
8025	Butter, unsalted	1	Tbs	14	3	102	0	0	0	12	7.2
8142	Butter, whipped	1	Tbs	9	2	68	0	0	0	8	4.8
8135	Butter/vegetable oil blend, Blue Bonnet spread	1	Tbs	14	2	102	0	0	0	12	4
5412	Butterbur (fuki), canned pieces	0.5	cup	62	61	2	0	0	—	0	—
5410	Butterbur (fuki), raw	0.5	cup	47	44	7	0	2	0.6	0	—
5411	Butterbur (fuki), stalks, cooked	3	each	45	44	4	0	1	0.6	0	—
7	Buttermilk, skim, cultured	1	cup	245	221	99	8	12	0	2	1.3
4643	Butternuts, dried	1	oz.	28	1	174	7	3	1.3	16	0.4
23184	Butterscotch morsels, Toll House	0.25	cup	42	0	243	0	30	0	12	12.3
5671	Cabbage, Chinese, steamed	0.5	cup	85	81	11	1	2	0.8	0	0
5608	Cabbage, Japanese, pickled	0.5	cup	75	69	16	1	3	2.3	0	0
5237	Cabbage, bok choy, cooked, drained	0.5	cup	85	81	10	1	2	1.4	0	0
5041	Cabbage, bok choy, shredded, raw	0.5	cup	35	33	5	1	1	0.4	0	0
5039	Cabbage, head, cooked, no added salt, drained	1	each	1262	1181	278	13	56	29	5	0.7
5037	Cabbage, head, raw	1	each	908	837	227	13	49	20.9	2	0.3
5535	Cabbage, kim chee style	0.5	cup	75	69	16	1	3	0.9	0	0
5609	Cabbage, mustard, salted	0.5	cup	64	59	13	1	3	2	0	0
5040	Cabbage, pe tsai, chopped, raw	0.5	cup	38	36	6	0	1	1.2	0	0

MonoF (g)	PolyF (g)	Choles (mg)	Calc (mg)	Phos (mg)	Sod (mg)	Pot (mg)	Zn (mg)	Iron (mg)	Magn (mg)	VitA (μg RE)	VitE (mg α-TE)	VitC (mg)	Thia (mg)	Ribo (mg)	Nia (mg)	B6 (mg)	Fola (μg)	B12 (μg)
0	0.1	0	47	51	22	166	0.3	0.6	18	174	1.52	37	0.05	0.08	0.4	0.12	52	0
0	0.1	0	21	29	12	143	0.2	0.4	11	68	0.73	41	0.03	0.05	0.3	0.07	31	0
0	0.1	0	30	41	17	201	0.2	0.5	16	91	0.3	49	0.04	0.07	0.4	0.09	37	0
0	0.1	0	37	51	21	253	0.3	0.7	20	108	0.37	62	0.05	0.09	0.5	0.12	44	0
0	0.3	0	83	106	47	526	0.7	1.5	43	250	3.04	134	0.1	0.2	1	0.26	90	0
0	0	0	15	16	7	54	0.1	0.2	6	57	0.31	12	0.02	0.02	0.1	0.04	9	0
0	0.3	0	72	100	41	491	0.6	1.3	38	233	2.51	141	0.1	0.18	1	0.24	107	0
—	—	—	—	—	—	—	—	—	—	186	—	32	—	—	—	—	—	0
1.1	2.4	8	34	35	31	121	0.2	0.5	10	51	1.05	27	0.04	0.07	0.4	0.06	22	0.03
2.4	1	15	148	128	365	269	0.7	0.8	24	176	0.76	57	0.06	0.17	0.5	0.13	41	0.18
0	0.1	0	21	29	12	143	0.2	0.4	11	18	0.73	41	0.03	0.05	0.3	0.07	31	0
0	0	0	0	—	76	93	—	0	—	0	—	2	—	—	0.5	—	—	—
0.1	0.1	1	9	9	1152	18	0	0.1	3	4	0.04	0	0.01	0.02	0.2	0	2	0.01
0.2	0.2	0	7	6	742	12	0	0	2	6	0.01	0	0	0.02	0.1	0	1	0.01
1	0.2	0	3	11	21	69	0	0.3	1	0	0.36	0	0.02	0.03	0.2	0	7	0
2	2.8	9	6	26	83	61	0.2	0.6	11	4	0.66	0	0.04	0.05	0.5	0.01	3	0.02
—	—	0	20	—	140	100	—	1.1	—	0	—	0	—	—	—	—	—	—
2.2	0.6	4	7	25	78	37	0.2	0.6	8	2	0.52	0	0.06	0.05	0.4	0.01	5	0.02
2.2	1.9	15	11	26	69	35	0.2	0.4	11	40	0.58	0	0.03	0.04	0.2	0.02	6	0.03
0	0.2	0	30	47	18	266	0.3	1	17	60	0.71	52	0.09	0.07	0.5	0.15	50	0
0	0.2	0	28	44	16	247	0.3	0.9	16	56	0.66	48	0.08	0.06	0.5	0.14	47	0
0	0.2	0	19	42	18	252	0.3	0.6	19	46	0.45	35	0.08	0.09	0.4	0.22	78	0
0	0.1	0	32	52	19	296	0.3	1.1	18	67	0.67	65	0.11	0.07	0.6	0.17	46	0
0	0.1	0	18	30	11	171	0.2	0.6	10	39	0.39	37	0.06	0.04	0.3	0.1	27	0
0.2	0.2	0	7	69	4	87	0.6	0.8	50	0	0.23	0	0.04	0.04	0.9	0.08	14	0
0.9	0.9	0	15	295	1	391	2	1.9	196	0	0.88	0	0.09	0.36	6	0.18	26	0
0	0.1	0	9	36	5	62	0.5	0.9	29	0	0.03	0	0.05	0.02	0.9	0.08	16	0
0.4	1.1	0	63	40	252	64	0.3	1.4	9	0	0.7	0	0.22	0.14	1.8	0.02	43	0.03
0.2	0.3	0	25	36	190	34	0.3	1.3	9	0	0.07	0	0.17	0.08	2.1	0.02	41	0.04
0.8	0.4	0	41	52	197	69	0.5	1.7	19	0	0.24	0	0.2	0.13	1.9	0.04	41	0
0.3	1	0	56	35	224	56	0.2	1.3	8	0	0.62	0	0.19	0.12	1.6	0.02	38	0.02
—	—	80	60	—	480	—	—	5.4	—	60	—	6	—	—	—	—	—	—
—	—	90	80	—	870	—	—	4.5	—	100	—	9	0.33	0.41	7	0.35	—	—
—	—	115	250	—	1350	—	—	4.5	—	150	—	9	0.34	0.48	7	0.33	—	—
—	—	137	203	—	1075	—	—	4.6	—	81	—	0	—	—	—	—	—	—
—	—	60	100	—	1400	—	—	3.6	—	0	—	0	—	—	—	—	—	—
—	—	90	60	—	980	—	—	2.7	—	20	—	1	—	—	—	—	—	—
—	—	76	153	—	783	—	—	3.7	—	81	—	5	—	—	—	—	—	—
—	—	62	62	—	543	—	—	3.7	—	41	—	5	—	—	—	—	—	—
7.2	2.2	8	33	31	443	219	0.8	2.2	16	78	—	2	0.36	0.37	3.9	0.16	51	1.07
2.5	1.8	28	214	180	1166	497	1.6	2.3	80	238	—	2	0.22	0.71	3.6	0.24	74	0.89
—	—	0	150	—	570	—	—	3.6	—	20	—	9	—	—	—	—	—	—
—	—	90	60	—	500	—	—	1.4	—	20	—	1	—	—	—	—	—	—
0	0	0	1	0	60	0	0	0.1	0	0	0	0	0	0	0	0	0	0
3.5	0.4	31	3	3	106	4	0	0	0	107	0.22	0	0	0	0	0	0	0.02
3.4	0.4	31	3	3	116	4	0	0	0	106	0.22	0	0	0	0	0	0	0.02
1.2	0.2	11	1	1	41	1	0	0	0	38	0.08	0	0	0	0	0	0	0.01
3.3	0.4	31	3	3	2	4	0	0	0	107	0.22	0	0	0	0	0	0	0.02
2.2	0.3	21	2	2	78	2	0	0	0	71	0.15	0	0	0	0	0	0	0.01
4.7	2.3	12	4	3	127	5	0	0	0	113	1.08	0	0	0	0	0	0	0.01
—	—	0	21	2	2	7	0	0.4	1	0	—	7	0	0	0.1	0.02	2	0
—	—	0	48	6	3	308	0.1	0	7	2	—	15	0.01	0.01	0.1	0.04	5	0
—	—	0	27	3	2	159	0	0	4	1	—	9	0	0	0	0.02	2	0
0.6	0.1	9	284	219	257	370	1	0.1	27	20	0.15	2	0.08	0.38	0.1	0.08	12	0.54
3	12.1	0	15	126	0	119	0.9	1.1	67	3	0.99	1	0.11	0.04	0.3	0.16	19	0
0	0	0	0	—	46	79	—	0	—	0	—	0	0.03	0.04	0	—	—	—
0	0.1	0	89	31	55	213	0.2	0.7	16	8	0.1	3	0.03	0.06	0.4	0.15	47	0
0	0	0	36	32	208	640	0.2	0.4	9	14	0.09	1	0	0.03	0.1	0.08	32	0
0	0.1	0	79	25	29	315	0.1	0.9	9	218	0.1	22	0.03	0.05	0.4	0.14	34	0
0	0	0	37	13	23	88	0.1	0.3	7	105	0.04	16	0.01	0.02	0.2	0.07	23	0
0.4	2.5	0	391	189	101	1224	1.1	2.2	101	164	1.33	254	0.72	0.69	3.6	1.43	252	0
0.2	1.1	0	427	209	163	2233	1.6	5.4	136	118	0.95	292	0.45	0.36	2.7	0.87	390	0
0	0.1	0	73	30	498	188	0.2	0.6	14	213	0.12	40	0.04	0.05	0.4	0.17	44	0
0	0	0	43	17	459	157	0.2	0.4	10	62	0.01	0	0.03	0.06	0.5	0.19	46	0
0	0	0	29	11	3	90	0.1	0.1	5	46	0.05	10	0.02	0.02	0.2	0.09	30	0

Esha Code	Food Item	Qty	Meas	Wgt (g)	Wtr (g)	Cals	Prot (g)	Carb (g)	Fib (g)	Fat (g)	SatF (g)
5235	Cabbage, pe tsai, cooked, drained	0.5	cup	60	57	8	1	1	1.6	0	0
5559	Cabbage, raw, fresh harvest	0.5	cup	35	32	8	0	2	0.8	0	0
5238	Cabbage, red, cooked, drained	0.5	cup	75	70	16	1	3	1.5	0	0
5533	Cabbage, red, pickled	0.5	cup	75	45	110	0	29	0.6	0	0
5042	Cabbage, red, raw	0.5	cup	35	32	9	0	2	0.7	0	0
5534	Cabbage, red, sweet & sour	0.5	cup	75	45	110	0	29	0.6	0	0
5044	Cabbage, savoy, cooked, drained	0.5	cup	72	67	17	1	4	2	0	0
5043	Cabbage, savoy, raw	0.5	cup	35	32	9	1	2	1.1	0	0
5038	Cabbage, shredded, cooked, no added salt, drained	0.5	cup	75	70	16	1	3	1.7	0	0
5036	Cabbage, shredded, raw	0.5	cup	35	32	9	1	2	0.8	0	0
5526	Cactus pad/nopales, cooked	1	each	29	25	12	0	3	1	0	0
5524	Cactus/nopales, raw	0.5	cup	59	52	24	0	6	2.1	0	0.1
26100	Cajun seasoning	0.25	tsp	1	0	2	0	0	0.1	0	—
46066	Cake, German chocolate, mix, prepared, w/frosting	1	piece	111	30	404	4	55	1.5	21	5.3
46004	Cake, angel food	1	piece	53	18	137	3	31	0.8	0	0.1
46050	Cake, angel food, mix, prepared	1	piece	50	16	129	3	29	0.1	0	0
46051	Cake, angel food, recipe	1	piece	53	17	142	4	32	0.2	0	0
46242	Cake, apple spice crumb, fat free, Entenmann's	1	piece	50	—	130	2	30	2	0	0
46102	Cake, applesauce w/nuts & icing	1	piece	108	21	399	3	70	1.5	13	3.2
46098	Cake, applesauce, no icing	1	piece	87	19	313	3	52	1.7	11	2.9
46099	Cake, apricot, no icing	1	piece	87	19	313	3	52	1.7	11	2.9
46244	Cake, banana loaf, fat free, Entenmann's	1	piece	57	—	150	2	34	1	0	0
46104	Cake, banana w/icing	1	piece	108	37	309	3	58	1.1	8	1.6
46103	Cake, banana, no icing	1	piece	87	32	245	3	43	1.1	7	1.6
46100	Cake, blackberry, no icing	1	piece	87	19	313	3	52	1.7	11	2.9
46010	Cake, carrot w/cream cheese frosting, recipe	1	piece	112	23	488	5	53	1.3	30	5.5
46054	Cake, carrot, mix, prepared, no frosting	1	piece	70	22	239	4	33	1.4	11	1.8
46055	Cake, cherry fudge, w/chocolate frosting	1	piece	71	33	187	2	27	0.9	9	3.6
46247	Cake, chocolate crunch, fat free, Entenmann's	1	piece	50	—	130	2	32	2	0	0
46120	Cake, chocolate w/fluffy white icing	1	piece	91	30	262	4	48	1	8	1.8
46061	Cake, chocolate, mix, low sodium, prepared	1	piece	38	9	116	1	23	0.6	3	1.4
46059	Cake, chocolate, mix, prepared	1	piece	65	21	198	4	32	1.4	8	1.8
46057	Cake, chocolate, mix, pudding type, prepared	1	piece	77	23	270	4	34	1.5	14	3
46062	Cake, chocolate, recipe, no frosting	1	piece	95	23	340	5	51	1.5	14	5.2
46013	Cake, chocolate, w/chocolate icing-commercial	1	piece	69	16	253	3	38	1.9	11	3.3
46117	Cake, chocolate, w/cream cheese icing	1	piece	103	26	355	4	57	1	14	3.7
46118	Cake, chocolate, w/vanilla icing	1	piece	103	26	358	4	58	1	14	3.6
46092	Cake, coffee, cheese	1	piece	76	24	258	5	34	0.8	12	4.1
46263	Cake, coffee, cheese, Entenmann's	1	piece	54	17	190	4	24	0	8	3.5
46093	Cake, coffee, cinnamon, w/crumb topping	1	piece	63	14	263	4	29	1.3	15	3.6
46095	Cake, coffee, cinnamon, w/crumb topping, recipe	1	piece	60	13	240	4	30	0.9	12	2.2
46096	Cake, coffee, creme filled, w/chocolate frosting	1	piece	90	26	298	4	48	1.8	10	2.6
46097	Cake, coffee, fruit	1	piece	50	16	156	3	26	1.2	5	1.2
46005	Cake, coffee, mix, prepared	1	piece	72	22	229	4	38	0.9	7	1.3
46106	Cake, date pudding	1	piece	42	14	131	2	19	0.9	6	3
46063	Cake, fruit, recipe	1	piece	43	8	155	2	28	1.6	5	0.6
45562	Cake, funnel, 6 inch diameter	1	each	90	37	285	7	29	0.9	15	3.9
46006	Cake, gingerbread, mix, prepared	1	piece	63	21	195	3	32	0.7	6	1.6
46000	Cake, gingerbread, recipe	1	piece	110	31	392	4	54	0.9	18	4.5
46254	Cake, golden loaf, fat free, Entenmann's	1	piece	48	—	120	2	28	0.5	0	0
46108	Cake, graham cracker	1	piece	45	13	156	3	22	0.4	7	1.7
46109	Cake, ice cream roll, chocolate	1	piece	34	13	102	1	14	0.3	5	2.2
46110	Cake, ice cream roll, chocolate	1	each	340	134	1015	14	136	3.5	50	22
46111	Cake, lemon, w/icing, 2-layer	1	piece	109	23	388	3	70	0.5	11	2.6
46119	Cake, marble w/chocolate icing	1	piece	111	28	404	3	59	0.9	19	4.4
46068	Cake, marble, mix, pudding type, dry	1	oz.	28	1	118	1	22	0.8	3	0.7
46389	Cake, mix, Angle Food, prepared	1	piece	53	5	192	5	43	0	0	0
46387	Cake, mix, Devil's Food, prep w/oil & egg	1	piece	44	6	210	3	25	0	10	3
46112	Cake, oatmeal w/icing	1	piece	110	21	410	3	70	1.5	14	3.4
46070	Cake, pineapple upside-down cake, recipe	1	piece	115	37	367	4	58	0.9	14	3.4
46107	Cake, plum pudding	1	piece	42	14	131	2	19	0.9	6	3
46114	Cake, poppyseed, no icing	1	piece	90	21	354	7	43	1	18	6.5
46016	Cake, pound w/butter	1	piece	29	7	113	2	14	0.1	6	3.4
46072	Cake, pound, commercial, not w/butter	1	piece	30	7	117	2	16	0.3	5	1.4
46075	Cake, pound, old fashion, w/butter	1	piece	53	11	229	3	25	0.4	13	7.6

MonoF (g)	PolyF (g)	Choles (mg)	Calc (mg)	Phos (mg)	Sod (mg)	Pot (mg)	Zn (mg)	Iron (mg)	Magn (mg)	VitA (μg RE)	VitE (mg α-TE)	VitC (mg)	Thia (mg)	Ribo (mg)	Nia (mg)	B6 (mg)	Fola (μg)	B12 (μg)
0	0	0	19	23	5	134	0.1	0.2	6	58	0.07	9	0.03	0.03	0.3	0.1	32	0
0	0	0	16	8	6	86	0.1	0.2	5	5	0.04	18	0.02	0.01	0.1	0.03	20	0
0	0.1	0	28	22	6	105	0.1	0.3	8	2	0.09	26	0.03	0.02	0.2	0.1	9	0
0	0	0	36	16	14	153	0.1	0.6	13	1	0.03	9	0.01	0.01	0.1	0.06	4	0
0	0	0	18	15	4	72	0.1	0.2	5	1	0.04	20	0.02	0.01	0.1	0.07	7	0
0	0	0	36	16	14	153	0.1	0.6	13	1	0.03	9	0.01	0.01	0.1	0.06	4	0
0	0	0	22	24	17	133	0.2	0.3	17	64	0.08	12	0.04	0.02	0	0.11	34	0
0	0	0	12	15	10	80	0.1	0.1	10	35	0.04	11	0.02	0.01	0.1	0.07	28	0
0	0.1	0	23	11	6	73	0.1	0.1	6	10	0.08	15	0.04	0.04	0.2	0.08	15	0
0	0	0	16	8	6	86	0.1	0.2	5	5	0.04	11	0.02	0.01	0.1	0.03	15	0
0	0.1	0	15	7	68	57	0	0.1	24	1	0	3	0	0.02	0.1	0.02	1	0
0.1	0.1	0	33	14	3	130	0.1	0.2	50	3	0.01	8	0.01	0.04	0.3	0.04	4	0
—	—	—	—	—	119	7	—	—	—	—	—	—	—	—	—	—	—	0
8.7	5.5	53	53	173	369	151	0.5	1.2	19	23	1.18	0	0.11	0.14	1.1	0.02	4	0.1
0	0.2	0	74	17	397	49	0	0.3	6	0	0.05	0	0.05	0.26	0.5	0.02	19	0.03
0	0.1	0	42	116	255	68	0.1	0.1	4	0	0	0	0.05	0.1	0.1	0	15	0.02
0	0	0	3	13	96	116	0.1	0.4	5	0	0.01	0	0.05	0.17	0.4	0	2	0.05
0	0	0	0	—	140	65	—	0	—	20	—	0	—	—	—	—	—	—
5.7	3.6	21	20	45	293	137	0.2	1.3	10	49	1.5	1	0.12	0.12	1	0.05	5	0.05
4.9	2.9	22	17	46	285	145	0.2	1.4	11	10	1.15	1	0.14	0.13	1.1	0.06	6	0.04
4.9	2.9	22	17	46	285	145	0.2	1.4	11	10	1.15	1	0.14	0.13	1.1	0.06	6	0.04
0	0	0	20	—	190	140	—	0	—	0	—	0	—	—	—	—	—	—
3.2	2.3	31	28	48	292	198	0.3	1	17	105	1.36	4	0.13	0.18	1.1	0.25	12	0.08
3.1	2.2	29	26	46	257	186	0.3	1	16	100	1.3	3	0.12	0.16	1	0.24	12	0.07
4.9	2.9	22	17	46	285	145	0.2	1.4	11	10	1.15	1	0.14	0.13	1.1	0.06	6	0.04
7.3	15.2	60	28	80	276	125	0.5	1.4	20	430	4.73	1	0.15	0.18	1.1	0.08	13	0.11
3.4	5	51	77	123	249	84	0.2	0.9	5	173	2.94	2	0.09	0.12	0.8	0.06	8	0.81
3.1	1.7	30	34	75	160	118	0.2	0.8	14	72	0.85	10	0.02	0.14	0.5	0.04	7	0.15
0	0	0	0	—	170	200	—	1.1	—	0	—	0	—	—	—	—	—	—
3.1	2.3	35	71	133	411	173	0.5	2.1	22	16	—	0	0.06	0.11	0.8	0.02	8	0.07
1.2	0.2	0	11	102	130	82	0.3	0.8	14	0	0.11	0	0.05	0.06	0.5	0	2	0.01
3.1	2.3	35	70	132	370	153	0.4	2.1	22	16	1.14	0	0.06	0.1	0.6	0.02	7	0.06
4.7	5.9	53	64	146	402	161	0.5	1.4	19	24	1.37	0	0.08	0.13	0.9	0.03	8	0.32
5.7	2.6	55	57	101	299	133	0.7	1.5	30	38	1.51	0	0.13	0.2	1.1	0.04	26	0.15
6	1.3	29	30	84	230	138	0.5	1.5	24	17	1.17	0	0.02	0.09	0.4	0.03	12	0.1
6.5	3.2	35	71	133	460	167	0.4	2.2	22	60	—	0	0.06	0.1	0.6	0.02	7	0.06
6.4	3.2	35	71	147	404	168	0.4	2.1	22	102	—	0	0.06	0.1	0.6	0.02	7	0.06
5.4	1.2	65	45	77	258	220	0.4	0.5	11	66	1.19	0	0.08	0.1	0.5	0.04	30	0.26
—	—	30	40	—	160	55	—	0	—	20	—	0	—	—	—	—	—	—
8.2	2	20	34	68	221	78	0.5	1.2	14	21	2.15	0	0.13	0.14	1.1	0.02	38	0.11
4.6	4.6	36	67	83	233	143	0.5	1.3	24	99	1.5	0	0.11	0.12	0.7	0.06	9	0.09
5.1	1.3	62	34	68	291	70	0.4	0.5	14	33	1.62	0	0.07	0.07	0.8	0.04	37	0.18
2.8	0.7	4	22	59	193	45	0.3	1.2	8	10	0.43	0	0.02	0.1	1.3	0.02	24	0.01
2.8	2.3	35	98	155	303	81	0.3	1	13	29	1.2	0	0.12	0.13	1.1	0.04	49	0.1
1.9	0.3	16	40	35	56	196	0.2	0.8	23	8	0.26	0	0.04	0.06	0.4	0.08	3	0.05
2	2	12	28	34	62	133	0.3	0.8	15	6	1.08	2	0.07	0.05	0.5	0.04	4	0.02
4.5	5.9	66	115	128	236	153	0.6	1.8	18	46	1	0	0.24	0.32	1.9	0.05	14	0.24
3.6	0.8	22	44	106	289	152	0.3	2.1	10	10	0.86	0	0.12	0.12	1	0.02	6	0.04
7.8	4.6	35	78	59	360	483	0.4	3.2	77	15	2.64	0	0.21	0.18	1.9	0.21	36	0.07
0	0	0	0	—	160	75	—	0	—	20	—	0	—	—	—	—	—	—
3	1.8	34	44	52	176	78	0.3	0.7	8	80	1.12	0	0.04	0.14	0.6	0.02	5	0.09
1.8	0.7	16	43	38	69	57	0.2	0.5	9	22	0.25	0	0.04	0.07	0.3	0.01	2	0.08
18.4	7	156	431	380	688	569	2.4	4.7	90	215	2.47	1	0.4	0.71	3	0.14	23	0.79
5.2	2.7	33	70	136	248	55	0.2	0.9	6	79	2.09	1	0.1	0.12	0.8	0.02	6	0.07
7.4	6.2	53	43	172	311	143	0.4	1.4	18	99	—	0	0.07	0.12	0.7	0.03	7	0.1
1.4	1.1	0	22	78	147	35	0.1	0.5	5	0	0.51	0	0.05	0.04	0.4	0.01	10	0
0	0	0	24	—	320	56	—	0	—	0	—	0	0	0	0	—	—	—
3	3.5	25	20	—	270	170	—	1.1	—	0	—	0	0.09	0.1	0.4	—	—	—
6.1	3.8	20	20	56	257	135	0.3	1.8	14	57	1.56	1	0.15	0.11	1.1	0.05	5	0.05
6	3.8	25	138	94	367	129	0.4	1.7	15	75	1.54	1	0.18	0.18	1.4	0.04	30	0.09
1.9	0.3	16	40	35	56	196	0.2	0.8	23	8	0.26	0	0.04	0.06	0.4	0.08	3	0.05
4.6	5.3	79	107	122	251	138	0.7	1.7	20	94	1.03	1	0.25	0.29	1.7	0.05	16	0.18
1.7	0.3	64	10	40	115	34	0.1	0.4	3	45	0.19	0	0.04	0.07	0.4	0.01	12	0.07
3	0.7	17	19	40	120	32	0.1	0.5	4	10	0.72	0	0.04	0.08	0.4	0.01	11	0.04
3.9	0.7	92	13	44	153	37	0.3	0.9	5	134	0.4	0	0.1	0.14	0.8	0.02	8	0.13

Esha Code	Food Item	Qty	Meas	Wgt (g)	Wtr (g)	Cals	Prot (g)	Carb (g)	Fib (g)	Fat (g)	SatF (g)
46076	Cake, pound, old fashion, w/margarine	1	piece	53	11	230	3	25	0.4	13	2.8
46074	Cake, pound, recipe, w/margarine	1	piece	54	13	206	3	28	0.4	9	2
46258	Cake, raisin loaf, fat free, Entenmann's	1	piece	53	—	140	2	33	1	0	0
46101	Cake, rhubarb, no icing	1	piece	87	19	313	3	52	1.7	11	2.9
46077	Cake, shortcake, biscuit type, recipe	1	each	65	18	225	4	32	0.8	9	2.5
46011	Cake, snack, chocolate, creme filled, w/icing	1	each	28	6	107	1	17	0.2	4	0.8
46008	Cake, snack, cream filled, Twinkie	1	each	42	8	153	1	27	0.2	5	1.1
46116	Cake, spice, w/icing	1	piece	109	27	374	4	65	1	11	3.8
46001	Cake, sponge, 1/12th	1	piece	65	19	188	4	40	0.4	2	0.5
46115	Cake, sponge, chocolate, no icing	1	piece	66	20	195	5	36	1	4	1.4
46105	Cake, sponge, fruit-cream filled, Twinkie	1	each	43	12	146	2	24	0.4	5	1.4
46078	Cake, sponge, recipe	1	piece	63	18	187	5	36	0.4	3	0.8
46084	Cake, white, mix, low sodium, prepared	1	piece	38	10	118	1	23	0.2	2	0.4
46082	Cake, white, mix, prepared, pkg	1	each	739	228	2261	30	409	4.9	57	8.6
46080	Cake, white, mix, pudding type, prepared	1	each	826	235	2915	30	427	3.7	122	23.1
46007	Cake, white, no yolk, chocolate icing	1	piece	109	22	397	3	70	1.2	12	5.7
46003	Cake, white, w/coconut frosting, recipe	1	piece	70	14	249	3	44	0.7	7	2.7
46017	Cake, white, w/white frosting	1	piece	71	14	266	2	45	0.7	10	4.3
46090	Cake, yellow, mix, prepared	1	piece	69	21	221	3	38	0.6	6	1.1
46012	Cake, yellow, w/chocolate frosting, commercial	1	piece	69	15	262	3	38	1.2	12	3.2
46015	Cake, yellow, w/vanilla frosting	1	piece	121	27	451	4	71	0.4	18	2.9
23021	Canduy, milk chocolate-covered peanuts	0.25	cup	42	1	221	6	21	2	14	6.2
23075	Candy, 3 Musketeers bar	1	each	60	4	251	2	46	1	8	3.9
23076	Candy, 3 Musketeers bar, snack size	1	each	18	1	75	1	14	0.3	2	1.2
23125	Candy, 5th Avenue bar	1	each	56	1	276	5	37	1.2	12	4.4
23049	Candy, Almond Joy bar	1	each	49	5	229	2	29	2.4	13	8.5
23077	Candy, Alpine White bar, w/almonds	1	each	35	0	193	3	18	1.9	13	7
23110	Candy, Baby Ruth bar	1	each	60	3	289	4	39	1.7	13	7.1
23111	Candy, Bar None bar	1	each	42	2	219	3	22	1.4	14	9.2
23112	Candy, Bit-o-Honey chews	6	piece	48	3	186	1	39	—	4	—
23066	Candy, Butterfinger bar	1	each	61	1	293	8	40	1.5	11	6.3
23067	Candy, Butterfinger bar, snack size	1	each	21	0	101	3	14	0.5	4	2.2
23116	Candy, Caramello bar	1	each	45	3	213	3	28	0.7	10	6.3
23122	Candy, Chunky bar, small	1	each	35	1	173	3	20	1.7	10	8.1
23098	Candy, Crisped Rice bar, almond	1	each	28	2	130	2	18	1	6	1.1
23099	Candy, Crisped Rice bar, chocolate chip	1	each	28	2	115	1	21	0.6	4	1.5
23123	Candy, Demet's Turtles	10	piece	170	10	825	11	99	4.4	47	18.4
23036	Candy, English toffee bar, Skor	1	each	39	1	217	2	22	0.6	13	8.5
23130	Candy, Golden Almond Solitaires	1	each	85	2	484	10	40	3.7	32	12.9
23129	Candy, Golden Almond bar	1	each	85	2	488	10	39	4.1	32	13.9
23131	Candy, Golden III bar	1	each	91	3	471	6	51	5.2	30	—
23060	Candy, Kit Kat bar	1	each	42	1	216	3	27	0.8	11	6.8
23061	Candy, Krackel bar	1	each	41	1	218	3	25	0.9	12	7.4
23048	Candy, M&M's, peanut, pieces	10	piece	20	0	103	2	12	0.7	5	2.1
23047	Candy, M&M's, peanut, pkg	1	each	49	1	254	5	30	1.7	13	5.1
23046	Candy, M&M's, plain, pieces	10	piece	7	0	34	0	5	0.2	1	0.9
23045	Candy, M&M's, plain, pkg	1	each	48	1	236	2	34	1.2	10	6.3
23037	Candy, Mars almond bar	1	each	50	2	234	4	31	1	12	3.6
23038	Candy, Milky Way bar	1	each	61	4	258	3	44	1	10	4.8
23039	Candy, Milky Way bar, snack size	1	each	18	1	76	1	13	0.3	3	1.4
23035	Candy, Mounds bar	1	each	53	6	253	2	31	3.1	13	10.8
23062	Candy, Mr. Goodbar bar	1	each	49	0	267	5	25	1.7	17	7.3
23136	Candy, Nestle 100 Grand bar	1	each	42	2	198	2	30	0.6	8	4.8
23133	Candy, Nestle Crunch bar	1	each	40	0	209	2	26	1	10	6.1
23134	Candy, Nestle Crunch bar, snack size	1	each	10	0	52	1	7	0.3	3	1.5
23135	Candy, Oh Henry! bar	1	each	57	3	246	6	37	2	10	3.8
23080	Candy, Planter's peanut bar	1.5	oz.	43	1	222	7	20	1.4	14	1.8
23140	Candy, Reese's Pieces	10	piece	8	0	39	1	5	0.2	2	1.4
23043	Candy, Reese's peanut butter cups	2	each	45	1	243	5	25	1.4	14	5
23141	Candy, Rolo chocolate-covered caramels	10	piece	55	11	225	3	29	0.4	11	6.7
23143	Candy, Skittles, bite size	10	piece	11	0	45	0	10	0	0	0.1
23040	Candy, Snickers bar, 2.2oz	1	each	59	3	281	5	35	1.5	14	5.3
23057	Candy, Special Dark Sweet bar	1	each	41	0	226	2	25	2	13	8.3
23144	Candy, Starburst fruit chews	6	piece	59	4	232	0	50	0	5	0.7
23146	Candy, Symphony bar	1	each	42	0	232	3	24	0.8	14	—

MonoF	PolyF	Choles	Calc	Phos	Sod	Pot	Zn	Iron	Magn	VitA	VitE	VitC	Thia	Ribo	Nia	B6	Fola	B12
(g)	(g)	(mg)	(mg)	(mg)	(mg)	(mg)	(mg)	(mg)	(mg)	(μg RE)	(mg α-TE)	(mg)	(mg)	(mg)	(mg)	(mg)	(μg)	(μg)
5.6	3.9	60	13	44	169	39	0.3	0.9	5	147	1.96	0	0.1	0.14	0.8	0.02	8	0.13
3.8	2.6	41	39	52	172	49	0.3	0.9	6	104	1.35	0	0.11	0.14	0.9	0.02	6	0.1
0	0	0	20	—	150	120	—	0	—	20	—	0	—	—	—	—	—	—
4.9	2.9	22	17	46	285	145	0.2	1.4	11	10	1.15	1	0.14	0.13	1.1	0.06	6	0.04
4	2.4	2	133	93	329	69	0.3	1.6	10	12	1.3	0	0.2	0.18	1.7	0.02	6	0.05
1.6	1.5	5	21	26	121	35	0.1	1	12	1	0.96	0	0.06	0.08	0.7	0.01	8	0.02
1.7	1.4	7	19	78	153	36	0.1	0.5	3	2	0.85	0	0.06	0.06	0.5	0.01	12	0.05
5.1	1.4	48	77	201	271	150	0.4	1.6	15	40	2.2	0	0.13	0.18	1.1	0.04	9	0.11
0.6	0.3	66	46	89	159	64	0.3	1.8	7	30	0.18	0	0.16	0.18	1.2	0.03	25	0.16
1.5	0.5	141	22	89	115	98	0.6	1.6	20	63	0.7	1	0.09	0.21	0.7	0.05	14	0.26
2.2	0.8	23	46	92	132	34	0.1	0.6	4	11	0.92	0	0.06	0.08	0.6	0.01	5	0.05
1	0.4	107	26	63	144	89	0.4	1	6	48	0.32	0	0.1	0.19	0.8	0.04	25	0.23
1	0.9	0	8	87	83	50	0.1	0.6	3	0	0.39	0	0.07	0.07	0.6	0	2	0.01
23.8	21.4	0	1019	1780	3591	702	2.5	7.3	66	1	9.53	1	0.99	1.19	5.2	0.13	37	0.66
45.4	48.9	0	421	1470	3650	504	1.4	7.2	58	0	14.1	1	1.18	1.25	11.6	0.11	33	0.58
3.9	1.9	20	84	144	336	78	0.2	0.7	6	64	1.06	0	0.08	0.1	0.4	0.01	3	0.07
2.6	1.5	1	63	49	199	69	0.2	0.8	8	8	0.5	0	0.09	0.13	0.7	0.02	15	0.04
3.8	1	6	34	46	166	41	0.1	0.6	4	23	1.28	0	0.07	0.09	0.6	0.01	4	0.04
2.7	2.2	40	70	165	327	50	0.2	0.9	6	17	1.07	0	0.08	0.13	0.8	0.05	6	0.13
6.6	1.5	38	26	111	233	123	0.4	1.4	21	23	1.57	0	0.08	0.11	0.9	0.02	15	0.12
7.4	6.2	67	75	173	416	64	0.3	1.3	7	23	2.3	0	0.12	0.08	0.6	0.03	33	0.18
5.5	1.8	4	44	90	17	213	0.8	0.6	40	0	1.08	0	0.05	0.07	1.8	0.09	3	0.12
2.6	0.3	7	51	55	117	80	0.3	0.4	18	14	0.38	0	0.02	0.08	0.1	0.01	0	0.1
0.8	0.1	2	15	16	35	24	0.1	0.1	5	4	0.11	0	0.01	0.02	0	0	0	0.03
5.6	1.9	3	41	86	92	166	0.7	0.7	36	8	1.29	0	0.08	0.07	1.9	0.05	21	0.07
3.2	0.7	2	30	69	72	121	0.4	0.7	32	2	1.1	0	0.02	0.07	0.2	0.03	—	0.06
5	0.9	4	81	82	26	146	0.4	0.2	13	9	1.33	0	0.03	0.15	0.3	0.03	5	0.3
3.7	1.9	2	25	91	136	238	0.8	0.1	48	0	1.13	0	0.06	0.06	1.7	0.04	19	0.03
3.3	0.9	7	61	84	44	164	0.5	0.5	30	10	0.63	0	0.02	0.11	0.7	0.03	12	0.18
—	—	0	27	32	124	60	0.2	0.1	10	0	—	0	0	0.12	0	0.01	2	0
3.4	1.7	1	16	80	121	232	0.7	0.5	48	0	0.99	0	0.05	0.04	1.5	0.04	16	0.01
1.2	0.6	0	6	28	42	80	0.2	0.2	17	0	0.34	0	0.02	0.02	0.5	0.01	6	0
3.2	0.3	12	83	72	62	153	0.4	0.3	19	35	0.76	0	0.02	0.18	0.5	0.02	—	0.28
0.1	1.5	4	50	73	19	187	0.6	0.4	26	4	0.52	0	0.03	0.14	0.7	0.04	8	0.13
2.1	2.2	0	21	47	66	65	1.5	1.8	20	75	—	3	0.37	0.42	5	0.5	0	0
1.1	1	0	6	38	79	48	0.2	1.8	14	50	0.03	0	0.15	0.17	2	0.2	40	0
18.9	7.9	37	269	335	160	524	2.4	2.3	89	58	—	1	0.26	0.41	0.6	0.09	17	0.68
4.3	0.5	20	51	58	108	93	0.3	0.2	13	27	0.53	0	0.01	0.13	0	0.01	—	0.11
15	3.6	11	160	255	48	428	1.6	2	100	8	1.93	0	0.05	0.42	0.9	0.04	—	0.4
15	3.3	13	190	230	57	400	1.4	1.5	94	32	0.51	0	0.05	0.45	0.9	0.04	—	0.37
—	—	17	275	200	79	413	1	0.5	61	20	1.18	1	0.06	0.26	0.1	0.1	11	0.41
3.1	0.3	3	69	100	32	122	0.5	0.4	16	20	0.34	0	0.07	0.23	1.1	0.05	60	0.07
3.9	0.4	8	72	91	57	140	0.5	0.4	23	5	0.53	0	0.02	0.12	0.2	0.01	—	0.24
2.2	0.8	2	20	46	10	69	0.5	0.2	15	5	0.49	0	0.02	0.03	0.8	0.02	7	0.04
5.4	2.1	4	50	112	24	171	1.1	0.6	36	12	1.2	0	0.05	0.08	1.8	0.04	17	0.09
0.5	0	1	7	10	4	19	0.1	0.1	3	4	0.06	0	0	0.02	0	0	0	0.02
3.3	0.3	7	50	72	29	127	0.5	0.5	20	25	0.41	0	0.03	0.1	0.1	0.01	3	0.13
5.4	2	8	84	117	85	163	0.6	0.6	36	25	2.33	0	0.02	0.16	0.5	0.03	10	0.18
3.7	0.4	9	79	88	146	147	0.4	0.5	21	20	0.4	1	0.02	0.14	0.2	0.03	6	0.2
1.1	0.1	3	23	26	43	43	0.1	0.1	6	6	0.12	0	0.01	0.04	0.1	0.01	2	0.06
2.3	0.3	1	8	48	79	131	0.5	1.1	30	1	0.36	0	0.02	0.03	0.2	0.05	2	0
5.7	2.4	4	53	122	73	219	0.9	0.6	42	18	1.34	0	0.08	0.12	1.6	0.04	19	0.15
2.5	0.3	8	48	57	88	96	0.4	0.1	16	10	0.31	0	0.12	0.18	1.4	0.14	30	0.11
3.4	0.3	5	68	81	53	138	0.6	0.2	23	8	0.44	0	0.14	0.22	1.6	0.16	32	0.15
0.9	0.1	1	17	20	13	34	0.1	0	6	2	0.11	0	0.03	0.06	0.4	0.04	8	0.04
3.8	1.6	5	62	94	135	185	0.7	0.3	35	5	1.08	0	0.01	0.09	1.6	0.04	17	0.12
7.1	4.5	3	33	65	102	173	0.6	0.4	32	22	0.41	0	0.04	0.06	3.4	0.04	26	0.01
0.2	0.1	0	7	11	12	18	0.1	0.1	4	0	0.17	0	0.01	0.01	0.2	0.01	2	0.02
5.9	2.5	2	35	91	143	158	0.8	0.5	40	9	1.83	0	0.11	0.08	2.1	0.07	25	0.07
3.4	0.3	10	84	82	96	136	0.5	0.3	21	20	0.46	0	0.03	0.12	0.1	0.02	3	0.15
0.3	0	0	0	0	2	1	0	0	0	0	0.03	7	0	0	0	0	0	0
6.2	2.9	8	55	130	156	190	1.4	0.4	42	23	0.9	0	0.06	0.09	2.5	0.05	24	0.09
4.6	0.4	0	11	62	3	123	0.6	1	46	2	0.18	0	0.01	0.03	0.2	0.01	1	0
2.1	1.8	0	2	4	33	1	0	0.1	1	0	0.89	31	0	0	0	0	0	0
—	—	9	90	105	39	162	0.5	0.5	23	5	0.52	0	0.04	0.16	0.1	0.02	—	0.16

A

Esha Code	Food Item	Qty	Meas	Wgt (g)	Wtr (g)	Cals	Prot (g)	Carb (g)	Fib (g)	Fat (g)	SatF (g)
23149	Candy, Twix Cookie bar, caramel	1	each	57	2	283	3	37	0.6	14	5
23150	Candy, Twix Cookie bar, peanut butter	1	each	48	1	257	5	26	1.6	16	5.5
23151	Candy, Whatchamacallit bar	1	each	48	5	214	4	29	1	9	4.5
23153	Candy, Y&S Nibs, cherry	1	oz.	28	0	106	1	26	0	1	—
23154	Candy, Y&S Twizzlers, strawberry	1	each	71	12	237	2	55	1	1	0.3
23152	Candy, York Peppermint Patty	1	each	42	4	165	1	34	0.8	3	1.8
23020	Candy, almonds, chocolate-coated	0.25	cup	41	1	234	5	16	3.5	18	3
23115	Candy, butterscotch	5	piece	30	0	119	0	29	0	1	0.3
23015	Candy, caramel, plain or chocolate	5	piece	40	3	153	2	31	0.5	3	2.6
23118	Candy, carob bar	1	each	87	1	470	7	49	3.3	27	25.2
23078	Candy, cherries, chocolate-covered	2	each	28	2	102	1	22	0.3	3	1.5
23082	Candy, chewing gum	1	piece	4	0	14	0	4	0	0	0
23083	Candy, chewing gum, uncoated, sugarless	1	piece	4	0	11	0	4	0	0	0
23063	Candy, chocolate Kisses	6	piece	28	0	145	2	17	0.8	9	5.2
23145	Candy, chocolate, sweet	1	each	41	0	207	2	24	2.3	14	8.2
23023	Candy, chocolate-covered mint patty	1	each	11	1	40	0	9	0.2	1	0.6
23053	Candy, divinity, no nuts	1	piece	20	2	70	0	18	0	0	0
23024	Candy, fondant/candy corn	1	cup	200	14	716	0	186	0	0	0
23124	Candy, fudge, brown sugar w/nuts, recipe	1	piece	14	1	55	0	11	0.1	1	0.2
23126	Candy, fudge, chocolate marshmallow, recipe	1	piece	20	2	84	0	14	0	3	2
23127	Candy, fudge, chocolate marshmallow, w/nuts, recipe	1	piece	22	2	96	1	15	0.4	4	2.1
23026	Candy, fudge, chocolate w/nuts, recipe	1	piece	19	1	81	1	14	0.2	3	1.1
23025	Candy, fudge, chocolate, recipe	1	piece	17	2	65	0	14	0.1	1	0.9
23128	Candy, fudge, peanut butter, recipe	1	piece	16	2	59	1	12	0.1	1	0.2
23027	Candy, fudge, vanilla, recipe	1	piece	16	2	59	0	13	0	1	0.5
23028	Candy, fudge, vanilla, w/nuts, recipe	1	piece	15	1	62	0	11	0.1	2	0.6
23029	Candy, gumdrops	10	piece	35	0	135	0	35	0	0	0
23030	Candy, gummy bears	10	each	35	0	135	0	35	0	0	0
23031	Candy, hard, all flavor	1	oz.	28	0	112	0	28	0	0	0
23074	Candy, hard, dietetic	1	piece	3	0	11	0	3	0	0	0
23033	Candy, jellybeans	10	piece	11	1	40	0	10	0	0	0
23189	Candy, licorice	1	oz.	28	1	120	0	24	0	3	3.1
23087	Candy, licorice, Good & Plenty	1.5	oz.	43	3	156	0	40	0	0	0.1
23032	Candy, lollipop	1	each	6	0	24	0	6	0	0	0
23084	Candy, malted milk balls, Whoppers	10	each	29	1	144	2	18	0.8	8	4.6
23016	Candy, milk chocolate bar	1	each	44	1	226	3	26	1.5	14	8.1
23018	Candy, milk chocolate bar w/almonds	1	each	41	1	216	4	22	2.5	14	7
23019	Candy, milk chocolate w/peanuts	1	each	43	1	238	7	17	2.4	18	5.2
23058	Candy, milk chocolate w/rice cereal	1	each	40	1	198	3	25	1.2	11	6.4
23132	Candy, milk chocolate-covered peanuts, Goobers	10	piece	10	0	51	1	5	0.6	3	1.2
23022	Candy, milk chocolate-covered raisins	0.25	cup	48	5	185	2	32	2	7	4.2
23214	Candy, milk chocolate-covered raisins,Raisinets	1	each	45	3	185	2	32	2.3	7	3.3
23081	Candy, peanut brittle, recipe	0.25	cup	37	1	166	3	26	0.7	7	1.8
23079	Candy, peanut butter cup, dietetic	2	each	16	1	88	2	7	1.1	6	5.1
23138	Candy, praline, recipe	1	piece	39	4	177	1	24	1	9	0.7
23142	Candy, sesame crunch	20	piece	35	1	181	4	18	2.8	12	1.6
23034	Candy, sugar-coated almonds, Jordan	7	each	28	1	129	2	20	1.3	5	0.4
23147	Candy, taffy, recipe	1	piece	15	1	56	0	14	0	0	0.3
23085	Candy, toffee, Almond Roca	1	piece	11	1	48	1	7	0.3	2	1.1
23173	Candy, toffee, recipe	4	piece	48	1	260	1	31	0	16	9.8
23117	Candy, tootsie roll, bite size	7	each	35	3	126	1	31	0.2	1	0.2
23088	Candy, yogurt-covered peanuts	0.25	cup	42	2	193	4	16	1.8	13	2.5
23089	Candy, yogurt-covered raisins	0.25	cup	48	4	190	2	34	1.5	6	3.6
23148	Candym, truffle, recipe	1	piece	12	2	59	1	5	0.3	4	2.1
3326	Cantaloupe Nectar	1	cup	250	210	151	1	38	0.8	0	0.2
5511	Capers	1	tsp	5	4	0	0	0	0.2	0	—
3240	Carambola, raw (starfruit)	1	each	127	115	42	1	10	3.4	0	0
26018	Caraway seed	0.25	tsp	1	0	2	0	0	0.2	0	0
26039	Cardamom, ground	0.25	tsp	0	0	1	0	0	0.1	0	0
3241	Carissa, raw (natal plum)	1	each	20	17	12	0	3	—	0	—
23246	Carob chips, unsweetened	0.25	cup	42	—	201	6	23	0	9	8.4
44	Carob flavor mix, prepared w/milk	1	cup	256	215	195	8	22	1	8	5.1
5517	Carrot chips, dried	0.5	cup	37	1	136	3	27	7.3	1	0.1
5226	Carrot juice, canned	1	cup	246	219	98	2	23	2	0	0.1
5047	Carrot slices, cooked, no added salt, drained	0.5	cup	78	68	35	1	8	2.6	0	0

MonoF	PolyF	Choles	Calc	Phos	Sod	Pot	Zn	Iron	Magn	VitA	VitE	VitC	Thia	Ribo	Nia	B6	Fola	B12
(g)	(g)	(mg)	(mg)	(mg)	(mg)	(mg)	(mg)	(mg)	(mg)	(μg RE)	(mg α-TE)	(mg)	(mg)	(mg)	(mg)	(mg)	(μg)	(μg)
7.6	0.5	3	51	68	109	115	0.4	0.5	18	14	0.69	0	0.09	0.13	0.7	0.02	14	0.1
7.2	2	2	37	92	132	173	0.7	0.4	36	9	0.54	0	0.05	0.07	2	0.07	12	0.06
2.8	1.5	5	55	87	99	148	0.6	0.3	29	9	0.71	0	0.22	0.29	3.5	0.27	5	0.16
—	—	0	18	88	67	18	0	0.2	2	1	0.17	0	0.01	0.01	0	0	0	0
—	—	0	5	220	175	45	0.1	0.2	4	0	—	0	0.01	0.03	0.1	0.01	—	0
1	0.1	0	6	40	10	54	0.3	0.4	26	0	0.13	0	0.01	0.04	0.4	0	—	0.01
12	3.2	0	83	141	24	225	1	1.2	91	0	5.21	0	0.05	0.22	0.7	0.03	32	0
0.2	0	3	1	1	110	1	0	0	0	10	0.02	0	0	0	0	0	0	0
0.3	0.1	3	55	46	98	86	0.2	0.1	7	3	0.18	0	0	0.07	0.1	0.01	2	0
0.4	0.3	3	264	110	93	551	3.1	1.1	31	7	1.37	0	0.09	0.16	0.9	0.11	24	0.87
0.9	0.1	0	5	27	7	47	0.1	0.4	18	1	0.1	0	0.01	0.02	0.2	0	0	0
0	0	0	0	0	0	0	0	0	0	0	0	0	0	0	0	0	0	0
0	0	0	1	0	0	0	0	0	0	0	0	0	0	0	0	0	0	0
2.8	0.3	6	54	61	23	109	0.4	0.4	17	14	0.35	0	0.02	0.08	0.1	0.01	2	0.11
4.6	0.4	0	10	60	7	119	0.6	1.1	46	1	0.49	0	0.01	0.1	0.3	0.02	1	0
0.3	0	0	2	10	3	18	0	0.2	7	0	0.04	0	0	0.01	0.1	0	0	0
0	0	0	0	1	9	4	0	0	0	0	—	0	0	0.01	0	0	0	0
0	0	0	4	4	80	32	0.1	0.1	2	1	0	0	0	0.03	0	0	0	0
0.3	0.8	1	16	12	14	52	0.1	0.3	7	2	—	0	0.01	0.01	0	0.02	2	0
1	0.1	5	9	13	21	28	0.1	0.2	7	16	—	0	0	0.02	0	0	0	0.01
1.3	0.7	5	11	18	21	37	0.2	0.2	10	16	—	0	0.01	0.02	0	0.01	2	0.01
0.8	1	3	10	18	11	30	0.1	0.1	9	9	0.08	0	0.01	0.02	0	0.02	2	0.01
0.4	0.1	2	7	10	10	18	0.1	0.1	4	8	0.02	0	0	0.01	0	0	0	0.01
0.5	0.3	1	7	10	12	21	0.1	0	4	2	—	0	0	0.01	0.2	0.01	2	0.01
0.2	0	3	6	5	11	8	0	0	1	8	0.03	0	0	0.01	0	0	0	0.01
0.5	0.8	2	7	11	9	17	0.1	0.1	4	7	0.07	0	0.01	0.01	0	0.01	2	0.01
0	0	0	1	0	15	2	0	0.1	0	0	0	0	0	0	0	0	0	0
0	0	0	1	0	15	2	0	0.1	0	0	0	0	0	0	0	0	0	0
0	0	0	1	1	11	1	0	0.1	1	0	0	0	0	0	0	0	0	0
0	0	0	0	0	0	0	0	0	0	0	0	0	0	0	0	0	0	0
0	0	0	0	0	3	4	0	0.1	0	0	0	0	0	0	0	0	0	0
—	—	0	0	—	80	54	0.1	0	3	0	—	0	—	—	—	—	—	—
0.1	0	0	1	2	11	16	0	0.5	1	0	0	0	0	0	0	0	0	0
0	0	0	0	0	2	0	0	0	0	0	0	0	0	0	0	0	0	0
2.5	0.2	6	50	56	42	100	0.3	0.2	14	3	0.36	0	0.02	0.08	0.1	0.02	3	0.11
4.4	0.5	10	84	95	36	169	0.6	0.6	26	24	0.55	0	0.04	0.13	0.1	0.02	4	0.17
5.5	0.9	8	92	108	30	182	0.5	0.7	37	6	0.78	0	0.02	0.18	0.3	0.02	5	0.14
7.8	3.9	4	50	126	17	230	1	0.8	53	9	1.99	0	0.12	0.08	3.2	0.07	36	0.08
3.5	0.3	8	68	77	58	137	0.4	0.3	20	4	0.44	0	0.02	0.12	0.2	0.02	4	0.14
1.5	0.5	1	13	30	4	50	0.2	0.1	12	0	0.26	0	0.01	0.02	0.5	0.02	1	0.03
2.2	0.2	1	41	68	17	244	0.4	0.8	21	3	0.46	0	0.04	0.08	0.2	0.04	2	0.09
2.7	0.9	2	49	65	16	231	0.4	0.5	20	4	0.47	0	0.04	0.1	0.2	0.05	2	0.1
3.1	1.7	5	11	41	166	76	0.4	0.5	18	17	0.6	0	0.07	0.02	1.3	0.04	26	0
0.7	0.1	1	48	53	17	97	0.4	0.2	21	0	0.63	0	0.03	0.08	0.4	0.03	10	0.12
5.9	2.4	0	12	42	24	82	0.8	0.5	20	2	0.58	0	0.12	0.02	0.1	0.03	5	0
4.4	5.1	0	229	148	58	113	1.3	1.5	88	0	0.53	0	0.19	0.06	1.3	0.19	23	0
3.6	1.1	0	28	47	6	72	0.5	0.5	46	0	0.52	0	0.01	0.08	0.3	0.02	16	0
0.1	0	1	0	0	13	1	0	0	0	5	0.08	0	0	0	0	0	0	0
0.6	0.2	1	16	19	20	34	0.1	0.1	5	2	0.17	0	0.01	0.02	0.2	0.01	3	0.01
4.6	0.6	50	16	16	90	24	0.1	0	2	153	0.96	0	0	0.03	0	0	1	0.03
0.4	0.3	0	9	14	28	36	0.2	0.1	11	1	0.08	0	0.01	0.03	0	0.01	0	0.02
6.4	3.5	1	17	63	14	107	0.9	0.5	25	10	2.04	1	0.05	0.03	2.4	0.05	48	0.17
1.9	0.2	4	55	65	21	269	0.2	0.6	10	13	0.64	1	0.05	0.08	0.3	0.08	4	0.15
1.8	0.2	6	19	21	9	37	0.1	0.1	6	17	0.14	0	0.01	0.03	0	0	0	0.04
0	0	0	13	18	13	279	0.2	0.2	12	242	0.15	30	0.03	0.02	0.5	0.1	8	0
—	—	0	2	—	105	—	—	0.1	—	1	—	0	—	—	—	—	—	0
0	0.2	0	5	20	3	207	0.1	0.3	11	62	0.47	27	0.04	0.03	0.5	0.13	18	0
0	0	0	4	3	0	8	0	0.1	1	0	0.01	0	0	0	0	0	0	0
0	0	0	2	1	0	5	0	0.1	1	0	—	0	0	0	0	—	—	0
—	—	0	2	1	1	52	—	0.3	3	1	—	8	0.01	0.01	0	—	—	0
—	—	4	269	—	187	—	—	0.4	—	5	—	2	—	—	—	—	—	—
2.4	0.3	33	292	228	133	369	0.9	0.7	33	77	0.1	2	0.1	0.39	0.3	0.12	12	0.87
0	0.3	0	81	125	111	921	0.6	1.5	45	3699	0.14	21	0.26	0.18	2.6	0.44	31	0
0	0.2	0	59	103	71	718	0.4	1.1	34	2693	0.02	21	0.23	0.14	1	0.53	9	0
0	0.1	0	24	23	52	177	0.2	0.5	10	1914	0.33	2	0.03	0.04	0.4	0.19	11	0

Esha Code	Food Item	Qty	Meas	Wgt (g)	Wtr (g)	Cals	Prot (g)	Carb (g)	Fib (g)	Fat (g)	SatF (g)
5655	Carrot slices, steamed	0.5	cup	78	68	34	1	8	2.3	0	0
5656	Carrot slices, stir fried	0.5	cup	78	68	34	1	8	2.3	0	0
5439	Carrot, baby, raw (2.75inch)	1	each	10	9	4	0	1	0.2	0	0
5633	Carrot, glazed	0.5	cup	80	56	117	1	17	2.1	6	1.1
5046	Carrot, raw, grated	0.5	cup	55	48	24	1	6	1.6	0	0
5045	Carrot, whole, raw	1	each	72	63	31	1	7	2.2	0	0
5199	Carrots, canned, drained	0.5	cup	73	68	18	0	4	1.1	0	0
5355	Carrots, canned, drained, low sodium	0.5	cup	73	68	18	0	4	1.1	0	0
5198	Carrots, canned, not drained	0.5	cup	123	114	28	1	7	2.2	0	0
5358	Carrots, frozen, cooked	0.5	cup	73	66	26	1	6	2.6	0	0
6174	Carrots, julienne	0.5	cup	55	48	24	1	6	1.7	0	0
5048	Carrots, whole, cooked, no added salt, drained	1	each	46	40	21	1	5	1.5	0	0
4662	Cashew butter, salted	1	Tbs	16	0	94	3	4	0.3	8	1.6
4537	Cashew butter, unsalted	2	Tbs	32	1	188	6	9	0.6	16	3.1
15930	Cashew chicken	1	cup	162	91	409	27	11	2	29	4.8
4519	Cashew, dry roasted, salted	0.25	cup	34	1	197	5	11	1	16	3.1
4621	Cashews, dry roasted, unsalted	0.25	cup	34	1	197	5	11	1	16	3.1
4596	Cashews, oil roasted, salted	0.25	cup	32	1	187	5	9	1.2	16	3.1
4622	Cashews, oil roasted, unsalted	0.25	cup	32	1	187	5	9	1.2	16	3.1
5625	Cassava (yuca blanca), pieces, cooked	0.5	cup	68	46	82	2	18	0.1	0	0.1
5356	Cassava, raw	4	oz.	113	68	181	2	43	2	0	0.1
27000	Catsup/ketchup	1	Tbs	15	10	16	0	4	0.2	0	0
27032	Catsup/ketchup, low sodium	1	Tbs	15	10	16	0	4	0.2	0	0
27001	Catsup/ketchup, packet	1	each	6	4	6	0	2	0.1	0	0
5052	Cauliflower flowerets, cooked, drained	3	each	54	50	12	1	2	1.5	0	0
5051	Cauliflower, cooked, drained, cup measure	0.5	cup	62	58	14	1	3	1.7	0	0
5539	Cauliflower, flowerets, batter-dipped, fried	5	piece	130	89	250	6	13	2.1	20	4.8
5607	Cauliflower, flowerets, pickled	3	each	81	71	34	1	8	1.5	0	0
5053	Cauliflower, frozen, cooked, drained	0.5	cup	90	85	17	1	3	2.4	0	0
5050	Cauliflower, raw flowerets	3	each	56	52	14	1	3	1.4	0	0
5049	Cauliflower, raw, cup measure	0.5	cup	50	46	12	1	3	1.2	0	0
5641	Cauliflower, w/cheese sauce	0.5	cup	81	67	73	3	5	0.9	5	2.2
5200	Celeriac/celery root, cooked	0.5	cup	78	72	21	1	5	0.9	0	0
5056	Celery pieces, cooked, no added salt	0.5	cup	75	71	14	1	3	1.2	0	0
26040	Celery seed	0.25	tsp	0	0	2	0	0	0.1	0	0
5054	Celery, chopped, raw	0.5	cup	60	57	10	0	2	1	0	0
5659	Celery, chopped, steamed	0.5	cup	75	71	12	1	3	1.3	0	0
5660	Celery, chopped, stir fried	0.5	cup	75	71	12	1	3	1.3	0	0
5606	Celery, pickled	0.5	cup	75	71	11	0	3	1.1	0	0
5055	Celery, raw, large outer stalk	1	each	40	38	6	0	1	0.7	0	0
56320	Celery, stuffed w/cheesey	1	piece	32	25	44	2	1	0.3	4	2.4
40059	Cereal, 100% Bran	0.5	cup	33	1	89	4	24	9.8	2	0.3
40063	Cereal, 100% Natural	0.5	cup	52	1	231	5	36	3.9	9	3.7
40064	Cereal, 100% Natural w/apple cinnamon	0.5	cup	52	1	239	6	35	3.4	10	7.8
40065	Cereal, 100% Natural w/raisins & dates	0.5	cup	55	2	248	6	36	3.6	10	6.8
40003	Cereal, All Bran	0.5	cup	43	1	114	5	33	13.9	1	0.3
40027	Cereal, Alpha Bits	1	cup	28	0	111	2	25	1.2	1	0.1
40123	Cereal, Amaranth flakes	0.5	cup	19	1	67	2	13	1.8	2	0.5
40028	Cereal, Apple Jacks	1	cup	28	1	109	1	25	0.5	0	0.1
40029	Cereal, Bran Buds	0.5	cup	43	1	119	4	34	17.1	1	0.2
40025	Cereal, Bran Chex	1	cup	49	1	156	5	39	7.9	1	0.2
40007	Cereal, Bran Flakes, Kellogg's	1	cup	39	1	128	4	31	6.2	1	0.2
40090	Cereal, Bran Flakes, Post	1	cup	47	1	152	5	37	9.2	1	0.1
40275	Cereal, Bran'ola raisin, Post	1	cup	110	3	400	8	88	10	6	1
40031	Cereal, C.W. Post w/raisins	1	cup	103	4	446	9	74	13.6	15	11
40030	Cereal, C.W. Post, plain	1	cup	97	2	421	9	73	7.2	13	1.7
40032	Cereal, Cap'n Crunch	1	cup	37	1	147	2	32	1.2	2	0.5
40034	Cereal, Cap'n Crunch, peanut butter	1	cup	35	1	146	3	28	1	3	0.7
40033	Cereal, Cap'n Crunchberries	1	cup	35	1	140	2	30	0.8	2	0.5
40004	Cereal, Cheerios	1	cup	23	1	83	2	17	2	1	0.3
40127	Cereal, Clusters	0.5	cup	28	1	111	4	20	2.9	3	0.4
40035	Cereal, Cocoa Krispies	1	cup	36	1	140	2	32	0.5	1	0.7
40037	Cereal, Cocoa Pebbles	1	cup	32	1	131	2	28	0.5	2	1.1
40036	Cereal, Corn Bran	1	cup	36	1	120	2	30	6.4	1	0.3
40038	Cereal, Corn Chex	1	cup	28	1	111	2	25	0.5	0	0

MonoF	PolyF	Choles	Calc	Phos	Sod	Pot	Zn	Iron	Magn	VitA	VitE	VitC	Thia	Ribo	Nia	B6	Fola	B12
(g)	(g)	(mg)	(mg)	(mg)	(mg)	(mg)	(mg)	(mg)	(mg)	(μg RE)	(mg α-TE)	(mg)	(mg)	(mg)	(mg)	(mg)	(μg)	(μg)
0	0.1	0	21	34	27	252	0.2	0.4	12	1977	0.33	5	0.07	0.04	0.7	0.11	10	0
0	0.1	0	21	34	27	252	0.2	0.4	12	1977	0.33	6	0.07	0.04	0.7	0.11	10	0
0	0	0	2	4	4	28	0	0.1	1	150	0.04	1	0	0	0.1	0.01	3	0
2.5	1.8	0	31	24	131	189	0.2	0.6	12	1717	1.16	2	0.02	0.04	0.3	0.17	9	0.01
0	0	0	15	24	19	178	0.1	0.3	8	1547	0.25	5	0.05	0.03	0.5	0.08	8	0
0	0.1	0	19	32	25	233	0.1	0.4	11	2025	0.33	7	0.07	0.04	0.7	0.11	10	0
0	0.1	0	18	18	177	131	0.2	0.5	6	1005	0.31	2	0.01	0.02	0.4	0.08	7	0
0	0.1	0	18	18	31	131	0.2	0.5	6	1005	0.31	2	0.01	0.02	0.4	0.08	7	0
0	0.1	0	38	25	295	213	0.4	0.6	11	1189	0.49	2	0.02	0.03	0.5	0.14	10	0
0	0	0	20	19	43	115	0.2	0.3	7	1292	0.31	2	0.02	0.03	0.3	0.09	8	0
0	0	0	15	24	19	178	0.1	0.3	8	1554	0.25	5	0.05	0.03	0.5	0.08	8	0
0	0	0	14	14	30	104	0.1	0.3	6	1129	0.19	1	0.02	0.03	0.2	0.11	6	0
4.7	1.3	0	7	73	98	87	0.8	0.8	41	0	0.25	0	0.05	0.03	0.3	0.04	11	0
9.3	2.7	0	14	146	5	175	1.6	1.6	83	0	0.5	0	0.1	0.06	0.5	0.08	22	0
13	9.1	60	47	249	988	415	1.4	1.9	60	93	3.65	9	0.14	0.14	12.5	0.56	40	0.24
9.4	2.7	0	15	168	219	194	1.9	2.1	89	0	0.2	0	0.07	0.07	0.5	0.09	24	0
9.4	2.7	0	15	168	5	194	1.9	2.1	89	0	0.2	0	0.07	0.07	0.5	0.09	24	0
9.2	2.6	0	13	138	203	172	1.5	1.3	83	0	0.51	0	0.14	0.06	0.6	0.08	22	0
9.2	2.6	0	13	138	6	172	1.5	1.3	83	0	0.51	0	0.14	0.06	0.6	0.08	22	0
0.1	0.1	0	60	43	165	473	0.2	2.4	43	1	0.13	22	0.12	0.06	0.9	0.19	10	0
0.1	0.1	0	18	31	16	307	0.4	0.3	24	2	0.22	23	0.1	0.05	1	0.1	31	0
0	0	0	3	6	182	74	0	0.1	3	16	0.22	2	0.01	0.01	0.2	0.03	2	0
0	0	0	3	6	3	72	0	0.1	3	15	0.22	2	0.01	0.01	0.2	0.03	2	0
0	0	0	1	2	71	29	0	0	1	6	0.09	1	0	0	0.1	0.01	1	0
0	0.1	0	9	17	8	77	0.1	0.2	5	1	0.02	24	0.02	0.03	0.2	0.09	24	0
0	0.1	0	10	20	9	88	0.1	0.2	6	1	0.02	28	0.03	0.03	0.3	0.11	27	0
5.2	9.1	30	167	173	239	332	0.6	0.9	19	45	3.43	47	0.1	0.16	0.7	0.19	40	0.17
0.1	0.1	0	20	28	129	192	0.1	0.4	10	30	0.08	35	0.04	0.03	0.3	0.12	24	0
0	0.1	0	15	22	16	125	0.1	0.4	8	2	0.04	28	0.03	0.05	0.3	0.08	37	0
0	0.1	0	12	25	17	170	0.2	0.2	8	1	0.02	26	0.03	0.04	0.3	0.12	32	0
0	0	0	11	22	15	152	0.1	0.2	8	1	0.02	23	0.03	0.03	0.3	0.11	28	0
1.7	0.8	10	88	73	258	183	0.4	0.2	10	41	0.29	21	0.04	0.1	0.3	0.1	22	0.17
0	0.1	0	20	51	47	134	0.2	0.3	9	0	0.16	3	0.02	0.03	0.3	0.08	3	0
0	0.1	0	32	19	68	213	0.1	0.3	9	10	0.27	5	0.03	0.04	0.2	0.06	16	0
0.1	0	0	9	3	1	7	0	0.2	2	0	0	0	0	0	0	0	0	0
0	0	0	24	15	52	172	0.1	0.2	7	8	0.22	4	0.03	0.03	0.2	0.05	17	0
0	0.1	0	30	19	65	216	0.1	0.3	8	10	0.27	4	0.1	0.03	0.2	0.06	18	0
0	0.1	0	30	19	65	215	0.1	0.3	8	9	0.27	4	0.1	0.03	0.2	0.06	17	0
0	0	0	26	15	183	177	0.1	0.3	8	8	0.24	3	0.02	0.03	0.2	0.05	12	0
0	0	0	16	10	35	115	0.1	0.2	4	5	0.14	3	0.02	0.02	0.1	0.04	11	0
1.1	0.1	12	45	50	110	75	0.2	0.2	4	46	0.16	2	0.01	0.04	0.1	0.02	7	0.06
0.3	0.9	0	23	401	229	326	2.9	4.1	156	0	0.77	31	0.79	0.89	10.5	1.06	23	3.14
3.7	1.1	1	50	161	14	228	1.2	1.6	55	1	0.59	0	0.18	0.08	0.9	0.09	13	0.06
0.9	0.7	0	78	175	26	257	1	1.4	36	3	0.36	1	0.17	0.29	0.9	0.05	8	0.15
1.9	0.9	0	80	174	24	269	1.1	1.6	62	3	0.38	0	0.15	0.32	1	0.08	23	0.07
0.3	0.8	0	152	422	87	490	5.4	6.4	185	323	0.79	22	0.56	0.6	7.2	0.73	129	2.15
0.2	0.2	0	8	51	180	55	1.5	2.7	17	376	0.02	0	0.37	0.43	5	0.51	100	1.51
0.4	0.9	0	3	63	7	67	0	0.3	5	2	1.61	0	0.01	0.02	0.5	0.01	2	0
0.1	0.2	0	3	28	127	30	3.5	4.2	8	213	0.05	14	0.37	0.4	4.7	0.48	100	0
0.2	0.6	0	29	238	286	386	9.2	6.4	119	323	0.68	22	0.56	0.6	7.2	0.73	129	0
0.3	0.7	0	29	173	345	216	6.5	14	69	11	0.56	26	0.64	0.26	8.6	0.88	173	2.6
0.2	0.5	0	19	202	304	236	5	10.9	81	488	7.22	20	0.51	0.58	6.7	0.66	138	1.95
0.1	0.4	0	21	296	431	251	2.5	13.4	102	622	0.54	0	0.61	0.7	8.3	0.85	166	2.49
—	—	0	0	200	440	440	3	9	80	751	—	0	0.75	0.85	10	1	200	3
1.7	1.4	0	50	232	161	261	1.6	16.4	74	1363	0.72	0	1.34	1.55	18.1	1.85	364	5.46
6	4.7	0	47	224	167	198	1.6	15.4	67	1284	0.68	0	1.26	1.46	17.1	1.75	342	5.14
0.4	0.3	0	7	39	286	47	5.1	6.2	13	5	0.18	0	0.51	0.58	6.8	0.68	137	0
1.1	0.7	0	4	67	264	80	4.9	5.8	24	5	0.19	0	0.49	0.55	6.5	0.65	130	0
0.4	0.3	0	9	40	256	49	5.4	6.1	13	6	0.25	0	0.5	0.57	6.7	0.67	135	0.01
0.5	0.2	0	42	86	215	67	2.8	6.1	25	284	0.16	11	0.28	0.32	3.8	0.38	76	0
1.4	1.4	0	51	106	135	137	0.4	4.5	27	373	0.97	16	0.39	0.48	6	0.52	100	0
0.1	0.1	0	5	34	244	70	1.7	2.1	13	261	0.17	17	0.43	0.5	5.8	0.58	108	0
0.4	0.1	0	5	25	180	53	1.7	2	13	424	0.04	0	0.42	0.48	5.6	0.58	113	1.7
0.3	0.4	0	27	48	338	75	5	10.1	19	5	0.19	0	0.1	0.56	6.7	0.67	134	0
0	0	0	3	11	310	23	0.1	8.1	4	14	0.07	15	0.37	0.07	5	0.51	100	1.5

A

Esha Code	Food Item	Qty	Meas	Wgt (g)	Wtr (g)	Cals	Prot (g)	Carb (g)	Fib (g)	Fat (g)	SatF (g)
40005	Cereal, Corn Flakes, USDA	1	cup	25	1	91	2	22	0.7	0	0
40067	Cereal, Corn Pops USDA	1	cup	28	1	108	1	26	0.4	0	0.1
40039	Cereal, Cracklin' Oat Bran	0.5	cup	30	1	123	3	22	3.6	4	1.6
40040	Cereal, Crispy Wheat `N Raisins	1	cup	43	3	150	3	35	2.7	1	0.1
40006	Cereal, Farina, enriched, cooked	0.5	cup	116	102	58	2	12	1.6	0	0
40042	Cereal, Froot Loops	1	cup	28	1	111	1	25	0.5	1	0.4
40020	Cereal, Frosted Flakes	1	cup	38	1	146	1	34	0.8	0	0.1
40085	Cereal, Fruit & Fibre, date-raisin-nut	0.5	cup	28	3	96	2	22	3.8	1	0.2
40046	Cereal, Fruity Pebbles	1	cup	32	1	130	1	28	0.4	2	1.4
40047	Cereal, Golden Grahams	1	cup	39	1	150	2	33	1.2	1	0.2
40008	Cereal, Granola, Nature Valley	0.5	cup	56	2	255	6	37	3.6	10	1.3
40137	Cereal, Granola, low fat	0.5	cup	47	1	182	5	38	3	3	0
40009	Cereal, Grape Nuts	0.5	cup	54	2	195	7	45	5.4	0	0
40049	Cereal, Grape Nuts Flakes	1	cup	39	1	144	4	32	3.9	1	0.6
40129	Cereal, Heartwise, plain	1	cup	39	1	113	4	31	8.6	1	0.2
40246	Cereal, Honey & Nut Corn Flakes .	667	cup	28	1	115	2	24	0.5	1	0.3
40052	Cereal, Honey Bran	1	cup	35	1	119	3	29	3.9	1	0.3
40084	Cereal, Honey Buckwheat Crisp	1	cup	38	2	147	4	31	3.4	1	0.2
40125	Cereal, Honey Bunches of Oats	1	cup	43	1	173	3	36	2.1	2	0.5
40053	Cereal, Honey Comb	1	cup	22	0	86	1	20	0.6	0	0.2
40051	Cereal, Honey Nut Cheerios	1	cup	33	1	126	3	27	1.7	1	0.3
40068	Cereal, Honey Smacks	1	cup	38	1	144	2	33	1.3	1	0.4
40134	Cereal, Just Right	1	cup	43	1	152	5	36	3	1	0.2
40054	Cereal, King Vitaman	1	cup	21	0	81	2	18	0.8	1	0.2
40010	Cereal, Kix	1	cup	19	0	72	1	16	0.5	0	0.1
40011	Cereal, Life, plain/cinnamon	1	cup	44	2	167	4	35	2.8	2	0.3
40055	Cereal, Lucky Charms	1	cup	32	1	124	2	27	1.3	1	0.2
40015	Cereal, Maypo, cooked, no salt added	0.5	cup	120	99	85	3	16	2.9	1	0.2
40056	Cereal, Most	1	cup	52	2	175	7	40	7.3	1	0.1
40124	Cereal, Mueslix Five Grain Muesli	0.5	cup	41	2	139	4	32	3.7	2	0.3
40138	Cereal, Multi-grain, cooked	0.5	cup	123	96	100	3	20	2	1	0.2
40041	Cereal, Oat flakes, fortified	1	cup	48	1	180	8	36	1.4	1	0.2
40072	Cereal, Oatmeal, instant, packet, prepared, plain	1	each	177	151	104	4	18	3	2	0.3
40092	Cereal, Post Toasties	1	cup	24	1	93	2	21	0.8	0	0
40012	Cereal, Product 19	1	cup	33	1	121	3	28	1.1	0	0
40066	Cereal, Quisp	1	cup	30	1	121	2	26	0.8	2	0.5
40013	Cereal, Raisin Bran, Kellogg's	1	cup	56	5	171	5	43	7.5	1	0
40091	Cereal, Raisin Bran, Post	1	cup	56	5	172	5	42	7.9	1	0.2
40133	Cereal, Raisin Nut Bran	1	cup	57	3	221	4	42	5.6	6	1
40088	Cereal, Ralston, cooked	0.5	cup	126	109	67	3	14	3	0	0.1
40026	Cereal, Rice Chex	1	cup	25	1	99	1	22	0.5	0	0
40017	Cereal, Rice Krispies	1	cup	28	1	111	2	25	0.3	0	0
40016	Cereal, Roman meal, cooked	0.5	cup	120	99	73	3	16	4.1	0	0.1
40062	Cereal, Shredded Wheat, large biscuit	1	each	24	1	85	3	19	2.3	0	0.1
40022	Cereal, Shredded Wheat, small	1	cup	43	2	152	5	34	4.2	1	0.1
40019	Cereal, Special K	1	cup	28	1	105	6	20	0.9	0	0
40069	Cereal, Super Golden Crisp	1	cup	33	0	123	2	30	0.5	0	0.1
40071	Cereal, Team Rice	1	cup	42	2	164	3	36	0.5	1	0.1
40021	Cereal, Total, wheat	1	cup	33	1	116	3	26	2.9	1	0.2
40060	Cereal, Trix	1	cup	28	1	114	1	24	0.7	2	0.4
40128	Cereal, Uncle Sam's High Fiber	0.5	cup	55	3	213	8	40	14.5	2	0.2
40061	Cereal, Wheat Chex	1	cup	46	1	169	5	38	4.1	1	0.2
40080	Cereal, Wheatena, cooked, unsalted	0.5	cup	122	104	68	2	14	3.3	1	0.1
40024	Cereal, Wheaties	1	cup	29	1	106	3	23	2	1	0.2
38156	Cereal, cream of rye, cooked	0.5	cup	126	111	54	1	12	2.2	0	0
40078	Cereal, cream of wheat, cooked	0.5	cup	122	107	63	1	14	0.1	0	0
40244	Cereal, cream of wheat, cooked	0.5	cup	122	106	66	2	14	0.6	0	0
40245	Cereal, cream of wheat, mix'n eat, prep, plain	1	each	142	117	102	3	21	0.4	0	0
40077	Cereal, farina, unenriched, cooked w/o salt	0.5	cup	116	102	58	2	12	1.6	0	0
40043	Cereal, frosted mini wheats, biscuits	4	each	31	2	105	3	26	3.3	0	0.1
40045	Cereal, frosted rice krispies	1	cup	19	0	71	1	17	0.2	0	0
40294	Cereal, honey cluster flake crunch, fat free	1	cup	41	1	173	4	35	5.3	0	0
40014	Cereal, malt-o-meal, plain, cooked	0.5	cup	120	105	61	2	13	0.5	0	0
40136	Cereal, oat bran, cooked, Mother's brand	0.5	cup	121	109	31	2	8	2	1	0.2
40000	Cereal, oatmeal, cooked	0.5	cup	117	100	72	3	13	2	1	0.2

MonoF	PolyF	Choles	Calc	Phos	Sod	Pot	Zn	Iron	Magn	VitA	VitE	VitC	Thia	Ribo	Nia	B6	Fola	B12
(g)	(g)	(mg)	(mg)	(mg)	(mg)	(mg)	(mg)	(mg)	(mg)	(μg RE)	(mg α-TE)	(mg)	(mg)	(mg)	(mg)	(mg)	(μg)	(μg)
0	0.1	0	1	10	266	23	0.2	7.8	3	188	0.03	12	0.32	0.35	4.2	0.42	88	0
0.1	0	0	2	6	113	21	1.4	1.7	2	213	0.03	14	0.37	0.4	4.7	0.48	100	0
1.8	0.4	0	14	102	107	139	0.9	1.1	42	138	0.2	9	0.23	0.26	3.1	0.31	83	0
0.1	0.1	0	54	110	223	180	0.8	3.5	33	293	0.45	0	0.29	0.33	3.9	0.39	78	0
0	0	0	2	14	0	15	0.1	0.6	2	0	0.02	0	0.09	0.06	0.6	0.01	27	0
0.2	0.3	0	3	20	133	30	3.5	4	8	200	0.1	13	0.37	0.4	4.7	0.48	85	0
0	0.1	0	1	10	244	25	0.2	5.5	3	274	0.05	18	0.45	0.53	6.1	0.6	113	0
0.6	0.5	0	15	110	134	167	1.5	5.1	40	361	0.66	0	0.38	0.43	5	0.5	100	1.5
0.1	0.1	0	4	19	178	24	1.7	2	9	424	0.03	0	0.42	0.48	5.6	0.58	113	1.7
0.4	0.2	0	19	47	357	69	4.9	5.8	12	293	0.29	20	0.49	0.55	6.5	0.65	130	0
6.7	1.9	0	42	164	92	188	1.1	1.8	54	0	3.98	0	0.18	0.06	0.6	0.08	8	0
—	—	0	—	121	91	144	5.7	2.7	36	227	7.61	—	0.57	0.64	7.6	0.76	152	2.27
0	0.1	0	5	137	379	182	1.2	15.6	36	722	0.14	0	0.71	0.82	9.6	0.98	192	2.89
0.1	0.2	0	16	116	220	136	0.8	11.2	43	516	0.1	0	0.51	0.58	6.9	0.7	138	2.07
0.3	0.4	0	30	154	168	265	2.1	6.2	55	310	0.02	0	0.52	0.58	7	0.69	137	1.95
0.6	0.4	0	3	19	191	31	0.2	2.3	3	116	0.07	8	0.2	0.23	2.6	0.26	57	0
0.1	0.3	0	16	132	202	151	0.9	5.6	46	463	0.81	19	0.46	0.52	6.2	0.63	24	1.86
0.3	0.6	0	53	107	359	141	0.7	10.8	43	908	8.94	36	0.9	1.02	12	1.87	11	3.6
1.4	0.3	0	8	66	272	77	0.7	6	24	838	0.3	0	0.55	0.74	8.3	1.04	196	3.67
0.1	0.1	0	4	22	124	25	1.2	2.1	7	291	0.09	0	0.29	0.33	3.9	0.4	78	1.17
0.5	0.2	0	22	113	285	94	4.1	5	32	248	0.34	16	0.41	0.47	5.5	0.55	110	0
0.1	0.3	0	4	56	71	59	0.5	2.5	22	315	0.19	21	0.53	0.6	7	0.72	140	0
0.2	0.4	0	11	94	288	98	22.8	27.3	29	341	45.6	0	2.27	2.58	30.3	3.03	607	9.1
0.3	0.2	0	3	54	176	58	2.6	5.9	18	212	1.42	8	0.26	0.3	3.5	0.35	71	1.06
0.1	0	0	27	26	166	26	2.4	5.1	6	236	0.05	9	0.24	0.27	3.2	0.32	63	0
0.6	0.8	0	134	187	240	109	5.5	12.3	43	2	0.22	0	0.55	0.62	7.4	0.73	147	0
0.4	0.2	0	35	81	217	58	4	4.8	21	240	0.14	16	0.4	0.45	5.3	0.53	107	0
0.4	0.4	0	62	124	5	106	0.7	4.2	25	352	0.84	14	0.36	0.36	4.7	0.48	5	1.44
0.2	0.3	0	79	361	276	340	2.8	33	103	2753	55	110	2.76	3.13	36.7	3.69	734	11
0.5	0.6	0	19	107	53	185	3.7	4.5	41	374	4.47	0	0.37	0.42	4.9	0.5	98	1.64
0.5	0.3	0	35	92	380	68	0.5	2.7	33	57	1.71	0	0.2	0.23	2.2	0.23	9	0
0.3	0.4	0	68	176	220	228	2.5	13.7	58	636	0.34	0	0.62	0.72	8.4	0.86	169	2.54
0.6	0.7	0	163	133	285	99	0.9	6.3	42	453	0.21	0	0.53	0.28	5.5	0.74	150	0
0	0	0	1	11	252	28	0.1	0.6	4	318	0.06	0	0.31	0.36	4.2	0.43	85	1.27
0.2	0.2	0	3	36	238	45	16.5	19.8	14	248	24.4	66	1.65	1.88	22	2.21	429	6.6
0.4	0.2	0	6	47	216	40	4.3	5.1	15	4	0.16	0	0.42	0.48	5.7	0.56	113	0
0.2	0.7	0	32	197	325	401	3.8	4.6	82	230	0.51	0	0.39	0.45	5.1	0.5	112	1.51
0.1	0.5	0	26	235	365	345	3	8.9	95	741	1.3	0	0.73	0.84	9.9	1.01	198	2.97
1.6	2.9	0	80	201	302	302	1.7	9	64	753	1.32	0	0.75	0.86	10.1	1	201	0
0.1	0.2	0	6	73	3	77	0.7	0.8	29	0	0.13	0	0.1	0.09	1	0.06	9	0.05
0	0	0	4	25	210	29	0.3	7.2	6	2	0.03	13	0.33	0.01	4.4	0.45	89	1.33
0	0	0	5	30	206	27	0.5	0.7	12	371	0.03	15	0.52	0.59	6.9	0.69	138	0.08
0.1	0.2	0	14	107	1	150	0.9	1.1	54	0	0.22	0	0.12	0.06	1.5	0.06	12	0
0.1	0.2	0	10	86	0	77	0.6	0.7	40	0	0.12	0	0.07	0.07	1.1	0.06	12	0
0.1	0.4	0	16	151	4	154	1.4	1.8	56	0	0.23	0	0.11	0.12	2.2	0.11	21	0
0	0.2	0	4	46	229	50	3.4	8	16	206	0.07	14	0.48	0.54	6.4	0.65	85	0
0.1	0.1	0	7	44	51	48	1.8	2.1	20	437	0.12	0	0.43	0.5	5.8	0.59	116	1.75
0.2	0.3	0	6	65	260	71	0.6	12	12	556	0.1	22	0.55	0.63	7.4	0.76	7	2.23
0.1	0.1	0	284	232	218	107	16.5	19.8	35	413	25.8	66	1.65	1.87	22.1	2.2	440	8.45
0.8	0.3	0	30	24	184	16	3.5	4.2	3	210	0.56	14	0.35	0.4	4.7	0.47	93	0
0.5	1.5	0	38	208	125	259	1.5	2	67	0	0.79	0	1.31	1.39	11.6	0.07	43	0
0.1	0.5	0	18	182	308	173	1.2	13.2	58	0	0.17	24	0.6	0.17	8.1	0.83	162	2.44
0.1	0.3	0	5	73	2	94	0.8	0.7	24	0	0.45	0	0.01	0.02	0.7	0.02	9	0
0.2	0.1	0	53	92	215	101	0.7	7.8	31	218	0.36	14	0.36	0.41	4.8	0.48	97	0
0	0.1	0	6	27	175	33	0.3	0.3	11	0	0.08	0	0.04	0.01	0.1	0.03	2	0
0	0	0	4	21	1	24	0.2	0.2	4	0	0.02	0	0	0	0.5	0.03	4	0
0	0.1	0	26	51	71	23	0.2	5.2	6	0	0.02	0	0.12	0	0.7	0.02	55	0
0	0.2	0	20	20	241	38	0.2	8.1	7	376	0.02	0	0.43	0.28	5	0.57	101	0
0	0	0	2	14	0	15	0.1	0	2	0	0.02	0	0.01	0.01	0.1	0.01	2	0
0.1	0.3	0	11	90	1	103	0.9	8.7	31	0	0.28	0	0.22	0.25	3	0.28	62	0.9
0	0.1	0	1	15	138	15	0.2	1.3	5	164	0.02	11	0.26	0.3	3.6	0.36	76	0
0	0	0	0	—	27	—	—	0.5	—	40	—	2	—	—	—	—	—	—
0	0	0	2	12	1	16	0.1	4.8	2	0	0.02	0	0.24	0.12	2.9	0.01	2	0
0.3	0.4	0	10	89	127	69	0.4	0.7	31	0	0.22	0	0.12	0.02	0.1	0.02	5	0
0.4	0.4	0	9	89	1	66	0.6	0.8	28	2	0.12	0	0.13	0.02	0.2	0.02	5	0

Esha Code	Food Item	Qty	Meas	Wgt (g)	Wtr (g)	Cals	Prot (g)	Carb (g)	Fib (g)	Fat (g)	SatF (g)
40073	Cereal, oatmeal, instant packet, prepared, apple-ci	1	each	149	117	125	3	26	2.5	1	0.3
40074	Cereal, oatmeal, instant packet, prepared, cinn-spi	1	each	161	118	177	5	35	2.6	2	0.4
40075	Cereal, oatmeal, instant packet, prepared, maple	1	each	155	116	153	4	32	2.6	2	0.4
40076	Cereal, oatmeal, instant, prepared, raisin-spice	1	each	158	119	161	4	32	2.2	2	0.3
40018	Cereal, puffed rice, fortified	1	cup	14	1	54	1	12	0.2	0	0
40023	Cereal, puffed wheat, fortified	1	cup	12	0	44	2	9	1.1	0	0
40002	Cereal, rolled wheat, cooked	0.5	cup	120	100	74	2	16	1.9	0	0.1
40070	Cerealm, Tasteeos	1	cup	24	1	94	3	19	2.5	1	0.2
5413	Chayote fruit, raw	1	each	203	191	39	2	9	3.4	0	0.1
5414	Chayote, cooked pieces	0.5	cup	80	75	19	0	4	2.2	0	0.1
1001	Cheese food, American cold pack	1	oz.	28	12	94	6	2	0	7	4.4
1071	Cheese food, swiss processed, slice	1	piece	21	9	68	5	1	0	5	3.3
1081	Cheese product, nonfat (Kraft Free Singles)	1	piece	19	12	30	4	3	0	0	0
44001	Cheese puffs (Cheetos)	1	cup	20	0	111	2	11	0.2	7	1.3
1002	Cheese spread, American	1	Tbs	15	7	44	2	1	0	3	2
1002	Cheese spread, American	2	Tbs	30	14	88	5	3	0	6	4.1
1272	Cheese spread, Velveeta	1	oz.	28	13	80	5	3	0	6	4
1020	Cheese spread, lowfat, low sodium (Velveeta)	1	Tbs	15	9	27	4	1	0	1	0.7
1094	Cheese spread, lowfat, low sodium (Velveeta)	1	piece	34	21	61	9	1	0	2	1.5
1072	Cheese, American food slice	1	piece	21	9	69	4	2	0	5	3.2
1000	Cheese, American processed	1	piece	21	8	79	5	0	0	7	4.1
1096	Cheese, American processed, lowfat	1	oz.	28	17	51	7	1	0	2	1.2
1132	Cheese, Gjetost	1	piece	28	4	132	3	12	0	8	5.4
1228	Cheese, Mexican, nonfat, Lifetime	1	oz.	28	18	40	8	1	0	0	0
1029	Cheese, asiago, shredded	0.25	cup	27	10	102	8	1	0	7	4.8
1039	Cheese, beer	1	oz.	28	12	105	7	1	0	8	5.3
1003	Cheese, blue	1	oz.	28	12	100	6	1	0	8	5.3
1109	Cheese, brick w/salami	1	oz.	28	12	102	6	1	0	8	5
1037	Cheese, brick, shredded	0.25	cup	28	12	105	7	1	0	8	5.3
1037	Cheese, brick, shredded	1	oz.	28	12	105	7	1	0	8	5.3
1004	Cheese, brie, sliced	1	oz.	28	14	95	6	0	0	8	4.9
1006	Cheese, camembert	0.25	cup	28	15	85	6	0	0	7	4.3
1006	Cheese, camembert	1	oz.	28	15	85	6	0	0	7	4.3
1045	Cheese, caraway	1	piece	28	11	107	7	1	0	8	5.3
1423	Cheese, cheddar, low fat, Alpine Lace	1	oz.	28	14	81	9	1	0	5	3
1105	Cheese, cheddar, low sodim	1	oz.	28	11	113	7	1	0	9	5.9
1091	Cheese, cheddar, lowfat, low sodium	0.25	cup	28	18	49	7	1	0	2	1.2
1224	Cheese, cheddar, nonfat, Lifetime	1	oz.	28	18	40	8	1	0	0	0
1008	Cheese, cheddar, shredded	0.25	cup	28	10	114	7	0	0	9	6
1046	Cheese, cheshire	1	oz.	28	11	110	7	1	0	9	5.5
1046	Cheese, cheshire	1	piece	28	11	110	7	1	0	9	5.5
1011	Cheese, colby, cubed	0.25	cup	33	13	130	8	1	0	11	6.7
1011	Cheese, colby, cubed	1	oz.	28	11	112	7	1	0	9	5.7
1107	Cheese, colby, low sodium	1	oz.	28	11	113	7	1	0	9	5.9
1089	Cheese, colby, lowfat, low sodium	1	oz.	28	18	49	7	1	0	2	1.3
1010	Cheese, colby, shredded	0.25	cup	28	11	111	7	1	0	9	5.7
1047	Cheese, cottage, 1% lowfat	0.5	cup	113	93	82	14	3	0	1	0.7
1014	Cheese, cottage, 2% lowfat	0.5	cup	113	18	810	1	0	0	92	57.2
1049	Cheese, cottage, creamed w/fruit	0.5	cup	113	82	140	11	15	0	4	2.4
1013	Cheese, cottage, creamed, large curd	0.5	cup	113	89	116	14	3	0	5	3.2
1099	Cheese, cottage, lowfat, low sodium	0.5	cup	112	94	81	14	3	0	1	0.7
1084	Cheese, cottage, nonfat (Knudsen)	0.5	cup	122	103	80	15	4	0	0	0
1084	Cheese, cottage, nonfat, Knudsen	0.5	cup	122	103	80	15	4	0	0	0
1012	Cheese, cottage, small curd	0.5	cup	105	83	108	13	3	0	5	3
1015	Cheese, cream	2	Tbs	29	16	101	2	1	0	10	6.4
1098	Cheese, cream, lowfat	2	Tbs	30	19	69	3	2	0	5	3.3
1115	Cheese, cream, nonfat (Philadelphia Free)	2	Tbs	33	26	30	5	2	0	0	0
1188	Cheese, cream, nonfat, Philadelphia	1	oz.	28	22	25	4	2	0	0	0
1083	Cheese, cream, soft (Philadelphia)	2	Tbs	30	17	100	2	1	0	10	7
1050	Cheese, edam	1	oz.	28	12	101	7	0	0	8	5
1016	Cheese, feta, shredded	0.25	cup	62	34	162	9	3	0	13	9.2
1016	Cheese, feta, shredded	1	oz.	28	16	75	4	1	0	6	4.2
1052	Cheese, fontina	1	oz.	28	11	110	7	0	0	9	5.4
1078	Cheese, goat, hard	1	oz.	28	8	128	9	1	0	10	7
1080	Cheese, goat, soft	0.5	cup	62	37	165	11	1	0	13	9

MonoF	PolyF	Choles	Calc	Phos	Sod	Pot	Zn	Iron	Magn	VitA	VitE	VitC	Thia	Ribo	Nia	B6	Fola	B12
(g)	(g)	(mg)	(mg)	(mg)	(mg)	(mg)	(mg)	(mg)	(mg)	(μg RE)	(mg α-TE)	(mg)	(mg)	(mg)	(mg)	(mg)	(μg)	(μg)
0.5	0.6	0	104	113	121	106	0.7	3.9	30	305	0.12	0	0.3	0.35	4.1	0.41	94	0
0.6	0.7	0	172	145	280	105	1	6.6	52	473	0.35	0	0.56	0.34	5.6	0.77	153	0
0.6	0.7	0	105	132	234	112	0.9	3.9	39	302	0.16	0	0.3	0.34	4	0.4	81	0
0.6	0.6	0	166	133	226	150	0.7	6.6	36	441	0.16	0	0.51	0.36	5.5	0.75	150	0
0	0	0	1	16	1	16	0.2	0.4	4	0	0.01	0	0.06	0.01	0.9	0	1	0
0	0.1	0	3	40	1	44	0.4	0.6	16	0	0.08	0	0.05	0.03	1.4	0.02	4	0.05
0.1	0.2	0	8	83	0	85	0.6	0.7	26	0	0.24	0	0.08	0.06	1.1	0.09	13	0
0.2	0.2	0	11	96	183	71	0.7	6.9	26	318	0.17	13	0.31	0.36	4.2	0.43	85	1.27
0	0.1	0	34	36	4	254	1.5	0.7	24	12	0.24	16	0.05	0.06	1	0.15	189	0
0	0.2	0	10	23	1	138	0.2	0.2	10	4	0.1	6	0.02	0.03	0.3	0.09	14	0
2	0.2	18	141	113	274	103	0.9	0.2	8	57	0.19	0	0.01	0.13	0	0.04	2	0.36
1.4	0.1	17	152	110	326	60	0.7	0.1	6	51	0.14	0	0	0.08	0	0.01	1	0.48
0	0	2	150	714	290	55	—	0	—	86	0	0	—	0.07	—	—	—	—
4.1	1	1	12	22	210	33	0.1	0.5	4	7	1.02	0	0.05	0.07	0.6	0.03	24	0.03
0.9	0.1	8	84	107	202	36	0.4	0	4	28	0.11	0	0.01	0.06	0	0.02	1	0.06
1.9	0.2	17	171	217	410	74	0.8	0.1	9	58	0.22	0	0.02	0.13	0	0.04	2	0.12
—	—	20	150	250	420	80	0.6	0	8	86	—	0	—	0.14	—	—	—	0.24
0.3	0	5	103	124	1	27	0.5	0.1	4	10	0.08	0	0	0.06	0	0.01	1	0.12
0.7	0.1	12	233	281	2	61	1.1	0.1	8	22	0.17	0	0.01	0.13	0	0.03	3	0.26
1.5	0.2	13	121	96	250	59	0.6	0.2	6	46	0.15	0	0.01	0.09	0	0.03	2	0.24
1.9	0.2	20	129	156	300	34	0.6	0.1	5	61	0.1	0	0.01	0.07	0	0.02	2	0.15
0.6	0.1	10	194	234	405	51	0.9	0.1	7	18	0.14	0	0.01	0.11	0	0.02	3	0.22
2.2	0.3	27	114	126	170	400	0.3	0.1	20	78	0.17	0	0.09	0.39	0.2	0.08	1	0.69
0	0	5	405	—	223	—	—	—	—	87	—	—	—	—	—	—	—	—
2	0.3	25	259	163	70	30	1	0	10	68	0.14	0	0.01	0.1	0	0.02	2	0.45
2.4	0.2	27	191	128	159	39	0.7	0.1	7	86	0.14	0	0	0.1	0	0.02	6	0.36
2.2	0.2	21	150	110	395	73	0.8	0.1	6	65	0.18	0	0.01	0.11	0.3	0.05	10	0.35
2.4	0.3	26	172	118	173	40	0.7	0.2	7	77	0.13	0	0.01	0.1	0.1	0.02	5	0.42
2.4	0.2	27	190	127	158	38	0.7	0.1	7	85	0.14	0	0	0.1	0	0.02	6	0.36
2.4	0.2	27	190	127	158	38	0.7	0.1	7	85	0.14	0	0	0.1	0	0.02	6	0.36
2.3	0.2	28	52	53	178	43	0.7	0.1	6	52	0.19	0	0.02	0.15	0.1	0.07	18	0.47
2	0.2	20	110	98	238	53	0.7	0.1	6	71	0.18	0	0.01	0.14	0.2	0.06	18	0.37
2	0.2	20	110	98	239	53	0.7	0.1	6	71	0.19	0	0.01	0.14	0.2	0.06	18	0.37
2.4	0.2	26	191	139	196	26	0.8	0.2	6	82	0.14	0	0.01	0.13	0.1	0.02	5	0.08
—	—	15	253	—	96	—	—	0.4	—	87	—	1	—	—	—	—	—	—
2.6	0.3	28	199	137	6	32	0.9	0.2	8	82	0.1	0	0.01	0.11	0	0.02	5	0.24
0.6	0.1	6	199	137	6	32	0.9	0.2	8	18	0.05	0	0.01	0.01	0	0.02	5	0.23
0	0	5	405	—	223	—	—	—	—	87	—	—	—	—	—	—	—	—
2.6	0.3	30	204	145	175	28	0.9	0.2	8	78	0.1	0	0.01	0.11	0	0.02	5	0.23
2.5	0.2	29	183	132	199	27	0.8	0.1	6	70	0.18	0	0.01	0.08	0	0.02	5	0.24
2.5	0.2	29	183	132	199	27	0.8	0.1	6	70	0.18	0	0.01	0.08	0	0.02	5	0.24
3.1	0.3	31	226	151	199	42	1	0.3	9	91	0.12	0	0	0.12	0	0.03	6	0.27
2.6	0.3	27	194	130	171	36	0.9	0.2	7	78	0.1	0	0	0.11	0	0.02	5	0.23
2.6	0.3	28	199	137	6	32	0.9	0.2	8	82	0.1	0	0.01	0.11	0	0.02	5	0.24
0.6	0.1	6	199	137	6	32	0.9	0.2	8	18	0.05	0	0.01	0.01	0	0.02	5	0.24
2.6	0.3	27	194	129	171	36	0.9	0.2	7	78	0.1	0	0	0.11	0	0.02	5	0.23
0.3	0	5	69	151	459	97	0.4	0.2	6	12	0.12	0	0.02	0.19	0.1	0.08	14	0.72
27.1	3.4	247	27	26	933	29	0.1	0.2	2	852	1.79	0	0.01	0.04	0	0	3	0.14
1.1	0.1	13	54	119	458	76	0.3	0.1	5	41	0.1	0	0.02	0.15	0.1	0.06	11	0.56
1.5	0.2	17	68	149	458	95	0.4	0.2	6	54	0.14	0	0.02	0.18	0.1	0.08	14	0.7
0.3	0	4	69	151	15	97	0.4	0.2	6	12	0.12	0	0.02	0.18	0.1	0.08	14	0.71
0	0	10	60	150	370	75	—	0	—	57	—	0	0	0.17	—	0.03	—	0.6
0	0	10	60	150	370	75	—	0	—	57	—	0	0	0.17	—	0.03	—	0.6
1.4	0.1	16	63	139	425	88	0.4	0.1	6	50	0.13	0	0.02	0.17	0.1	0.07	13	0.65
2.8	0.4	32	23	30	86	34	0.2	0.3	2	111	0.27	0	0	0.06	0	0.01	4	0.12
1.7	0.2	17	34	44	89	50	0.2	0.5	2	66	0.14	0	0.01	0.08	0	0.02	5	0.18
0	0	2	100	150	160	65	0.3	0	0	143	—	0	—	0.34	—	—	—	0.12
0	0	3	81	101	137	51	0.3	0	0	145	—	0	—	0.07	—	—	—	0.12
—	—	30	20	20	100	40	0	0	0	86	—	0	—	0.03	—	—	—	0
2.3	0.2	25	207	152	274	53	1.1	0.1	8	72	0.21	0	0.01	0.11	0	0.02	5	0.44
2.8	0.4	55	303	207	686	38	1.8	0.4	12	79	0.02	0	0.1	0.52	0.6	0.26	20	1.04
1.3	0.2	25	140	96	316	18	0.8	0.2	5	36	0.01	0	0.04	0.24	0.3	0.12	9	0.48
2.5	0.5	33	156	98	227	18	1	0.1	4	82	0.1	0	0.01	0.06	0	0.02	2	0.48
2.3	0.2	30	254	207	98	14	0.5	0.5	15	135	0.22	0	0.04	0.34	0.7	0.02	1	0.03
3	0.3	28	86	157	226	16	0.6	1.2	10	174	0.28	0	0.04	0.23	0.3	0.15	7	0.12

Esha Code	Food Item	Qty	Meas	Wgt (g)	Wtr (g)	Cals	Prot (g)	Carb (g)	Fib (g)	Fat (g)	SatF (g)
1080	Cheese, goat, soft	1	oz.	28	17	76	5	0	0	6	4.1
1054	Cheese, gouda	1	oz.	28	12	101	7	1	0	8	5
1074	Cheese, gruyere	1	oz.	28	9	117	8	0	0	9	5.4
1038	Cheese, havarti	1	oz.	28	12	105	7	1	0	8	5.3
1092	Cheese, imitation mozzarella, shredded	0.25	cup	28	17	51	4	3	0	2	1.3
1082	Cheese, light neufchatel (Kraft Philadelphia)	1	oz.	28	18	71	3	1	0	6	4
1055	Cheese, limburger	1	oz.	28	14	93	6	0	0	8	4.7
1018	Cheese, monterey jack, cubed	0.25	cup	33	14	123	8	0	0	10	6.3
1223	Cheese, monterey jack, nonfat, Lifetime	1	oz.	28	18	40	8	1	0	0	0
1017	Cheese, monterey jack, shredded	0.25	cup	28	12	105	7	0	0	9	5.4
56701	Cheese, mozzarella nuggets, Banquet	8	piece	35	15	110	5	8	1	6	2.5
1059	Cheese, mozzarella sting/stick	1	each	28	15	72	7	1	0	5	2.9
1100	Cheese, mozzarella, low sodium	1	oz.	28	14	79	8	1	0	5	3.1
1101	Cheese, mozzarella, low sodium string/stick	1	each	28	14	79	8	1	0	5	3.1
1020	Cheese, mozzarella, lowfat, shredded	0.25	cup	28	14	79	8	1	0	5	3.1
1226	Cheese, mozzarella, nonfat, Lifetime	1	oz.	28	18	40	8	1	0	0	0
1019	Cheese, mozzarella, part skim, low moisture	0.25	cup	28	14	79	8	1	0	5	3.1
1058	Cheese, mozzarella, part skim, shredded	0.25	cup	28	15	72	7	1	0	4	2.8
1057	Cheese, mozzarella, whole milk, low moisture	0.25	cup	28	14	90	6	1	0	7	4.4
1056	Cheese, mozzarella, whole milk, shredded	0.25	cup	28	15	79	5	1	0	6	3.7
1021	Cheese, muenster	0.25	cup	28	12	104	7	0	0	8	5.4
1102	Cheese, muenster, low sodium	1	oz.	28	12	104	7	0	0	9	5.4
1060	Cheese, neufchatel	1	oz.	28	18	74	3	1	0	7	4.2
1075	Cheese, parmesan, grated	1	Tbs	6	1	28	3	0	0	2	1.2
1061	Cheese, parmesan, hard, cubed	1	each	10	3	40	4	0	0	3	1.7
1103	Cheese, parmesan, low sodium, grated	0.25	cup	25	6	114	10	1	0	8	4.9
1112	Cheese, parmesan, shredded	2	oz.	57	14	235	22	2	0	16	9.9
1069	Cheese, pimento processed	1	oz.	28	11	106	6	0	0	9	5.6
1062	Cheese, port du salut	1	oz.	28	13	100	7	0	0	8	4.7
1023	Cheese, provolone	0.25	cup	33	14	116	8	1	0	9	5.6
1024	Cheese, ricotta, part skim	1	oz.	28	21	39	3	1	0	2	1.4
1064	Cheese, ricotta, whole milk	0.33	cup	82	59	143	9	2	0	11	6.8
1066	Cheese, romano, grated	0.33	cup	33	10	128	10	1	0	9	5.6
1026	Cheese, roquefort, crumbled	0.25	cup	34	13	125	7	1	0	10	6.5
1025	Cheese, roquefort, cubed	1	each	17	7	64	4	0	0	5	3.3
1025	Cheese, roquefort, cubed	1	oz.	28	11	105	6	1	0	9	5.5
1227	Cheese, sharp cheddar, nonfat, Lifetime	1	oz.	28	18	40	8	1	0	0	0
1035	Cheese, swiss	1	oz.	28	10	107	8	1	0	8	5
1428	Cheese, swiss, low fat, Alpine Lace	1	oz.	28	12	91	8	1	0	6	4
1104	Cheese, swiss, low sodium	1	oz.	28	11	107	8	1	0	8	5
1225	Cheese, swiss, nonfat, Lifetime	1	oz.	28	18	40	8	1	0	0	0
1027	Cheese, swiss, shredded	0.25	cup	27	10	102	8	1	0	7	4.8
1067	Cheese, tilsit, whole milk	1	oz.	28	12	96	7	1	0	7	4.8
1420	Cheese, white, fat free, Apine Lace	1	oz.	28	18	25	5	1	0	0	0
1085	Cheese, yogurt	1	oz.	28	21	22	2	3	0	0	0
3242	Cherimoya, raw	1	each	547	402	514	7	131	13.1	2	—
3247	Cherries, ground, raw	0.5	cup	70	60	37	1	8	1.9	0	—
3459	Cherries, maraschino	0.5	cup	80	56	93	0	24	—	0	0
3335	Cherries, sour, canned in extra heavy syrup	0.5	cup	130	91	149	1	38	1	0	0
3035	Cherries, sour, canned in water	0.5	cup	122	110	44	1	11	1.3	0	0
3159	Cherries, sour, frozen, unsweetened	0.5	cup	78	68	36	1	9	1.2	0	0.1
3334	Cherries, sour, red, fresh, pitted	0.5	cup	78	67	39	1	9	1.2	0	0.1
3038	Cherries, sweet, canned in heavy syrup	0.5	cup	128	100	107	1	27	1.9	0	0
3336	Cherries, sweet, canned in juice	0.5	cup	125	106	68	1	17	1.9	0	0
3036	Cherries, sweet, fresh	10	each	68	55	49	1	11	1.6	1	0.1
3037	Cherries, sweet, fresh, cup measure	0.5	cup	72	59	52	1	12	1.7	1	0.2
3158	Cherries, sweet, frozen, sweetened	0.5	cup	130	98	115	1	29	2.7	0	0
49023	Cherry crisp	1	cup	246	97	710	5	112	2.3	28	6.2
49007	Cherry crisp, piece, 3x3 in	1	piece	138	106	146	2	24	1.3	5	0.9
45552	Cherry turnover	1	each	78	32	238	3	31	0.9	12	2.9
26108	Chervil, dried	0.25	tsp	0	0	0	0	0	0	0	0
4646	Chestnuts, Chinese, cooked	1	oz.	28	18	43	1	10	0.3	0	0
4645	Chestnuts, Chinese, dried	1	oz.	28	3	103	2	23	0.6	1	0.1
4644	Chestnuts, Chinese, raw	1	oz.	28	12	64	1	14	0.4	0	0
4647	Chestnuts, Chinese, roasted	1	oz.	28	11	68	1	15	0.4	0	0

MonoF	PolyF	Choles	Calc	Phos	Sod	Pot	Zn	Iron	Magn	VitA	VitE	VitC	Thia	Ribo	Nia	B6	Fola	B12
(g)	(g)	(mg)	(mg)	(mg)	(mg)	(mg)	(mg)	(mg)	(mg)	(μg RE)	(mg α-TE)	(mg)	(mg)	(mg)	(mg)	(mg)	(μg)	(μg)
1.4	0.1	13	40	73	104	7	0.3	0.5	5	80	0.13	0	0.02	0.11	0.1	0.07	3	0.05
2.2	0.2	32	198	155	232	34	1.1	0.1	8	49	0.1	0	0.01	0.1	0	0.02	6	0.44
2.8	0.5	31	287	172	95	23	1.1	0	10	85	0.1	0	0.02	0.08	0	0.02	3	0.45
2.4	0.2	27	191	128	159	39	0.7	0.1	7	86	0.14	0	0	0.1	0	0.02	6	0.36
0.6	0.1	5	161	206	324	65	0.7	0	8	23	0.05	0	0.01	0.11	0.1	0.04	1	0.13
—	—	20	20	40	122	30	0	0	0	58	—	0	—	0.03	—	—	—	0
2.4	0.1	26	141	111	227	36	0.6	0	6	90	0.18	0	0.02	0.14	0	0.02	16	0.3
2.9	0.3	29	246	147	177	27	1	0.2	9	84	0.11	0	0	0.13	0	0.03	6	0.27
0	0	5	405	—	223	—	—	—	—	87	—	—	—	—	—	—	—	—
2.5	0.3	25	211	125	151	23	0.8	0.2	8	72	0.1	0	0	0.11	0	0.02	5	0.23
—	—	10	100	290	200	60	—	0.4	—	0	—	0	0.06	0.1	0.2	—	—	—
1.3	0.1	16	183	131	132	24	0.8	0.1	7	50	0.12	0	0	0.09	0	0.02	2	0.23
1.4	0.1	15	207	149	5	27	0.9	0.1	7	54	0.13	0	0.01	0.1	0	0.02	3	0.26
1.4	0.1	15	207	149	5	27	0.9	0.1	7	54	0.13	0	0.01	0.1	0	0.02	3	0.26
1.4	0.1	15	207	148	149	27	0.9	0.1	7	54	0.13	0	0.01	0.1	0	0.02	3	0.26
0	0	5	405	—	223	—	—	—	—	87	—	—	—	—	—	—	—	—
1.4	0.1	15	207	148	149	27	0.9	0.1	7	54	0.13	0	0.01	0.1	0	0.02	3	0.26
1.3	0.1	16	182	131	132	24	0.8	0.1	7	50	0.12	0	0	0.09	0	0.02	2	0.23
2	0.2	25	162	116	117	21	0.7	0.1	6	77	0.19	0	0	0.08	0	0.02	2	0.2
1.9	0.2	22	146	105	105	19	0.6	0.1	5	68	0.1	0	0	0.07	0	0.02	2	0.18
2.5	0.2	27	203	132	177	38	0.8	0.1	8	89	0.13	0	0	0.09	0	0.02	3	0.42
2.5	0.2	27	203	133	5	38	0.8	0.1	8	90	0.13	0	0	0.09	0	0.02	3	0.42
1.9	0.2	22	21	39	113	32	0.1	0.1	2	85	0.27	0	0	0.06	0	0.01	3	0.08
0.5	0	5	86	50	116	7	0.2	0.1	3	11	0.05	0	0	0.02	0	0.01	0	0.09
0.8	0.1	7	122	72	165	10	0.3	0.1	4	15	0.08	0	0	0.03	0	0.01	1	0.12
2.2	0.2	20	344	202	16	27	0.8	0.2	13	43	0.2	0	0.01	0.1	0.1	0.02	2	0.35
5	0.4	41	710	417	962	55	1.8	0.5	29	98	0.48	0	0.02	0.2	0.2	0.06	5	0.79
2.5	0.3	27	174	211	405	46	0.8	0.1	6	91	0.13	1	0.01	0.1	0	0.02	2	0.2
2.6	0.2	35	184	102	151	39	0.7	0.1	7	105	0.14	0	0	0.07	0	0.02	5	0.42
2.4	0.3	23	249	164	289	46	1.1	0.2	9	87	0.12	0	0.01	0.11	0.1	0.02	3	0.48
0.7	0.1	9	77	52	35	35	0.4	0.1	4	32	0.06	0	0.01	0.05	0	0.01	4	0.08
3	0.3	42	170	130	69	86	1	0.3	9	110	0.29	0	0.01	0.16	0.1	0.04	10	0.28
2.6	0.2	34	351	251	396	28	0.9	0.3	14	46	0.24	0	0.01	0.12	0	0.03	2	0.37
2.9	0.4	30	223	132	611	31	0.7	0.2	10	101	0.26	0	0.01	0.2	0.2	0.04	16	0.22
1.5	0.2	16	115	68	313	16	0.4	0.1	5	52	0.13	0	0.01	0.1	0.1	0.02	8	0.11
2.4	0.4	26	188	111	513	26	0.6	0.2	8	85	0.22	0	0.01	0.17	0.2	0.04	14	0.18
0	0	5	405	—	223	—	—	—	—	87	—	—	—	—	—	—	—	—
2.1	0.3	26	272	172	74	32	1.1	0	10	72	0.14	0	0.01	0.1	0	0.02	2	0.48
—	—	20	253	—	35	—	—	0.4	—	87	—	1	—	—	—	—	—	—
2.1	0.3	26	272	172	4	32	1.1	0	10	72	0.14	0	0.01	0.1	0	0.02	2	0.48
0	0	5	405	—	223	—	—	—	—	87	—	—	—	—	—	—	—	—
2	0.3	25	259	163	70	30	1	0	10	68	0.14	0	0.01	0.1	0	0.02	2	0.45
2	0.2	29	198	142	213	18	1	0.1	4	82	0.2	0	0.02	0.1	0.1	0.02	6	0.6
0	0	5	150	—	420	—	—	0.4	—	57	—	1	—	—	—	—	—	—
0	0	1	56	44	22	72	0.3	0	5	1	0	0	0.01	0.06	0	0.01	3	0.17
—	—	0	126	219	16	—	—	2.7	—	5	—	49	0.55	0.6	7.1	—	—	0
—	—	0	6	28	1	191	—	0.7	—	50	0.31	8	0.08	0.03	2	—	—	0
0	0	0	12	10	1	101	—	0.2	—	0	0.1	0	0	0	0	—	—	0
0	0	0	13	12	9	119	0.1	1.6	7	91	0.16	2	0.02	0.05	0.2	0.06	10	0
0	0	0	13	12	9	120	0.1	1.7	7	92	0.16	3	0.02	0.05	0.2	0.05	10	0
0.1	0.1	0	10	12	1	96	0.1	0.4	7	67	0.1	1	0.03	0.03	0.1	0.05	3	0
0.1	0.1	0	12	12	2	134	0.1	0.2	7	99	0.1	8	0.02	0.03	0.3	0.03	6	0
0.1	0.1	0	12	23	4	186	0.1	0.4	12	19	0.08	5	0.03	0.05	0.5	0.04	5	0
0	0	0	18	28	4	164	0.1	0.7	15	16	0.12	3	0.02	0.03	0.5	0.04	5	0
0.2	0.2	0	10	13	0	152	0	0.3	7	14	0.09	5	0.03	0.04	0.3	0.02	3	0
0.2	0.2	0	11	14	0	162	0	0.3	8	15	0.09	5	0.04	0.04	0.3	0.03	3	0
0	0.1	0	16	21	1	258	0.1	0.5	13	25	0.17	1	0.04	0.06	0.2	0.05	5	0
13.2	7.3	0	157	284	592	223	0.3	3.7	20	305	5.26	3	0.27	0.27	2.2	0.09	16	0.02
2.5	1.8	0	26	23	74	154	0.2	2.1	11	150	0.93	3	0.06	0.08	0.6	0.06	11	0.01
5.1	3.1	0	8	28	212	58	0.2	1.6	7	27	1.09	1	0.14	0.11	1.2	0.02	6	0
0	0	0	2	1	0	8	0	0.1	0	1	0	0	0	0	0	0	0	0
0.1	0.1	0	3	19	1	87	0.2	0.3	16	4	0.11	7	0.03	0.04	0.2	0.08	13	0
0.3	0.1	0	8	44	1	206	0.4	0.6	39	9	0.26	17	0.07	0.08	0.4	0.19	31	0
0.2	0.1	0	5	27	1	127	0.2	0.4	24	6	0.17	10	0.04	0.05	0.2	0.12	19	0
0.2	0.1	0	5	29	1	135	0.3	0.4	26	0	0.17	11	0.04	0.03	0.4	0.12	20	0

A

Esha Code	Food Item	Qty	Meas	Wgt (g)	Wtr (g)	Cals	Prot (g)	Carb (g)	Fib (g)	Fat (g)	SatF (g)
4648	Chestnuts, European, cooked	1	oz.	28	19	37	1	8	1.4	0	0.1
4530	Chestnuts, European, raw, peeled	1	oz.	28	15	56	0	12	2.2	0	0.1
4538	Chestnuts, European, roasted, cup measure	0.25	cup	36	14	88	1	19	1.8	1	0.1
4539	Chestnuts, European, roasted, whole	17	each	143	58	350	5	76	7.3	3	0.6
25125	Chewing gum, Care Free sugarless	1	piece	2	—	5	0	2	—	0	0
44032	Chex party mix	1	oz.	28	1	120	3	18	1.6	5	1.5
4610	Chia seeds, dried	1	oz.	28	2	134	5	14	7.2	7	3
56213	Chicken & dumplings, Chicken Helper	0.5	cup	122	87	187	13	10	0.3	10	2.9
56090	Chicken & noodles, recipe	1	cup	240	171	367	22	26	1.8	18	5.9
15023	Chicken hearts, simmered	1	each	3	2	6	1	0	0	0	0.1
15065	Chicken nuggets, fast food serving	1	each	102	52	276	17	15	0	16	3.5
15927	Chicken parmigiana	1	piece	182	120	317	28	15	1.4	16	5.4
15902	Chicken patty, breaded, cooked	1	each	75	37	213	12	11	0.3	13	4.1
16233	Chicken pot pie, Banquet	1	each	198	133	350	10	36	3	18	7
56002	Chicken salad, w/celery	0.5	cup	78	41	268	11	1	0.2	25	3.1
15915	Chicken teriyaki, breast	1	each	128	85	176	26	7	0.2	4	0.9
15916	Chicken teriyaki, drumstick	1	each	68	45	93	14	4	0.1	2	0.5
15050	Chicken, back, skinless, fried	0.5	each	58	28	167	17	3	0	9	2.4
15051	Chicken, back, skinless, roasted	0.5	each	40	24	96	11	0	0	5	1.4
15014	Chicken, back, w/skin, flour fried	1	each	72	32	238	20	5	0.1	15	4
15015	Chicken, back, w/skin, roasted	1	each	53	28	159	14	0	0	11	3.1
15016	Chicken, boned, w/broth, can	1	each	142	98	234	31	0	0	11	3.1
15039	Chicken, breast meat, skinless, stewed	1	each	95	65	143	28	0	0	3	0.8
15001	Chicken, breast w/skin, roasted	1	each	98	61	193	29	0	0	8	2.2
15057	Chicken, breast, skinless, fried	1	each	86	52	161	29	0	0	4	1.1
15004	Chicken, breast, skinless, roasted	1	each	86	56	142	27	0	0	3	0.9
15003	Chicken, breast, w/skin, flour fried	1	each	98	56	218	31	2	0.1	9	2.4
15038	Chicken, breast, w/skin, stewed	1	each	110	73	202	30	0	0	8	2.3
15208	Chicken, canned in water, Swanson	0.5	cup	124	94	131	24	2	0	2	1.1
15018	Chicken, canned, diced, dark meat	0.5	cup	102	70	169	22	0	0	8	2.3
15020	Chicken, canned, diced, light & dark meat	0.5	cup	102	70	169	22	0	0	8	2.3
15022	Chicken, canned, diced, light meat	0.5	cup	102	70	169	22	0	0	8	2.3
15026	Chicken, dark meat, skinless, fried	4	oz.	113	63	271	33	3	0	13	3.5
15027	Chicken, dark meat, skinless, roasted	4	oz.	113	72	232	31	0	0	11	3
15030	Chicken, drumstick, batter fried	1	each	72	38	193	16	6	0.2	11	3
15007	Chicken, drumstick, flour fried	1	each	49	28	120	13	1	0	7	1.8
15008	Chicken, drumstick, roasted	1	each	52	33	112	14	0	0	6	1.6
15042	Chicken, drumstick, skinless, fried	1	each	42	26	82	12	0	0	3	0.9
15035	Chicken, drumstick, skinless, roasted	1	each	44	29	76	12	0	0	2	0.7
15063	Chicken, fried, dark meat, 2 piece serving	1	each	148	72	431	30	16	0.9	27	7
15064	Chicken, fried, white meat, 2 piece serving	1	each	163	74	494	36	20	1.1	30	7.8
15025	Chicken, gizzard, simmered	1	each	22	15	34	6	0	0	1	0.2
15031	Chicken, light meat, skinless, fried	4	oz.	113	68	218	37	0	0	6	1.7
15032	Chicken, light meat, skinless, roasted	4	oz.	113	74	196	35	0	0	5	1.4
15092	Chicken, liver pate, canned	0.5	cup	104	68	209	14	7	0.2	14	4.2
15005	Chicken, liver, simmered	7	each	140	96	220	34	1	0	8	2.6
15028	Chicken, meat, all types, skinless, fried	4	oz.	113	65	248	35	2	0.1	10	2.8
15000	Chicken, meat, all types, skinless, roasted	4	oz.	113	72	215	33	0	0	8	2.3
15006	Chicken, meat, all types, skinless, stewed	0.5	cup	70	47	124	19	0	0	5	1.3
15131	Chicken, roaster, skinless, roasted	4	oz.	113	76	189	28	0	0	8	2
15087	Chicken, skinless, stewed	0.5	cup	70	40	166	21	0	0	8	2.2
15088	Chicken, stewer w/giblets, cooked	1	each	593	322	1636	157	0	0	107	29.1
15011	Chicken, thigh, skinless, fried	1	each	52	31	113	15	1	0	5	1.4
15012	Chicken, thigh, skinless, roasted	1	each	52	33	109	14	0	0	6	1.6
15009	Chicken, thigh, w/skin, flour fried	1	each	62	34	162	17	2	0.1	9	2.5
15010	Chicken, thigh, w/skin, roasted	1	each	62	37	153	16	0	0	10	2.7
15074	Chicken, whole, roasted	1	each	598	356	1429	163	0	0	81	22.7
15075	Chicken, whole, stewed	1	each	668	427	1462	165	0	0	84	23.4
15029	Chicken, wing, flour fried	1	each	32	16	103	8	1	0	7	1.9
15048	Chicken, wing, skinless, fried	1	each	20	12	42	6	0	0	2	0.5
15059	Chicken, wing, skinless, roasted	1	each	21	13	43	6	0	0	2	0.5
15002	Chicken, wing, w/skin, roasted	3	each	102	56	296	27	0	0	20	5.6
15903	Chicken, wings, buffalo type/spicy	1	piece	16	8	49	4	0	0	3	0.9
6119	Chile, banana, cooked	4	oz.	113	101	17	1	4	1.8	0	—
6118	Chile, banana, raw	0.5	cup	75	68	10	1	3	1	0	—

MonoF (g)	PolyF (g)	Choles (mg)	Calc (mg)	Phos (mg)	Sod (mg)	Pot (mg)	Zn (mg)	Iron (mg)	Magn (mg)	VitA (μg RE)	VitE (mg α-TE)	VitC (mg)	Thia (mg)	Ribo (mg)	Nia (mg)	B6 (mg)	Fola (μg)	B12 (μg)
0.1	0.2	0	13	28	8	203	0.1	0.5	15	1	0.2	8	0.04	0.03	0.2	0.07	11	0
0.1	0.1	0	5	11	1	137	0.1	0.3	9	1	0.2	11	0.04	0	0.3	0.1	16	0
0.3	0.3	0	10	38	1	212	0.2	0.3	12	1	0.43	9	0.09	0.06	0.5	0.18	25	0
1.1	1.2	0	42	153	3	847	0.8	1.3	47	3	1.72	37	0.35	0.25	1.9	0.71	100	0
0	0	—	—	—	0	0	—	—	—	—	—	—	—	—	—	—	—	—
2.6	0.7	0	10	53	288	76	0.6	7	18	4	0.07	14	0.44	0.14	4.8	0.44	0	3.52
2.1	2.1	0	150	171	11	292	1.5	2.8	22	1	—	4	0.25	0.05	1.6	0.2	32	0
4	2.2	47	55	125	503	151	1	1.1	17	24	0.37	1	0.11	0.15	4.8	0.15	5	0.16
7.1	3.5	96	26	247	600	149	1.5	2.2	26	10	—	0	0.05	0.17	4.3	0.19	10	0.25
0.1	0.1	8	1	7	2	4	0.2	0.3	1	0	0.05	0	0	0.02	0.1	0.01	3	0.24
7.1	3.4	59	13	278	494	294	1	0.9	24	0	1.35	0	0.11	0.15	7.2	0.3	30	0.3
4.4	4.3	138	189	317	767	463	2.3	2.1	44	146	1.84	9	0.15	0.33	8.2	0.36	18	0.43
6.4	1.6	45	12	150	399	185	0.8	0.9	15	22	1.46	0	0.07	0.1	5	0.23	8	0.22
—	—	40	20	—	950	—	—	1.1	—	200	—	0	—	—	—	—	—	—
4.5	15.8	48	16	80	201	138	0.8	0.6	11	31	6.27	1	0.03	0.07	3.3	0.34	8	0.19
1	0.9	80	27	199	1866	309	1.9	1.8	36	16	0.35	3	0.08	0.2	8.7	0.46	13	0.28
0.6	0.5	43	14	105	991	164	1	0.9	19	8	0.18	2	0.04	0.1	4.6	0.24	7	0.15
3.3	2.1	54	15	102	57	146	1.6	1	14	17	0.34	0	0.06	0.15	4.4	0.2	5	0.18
1.9	1.2	36	10	66	38	95	1.1	0.6	9	11	0.11	0	0.03	0.09	2.8	0.14	3	0.12
5.9	3.5	64	17	120	65	163	1.8	1.2	17	27	0.6	0	0.08	0.17	5.3	0.22	11	0.2
4.4	2.4	47	11	82	46	111	1.2	0.8	11	52	0.14	0	0.03	0.1	3.6	0.14	3	0.14
4.5	2.5	88	20	158	714	196	2	2.2	17	48	0.3	3	0.02	0.18	9	0.5	6	0.41
1	0.6	73	12	157	60	178	0.9	0.8	23	6	0.25	0	0.04	0.11	8	0.31	3	0.22
3	1.6	82	14	210	70	240	1	1	26	26	0.26	0	0.06	0.12	12.4	0.55	4	0.31
1.5	0.9	78	14	212	68	237	0.9	1	27	6	0.36	0	0.07	0.11	12.7	0.55	3	0.32
1.1	0.7	73	13	196	64	220	0.9	0.9	25	5	0.23	0	0.06	0.1	11.8	0.52	3	0.29
3.4	1.9	87	16	228	74	254	1.1	1.2	29	15	0.56	0	0.08	0.13	13.4	0.57	6	0.33
3.2	1.7	82	14	172	68	196	1.1	1	24	26	0.29	0	0.04	0.13	8.6	0.32	3	0.23
—	—	54	0	—	500	—	—	0	—	0	—	0	—	—	—	—	—	—
3.2	1.8	64	14	114	516	141	1.4	1.6	12	35	0.22	2	0.02	0.13	6.5	0.36	4	0.3
3.2	1.8	64	14	114	516	141	1.4	1.6	12	35	0.22	2	0.02	0.13	6.5	0.36	4	0.3
3.2	1.8	64	14	114	516	141	1.4	1.6	12	35	0.22	2	0.02	0.13	6.5	0.36	4	0.3
4.9	3.1	109	20	212	110	287	3.3	1.7	28	27	0.66	0	0.1	0.28	8	0.42	10	0.37
4	2.6	105	17	203	105	272	3.2	1.5	26	25	0.3	0	0.08	0.26	7.4	0.41	9	0.36
4.6	2.7	62	12	106	194	134	1.7	1	14	19	0.88	0	0.08	0.16	3.7	0.19	13	0.2
2.7	1.6	44	6	86	44	112	1.4	0.7	11	12	0.41	0	0.04	0.11	3	0.17	5	0.16
2.2	1.3	47	6	91	47	119	1.5	0.7	12	16	0.14	0	0.04	0.11	3.1	0.18	4	0.17
1.2	0.8	40	5	78	40	105	1.4	0.6	10	8	0.21	0	0.03	0.1	2.6	0.16	4	0.15
0.8	0.6	41	5	81	42	108	1.4	0.6	11	8	0.12	0	0.03	0.1	2.7	0.17	4	0.15
10.9	6.3	166	36	240	755	445	3.2	1.6	37	67	1.33	0	0.13	0.43	7.2	0.33	25	0.83
12.2	6.8	148	60	306	975	566	1.6	1.5	38	59	1.52	0	0.15	0.29	12	0.57	29	0.67
0.2	0.2	43	2	34	15	39	1	0.9	4	12	0.26	0	0.01	0.05	0.9	0.03	12	0.43
2.2	1.4	102	18	262	92	298	1.4	1.3	33	10	0.34	0	0.08	0.14	15.2	0.71	5	0.41
1.8	1.1	96	17	245	87	280	1.4	1.2	31	10	0.3	0	0.07	0.13	14.1	0.68	5	0.39
5.5	2.6	407	10	182	401	99	2.2	9.6	14	226	1.02	10	0.05	1.46	7.8	0.27	334	8.4
1.9	1.3	883	20	437	71	196	6.1	11.9	29	6878	2.02	22	0.21	2.45	6.2	0.81	1078	27.2
3.8	2.4	107	19	232	103	291	2.5	1.5	31	20	0.52	0	0.1	0.22	11	0.54	8	0.39
3	1.9	101	17	221	98	276	2.4	1.4	28	18	0.3	0	0.08	0.2	10.4	0.53	7	0.37
1.7	1.1	58	10	105	49	126	1.4	0.8	15	10	0.19	0	0.03	0.11	4.3	0.18	4	0.15
2.8	1.7	85	14	218	85	260	1.7	1.4	24	14	0.47	0	0.07	0.17	8.9	0.46	6	0.33
2.8	2	58	9	143	55	141	1.4	1	15	23	0.21	0	0.08	0.19	4.5	0.22	4	0.18
40.5	23.8	605	77	1079	421	1049	12	10.9	119	1630	2.09	3	0.55	1.8	33.4	1.54	213	5.93
2	1.3	53	7	103	49	135	1.4	0.8	14	11	0.3	0	0.05	0.13	3.7	0.2	5	0.17
2.2	1.3	49	6	95	46	124	1.3	0.7	12	10	0.14	0	0.04	0.12	3.4	0.18	4	0.16
3.6	2.1	60	9	116	55	147	1.6	0.9	16	18	0.52	0	0.06	0.15	4.3	0.2	7	0.19
3.8	2.1	58	7	108	52	138	1.5	0.8	14	30	0.16	0	0.04	0.13	4	0.19	4	0.18
31.9	17.8	526	90	1088	490	1333	11.6	7.5	138	281	1.58	0	0.38	1	50.8	2.39	30	1.79
32.9	18.3	521	87	929	448	1108	11.8	7.8	127	281	1.77	0	0.31	0.99	37.3	1.47	33	1.34
2.8	1.6	26	5	48	25	57	0.6	0.4	6	12	0.18	0	0.02	0.04	2.1	0.13	2	0.09
0.6	0.4	17	3	33	18	42	0.4	0.2	4	4	0.06	0	0.01	0.03	1.4	0.12	1	0.07
0.5	0.4	18	3	35	19	44	0.4	0.2	4	4	0.06	0	0.01	0.03	1.5	0.12	1	0.07
7.8	4.2	86	15	154	84	188	1.9	1.3	19	48	0.27	0	0.04	0.13	6.8	0.43	3	0.3
1.4	0.8	13	2	24	30	29	0.3	0.2	3	9	0.12	0	0.01	0.02	1	0.07	0	0.04
—	—	0	23	—	5	255	0.5	0.5	19	10	—	136	0.06	0.04	0.7	—	—	0
—	—	0	16	—	3	188	0.3	0.3	14	8	—	113	0.04	0.03	0.5	—	—	0

A

Esha Code	Food Item	Qty	Meas	Wgt (g)	Wtr (g)	Cals	Prot (g)	Carb (g)	Fib (g)	Fat (g)	SatF (g)
56112	Chiles rellenos	1	each	143	75	425	23	7	1	35	17
56001	Chili & beans, canned	1	cups	255	193	286	15	30	11.2	14	6
26072	Chili pepper, dried, Foran Spice	0.5	gram	0	0	2	0	0	0.1	0	—
26002	Chili powder	1	Tbs	8	1	24	1	4	2.6	1	0.2
6532	Chilies, green, canned, Santiago	1	each	62	58	13	0	3	0.7	0	0
6415	Chilies, green, whole, Old El Paso	1	each	35	33	10	0	2	1	0	0
56634	Chimichanga, beef	1	each	174	88	425	20	43	2	20	8.5
56121	Chimichanga, beef & bean	1	each	118	68	249	11	26	3.1	12	3.4
26042	Chives, freeze dried	0.25	cup	1	0	2	0	1	0.2	0	0
5359	Chives, fresh	1	Tbs	3	3	1	0	0	0.1	0	0
47151	Chocolate brownie, Weight Watchers	1	each	182	136	190	6	35	4	4	1
23017	Chocolate chips, milk chocolate	0.25	cup	42	1	218	3	25	1.4	13	7.9
23012	Chocolate chips, semi-sweet	0.25	cup	42	0	204	2	27	2.5	13	7.6
85	Chocolate drink (syrup w/whole milk)	1	cup	250	203	205	8	30	0.5	8	4.7
86	Chocolate drink, syrup w/lowfat milk	1	cup	250	206	181	8	30	0.6	4	2.8
87	Chocolate drink, syrup w/skim milk	1	cup	250	209	149	8	30	0.6	1	0.4
62186	Chocolate fudge shake, Weight Watchers	1	cup	250	206	158	10	30	4.8	2	0
23181	Chocolate morsels, milk chocolate, Toll House	0.25	cup	42	1	213	0	27	0	14	7.6
23182	Chocolate morsels, semi-sweet, Toll House	0.25	cup	42	2	213	0	27	0.1	12	6
23183	Chocolate morsels, semi-sweet, Toll House mini	0.25	cup	42	2	213	0	27	0.1	12	6
23011	Chocolate, baking, unsweetened, grated	0.25	cup	33	0	172	3	9	5.1	18	10.8
23010	Chocolate, baking, unsweetened, square	1	each	28	0	148	3	8	4.4	16	9.2
23044	Chocolate, bittersweet, square	1	each	28	1	135	2	13	0.9	11	6.3
83002	Chow mein entree, chicken, Chun King	1	each	369	292	370	16	45	4	14	5
56092	Chow mein, chicken, canned	1	cup	250	222	95	6	18	2	1	0
56248	Chow mein, pork, no noodles	0.5	cup	110	83	144	11	6	1.2	8	2.2
50093	Chowder, Manhattan clam, chunky, RTS	0.5	cup	120	103	67	4	9	1.4	2	1.1
50094	Chowder, Manhattan clam, chunky, RTS, can	1	each	539	464	302	16	42	6.5	8	4.7
50021	Chowder, Manhattan clam, w/water	0.5	cup	122	112	39	1	6	0.7	1	0.2
50008	Chowder, New England clam, w/milk	0.5	cup	124	106	82	5	8	0.7	3	1.5
50195	Chowder, New England clam, w/water	0.5	cup	122	110	48	2	6	0.7	1	0.2
50211	Chowder, fish/seafood	0.5	cup	122	100	98	12	6	0.3	3	1.5
27036	Chutney	1	Tbs	17	10	26	0	7	0.4	0	0
26003	Cinnamon	0.25	tsp	1	0	1	0	0	0.3	0	0
23001	Citron, candied, chopped	2	Tbs	28	5	89	0	23	0.4	0	0
20052	Citrus drink, concentrate, frozen, prepared	1	cup	252	221	116	1	29	0	0	0
20098	Citrus fruit juice drink, frozen concentrate	0.5	cup	141	81	228	2	57	0.1	0	0
20123	Citrus juice drink, Citrus Hill	1	cup	240	210	112	1	28	0.1	0	0
19021	Clam nectar, canned	1	cup	240	234	5	1	0	0	0	0
19415	Clam patty	1	each	120	33	429	24	40	1.2	18	4.4
19049	Clam, baked/broiled, small	15	each	150	108	209	22	5	0	10	1.9
26019	Cloves, ground	0.25	tsp	1	0	2	0	0	0.2	0	0
49003	Cobbler, apple, piece, 3 x 3	1	piece	104	59	199	2	35	2.1	6	1.2
49019	Cobbler, berry	1	cup	217	103	506	6	92	3.8	14	3.7
49020	Cobbler, cherry	1	cup	217	120	430	5	78	2	12	3.1
49002	Cobbler, cherry, piece, 3 x 3	1	piece	129	85	198	2	34	1.2	6	1.2
49008	Cobbler, peach, piece, 3x3 in	1	piece	130	84	204	2	36	1.7	6	1.2
49021	Cobbler, plum	1	cup	217	115	446	5	84	3	11	2.9
49022	Cobbler, rhubarb	1	cup	217	93	548	5	102	2.9	15	3.6
46	Cocoa mix, prep w/water, sugar free	1	cup	250	231	62	5	11	0.5	0	0.3
73	Cocoa mix, w/water (fortified)	1	cup	279	237	159	3	32	1.1	4	2.4
28209	Cocoa powder unsweetened, European	1	Tbs	5	0	21	1	3	1.6	0	0.3
83	Cocoa powder w/lowfat milk added	1	cup	250	205	186	8	30	1.2	5	3.1
84	Cocoa powder w/skim milk added	1	cup	250	208	152	8	30	1.2	1	0.6
28210	Cocoa powder, dutch processed, unsweetened	1	Tbs	5	0	12	1	3	1.6	1	0.4
28200	Cocoa powder, unsweetened	1	Tbs	5	0	12	1	3	1.8	1	0.4
28211	Cocoa, baking type	1	oz.	28	1	85	6	16	11.3	3	0
28214	Cocoa, dry, low fat	1	oz.	28	1	53	6	16	—	2	1.1
92	Cocoa, sugar free w/lowfat milk (Swiss Miss)	1	cup	250	218	136	9	14	1.5	6	3.3
4649	Coconut cream, canned	0.5	cup	148	105	284	4	12	3.3	26	23.2
4528	Coconut milk, raw	1	cup	240	162	552	6	13	5.3	57	50.6
4527	Coconut water, raw	1	cup	240	228	46	2	9	2.6	0	0.4
4511	Coconut, dried, sweetened, shredded	0.25	cup	23	3	116	1	11	1	8	7.3
4575	Coconut, dried, toasted	1	oz.	28	0	168	2	13	1.8	13	11.8
4510	Coconut, dried, unsweetened	0.25	cup	20	1	129	1	5	3.2	13	11.2

MonoF (g)	PolyF (g)	Choles (mg)	Calc (mg)	Phos (mg)	Sod (mg)	Pot (mg)	Zn (mg)	Iron (mg)	Magn (mg)	VitA (μg RE)	VitE (mg α-TE)	VitC (mg)	Thia (mg)	Ribo (mg)	Nia (mg)	B6 (mg)	Fola (μg)	B12 (μg)
10.2	5.4	165	595	409	620	337	2.8	1.6	39	641	1.84	88	0.07	0.46	0.8	0.22	29	0.54
5.9	0.9	43	120	393	1331	931	5.1	8.8	115	87	1.87	4	0.12	0.27	0.9	0.34	58	0
—	—	0	0	2	0	10	—	0	—	26	—	0	0	0.01	0.1	—	—	0
0.3	0.6	0	21	23	76	144	0.2	1.1	13	262	0.08	5	0.03	0.06	0.6	0.14	8	0
0	0.1	0	39	9	122	77	—	0.8	—	35	—	23	0.01	0.01	0.3	0.3	—	0
0	0	0	0	—	230	—	—	—	—	20	—	9	—	—	—	—	—	0
8.1	1.1	9	63	124	910	586	5	4.5	63	16	—	5	0.49	0.64	5.8	0.28	84	1.51
4.9	2.3	24	46	132	242	386	1.8	2.6	34	40	1.73	9	0.2	0.17	2.8	0.18	55	0.69
0	0	0	6	4	1	24	0	0.2	5	55	0.02	5	0.01	0.01	0	0.02	1	0
0	0	0	3	2	0	9	0	0	1	13	0.01	2	0	0	0	0	3	0
2	1	5	80	—	160	230	—	1.1	—	0	—	0	0.06	0.03	0.2	0.03	—	—
4.2	0.5	9	81	92	35	164	0.6	0.6	26	23	0.53	0	0.03	0.13	0.1	0.02	3	0.17
4.2	0.4	0	14	56	5	155	0.7	1.3	49	1	0.51	0	0.02	0.04	0.2	0.02	1	0
2.2	0.3	30	263	245	138	403	1.1	0.8	50	68	0.2	2	0.08	0.37	0.3	0.09	12	0.78
1.3	0.2	16	268	249	140	410	1.1	0.8	52	124	0.16	2	0.09	0.38	0.3	0.1	12	0.79
0.2	0	4	272	262	144	434	1.1	0.8	46	133	0.1	2	0.08	0.32	0.3	0.09	13	0.82
2.2	0.2	5	396	278	175	443	4.3	5	110	277	5.53	16	0.43	0.48	5.5	0.55	110	1.65
—	—	9	0	—	0	123	—	0	—	0	—	0	0.03	0.08	0.1	—	—	—
—	—	0	0	67	0	136	—	0	—	0	—	0	0.03	—	0.2	—	—	—
4.4	0.5	0	0	67	0	136	—	0	—	0	—	0	0.03	—	0.2	—	—	—
6.1	0.6	0	24	138	5	275	1.3	2.1	102	3	0.41	0	0.03	0.06	0.4	0.03	2	0
5.2	0.5	0	21	118	4	236	1.1	1.8	88	3	0.35	0	0.02	0.05	0.3	0.03	2	0
4.2	0.2	0	16	80	1	174	1.1	1.4	28	3	0.35	0	0.01	0.05	0.3	0.01	3	0
—	—	45	40	200	2010	260	—	1.4	—	100	—	9	1.5	0.17	3	—	—	—
0.1	0.8	8	45	85	725	418	1.3	1.2	14	28	0.05	12	0.05	0.1	1	0.09	12	0.05
3.7	1.9	28	24	113	385	264	1.2	0.9	20	77	1.07	12	0.32	0.17	2.4	0.22	20	0.24
0.5	0.1	7	34	42	500	192	0.8	1.3	10	164	0.05	6	0.03	0.03	0.9	0.13	5	3.96
2.2	0.3	32	151	189	2247	862	3.8	5.9	43	738	0.22	28	0.13	0.14	4.2	0.59	21	17.8
0.2	0.6	1	13	21	289	94	0.5	0.8	6	49	0.37	2	0.02	0.02	0.4	0.05	5	2.03
1.1	0.5	11	93	78	496	150	0.4	0.7	11	20	0.07	2	0.03	0.12	0.5	0.06	5	5.12
0.6	0.5	2	22	27	458	73	0.4	0.7	4	0	0.04	1	0.01	0.02	0.5	0.04	2	4
1	0.3	30	73	146	251	351	0.5	0.3	24	22	0.19	4	0.08	0.13	1.4	0.18	8	0.61
0	0	0	5	7	38	65	0	0.2	4	8	0.1	3	0.01	0.01	0.1	0.02	2	0
0	0	0	7	0	0	3	0	0.2	0	0	0	0	0	0	0	0	0	0
0	0	0	24	7	82	34	—	0.2	—	0	—	0	0	0	0	0	—	0
0	0	0	23	25	8	282	0.1	2.8	15	10	0	68	0.04	0.03	0.5	0.06	5	0
0	0	0	35	51	4	554	0.2	5.6	28	21	0	134	0.07	0.05	0.9	0.12	10	0
0	0	0	316	20	4	196	0.1	0.2	17	1	0.07	80	0.06	0.03	0.3	0.06	5	0
0	0	7	31	274	516	358	0.2	0.7	26	22	2.4	2	0.02	0.05	0.4	0.02	5	12
7.5	4.8	117	191	336	567	496	2.4	21.2	24	168	2.57	12	0.37	0.56	4.6	0.11	29	56.7
4.1	3.3	60	84	299	622	556	2.4	24.5	16	253	3.16	22	0.13	0.3	2.9	0.1	27	82.4
0	0	0	4	1	1	6	0	0	1	0	0.01	0	0	0	0	0.01	1	0
2.8	2	1	22	30	288	106	0.2	0.8	6	76	1.11	0	0.1	0.09	0.7	0.04	3	0.04
5.8	3.6	4	141	105	347	189	0.5	2	19	18	2.35	12	0.29	0.28	2.4	0.06	12	0.06
5	3	3	118	86	354	195	0.4	3.4	18	106	1.29	2	0.21	0.23	1.8	0.08	12	0.05
2.8	2	1	28	34	294	133	0.2	1.8	9	135	1.01	2	0.1	0.11	0.8	0.05	9	0.04
2.8	1.9	1	24	40	291	159	0.2	0.9	10	105	1.16	3	0.09	0.09	1.2	0.03	6	0.04
4.9	2.7	3	107	85	258	291	0.4	1.5	20	42	1.74	10	0.24	0.3	2.2	0.12	8	0.05
6.2	4	3	184	89	408	356	0.4	1.9	24	83	1.84	6	0.24	0.23	2.1	0.04	11	0.05
0.2	0	2	118	175	225	528	0.7	1	42	0	0.08	0	0.05	0.27	0.2	0.06	3	0.38
1.3	0.1	0	139	148	276	541	0.4	2.4	31	201	0.11	8	0.2	0.23	2.7	0.05	0	0.56
0.2	0	0	8	45	3	273	0.4	2.2	30	0	0.02	0	0	0.01	0.2	0.01	—	0
1.5	0.2	17	287	245	158	476	1.2	0.8	52	131	0.24	2	0.1	0.41	0.3	0.1	13	0.84
0.3	0	4	291	258	162	502	1.2	0.7	46	140	0.18	2	0.09	0.35	0.3	0.1	13	0.87
0.2	0	0	6	39	1	135	0.3	0.8	26	0	0.02	0	0.01	0.02	0.1	0.01	2	0
0.2	0	0	7	40	1	82	0.4	0.7	27	0	0.02	0	0	0.01	0.1	0.01	2	0
0.9	0.1	0	0	—	0	493	—	2	—	0	—	0	0.05	0.07	0.7	—	—	—
0.9	0.2	0	43	213	2	431	—	3	—	0	—	0	0.03	0.13	0.7	—	—	—
1.6	0.3	18	303	268	160	495	1.3	0.8	56	140	0.22	2	0.1	0.44	0.3	0.12	14	0.9
1.1	0.3	0	1	33	74	149	0.9	0.8	25	0	1.08	3	0.03	0.06	0.1	0.04	21	0
2.4	0.6	0	38	240	36	631	1.6	3.9	89	0	1.75	7	0.06	0	1.8	0.08	39	0
0	0	0	58	48	252	600	0.2	0.7	60	0	0	6	0.07	0.14	0.2	0.08	6	0
0.4	0.1	0	3	25	61	78	0.4	0.4	12	0	0.31	0	0.01	0	0.1	0.06	2	0
0.6	0.1	0	8	60	10	157	0.6	1	26	0	0.28	0	0.02	0.03	0.2	0.09	3	0
0.5	0.1	0	5	40	7	106	0.4	0.6	18	0	0.26	0	0.01	0.02	0.1	0.06	2	0

Esha Code	Food Item	Qty	Meas	Wgt (g)	Wtr (g)	Cals	Prot (g)	Carb (g)	Fib (g)	Fat (g)	SatF (g)
4508	Coconut, fresh piece, 2.5 x 2 inch	1	piece	45	21	159	2	7	4	15	13.4
4507	Coconut, fresh, grated	0.25	cup	20	9	71	1	3	1.8	7	5.9
20097	Coffee substitute, cereal grain, dry	1	Tbs	7	0	23	0	6	0.6	0	0
20048	Coffee substitute, dry, prepared, Postum	1	cup	240	237	12	0	2	0	0	0
20012	Coffee, brewed	1	cup	240	238	5	0	1	0	0	0
20065	Coffee, brewed. decaffeinated	1	cup	240	238	5	0	1	0	0	0
20044	Coffee, cappuccino, mix, prepared	1	cup	256	237	82	1	14	0	3	2.4
20092	Coffee, chicory, instant, dry	1	Tbs	3	0	9	0	2	0	0	0
20093	Coffee, chicory, instant, prepared	1	cup	239	236	10	0	2	0	0	0
20091	Coffee, decaffeinated, instant, prepared	1	cup	239	236	5	0	1	0	0	0
20062	Coffee, demi tasse	1	cup	240	238	5	0	1	0	0	0
20063	Coffee, espresso	1	cup	240	238	5	0	1	0	0	0
20064	Coffee, espresso, decaffeinated	1	cup	240	238	5	0	1	0	0	0
20108	Coffee, french, mix, prepared	1	cup	252	237	76	1	9	0	5	3.9
20094	Coffee, mocha, instant, dry	1	Tbs	9	0	38	0	6	0.1	1	1.2
20109	Coffee, mocha, mix, prepared	1	cup	251	236	68	1	11	0.3	3	2.2
20023	Coffee, prepared from instant	1	cup	240	238	5	0	1	0	0	0
20043	Coffee, swiss mocha, mix, prepared	1	cup	251	235	67	1	11	0.2	2	2.2
20089	Coffee, vending machine, creamer	1	each	180	174	27	0	3	0	2	1.5
20087	Coffee, vending machine, sugared	1	each	180	172	28	0	7	0	0	0
20088	Coffee, vending machine, sugared, creamed	1	each	180	168	51	0	9	0	2	1.4
5461	Coleslaw salad	0.5	cup	60	44	89	1	8	1	7	1
5061	Collard greens, cooked, no added salt	0.5	cup	64	59	17	1	3	1.8	0	0
5062	Collard greens, frozen, cooked, no added salt	0.5	cup	85	75	31	3	6	2.4	0	0.1
5060	Collard greens, raw	0.5	cup	18	16	5	0	1	0.6	0	0
26305	Comfrey leaves	1	oz.	28	25	9	1	2	—	0	—
50098	Consomme, beef, w/gelatin, prep w/water	0.5	cup	120	116	14	3	1	0	0	0
45530	Cookie crust, chocolate, recipe, baked	1	each	219	12	1130	11	122	3.4	69	15
47013	Cookie dough, chocolate chip, refrigerated	4	each	48	6	213	2	30	0.7	10	3.2
47050	Cookie mix, oatmeal, dry	8	oz.	227	12	1047	15	153	6.4	44	10.8
47051	Cookie mix, oatmeal, dry, prepared	2	each	32	2	148	2	21	1.2	6	1.6
47012	Cookie, Fig bar	4	each	56	9	195	2	40	2.6	4	0.6
47009	Cookie, Ladyfinger	2	each	22	4	80	2	13	0.2	2	0.7
47171	Cookie, Nilla wafers	7	each	28	—	124	1	21	0.4	4	0.9
47073	Cookie, almond	2	each	20	1	104	2	10	0.5	6	1
47015	Cookie, animal, small box	1	each	67	3	299	4	50	—	9	3.5
47514	Cookie, apple filled oatmeal, Archway	1	each	28	4	111	1	18	0.6	4	0.8
47074	Cookie, applesauce, large	2	each	36	6	133	2	23	1.1	4	0.9
47516	Cookie, apricot filled, Archway	1	each	28	4	112	1	18	0.4	4	1.5
47517	Cookie, blueberry filled, Archway	1	each	28	—	110	1	19	0.5	4	1.5
47005	Cookie, butter, commercially prepared	5	each	25	1	117	2	17	0.2	5	2.8
47075	Cookie, butterscotch brownie	1	each	34	4	149	2	22	0.3	7	1.2
47076	Cookie, carob	2	each	26	1	103	2	17	1.6	4	0.8
47213	Cookie, chocolate brownie, fat free, Entenmann's	1	each	12	1	40	0	10	0.5	0	0
47213	Cookie, chocolate brownie, fat-free, Entenmann's	2	each	24	2	80	1	20	1	0	0
47520	Cookie, chocolate chip, Archway	3	each	27	—	130	1	17	0	7	2
47032	Cookie, chocolate chip, commercial	1	each	10	0	45	1	7	0.4	2	0.4
47022	Cookie, chocolate chip, dietetic	5	each	25	1	125	1	16	1.2	7	2.2
47037	Cookie, chocolate chip, homemade, w/butter	2	each	32	2	156	2	19	0.8	9	4.5
47002	Cookie, chocolate chip, homemade, w/margarine	2	each	20	1	98	1	12	0.6	6	1.6
47035	Cookie, chocolate chip, mix, prepared	2	each	32	1	159	2	20	0.4	8	2.7
47033	Cookie, chocolate chip, no sodium, w/fructose	4	each	28	1	126	1	21	0.4	5	1.2
47036	Cookie, chocolate chip, refrigerated dough, baked	2	each	24	1	118	1	16	0.4	5	1.9
47031	Cookie, chocolate chip, rich	1	each	10	0	48	1	7	0.2	2	0.7
47016	Cookie, chocolate chip, small box	1	each	55	3	233	3	36	—	12	5.3
47001	Cookie, chocolate chip, soft	2	each	21	2	96	1	12	0.7	5	1.6
47164	Cookie, chocolate sandwich, Snackwell's	1	oz.	28	1	116	1	22	0.7	3	0.7
47006	Cookie, chocolate sandwich, creme-filled	2	each	20	0	94	1	14	0.6	4	0.7
47039	Cookie, chocolate sandwich, low sodium, w/fructose	3	each	30	1	138	1	20	1.2	7	1.2
47038	Cookie, chocolate sandwich, w/chocolate icing	2	each	34	1	164	1	22	1.8	9	2.5
47040	Cookie, chocolate sandwich, w/extra creme	2	each	26	0	130	1	18	0.5	7	1
47041	Cookie, chocolate wafer	4	each	24	1	104	2	17	0.8	3	1
47502	Cookie, cinnamon honey, fat free, Archway	3	each	30	3	106	1	25	0.4	0	0.1
47526	Cookie, coconut macaroon, Archway	1	each	23	2	111	1	13	0.5	6	5.7
47042	Cookie, coconut macaroon, recipe	1	each	24	3	97	1	17	0.4	3	2.7

MonoF	PolyF	Choles	Calc	Phos	Sod	Pot	Zn	Iron	Magn	VitA	VitE	VitC	Thia	Ribo	Nia	B6	Fola	B12
(g)	(g)	(mg)	(mg)	(mg)	(mg)	(mg)	(mg)	(mg)	(mg)	(μg RE)	(mg α-TE)	(mg)	(mg)	(mg)	(mg)	(mg)	(μg)	(μg)
0.6	0.2	0	6	51	9	160	0.5	1.1	14	0	0.33	1	0.03	0.01	0.2	0.02	12	0
0.3	0.1	0	3	23	4	71	0.2	0.5	6	0	0.15	1	0.01	0	0.1	0.01	5	0
0	0.1	0	4	40	5	127	0	0.3	17	0	0.07	0	0.04	0.01	1.2	0.06	2	0
0	0	0	7	17	10	58	0.1	0.1	10	0	0	0	0.02	0	0.5	0.03	1	0
0	0	0	5	2	5	130	0	0.1	12	0	0	0	0	0	0.5	0	0	0
0	0	0	5	2	5	130	0	0.1	12	0	0	0	0	0	0.5	0	0	0
0.2	0.1	0	10	36	138	159	0.1	0.2	13	0	0.1	0	0.02	0.01	0.4	0	0	0
0	0	0	3	7	7	92	0	0.1	6	0	0	0	0	0.01	0.6	0	0	0
0	0	0	7	7	14	81	0.1	0.1	7	0	0	0	0	0.01	0.5	0	0	0
0	0	0	7	7	7	84	0.1	0.1	10	0	0	0	0	0.03	0.7	0	0	0
0	0	0	5	2	5	130	0	0.1	12	0	0	0	0	0	0.5	0	0	0
0	0	0	5	2	5	130	0	0.1	12	0	0	0	0	0	0.5	0	0	0
0	0	0	5	2	5	130	0	0.1	12	0	0	0	0	0	0.5	0	0	0
0.3	0.1	0	10	55	40	181	0	0	3	0	0	0	0	0	0.9	0	0	0
0.1	0	0	3	22	23	89	0.1	0.2	6	0	0	0	0	0	0.2	0	0	0
0.1	0	0	10	38	48	158	0.2	0.3	12	0	0.02	0	0	0	0.3	0	0	0
0	0	0	7	7	7	86	0.1	0.1	10	0	0	0	0	0	0.7	0	0	0
0.1	0	0	10	38	48	158	0.2	0.3	13	0	0	0	0	0	0.3	0	0	0
0	0	0	6	22	14	72	0.1	0.1	5	1	0.01	0	0	0.01	0.3	0	0	0
0	0	0	5	3	6	35	0.1	0.1	5	0	0	0	0	0	0.3	0	0	0
0	0	0	6	21	13	70	0.1	0.1	5	1	0.01	0	0	0.01	0.3	0	0	0
1.5	3.9	3	20	22	162	107	0.1	0.4	5	30	2.4	5	0.02	0.02	0	0.07	23	0.11
0	0.1	0	76	17	6	166	0.3	0.3	11	200	0.56	12	0.03	0.07	0.4	0.08	60	0
0	0.2	0	179	23	42	213	0.2	1	26	508	0.42	22	0.04	0.1	0.5	0.1	65	0
0	0	0	26	2	4	30	0	0	2	69	0.41	6	0.01	0.02	0.1	0.03	30	0
—	—	—	90	15	—	—	—	0.9	—	275	—	7	0.03	0.06	0.4	—	—	0
0	0	0	5	16	318	77	0.2	0.3	0	0	0.01	0	0.01	0.01	0.4	0.01	1	0
32.9	17.2	4	68	234	1502	374	1.8	6.7	90	488	—	0	0.34	0.46	4.8	0	0	0.04
5	1	12	12	33	100	86	0.2	1.1	12	8	1.11	0	0.09	0.09	1	0.02	27	0.04
24	6.3	0	57	370	1072	415	1.8	5	109	5	5.9	0	0.32	0.32	3	0.1	113	0
3.4	0.9	13	9	56	150	60	0.3	0.7	15	7	0.9	0	0.09	0.05	0.4	0.02	4	0.03
1.7	1.6	0	36	35	196	116	0.2	1.6	15	2	0.7	0	0.09	0.12	1	0.04	15	0.05
0.9	0.3	80	10	38	32	25	0.3	0.8	3	37	0.28	1	0.06	0.09	0.5	0.03	17	0.16
1.3	0	2	18	—	89	27	—	1	—	—	—	—	—	—	—	—	—	—
3.2	1.8	9	15	34	49	42	0.2	0.5	14	57	1.7	0	0.05	0.07	0.5	0.01	4	0.02
3.8	1	11	11	64	273	56	0.3	1.5	11	8	0.32	1	0.25	0.24	2.5	0.02	81	0.05
1.4	0.3	2	8	—	116	51	—	0.9	—	1	—	0	0.07	0.04	0.5	—	15	—
1.9	1.4	9	22	44	109	76	0.2	0.7	11	55	0.74	0	0.07	0.05	0.4	0.03	3	0.02
1.2	0.2	8	6	—	9	35	—	0.6	—	3	—	0	0.07	0.06	0.5	—	—	—
—	—	5	0	—	115	—	—	0.7	—	0	—	0	—	—	—	—	—	—
1.4	0.2	29	7	26	88	28	0.1	0.6	3	42	0.13	0	0.09	0.08	0.8	0.01	10	0.09
2.6	2.3	18	24	26	96	80	0.2	0.7	10	76	0.96	0	0.05	0.06	0.4	0.02	4	0.04
2	1.4	16	70	59	80	140	0.4	0.6	17	7	0.7	0	0.04	0.09	0.5	0.05	6	0.08
0	0	0	0	—	45	62	—	0.4	—	0	—	0	—	—	—	—	—	—
0	0	0	0	—	90	125	—	0.7	—	0	—	0	—	—	—	—	—	—
—	—	10	0	—	70	—	—	0.7	—	0	—	0	—	—	—	—	—	—
0.6	0.5	0	2	8	38	12	0.1	0.3	3	0	0.18	0	0.03	0.03	0.3	0.03	7	0
2.2	1.9	3	8	14	3	21	0.2	0.3	6	2	0.64	0	0.04	0.04	0.3	0.02	2	0.03
2.6	1.4	22	12	32	109	71	0.3	0.8	18	47	0.29	0	0.06	0.06	0.4	0.03	11	0.03
2.1	1.7	6	8	20	72	45	0.2	0.5	11	33	0.57	0	0.04	0.04	0.3	0.02	7	0.02
4.2	0.9	13	15	30	94	68	0.2	0.7	12	6	0.83	0	0.05	0.07	0.6	0.01	3	0.03
1.9	1.4	0	13	30	3	56	0.1	1	6	0	0.69	0	0.1	0.05	0.8	0	13	0
2.7	0.6	6	7	18	56	48	0.1	0.6	6	4	0.49	0	0.04	0.05	0.5	0	2	0.02
1.2	0.2	0	2	11	32	14	0.1	0.3	3	0	0.26	0	0.02	0.03	0.3	0.01	4	0
5	1	12	20	52	188	82	0.3	1.5	16	15	0.37	1	0.09	0.19	1.4	0.03	33	0.1
2.7	0.7	0	3	10	68	20	0.1	0.5	7	0	0.61	0	0.02	0.04	0.3	0.03	8	0
0.8	0.2	0	16	58	217	45	0.2	0.8	13	0	—	0	0.04	0.05	0.6	0.01	—	0
1.7	1.4	0	5	20	121	35	0.2	0.8	9	0	0.69	0	0.02	0.04	0.4	0	9	0.01
2.8	2.4	0	29	60	73	88	0.2	1.4	8	0	1.13	0	0.16	0.09	1.2	0.01	19	0.01
5	1	0	12	31	111	82	0.2	1.1	13	0	1.13	0	0.03	0.07	0.5	0.02	6	0.02
2.8	2.4	0	6	24	128	32	0.2	0.7	9	0	1.17	0	0.02	0.04	0.4	0.01	11	0
1.2	1	0	7	32	139	50	0.3	1	13	1	0.38	0	0.05	0.06	0.7	0.01	12	0.02
0.1	0.1	0	6	—	123	20	—	0.8	—	0	—	0	0.1	0.06	0.8	—	24	—
0.4	0.1	0	4	—	40	6	—	0.4	—	0	—	0	0.01	0.01	0.1	—	1	—
0.1	0	0	2	10	59	37	0.2	0.2	5	0	0.07	0	0	0.03	0	0.02	1	0.01

Esha Code	Food Item	Qty	Meas	Wgt (g)	Wtr (g)	Cals	Prot (g)	Carb (g)	Fib (g)	Fat (g)	SatF (g)
47530	Cookie, date filled oatmeal, Archway	1	each	28	4	111	1	19	0.8	3	0.8
47153	Cookie, devil's food, Snackwell's	1	oz.	28	5	97	1	22	0.4	0	0
47324	Cookie, double fudge, fat free, Snackwell's	1	oz.	28	4	94	1	21	0.5	0	0.2
47043	Cookie, fortune	4	each	32	3	121	1	27	0.5	1	0.2
47376	Cookie, fruit bar, no fat, Archway	1	each	28	—	90	2	21	0	0	0
47044	Cookie, fudge cake type	1	each	21	2	73	1	16	0.6	1	0.2
47324	Cookie, fudge, fat free, Snackwell's	2	each	32	5	106	2	24	0.6	0	0.2
47509	Cookie, gingerbread, iced, Archway	3	each	32	1	149	1	23	0.4	6	1.8
47045	Cookie, gingersnap	4	each	28	1	116	2	22	0.6	3	0.7
43527	Cookie, graham cracker, chocolate-coated	2	each	28	1	136	2	19	0.9	6	3.8
47077	Cookie, granola	2	each	26	1	119	2	17	1.1	4	3.7
47078	Cookie, lemon bar	2	each	32	4	139	2	20	0.3	6	1.2
47046	Cookie, marshmallow, chocolate-coated	2	each	26	3	109	1	18	0.5	4	1.2
47109	Cookie, molasses	2	each	30	2	129	2	22	0.3	4	1
47546	Cookie, molasses, old fashioned, Archway	1	each	28	3	113	1	20	0.3	3	0.8
47047	Cookie, oatmeal	2	each	36	2	162	2	25	1	7	1.6
47369	Cookie, oatmeal chocolate chip, fat free, Entenmann	1	each	12	—	40	0	10	0.5	0	0
47496	Cookie, oatmeal raisin, Archway	1	each	28	—	110	2	19	0.5	4	1
47212	Cookie, oatmeal raisin, fat free, Entenmann's	1	each	24	4	80	1	18	0.5	0	0
47500	Cookie, oatmeal raisin, no fat, Archway	1	each	28	4	96	1	22	0.9	0	0.1
47003	Cookie, oatmeal raisin, recipe	2	each	26	2	113	2	18	0.8	4	0.8
47049	Cookie, oatmeal raisin, w/fructose, no sodium	4	each	28	2	126	1	20	0.8	5	0.8
47023	Cookie, oatmeal w/raisins, dietetic	3	each	33	3	144	2	21	0.8	6	1.5
47541	Cookie, oatmeal, Archway	1	each	27	3	115	2	18	0.8	4	0.9
47053	Cookie, oatmeal, chilled dough, baked	2	each	24	1	113	1	16	0.7	5	1.3
47054	Cookie, oatmeal, recipe	2	each	30	2	134	2	20	0.9	5	1.1
47048	Cookie, oatmeal, soft	2	each	30	3	123	2	20	0.8	4	1.1
47180	Cookie, oreo sandwich	2	each	28	—	138	2	20	0.9	6	1.3
47059	Cookie, peanut butter sandwich	2	each	28	1	134	2	18	0.5	6	1.4
47060	Cookie, peanut butter sandwich, low sodium, w/fruct	3	each	30	1	161	3	15	0.5	10	1.5
47549	Cookie, peanut butter, Archway	1	each	28	2	134	3	16	0.8	7	1.5
47058	Cookie, peanut butter, chilled dough, baked	2	each	24	1	121	2	14	0.3	7	1.5
47010	Cookie, peanut butter, homemade	2	each	24	1	114	2	14	0.5	6	1.1
47056	Cookie, peanut butter, soft type	2	each	30	3	137	2	17	0.5	7	1.8
47079	Cookie, pecan sandies	2	each	30	1	149	2	20	0.5	7	1.8
47062	Cookie, pecan shortbread	2	each	28	1	152	1	16	0.5	9	2.3
47554	Cookie, raisin oatmeal, Archway	3	each	28	—	130	2	19	1	6	1.5
47061	Cookie, raisin, soft type	2	each	30	4	120	1	20	0.4	4	1
47555	Cookie, raspberry filled, Archway	1	each	28	4	113	1	18	0.4	4	1.5
47499	Cookie, raspberry oatmeal, no fat, Archway	1	each	28	3	98	1	22	0.9	0	0.1
47024	Cookie, sandwich-type, dietetic	3	each	33	4	151	2	18	0.3	8	2
47007	Cookie, shortbread, commercial, plain	4	each	32	1	161	2	21	0.6	8	2
47014	Cookie, shortbread, homemade, w/butter	2	each	28	1	155	2	16	0.4	9	5.8
47063	Cookie, shortbread, homemade, w/margarine	3	each	33	1	180	2	19	0.5	11	2.1
47011	Cookie, snickerdoodle	1	each	20	4	81	1	12	0.4	3	2.1
47064	Cookie, sugar	2	each	30	1	143	2	20	0.2	6	1.6
47070	Cookie, sugar wafer, cream-filled w/fructose, no so	7	each	28	1	141	1	18	0.5	7	1.1
47069	Cookie, sugar wafer, creme-filled	8	each	28	0	143	1	20	0.2	7	1
47561	Cookie, sugar, Archway	1	each	28	—	120	2	20	0	4	1
47067	Cookie, sugar, homemade, w/butter	2	each	28	2	132	2	17	0.4	7	4
47068	Cookie, sugar, homemade, w/margarine	2	each	28	2	132	2	17	0.3	7	1.3
47065	Cookie, sugar, no sodium, w/fructose	4	each	28	2	121	1	22	0.2	4	0.5
47004	Cookie, sugar, refrigerated dough, baked	2	each	24	1	116	1	16	0.2	6	1.4
47559	Cookie, sugar, soft, Archway	1	each	28	3	115	1	19	0.3	4	0.9
47025	Cookie, sugar/plain, dietetic	5	each	30	3	139	1	18	0.1	7	1.4
47071	Cookie, vanilla sandwich	3	each	30	1	145	1	22	0.4	6	0.9
47160	Cookie, vanilla sandwich, Snackwell's	1	oz.	28	1	119	1	23	0.6	3	0.6
47562	Cookie, vanilla wafer, Archway	5	each	30	—	130	2	22	0	4	1
47008	Cookie, vanilla wafer, made w/egg	7	each	28	1	123	1	21	0.5	4	1.1
47072	Cookie, vanilla wafer, no egg	4	each	24	1	114	1	17	0.5	5	1.2
47020	Cookie, whole wheat fruit & nut	2	each	28	4	121	2	16	1.3	6	1
22608	Cooking wine, red, Fleischmann's	1	Tbs	15	13	10	0	0	0	0	0
22609	Cooking wine, white, Fleischmann's	1	Tbs	15	13	10	0	0	0	0	0
26020	Coriander leaf, dried	0.25	tsp	0	0	0	0	0	0	0	0
26041	Coriander seed	0.25	tsp	0	0	1	0	0	0.2	0	0

MonoF (g)	PolyF (g)	Choles (mg)	Calc (mg)	Phos (mg)	Sod (mg)	Pot (mg)	Zn (mg)	Iron (mg)	Magn (mg)	VitA (μg RE)	VitE (mg α-TE)	VitC (mg)	Thia (mg)	Ribo (mg)	Nia (mg)	B6 (mg)	Fola (μg)	B12 (μg)
1.3	0.3	4	10	—	110	59	—	0.6	—	1	—	0	0.07	0.05	0.5	—	—	—
0.2	0	0	9	22	48	30	0.1	0.4	6	0	—	0	0.03	0.04	0.4	0.01	—	0.02
0.1	0.1	0	5	20	125	47	0.1	0.5	9	0	0	0	0.03	0.03	0.5	0.01	—	0
0.4	0.1	1	4	11	88	13	0.1	0.5	2	0	0.11	0	0.06	0.04	0.6	0	18	0
0	0	0	0	—	95	—	—	0.4	—	0	0.01	0	—	—	—	—	—	—
0.4	0.1	0	7	17	40	29	0.1	0.5	7	0	0.12	0	0.05	0.04	0.3	0.01	9	0.02
0.1	0.1	0	6	22	141	53	0.2	0.6	10	0	0	0	0.03	0.04	0.5	0.01	—	0
1.9	0.7	0	7	—	114	22	—	0.1	—	0	—	0	0.06	0.09	0.8	—	22	—
1.5	0.4	0	22	23	183	97	0.2	1.8	14	0	0.36	0	0.06	0.08	0.9	0.03	20	0
2.2	0.3	0	16	38	82	58	0.3	1	16	0	0.32	0	0.04	0.06	0.6	0.02	5	0
0.3	0.1	0	18	93	86	94	0.4	0.8	26	0	0.03	0	0.16	0.06	0.5	0.09	21	0
2.6	1.8	25	12	22	78	22	0.1	0.5	3	83	1	1	0.06	0.07	0.4	0.01	4	0.05
2.4	0.5	0	12	25	44	47	0.2	0.7	9	0	0.56	0	0.02	0.05	0.2	0.02	5	0.04
2.1	0.5	0	22	28	138	104	0.1	1.9	16	0	0.51	0	0.11	0.08	0.9	0.03	22	0
1.2	0.2	9	10	—	148	32	—	1.3	—	3	—	0	0.08	0.07	0.7	—	—	—
3.6	0.9	0	13	50	138	51	0.3	0.9	12	1	0.91	0	0.1	0.08	0.8	0.02	16	0
0	0	0	0	—	55	40	—	0.2	—	0	—	0	—	—	—	—	—	—
—	—	2	0	—	115	—	—	1.1	—	0	—	0	—	—	—	—	—	—
0	0	0	0	—	120	60	—	0	—	0	—	0	—	—	—	—	—	—
0.1	0.2	0	10	—	149	79	—	0.9	—	0	—	0	0.07	0.04	0.5	—	13	—
1.8	1.3	9	26	42	140	62	0.2	0.7	11	43	0.65	0	0.06	0.04	0.3	0.02	8	0.02
2.1	1.9	0	15	34	3	49	0.1	1.1	5	0	0.9	0	0.13	0.06	0.9	0.01	15	0
2.6	1.6	1	7	46	1	55	0.3	0.7	9	0	0.82	0	0.08	0.03	0.3	0.01	4	0.04
1.5	0.4	3	8	—	94	50	—	0.6	—	1	—	0	0.08	0.05	0.5	—	—	—
2.8	0.7	6	8	28	78	39	0.2	0.6	8	3	0.72	0	0.05	0.04	0.4	0.01	2	0.01
2.3	1.7	11	32	50	179	55	0.3	0.8	13	55	0.81	0	0.08	0.05	0.4	0.02	10	0.03
2.4	0.7	2	27	63	105	40	0.1	0.8	9	2	0.6	0	0.06	0.07	0.5	0.03	10	0
2.6	0.4	0	—	—	189	52	—	0.6	—	—	—	—	—	—	—	—	—	—
3.1	1.1	0	15	53	103	54	0.3	0.7	14	0	0.91	0	0.09	0.07	1	0.04	12	0.06
4.6	3.6	0	13	46	124	88	0.3	0.8	15	0	1.72	0	0.1	0.04	1.6	0.02	16	0
2.9	1.2	10	10	—	113	59	—	0.8	—	3	—	0	0.07	0.06	1.2	—	—	—
3.5	1.2	7	27	63	105	81	0.2	0.4	10	3	0.96	0	0.04	0.04	1	0.02	2	0.01
2.6	1.7	7	9	28	124	55	0.2	0.5	9	37	0.91	0	0.05	0.05	0.8	0.02	13	0.02
4.1	1	0	4	26	101	32	0.2	0.3	10	0	1.17	0	0.07	0.05	0.6	0.01	20	0
3.9	0.9	10	21	47	18	20	0.1	0.9	5	7	0.89	0	0.14	0.08	0.9	0.01	3	0.02
5.2	1.2	9	8	24	79	20	0.2	0.7	5	0	1.06	0	0.08	0.06	0.7	0.01	18	0
—	—	10	0	—	55	—	—	0.7	—	0	—	0	—	—	—	—	—	—
2.3	0.5	1	14	25	101	42	0.1	0.7	6	0	0.58	0	0.06	0.06	0.6	0.02	13	0.01
1.2	0.2	8	7	—	94	35	—	0.6	—	2	—	0	0.09	0.06	0.5	—	—	—
0.2	0.2	0	11	—	150	80	—	0.9	—	0	—	0	0.08	0.04	0.5	—	13	—
3.6	2.2	0	12	21	4	32	0.2	0.4	10	0	1.32	0	0.05	0.05	0.4	0.01	2	0
4.3	1	6	11	35	146	32	0.2	0.9	5	4	1.03	0	0.11	0.1	1.1	0.03	19	0.03
2.7	0.4	25	5	20	132	20	0.1	0.7	4	87	0.23	0	0.1	0.07	0.8	0.01	3	0.01
4.8	3.5	0	7	23	169	25	0.1	0.9	4	114	1.65	0	0.12	0.08	1	0.01	4	0.01
1	0.2	9	8	10	74	24	0.1	0.5	2	32	0.1	0	0.05	0.04	0.4	0.01	2	0.02
3.5	0.8	15	6	24	107	19	0.1	0.6	4	8	0.85	0	0.07	0.06	0.8	0.02	14	0.06
3	2.7	0	15	10	3	17	0.1	0.4	2	0	1.13	0	0.05	0.03	0.4	0	12	0
2.9	2.6	0	5	16	41	16	0.1	0.5	3	0	1.23	0	0.03	0.06	0.7	0	12	0
—	—	2	0	—	190	—	—	0.7	—	0	—	0	—	—	—	—	—	—
1.9	0.3	24	20	25	129	20	0.1	0.7	3	62	0.2	0	0.08	0.07	0.7	0.01	3	0.02
2.9	2	7	20	25	137	22	0.1	0.7	3	70	1.02	0	0.08	0.07	0.7	0.01	15	0.02
1.5	1.3	0	7	20	1	29	0.1	1.1	3	0	0.62	0	0.14	0.06	1	0	16	0
3.1	0.7	8	22	45	112	39	0.1	0.4	2	3	0.77	0	0.04	0.03	0.6	0.01	13	0.02
1.3	0.2	6	9	—	189	23	—	0.6	—	2	—	0	0.09	0.06	0.7	—	—	—
3.1	2.2	18	2	11	0	12	0.1	0.4	4	0	0.96	0	0.06	0.03	0.4	0.01	3	0.03
2.5	2.3	0	8	22	105	27	0.1	0.7	4	0	1.08	0	0.08	0.07	0.8	0	18	0
0.8	0.2	0	19	40	104	31	0.2	0.7	5	0	—	0	0.05	0.07	0.7	0.01	—	0.02
—	—	5	0	—	130	—	—	1.1	—	0	—	0	—	—	—	—	—	—
1.8	1.1	14	13	29	87	27	0.1	0.7	4	2	0.36	0	0.08	0.09	0.9	0.02	14	0.04
2.7	0.6	0	6	15	73	26	0.1	0.5	3	0	0.34	0	0.09	0.05	0.7	0.01	10	0.01
2.2	2.7	15	18	49	59	111	0.4	0.7	20	50	0.81	0	0.05	0.04	0.5	0.06	6	0.03
0	0	—	1	2	90	12	—	0.1	—	0	—	0	0.08	0.08	0.1	—	—	0
0	0	—	1	2	90	13	—	0.1	—	0	—	0	0.08	0.08	0.1	—	—	0
0	0	0	2	1	0	7	0	0.1	1	1	0	1	0	0	0	0	0	0
0.1	0	0	3	2	0	5	0	0.1	1	0	—	0	0	0	0	—	0	0

Esha Code	Food Item	Qty	Meas	Wgt (g)	Wtr (g)	Cals	Prot (g)	Carb (g)	Fib (g)	Fat (g)	SatF (g)
26038	Coriander/cilantro, fresh	0.25	cup	4	4	1	0	0	0.1	0	0
38074	Corn bran, crude	0.25	cup	19	1	43	2	16	16.2	0	0
44026	Corn chips, BBQ flavor	10	piece	18	0	94	1	10	0.9	6	0.8
44002	Corn chips/Fritos	1	cup	26	0	140	2	15	1.3	9	1.2
44003	Corn chips/Fritos, grab bag	1	each	85	1	458	6	48	4.2	28	3.9
44030	Corn cones, nacho flavor, Bugles	1	oz.	28	1	152	2	16	0.3	9	7.6
44029	Corn cones, plain, Bugles	1	oz.	28	1	145	2	18	0.3	8	6.5
42208	Corn flour patties, fried	1	each	10	4	23	0	5	0.7	0	0.1
40243	Corn grits, instant, w/imitation bacon bits, prepar	0.5	cup	105	86	70	2	16	1	0	0
40093	Corn grits, white, enriched, cooked	0.5	cup	121	103	73	2	16	0.2	0	0
40089	Corn grits, white, packet, prepared	1	each	137	113	89	2	21	1.2	0	0
40094	Corn grits, white, unenriched, cooked	0.5	cup	121	103	73	2	16	0.2	0	0
38007	Corn grits, yellow, enriched, cooked	0.5	cup	121	103	73	2	16	0.2	0	0
38006	Corn grits, yellow, enriched, dry	0.5	cup	78	8	289	7	62	1.2	1	0.1
40081	Corn grits, yellow, unenriched, cooked	0.5	cup	121	103	73	2	16	0.2	0	0
5364	Corn on cob, small, frozen, cooked	1	each	77	56	72	2	17	2.2	1	0.1
5515	Corn w/sweet peppers, canned, w/liquid	0.5	cup	114	88	85	3	21	2.3	1	0.1
5201	Corn, canned, not drained	0.5	cup	128	104	82	2	20	2.2	1	0.1
5068	Corn, creamed, canned	0.5	cup	128	101	92	2	23	1.5	1	0.1
5066	Corn, sweet, yellow, canned, drained	0.5	cup	82	63	66	2	15	1.6	1	0.1
5563	Corn, white, canned, drained, salted	0.5	cup	82	63	66	2	15	1.6	1	0.1
5561	Corn, white, canned, w/liquid, salted	0.5	cup	128	104	82	2	20	2.2	1	0.1
5562	Corn, white, canned, w/liquid, unsalted	0.5	cup	128	104	82	2	20	0.9	1	0.1
5566	Corn, white, cream style, canned, drained, salted	0.5	cup	128	101	92	2	23	1.5	1	0.1
5564	Corn, white, cream style, canned, w/salt	0.5	cup	128	101	92	2	23	1.5	1	0.1
5565	Corn, white, creamed, canned w/liquid, salted	0.5	cup	128	101	92	2	23	1.5	1	0.1
5560	Corn, white, fresh, cooked	0.5	cup	82	57	89	3	21	2.2	1	0.2
5393	Corn, white, kernel, frozen, cooked	0.5	cup	82	63	66	2	16	2	0	0.1
5244	Corn, yellow, canned, not drained, low sodium	0.5	cup	128	104	82	2	20	2.2	1	0.1
5287	Corn, yellow, creamed, low sodium	0.5	cup	128	101	92	2	23	1.5	1	0.1
5379	Corn, yellow, fresh, cooked	0.5	cup	82	57	89	3	21	2.3	1	0.2
5065	Corn, yellow, frozen, cooked, no added salt	0.5	cup	82	63	66	2	16	2	0	0.1
5380	Corn, yellow, on cob, cooked ear	1	each	77	54	83	3	19	2.2	1	0.2
42114	Cornbread mix, dry, 8.5 oz pkg	1	each	241	19	1007	17	167	15.7	29	7.4
42115	Cornbread mix, dry, prepared	1	piece	60	19	188	4	29	1.4	6	1.6
42116	Cornbread, dry, recipe, w/2% milk, 1/6th	1	piece	60	24	160	4	26	1.7	4	0.9
42117	Cornbread, dry, recipe, w/whole milk, 1/9th	1	piece	65	25	176	4	28	2.3	5	1.2
42207	Cornbread, jalapeno, piece	1	piece	65	31	161	4	23	1.9	6	2.1
56668	Corndog (hotdog w/coating)	1	each	175	82	460	17	56	—	19	5.2
15181	Corndog, chicken	1	each	113	59	272	13	26	—	13	—
56070	Corned beef hash, canned	0.5	cup	110	74	199	10	12	0.6	12	6
15069	Cornish game hen, whole, roasted (20oz hen)	1	each	306	181	727	83	0	0	41	11.5
15070	Cornish game hen, whole, skinless, roasted	1	each	249	158	470	72	0	0	18	5
38154	Cornmeal mush, fried slice	1	piece	51	32	84	2	15	0.8	2	0.4
38155	Cornmeal mush, made w/milk	0.5	cup	120	80	180	7	25	1.2	6	3.3
38183	Cornmeal, white, degermed, enriched	1	cup	138	16	505	12	107	10.2	2	0.3
38162	Cornmeal, white, whole grain	1	cup	122	13	442	10	94	8.9	4	0.6
38004	Cornmeal, yellow, degermed, enriched	0.5	cup	69	8	253	6	54	5.1	1	0.2
38041	Cornmeal, yellow, enriched, baked value	1	cup	138	16	505	12	107	10.2	2	0.3
38075	Cornmeal, yellow, self rising, degermed	1	cup	138	14	490	12	103	9.8	2	0.3
38059	Cornmeal, yellow, whole grain	0.5	cup	61	6	221	5	47	4.4	2	0.3
44034	Cornnuts, BBQ flavor	10	piece	18	0	78	2	13	1.5	3	0.5
44031	Cornnuts, plain	10	piece	18	0	79	2	13	1.2	3	0.5
30000	Cornstarch	1	tsp	3	0	10	0	2	0	0	0
38076	Couscous, cooked	0.5	cup	90	65	100	3	21	1.2	0	0
7056	Cowpea, catjang, dry, cooked	0.5	cup	86	60	101	7	18	3.1	1	0.2
19420	Crab cake, blue crab	1	each	60	43	93	12	0	0	5	0.9
19404	Crab imperial	0.5	cup	130	94	196	20	4	0.2	10	2.5
56253	Crab salad	0.5	cup	104	76	142	14	6	0.3	7	1
19409	Crab thermidor	0.5	cup	122	75	306	15	5	0.1	25	14.8
19079	Crab, deviled	0.5	cup	88	54	171	11	12	0.7	9	1.8
3243	Crabapple, raw, slices	0.5	cup	55	43	42	0	11	0.6	0	0
43556	Cracker bread, Armenian/Ak Mak	4	piece	24	1	94	3	20	0.7	0	0
43550	Cracker meal	1	cup	115	9	440	11	93	2.9	2	0.3
43555	Cracker, Better Cheddar, low sodium	4	each	5	0	25	1	3	0	1	0.4

MonoF	PolyF	Choles	Calc	Phos	Sod	Pot	Zn	Iron	Magn	VitA	VitE	VitC	Thia	Ribo	Nia	B6	Fola	B12
(g)	(g)	(mg)	(mg)	(mg)	(mg)	(mg)	(mg)	(mg)	(mg)	(μg RE)	(mg α-TE)	(mg)	(mg)	(mg)	(mg)	(mg)	(μg)	(μg)
0	0	0	4	1	1	22	0	0.1	1	11	0.1	0	0	0	0	0	0	0
0	0.1	0	8	14	1	8	0.3	0.5	12	1	0.44	0	0	0.02	0.5	0.03	1	0
1.7	2.9	0	24	37	137	42	0.2	0.3	14	11	0.24	0	0.01	0.04	0.3	0.04	7	0
2.5	4.3	0	33	48	164	37	0.3	0.3	20	2	0.35	0	0.01	0.04	0.3	0.06	5	0
8.2	14	0	108	157	536	121	1.1	1.1	65	8	1.16	0	0.02	0.12	1	0.21	17	0
0.6	0.2	1	10	22	270	35	0.1	0.4	7	11	0.6	0	0.06	0.03	0.4	0.03	1	0
0.5	0.2	0	1	12	290	23	0.1	0.7	3	9	0.54	0	0.09	0.07	0.4	0.01	1	0
0.1	0.2	0	8	12	40	16	0.1	0.4	6	0	0.06	0	0.06	0.04	0.5	0.02	1	0
0.1	0.1	0	9	28	247	50	0.2	6	7	0	0.02	0	0.12	0.06	1	0.05	34	0
0.1	0.1	0	0	14	0	27	0.1	0.8	5	0	0.06	0	0.12	0.07	1	0.03	38	0
0	0.1	0	8	29	289	38	0.2	8.2	11	0	0.03	0	0.15	0.08	1.4	0.06	47	0
0.1	0.1	0	0	14	0	27	0.1	0.2	5	0	0.06	0	0.02	0.01	0.2	0.03	1	0
0.1	0.1	0	0	14	0	27	0.1	0.8	5	7	0.06	0	0.12	0.07	1	0.03	38	0
0.2	0.4	0	2	57	1	107	0.3	3	21	34	0.2	0	0.5	0.3	3.9	0.12	146	0
0.1	0.1	0	0	14	0	27	0.1	0.2	5	7	0.06	0	0.02	0.01	0.2	0.03	1	0
0.2	0.3	0	2	58	3	193	0.5	0.5	22	16	0.07	4	0.13	0.05	1.2	0.17	24	0
0.2	0.3	0	6	70	394	174	0.4	0.9	28	26	1.25	10	0.02	0.09	1.1	0.11	38	0
0.2	0.3	0	5	65	273	210	0.5	0.5	20	19	0.15	7	0.03	0.08	1.2	0.05	49	0
0.2	0.3	0	4	65	365	172	0.7	0.5	22	13	0.12	6	0.03	0.07	1.2	0.08	57	0
0.2	0.4	0	4	53	175	160	0.3	0.7	16	13	0.12	7	0.03	0.06	1	0.04	40	0
0.2	0.4	0	4	53	265	160	0.3	0.7	16	0	0.07	7	0.03	0.06	1	0.04	40	0
0.2	0.3	0	5	65	273	210	0.5	0.5	20	0	0.09	7	0.03	0.08	1.2	0.05	49	0
0.2	0.3	0	5	65	15	210	0.5	0.5	20	0	0.09	7	0.03	0.08	1.2	0.05	49	0
0.2	0.3	0	4	65	4	172	0.7	0.5	22	0	0.12	6	0.03	0.07	1.2	0.08	57	0
0.2	0.3	0	4	65	365	172	0.7	0.5	22	0	0.12	6	0.03	0.07	1.2	0.08	57	0
0.2	0.3	0	4	65	365	172	0.7	0.5	22	0	0.12	6	0.03	0.07	1.2	0.08	57	0
0.3	0.5	0	2	84	14	204	0.4	0.5	26	0	0.07	5	0.18	0.06	1.3	0.05	38	0
0.1	0.2	0	3	47	4	121	0.3	0.3	16	0	0.07	3	0.07	0.06	1.1	0.11	25	0
0.2	0.3	0	5	65	15	210	0.5	0.5	20	19	0.15	7	0.03	0.08	1.2	0.05	49	0
0.2	0.3	0	4	65	4	172	0.7	0.5	22	13	0.12	6	0.03	0.07	1.2	0.08	57	0
0.3	0.5	0	2	84	14	204	0.4	0.5	26	18	0.07	5	0.18	0.06	1.3	0.05	38	0
0.1	0.2	0	3	47	4	121	0.3	0.3	16	18	0.07	3	0.07	0.06	1.1	0.11	25	0
0.3	0.5	0	2	79	13	192	0.4	0.5	25	17	0.07	5	0.17	0.06	1.2	0.05	36	0
16.2	4	5	137	1178	2677	272	1.4	6	58	29	3.98	0	1.03	0.66	8	0.31	253	0.22
3.1	0.7	37	44	226	467	77	0.4	1.1	12	26	0.72	0	0.15	0.16	1.2	0.06	7	0.1
1.1	1.9	24	149	101	395	88	0.4	1.5	15	32	0.54	0	0.18	0.18	1.4	0.07	38	0.09
1.3	2.1	28	161	109	428	95	0.4	1.6	16	28	0.65	0	0.19	0.19	1.5	0.07	12	0.1
2.1	1	40	61	188	369	94	0.4	0.8	15	39	0.95	0	0.09	0.15	0.7	0.06	7	0.17
9.1	3.5	79	102	166	973	263	1.3	6.2	18	37	0.7	0	0.28	0.7	4.2	0.09	103	0.44
—	—	65	—	—	670	—	—	—	—	—	—	—	—	—	—	—	—	—
5.5	0.4	36	14	74	594	220	1.6	2.2	18	0	0.24	0	0.01	0.1	2.3	0.22	10	0.67
16.2	9	268	46	554	957	678	5.9	3.8	70	143	0.8	0	0.19	0.51	25.8	1.22	15	0.91
6.6	4.2	220	38	483	788	602	5.2	3	62	40	0.66	0	0.17	0.44	22.7	1.16	15	0.82
0.8	0.5	0	2	20	265	23	0.3	0.8	11	7	0.31	0	0.06	0.05	0.6	0.04	3	0
1.6	0.4	21	187	165	262	273	0.8	1	30	57	0.23	1	0.18	0.34	1.2	0.11	14	0.44
0.6	1	0	7	116	4	224	1	5.7	55	0	0.46	0	0.99	0.56	6.9	0.36	258	0
1.2	2	0	7	294	43	350	2.2	4.2	155	0	0.4	0	0.47	0.24	4.4	0.37	31	0
0.3	0.5	0	3	58	2	112	0.5	2.8	28	28	0.23	0	0.49	0.28	3.5	0.18	129	0
0.6	1	0	7	116	4	224	1	5.7	55	57	0.5	0	0.79	0.5	6.2	0.32	181	0
0.6	1	0	483	860	1860	235	1.4	6.5	68	57	0.28	0	0.94	0.53	6.3	0.54	258	0
0.6	1	0	4	147	21	175	1.1	2.1	78	29	0.41	0	0.24	0.12	2.2	0.18	16	0
1.3	0.6	0	3	51	176	52	0.3	0.3	20	6	0.18	0	0.06	0.03	0.3	0.03	0	0
1.3	0.6	0	2	50	99	50	0.3	0.3	20	0	0.18	0	0.01	0.02	0.3	0.04	0	0
0	0	0	0	0	0	0	0	0	0	0	0	0	0	0	0	0	0	0
0	0.1	0	7	20	4	52	0.2	0.3	7	0	0.01	0	0.06	0.02	0.9	0.05	13	0
0.1	0.3	0	22	122	16	323	1.6	2.6	83	1	0.32	0	0.14	0.04	0.6	0.08	122	0
1.7	1.4	90	63	128	198	194	2.4	0.6	20	49	0.9	2	0.05	0.05	1.7	0.1	32	3.56
4	2.8	162	125	229	336	345	3.8	1.2	34	125	2.23	7	0.13	0.19	2.8	0.19	49	6.27
1.8	3.6	72	79	147	513	266	2.9	0.7	24	18	1.43	3	0.08	0.05	2.3	0.14	40	4.93
7.3	1.3	212	124	193	446	266	2	1.2	27	263	1.49	1	0.07	0.2	1.5	0.11	22	2.48
3.5	2.6	81	70	126	576	255	2	1.1	23	121	1.91	6	0.11	0.12	2	0.12	31	3.17
0	0	0	10	8	1	107	—	0.2	4	2	0.32	4	0.02	0.01	0.1	—	—	0
0	0.1	0	4	28	120	27	0.2	1.2	6	0	0.1	0	0.16	0.11	1.4	0.01	5	0
0.2	0.8	0	26	120	32	132	0.8	5.3	28	0	0.06	0	0.8	0.54	6.6	0.04	132	0
0.5	0.1	2	18	16	24	6	0	0.2	1	2	0.03	0	0.02	0.02	0.2	0.01	1	0.02

Esha Code	Food Item	Qty	Meas	Wgt (g)	Wtr (g)	Cals	Prot (g)	Carb (g)	Fib (g)	Fat (g)	SatF (g)
43551	Cracker, Cuban	4	each	20	1	80	2	15	0.4	1	0.3
43529	Cracker, Finn Ry Krisp, thin	3	each	6	0	21	1	5	0.5	0	0
43535	Cracker, Matzoh, egg	1	each	28	2	111	3	22	0.8	1	0.2
43536	Cracker, Matzoh, egg & onion	1	each	28	2	111	3	22	1.4	1	0.3
43534	Cracker, Matzoh, plain	1	each	28	1	112	3	24	0.9	0	0.1
43510	Cracker, Matzoh, whole wheat	1	each	28	1	100	4	22	3.4	0	0.1
43566	Cracker, Melba Toast, unsalted	4	piece	20	1	78	2	15	1.3	1	0.1
43538	Cracker, Melba Toast, wheat	2	piece	10	1	37	1	8	0.7	0	0
43509	Cracker, Melba toast, plain	1	piece	5	0	20	1	4	0.3	0	0
43533	Cracker, Norwegian flatbread	4	each	23	1	85	2	19	3.8	0	0
43586	Cracker, Premium, unsalted tops	4	each	12	—	50	2	8	0	1	0
43553	Cracker, Saltine, unsalted top	4	each	20	1	87	2	14	0.6	2	0.6
43561	Cracker, Saltine, whole wheat	4	each	12	0	52	1	8	0.8	2	0.4
43530	Cracker, Wasa rye crispbread	2	piece	17	1	58	2	13	1.5	0	0
43565	Cracker, Wheatsworth	6	each	18	1	86	1	12	1	4	1.6
43543	Cracker, buttery, Ritz	10	each	30	1	151	2	18	0.5	8	1.1
43501	Cracker, cheese w/peanut butter filling	4	each	30	1	145	4	17	0.8	7	1.6
43558	Cracker, crispbread, Wasa extra crisp	4	each	24	1	95	3	18	1.7	2	0.4
43557	Cracker, crispbread, wheat	4	each	24	1	94	3	20	0.7	0	0
43559	Cracker, crispbread, white/rye, fat added	4	each	24	1	95	3	18	1.7	2	0.4
43503	Cracker, graham, crumbs	0.25	cup	30	1	127	2	23	0.8	3	0.5
45500	Cracker, graham, crust, baked	1	piece	54	2	268	2	35	0.8	14	2.8
43502	Cracker, graham, plain/honey	2	each	14	1	59	1	11	0.4	1	0.2
43539	Cracker, milk, New England Biscuit	2	each	22	1	100	2	15	0.4	3	0.7
43528	Cracker, oat bran-oat thins	3	each	6	0	26	1	4	0.3	1	0.1
43540	Cracker, rusk toast	2	each	20	1	81	3	14	0.4	1	0.3
43532	Cracker, rye crispbread	3	each	30	2	110	2	25	5	0	0
43531	Cracker, rye crispbread, low sodium	2	piece	14	1	48	2	11	2.3	0	0
43537	Cracker, rye, Melba Toast	2	each	10	0	39	1	8	0.8	0	0
43541	Cracker, rye, cheese filled	4	each	28	1	135	3	17	1	6	1.7
43542	Cracker, rye, seasoned, triple	1	each	22	1	84	2	16	4.6	2	0.3
43544	Cracker, sesame seed	8	each	24	1	120	2	15	0.4	6	0.9
43545	Cracker, snack type, cheese-filled	4	each	28	1	134	3	17	0.5	6	1.7
43546	Cracker, snack type, peanut butter-filled	4	each	28	1	137	3	16	0.8	7	1.6
43547	Cracker, wheat	15	each	30	1	142	3	20	1.4	6	1.6
43554	Cracker, wheat thin type, low sodium	10	each	20	1	92	2	14	0.4	4	1.1
43563	Cracker, wheat'n bran, Triscuits	4	each	16	1	64	1	11	1.7	2	0.4
43562	Cracker, wheat, 100% stoned wheat	4	each	16	1	64	1	11	1.7	2	0.4
43548	Cracker, wheat, cheese-filled	4	each	28	1	139	3	16	0.9	7	1.2
43549	Cracker, wheat, peanut butter-filled	4	each	28	1	139	4	15	1.2	7	1.3
43564	Cracker, wheat, thin type	10	each	20	1	95	1	13	1.1	4	1.8
43508	Cracker, whole wheat, Triscuit	2	each	9	0	40	1	6	0.9	2	0.3
43596	Crackers, Cracked Pepper, Snackwell's	1	oz.	28	0	113	3	24	0.9	1	0.2
43646	Crackers, Fire, chilis and cheese, fat free, Health	6	each	15	1	50	2	11	2	0	0
43643	Crackers, Pizza, zesty cheese, fat free, Health Val	6	each	15	1	50	2	11	2	0	0
139	Crackers, buttery snack type (Club/Waverly)	7	each	28	1	141	2	17	0.4	7	1.1
43500	Crackers, cheese, Cheez-its	10	each	10	0	50	1	6	0.2	3	0.9
47369	Crackers, cheese, reduced fat, Snackwell's	1	oz.	28	1	119	3	22	0.9	2	0.6
43595	Crackers, classic golden, reduced fat, Snackwell's	1	oz.	28	0	117	2	23	0.7	2	0.4
43596	Crackers, cracked pepper, Snackwell's	1	each	15	0	60	2	12	0.5	0	0.1
43507	Crackers, oyster	1	each	1	0	4	0	1	0	0	0
43505	Crackers, oyster, crushed	0.25	cup	18	1	76	2	12	0.5	2	0.5
43506	Crackers, saltine	4	each	12	0	52	1	9	0.4	1	0.4
43593	Crackers, wheat, fat free, Snackwell's	1	oz.	28	0	113	3	23	1.2	1	0.2
43504	Crackers, whole grain rye, Ry Krisp	2	each	14	1	47	1	11	3.2	0	0
3039	Cranberries, fresh	0.5	cup	48	41	23	0	6	2	0	0
3041	Cranberries, fresh, cooked, sauce	0.5	cup	138	84	209	0	54	1.4	0	0
3042	Cranberry juice cocktail	1	cup	253	216	144	0	36	0.3	0	0
20115	Cranberry juice cocktail, frozen, prepared	1	cup	249	214	137	0	35	0.2	0	0
3276	Cranberry juice, low calorie, bottled	1	cup	237	226	45	0	11	0	0	0
3040	Cranberry sauce, sweetened, canned	0.5	cup	138	84	209	0	54	1.4	0	0
3223	Cranberry-apple drink, w/vitamin C, bottled	1	cup	253	209	170	0	43	0.3	0	0
20071	Cranberry-apple juice drink, low calorie	1	cup	240	228	46	0	11	0.2	0	0
20074	Cranberry-apricot juice drink, low calorie	1	cup	240	228	46	0	11	0.2	0	0
20073	Cranberry-blackberry juice drink, low calorie	1	cup	240	228	46	0	11	0.2	0	0

MonoF (g)	PolyF (g)	Choles (mg)	Calc (mg)	Phos (mg)	Sod (mg)	Pot (mg)	Zn (mg)	Iron (mg)	Magn (mg)	VitA (μg RE)	VitE (mg α-TE)	VitC (mg)	Thia (mg)	Ribo (mg)	Nia (mg)	B6 (mg)	Fola (μg)	B12 (μg)
0.7	0.2	0	15	18	52	52	0.1	0.3	9	0	0.22	0	0.02	0.01	0.2	0.02	3	0
0	0	0	3	23	53	36	0.2	0.2	7	0	0.11	0	0.02	0.02	0.1	0.02	3	0
0.2	0.1	24	11	42	6	42	0.2	0.8	7	4	0.28	0	0.22	0.18	1.4	0.02	33	0.05
0.3	0.3	13	10	25	81	24	0.2	1.2	9	2	0.17	0	0.16	0.12	1.4	0.03	45	0.06
0	0.2	0	4	25	1	32	0.2	0.9	7	0	0.02	0	0.11	0.08	1.1	0.03	33	0
0.1	0.2	0	7	86	1	90	0.7	1.3	38	0	0.38	0	0.1	0.08	1.5	0.04	14	0
0.2	0.3	0	19	39	4	40	0.4	0.7	12	0	0.01	0	0.08	0.06	0.8	0.02	25	0
0.1	0.1	0	4	16	84	15	0.2	0.4	6	0	0.04	0	0.04	0.03	0.5	0.01	13	0
0	0.1	0	5	10	42	10	0.1	0.2	3	0	0	0	0.02	0.01	0.2	0	6	0
0	0.1	0	7	62	61	74	0.6	0.6	18	0	0.31	0	0.06	0.03	0.2	0.05	11	0
0	0	0	—	—	100	10	—	0.7	—	—	0.2	—	—	—	—	—	—	—
1.3	0.3	0	24	21	127	145	0.2	1.1	5	0	0.31	0	0.11	0.09	1	0.01	25	0
0.9	0.2	0	3	23	124	26	0.2	0.5	8	0	0.28	0	0.06	0.04	0.6	0.02	3	0
0	0.1	0	9	66	150	102	0.5	0.7	20	0	0.32	0	0.05	0.04	0.2	0.05	8	0
1.8	0.4	4	6	32	157	36	0.3	0.6	11	1	0.05	0	0.09	0.06	0.8	0.02	3	0.08
3.2	2.9	0	36	68	254	40	0.2	1.1	8	0	1.36	0	0.12	0.1	1.2	0.02	23	0
3.5	1.4	2	24	97	298	74	0.3	0.9	17	10	1.12	0	0.12	0.1	2	0.45	26	0
0.8	0.3	0	20	45	153	68	0.3	0.8	11	0	0.34	0	0.1	0.08	0.8	0.03	4	0.03
0	0.1	0	4	28	120	27	0.2	1.2	6	0	0.1	0	0.16	0.11	1.4	0.01	5	0
0.8	0.3	0	20	45	153	68	0.3	0.8	11	0	0.34	0	0.1	0.08	0.8	0.03	4	0.03
1.2	1.2	0	7	31	182	40	0.2	1.1	9	0	0.61	0	0.07	0.09	1.2	0.02	18	0
6.2	3.8	0	11	35	309	48	0.3	1.2	10	109	2.21	0	0.06	0.1	1.2	0.02	13	0.01
0.6	0.5	0	3	15	85	19	0.1	0.5	4	0	0.29	0	0.03	0.04	0.6	0.01	8	0
1.9	0.5	2	38	67	130	25	0.1	0.8	5	2	0.6	0	0.12	0.09	1	0.01	18	0.02
0.3	0.3	0	5	17	36	12	0.1	0.2	4	0	0.14	0	0.03	0.02	0.2	0	1	0
0.6	0.5	16	5	31	51	49	0.2	0.5	7	2	0.1	0	0.08	0.08	0.9	0.01	17	0.04
0	0.2	0	9	81	79	96	0.7	0.7	23	0	0.4	0	0.07	0.04	0.3	0.06	14	0
0	0.1	0	7	54	33	84	0.4	0.5	17	0	0.26	0	0.04	0.04	0.2	0.04	6	0
0.1	0.1	0	8	18	90	19	0.1	0.4	4	0	0.06	0	0.05	0.03	0.5	0.01	8	0
3.4	0.8	3	62	95	292	96	0.2	0.7	10	11	0.56	0	0.17	0.14	1	0.02	23	0.03
0.7	0.8	0	10	68	195	100	0.6	0.7	23	0	0.44	0	0.07	0.05	0.5	0.04	3	0
2.5	2.3	0	29	55	203	32	0.2	0.9	6	0	1.08	0	0.1	0.08	1	0.01	18	0
3.2	0.7	1	72	114	392	120	0.2	0.7	10	5	0.14	0	0.12	0.19	1.1	0.01	24	0.03
3.5	1.2	0	27	68	264	62	0.3	0.9	15	0	1.04	0	0.12	0.09	1.6	0.03	24	0
3.4	0.8	0	15	66	239	55	0.5	1.3	19	0	0.97	0	0.15	0.1	1.5	0.04	13	0
1.3	0.9	0	6	38	50	43	0.2	0.8	10	3	0.12	0	0.1	0.07	0.9	0.03	5	0
1.2	0.3	0	4	32	86	22	0.2	0.5	11	0	0.59	0	0.08	0.05	0.7	0.02	4	0.15
1.2	0.3	0	4	30	88	19	0.2	0.5	10	0	0.59	0	0.08	0.05	0.7	0.02	4	0.16
2.9	2.6	2	57	107	256	86	0.2	0.7	15	3	0.17	0	0.1	0.12	0.9	0.07	18	0.03
3.3	2.5	0	48	97	226	83	0.2	0.7	11	0	0.17	0	0.11	0.08	1.6	0.04	20	0
2	0.5	4	6	36	174	40	0.3	0.7	13	1	0.05	0	0.1	0.07	0.8	0.03	4	0.08
0.5	0.6	0	4	27	59	27	0.2	0.3	9	0	0.1	0	0.02	0.01	0.4	0.02	4	0
0.1	0.3	0	49	96	280	36	0.3	1.4	7	0	—	0	0.1	0.12	1.5	0.02	—	—
0	0	0	0	—	80	—	—	0	—	20	—	1	—	—	—	—	—	—
0	0	0	0	—	140	—	—	0	—	20	—	1	—	—	—	—	—	—
3	2.7	0	34	64	237	37	0.2	1	8	0	1.27	0	0.11	0.1	1.1	0.02	22	0
1.2	0.2	1	15	22	100	14	0.1	0.5	4	3	0.26	0	0.06	0.04	0.5	0.06	8	0.05
0.6	0.2	2	18	45	320	43	0.3	1.4	8	12	—	0	0.11	0.16	1.8	0.03	—	0.01
0.6	0.2	0	56	104	292	31	0.2	1.2	6	0	—	0	0.18	0.12	1.4	0.02	—	0.01
0	0.1	0	26	51	148	19	0.1	0.7	4	0	—	0	0.05	0.06	0.8	0.01	—	—
0.1	0	0	1	1	13	1	0	0.1	0	0	0.02	0	0.01	0	0.1	0	1	0
1.1	0.3	0	21	18	228	22	0.1	0.9	5	0	0.27	0	0.1	0.08	0.9	0.01	22	0
0.8	0.2	0	14	13	156	15	0.1	0.6	3	0	0.19	0	0.07	0.06	0.6	0	15	0
0.2	0.3	0	52	116	320	81	0.4	1.1	13	0	—	0	0.08	0.14	1.4	0.03	—	0.04
0	0.1	0	6	47	111	69	0.4	0.8	17	0	0.2	0	0.06	0.04	0.2	0.04	2	0
0	0	0	3	4	0	34	0.1	0.1	2	2	0.05	6	0.01	0.01	0	0.03	1	0
0	0.1	0	6	8	40	36	0.1	0.3	4	3	0.14	3	0.02	0.03	0.1	0.02	1	0
0	0.1	0	8	5	5	46	0.2	0.4	5	1	0	90	0.02	0.02	0.1	0.05	1	0
0	0	0	12	2	7	35	0.1	0.2	5	2	0.02	25	0.02	0.02	0	0.04	0	0
0	0	0	21	2	7	52	0	0.1	5	1	0	76	0.02	0.02	0.1	0.04	0	0
0	0.1	0	6	8	40	36	0.1	0.3	4	3	0.14	3	0.02	0.03	0.1	0.02	1	0
0	0	0	18	8	5	68	0.1	0.2	5	1	0	81	0.01	0.05	0.2	0.05	1	0
0	0	0	17	7	5	65	0.1	0.1	5	1	0	77	0	0.05	0.1	0.05	0	0
0	0	0	17	7	5	65	0.1	0.1	5	1	0	77	0	0.05	0.1	0.05	0	0
0	0	0	17	7	5	65	0.1	0.1	5	1	0	77	0	0.05	0.1	0.05	0	0

Esha Code	Food Item	Qty	Meas	Wgt (g)	Wtr (g)	Cals	Prot (g)	Carb (g)	Fib (g)	Fat (g)	SatF (g)
20075	Cranberry-grape juice drink, low calorie	1	cup	240	228	46	0	11	0.2	0	0
20072	Cranberry-raspberry juice drink, low calorie	1	cup	240	228	46	0	11	0.2	0	0
26017	Cream of tartar	0.25	tsp	1	0	2	0	1	0	0	0
28030	Cream of tartar	0.25	tsp	1	0	1	0	0	0	0	0
45521	Cream puff shell, recipe	1	each	66	27	239	6	15	0.5	17	3.7
45509	Cream puff, custard-filled	1	each	110	59	284	7	25	0.4	17	4
501	Cream, coffee/table	1	Tbs	15	11	29	0	1	0	3	1.8
500	Cream, half & half	2	Tbs	30	24	39	1	1	0	3	2.2
527	Cream, medium, 25% fat	1	Tbs	15	10	36	0	1	0	4	2.3
504	Cream, sour, cultured	2	Tbs	29	20	62	1	1	0	6	3.7
505	Cream, sour, imitation, IMO	2	Tbs	29	20	60	1	2	0	6	5.1
515	Cream, sour, low cal, half & half	2	Tbs	30	24	40	1	1	0	4	2.2
510	Cream, whipped, pressurized	2	Tbs	8	5	19	0	1	0	2	1
502	Cream, whipping, heavy	2	Tbs	30	17	103	1	1	0	11	6.8
503	Cream, whipping, heavy	2	Tbs	15	9	51	0	0	0	6	3.4
511	Cream, whipping, light	1	Tbs	30	19	87	1	1	0	9	5.8
512	Cream, whipping, light	2	Tbs	15	9	44	0	0	0	5	2.9
540	Creamer, non-dairy, Cremora	1	tsp	2	—	10	0	1	—	0	0.5
517	Creamer, non-dairy, Mocha Mix	1	Tbs	14	11	19	0	1	0	2	0.3
506	Creamer, non-dairy, powdered coffee whitener	1	tsp	2	0	11	0	1	0	1	0.6
45033	Crepe suzette w/sauce	1	each	66	36	161	4	16	0.3	9	4.2
45031	Crepe, chocolate-filled	1	each	78	53	119	4	15	0.6	5	2
45032	Crepe, fruit-filled	1	each	78	49	131	4	21	0.9	4	1.2
5374	Cress, garden, cooked, drained	0.5	cup	68	62	16	1	3	0.5	0	0
5372	Cress, garden, raw	0.5	cup	25	22	8	1	1	0.3	0	0
5373	Cress, garden, raw sprigs	20	each	20	18	6	1	1	0.2	0	0
45522	Croissant, apple	1	each	57	26	145	4	21	1.4	5	2.8
42015	Croissant, butter	1	each	57	13	231	5	26	1.5	12	6.7
45523	Croissant, cheese	1	each	57	12	236	5	27	1.5	12	6
45545	Croissant, chocolate	1	each	56	12	233	5	23	1.6	14	8.2
56606	Croissant, egg & cheese	1	each	127	58	368	13	24	—	25	14.1
42016	Croutons, dry	0.25	cup	8	0	30	1	6	0.4	0	0.1
42148	Croutons, seasoned	3	Tbs	7	0	33	1	4	0.4	1	0.4
5638	Cucumber salad, cucumber & vinegar	0.5	cup	80	72	24	0	6	0.6	0	0
5610	Cucumber, kim chee	0.5	cup	75	68	16	1	4	1.1	0	0
5071	Cucumber, w/peel, raw slices	0.5	cup	52	50	7	0	1	0.4	0	0
5070	Cucumber, w/peel, raw, whole	1	each	301	289	39	2	8	2.4	0	0.1
26036	Cumin seed	0.25	tsp	0	0	2	0	0	0.1	0	0
46014	Cupcake, chocolate w/chocolate icing-commercial	1	each	42	10	154	2	23	1.2	7	2
3190	Currants, black, fresh	0.5	cup	56	46	35	1	9	4.1	0	0
3192	Currants, dried (Zante)	0.5	cup	72	14	204	3	53	4.9	0	0
3191	Currants, red/white, fresh	0.5	cup	56	47	31	1	8	2.4	0	0
26004	Curry powder	0.25	tsp	1	0	2	0	0	0.2	0	0
3244	Custard apple, raw	4	oz.	113	81	115	2	29	4.2	1	0.1
2600	Custard, egg, baked, recipe	0.5	cup	141	111	148	7	15	0	7	3.3
2622	Custard, egg, mix, w/2% milk	0.5	cup	133	99	149	6	24	0	4	1.9
2613	Custard, egg, prepared mix w/whole milk	0.5	cup	133	97	162	5	23	0	5	3
2132	Dairy Queen blizzard, heath, regular size	1	each	404	236	820	14	119	1	33	20
2239	Dairy Queen breeze, heath, frozen yogurt	1	each	379	229	666	14	115	0.9	17	10.3
2224	Dairy Queen shake, chocolate	1	each	397	273	567	12	96	0	15	9.6
2133	Dairy Queen, Buster bar	1	each	149	67	450	10	41	2	28	12
2135	Dairy Queen, Dilly Bar	1	each	85	47	210	3	21	0	13	7
2147	Dairy Queen, Mr. Misty, regular size	1	each	330	267	250	0	63	0	0	0
2131	Dairy Queen, banana split	1	each	369	249	510	8	96	3	12	8
2227	Dairy Queen, blizzard, strawberry	1	each	383	259	570	12	95	1	16	11
2237	Dairy Queen, breeze, strawberry frozen yogurt	1	each	354	246	425	12	92	0.9	1	0.9
56371	Dairy Queen, cheeseburger, single	1	each	156	86	349	20	30	2	17	8.2
2136	Dairy Queen, choc dipped vanilla cone, regular	1	each	156	92	340	6	42	0.7	17	8.7
2222	Dairy Queen, chocolate cone, regular	1	each	142	90	240	6	37	0	7	5.3
56368	Dairy Queen, hamburger, single	1	each	142	80	298	18	30	2.1	12	5.1
2141	Dairy Queen, hot fudge brownie delight	1	each	305	160	710	11	102	0.6	29	14
56374	Dairy Queen, hotdog	1	each	99	57	240	9	19	1	14	5
56375	Dairy Queen, hotdog, w/cheese	1	each	113	62	290	12	20	1	18	8
2145	Dairy Queen, malt, vanilla, regular size	1	each	418	285	610	13	106	0.3	14	8
2151	Dairy Queen, peanut buster parfait	1	each	305	156	730	16	99	2	31	17

MonoF	PolyF	Choles	Calc	Phos	Sod	Pot	Zn	Iron	Magn	VitA	VitE	VitC	Thia	Ribo	Nia	B6	Fola	B12
(g)	(g)	(mg)	(mg)	(mg)	(mg)	(mg)	(mg)	(mg)	(mg)	(μg RE)	(mg α-TE)	(mg)	(mg)	(mg)	(mg)	(mg)	(μg)	(μg)
0	0	0	17	7	5	65	0.1	0.1	5	1	0	77	0	0.05	0.1	0.05	0	0
0	0	0	17	7	5	65	0.1	0.1	5	1	0	77	0	0.05	0.1	0.05	0	0
0	0	0	0	0	0	137	0	0	0	0	0	0	0	0	0	0	0	0
0	0	0	0	0	58	30	—	0	—	0	—	0	0	0	0	—	—	—
7.3	4.9	129	24	78	368	64	0.5	1.3	8	203	2.54	0	0.14	0.24	1	0.05	32	0.26
7.2	4.6	147	73	120	375	127	0.7	1.3	13	219	2.43	0	0.13	0.31	0.9	0.07	31	0.4
0.8	0.1	10	14	12	6	18	0	0	1	27	0.02	0	0	0.02	0	0	0	0.03
1	0.1	11	32	29	12	39	0.2	0	3	32	0.03	0	0.01	0.04	0	0.01	1	0.1
1.1	0.1	13	14	10	6	17	0	0	1	35	0.09	0	0	0.02	0	0	0	0.03
1.7	0.2	13	33	24	15	41	0.1	0	3	56	0.16	0	0.01	0.04	0	0	3	0.09
0.2	0	0	1	13	29	46	0.3	0.1	2	0	0.04	0	0	0	0	0	0	0
1	0.1	12	31	28	12	39	0.2	0	3	34	0.1	0	0.01	0.04	0	0	3	0.09
0.5	0.1	6	8	7	10	11	0	0	1	16	0.04	0	0	0	0	0	0	0.02
3.2	0.4	41	19	19	11	22	0.1	0	2	125	0.19	0	0.01	0.03	0	0.01	1	0.05
1.6	0.2	20	10	9	6	11	0	0	1	63	0.09	0	0	0.02	0	0	1	0.03
2.7	0.3	33	21	18	10	29	0.1	0	2	88	0.18	0	0.01	0.04	0	0.01	1	0.06
1.4	0.1	17	10	9	5	14	0	0	1	44	0.09	0	0	0.02	0	0	1	0.03
—	—	—	—	—	5	15	—	—	—	—	—	—	—	—	—	—	—	—
0	0.7	0	1	8	7	20	—	—	0	—	—	—	—	—	—	—	—	—
0	0	0	0	8	4	16	0	0	0	0	0	0	0	0	0	0	0	0
3.2	1.2	84	45	68	163	84	0.4	0.8	8	76	0.72	3	0.08	0.17	0.6	0.04	11	0.22
1.7	0.7	58	81	89	148	126	0.5	0.7	12	58	0.52	0	0.07	0.2	0.4	0.04	8	0.27
1.5	0.8	63	38	59	124	90	0.3	0.7	8	59	0.92	4	0.08	0.16	0.6	0.04	9	0.19
0.1	0.1	0	41	32	5	238	0.1	0.5	18	520	0.47	16	0.04	0.11	0.5	0.11	25	0
0.1	0.1	0	20	19	4	152	0.1	0.3	10	233	0.18	17	0.02	0.06	0.2	0.06	20	0
0	0	0	16	15	3	121	0	0.3	8	186	0.14	14	0.02	0.05	0.2	0.05	16	0
1.4	0.4	18	17	33	156	51	0.6	0.6	7	56	0.11	0	0.13	0.09	0.9	0.02	32	0.11
3.2	0.6	38	21	60	424	67	0.4	1.2	9	106	0.25	0	0.22	0.14	1.2	0.03	35	0.09
3.7	1.4	32	30	74	316	75	0.5	1.2	14	112	0.59	0	0.3	0.18	1.2	0.04	42	0.18
4.2	0.7	56	31	82	257	113	0.6	1.7	28	105	0.42	0	0.19	0.21	2	0.05	19	0.1
7.5	1.4	216	244	348	551	174	1.8	2.2	22	255	—	0	0.19	0.38	1.5	0.1	47	0.78
0.2	0.1	0	6	9	52	9	0.1	0.3	2	0	0.02	0	0.05	0.02	0.4	0	10	0
0.4	0.2	0	7	10	87	13	0.1	0.2	3	1	0.15	0	0.04	0.03	0.3	0.01	6	0.01
0	0	0	10	13	175	105	0.1	0.3	10	2	0.05	3	0.02	0.01	0.2	0.04	8	0
0	0	0	7	10	766	88	0.4	3.6	6	25	0.12	3	0.02	0.02	0.3	0.08	17	0
0	0	0	7	10	1	75	0.1	0.1	6	11	0.04	3	0.01	0.01	0.1	0.02	7	0
0	0.2	0	42	60	6	433	0.6	0.8	33	63	0.24	16	0.07	0.07	0.7	0.13	39	0
0.1	0	0	5	2	1	9	0	0.3	2	1	0	0	0	0	0	0	0	0
3.7	0.8	18	18	51	140	84	0.3	0.9	14	10	0.71	0	0.01	0.06	0.2	0.02	7	0.06
0	0.1	0	31	33	1	180	0.2	0.9	13	13	0.06	101	0.03	0.03	0.2	0.04	2	0
0	0.1	0	62	90	6	642	0.5	2.4	30	5	0.07	3	0.12	0.1	1.2	0.21	7	0
0	0	0	18	25	1	154	0.1	0.6	7	7	0.06	23	0.02	0.03	0.1	0.04	4	0
0	0	0	2	2	0	8	0	0.2	1	1	0	0	0	0	0	0	1	0
0.2	0.1	0	34	24	5	433	0.5	0.8	20	3	—	22	0.09	0.11	0.6	0.25	—	0
2.1	0.5	123	158	159	109	216	0.7	0.4	20	85	0.34	1	0.05	0.32	0.1	0.07	14	0.44
1.2	0.3	74	197	176	200	287	0.7	0.3	27	74	0.27	1	0.07	0.29	0.2	0.08	11	0.61
1.7	0.3	81	194	174	198	283	0.7	0.3	25	44	0.13	1	0.07	0.29	0.2	0.08	11	0.6
—	—	60	450	450	580	730	—	1.8	—	300	—	1	0.15	0.76	—	—	—	—
—	—	19	422	449	544	539	—	2.5	—	19	—	2	0.12	0.76	—	—	—	—
—	—	52	442	400	309	600	—	2	—	295	—	2	0.12	0.59	0.8	—	—	—
—	—	15	150	250	280	400	—	1.1	—	80	—	0	0.09	0.17	3	0.08	—	—
3	3	10	100	80	75	170	—	0.4	—	60	—	0	0.03	0.14	—	0.06	—	—
0	0	0	0	—	10	—	—	0	—	0	—	2	0	0	—	0	—	—
—	—	30	250	40	180	860	—	1.8	—	200	—	15	0.15	0.26	0.4	0.2	—	—
—	—	50	450	350	260	700	—	1.8	—	300	—	9	0.15	0.68	—	—	—	—
0	0	9	416	349	250	490	—	2.5	—	0	—	8	0.12	0.68	—	—	—	—
—	—	56	154	249	872	270	—	3.7	—	62	—	4	0.3	0.34	4	—	—	—
—	—	20	200	150	133	290	—	1.2	—	100	—	2	0.06	0.26	0.1	0.09	—	—
—	—	20	167	200	120	350	—	1.2	—	133	—	1	0.06	0.26	—	—	—	—
6.2	1	46	62	149	648	259	—	2.8	—	41	—	4	0.3	0.25	4	—	—	—
12	2	35	300	600	340	510	—	5.4	—	80	—	1	0.15	0.68	0.3	0.18	—	—
—	—	25	60	60	730	170	—	1.8	—	20	—	4	0.22	0.14	2	—	—	—
8	2	40	150	150	950	180	—	1.8	—	60	—	4	0.22	0.17	2	—	—	—
2	2	45	400	350	230	570	—	1.4	—	80	—	0	0.12	0.6	0.8	0.19	—	—
—	—	35	300	450	400	660	—	1.8	—	150	—	1	0.15	0.51	3	0.22	—	—

A

Esha Code	Food Item	Qty	Meas	Wgt (g)	Wtr (g)	Cals	Prot (g)	Carb (g)	Fib (g)	Fat (g)	SatF (g)
13236	Dairy Queen, quarter pound super hotdog	1	each	198	98	590	20	41	—	38	16
2154	Dairy Queen, sundae, chocolate, regular	1	each	177	110	301	6	54	0	7	4.4
2225	Dairy Queen, sundae, nutty double fudge	1	each	276	—	570	10	85	—	22	10
69027	Dairy Queen, ultimate burger, double bacon-cheese	1	each	276	159	687	41	30	2	44	19.5
5242	Dandelion greens, cooked, drained	0.5	cup	52	47	17	1	3	1.5	0	0.1
45588	Danish pastry, cheese	1	each	91	31	353	6	29	—	25	5.1
45512	Danish pastry, cinnamon	1	each	88	18	349	5	47	0.3	17	3.5
45512	Danish pastry, cinnamon	1	each	88	18	349	5	47	0.3	17	3.5
45513	Danish pastry, fruit filled	1	each	94	27	335	5	45	—	16	3.3
3043	Dates, chopped	0.5	cup	89	20	245	2	65	6.7	0	0.2
3044	Dates, whole	10	each	83	19	228	2	61	6.2	0	0.2
14032	Deer/venison steak, fried	1	each	85	52	146	28	0	0	3	1.2
14013	Deer/venison, roasted	4	oz.	113	74	179	34	0	0	4	1.4
526	Dessert topping, low cal, mix, prepared	1	Tbs	5	4	3	0	1	0	0	0.3
526	Dessert topping, low cal, mix, prepared	2	Tbs	10	8	5	0	1	0	1	0.6
509	Dessert topping, mix w/whole milk (Dream Whip)	1	Tbs	5	3	9	0	1	0	1	0.5
509	Dessert topping, mix w/whole milk (Dream Whip)	2	Tbs	10	7	19	0	2	0	1	1.1
508	Dessert topping, non-dairy, frozen (Cool Whip)	1	Tbs	5	2	15	0	1	0	1	1
508	Dessert topping, non-dairy, frozen (Cool Whip)	2	Tbs	9	5	30	0	2	0	2	2
514	Dessert topping, non-dairy, pressurized	1	Tbs	4	3	12	0	1	0	1	0.8
514	Dessert topping, non-dairy, pressurized	2	Tbs	9	5	23	0	1	0	2	1.6
26109	Dill seed	1	tsp	2	0	7	0	1	0.5	0	0
26021	Dill weed, dried	0.25	tsp	0	0	1	0	0	0	0	0
26047	Dill weed, fresh sprig	0.25	cup	2	2	1	0	0	0	0	0
7083	Dip, Jalapeno pepper bean	1	Tbs	33	22	46	2	6	2.2	2	0.2
23247	Dip, caramel, Marie's	2	cup	35	5	150	0	24	1	5	4
8136	Dip, sour cream, buttermilk/onion	2	Tbs	30	20	67	1	2	0.2	6	3.7
8137	Dip, sour cream, low calorie	2	Tbs	30	22	44	1	2	0.2	3	2.1
22543	Distilled spirits, 100 proof	1	oz.	28	16	84	0	0	0	0	0
22514	Distilled spirits, 80 proof, all	1	oz.	28	19	66	0	0	0	0	0
22516	Distilled spirits, 86 proof, all	1	oz.	28	18	71	0	0	0	0	0
22517	Distilled spirits, 90 proof, all	1	oz.	28	18	75	0	0	0	0	0
22542	Distilled spirits, 94 proof	1	oz.	28	17	78	0	0	0	0	0
5418	Dock/sorrel greens, cooked	0.5	cup	50	47	10	1	1	1.3	0	—
57025	Domino's pizza, pepperoni, deep dish	2	piece	218	94	622	26	63	3.3	29	11.3
57016	Domino's pizza, pepperoni, hand tossed	2	piece	159	72	406	18	50	2.6	15	6.5
57019	Domino's pizza, pepperoni, thin crust	1	piece	59	26	169	7	15	0.8	9	3.5
57028	Domino's pizza, sausage mushroom, deep dish	2	piece	236	111	618	26	66	3.8	28	10.8
57017	Domino's pizza, vegetarian, hand tossed	2	piece	176	95	360	15	52	3	10	4.6
57029	Domino's pizza, veggie, deep dish	2	piece	236	117	576	24	65	3.8	25	9.2
57023	Domino's pizza, veggie, thin crust	1	piece	68	37	146	6	16	1	6	2.4
44035	Doo Dads, original flavor	0.5	cup	28	1	129	3	18	1.9	5	1
45508	Doughnut, Eclair, chocolate, custard-filled	1	each	94	49	246	6	23	0.6	15	3.9
45527	Doughnut, French cruller, glazed	1	each	41	7	169	1	24	0.5	8	1.9
45559	Doughnut, Mexican crueller	1	each	26	6	116	1	12	0.2	7	1.4
45518	Doughnut, cake, chocolate w/choc icing	1	each	42	7	175	2	24	0.9	8	2.2
45524	Doughnut, cake, chocolate-iced	1	each	43	6	204	2	21	0.9	13	3.5
45505	Doughnut, cake, plain	1	each	50	10	211	2	25	0.8	12	1.8
45525	Doughnut, cake, sugared/glazed	1	each	45	9	192	2	23	0.7	10	2.7
45519	Doughnut, custard filled, Bismarck	1	each	70	20	261	3	34	1	13	5.9
45561	Doughnut, eggless, carob-coated, raised	1	each	78	21	285	5	32	5.4	18	2.6
45515	Doughnut, fritter, apple	1	each	24	9	87	1	8	0.3	6	1.6
45560	Doughnut, oriental, Okinawan	1	each	18	3	75	1	10	0.2	4	0.9
45526	Doughnut, wheat, sugared/glazed	1	each	45	13	162	3	19	1	9	1.4
45517	Doughnut, yeast, chocolate, w/choc icing	1	each	71	20	273	4	30	2.5	16	7.5
45563	Doughnut, yeast, creme-filled	1	each	85	32	307	5	26	0.7	21	4.6
45506	Doughnut, yeast, glazed	1	each	60	15	242	4	27	0.7	14	3.5
45507	Doughnut, yeast, jelly-filled	1	each	65	23	221	4	25	0.6	12	3.2
20314	Drink mix, citrus, Crystal Light	1	cup	238	237	5	0	0	0	0	0
14000	Duck meat, skinless, roasted	4	oz.	113	73	228	27	0	0	13	4.7
14001	Duck, domestic, w/skin, roasted	4	oz.	113	59	382	22	0	0	32	11
49006	Dumpling, apple	1	each	151	78	357	2	53	2.5	16	3.6
45520	Dumpling, plain, medium	1	each	32	22	42	1	7	0.2	1	0.4
19581	Egg Beaters, Fleischmann's	0.5	cup	122	—	60	12	2	0	0	0
19550	Egg Delight, frozen, prepared	0.5	cup	70	51	92	9	5	0	4	0.7

MonoF	PolyF	Choles	Calc	Phos	Sod	Pot	Zn	Iron	Magn	VitA	VitE	VitC	Thia	Ribo	Nia	B6	Fola	B12
(g)	(g)	(mg)	(mg)	(mg)	(mg)	(mg)	(mg)	(mg)	(mg)	(μg RE)	(mg α-TE)	(mg)	(mg)	(mg)	(mg)	(mg)	(μg)	(μg)
16	4	60	100	150	1360	340	—	2.7	—	—	—	—	0.45	0.34	5	—	—	—
—	—	22	184	150	154	289	—	1.1	—	110	—	0	0.06	0.26	0.3	0.14	—	—
9	3	35	300	300	170	450	—	3.6	—	60	—	—	0.12	0.6	—	—	—	—
—	—	139	616	399	1241	479	—	2.8	—	41	—	4	0.44	0.5	7.9	—	—	—
0	0.1	0	74	22	23	122	0.1	0.9	13	614	1.31	9	0.07	0.09	0.3	0.08	7	0
15.6	2.4	20	70	80	319	116	0.6	1.8	16	43	—	3	0.26	0.21	2.6	0.06	55	0.23
10.6	1.6	27	37	74	326	96	0.5	1.8	14	5	0.79	3	0.26	0.19	2.2	0.05	55	0.22
10.6	1.6	27	37	74	326	96	0.5	1.8	14	5	0.79	3	0.26	0.19	2.2	0.05	55	0.22
10.1	1.6	19	22	69	333	110	0.5	1.4	14	24	0.85	2	0.29	0.21	1.8	0.06	31	0.24
0.1	0	0	28	36	3	580	0.3	1	31	4	0.09	0	0.08	0.09	2	0.17	11	0
0.1	0	0	27	33	2	541	0.2	1	29	4	0.08	0	0.08	0.08	1.8	0.16	10	0
0.9	0.6	102	6	206	331	305	2.5	4.1	24	0	0.24	0	0.14	0.55	5.7	0.22	5	5.3
1	0.7	127	8	256	61	380	3.1	5.1	27	0	0.28	0	0.2	0.68	7.6	0.43	5	3.61
0	0	0	0	2	5	1	0	0	0	0	0	0	0	0	0	0	0	0
0	0	0	0	3	11	3	0	0	0	0	0	0	0	0	0	0	0	0
0	0	0	5	4	3	8	0	0	0	2	0.01	0	0	0.01	0	0	0	0.01
0.1	0	1	9	9	7	15	0	0	1	5	0.01	0	0	0.01	0	0	0	0.03
0.1	0	0	0	0	1	1	0	0	0	4	0.01	0	0	0	0	0	0	0
0.2	0	0	1	1	2	2	0	0	0	8	0.02	0	0	0	0	0	0	0
0.1	0	0	0	1	3	1	0	0	0	2	0.01	0	0	0	0	0	0	0
0.2	0	0	0	2	5	2	0	0	0	4	0.02	0	0	0	0	0	0	0
0.2	0	0	33	6	0	26	0.1	0.4	6	0	0.02	0	0.01	0.01	0.1	0.01	0	0
0	0	0	5	1	1	9	0	0.1	1	2	—	0	0	0	0	0	—	0
0	0	0	5	1	1	16	0	0.1	1	17	—	2	0	0.01	0	0	3	0
0.4	1	0	11	34	382	96	0.2	0.5	12	18	0.38	4	0.03	0.02	0.1	0.03	23	0
—	—	5	20	—	75	—	—	0	—	0	—	0	—	—	—	—	—	—
1.8	0.2	13	36	32	228	56	0.1	0.1	5	55	0.18	0	0.02	0.06	0.1	0.01	3	0.08
1	0.1	11	32	34	212	51	0.2	0.1	4	31	0.11	0	0.02	0.06	0.1	0.01	3	0.08
0	0	0	0	1	0	1	0	0	0	0	0	0	0	0	0	0	0	0
0	0	0	0	1	0	1	0	0	0	0	0	0	0	0	0	0	0	0
0	0	0	0	1	0	1	0	0	0	0	0	0	0	0	0	0	0	0
0	0	0	0	1	0	1	0	0	0	0	0	0	0	0	0	0	0	0
0	0	0	0	1	0	1	0	0	0	0	0	0	0	0	0	0	0	0
—	—	0	19	26	2	161	0.1	1	44	174	0.5	13	0.02	0.04	0.2	0.05	4	0
—	—	44	456	—	1382	—	—	5	—	155	—	3	—	—	—	—	—	—
—	—	32	282	—	1179	—	—	4.3	—	94	—	3	—	—	—	—	—	—
—	—	16	162	—	484	—	—	0.7	—	44	—	1	—	—	—	—	—	—
—	—	43	460	—	1355	—	—	5.2	—	158	—	4	—	—	—	—	—	—
—	—	19	286	—	1028	—	—	4.4	—	99	—	13	—	—	—	—	—	—
—	—	32	460	—	1232	—	—	5.2	—	160	—	13	—	—	—	—	—	—
—	—	10	164	—	408	—	—	0.7	—	47	—	6	—	—	—	—	—	—
3.2	0.9	0	21	84	360	78	0.6	0.7	17	12	0.04	0	0.1	0.07	1.5	0.06	11	0
6.1	3.7	119	59	101	317	110	0.6	1.1	14	180	1.97	0	0.11	0.25	0.8	0.06	26	0.32
4.3	0.9	5	11	50	141	32	0.1	1	5	1	1.02	0	0.07	0.09	0.9	0.01	14	0.02
3	2.6	2	2	8	37	8	0.1	0.3	2	6	1.11	0	0.04	0.03	0.4	0	1	0
4.8	1	24	90	68	143	44	0.2	1	14	5	1.13	0	0.02	0.03	0.2	0.01	16	0.04
7.5	1.6	26	15	87	184	84	0.3	1.1	17	5	1.79	0	0.06	0.04	0.6	0.02	12	0.1
4.6	3.9	18	22	135	273	64	0.3	1	10	8	1.92	0	0.11	0.12	0.9	0.03	24	0.14
5.7	1.3	14	27	53	181	46	0.2	0.5	8	1	0.45	0	0.1	0.09	0.7	0.01	21	0.11
5.3	0.9	20	27	43	125	50	0.6	1	13	4	1.91	0	0.11	0.12	0.9	0.04	13	0.17
6.4	7.4	0	77	146	74	218	1.1	1.6	56	0	2.74	0	0.14	0.13	2.3	0.16	30	0
2.4	1.4	21	13	22	10	34	0.1	0.3	3	12	0.55	0	0.04	0.06	0.3	0.02	3	0.06
1.5	0.9	13	19	19	49	15	0.1	0.4	2	7	0.34	0	0.04	0.05	0.4	0.01	2	0.03
3.6	3.2	9	22	47	160	67	0.3	0.5	10	7	1.62	0	0.1	0.11	0.8	0.04	9	0.08
6.5	1.2	22	31	74	129	110	0.9	1.6	35	10	2.17	0	0.12	0.14	1	0.04	15	0.18
10.3	2.6	20	21	65	263	68	0.7	1.6	17	16	2.35	0	0.29	0.13	1.9	0.06	54	0.12
7.7	1.7	4	26	56	205	65	0.5	1.2	13	2	1.84	0	0.22	0.13	1.7	0.03	26	0.05
6.6	1.6	17	16	55	190	51	0.5	1.1	13	10	1.6	0	0.2	0.09	1.4	0.06	40	0.14
0	0	0	0	—	0	45	—	0	—	0	—	6	—	—	—	—	—	0
4.2	1.6	101	14	230	74	286	3	3.1	23	26	0.79	0	0.3	0.53	5.8	0.28	11	0.45
14.6	4.1	95	12	177	67	231	2.1	3.1	18	71	0.79	0	0.2	0.3	5.5	0.2	7	0.34
8.2	3.4	0	50	38	302	212	0.2	1.3	16	94	3.24	5	0.1	0.07	0.8	0.07	6	0.01
0.4	0.2	1	33	22	105	21	0.1	0.4	3	2	0.1	0	0.06	0.05	0.5	0.01	2	0.02
0	0	0	80	—	200	170	—	2.2	—	80	0.59	—	—	—	—	—	—	—
1.6	1.2	46	12	21	113	103	0.1	0.2	7	172	0.59	0	0.01	0.21	0.1	0.01	12	0.12

Esha Code	Food Item	Qty	Meas	Wgt (g)	Wtr (g)	Cals	Prot (g)	Carb (g)	Fib (g)	Fat (g)	SatF (g)
56132	Egg foo yung patty	1	each	86	67	113	6	3	0.6	8	1.9
19535	Egg omelet, ham & cheese, 1 egg	1	each	78	55	142	10	1	0	11	3.9
19543	Egg omelet, mushroom, 1 egg	1	each	69	54	91	6	1	0.1	7	2.6
19537	Egg omelet, onion, peppper, tomato, mushroom, 3 egg	1	each	145	122	125	5	7	1.6	9	2
19534	Egg omelet, plain, 1 large egg	1	each	59	45	90	6	1	0	7	1.9
19544	Egg omelet, sausage & mushroom, 1 egg	1	each	95	68	172	11	1	0.2	13	4.9
19536	Egg omelet, spanish, 1 egg	1	each	145	122	125	5	7	1.6	9	2
19542	Egg omelet, spinach, 1 egg	1	each	84	68	95	7	2	0.7	7	2.2
83000	Egg roll, chicken, Chun King	6	piece	106	62	210	6	30	3	7	1.5
83001	Egg roll, shrimp, Chun King	6	piece	106	65	190	5	29	3	6	1
56003	Egg salad	0.5	cup	92	52	293	8	1	0	28	5.3
19524	Egg substitute, frozen	0.25	cup	60	44	96	7	2	0	7	1.2
19525	Egg substitute, liquid	0.25	cup	63	52	53	8	0	0	2	0.4
19552	Egg substitute, liquid, prepared	0.5	cup	105	84	100	14	1	0	4	0.8
19526	Egg substitute, powder	1	oz.	28	1	126	16	6	0	4	1.1
19551	Egg substitute, w/cholesterol, frozen, prepared	0.5	cup	70	51	92	9	5	0	4	0.7
19522	Egg white, cooked	1	each	33	29	17	4	0	0	0	0
19507	Egg white, fresh or frozen, raw	2	each	67	59	33	7	1	0	0	0
19506	Egg white, fresh or frozen, raw, large	1	each	33	29	17	4	0	0	0	0
19523	Egg yolk, cooked	1	each	17	8	59	3	0	0	5	1.6
19508	Egg yolk, fresh, raw, large	1	each	17	8	59	3	0	0	5	1.6
19532	Egg yolk, frozen, raw, salted	0.5	cup	122	62	333	17	2	0	28	8.5
19553	Egg, Second Nature, prepared	0.5	cup	105	84	100	14	1	0	4	0.8
19538	Egg, creamed	1	each	145	107	230	11	8	0.2	17	5.2
19539	Egg, deviled	2	each	62	43	125	7	1	0	10	2.5
19512	Egg, hard cooked, extra large	1	each	58	43	90	7	1	0	6	1.9
19511	Egg, hard cooked/boiled, chopped, large	1	cup	136	101	211	17	2	0	14	4.4
19510	Egg, hard cooked/boiled, large	1	each	50	37	78	6	1	0	5	1.6
19514	Egg, hard cooked/boiled, medium	1	each	44	33	68	6	0	0	5	1.4
19518	Egg, poached, extra large	1	each	57	43	85	7	1	0	6	1.8
19517	Egg, poached, large	1	each	50	38	74	6	1	0	5	1.6
19520	Egg, poached, medium size	1	each	44	33	66	5	1	0	4	1.4
19540	Egg, scrambled, dry, prepared	0.5	cup	107	73	238	10	1	0	21	5.1
19547	Egg, scrambled, frozen, prepared, no cholesterol	0.5	cup	76	53	139	10	3	0	10	1.7
19549	Egg, scrambled, w/cheese, no chol, frozen, prepared	0.5	cup	76	62	64	10	2	0	2	1
19516	Egg, scrambled, w/milk & margarine, large	1	each	61	45	101	7	1	0	7	2.2
19546	Egg, substitute, dry, prepared	0.5	cup	94	64	181	11	4	0	13	2.8
19548	Egg, substitute, frozen, prepared	0.5	cup	76	53	139	10	3	0	10	1.7
19527	Egg, whole, dried	0.5	cup	42	1	252	20	2	0	17	5.4
19500	Egg, whole, fresh or frozen, raw	1	each	50	38	74	6	1	0	5	1.6
19503	Egg, whole, fresh or frozen, raw, jumbo	1	each	65	49	97	8	1	0	6	2
19504	Egg, whole, fresh or frozen, raw, medium	1	each	44	33	66	6	1	0	4	1.4
19505	Egg, whole, fresh or frozen, raw, small	1	each	37	28	55	5	0	0	4	1.2
19502	Egg, whole, fresh or frozen, raw, xtra large	1	each	58	44	86	7	1	0	6	1.8
19509	Egg, whole, fried in margarine, large	1	each	46	32	92	6	1	0	7	1.9
98	Eggnog, made w/2% lowfat milk	1	cup	254	215	189	12	17	0	8	3.8
17	Eggnog, w/whole milk, commercial	1	cup	254	189	343	10	34	0	19	11.3
5642	Eggplant slices, batter-dipped, fried	1	piece	50	37	75	1	6	1.2	5	1.3
5073	Eggplant slices, cooked, drained, no added salt	1	piece	54	50	15	0	4	1.4	0	0
5673	Eggplant, pieces, steamed	0.5	cup	48	44	12	0	3	1.2	0	0
5674	Eggplant, pieces, stir fried, no oil	0.5	cup	48	44	12	0	3	1.2	0	0
5371	Eggplant, raw, cubes	0.5	cup	41	38	11	0	2	1	0	0
5074	Eggplant, whole, cooked, drained, no added salt	1	each	538	494	151	4	36	13.5	1	0.2
19567	Eggs, scrambled, plain	2	each	100	75	155	13	1	0	11	3.3
3310	Elderberries, cooked or canned	0.5	cup	128	87	152	1	39	6.6	0	0
3245	Elderberries, raw	0.5	cup	72	58	53	0	13	5.1	0	0
14014	Elk, roasted	4	oz.	113	75	166	34	0	0	2	0.8
16289	Emu, thigh, raw	4	oz.	113	—	105	23	—	—	2	—
16194	Enchilada suiza, chicken, Stouffer's Lean Cuisine	1	each	255	187	290	12	48	5	5	2
15978	Enchilada suiza, chicken, Weight Watchers	1	each	255	203	250	15	28	4	8	3
66021	Enchilada, cheese	1	each	163	103	319	10	28	—	19	10.6
56866	Enchilada, cheese, Stouffer's Entrees	1	each	276	197	370	12	48	5	14	5
56060	Enchilada, chicken	1	each	120	81	192	13	16	1.9	9	3.5
66020	Enchirito, beef-bean-cheese	1	each	193	121	344	18	34	5.5	16	8
42214	English muffin, cheese	1	each	63	28	148	6	25	1.5	2	1

MonoF (g)	PolyF (g)	Choles (mg)	Calc (mg)	Phos (mg)	Sod (mg)	Pot (mg)	Zn (mg)	Iron (mg)	Magn (mg)	VitA (μg RE)	VitE (mg α-TE)	VitC (mg)	Thia (mg)	Ribo (mg)	Nia (mg)	B6 (mg)	Fola (μg)	B12 (μg)
3.4	2.1	184	31	93	310	118	0.7	1	12	86	1.57	5	0.04	0.26	0.4	0.09	30	0.37
4.1	1.6	231	70	163	368	98	1	0.8	9	138	1.69	0	0.08	0.29	0.4	0.1	19	0.54
2.6	1.3	204	25	97	158	99	0.6	0.8	6	109	1.53	0	0.04	0.28	0.5	0.07	19	0.41
3.6	2.3	126	28	118	251	325	0.7	1.2	15	147	1.88	14	0.09	0.34	1.9	0.15	28	0.26
2.7	1.3	207	25	87	159	60	0.5	0.7	5	110	0.76	0	0.03	0.24	0	0.06	17	0.41
5.6	2.2	254	35	140	454	145	1.1	1.1	10	128	1.82	0	0.17	0.32	1	0.14	21	0.79
3.6	2.3	126	28	118	251	325	0.7	1.2	15	147	1.88	14	0.09	0.34	1.9	0.15	28	0.26
3	1.4	201	44	101	201	152	0.7	1.2	16	198	1.69	16	0.04	0.27	0.2	0.11	38	0.4
—	—	10	20	90	260	120	—	0.4	—	3	—	1	0.1	0.06	0.7	—	—	—
—	—	10	20	50	360	80	—	0.4	—	20	—	4	0.09	0.03	0.4	—	—	—
8.7	12.1	287	37	117	333	90	0.7	0.9	7	130	4.44	0	0.04	0.33	0	0.23	31	0.79
1.5	3.7	1	44	43	119	128	0.6	1.2	9	81	1.27	0	0.07	0.23	0.1	0.08	10	0.2
0.6	1	1	33	76	111	207	0.8	1.3	5	136	0.3	0	0.07	0.19	0.1	0	9	0.19
1.1	1.9	1	63	144	211	394	1.6	2.5	10	258	0.58	0	0.11	0.34	0.1	0	13	0.3
1.5	0.5	162	92	136	227	211	0.5	0.9	18	105	0.46	0	0.06	0.5	0.2	0.04	35	1
1.6	1.2	46	12	21	113	103	0.1	0.2	7	172	0.59	0	0.01	0.21	0.1	0.01	12	0.12
0	0	0	2	4	106	48	0	0	4	0	0	0	0	0.14	0	0	1	0.06
0	0	0	4	9	110	96	0	0	7	0	0	0	0	0.3	0.1	0	2	0.13
0	0	0	2	4	55	48	0	0	4	0	0	0	0	0.15	0	0	1	0.07
1.9	0.7	212	23	81	33	16	0.5	0.6	1	97	0.49	0	0.02	0.1	0	0.06	18	0.44
1.9	0.7	213	23	81	7	16	0.5	0.6	1	97	0.52	0	0.03	0.11	0	0.06	24	0.52
10.8	3.8	1160	139	524	4592	142	3.4	4.6	12	434	2.74	0	0.16	0.52	0	0.32	130	3.06
1.1	1.9	1	63	144	211	394	1.6	2.5	10	258	0.58	0	0.11	0.34	0.1	0	13	0.3
6.7	3.4	281	125	185	484	193	1	0.9	16	216	2.33	1	0.08	0.46	0.3	0.11	33	0.98
3.5	3	242	29	98	187	73	0.6	0.7	6	99	1.72	0	0.04	0.29	0	0.1	26	0.65
2.4	0.8	246	29	100	72	73	0.6	0.7	6	97	0.61	0	0.04	0.3	0	0.07	26	0.64
5.6	1.9	577	68	234	169	171	1.4	1.6	14	228	1.43	0	0.09	0.7	0.1	0.16	60	1.51
2	0.7	212	25	86	62	63	0.5	0.6	5	84	0.52	0	0.03	0.26	0	0.06	22	0.56
1.8	0.6	187	22	76	55	55	0.5	0.5	4	74	0.46	0	0.03	0.23	0	0.05	19	0.49
2.2	0.8	241	28	101	160	68	0.6	0.8	6	108	0.6	0	0.03	0.24	0	0.07	20	0.46
1.9	0.7	212	24	88	140	60	0.6	0.7	5	95	0.52	0	0.02	0.22	0	0.06	18	0.4
1.7	0.6	186	22	78	123	53	0.5	0.6	4	84	0.46	0	0.02	0.19	0	0.05	15	0.35
9.3	5.1	411	52	149	468	111	1.2	1.7	11	291	3.13	0	0.06	0.24	0.1	0.08	30	1.83
2.1	5.4	2	63	62	173	185	0.9	1.7	13	117	1.84	0	0.09	0.32	0.1	0.11	11	0.25
0.4	0	4	66	87	271	135	0.3	0.1	12	14	0.04	0	0.01	0.37	0.1	0.01	2	0.15
2.9	1.3	215	43	104	171	84	0.6	0.7	7	119	0.8	0	0.03	0.27	0	0.07	18	0.47
6.1	3.9	108	67	93	281	146	0.4	0.6	13	216	2.04	0	0.04	0.32	0.1	0.03	18	0.58
2.1	5.4	2	63	62	173	185	0.9	1.7	13	117	1.84	0	0.09	0.32	0.1	0.11	11	0.25
6.5	2.5	729	98	353	222	210	2.2	2.9	18	115	1.86	0	0.08	0.66	0.1	0.16	73	1.68
1.9	0.7	213	24	89	63	60	0.6	0.7	5	96	0.52	0	0.03	0.25	0	0.07	24	0.5
2.5	0.9	276	32	116	82	79	0.7	0.9	6	124	0.68	0	0.04	0.33	0	0.09	31	0.65
1.7	0.6	187	22	78	55	53	0.5	0.6	4	84	0.46	0	0.03	0.22	0	0.06	21	0.44
1.4	0.5	157	18	66	47	45	0.4	0.5	4	71	0.39	0	0.02	0.19	0	0.05	17	0.37
2.2	0.8	247	28	103	73	70	0.6	0.8	6	111	0.61	0	0.04	0.3	0	0.08	27	0.58
2.8	1.3	211	25	89	162	61	0.5	0.7	5	114	0.75	0	0.03	0.24	0	0.07	18	0.42
2.7	0.7	194	269	269	155	367	1.3	0.7	32	197	1.01	2	0.11	0.55	0.2	0.15	30	1.17
5.7	0.9	149	330	277	138	419	1.2	0.5	47	203	0.58	4	0.09	0.48	0.3	0.13	2	1.14
2.3	1.5	9	27	26	31	107	0.1	0.5	6	5	0.45	1	0.06	0.04	0.5	0.04	7	0.06
0	0	0	3	12	2	134	0.1	0.2	7	3	0.02	1	0.04	0.01	0.3	0.05	8	0
0	0	0	3	11	1	104	0.1	0.1	5	3	0.01	1	0.04	0.01	0.3	0.04	9	0
0	0	0	3	11	1	104	0.1	0.1	5	3	0.01	1	0.04	0.01	0.3	0.04	9	0
0	0	0	3	9	1	89	0.1	0.1	6	3	0.01	1	0.02	0.01	0.2	0.03	8	0
0.1	0.5	0	32	118	16	1334	0.8	1.9	70	32	0.16	7	0.41	0.11	3.2	0.46	78	0
4.1	1.4	424	50	172	124	126	1	1.2	10	168	1.05	0	0.07	0.51	0.1	0.12	44	1.11
0.1	0.2	0	34	37	6	236	0.1	1.5	5	42	0.94	24	0.05	0.06	0.4	0.19	3	0
0.1	0.2	0	28	28	4	203	0.1	1.2	4	44	0.72	26	0.05	0.04	0.4	0.17	4	0
0.5	0.5	83	6	204	69	372	3.6	4.1	27	0	0.03	0	0.25	0.91	6.6	0.28	5	7.37
—	—	56	—	—	—	—	—	5.7	—	—	—	—	—	—	—	—	—	—
1.5	1.5	25	150	—	530	360	—	0.7	—	60	—	4	—	—	—	—	—	—
—	—	25	300	—	570	470	—	1.4	—	40	—	1	0.15	0.26	4	—	—	—
6.3	0.8	44	324	134	784	240	2.5	1.3	50	186	1.47	1	0.08	0.42	1.9	0.39	65	0.75
—	—	25	200	—	890	310	—	1.4	—	200	—	12	—	—	—	—	—	—
2.5	2	36	159	212	307	199	1.3	1	34	108	0.73	16	0.08	0.13	3.1	0.25	15	0.2
6.5	0.3	50	218	224	1250	560	2.8	2.4	71	133	1.54	5	0.17	0.7	3	0.21	60	1.62
0.7	0.5	3	118	78	184	80	0.6	1.8	14	10	0.1	0	0.26	0.27	3	0.1	55	0.02

A

Esha Code	Food Item	Qty	Meas	Wgt (g)	Wtr (g)	Cals	Prot (g)	Carb (g)	Fib (g)	Fat (g)	SatF (g)
42215	English muffin, cheese, toasted	1	each	56	21	151	6	26	1.5	2	1
42149	English muffin, mixed grain	1	each	61	24	143	6	28	1.7	1	0.1
42150	English muffin, mixed grain, toasted	1	each	61	21	156	6	31	1.8	1	0.2
42059	English muffin, plain	1	each	57	24	134	4	26	1.5	1	0.1
42151	English muffin, raisin cinnamon	1	each	57	22	139	4	28	1.6	2	0.2
42152	English muffin, raisin cinnamon, toasted	1	each	52	17	137	4	28	1.6	2	0.2
42060	English muffin, sourdough	1	each	56	24	132	4	26	1.5	1	0.1
42062	English muffin, sourdough, toasted	1	each	50	19	128	4	25	1.4	1	0.1
42061	English muffin, toasted	1	each	50	19	128	4	25	1.4	1	0.1
42064	English muffin, w/butter, fast food	1	each	63	20	189	5	30	1.9	6	2.4
42153	English muffin, wheat	1	each	57	24	127	5	26	2.6	1	0.2
42154	English muffin, wheat, toasted	1	each	52	19	126	5	25	2.6	1	0.2
42082	English muffin, whole wheat	1	each	50	23	102	4	20	3.4	1	0.6
42083	English muffin, whole wheat, toasted	1	each	50	20	111	5	22	3.6	1	0.2
5202	Escarole/curly endive, raw, chopped	0.5	cup	25	24	4	0	1	0.8	0	0
19067	Escarot, snail, steamed	2	each	10	6	18	3	0	0	0	0.1
56124	Fajita, w/beef	1	each	223	140	409	17	46	3.8	18	5.1
56102	Falafel, fava bean patty	1	piece	17	6	57	2	5	0.9	3	0.4
8471	Fat replacer, plum puree	0.5	cup	124	25	391	2	95	7.2	0	0
8004	Fat, beef/tallow, drippings	1	Tbs	13	0	116	0	0	0	13	6.4
8005	Fat, chicken	1	Tbs	13	0	115	0	0	0	13	3.8
3271	Feijoa fruit, raw	1	each	50	43	24	1	5	2.1	0	0.1
26105	Fennel seed	0.25	tsp	0	0	2	0	0	0.2	0	0
26022	Fenugreek seed	0.25	tsp	1	0	3	0	1	0.2	0	0
3161	Fig, canned in heavy syrup	3	each	85	65	75	0	20	1.9	0	0
3337	Figs, canned in water	3	each	80	68	42	0	11	1.8	0	0
3162	Figs, dried	10	each	187	53	477	6	122	22.8	2	0.4
3575	Figs, dried DFA	10	each	187	52	527	6	124	22.8	1	0
3314	Figs, dried, cooked, unsweetened	0.5	cup	130	90	140	2	36	6.6	1	0.1
3160	Figs, fresh	1	each	50	40	37	0	10	1.6	0	0
4515	Filbert/hazelnut, dried, ground	0.25	cup	19	1	119	2	3	1.1	12	0.9
4514	Filbert/hazelnut, dried, unblanched, chopped	0.25	cup	29	2	182	4	4	1.8	18	1.3
4513	Filbert/hazelnut, dried, unblanched, whole	0.25	cup	34	2	213	4	5	2.1	21	1.6
4651	Filberts/hazelnuts, dry roasted, unsalted	1	oz.	28	1	188	3	5	2	19	1.4
4663	Filberts/hazelnuts, dry roasted, w/salt	1	oz.	28	1	188	3	5	2.2	19	1.4
4664	Filberts/hazelnuts, oil roasted, salted	1	oz.	28	0	187	4	5	1.8	18	1.3
4652	Filberts/hazelnuts, oil roasted, unsalted	1	oz.	28	0	187	4	5	1.8	18	1.3
18805	Fish ball, cod	1	each	63	39	125	9	8	0.7	7	1.7
18806	Fish cake, cod	1	each	120	74	239	16	15	1.4	13	3.3
17039	Fish cake, fried	1	each	69	41	150	14	5	0.3	8	2
17040	Fish cake, fried, frozen, heated	1	each	85	45	230	8	15	0.8	15	6
18825	Fish dinner, lemon pepper, Healthy Choice	1	each	303	236	320	14	50	5	7	2
17003	Fish patty, heated from frozen	1	each	57	26	155	9	14	0	7	1.8
17002	Fish stick/portion, heated, from frozen	2	each	57	26	155	9	14	0	7	1.8
19019	Fish, Abalone, canned	4	oz.	113	91	91	18	3	0	6	0.3
17124	Fish, Anchovies, canned in oil, drained	10	each	40	20	84	12	0	0	4	0.9
17103	Fish, Gefiltefish, sweet, commercial	1	piece	42	34	35	4	3	0	1	0.2
18814	Fish, Kamaboko (Japanese fish cake)	1	piece	16	11	18	2	2	0	0	0
19054	Fish, King Crab leg, baked/broiled	1	each	119	87	164	23	0	0	8	1.4
17114	Fish, Lingcod, baked/broiled fillet	0.5	each	151	114	165	34	0	0	2	0.4
19083	Fish, Queen crab, baked/broiled	0.5	cup	59	44	68	14	0	0	1	0.1
19053	Fish, Snow Crab leg, baked/broiled	1	each	10	7	14	2	0	0	1	0.1
19084	Fish, Spiny lobster, steamed	1	each	229	153	327	60	7	0	4	0.7
19041	Fish, abalone, floured, fried	4	oz.	113	68	214	22	13	0	8	1.9
19042	Fish, abalone, fried	4	oz.	113	68	214	22	13	0	8	1.9
19018	Fish, abalone, mixed species, raw	4	oz.	113	85	119	19	7	0	1	0.2
19086	Fish, abalone, steamed/poached	4	oz.	113	56	238	39	14	0	2	0.3
17125	Fish, anchovies, cooked	10	each	40	20	84	12	0	0	4	0.9
17106	Fish, butterfish, baked/broiled fillet	1	each	25	17	47	6	0	0	3	0.8
17106	Fish, butterfish, baked/broiled fillet	3	oz.	85	57	159	19	0	0	9	2.6
19073	Fish, calamari, dried	1	oz.	28	6	95	16	3	0	1	0.4
17087	Fish, carp, baked/broiled fillet	1	each	170	118	275	39	0	0	12	2.4
17087	Fish, carp, baked/broiled fillet	3	oz.	85	59	138	20	0	0	6	1.2
17088	Fish, catfish, breaded fried fillet	1	each	87	51	199	16	7	0.7	12	2.9
17088	Fish, catfish, breaded fried fillet	3	oz.	85	50	195	15	7	0.6	11	2.8

MonoF	PolyF	Choles	Calc	Phos	Sod	Pot	Zn	Iron	Magn	VitA	VitE	VitC	Thia	Ribo	Nia	B6	Fola	B12
(g)	(g)	(mg)	(mg)	(mg)	(mg)	(mg)	(mg)	(mg)	(mg)	(μg RE)	(mg α-TE)	(mg)	(mg)	(mg)	(mg)	(mg)	(μg)	(μg)
0.7	0.5	3	121	79	188	82	0.6	1.9	15	9	0.1	0	0.21	0.28	3	0.1	48	0.02
0.5	0.3	0	120	49	254	95	0.8	1.8	25	0	0.17	0	0.26	0.19	2.2	0.02	49	0
0.5	0.4	0	130	99	276	103	0.6	2	29	1	0.76	0	0.23	0.19	2.1	0.06	41	0
0.2	0.5	0	99	76	264	75	0.4	1.4	12	0	0.1	0	0.25	0.16	2.2	0.02	46	0.02
0.3	0.8	0	84	39	255	119	0.6	1.4	9	0	0.23	0	0.22	0.17	2	0.04	46	0
0.3	0.8	0	83	44	253	118	0.6	1.4	9	0	0.1	0	0.17	0.15	1.8	0.04	36	0
0.2	0.5	0	97	74	260	73	0.4	1.4	12	0	0.1	0	0.25	0.16	2.2	0.02	45	0.02
0.2	0.5	0	94	72	252	72	0.4	1.4	11	0	0.09	0	0.19	0.14	1.9	0.02	37	0.02
0.2	0.5	0	94	72	252	72	0.4	1.4	11	0	0.09	0	0.19	0.14	1.9	0.02	37	0.02
1.5	1.4	13	103	85	386	69	0.4	1.6	13	33	0.13	1	0.25	0.32	2.6	0.04	57	0.02
0.2	0.5	0	101	61	218	106	0.6	1.6	21	0	0.28	0	0.25	0.17	1.9	0.05	31	0
0.2	0.5	0	100	65	216	105	0.6	1.6	22	0	0.18	0	0.2	0.15	1.7	0.05	24	0
0.4	0	0	133	141	319	105	0.8	1.2	36	0	0.35	0	0.15	0.07	1.7	0.08	21	0
0.3	0.5	0	144	154	346	114	0.9	1.3	38	0	0.38	0	0.13	0.07	1.7	0.08	18	0
0	0	0	13	7	6	78	0.2	0.2	4	51	0.11	2	0.02	0.02	0.1	0	36	0
0.1	0.1	10	2	38	12	54	0.2	0.6	42	5	1	0	0	0.02	0.2	0.02	1	0.06
7.6	3.9	26	76	200	850	427	2.4	3.7	38	52	2.08	29	0.46	0.3	4.7	0.32	25	1.18
1.7	0.7	0	9	33	50	100	0.3	0.6	14	0	0.19	0	0.02	0.03	0.2	0.02	16	0
—	—	—	16	—	45	443	—	1	—	27	—	4	—	—	—	—	—	—
5.4	0.5	14	0	0	0	0	0	0	0	0	0.35	0	0	0	0	0	0	0
5.7	2.7	11	0	0	0	0	0	0	0	0	0.35	0	0	0	0	0	0	0
0	0.2	0	8	10	2	78	0	0	4	0	—	10	0	0.02	0.1	0.02	19	0
0	0	0	6	2	0	8	0	0.1	2	0	—	0	0	0	0	—	—	0
—	—	0	2	3	1	7	0	0.3	2	0	—	0	0	0	0	—	1	0
0	0	0	23	8	1	84	0.1	0.2	8	3	0.76	1	0.02	0.03	0.4	0.06	2	0
0	0	0	22	8	1	82	0.1	0.2	8	3	0.71	1	0.02	0.03	0.4	0.06	2	0
0.5	1	0	269	127	21	1331	1	4.2	110	24	0	2	0.13	0.16	1.3	0.42	14	0
—	—	0	249	134	23	1138	1	5.7	115	2	—	1	0.14	0.17	1.4	0.63	33	0
0.1	0.3	0	79	38	6	390	0.3	1.2	32	21	0	6	0.01	0.14	0.8	0.17	1	0
0	0.1	0	18	7	0	116	0.1	0.2	8	7	0.44	1	0.03	0.02	0.2	0.06	3	0
9.2	1.1	0	35	58	1	83	0.4	0.6	53	1	4.48	0	0.09	0.02	0.2	0.12	14	0
14.1	1.7	0	54	90	1	128	0.7	0.9	82	2	6.87	0	0.14	0.03	0.3	0.18	21	0
16.6	2	0	64	105	1	150	0.8	1.1	96	2	8.07	0	0.17	0.04	0.4	0.21	24	0
14.7	1.8	0	55	92	1	131	0.7	1	84	2	6.78	0	0.06	0.06	0.8	0.18	21	0
14.7	1.8	0	55	92	221	131	0.7	1	84	0	7.09	0	0.06	0.06	0.8	0.18	21	0
14.1	1.7	0	56	92	223	132	0.7	1	84	2	7.09	0	0.06	0.06	0.8	0.18	21	0
14.1	1.7	0	56	92	1	132	0.7	1	84	2	6.78	0	0.06	0.06	0.8	0.18	21	0
2.8	1.7	35	18	108	175	274	0.3	0.4	20	13	0.64	2	0.07	0.07	1.3	0.16	7	0.33
5.3	3.2	66	34	206	333	522	0.7	0.8	38	25	1.21	5	0.13	0.13	2.5	0.31	13	0.63
3.2	2	47	24	139	267	255	0.4	0.6	24	13	1.89	1	0.07	0.09	2.2	0.13	8	0.94
3.4	3.4	22	9	142	150	296	0.3	0.3	15	17	0.51	0	0.03	0.06	1.4	0.04	10	0.85
—	—	30	20	—	480	—	—	1.1	—	100	—	30	—	—	—	—	—	—
2.9	1.8	64	11	103	332	149	0.4	0.4	14	18	0.78	0	0.07	0.1	1.2	0.03	10	1.03
2.9	1.8	64	11	103	332	149	0.4	0.4	14	18	0.78	0	0.07	0.1	1.2	0.03	10	1.03
2.6	3.6	91	16	145	794	318	1	2.6	57	2	5.67	1	0.14	0.08	2	0.17	2	0.79
1.5	1	34	93	101	1467	218	1	1.8	28	8	2	0	0.03	0.14	8	0.08	5	0.35
0.3	0.1	13	10	31	220	38	0.3	1	4	11	0.06	0	0.03	0.02	0.4	0.03	1	0.35
0	0.1	8	7	24	135	39	0.1	0.1	7	1	0.02	0	0	0.02	0.4	0.03	0	0.33
2.8	2.5	111	118	231	642	364	4.7	1	37	78	2.01	4	0.11	0.06	3.7	0.2	57	8.13
0.7	0.6	101	27	390	115	846	0.9	0.6	50	26	0.44	0	0.05	0.21	3.5	0.52	15	6.27
0.2	0.3	42	20	76	408	118	2.1	1.7	37	31	0.67	4	0.06	0.14	1.7	0.1	25	6.14
0.2	0.2	9	10	19	54	31	0.4	0.1	3	7	0.17	0	0.01	0	0.3	0.02	5	0.68
0.8	1.7	206	144	524	520	476	16.6	3.2	117	14	4.58	5	0.02	0.13	11.2	0.4	2	9.25
3.1	1.9	107	42	246	670	322	1.1	4.3	64	2	6.8	2	0.25	0.15	2.2	0.17	16	0.78
3.1	1.9	107	42	246	670	322	1.1	4.3	64	2	6.8	2	0.25	0.15	2.2	0.17	16	0.78
0.1	0.1	96	35	215	341	284	0.9	3.6	54	2	4.54	2	0.22	0.11	1.7	0.17	6	0.83
0.2	0.2	193	67	302	580	397	1.9	6.5	92	4	9.07	3	0.39	0.17	2.6	0.29	9	0.99
1.5	1	34	93	101	1467	218	1	1.8	28	8	2	0	0.03	0.14	8	0.08	5	0.35
0.9	0.8	21	7	77	28	120	0.2	0.2	8	8	0.15	0	0.04	0.05	1.4	0.09	4	0.46
3.1	2.7	71	24	262	97	409	0.8	0.5	27	28	0.52	0	0.12	0.16	4.9	0.29	14	1.56
0.1	0.5	240	33	228	165	253	1.6	0.7	34	9	1.24	4	0.02	0.42	2.2	0.06	5	1.27
5.1	3.1	143	88	903	107	726	3.2	2.7	65	15	1.82	3	0.24	0.12	3.6	0.37	29	2.5
2.5	1.6	71	44	451	54	363	1.6	1.4	32	8	0.91	1	0.12	0.06	1.8	0.19	15	1.25
4.9	2.9	70	38	188	244	296	0.7	1.2	24	7	1.11	0	0.06	0.12	2	0.16	26	1.65
4.8	2.8	69	37	184	238	289	0.7	1.2	23	7	1.09	0	0.06	0.11	1.9	0.16	26	1.62

Esha Code	Food Item	Qty	Meas	Wgt (g)	Wtr (g)	Cals	Prot (g)	Carb (g)	Fib (g)	Fat (g)	SatF (g)
17128	Fish, catfish, steamed/poached	4	oz.	113	78	191	22	0	0	11	2.5
17034	Fish, caviar, black/red, granular	2	Tbs	32	15	81	8	1	0	6	1.3
19081	Fish, clam, breaded, fried	0.5	cup	75	46	152	11	8	0.1	8	2
19080	Fish, clam, breaded, fried, small	0.5	cup	75	46	152	11	8	0.1	8	2
19051	Fish, clam, smoked, canned in oil	10	each	100	69	175	14	3	0	12	2.7
19002	Fish, clams, canned, drained	4	oz.	113	72	168	29	6	0	2	0.2
19020	Fish, clams, minced, w/liquid, small can	1	each	183	146	145	25	5	0	2	0.2
19001	Fish, clams, steamed, large	8	each	150	95	222	38	8	0	3	0.3
19000	Fish, clams, steamed, small	20	each	90	57	133	23	5	0	2	0.2
17107	Fish, cod, Pacific, baked/broiled fillet	1	each	90	68	94	21	0	0	1	0.1
17107	Fish, cod, Pacific, baked/broiled fillet	3	oz.	85	65	89	20	0	0	1	0.1
17000	Fish, cod, batter fried pieces	3	piece	48	32	83	8	3	0.1	4	0.9
17001	Fish, cod, steamed/poached	4	oz.	113	87	116	25	0	0	1	0.2
19036	Fish, crab leg, Alaskan King, steamed	1	each	134	104	130	26	0	0	2	0.2
19052	Fish, crab, baked/broiled	0.5	cup	59	43	81	11	0	0	4	0.7
19005	Fish, crab, blue, canned meat	4	oz.	113	86	112	23	0	0	1	0.3
19033	Fish, crab, blue, steamed	1	cup	118	91	120	24	0	0	2	0.3
19034	Fish, crab, blue, steamed, whole	1	each	48	37	49	10	0	0	1	0.1
19003	Fish, crab, dungeness, steamed	4	oz.	113	83	125	25	1	0	1	0.2
19004	Fish, crab, dungeness, whole, steamed	1	each	127	93	140	28	1	0	2	0.2
19037	Fish, crab, imitation	4	oz.	113	84	116	14	12	0	1	0.3
19055	Fish, crab, soft shell, floured/breaded, fried	1	each	65	26	217	13	11	0.5	13	3.2
19038	Fish, crayfish/Crawdads, steamed	4	oz.	113	90	93	19	0	0	1	0.2
19022	Fish, crayfish/crawdads wild, raw	8	each	27	22	21	4	0	0	0	0
19058	Fish, ctopus, dried, cooked	0.5	cup	53	30	97	16	3	0	1	0.4
19085	Fish, cuttlefish, steamed	4	oz.	113	69	179	37	2	0	2	0.3
17102	Fish, eel, baked/broiled fillet	1	each	159	94	375	38	0	0	24	4.8
17130	Fish, eel, steamed/poached	4	oz.	113	68	261	26	0	0	16	3.3
17071	Fish, grouper, baked/broiled fillet	1	each	202	148	238	50	0	0	3	0.6
17071	Fish, grouper, baked/broiled fillet	3	oz.	85	62	100	21	0	0	1	0.3
18813	Fish, haddock patty	1	each	120	74	239	16	15	1.4	13	3.3
17090	Fish, haddock, baked/broiled fillet	1	each	150	111	168	36	0	0	1	0.3
17090	Fish, haddock, baked/broiled fillet	3	oz.	85	63	95	21	0	0	1	0.1
17007	Fish, haddock, breaded, fried fillet	1	each	81	45	189	16	10	0.6	9	2.3
17007	Fish, haddock, breaded, fried fillet	3	oz.	85	47	199	16	11	0.6	10	2.4
17008	Fish, haddock, steamed/poached	3	oz.	85	64	92	20	0	0	1	0.1
17008	Fish, haddock, steamed/poached	4	oz.	113	85	123	27	0	0	1	0.2
17011	Fish, halibut, Pacific, steamed	4	oz.	113	81	159	30	0	0	3	0.5
17047	Fish, herring, Atlantic, baked/broiled fillet	1	each	143	92	290	33	0	0	17	3.8
17047	Fish, herring, Atlantic, baked/broiled fillet	3	oz.	85	55	173	20	0	0	10	2.2
17012	Fish, herring, Atlantic, pickled	6	piece	90	50	236	13	9	0	16	2.1
17112	Fish, herring, Pacific, baked/broiled fillet	1	each	144	91	360	30	0	0	26	6
19071	Fish, jellyfish, pickled	0.5	cup	29	20	10	2	0	0	0	0.1
19057	Fish, lobster pieces, baked/broiled	0.5	cup	72	54	84	14	1	0	2	1.2
19056	Fish, lobster tail, baked/broiled	1	each	125	92	145	25	2	0	4	2
19075	Fish, lobster, battered, fried	1	each	111	67	235	21	9	0.2	12	3
19075	Fish, lobster, battered, fried	3	oz.	85	51	180	16	7	0.2	9	2.3
19023	Fish, lobster, northern, raw	1	each	150	115	135	28	1	0	1	0.3
19023	Fish, lobster, northern, raw	3	oz.	85	65	76	16	0	0	1	0.2
19006	Fish, lobster, northern, steamed	4	oz.	113	86	111	23	1	0	1	0.1
19407	Fish, lobster, w/butter sauce	0.5	cup	94	59	224	15	1	0	18	10.9
18812	Fish, mackerel patty	1	each	120	65	298	19	16	1.5	18	4.8
17049	Fish, mackerel, Atlantic, baked/broiled fillet	1	each	88	47	231	21	0	0	16	3.7
17049	Fish, mackerel, Atlantic, baked/broiled fillet	3	oz.	85	45	223	20	0	0	15	3.6
17050	Fish, mackerel, Jack, canned, drained	1	cup	190	131	296	44	0	0	12	3.5
17115	Fish, mackerel, king, baked/broiled fillet	0.5	piece	154	106	206	40	0	0	4	0.7
17150	Fish, moochim, Korean (dried fish & soy sauce)	0.5	cup	40	9	133	15	4	0.2	6	0.9
17072	Fish, mullet, baked/broiled fillet	1	each	93	66	140	23	0	0	5	1.3
17072	Fish, mullet, baked/broiled fillet	3	oz.	85	60	128	21	0	0	4	1.2
19024	Fish, mussels, blue, raw	4	oz.	113	91	98	14	4	0	3	0.5
19044	Fish, mussels, blue, steamed	4	oz.	113	69	195	27	8	0	5	1
19102	Fish, mussels, smoked, canned, in oil, drained	0.5	cup	75	46	146	16	3	0	8	—
19412	Fish, mussels, w/tomato-based sauce	0.5	cup	120	87	134	15	12	1.8	3	0.6
19048	Fish, octopus, cooked	4	oz.	113	69	186	34	5	0	2	0.5
19072	Fish, octopus, dried	0.5	cup	26	5	90	15	3	0	1	0.3

MonoF	PolyF	Choles	Calc	Phos	Sod	Pot	Zn	Iron	Magn	VitA	VitE	VitC	Thia	Ribo	Nia	B6	Fola	B12
(g)	(g)	(mg)	(mg)	(mg)	(mg)	(mg)	(mg)	(mg)	(mg)	(μg RE)	(mg α-TE)	(mg)	(mg)	(mg)	(mg)	(mg)	(μg)	(μg)
5.1	2.2	67	13	258	68	360	1	0.7	29	17	1.7	1	0.41	0.1	2.8	0.21	11	2.98
1.5	2.4	188	88	114	480	58	0.3	3.8	96	179	2.24	0	0.06	0.2	0	0.1	16	6.4
3.4	2.2	46	47	141	273	245	1.1	10.4	10	68	1.88	8	0.08	0.18	1.6	0.04	27	30.2
3.4	2.2	46	47	141	273	245	1.1	10.4	10	68	1.88	8	0.08	0.18	1.6	0.04	27	30.2
4.8	3.1	38	52	188	321	349	1.5	15.6	10	100	1.97	14	0.08	0.24	2	0.07	18	55
0.2	0.6	76	104	383	127	712	3.1	31.8	20	194	1.13	25	0.17	0.48	3.8	0.12	33	112
0.2	0.5	65	101	328	293	609	2.8	27.1	28	166	1.46	3	0.01	0.41	3.3	0.08	4	98.8
0.3	0.8	101	138	507	168	942	4.1	42	27	257	2.94	33	0.22	0.64	5	0.16	43	148
0.2	0.5	60	83	304	101	565	2.5	25.2	16	154	1.76	20	0.14	0.38	3	0.1	26	89
0.1	0.3	42	8	201	82	465	0.5	0.3	28	9	0.31	3	0.02	0.05	2.2	0.42	7	0.94
0.1	0.3	40	8	190	77	439	0.4	0.3	26	8	0.29	3	0.02	0.04	2.1	0.39	7	0.88
1.5	1.1	27	18	98	52	188	0.3	0.4	15	7	0.39	0	0.05	0.06	1.1	0.1	4	0.41
0.1	0.3	61	23	259	69	498	0.6	0.5	41	14	0.32	1	0.09	0.08	2.5	0.28	8	1.09
0.2	0.7	71	79	375	1436	351	10.2	1	84	12	1.21	10	0.07	0.07	1.8	0.24	68	15.4
1.4	1.2	55	59	115	319	180	2.3	0.5	18	38	0.99	2	0.06	0.03	1.8	0.1	28	4.03
0.2	0.5	101	115	295	378	424	4.6	1	44	2	1.13	3	0.09	0.1	1.6	0.17	48	0.52
0.3	0.8	118	123	243	329	382	5	1.1	39	2	1.18	4	0.12	0.06	3.9	0.21	60	8.61
0.1	0.3	48	50	99	134	156	2	0.4	16	1	0.48	2	0.05	0.02	1.6	0.09	24	3.5
0.2	0.5	86	67	198	429	463	6.2	0.5	66	35	1.28	4	0.06	0.23	4.1	0.2	48	11.8
0.3	0.5	96	75	222	480	518	7	0.5	74	39	1.44	5	0.07	0.26	4.6	0.22	53	13.2
0.2	0.8	23	15	320	954	102	0.4	0.4	49	23	0.11	0	0.04	0.03	0.2	0.03	2	1.81
5.4	3.4	80	71	141	336	203	2.4	1.2	23	14	1.63	1	0.13	0.12	2.4	0.1	28	3.34
0.3	0.4	151	68	306	107	336	2	0.9	37	17	1.7	1	0.06	0.1	2.6	0.09	50	2.44
0	0.1	31	7	69	16	82	0.4	0.2	7	4	0.77	0	0.02	0.01	0.6	0.03	10	0.54
0.1	0.6	246	34	233	169	259	1.6	0.7	35	9	1.26	4	0.02	0.43	2.3	0.06	5	1.3
0.2	0.3	254	204	658	844	722	3.9	12.2	68	230	5.1	10	0.02	1.96	2.5	0.31	27	6.12
14.7	1.9	256	41	440	103	555	3.3	1	41	1806	8.11	3	0.29	0.08	7.1	0.12	28	4.6
10.2	1.3	179	28	276	65	328	2.3	0.7	26	1256	5.67	2	0.17	0.05	4.2	0.08	17	3.61
0.5	0.8	95	42	289	107	960	1	2.3	75	101	1.26	0	0.16	0.01	0.8	0.71	21	1.4
0.2	0.3	40	18	122	45	404	0.4	1	32	42	0.53	0	0.07	0	0.3	0.3	9	0.59
5.3	3.2	66	34	206	333	522	0.7	0.8	38	25	1.21	5	0.13	0.13	2.5	0.31	13	0.63
0.2	0.5	111	63	362	131	599	0.7	2	75	28	0.73	0	0.06	0.07	7	0.52	20	2.09
0.1	0.3	63	36	205	74	339	0.4	1.2	42	16	0.42	0	0.03	0.04	3.9	0.29	11	1.18
3.8	2.4	68	45	163	375	247	0.4	1.4	33	24	1.12	0	0.06	0.1	3.2	0.2	14	0.81
4	2.5	72	48	171	393	259	0.4	1.4	35	25	1.17	0	0.06	0.11	3.4	0.21	15	0.85
0.1	0.3	61	35	180	65	281	0.4	1.1	37	14	0.41	0	0.03	0.04	3.4	0.26	10	1.09
0.2	0.3	81	47	240	87	375	0.5	1.5	50	19	0.55	0	0.04	0.05	4.6	0.34	13	1.45
1.1	1.1	46	68	323	78	653	0.6	1.2	121	61	1.24	0	0.08	0.1	8.1	0.45	16	1.55
6.8	3.9	110	106	433	164	599	1.8	2	59	44	1.92	1	0.16	0.43	5.9	0.5	16	18.7
4.1	2.3	66	63	258	98	356	1.1	1.2	35	26	1.14	1	0.1	0.25	3.5	0.3	10	11.1
10.7	1.5	12	69	80	783	62	0.5	1.1	7	232	0.9	0	0.03	0.12	3	0.15	2	3.84
12.7	4.5	143	153	420	137	780	1	2.1	59	50	1.87	0	0.1	0.37	4.1	0.75	9	13.9
0.1	0.2	1	1	6	2809	1	0.1	0.7	1	1	0.01	0	0	0	0.1	0	0	0.01
0.6	0.1	55	43	130	451	247	2	0.3	24	35	0.73	0	0	0.05	0.7	0.05	8	2.18
1.1	0.2	95	75	224	777	425	3.5	0.5	42	60	1.27	0	0.01	0.08	1.3	0.09	14	3.75
5.2	3.4	88	83	203	426	363	2.9	0.9	37	30	1.91	0	0.06	0.12	1.5	0.08	12	2.64
4	2.6	68	64	155	326	278	2.2	0.7	28	23	1.46	0	0.05	0.1	1.1	0.06	9	2.02
0.4	0.2	143	72	216	444	413	4.5	0.4	40	32	2.21	0	0.01	0.07	2.2	0.1	14	1.39
0.2	0.1	81	41	122	252	234	2.6	0.3	23	18	1.25	0	0	0.04	1.2	0.05	8	0.79
0.2	0.1	82	69	210	431	399	3.3	0.4	40	30	1.13	0	0.01	0.08	1.2	0.09	13	3.53
5.1	0.7	99	49	139	453	261	2.1	0.3	26	180	1.06	0	0.01	0.06	0.8	0.06	9	2.29
7.3	4.5	91	193	265	478	349	1	2	40	97	2.18	5	0.12	0.24	5.4	0.3	12	3.76
6.2	3.8	66	13	245	73	353	0.8	1.4	85	48	1.63	0	0.14	0.36	6	0.4	1	16.7
6	3.7	64	13	236	71	341	0.8	1.3	82	46	1.57	0	0.14	0.35	5.8	0.39	1	16.2
4.2	3.1	150	458	572	720	369	1.9	3.9	70	247	2.66	2	0.08	0.4	11.7	0.4	10	13.2
1.5	0.9	105	62	490	313	859	1.1	3.5	63	388	2.66	2	0.18	0.89	16.2	0.78	14	27.7
2.3	2.5	34	54	230	2015	349	0.5	1	38	9	0.37	1	0.08	0.07	2	0.22	8	2.22
1.3	0.9	59	29	227	66	426	0.8	1.3	31	39	1.13	1	0.09	0.09	5.9	0.46	9	0.23
1.2	0.8	54	26	207	60	389	0.7	1.2	28	36	1.04	1	0.08	0.08	5.4	0.42	8	0.21
0.6	0.7	32	30	223	324	363	1.8	4.5	39	54	0.84	9	0.18	0.24	1.8	0.06	48	13.6
1.2	1.4	64	37	323	418	304	3	7.6	42	103	1.64	15	0.34	0.48	3.4	0.11	86	27.2
—	—	69	51	—	341	104	2.8	7	74	90	—	0	—	0.36	1.7	—	—	—
0.6	0.7	34	37	193	745	457	2	4.5	44	72	1.91	12	0.21	0.26	2.2	0.1	52	13
0.4	0.5	109	120	316	522	714	3.8	10.8	68	92	1.36	9	0.06	0.09	4.3	0.74	27	40.8
0.1	0.5	227	31	215	156	240	1.5	0.7	32	9	1.17	4	0.02	0.4	2.1	0.05	5	1.2

Esha Code	Food Item	Qty	Meas	Wgt (g)	Wtr (g)	Cals	Prot (g)	Carb (g)	Fib (g)	Fat (g)	SatF (g)
19025	Fish, octopus, raw	4	oz.	113	91	93	17	2	0	1	0.3
19059	Fish, octopus, smoked	4	oz.	113	75	158	29	4	0	2	0.4
17121	Fish, orange roughy baked/broiled	0.5	cup	66	46	59	12	0	0	1	0
19009	Fish, oyster, Eastern, breaded, fried	6	each	88	57	173	8	10	0.1	11	2.8
19010	Fish, oyster, Eastern, breaded, fried, cup measure	1	cup	131	85	258	12	15	0.2	16	4.2
19045	Fish, oyster, Pacific, raw	1	each	50	41	40	5	2	0	1	0.3
19060	Fish, oyster, baked/broiled	4	oz.	113	94	82	9	5	0	2	0.6
19028	Fish, oyster, eastern, canned, w/liquid	0.5	cup	124	106	86	9	5	0	3	0.8
19026	Fish, oyster, eastern, raw	4	oz.	113	97	77	8	4	0	3	0.9
19027	Fish, oyster, eastern, steamed	6	each	42	30	58	6	3	0	2	0.6
19008	Fish, oysters, Pacific, steamed/boiled	4	oz.	113	73	185	21	11	0	5	1.2
17094	Fish, perch, mixed, baked/broiled fillet	1	each	46	34	54	12	0	0	1	0.1
17094	Fish, perch, mixed, baked/broiled fillet	3	oz.	85	62	100	21	0	0	1	0.2
17096	Fish, pollock, walleye, baked/broiled	1	each	60	44	68	14	0	0	1	0.1
17096	Fish, pollock, walleye, baked/broiled	3	oz.	85	63	96	20	0	0	1	0.2
18808	Fish, salmon cake/patty	1	each	120	71	261	16	14	1.3	16	4.1
18807	Fish, salmon croquette	1	each	63	37	137	9	7	0.7	8	2.2
18809	Fish, salmon loaf	1	each	105	63	210	16	9	0.4	12	3.1
18809	Fish, salmon loaf	3	oz.	85	51	170	13	7	0.3	9	2.5
17123	Fish, salmon, Atlantic, baked/broiled fillet	0.5	each	154	92	280	39	0	0	12	1.9
17123	Fish, salmon, Atlantic, baked/broiled fillet	3	oz.	85	51	155	22	0	0	7	1.1
17169	Fish, salmon, chinook, baked/broiled	4	oz.	113	74	262	29	0	0	15	3.6
17019	Fish, salmon, chinook, smoked/lox	4	oz.	113	82	133	21	0	0	5	1
17152	Fish, salmon, chinook, smoked/lox	4	oz.	113	82	133	21	0	0	5	1
17170	Fish, salmon, chum, baked/broiled	4	oz.	113	78	175	29	0	0	5	1.2
17098	Fish, salmon, chum, canned, drained	0.5	cup	75	53	106	16	0	0	4	1.1
17016	Fish, salmon, coho, steamed/poached fillet	3	oz.	85	56	156	23	0	0	6	1.4
17016	Fish, salmon, coho, steamed/poached fillet	4	oz.	113	74	209	31	0	0	9	1.8
17171	Fish, salmon, pink, baked/broiled	4	oz.	113	79	169	29	0	0	5	0.8
17018	Fish, salmon, pink, w/bone, #1 can, drained	1	cup	150	103	209	30	0	0	9	2.3
17099	Fish, salmon, sockeye, baked/broiled fillet	1	each	155	96	335	42	0	0	17	3
17059	Fish, salmon, sockeye, canned, drained	0.5	cup	75	52	115	15	0	0	5	1.2
17060	Fish, sardine, Atlantic, canned in oil, drained	4	each	48	29	100	12	0	0	6	0.7
18827	Fish, sardines in soy oil	1	each	84	—	150	18	1	0	8	4
17061	Fish, sardines, Pacific, canned in tomato sauce	2	each	76	52	135	12	0	0	9	2.4
17021	Fish, sardines, canned, w/mustard	4	oz.	113	73	222	21	2	0	14	4.4
17133	Fish, sardines, skinless, water pack	4	each	84	50	182	21	0	0	10	2.3
19070	Fish, scallop, battered, fried	10	each	80	44	184	14	11	0.4	9	2.2
19029	Fish, scallop, raw, small	5	each	30	24	26	5	1	0	0	0
19061	Fish, scallops, baked/broiled	4	each	100	70	133	21	3	0	4	0.7
19030	Fish, scallops, breaded, fried, large	2	each	31	18	67	6	3	0	3	0.8
19046	Fish, scallops, imitation, from surimi	4	oz.	113	84	112	14	12	0	0	0.1
19011	Fish, scallops, steamed	4	oz.	113	86	121	18	3	0	4	0.6
17086	Fish, sea bass, baked/broiled fillet	1	each	101	73	125	24	0	0	3	0.7
17086	Fish, sea bass, baked/broiled fillet	3	oz.	85	61	105	20	0	0	2	0.6
17104	Fish, sea bass, striped, baked/broiled	4	oz.	113	83	141	26	0	0	3	0.7
17134	Fish, shark, baked/broiled w/marg, lemon juice, sal	4	oz.	113	74	203	28	0	0	9	1.9
17076	Fish, shark, batter fried	4	oz.	113	68	259	21	7	0	16	3.6
19401	Fish, shrimp cocktail	0.5	cup	115	89	98	13	10	2.1	1	0.3
19411	Fish, shrimp w/butter sauce	0.5	cup	68	47	110	15	1	0	5	2.6
19065	Fish, shrimp, baked/broiled, medium size	2	each	10	7	16	2	0	0	1	0.1
19062	Fish, shrimp, batter fried	12	each	90	48	218	19	10	0.3	11	1.9
19017	Fish, shrimp, canned, drained	10	each	32	23	38	7	0	0	1	0.1
19016	Fish, shrimp, canned, drained, cup	1	cup	128	93	154	30	1	0	3	0.5
19078	Fish, shrimp, dried	1	cup	38	12	115	22	1	0	2	0.4
19077	Fish, shrimp, dried, whole	60	each	30	9	91	18	1	0	1	0.3
19039	Fish, shrimp, imitation, made from surimi	4	oz.	113	85	115	14	10	0	2	0.3
19014	Fish, shrimp, large/prawns, breaded, fried	5	each	85	45	206	18	10	0.3	10	1.8
19012	Fish, shrimp, large/prawns, steamed	10	each	55	42	54	12	0	0	1	0.2
19066	Fish, shrimp, popcorn, baked/broiled	15	each	15	10	23	4	0	0	1	0.1
19032	Fish, shrimp, raw (1 large=7 gram)	4	each	28	21	30	6	0	0	0	0.1
19015	Fish, shrimp, small, breaded, fried	12	each	72	38	174	15	8	0.3	9	1.5
19013	Fish, shrimp, small, steamed	10	each	40	31	40	8	0	0	0	0.1
19400	Fish, shrimp, sweet & sour	0.5	cup	88	42	240	9	21	0.4	14	2.1
17100	Fish, smelt, rainbow, baked/broiled	4	oz.	113	83	141	26	0	0	4	0.7

MonoF (g)	PolyF (g)	Choles (mg)	Calc (mg)	Phos (mg)	Sod (mg)	Pot (mg)	Zn (mg)	Iron (mg)	Magn (mg)	VitA (μg RE)	VitE (mg α-TE)	VitC (mg)	Thia (mg)	Ribo (mg)	Nia (mg)	B6 (mg)	Fola (μg)	B12 (μg)
0.2	0.3	54	60	211	261	397	1.9	6	34	51	1.36	6	0.03	0.04	2.4	0.41	18	22.7
0.3	0.5	93	102	359	444	676	3.2	10.2	58	78	2.32	8	0.06	0.08	4.1	0.66	29	36.7
0.4	0	17	25	169	54	254	0.6	0.2	25	16	0.42	0	0.08	0.12	2.4	0.23	5	1.52
4.1	2.9	71	55	140	367	215	76.6	6.1	51	79	2.01	3	0.13	0.18	1.4	0.06	27	13.7
6.2	4.3	106	81	208	546	320	114	9.1	76	118	2.99	5	0.2	0.26	2.2	0.08	41	20.4
0.2	0.4	25	4	80	53	83	8.2	2.5	11	40	0.42	4	0.03	0.12	1	0.02	5	7.94
0.3	0.9	56	51	154	277	191	83.5	4.9	52	0	0.96	5	0.1	0.09	1.9	0.11	20	31.5
0.3	0.9	68	56	172	139	284	113	8.3	67	112	1.05	6	0.19	0.21	1.5	0.12	11	23.7
0.4	1.1	60	51	153	239	177	103	7.6	53	34	0.96	4	0.11	0.11	1.6	0.07	11	22.1
0.3	0.8	44	38	85	177	118	76.4	5	40	23	0.67	3	0.08	0.08	1	0.05	6	14.7
0.8	2	113	18	276	240	342	37.6	10.4	50	166	2.01	14	0.14	0.5	4.1	0.1	17	32.7
0.1	0.2	53	47	118	36	158	0.7	0.5	18	5	0.7	1	0.04	0.06	0.9	0.06	3	1.01
0.2	0.4	98	87	218	67	292	1.2	1	32	8	1.28	1	0.07	0.1	1.6	0.12	5	1.87
0.1	0.3	58	4	289	70	232	0.4	0.2	44	14	0.12	0	0.04	0.05	1	0.04	2	2.52
0.1	0.4	82	5	410	99	329	0.5	0.2	62	20	0.17	0	0.06	0.06	1.4	0.06	3	3.57
6.4	4	56	180	275	657	385	0.9	0.9	32	27	2.11	4	0.09	0.18	5.4	0.37	20	2.19
3.4	2.1	30	95	144	345	202	0.5	0.5	17	14	1.11	2	0.05	0.1	2.9	0.2	10	1.15
4.3	3.2	122	188	276	791	289	1	1.3	30	120	2.01	2	0.09	0.3	4.5	0.22	22	2.35
3.5	2.6	99	153	223	640	234	0.8	1	25	97	1.63	2	0.07	0.24	3.7	0.18	18	1.9
4.2	5	109	23	394	86	967	1.3	1.6	57	20	1.94	0	0.42	0.75	15.6	1.45	45	4.7
2.3	2.8	60	13	218	48	534	0.7	0.9	32	11	1.07	0	0.23	0.41	8.6	0.8	25	2.59
6.5	3	96	32	421	68	573	0.6	1	138	169	1.94	5	0.05	0.18	11.3	0.52	40	3.25
2.3	1.1	26	12	186	889	198	0.4	1	20	30	1.53	0	0.03	0.12	5.4	0.32	2	3.7
2.3	1.1	26	12	186	2268	198	0.4	1	20	30	1.53	0	0.03	0.12	5.4	0.32	2	3.7
2.2	1.3	108	16	412	73	624	0.7	0.8	32	39	1.94	0	0.1	0.25	9.7	0.52	6	3.92
1.4	1.1	29	187	266	365	225	0.8	0.5	22	14	1.2	0	0.02	0.12	5.2	0.28	15	3.3
2.3	2.1	48	39	253	45	387	0.4	0.6	30	27	0.69	1	0.1	0.14	6.6	0.47	8	3.81
3.1	2.9	65	52	338	60	516	0.6	0.8	40	36	0.92	1	0.13	0.18	8.8	0.63	10	5.08
1.4	2	76	19	335	98	469	0.8	1.1	37	46	1.43	0	0.22	0.08	9.7	0.26	6	3.92
2.7	3.1	82	320	494	831	489	1.4	1.3	51	26	2.03	0	0.04	0.28	9.8	0.45	23	6.6
8.2	3.7	135	11	428	102	581	0.8	0.9	48	98	1.95	0	0.33	0.26	10.3	0.34	8	8.99
2.4	1.4	33	179	245	404	283	0.8	0.8	22	40	1.2	0	0.01	0.14	4.1	0.22	7	0.22
1.9	2.5	68	183	235	242	191	0.6	1.4	19	32	0.14	0	0.04	0.11	2.5	0.08	6	4.29
—	—	100	250	—	310	—	—	1.4	—	0	—	0	—	—	—	—	—	—
4.2	1.8	46	182	278	315	259	1.1	1.8	26	53	2.81	1	0.03	0.18	3.2	0.09	18	6.84
4.8	3.2	125	344	401	862	295	0.6	5.9	11	10	1.13	0	0.03	0.23	6.1	0.14	18	7.94
4.3	2.4	69	71	273	771	375	1.1	1.3	39	33	0.84	1	0.11	0.27	3.7	0.35	12	15.7
3.7	2.3	65	29	182	374	248	0.8	0.9	43	29	1.55	2	0.07	0.14	1.3	0.11	15	0.98
0	0.1	10	7	66	48	97	0.3	0.1	17	4	0.3	1	0	0.02	0.3	0.04	5	0.46
1.4	1.3	40	30	265	511	390	1.2	0.4	68	56	1.69	3	0.01	0.06	1.3	0.17	18	1.75
1.4	0.9	19	13	73	144	103	0.3	0.3	18	7	0.59	1	0.01	0.03	0.5	0.04	12	0.41
0.1	0.2	25	9	320	902	117	0.4	0.4	49	23	0.12	0	0.01	0.02	0.4	0.03	2	1.81
1.3	1.2	36	28	180	465	318	1	0.3	61	52	1.53	3	0.01	0.07	1.1	0.16	13	1.51
0.5	1	54	13	250	88	331	0.5	0.4	54	65	0.64	0	0.13	0.15	1.9	0.46	6	0.3
0.5	0.8	45	11	211	74	279	0.4	0.3	45	54	0.54	0	0.11	0.13	1.6	0.39	5	0.26
1	1.2	117	22	288	100	372	0.6	1.2	58	35	0.69	0	0.13	0.04	2.9	0.39	11	5
3.5	3	68	47	279	455	219	0.6	1.1	65	124	1.86	2	0.05	0.08	3.9	0.48	4	1.48
6.7	4.2	67	57	220	138	176	0.5	1.3	49	61	1.19	0	0.08	0.11	3.2	0.34	17	1.37
0.2	0.4	87	43	138	496	277	0.7	1.7	27	36	2.32	12	0.05	0.05	1.9	0.12	27	0.56
1.3	0.6	120	38	149	146	134	0.8	1.7	26	47	1.66	1	0.02	0.02	1.8	0.07	1	0.72
0.2	0.2	18	6	25	50	22	0.1	0.3	4	10	0.39	0	0	0	0.3	0.01	0	0.13
3.4	4.6	159	60	196	310	203	1.2	1.1	36	50	1.35	1	0.12	0.12	2.8	0.09	7	1.68
0.1	0.2	55	19	75	54	67	0.4	0.9	13	6	0.3	1	0.01	0.01	0.9	0.04	1	0.36
0.4	1	221	76	298	216	269	1.6	3.5	52	23	1.19	3	0.04	0.05	3.5	0.14	2	1.43
0.3	0.7	166	57	224	163	202	1.2	2.6	39	17	2.41	2	0.03	0.04	2.6	0.11	2	1.08
0.2	0.6	131	45	177	128	159	1	2.1	31	14	1.9	2	0.02	0.03	2.1	0.08	1	0.85
0.2	0.9	41	22	320	799	101	0.4	0.7	49	23	0.12	0	0.03	0.04	0.2	0.03	2	1.81
3.2	4.3	150	57	185	292	191	1.2	1.1	34	48	1.28	1	0.11	0.12	2.6	0.08	7	1.59
0.1	0.2	107	22	75	123	100	0.9	1.7	19	36	0.28	1	0.02	0.02	1.4	0.07	2	0.82
0.2	0.3	28	10	37	75	34	0.2	0.4	7	14	0.59	0	0	0	0.4	0.02	1	0.2
0.1	0.2	43	15	57	41	52	0.3	0.7	10	15	0.23	1	0.01	0.01	0.7	0.03	1	0.32
2.7	3.7	127	48	157	248	162	1	0.9	29	40	1.08	1	0.09	0.1	2.2	0.07	6	1.35
0.1	0.2	78	16	55	90	73	0.6	1.2	14	26	0.2	1	0.01	0.01	1	0.05	1	0.6
3.3	8.2	60	29	98	409	183	0.6	1.5	23	25	2.07	5	0.03	0.04	1.4	0.1	3	0.39
0.9	1.3	102	87	335	87	422	2.4	1.3	43	19	0.71	0	0.01	0.17	2	0.19	5	4.5

A

Esha Code	Food Item	Qty	Meas	Wgt (g)	Wtr (g)	Cals	Prot (g)	Carb (g)	Fib (g)	Fat (g)	SatF (g)
17022	Fish, snapper, baked/broiled fillet	4	oz.	113	80	145	30	0	0	2	0.4
17068	Fish, sole/flounder, baked/broiled fillet	1	each	127	93	149	31	0	0	2	0.5
17068	Fish, sole/flounder, baked/broiled fillet	3	oz.	85	62	100	21	0	0	1	0.3
17005	Fish, sole/flounder, batter fried pieces	4	piece	64	42	121	13	5	0.1	5	1
17004	Fish, sole/flounder, breaded, fried fillet	1	each	81	48	176	16	6	0.4	9	2.3
17004	Fish, sole/flounder, breaded, fried fillet	3	oz.	85	50	185	17	7	0.4	10	2.4
17006	Fish, sole/flounder, steamed/poached	4	oz.	113	84	129	27	0	0	2	0.4
19074	Fish, squid, canned	0.5	cup	94	70	99	17	3	0	1	0.4
19047	Fish, squid, flour fried	0.5	cup	75	48	131	13	6	0	6	1.4
19069	Fish, squid, pickled	4	oz.	113	85	104	17	5	0	2	0.4
19068	Fish, squid/calamari, baked/broiled	4	oz.	113	80	156	21	4	0	5	1.2
17023	Fish, steelhead, baked/broiled fillet	3	oz.	85	61	113	18	0	0	4	1.1
17023	Fish, steelhead, baked/broiled fillet	4	oz.	113	82	151	24	0	0	5	1.5
17078	Fish, sturgeon, baked/broiled	4	oz.	113	79	153	24	0	0	6	1.3
17079	Fish, sturgeon, smoked	4	oz.	113	71	196	35	0	0	5	1.2
17080	Fish, surimi (processed pollock)	4	oz.	113	86	112	17	8	0	1	0.2
17066	Fish, swordfish, broiled/baked	1	piece	106	73	164	27	0	0	5	1.5
17066	Fish, swordfish, broiled/baked	3	oz.	85	58	132	22	0	0	4	1.2
17136	Fish, swordfish, steamed/poached	4	oz.	113	78	174	28	0	0	6	1.6
17138	Fish, trout, floured/breaded, fried	1	each	125	63	334	29	12	0.7	18	4
17175	Fish, trout, mixed, baked/broiled	4	oz.	113	72	215	30	0	0	10	1.7
17082	Fish, trout, rainbow, baked/broiled fillet	1	each	62	44	93	14	0	0	4	1
17082	Fish, trout, rainbow, baked/broiled fillet	3	oz.	85	60	128	20	0	0	5	1.4
18810	Fish, tuna cake/patty	1	each	120	64	300	22	14	1.3	17	4.2
17101	Fish, tuna, bluefin, baked/broiled	4	oz.	113	67	209	34	0	0	7	1.8
17025	Fish, tuna, light, canned in oil, drained	1	cup	146	87	289	42	0	0	12	2.2
17176	Fish, tuna, skipjack, baked/broiled	4	oz.	113	71	150	32	0	0	1	0.5
17141	Fish, tuna, smoked pieces	4	piece	64	38	140	15	0	0	8	2.2
17177	Fish, tuna, yellowfin, baked/broiled	4	oz.	113	71	158	34	0	0	1	0.3
19040	Fish, whelk, steamed	4	oz.	113	36	312	54	18	0	1	0.1
17145	Fish, whiting, baked/broiled	4	oz.	113	85	132	27	0	0	2	0.5
2624	Flan caramel custard mix w/2% milk	0.5	cup	133	100	136	4	26	0.1	2	1.5
2625	Flan caramel custard mix w/whole milk	0.5	cup	133	99	150	4	25	0.1	4	2.5
56119	Flauta, beef	1	each	113	55	360	16	13	1.7	27	4.9
56120	Flauta, chicken	1	each	113	59	343	14	13	1.7	27	4.3
7502	Flour, Soy, lowfat	1	cup	88	2	325	45	30	9	6	0.9
38071	Flour, arrowroot	1	cup	128	15	457	0	113	4.4	0	0
38171	Flour, bread, white, Pillsbury	1	cup	113	16	396	14	81	2.7	1	0.3
38091	Flour, brown rice	1	cup	158	19	574	11	121	7.3	4	0.9
38053	Flour, buckwheat, whole groat	1	cup	98	11	328	12	69	9.8	3	0.7
38063	Flour, carob	1	cup	103	4	229	5	92	41	1	0.1
7109	Flour, chickpea	1	cup	85	8	313	17	51	3.1	6	—
38096	Flour, corn, white, whole grain	1	cup	117	13	422	8	90	11.2	5	0.6
38161	Flour, corn, yellow	1	cup	114	10	416	11	87	15.3	4	0.6
38049	Flour, corn, yellow, whole grain	1	cup	117	13	422	8	90	15.7	5	0.6
38005	Flour, corn/masa harina, enriched	1	cup	114	10	416	11	87	10.9	4	0.6
38065	Flour, gluten	1	cup	140	12	529	58	66	1.2	3	0
38042	Flour, masa harina, enriched, baked value	1	cup	114	10	416	11	87	10.9	4	0.6
5262	Flour, potato	1	cup	179	12	639	12	149	10.6	1	0.2
38022	Flour, rye, dark	1	cup	128	14	415	18	88	28.9	3	0.4
38023	Flour, rye, light	1	cup	102	9	374	9	82	14.9	1	0.1
38044	Flour, rye, light, baked value	1	cup	102	9	374	9	82	14.9	1	0.1
38056	Flour, rye, medium	1	cup	102	10	361	10	79	14.9	2	0.2
38058	Flour, rye, medium, baked value	1	cup	102	10	361	10	79	14.9	2	0.2
38172	Flour, rye-wheat, bohemian style, Pillsbury	1	cup	113	16	395	13	82	6.5	2	0.3
38054	Flour, semolina, enriched	1	cup	167	21	601	21	122	6.5	2	0.3
4615	Flour, sesame, high fat	1	oz.	28	0	149	9	8	1.8	10	1.5
4617	Flour, sesame, lowfat	1	oz.	28	2	94	14	10	1.4	0	0.1
4616	Flour, sesame, partially defatted	1	oz.	28	2	108	11	10	1.7	3	0.5
38173	Flour, shake and blend, Pillsbury	1	cup	216	30	756	23	158	5.8	3	1.1
7501	Flour, soy, whole fat	1	cup	85	4	369	32	27	8.2	18	2.5
4638	Flour, sunflower seed, partially defatted	1	cup	80	6	261	38	29	4.2	1	0.1
38087	Flour, triticale, whole grain	1	cup	130	13	439	17	95	19	2	0.4
38158	Flour, white rice	1	cup	158	19	578	9	127	3.8	2	0.6
38030	Flour, white, all purpose, enriched	1	cup	125	15	455	13	95	3.4	1	0.2

MonoF	PolyF	Choles	Calc	Phos	Sod	Pot	Zn	Iron	Magn	VitA	VitE	VitC	Thia	Ribo	Nia	B6	Fola	B12
(g)	(g)	(mg)	(mg)	(mg)	(mg)	(mg)	(mg)	(mg)	(mg)	(μg RE)	(mg α-TE)	(mg)	(mg)	(mg)	(mg)	(mg)	(μg)	(μg)
0.4	0.7	53	45	228	65	592	0.5	0.3	42	40	0.71	2	0.06	0	0.4	0.52	7	3.97
0.3	0.8	86	23	367	133	437	0.8	0.4	74	14	2.4	0	0.1	0.14	2.8	0.3	12	3.19
0.2	0.5	58	15	246	89	292	0.5	0.3	49	9	1.61	0	0.07	0.1	1.8	0.2	8	2.13
2	1.8	31	44	145	105	277	0.3	0.8	50	66	1.04	0	0.07	0.08	3.7	0.18	9	0.7
3.8	2.4	56	28	163	314	300	0.5	0.7	28	15	2.22	1	0.08	0.1	2.6	0.15	10	1.1
4	2.5	58	30	171	329	315	0.5	0.7	29	16	2.33	1	0.09	0.11	2.8	0.16	10	1.16
0.3	0.5	68	26	235	103	435	0.6	0.5	40	11	2.68	2	0.1	0.1	3.5	0.24	9	1.83
0.1	0.6	250	35	190	292	211	1.6	0.7	32	9	1.29	4	0.02	0.35	1.9	0.04	4	1.05
2.1	1.6	195	29	188	230	209	1.3	0.8	28	8	1.39	3	0.04	0.34	2	0.04	10	0.92
0.1	0.6	254	37	229	1585	273	1.7	0.7	36	10	1.31	4	0.02	0.45	2.2	0.05	5	1.35
1.7	1.8	318	45	303	420	338	2.1	0.9	45	58	2.19	6	0.02	0.45	2.8	0.07	6	1.69
1	0.8	90	19	273	63	371	0.5	0.3	34	30	0.21	0	0.06	0.18	2.5	0.39	5	2.94
1.3	1	120	25	364	84	496	0.7	0.4	45	40	0.28	0	0.08	0.24	3.3	0.52	7	3.92
2.8	1	87	19	307	78	413	0.6	1	51	274	0.85	0	0.09	0.1	11.5	0.26	20	2.84
2.7	0.5	91	19	319	838	430	0.6	1	53	318	0.57	0	0.1	0.1	12.6	0.31	23	3.29
0.2	0.5	34	10	320	162	127	0.4	0.3	49	23	0.28	0	0.02	0.02	0.2	0.03	2	1.81
2.1	1.2	53	6	357	122	391	1.6	1.1	36	44	0.67	1	0.05	0.12	12.5	0.4	2	2.14
1.7	1	42	5	286	98	314	1.2	0.9	29	35	0.54	1	0.04	0.1	10	0.32	2	1.72
2.2	1.3	56	6	340	116	351	1.6	1.2	35	44	0.72	1	0.04	0.12	11.8	0.38	2	2.14
7.4	5.5	106	80	341	530	484	1	2.6	34	34	1.24	1	0.41	0.48	6.2	0.24	23	8.74
4.7	2.2	84	62	356	76	525	1	2.2	32	22	0.3	1	0.48	0.48	6.5	0.26	17	8.49
1.1	1.1	43	53	167	35	278	0.3	0.2	19	9	0.31	1	0.09	0.06	3.6	0.22	12	3.91
1.5	1.6	59	73	229	48	381	0.4	0.3	26	13	0.43	2	0.13	0.08	4.9	0.29	16	5.36
7.2	4.9	43	28	252	421	325	0.9	1.4	33	30	1.87	4	0.1	0.15	9.2	0.21	11	1.38
2.3	2.1	56	11	370	57	366	0.9	1.5	73	857	1.43	0	0.32	0.35	11.9	0.6	2	12.4
4.3	4.2	26	19	454	517	302	1.3	2	45	34	1.75	0	0.06	0.18	18.1	0.16	8	3.21
0.3	0.5	68	42	323	53	592	1.2	1.8	50	20	1.43	1	0.04	0.14	21.3	1.11	11	2.48
3.3	2.2	61	42	163	179	192	0.4	0.9	19	30	0.96	0	0.01	0.18	2.1	0.32	6	4.48
0.2	0.4	66	24	278	53	645	0.8	1.1	73	23	0.71	1	0.57	0.06	13.5	1.18	2	0.68
0.1	0.1	147	128	320	467	787	3.7	11.5	195	56	0.3	8	0.06	0.24	2.3	0.74	13	20.5
0.5	0.7	95	70	323	150	492	0.6	0.5	31	39	0.34	0	0.08	0.07	1.9	0.2	17	2.95
0.7	0.1	9	153	116	66	194	0.5	0.1	17	62	0.07	1	0.04	0.2	0.1	0.05	5	0.36
1.2	0.2	16	150	114	65	192	0.5	0.1	16	35	0.13	1	0.04	0.2	0.1	0.05	5	0.35
11.6	9.1	45	50	199	187	292	4.2	2.2	29	15	4	14	0.07	0.15	2.1	0.25	10	1.45
11.1	9.6	37	52	146	189	243	1.2	1	28	22	4.06	14	0.05	0.1	3.2	0.22	8	0.09
1.3	3.3	0	165	522	16	2261	1	5.3	202	4	0.17	0	0.33	0.25	1.9	0.46	361	0
0	0.1	0	51	6	3	14	0.1	0.4	4	0	—	0	0	0	0	0.01	9	0
—	—	0	23	—	1	—	—	5	—	0	—	0	0.68	0.45	6	—	175	—
1.6	1.6	0	17	532	13	457	3.9	3.1	177	0	1.14	0	0.7	0.13	10	1.16	25	0
0.9	0.9	0	40	330	11	565	3.1	4	246	0	1.01	0	0.41	0.19	6	0.57	53	0
0.2	0.2	0	358	81	36	852	0.9	3	56	1	0.65	0	0.06	0.48	2	0.38	30	0
—	—	—	85	296	—	—	—	6	92	—	—	—	0.1	0.28	0.6	—	—	0
1.2	2.1	0	8	318	6	369	2	2.8	109	0	0.29	0	0.29	0.09	2.2	0.43	29	0
1.1	2	0	161	254	6	340	2	8.2	125	54	0.95	0	1.63	0.86	11.2	0.42	213	0
1.2	2.1	0	8	318	6	369	2	2.8	109	55	0.29	0	0.29	0.09	2.2	0.43	29	0
1.1	2	0	161	254	6	340	2	8.2	125	0	0.28	0	1.63	0.86	11.2	0.42	213	0
0	0	0	56	196	3	84	—	0.6	—	0	—	0	0.04	0.04	0.7	—	30	0
1.1	2	0	161	254	6	340	2	8.2	125	0	0.95	0	1.63	0.77	10.1	0.38	149	0
0	0.3	0	116	301	98	1791	1	2.5	116	0	0.45	7	0.41	0.09	6.3	1.38	45	0
0.4	1.5	0	72	809	1	934	7.2	8.3	317	0	3.3	0	0.4	0.32	5.5	0.57	77	0
0.2	0.6	0	21	198	2	238	1.8	1.8	71	0	0.57	0	0.34	0.09	0.8	0.24	22	0
0.2	0.6	0	21	198	2	238	1.8	1.8	71	0	0.57	0	0.27	0.08	0.7	0.22	16	0
0.2	0.8	0	24	211	3	347	2	2.2	76	0	1.36	0	0.29	0.12	1.8	0.27	19	0
0.2	0.8	0	24	211	3	347	2	2.2	76	0	0.81	0	0.24	0.1	1.6	0.25	14	0
—	—	0	22	—	0	—	—	5	—	0	—	0	0.68	0.45	6	—	—	—
0.2	0.7	0	28	227	2	311	1.8	7.3	78	0	0.1	0	1.35	0.95	10	0.17	257	0
4	4.6	0	45	229	12	120	3	4.3	102	2	0.44	0	0.76	0.08	3.8	0.04	9	0
0.2	0.2	0	42	215	11	113	2.8	4	96	2	0.02	0	0.71	0.08	3.5	0.04	8	0
1.2	1.4	0	42	230	12	120	3	4	103	2	0.16	0	0.72	0.08	3.6	0.04	8	0
—	—	0	43	—	2	—	—	9.5	—	0	—	0	1.3	0.86	11.4	—	—	—
3.9	10	0	175	420	11	2137	3.3	5.4	365	10	1.66	0	0.49	0.99	3.7	0.39	293	0
0.2	0.7	0	91	551	2	54	4	5.3	277	4	1.3	1	2.55	0.21	5.8	0.6	178	0
0.2	1	0	46	417	3	606	3.5	3.4	199	0	2.48	0	0.49	0.17	3.7	0.52	96	0
0.7	0.6	0	16	155	0	120	1.3	0.6	55	0	0.2	0	0.22	0.03	4.1	0.69	6	0
0.1	0.5	0	19	135	2	134	0.9	5.8	28	0	0.08	0	0.98	0.62	7.4	0.06	193	0

Esha Code	Food Item	Qty	Meas	Wgt (g)	Wtr (g)	Cals	Prot (g)	Carb (g)	Fib (g)	Fat (g)	SatF (g)
38037	Flour, white, all purpose, enriched, baked value	1	cup	125	15	455	13	95	4.1	1	0.2
38318	Flour, white, all purpose, enriched, unbleached	1	cup	125	15	455	13	95	3.4	1	0.2
38031	Flour, white, all purpose, sifted	1	cup	115	14	419	12	88	3.1	1	0.2
38039	Flour, white, cake, baked value	1	cup	109	14	395	9	85	1.8	1	0.1
38035	Flour, white, cake, enriched, sifted	1	cup	96	12	348	8	75	1.6	1	0.1
38036	Flour, white, cake, sifted, baked value	1	cup	96	12	348	8	75	1.6	1	0.1
38033	Flour, white, self-rising, enriched	1	cup	125	13	443	12	93	3.4	1	0.2
38032	Flour, whole wheat	1	cup	120	12	407	16	87	14.6	2	0.4
38174	Flour, whole wheat, Pillsbury	1	cup	113	16	397	16	77	13.4	3	0.6
38040	Flour, whole wheat, baked value	1	cup	120	12	407	16	87	14.6	2	0.4
62207	Forza energy bar	1	each	70	12	231	10	45	4	1	—
42156	French toast, homemade, w/2% milk	1	piece	65	36	149	5	16	0.6	7	1.8
42040	French toast, recipe, w/whole milk	1	piece	65	35	151	5	16	0.5	7	2
45547	Fritter, banana	1	each	34	13	116	2	11	0.4	7	2
45546	Fritter, berry	1	each	34	15	111	2	10	0.6	7	1.9
45548	Fritter, wheat, no syrup	1	each	22	8	99	2	4	0.1	9	2
14029	Frog legs, steamed	2	each	100	74	106	24	0	0	0	0.1
46036	Frosting, chocolate cream, recipe, w/margarine	2	Tbs	34	3	138	0	27	0.6	4	0.9
46312	Frosting, chocolate supreme, Pillsbury	2	Tbs	35	7	139	0	21	0.2	6	1.7
46037	Frosting, chocolate, creamy, ready to eat, can	1	each	462	78	1834	5	292	2.8	81	25.5
46034	Frosting, chocolate, creamy, w/butter	2	Tbs	34	5	131	0	25	0.6	4	1.9
46035	Frosting, chocolate, creamy, w/margarine	2	Tbs	34	5	132	0	25	0.6	4	0.6
46038	Frosting, coconut nut, ready to eat, can	1	each	462	97	1903	7	244	6.5	111	32.5
46039	Frosting, cream cheese flavor, ready to eat	1	each	462	70	1908	0	308	0	80	23.3
46032	Frosting, creamy chocolate butter, recipe	2	Tbs	34	3	138	0	27	0.6	4	2.4
46315	Frosting, french vanilla supreme, Pillsbury	2	Tbs	38	6	158	0	26	0	6	1.7
46162	Frosting, lite, milk chocolate, Pillsbury	2	Tbs	58	11	209	1	41	1.6	5	1.4
46163	Frosting, lite, vanilla, Pillsbury	2	Tbs	32	5	121	0	24	0.1	3	0.7
46041	Frosting, seven minute, recipe	0.25	cup	80	14	254	1	64	0	0	0
46042	Frosting, sour cream flavor, ready to eat, can	1	each	462	66	1903	0	312	0.5	80	23.1
46045	Frosting, vanilla cream, recipe, w/butter	2	Tbs	40	7	137	0	31	0	2	1
46046	Frosting, vanilla cream, recipe, w/margarine	2	Tbs	40	4	162	0	32	0	4	0.9
46044	Frosting, vanilla, creamy, mix w/water & butter	2	Tbs	40	5	169	0	28	0	7	2.8
46048	Frosting, white, fluffy, mix w/water, pkg	1	each	315	111	769	5	197	0	0	0
46388	Frosting/Icing, chocolate, ready to spread	1	oz.	28	5	120	0	18	0	5	2
46040	Frosting/glaze, recipe	0.25	cup	80	14	287	0	59	0	6	1.4
46009	Frosting/icing, creamy vanilla, canned	2	Tbs	31	4	131	0	22	0	5	1.5
46018	Frosting/icing, creamy, mix, prepared	2	Tbs	40	5	169	0	28	0	7	1.3
2062	Frozen dessert bar, Treat, Weight Watchers	1	each	81	58	88	2	19	0	1	0.2
2061	Frozen dessert, Weight Watchers	0.5	cup	66	47	73	3	14	0	1	0.3
2045	Frozen yogurt cone, chocolate	1	each	78	44	157	4	22	1.1	7	3.9
2047	Frozen yogurt cone, not chocolate	1	each	78	47	143	3	22	0.5	5	2.6
2212	Frozen yogurt, Cherry Garcia Ben & Jerry's	0.5	cup	106	—	170	4	31	0	3	2
2071	Frozen yogurt, chocolate	0.5	cup	96	67	110	5	21	1.5	2	1.2
2043	Frozen yogurt, chocolate-coated	1	each	41	21	109	1	12	0.1	7	5.4
2039	Frozen yogurt, nonfat, chocolate	0.5	cup	96	67	104	5	21	1.5	1	0.5
2079	Frozen yogurt, nonfat, fruit	0.5	cup	96	72	95	5	19	0	0	0.1
2035	Frozen yogurt, soft serve, chocolate	0.5	cup	72	46	115	3	18	1.6	4	2.6
2064	Frozen yogurt, soft serve, vanilla	0.5	cup	72	47	114	3	17	0	4	2.5
2068	Frozen yogurt, vanilla	0.5	cup	96	71	102	4	18	0	1	0.8
2075	Frozen yogurt, vanilla/fruit	0.5	cup	96	71	102	4	18	0	1	0.8
3163	Fruit cocktail in light syrup	0.5	cup	126	106	72	1	19	1.3	0	0
3045	Fruit cocktail, canned in heavy syrup	0.5	cup	128	103	93	0	24	1.3	0	0
3164	Fruit cocktail, juice pack	0.5	cup	124	108	57	1	15	1.2	0	0
3313	Fruit cocktail, water pack	0.5	cup	122	111	39	1	10	1.2	0	0
20124	Fruit drink, Crystal Light, prepared	1	cup	240	239	3	0	0	0	0	0
20018	Fruit drink, low cal (Wylers/Koolaid)	1	cup	240	228	43	0	11	0	0	0
20060	Fruit drink, low calorie, dry mix (Crystal Light)	1	Tbs	12	1	27	1	12	0	0	0
20017	Fruit drink, low calorie, powder, prepared	1	cup	240	228	43	0	11	0	0	0
20016	Fruit drink, powder, prepared (Koolade)	1	cup	240	217	89	0	23	0	0	0
20019	Fruit drink, punch flavor (Hi C)	1	cup	240	228	43	0	11	0	0	0
23174	Fruit juice bar, frozen	1	each	77	60	63	1	16	0	0	0
23094	Fruit juice bar, w/cream, frozen	1	each	65	43	86	1	19	0.1	1	0.8
23086	Fruit leather/roll ups, small	1	each	14	2	49	0	12	0.5	0	0.1
20024	Fruit punch drink, canned	1	cup	253	223	119	0	30	0.3	0	0

MonoF	PolyF	Choles	Calc	Phos	Sod	Pot	Zn	Iron	Magn	VitA	VitE	VitC	Thia	Ribo	Nia	B6	Fola	B12
(g)	(g)	(mg)	(mg)	(mg)	(mg)	(mg)	(mg)	(mg)	(mg)	(μg RE)	(mg α-TE)	(mg)	(mg)	(mg)	(mg)	(mg)	(μg)	(μg)
0.1	0.5	0	19	135	2	134	0.9	5.8	28	0	0.46	0	0.78	0.56	6.6	0.05	135	0
0.1	0.5	0	19	135	2	134	0.9	5.8	28	0	0.46	0	0.98	0.62	7.4	0.06	193	0
0.1	0.5	0	17	124	2	123	0.8	5.3	25	0	0.07	0	0.9	0.57	6.8	0.05	177	0
0.1	0.4	0	15	93	2	114	0.7	8	17	0	0.08	0	0.78	0.42	6.7	0.03	118	0
0.1	0.4	0	13	82	2	101	0.6	7	15	0	0.06	0	0.86	0.41	6.5	0.03	148	0
0.1	0.4	0	13	82	2	101	0.6	7	15	0	0.06	0	0.86	0.41	6.5	0.03	148	0
0.1	0.5	0	423	744	1587	155	0.8	5.8	24	0	0.08	0	0.84	0.52	7.3	0.06	193	0
0.3	0.9	0	41	415	6	486	3.5	4.7	166	0	1.48	0	0.54	0.26	7.6	0.41	53	0
—	—	0	45	—	1	—	—	5.6	—	0	—	0	0.57	0.11	5.8	—	—	—
0.3	0.9	0	41	415	6	486	3.5	4.7	166	0	0.5	0	0.43	0.23	6.9	0.37	37	0
—	—	0	300	350	65	220	5.2	6.3	160	—	20	60	1.5	1.7	20	2	400	6
2.9	1.7	75	65	76	311	87	0.4	1.1	11	86	0.72	0	0.13	0.21	1.1	0.05	28	0.2
3	1.7	76	64	76	311	86	0.4	1.1	11	81	0.31	0	0.13	0.21	1.1	0.05	15	0.2
3.1	1.8	25	16	29	19	86	0.2	0.4	8	23	0.75	1	0.05	0.09	0.4	0.1	5	0.07
3.1	1.8	25	16	27	20	41	0.2	0.4	4	23	0.87	2	0.05	0.08	0.4	0.02	4	0.08
3.8	2.4	36	6	21	56	17	0.1	0.3	2	67	1.11	0	0.03	0.06	0.3	0.01	4	0.08
0.1	0.2	72	26	160	84	372	1.4	2	29	20	1.45	0	0.19	0.34	1.6	0.16	16	0.52
1.7	1.1	0	6	16	70	32	0.1	0.3	9	38	0.69	0	0	0.01	0	0	1	0.01
—	—	0	4	—	78	—	—	0.6	—	0	—	0	—	—	—	—	—	—
41.7	9.8	0	37	365	845	906	1.3	6.6	97	915	10.9	0	0.06	0.08	0.6	0.02	0	0
0.9	0.1	8	4	17	52	49	0.2	0.3	10	21	0.69	0	0	0.01	0	0.02	0	0
1.4	1	0	4	17	56	50	0.2	0.3	10	23	0.69	0	0	0.01	0	0.02	0	0
56.4	15.8	0	60	291	901	859	1.9	2.5	88	0	5.27	1	0.16	0.09	1	0.25	28	0
41.7	10.9	0	14	14	1094	162	0	0.7	9	536	9.33	0	0	0.03	0.1	0	0	0
1.1	0.1	10	6	16	65	31	0.1	0.3	9	34	0.69	0	0	0.01	0	0	1	0.01
—	—	0	1	—	76	—	—	0	—	0	—	0	—	—	—	—	—	—
—	—	0	5	—	144	—	—	0.9	—	0	—	0	—	—	—	—	—	—
—	—	0	1	—	58	—	—	0	—	0	—	0	—	—	—	—	—	—
0	0	0	2	2	136	51	0	0.1	2	0	0	0	0	0.07	0	0	0	0.02
41.5	10.8	0	9	18	942	896	0	0.3	9	564	9.33	0	0.05	0.09	3.1	0.02	5	0.05
0.5	0.1	5	9	7	26	12	0	0	1	15	0.81	0	0	0.01	0	0	0	0.03
1.9	1.3	0	5	4	82	7	0	0	1	45	0.81	0	0	0.01	0	0	0	0.02
2.2	1.3	10	4	11	83	8	0	0.1	1	38	0.28	0	0.01	0.01	0.1	0	0	0
0	0	0	13	16	491	243	0.1	0.2	6	0	0	0	0	0.08	2.1	0	6	0.03
2	0	0	0	—	40	40	—	0	—	0	—	0	0	0	0	—	—	—
2.7	1.8	2	18	14	75	24	0.1	0	2	65	0.61	0	0.01	0.02	0	0.01	1	0.06
2.7	0.7	0	1	12	28	12	0	0	0	70	1.47	0	0	0	0	0	0	0
2.7	2.3	0	4	11	88	9	0	0.1	1	43	0.81	0	0.01	0.01	0.1	0	0	0
0.1	0.4	1	82	66	47	111	0.3	0.1	10	38	0.07	1	0.03	0.11	0.1	0.03	3	0.24
0.2	0	3	111	88	61	156	0.3	0.1	10	5	0.01	0	0.03	0.13	0.1	0.03	1	0.44
2.5	0.5	1	115	119	70	193	0.5	0.6	29	42	0.34	1	0.05	0.17	0.3	0.08	6	0.2
1.8	0.4	1	118	107	74	167	0.4	0.4	17	44	0.3	1	0.04	0.17	0.3	0.08	6	0.21
—	—	10	150	—	70	—	—	0.4	—	40	—	1	—	—	—	—	—	—
0.6	0.1	5	150	150	56	311	1	0.8	38	13	0.05	1	0.04	0.19	0.2	0.04	10	0.44
0.8	0.2	1	46	43	28	74	0.2	0.1	6	18	0.05	0	0.01	0.07	0.1	0.03	2	0.09
0.3	0	1	163	160	62	327	1.1	0.9	39	2	0.02	1	0.04	0.21	0.2	0.05	11	0.48
0	0	2	167	132	64	214	0.8	0.1	16	2	0	1	0.04	0.2	0.1	0.04	10	0.51
1.3	0.2	4	106	100	71	188	0.4	0.9	19	31	0.1	0	0.03	0.15	0.2	0.05	8	0.21
1.1	0.2	1	103	93	63	152	0.3	0.2	10	41	0.04	1	0.03	0.16	0.2	0.06	4	0.21
0.4	0	5	153	121	59	197	0.8	0.1	15	13	0.04	1	0.04	0.18	0.1	0.04	9	0.47
0.4	0	5	153	121	59	197	0.8	0.1	15	13	0.04	1	0.04	0.18	0.1	0.04	9	0.47
0	0	0	8	14	8	112	0.1	0.4	6	26	0.36	2	0.02	0.02	0.5	0.06	3	0
0	0	0	8	14	8	112	0.1	0.4	6	26	0.37	2	0.02	0.02	0.5	0.06	3	0
0	0	0	10	17	5	118	0.1	0.3	9	38	0.25	3	0.02	0.02	0.5	0.06	3	0
0	0	0	6	14	5	115	0.1	0.3	9	31	0.36	3	0.02	0.01	0.4	0.06	3	0
0	0	0	38	15	7	45	0.1	0	2	0	0	6	0	0	0	0	0	0
0	0	0	17	5	50	50	0.3	0.6	5	2	0	78	0.02	0.05	0	0	5	0
0	0	0	342	156	1	465	0	0	0	0	0	62	0	0	0	0	0	0
0	0	0	17	5	50	50	0.3	0.6	5	2	0	78	0.02	0.05	0	0	5	0
0	0	0	38	48	34	2	0.1	0.1	2	0	0	28	0	0	0	0	0	0
0	0	0	17	5	50	50	0.3	0.6	5	2	0	78	0.02	0.05	0	0	5	0
0	0	0	4	5	3	41	0	0.1	3	2	0	7	0.01	0.01	0.1	0.02	5	0
0.4	0	5	29	5	20	64	0	0.1	2	8	0.03	8	0.01	0.06	0.1	0.03	3	0.05
0.2	0.1	0	4	4	9	41	0	0.1	3	2	0.04	1	0.01	0	0	0.04	1	0
0	0	0	20	3	56	63	0.3	0.5	5	4	0	75	0.06	0.06	0.1	0	3	0

Esha Code	Food Item	Qty	Meas	Wgt (g)	Wtr (g)	Cals	Prot (g)	Carb (g)	Fib (g)	Fat (g)	SatF (g)
20035	Fruit punch drink, frozen concentrate, prepared	1	cup	247	218	114	0	29	0.2	0	0
20106	Fruit punch juice drink, frozen, prepared	1	cup	248	217	124	0	30	0.2	0	0.1
20099	Fruit punch, powder	1	Tbs	6	0	24	0	6	0	0	0
3246	Fruit salad, canned in light syrup	0.5	cup	126	106	73	0	19	1.3	0	0
3312	Fruit salad, includes citrus	0.5	cup	88	74	50	0	13	1.2	0	0.1
3311	Fruit salad, no citrus	0.5	cup	88	73	51	1	13	1.5	0	0.1
3355	Fruit salad, tropical, canned in heavy syrup	0.5	cup	128	99	111	1	29	1.7	0	0
23278	Fruit spread, strawberry, low calorie, Kraft	1	Tbs	20	—	20	0	5	0	0	0
26005	Garlic clove, fresh	1	each	3	2	4	0	1	0.1	0	0
26006	Garlic clove, fresh, chopped	0.25	cup	34	20	51	2	11	0.7	0	0
26007	Garlic powder	0.25	tsp	1	0	2	0	1	0.1	0	0
6553	Garlic, dehydrated	0.25	tsp	1	0	2	0	1	0.1	0	—
1358	Gatorade	1	cup	241	93	60	0	15	0	0	0
23052	Gelatin dessert/Jello, prepared	0.5	cup	135	114	80	2	19	0	0	0
23093	Gelatin dessert/Jello, sugar-free	0.5	cup	117	115	8	1	1	0	0	0
23155	Gelatin, dry mix, sweetened, pkg	1	each	85	1	324	7	77	0	0	0
23009	Gelatin, dry, unsweetened, envelope	1	each	7	1	24	6	0	0	0	0
23156	Gelatin/Jello dessert w/fruit (Jello)	0.5	cup	106	86	73	1	18	0.6	0	0.1
23158	Gelatin/Jello frozen fruit bar	1	each	44	36	31	1	7	0	0	—
6117	Gherkin in sweetened brine	1	each	19	14	19	0	5	0.4	0	0
26043	Ginger root, raw slices	1	piece	2	2	2	0	0	0	0	0
26044	Ginger root, raw, chopped	0.25	cup	24	20	17	0	4	0.5	0	0
26023	Ginger, ground	0.25	tsp	0	0	2	0	0	0.1	0	0
49029	Gnocchi, cheese	0.5	cup	35	24	62	3	3	0.1	4	1.6
49030	Gnocchi, potato	0.5	cup	94	68	136	2	17	0.9	7	4.2
13530	Goat meat, cooked	4	oz.	113	66	237	37	0	0	9	3.7
14016	Goat ribs, cooked	1	each	46	31	66	12	0	0	1	0.4
16048	Goose, liver pate, smoked, canned	0.5	cup	104	38	480	12	5	0	46	15.1
14003	Goose, roasted	4	oz.	113	59	346	29	0	0	25	7.8
14002	Goose, skinless, roasted	4	oz.	113	65	270	33	0	0	14	5.2
3204	Gooseberries canned in light syrup	0.5	cup	126	101	92	1	24	3	0	0
3205	Gooseberries, cooked	0.5	cup	126	101	92	1	24	3	0	0
3203	Gooseberries, fresh	0.5	cup	75	66	33	1	8	3.2	0	0
45531	Graham cracker crust, chilled, not baked	1	oz.	28	2	137	1	18	0.4	7	1.4
23168	Granola bar, New Trail, raisin-coconut, soft	1	each	40	2	182	4	27	1.2	7	4.6
23100	Granola bar, hard, almond	1	each	24	1	117	2	15	1.1	6	3
23101	Granola bar, hard, chocolate chip	1	each	24	1	103	2	17	1	4	2.7
23103	Granola bar, hard, peanut butter	1	each	24	1	114	2	15	0.7	6	0.8
23059	Granola bar, hard, plain	1	each	28	1	134	3	18	1.5	6	0.7
23170	Granola bar, high fiber, yogurt coating, Fi-Bar	1	each	28	3	96	3	19	2.2	3	1
23106	Granola bar, soft, choc chip w/granola&marshmallow	1	each	28	2	121	2	20	1.1	4	2.6
23096	Granola bar, soft, chocolate chocolate chip	1	each	35	1	165	2	23	1.2	9	5
23095	Granola bar, soft, chocolate peanut butter	1	each	37	1	187	4	20	1	11	6.2
23097	Granola bar, soft, chocolate raisin	1	each	42	3	190	3	28	1.8	8	4.1
23107	Granola bar, soft, nut & raisin	1	each	28	2	129	2	18	1.6	6	2.7
23108	Granola bar, soft, peanut butter	1	each	24	2	101	2	15	1	4	0.9
23109	Granola bar, soft, peanut butter chocolate chip	1	each	28	2	122	3	18	1.2	6	1.6
23105	Granola bar, soft, uncoated, chocolate	1	each	42	2	179	3	29	2	7	4.3
23104	Granola bar, soft, uncoated, plain	1	each	28	2	126	2	19	1.3	5	2
23169	Granola clusters, Nature Valley	1	each	34	1	140	2	24	1.4	5	1.9
20101	Grape drink, canned	1	cup	251	222	113	0	29	0	0	0
20082	Grape drink, low calorie	1	cup	240	228	43	0	11	0	0	0
20026	Grape juice drink, canned	1	cup	250	218	125	0	32	0.2	0	0
3062	Grape juice, bottle/canned, unsweetened	1	cup	253	213	154	1	38	0.3	0	0.1
3064	Grape juice, frozen conc w/vit C, prepared	1	cup	250	217	128	0	32	0.2	0	0.1
5541	Grape leaves. raw	1	oz.	28	22	19	1	4	—	0	—
3059	Grape, American type/slip skin, no seeds	0.5	cup	46	37	31	0	8	0.5	0	0.1
3054	Grape, Thompson seedless, cup measure	0.5	cup	80	64	57	1	14	0.8	0	0.2
3057	Grape, Tokay/Red Flame, seedless, cup measure	0.5	cup	80	64	57	1	14	0.8	0	0.2
3058	Grape, adherent skin type	0.5	cup	80	64	57	1	14	0.8	0	0.2
3052	Grapefruit juice, canned, unsweetened	1	cup	247	223	94	1	22	0.2	0	0
3051	Grapefruit juice, fresh	1	cup	247	222	96	1	23	0.2	0	0
3053	Grapefruit juice, frozen concentrate, prepared	1	cup	247	221	101	1	24	0.2	0	0
3342	Grapefruit sections canned in juice	0.5	cup	124	112	46	1	12	0.5	0	0
3050	Grapefruit sections, canned in light syrup	0.5	cup	127	106	76	1	20	0.5	0	0

MonoF	PolyF	Choles	Calc	Phos	Sod	Pot	Zn	Iron	Magn	VitA	VitE	VitC	Thia	Ribo	Nia	B6	Fola	B12
(g)	(g)	(mg)	(mg)	(mg)	(mg)	(mg)	(mg)	(mg)	(mg)	(μg RE)	(mg α-TE)	(mg)	(mg)	(mg)	(mg)	(mg)	(μg)	(μg)
0	0	0	10	2	10	32	0.1	0.2	5	2	0	108	0.02	0.03	0.1	0.02	2	0
0.1	0.1	0	17	0	12	191	0.5	0.6	10	2	0	14	0	0.16	0.1	0.03	0	0
0	0	0	9	13	8	0	0	0	0	0	0	8	0	0	0	0	0	0
0	0	0	9	11	8	103	0.1	0.4	6	54	0.82	3	0.02	0.02	0.5	0.04	3	0
0	0.1	0	8	9	0	154	0.1	0.2	9	7	0.39	14	0.03	0.03	0.2	0.12	7	0
0	0.1	0	7	10	0	164	0.1	0.2	10	17	0.39	7	0.04	0.04	0.4	0.1	7	0
0	0	0	17	9	3	168	0.1	0.7	17	17	0.64	22	0.07	0.06	0.7	0.15	12	0
0	0	0	0	—	20	25	—	0	—	0	—	0	—	—	—	—	—	—
0	0	0	5	5	1	12	0	0.1	1	0	0	1	0.01	0	0	0.04	0	0
0	0.1	0	62	52	6	136	0.4	0.6	8	0	0	11	0.07	0.04	0.2	0.42	1	0
0	0	0	1	3	0	8	0	0	0	0	0	0	0	0	0	0.02	0	0
—	—	—	1	0	0	10	0	0	1	0	—	0	0	0	—	—	—	0
0	0	0	0	22	96	26	.05	.12	2	0	0	0	.01	0	0	0	0	0
0	0	0	3	30	57	1	0	0	1	0	0	0	0	0	0	0	0	0
0	0	0	2	32	56	0	0	0	1	0	0	0	0	0	0	0	0	0
0	0	0	3	121	216	6	0	0.1	2	0	0	0	0	0.02	0	0.01	3	0
0	0	0	4	3	14	1	0	0.1	2	0	0	0	0	0.02	0	0	2	0
0	0.1	0	5	22	30	110	0.1	0.1	7	3	0.11	4	0.03	0.03	0.2	0.13	4	0
—	—	0	1	0	20	1	0	0	0	0	—	0	0	0	0	0	0	0
0	0	0	4	—	99	2	—	0.1	—	1	—	0	0	0	—	0.01	3	0
0	0	0	0	1	0	10	0	0	1	0	0.01	0	0	0	0	0	0	0
0	0	0	4	6	3	100	0.1	0.1	10	0	0.06	1	0.01	0.01	0.2	0.04	3	0
0	0	0	1	1	0	6	0	0.1	1	0	0	0	0	0	0	0	0	0
1.6	0.8	24	68	52	92	25	0.3	0.3	4	52	0.47	0	0.02	0.06	0.2	0.01	4	0.1
1.9	0.3	18	22	39	71	121	0.2	0.7	10	65	0.2	2	0.11	0.09	1.1	0.08	5	0.05
3.3	0.5	192	42	271	368	320	4.9	1.5	30	0	0.44	0	0.07	0.41	11.3	0.29	18	1.83
0.6	0.1	34	8	92	40	186	2.4	1.7	0	0	0.02	0	0.04	0.28	1.8	0	2	0.55
26.6	0.9	156	73	208	725	144	1	5.7	14	1040	1.79	2	0.09	0.31	2.6	0.06	62	9.78
11.7	2.9	103	15	306	79	373	3	3.2	25	24	1.97	0	0.09	0.37	4.7	0.42	2	0.46
4.9	1.8	109	16	350	86	440	3.6	3.2	28	14	1.76	0	0.1	0.44	4.6	0.53	14	0.56
0	0.1	0	20	9	3	97	0.1	0.4	8	18	0.47	13	0.02	0.07	0.2	0.02	4	0
0	0.1	0	20	9	3	97	0.1	0.4	8	18	0.47	13	0.02	0.07	0.2	0.02	4	0
0	0.2	0	19	20	1	149	0.1	0.2	8	22	0.28	21	0.03	0.02	0.2	0.06	4	0
3.2	1.9	0	6	18	159	24	0.1	0.6	5	56	1.15	0	0.03	0.05	0.6	0.01	10	0.01
1	1	0	24	111	111	130	0.6	1.3	40	0	0.28	0	0.11	0.04	0.7	0.14	32	0
1.8	0.9	0	8	54	60	64	0.4	0.6	19	1	0.42	0	0.07	0.02	0.1	0.01	3	0
0.6	0.3	0	18	48	81	59	0.5	0.7	17	1	0.21	0	0.04	0.02	0.1	0.01	3	0
1.6	2.9	0	10	33	67	69	0.3	0.6	13	0	0.31	0	0.05	0.02	0.5	0.02	4	0
1.2	3.4	0	17	79	84	95	0.6	0.8	28	4	0.38	0	0.08	0.03	0.4	0.02	7	0
1	0.7	0	15	107	6	107	0.6	0.7	36	0	0.56	0	0.12	0.05	0.8	0.04	8	0.01
0.8	0.7	0	25	57	90	78	0.4	0.7	20	1	0.26	0	0.04	0.04	0.3	0.01	6	0
2.8	0.6	2	36	70	71	111	0.5	0.8	23	2	0.35	0	0.03	0.09	0.3	0.04	9	0.2
2.4	0.7	4	40	83	71	124	0.5	0.5	25	13	0.48	0	0.04	0.08	1.2	0.04	9	0
1.2	1.4	0	43	94	120	154	0.6	1	31	0	0.47	0	0.1	0.07	0.5	0.04	9	0.08
1.2	1.6	0	24	68	72	111	0.5	0.6	26	1	0.31	0	0.05	0.05	0.7	0.03	9	0.07
1.6	1	0	22	59	96	69	0.4	0.5	20	0	0.29	0	0.05	0.04	0.7	0.02	8	0.05
2.4	1.3	0	23	74	93	107	0.5	0.6	25	1	0.37	0	0.03	0.03	0.9	0.03	9	0.13
1.5	0.8	0	40	98	116	145	0.6	1.1	33	2	0.42	0	0.1	0.06	0.4	0.04	9	0.07
1.1	1.5	0	30	65	79	92	0.4	0.7	21	0	0.35	0	0.08	0.05	0.1	0.03	7	0.11
1.1	1.6	0	15	55	48	77	0.5	0.6	16	2	0.58	0	0.08	0.05	0.3	0.05	10	0.01
0	0	0	8	3	15	12	0.3	0.4	5	0	0	86	0.01	0.01	0.1	0.02	1	0
0	0	0	17	5	50	50	0.3	0.6	5	2	0	78	0.02	0.05	0	0	5	0
0	0	0	8	10	2	88	0.1	0.2	10	0	0	40	0.02	0.02	0.2	0.05	2	0
0	0.1	0	23	28	8	334	0.1	0.6	25	3	0	0	0.07	0.09	0.7	0.16	7	0
0	0.1	0	10	10	5	52	0.1	0.2	10	2	0.12	60	0.04	0.06	0.3	0.1	3	0
—	—	0	203	11	6	72	—	2	—	765	—	3	0.06	0.02	0.3	—	—	0
0	0	0	6	5	1	88	0	0.1	2	5	0.16	2	0.04	0.03	0.1	0.05	2	0
0	0.1	0	9	10	2	148	0	0.2	5	6	0.56	9	0.07	0.05	0.2	0.09	3	0
0	0.1	0	9	10	2	148	0	0.2	5	6	0.56	9	0.07	0.05	0.2	0.09	3	0
0	0.1	0	9	10	2	148	0	0.2	5	6	0.56	9	0.07	0.05	0.2	0.09	3	0
0	0.1	0	17	27	2	378	0.2	0.5	25	2	0.12	72	0.1	0.05	0.6	0.05	26	0
0	0.1	0	22	37	2	400	0.1	0.5	30	2	0.12	94	0.1	0.05	0.5	0.11	25	0
0	0.1	0	20	35	2	336	0.1	0.3	27	2	0.12	83	0.1	0.05	0.5	0.11	9	0
0	0	0	19	15	9	210	0.1	0.3	14	0	0.31	42	0.04	0.02	0.3	0.02	11	0
0	0	0	18	13	3	164	0.1	0.5	13	0	0.32	27	0.05	0.02	0.3	0.02	11	0

Esha Code	Food Item	Qty	Meas	Wgt (g)	Wtr (g)	Cals	Prot (g)	Carb (g)	Fib (g)	Fat (g)	SatF (g)
3049	Grapefruit sections, fresh	1	piece	15	14	5	0	1	0.2	0	0
3048	Grapefruit sections, fresh, cup measure	0.5	cup	115	105	37	1	9	1.3	0	0
3046	Grapefruit, pink/red	0.5	each	123	112	37	1	9	1.7	0	0
3340	Grapefruit, pink/red	0.5	each	123	110	46	1	12	1.6	0	0
3047	Grapefruit, white	0.5	each	118	107	39	1	10	1.3	0	0
3338	Grapefruit, white, California	0.5	each	118	106	44	1	11	1.5	0	0
3060	Grapes, Concord	0.5	cup	46	37	31	0	8	0.5	0	0.1
3206	Grapes, Thompson seedless, canned in heavy syrup	0.5	cup	128	102	93	1	25	0.5	0	0
53034	Gravy, au jus, canned	0.25	cup	60	56	10	1	1	0	0	0.1
53035	Gravy, au jus, dry w/water	0.25	cup	62	59	8	0	1	0	0	0.2
53023	Gravy, beef, canned	0.25	cup	58	51	31	2	3	0.2	1	0.7
53006	Gravy, beef, recipe	0.25	cup	34	29	22	1	2	0.1	1	0.4
53027	Gravy, brown, from dry, w/water	0.25	cup	64	59	19	1	3	0.1	0	0.2
53005	Gravy, chicken giblet, recipe	0.25	cup	32	28	24	2	2	0.1	1	0.3
53022	Gravy, chicken, canned	0.25	cup	60	51	47	1	3	0.2	3	0.8
53028	Gravy, chicken, dry mix w/water	0.25	cup	65	59	21	1	4	0.1	0	0.1
53026	Gravy, mushroom, canned	0.25	cup	60	53	30	1	3	0.2	2	0.2
53039	Gravy, mushroom, dry mix w/water	0.25	cup	64	59	17	1	3	0.3	0	0.1
53024	Gravy, swiss steak	0.25	cup	58	51	31	2	3	0.2	1	0.7
53033	Gravy, turkey, canned	0.25	cup	60	53	30	2	3	0.2	1	0.4
53045	Gravy, turkey, dry, w/water	0.25	cup	65	59	22	1	4	0.3	0	0.1
56074	Green pepper, stuffed	1	each	172	128	229	11	20	1.8	12	5
7579	Grits, Soy HS	0.5	cup	78	7	218	41	23	—	1	—
3305	Guava juice drink, vitamin C added	1	cup	253	218	132	0	34	2	0	0.1
3304	Guava nectar	1	cup	250	211	149	0	38	2	0	0.1
3208	Guava sauce, cooked	0.5	cup	119	107	43	0	11	4.3	0	0
45555	Guava turnover	1	each	78	33	240	3	29	2.6	13	3.2
3207	Guava, raw	1	each	90	78	46	1	11	4.9	1	0.2
3343	Guava, strawberry, raw	1	each	6	5	4	0	1	0.4	0	0
12134	Ham hocks, diced meat, cooked	0.5	cup	70	33	229	20	0	0	16	5.9
13033	Ham patty, cured, grilled	1	each	70	36	238	9	1	0	22	7.7
13034	Ham salad spread	0.5	cup	120	75	259	10	13	0	19	6.1
12225	Ham, canned, unheated, extra lean (7% fat)	0.5	cup	70	50	101	13	0	0	5	1.7
12251	Ham, smoked, sliced, 95% fat free	1	oz.	28	—	31	5	0	—	1	0.3
12006	Ham, whole, roasted, lean	4	oz.	28	19	44	7	0	0	2	0.5
12005	Ham, whole, roasted, lean & fat	4	oz.	113	66	276	24	0	0	19	6.8
56310	Hamburger macaroni & cheese, Hamburger Helper	0.5	cup	122	85	178	17	8	0.7	8	4
56407	Hardee's Big Country Breakfast, bacon	1	each	217	66	740	25	81	—	43	13
56411	Hardee's Biscuit 'n gravy	1	each	221	126	510	10	55	—	28	9
56420	Hardee's ham'n cheese sandwich, hot	1	each	201	101	530	18	49	—	30	9
56417	Hardee's mushroom & swiss hamburger	1	each	203	107	520	30	37	—	27	13
56418	Hardee's roast beef sandwich, regular	1	each	124	68	270	15	28	—	11	5
2158	Hardee's sundae, Cool Twist, hot fudge	1	each	156	91	290	7	51	—	6	3
69061	Hardee's, Frisco hamburger	1	each	242	—	760	36	43	—	50	18
2247	Hardee's, ice cream cone, Cool Twist, vanilla/choc	1	each	118	77	180	4	34	—	2	0.7
2250	Hardee's, shake, peach	1	each	345	—	390	10	77	—	4	3
83019	Healthy Choice Meal, Beef Broccoli Bejing	1	each	340	261	300	21	45	5	4	1.5
82031	Healthy Choice Meal, Beef Burrito Ranchero, mild	1	each	306	240	300	13	45	7	7	2.5
11112	Healthy Choice Meal, Beef Macaroni Casserole	1	each	241	191	210	14	34	5	2	0.5
11113	Healthy Choice Meal, Beef Tips Francais	1	each	262	196	280	20	40	4	5	1.5
11117	Healthy Choice Meal, Beef/Peppers Cantonese	1	each	326	264	270	22	32	5	6	2.5
81084	Healthy Choice Meal, Cacciatore Chicken	1	each	354	292	270	22	36	5	4	1
53230	Healthy Choice Meal, Cheddar Broccoli Potatoes	1	each	298	226	330	13	53	6	7	3
81081	Healthy Choice Meal, Cheese Ravioli Parmigiana	1	each	255	195	260	11	44	6	5	2.5
16250	Healthy Choice Meal, Chicken & Vegetable Marsala	1	each	326	270	240	20	32	3	4	2
16260	Healthy Choice Meal, Chicken Broccoli Alfredo	1	each	326	259	300	25	34	2	7	3
16259	Healthy Choice Meal, Chicken Cantonese	1	each	305	242	280	22	34	2	6	3
16255	Healthy Choice Meal, Chicken Con Queso Burrito	1	each	299	218	350	14	60	6	6	2.5
82034	Healthy Choice Meal, Chicken Enchilada Suprema	1	each	320	253	300	13	46	4	7	3
82030	Healthy Choice Meal, Chicken Enchiladas Suiza	1	tsp	284	217	280	14	43	5	6	3
16252	Healthy Choice Meal, Chicken Fettuccini Alfredo	1	each	241	183	260	22	35	3	4	2
16257	Healthy Choice Meal, Chicken Francesca Classic	1	each	354	270	330	23	46	4	6	2.5
16263	Healthy Choice Meal, Country Herb Chicken	1	each	344	293	310	18	44	3	6	2.5
16933	Healthy Choice Meal, Country Inn Roast Turkey	1	each	284	224	250	20	28	4	6	2
16930	Healthy Choice Meal, Country Roast Turkey with Mush	1	each	241	189	230	19	26	2	5	1.5

A

MonoF (g)	PolyF (g)	Choles (mg)	Calc (mg)	Phos (mg)	Sod (mg)	Pot (mg)	Zn (mg)	Iron (mg)	Magn (mg)	VitA (μg RE)	VitE (mg α-TE)	VitC (mg)	Thia (mg)	Ribo (mg)	Nia (mg)	B6 (mg)	Fola (μg)	B12 (μg)
0	0	0	2	1	0	21	0	0	1	2	0.04	5	0	0	0	0.01	2	0
0	0	0	14	9	0	160	0.1	0.1	9	14	0.29	40	0.04	0.02	0.3	0.05	12	0
0	0	0	14	11	0	159	0.1	0.1	10	32	0.31	47	0.04	0.02	0.2	0.05	15	0
0	0	0	14	15	1	181	0.1	0.1	11	32	0.31	47	0.04	0.02	0.2	0.05	15	0
0	0	0	14	9	0	175	0.1	0.1	11	1	0.3	39	0.04	0.02	0.3	0.05	12	0
0	0	0	14	14	0	169	0.1	0.1	11	1	0.3	39	0.04	0.02	0.3	0.05	14	0
0	0	0	6	5	1	88	0	0.1	2	5	0.16	2	0.04	0.03	0.1	0.05	2	0
0	0	0	13	22	6	132	0.1	1.2	8	8	0.9	1	0.04	0.03	0.2	0.08	3	0
0	0	0	2	18	30	48	0.6	0.4	1	0	0	1	0.01	0.04	0.5	0.01	1	0.06
0.1	0	1	6	0	241	0	0	0	2	0	0	0	0	0	0	0	0	0
0.6	0	2	4	18	326	47	0.6	0.4	1	0	0.04	0	0.02	0.02	0.4	0.01	1	0.06
0.6	0.2	1	4	10	192	32	0.3	0.2	1	19	0.04	0	0.01	0.01	0.2	0	1	0.03
0.2	0	1	17	11	269	14	0.1	0.1	3	0	0.01	0	0.01	0.02	0.2	0	0	0
0.5	0.3	14	4	16	171	38	0.4	0.4	1	82	0.08	0	0.01	0.05	0.4	0.01	12	0.58
1.5	0.9	1	12	17	343	65	0.5	0.3	1	66	0.09	0	0.01	0.03	0.3	0.01	1	0.06
0.2	0.1	1	10	12	283	16	0.1	0.1	3	0	0.01	1	0.01	0.04	0.2	0.01	1	0.04
0.7	0.6	0	4	9	339	63	0.4	0.4	1	0	0.05	0	0.02	0.04	0.4	0.01	7	0
0.1	0	0	12	11	350	14	0.1	0.1	2	0	0.01	0	0.01	0.02	0.2	0.01	1	0.04
0.6	0	2	4	18	326	47	0.6	0.4	1	0	0.04	0	0.02	0.02	0.4	0.01	1	0.06
0.5	0.3	1	2	17	343	65	0.5	0.4	1	0	0.04	0	0.01	0.05	0.8	0.01	1	0.06
0.2	0.1	1	12	12	374	16	0.1	0.1	3	0	0.01	0	0.01	0.03	0.3	0.01	1	0.06
4.9	0.5	34	16	85	201	233	2.3	1.8	20	44	0.75	55	0.15	0.1	2.7	0.3	17	0.67
—	—	0	250	569	8	1926	4.1	7.8	244	0	0	0	0.47	0.24	2	0.39	0	0
0	0.1	0	11	10	7	105	0.1	0.1	6	29	0.41	85	0.02	0.02	0.4	0.05	5	0
0	0.1	0	11	10	7	93	0.1	0.2	5	22	0.4	46	0.02	0.02	0.4	0.05	3	0
0	0.1	0	8	13	5	268	0.2	0.2	8	33	0	174	0.03	0.02	0.5	0.11	6	0
5.6	3.5	0	14	34	105	124	0.2	1.1	9	36	1.59	49	0.15	0.12	1.5	0.06	7	0
0	0.2	0	18	22	3	256	0.2	0.3	9	71	1.01	166	0.04	0.04	1.1	0.13	13	0
0	0	0	1	2	2	18	0	0	1	1	0.03	2	0	0	0	0	0	0
7.2	1.6	76	13	147	223	257	2.9	1.1	13	2	0.18	0	0.38	0.21	3.6	0.24	3	0.45
10.2	2.3	50	6	70	739	170	1.3	1.1	7	0	0.18	0	0.24	0.13	2.3	0.11	2	0.49
8.6	3.2	44	10	144	1094	180	1.3	0.7	12	0	2.09	0	0.52	0.14	2.5	0.18	1	0.91
2.5	0.5	27	4	145	893	234	1.3	0.6	11	0	0.18	0	0.62	0.16	3.2	0.32	4	0.56
0.6	0.3	14	—	—	357	—	—	—	—	—	—	—	—	—	—	—	—	—
0.7	0.2	16	2	64	376	90	0.7	0.3	6	0	0.07	0	0.19	0.07	1.4	0.13	1	0.2
8.9	2	70	8	243	1346	324	2.6	1	22	0	0.3	0	0.68	0.25	5.1	0.43	3	0.73
2.9	0.4	54	86	181	952	223	2.8	1.9	20	34	0.14	0	0.1	0.17	2.4	0.21	8	1.3
22	8	305	166	—	1800	530	—	5	—	—	—	—	—	—	—	—	—	—
14	5	15	150	—	1500	210	—	2	—	—	—	—	—	—	—	—	—	—
—	—	65	288	—	—	300	—	3	—	—	—	—	—	—	—	—	—	—
12	2	45	294	—	890	370	—	5	—	—	—	—	—	—	—	—	—	—
4	2	25	105	—	780	260	—	4	—	—	—	—	—	—	—	—	—	—
1.6	0.2	20	152	—	310	173	—	0.4	—	—	—	—	—	—	—	—	—	—
—	—	70	—	—	1280	—	—	—	—	—	—	—	—	—	—	—	—	—
1.3	0	10	123	—	120	180	—	2	—	—	—	—	—	—	—	—	—	—
—	—	25	—	—	290	—	—	—	—	—	—	—	—	—	—	—	—	—
—	—	25	40	—	420	—	—	2.7	—	200	—	12	—	—	—	—	—	—
—	—	15	20	—	480	—	—	1.1	—	40	—	5	—	—	—	—	—	—
—	—	15	40	—	450	—	—	2.7	—	100	—	54	—	—	—	—	—	—
—	—	30	20	—	520	—	—	1.8	—	0	—	0	—	—	—	—	—	—
—	—	55	40	—	480	—	—	1.8	—	100	—	21	—	—	—	—	—	—
—	—	35	40	—	550	—	—	1.8	—	40	—	6	—	—	—	—	—	—
—	—	25	200	—	550	—	—	1.1	—	60	—	27	—	—	—	—	—	—
—	—	30	150	—	290	—	—	1.8	—	60	—	0	—	—	—	—	—	—
—	—	30	40	—	440	—	—	0.7	—	100	—	4	—	—	—	—	—	—
—	—	50	100	—	530	—	—	1.8	—	20	—	2	—	—	—	—	—	—
—	—	50	40	—	480	—	—	1.8	—	600	—	6	—	—	—	—	—	—
—	—	35	40	—	590	—	—	1.8	—	300	—	15	—	—	—	—	—	—
—	—	40	100	—	560	—	—	0.7	—	150	—	18	—	—	—	—	—	—
—	—	40	150	—	440	—	—	1.1	—	60	—	6	—	—	—	—	—	—
—	—	40	100	—	410	—	—	1.4	—	0	—	0	—	—	—	—	—	—
—	—	30	100	—	600	—	—	1.8	—	20	—	15	—	—	—	—	—	—
—	—	45	40	—	540	—	—	0.7	—	250	—	0	—	—	—	—	—	—
—	—	40	40	—	530	—	—	1.8	—	100	—	0	—	—	—	—	—	—
—	—	45	0	—	440	—	—	0.7	—	150	—	0	—	—	—	—	—	—

Esha Code	Food Item	Qty	Meas	Wgt (g)	Wtr (g)	Cals	Prot (g)	Carb (g)	Fib (g)	Fat (g)	SatF (g)
82029	Healthy Choice Meal, Fiesta Chicken Fajitas	1	each	198	136	260	21	36	5	4	1
53229	Healthy Choice Meal, Garden Potato Casserole	1	each	262	216	210	11	30	6	5	1.5
16256	Healthy Choice Meal, Ginger Chicken Hunan	1	each	357	271	380	24	59	5	5	1
16253	Healthy Choice Meal, Honey Mustard Chicken	1	each	269	205	270	21	38	2	4	1.5
16249	Healthy Choice Meal, Imperial Chicken	1	each	255	201	240	17	31	3	5	1.5
66047	Healthy Choice Meal, Macaroni and Cheese	1	each	255	189	320	15	50	4	7	2.5
16251	Healthy Choice Meal, Mandarin Chicken	1	each	284	216	280	20	44	4	2	0
11114	Healthy Choice Meal, Mesquite Beef Barbeque	1	each	312	239	320	21	38	5	9	3
16262	Healthy Choice Meal, Mesquite Chicken Barbeque	1	each	298	221	310	18	48	6	5	2
81083	Healthy Choice Meal, Pasta Shells Marinara	1	each	340	252	380	25	55	5	6	3.5
11115	Healthy Choice Meal, Salisbury Steak Classics	1	each	312	255	310	16	40	4	9	3
16258	Healthy Choice Meal, Sesame Chicken Shanghai	1	each	340	268	300	24	40	6	5	1
81085	Healthy Choice Meal, Shrimp & Vegetable Maria	1	each	354	290	290	15	46	5	5	2
19426	Healthy Choice Meal, Shrimp Marinara	1	each	298	243	250	10	44	5	4	2
16261	Healthy Choice Meal, Smokey Chicken Barbeque	1	each	361	273	290	25	57	7	5	3
81080	Healthy Choice Meal, Three Cheese Manicotti	1	each	312	245	300	15	40	5	9	3
11116	Healthy Choice Meal, Traditional Beef Tips	1	each	319	261	280	20	32	4	8	3
81082	Healthy Choice Meal, Vegetable Pasta Italiano	1	each	284	230	250	9	48	6	3	1.5
11118	Healthy Choice Meal, Yankee Pot Roast	1	each	312	249	290	19	38	4	7	3
81079	Healthy Choice Meal, Zucchini Lasagna	1	each	383	318	280	13	47	5	4	2.5
20158	Hi-C, punch	1	cup	240	207	125	0	33	0	0	0
4618	Hickory nuts, dried	1	oz.	28	1	186	4	5	1.8	18	2
5640	Hominy, cooked	0.5	cup	82	62	73	2	17	4.7	1	0.1
38077	Hominy, white, canned	0.5	cup	80	66	58	1	11	2	1	0.1
5470	Hominy, yellow, canned	0.5	cup	80	66	58	1	11	2	1	0.1
25001	Honey	1	Tbs	21	4	64	0	18	0	0	0
27004	Horseradish, prepared	1	tsp	5	4	2	0	1	0.2	0	0
21	Hot cocoa, homemade, w/whole milk	1	cup	250	203	193	10	30	2	6	3.6
13250	Hot dog, beef, fat free, Oscar Mayer	1	piece	50	39	39	7	3	0	0	0.1
13012	Hot dog, turkey	1	oz.	28	18	64	4	0	0	5	1.7
56667	Hotdog, w/chili	1	each	114	54	296	14	31	—	14	4.9
13009	Hotdog/frankfurter, beef & pork, 8 per pkg	1	each	57	31	182	6	1	0	17	6.2
13008	Hotdog/frankfurter, beef, 8 per pkg	1	each	57	31	180	7	1	0	16	6.9
13012	Hotdog/frankfurter, turkey	1	each	45	28	102	6	1	0	8	2.6
7081	Hummus/hummous	0.5	cup	123	80	210	6	25	6.3	10	1.6
70767	Hungry Man dinner, Mexican	1	each	567	420	690	26	87	13	27	9
49012	Hush puppies, recipe	1	each	22	6	74	2	10	0.6	3	0.5
2032	Ice Cream sundae, hot fudge	1	each	158	94	284	6	48	0	9	5
2033	Ice Cream sundae, strawberry	1	each	153	93	268	6	45	0	8	3.7
2028	Ice cream bar, Creamsicle	1	each	66	44	92	2	18	0	2	1.2
2029	Ice cream bar, Drumstick	1	each	60	29	157	3	18	0.7	9	4.3
2030	Ice cream bar, Fudgesicle	1	each	73	49	90	4	19	0.1	0	0.1
2084	Ice cream bar, Heath	1	each	68	33	206	2	17	0.2	15	11.6
2091	Ice cream bar, Nutty Buddy	1	each	78	37	215	4	23	1.3	13	5.5
2085	Ice cream bar, chocolate coated w/nuts	1	each	54	23	171	2	17	0.3	11	6.4
49013	Ice cream cone, cake/wafer type	1	each	4	0	17	0	3	0.1	0	0
2113	Ice cream cone, chocolate	1	each	78	42	171	3	25	0.6	7	4.4
49014	Ice cream cone, sugar/rolled type	1	each	10	0	40	1	8	0.2	0	0.1
2093	Ice cream cone, vanilla	1	each	78	44	167	3	22	0.1	8	4.9
2092	Ice cream cone, vanilla, choc dipped	1	each	78	41	185	3	24	0.4	9	5.6
2089	Ice cream cookie sandwich, Chipwich	1	each	59	28	144	3	22	0.6	6	3.2
2056	Ice cream pie, cookie crust, fudge topping	1	each	1836	723	5579	70	723	11	297	141
2087	Ice cream sandwich	1	each	59	28	144	3	22	0.6	6	3.2
2088	Ice cream sandwich, mini Oreo	1	each	29	14	71	1	11	0.3	3	1.6
2216	Ice cream, Choc Chip Cookie Dough, Ben & Jerry's	0.5	cup	106	—	270	4	30	0	17	9
2202	Ice cream, Chunky Monkey, Ben & Jerry's	0.5	cup	106	—	280	4	29	1	19	10
70661	Ice cream, brandied cherry, HaagenDaz	0.5	cup	106	—	250	4	24	—	15	0.5
2055	Ice cream, chocolate Dove bar	1	each	101	38	339	3	36	2.1	23	13.8
2185	Ice cream, chocolate chip, low fat, Healthy Choice	0.5	cup	71	44	120	3	21	0.5	2	1
2017	Ice cream, chocolate, Breyers	0.5	cup	70	38	160	3	20	0.5	8	5
2050	Ice cream, chocolate, regular	0.5	cup	66	37	143	3	19	0.8	7	4.5
2105	Ice cream, cookie & cream, Healthy Choice	0.5	cup	71	44	120	3	21	0.5	2	1.5
70650	Ice cream, deep choc pnut butter, HaagenDaz	0.5	cup	106	—	330	7	25	—	19	—
2054	Ice cream, imitation, chocolate, Mellorine	0.5	cup	66	40	134	3	16	0.5	7	6
2053	Ice cream, imitation, strawberry, Mellorine	0.5	cup	66	41	132	2	16	0	7	5.9

MonoF (g)	PolyF (g)	Choles (mg)	Calc (mg)	Phos (mg)	Sod (mg)	Pot (mg)	Zn (mg)	Iron (mg)	Magn (mg)	VitA (μg RE)	VitE (mg α-TE)	VitC (mg)	Thia (mg)	Ribo (mg)	Nia (mg)	B6 (mg)	Fola (μg)	B12 (μg)
—	—	30	20	—	410	—	—	1.8	—	150	—	36	—	—	—	—	—	—
—	—	10	100	—	520	—	—	0.7	—	250	—	21	—	—	—	—	—	—
—	—	30	60	—	430	—	—	2.7	—	100	—	0	—	—	—	—	—	—
—	—	40	20	—	520	—	—	0.4	—	200	—	0	—	—	—	—	—	—
—	—	50	20	—	470	—	—	1.4	—	150	—	6	—	—	—	—	—	—
—	—	25	250	—	580	—	—	1.4	—	0	—	0	—	—	—	—	—	—
—	—	35	20	—	520	—	—	0.7	—	150	—	15	—	—	—	—	—	—
—	—	55	40	—	490	—	—	1.1	—	250	—	0	—	—	—	—	—	—
—	—	55	40	—	480	—	—	1.4	—	350	—	9	—	—	—	—	—	—
—	—	25	400	—	390	—	—	1.8	—	100	—	0	—	—	—	—	—	—
—	—	45	20	—	550	—	—	1.8	—	200	—	0	—	—	—	—	—	—
—	—	40	40	—	550	—	—	1.8	—	150	—	5	—	—	—	—	—	—
—	—	40	40	—	540	—	—	2.7	—	20	—	12	—	—	—	—	—	—
—	—	55	60	—	260	—	—	1.8	—	60	—	1	—	—	—	—	—	—
—	—	50	40	—	450	—	—	1.8	—	450	—	6	—	—	—	—	—	—
—	—	35	250	—	550	—	—	0.2	—	150	—	0	—	—	—	—	—	—
—	—	50	20	—	480	—	—	1.8	—	600	—	42	—	—	—	—	—	—
—	—	10	60	—	480	—	—	2.7	—	100	—	2	—	—	—	—	—	—
—	—	55	40	—	460	—	—	1.8	—	450	—	6	—	—	—	—	—	—
—	—	10	200	—	310	—	—	1.8	—	250	—	0	—	—	—	—	—	—
0	0	—	—	—	29	—	—	—	—	0	—	96	—	—	—	—	—	0
9.2	6.2	0	17	95	0	124	1.2	0.6	49	4	1.48	1	0.25	0.04	0.3	0.05	11	0
0.2	0.5	0	8	35	146	8	0.9	0.8	14	0	0.04	0	0	0	0	0.01	1	0
0.2	0.3	0	8	28	168	7	0.8	0.5	13	0	0.04	0	0	0	0	0	1	0
0.2	0.3	0	8	28	168	7	0.8	0.5	13	9	0.08	0	0	0	0	0	1	0
0	0	0	1	1	1	11	0	0.1	0	0	0	0	0	0.01	0	0	0	0
0	0	0	3	2	16	12	0	0	1	0	0	1	0	0	0	0	3	0
1.7	0.2	20	315	293	128	500	1.5	1.2	70	138	0.26	2	0.1	0.44	0.4	0.12	15	0.92
0.1	0.1	15	10	64	484	234	1.2	1	10	0	—	0	—	—	—	—	—	—
1.6	1.4	30	30	38	404	51	0.9	0.5	4	0	0.18	0	0.01	0.05	1.2	0.06	2	0.08
6.6	1.2	51	19	192	480	166	0.8	3.3	10	6	—	3	0.22	0.4	3.7	0.05	73	0.3
7.8	1.6	28	6	49	638	95	1	0.7	6	0	0.14	0	0.11	0.07	1.5	0.07	2	0.74
7.8	0.8	35	11	50	585	95	1.2	0.8	2	0	0.11	0	0.03	0.06	1.4	0.07	2	0.88
2.5	2.2	48	48	60	642	81	1.4	0.8	6	0	0.28	0	0.02	0.08	1.9	0.1	4	0.13
4.4	3.9	0	62	138	300	214	1.4	1.9	36	2	1.23	10	0.11	0.06	0.5	0.49	73	0
—	—	35	300	—	2170	—	—	3.6	—	300	—	36	—	—	—	—	—	—
0.7	1.6	10	61	42	147	32	0.1	0.7	5	9	0.52	0	0.08	0.07	0.6	0.02	16	0.04
2.3	0.8	20	207	228	182	395	0.9	0.6	33	57	0.66	2	0.06	0.3	1.1	0.13	9	0.65
2.7	1	21	161	155	92	271	0.7	0.3	24	58	0.78	2	0.06	0.28	0.9	0.08	18	0.64
0.6	0.1	7	62	48	42	102	0.4	0.1	7	22	0	1	0.02	0.1	0.1	0.02	4	0.24
3	1	21	72	86	48	151	0.7	0.4	21	55	0.4	0	0.04	0.14	0.9	0.04	7	0.18
0.1	0	1	129	99	55	173	0.3	0.1	14	2	0.01	0	0.03	0.18	0.1	0.05	1	0.62
2.3	0.4	24	70	62	43	126	0.4	0.2	11	63	0.07	0	0.02	0.13	0.1	0.03	3	0.21
5.4	1.3	26	104	123	60	206	0.9	0.6	40	69	0.53	0	0.05	0.25	0.6	0.04	9	0.23
2.6	0.8	1	136	62	50	129	0.3	0.4	16	25	0.36	0	0.02	0.1	0.5	0.12	6	0.2
0.1	0.1	0	1	4	6	4	0	0.1	1	0	0.07	0	0.01	0.01	0.2	0	4	0
2	0.3	18	96	89	51	176	0.4	0.4	17	62	0.22	0	0.04	0.14	0.3	0.03	4	0.27
0.1	0.1	0	4	10	32	14	0.1	0.4	3	0	0.05	0	0.05	0.04	0.5	0	8	0
2.3	0.4	32	102	88	72	158	0.5	0.2	11	84	0.03	0	0.04	0.2	0.3	0.04	4	0.28
2.8	0.4	29	95	89	66	169	0.6	0.4	18	77	0.1	0	0.04	0.19	0.3	0.04	4	0.26
1.7	0.4	20	60	64	36	122	0.4	0.3	13	53	0.09	0	0.03	0.12	0.2	0.03	5	0.18
94.1	45.4	505	1733	2076	2765	3607	11.6	13.5	441	1377	8.17	7	0.75	4.33	8.9	0.75	94	4.98
1.7	0.4	20	60	64	36	122	0.4	0.3	13	53	0.09	0	0.03	0.12	0.2	0.03	5	0.18
0.8	0.2	10	30	31	18	60	0.2	0.1	6	26	0.05	0	0.02	0.06	0.1	0.01	2	0.09
—	—	80	100	—	95	—	—	1.1	—	150	—	1	—	—	—	—	—	—
—	—	70	100	—	50	—	—	1.1	—	100	—	1	—	—	—	—	—	—
7.5	7	100	107	107	80	170	—	—	—	160	—	—	0.16	0.18	—	—	—	—
7.1	0.7	38	74	139	56	260	1.1	1.1	63	95	0.72	0	0.03	0.21	0.3	0.04	2	0.23
1	0	2	100	141	50	240	—	0	—	40	—	0	—	—	—	—	—	—
2	0	20	48	32	30	150	—	—	—	40	0.21	—	—	0.1	—	—	—	0.04
2.1	0.3	22	72	71	50	164	0.4	0.6	19	78	0.22	0	0.03	0.13	0.1	0.04	11	0.19
0.5	0	2	100	141	90	254	—	—	—	60	—	2	0.03	0.15	—	—	—	—
—	—	—	107	213	90	300	—	1.2	—	21	—	—	0.1	0.14	2.1	—	—	—
0.5	0.1	0	90	81	48	179	0.8	0.3	17	0	0.06	0	0.03	0.15	0.1	0.04	2	0.38
0.4	0.1	0	90	71	48	144	0.7	0.1	10	0	0.05	0	0.03	0.15	0.1	0.04	1	0.39

Esha Code	Food Item	Qty	Meas	Wgt (g)	Wtr (g)	Cals	Prot (g)	Carb (g)	Fib (g)	Fat (g)	SatF (g)
2052	Ice cream, imitation, vanilla, Mellorine	0.5	cup	66	41	132	2	16	0	7	5.9
70308	Ice cream, orange sorbet & vanilla, HaagenDaz	0.5	cup	106	62	199	3	30	—	8	4
2107	Ice cream, praline & cream, Healthy Choice	0.5	cup	71	40	130	3	25	0.5	2	0.5
2123	Ice cream, rocky road, low fat, Healthy Choice	0.5	cup	71	37	140	3	28	2	2	1
2051	Ice cream, soft serve, chocolate	0.5	cup	173	100	355	6	48	1.4	17	10.4
2008	Ice cream, soft serve, french vanilla	0.5	cup	86	51	185	4	19	0	11	6.4
2063	Ice cream, strawberry	0.5	cup	66	40	127	2	18	0.2	6	3.4
2018	Ice cream, strawberry, Breyers	0.5	cup	70	45	130	2	16	0.1	6	4
2330	Ice cream, triple choc chunk, Healthy Choice	0.5	cup	71	44	110	3	21	1	2	1
2004	Ice cream, vanilla	0.5	cup	66	40	133	2	16	0	7	4.5
2019	Ice cream, vanilla, Breyers	0.5	cup	70	43	150	3	15	0.1	8	5
2110	Ice cream, vanilla, Healthy Choice	0.5	cup	71	47	100	3	18	1	2	0.5
2006	Ice cream, vanilla, rich, 16% fat	0.5	cup	74	42	178	3	17	0	12	7.4
2057	Ice milk, chocolate	0.5	cup	66	43	94	3	17	0.3	2	1.3
2060	Ice milk, chocolate, Breyer's Light	0.5	cup	68	41	122	3	19	0.3	4	2.6
2059	Ice milk, premium, strawberry, Breyer's Light	0.5	cup	68	41	122	3	19	0	4	2.5
2058	Ice milk, vanilla, Breyer's Light	0.5	cup	68	41	122	3	19	0	4	2.5
2009	Ice milk, vanilla, hard	0.5	cup	66	45	92	3	15	0	3	1.7
2010	Ice milk, vanilla, soft, 3% fat	0.5	cup	88	61	111	4	19	0	2	1.4
23051	Ice slushy	1	cup	193	129	151	1	63	0	0	0
23160	Ices, fruit flavor, sugar-free	1	each	51	48	12	0	3	0	0	0
23159	Ices, lime	1	cup	192	128	246	1	63	0	0	0
42202	Injera (Ethiopian bread), 12 inch loaf	1	piece	21	13	29	1	6	0.2	0	0.1
62177	Instant breakfast, vanilla, Carnation	1	cup	281	—	975	56	167	0	0	0
101	Instant breakfast, w/1% milk	1	cup	281	222	233	15	36	0.2	3	2
26	Instant breakfast, w/2% milk	1	cup	281	220	252	16	36	0.2	5	3.3
27	Instant breakfast, w/nonfat milk	1	cup	282	225	216	16	36	0.2	1	0.7
25	Instant breakfast, w/whole milk	1	cup	281	217	280	15	36	0.2	9	5.4
56430	Jack in the Box, BreakfastJack sandwich	1	each	121	59	300	18	30	0	12	4.8
56436	Jack in the Box, Jumbo Jack	1	each	229	126	560	26	41	0	32	10
56437	Jack in the Box, Jumbo Jack w/cheese	1	each	242	133	610	29	41	0	36	12
69032	Jack in the Box, bacon cheeseburger	1	each	242	119	710	35	41	0	45	15
69063	Jack in the Box, chicken caesar pita sandwich	1	each	237	139	520	27	44	4	26	6
69035	Jack in the Box, chicken sandwich	1	each	160	83	400	20	38	0	18	4
90094	Jack in the Box, cinnamon churritos, serving	1	each	75	16	330	3	34	3	21	5
56441	Jack in the Box, fajita, chicken pita	1	each	189	127	290	24	29	3	8	3
69036	Jack in the Box, fried steak sandwich	1	each	153	70	450	14	42	0	25	7
69033	Jack in the Box, hamburger, sourdough, grilled	1	each	223	107	670	32	39	0	43	16
69064	Jack in the Box, monterey roast beef sandwich	1	each	238	135	540	30	40	3	30	9
69040	Jack in the Box, sourdough breakfast sandwich	1	each	147	73	380	21	31	0	20	7
69065	Jack in the Box, ultimate breakfast sandwich	1	each	242	128	620	36	39	—	35	11
3248	Jackfruit, raw	4	oz.	113	83	107	2	27	1.8	0	0.1
23175	Jam, cherry/strawberry	1	Tbs	20	6	54	0	14	—	0	0
23002	Jam, not cherry/strawberry	1	Tbs	20	6	54	0	14	0.2	0	0
23166	Jam/marmalade, artificially sweetened	1	Tbs	20	9	2	0	11	0.5	0	0
23054	Jam/preserves, 1 pkt	1	Tbs	20	7	48	0	13	0.2	0	0
23167	Jam/preserves/marmalade, reduced sugar	1	Tbs	20	10	36	0	9	0.6	0	0
3249	Java plum/jambolan, fresh	3	each	9	7	5	0	1	0.1	0	—
23003	Jelly	1	Tbs	18	5	49	0	13	0.2	0	0
23092	Jelly, dietetic	1	Tbs	19	8	6	0	11	0.2	0	0
23004	Jelly, packet	1	each	14	4	38	0	10	0.1	0	0
23165	Jelly, reduced sugar, all flavors	1	Tbs	19	10	34	0	9	0.2	0	0
5224	Jicama, raw	0.5	cup	60	54	23	1	5	2.9	0	0
5436	Jicama/Yambean tuber, sliced, cooked	0.5	cup	50	45	19	0	4	2.4	0	0
5435	Jicama/Yambean tuber, sliced, raw	0.5	cup	60	54	23	0	5	2.9	0	0
3226	Juice drink, cranberry apricot, w/vitamin C	1	cup	253	209	170	0	43	0.3	0	0
3225	Juice drink, cranberry blueberry, w/vitamin C	1	cup	253	209	170	0	43	0.3	0	0
3227	Juice drink, cranberry grape, w/vitamin C	1	cup	253	209	170	0	43	0.3	0	0
3224	Juice drink, cranberry raspberry, w/vitamin C	1	cup	253	209	170	0	43	0.3	0	0
20280	Juice drink, orange, CapriSun Natural	1	cup	176	—	83	0	22	0	0	0
3238	Juice, acerola, fresh	1	cup	242	228	56	1	12	0.7	1	0.2
3327	Juice, apple, frozen w/vit C, prepared	1	cup	239	210	112	0	28	0.2	0	0
3328	Juice, apple, w/vit C, canned/bottled	1	cup	248	218	117	0	29	0.2	0	0
3319	Juice, apple-cherry	1	cup	250	219	117	1	29	0.8	0	0.1
3321	Juice, apple-grape	1	cup	244	211	128	1	32	0.2	0	0.1

MonoF	PolyF	Choles	Calc	Phos	Sod	Pot	Zn	Iron	Magn	VitA	VitE	VitC	Thia	Ribo	Nia	B6	Fola	B12
(g)	(g)	(mg)	(mg)	(mg)	(mg)	(mg)	(mg)	(mg)	(mg)	(μg RE)	(mg α-TE)	(mg)	(mg)	(mg)	(mg)	(mg)	(μg)	(μg)
0.4	0.1	0	90	71	48	144	0.7	0.1	10	0	0.05	0	0.03	0.15	0.1	0.04	1	0.39
—	—	60	64	64	30	114	—	0	—	85	—	6	0.03	0.11	0.8	—	—	—
0.1	1.4	2	100	141	70	226	—	0	—	40	—	0	0.03	0.15	—	—	—	—
0.5	0	2	100	9	60	168	—	0	—	40	—	0	0.03	0.15	—	—	—	—
4.9	0.6	43	206	184	89	384	1	0.7	37	147	0.46	1	0.07	0.27	0.2	0.06	9	0.64
3	0.4	78	113	100	52	152	0.4	0.2	10	132	0.32	1	0.04	0.16	0.1	0.04	8	0.43
1.6	0.2	19	79	66	40	124	0.2	0.1	9	52	0.13	5	0.03	0.17	0.1	0.03	8	0.2
2	0	20	64	48	40	125	—	—	—	40	0.14	—	0.03	0.14	—	—	—	0.08
—	—	2	100	—	60	—	—	0.4	—	8	—	0	—	—	—	—	—	—
2.1	0.3	29	84	69	53	131	0.5	0.1	9	77	0	0	0.03	0.16	0.1	0.03	3	0.26
2	0.3	25	80	80	50	140	—	0.1	—	60	0.21	—	0.03	0.15	—	—	—	0.12
1.5	0	5	100	141	50	254	—	—	—	60	—	2	0.05	0.22	—	—	—	—
3.4	0.4	45	87	70	41	118	0.3	0	8	136	0	1	0.03	0.12	0.1	0.03	4	0.27
0.6	0.1	6	94	78	41	155	0.4	0.2	13	18	0.06	0	0.03	0.12	0.1	0.03	4	0.3
1.2	0.2	12	105	87	46	172	0.4	0.2	14	37	0.12	1	0.04	0.13	0.1	0.03	4	0.33
0.8	0.2	16	109	80	63	162	0.3	0.1	11	27	0.08	0	0.05	0.2	0.1	0.05	2	0.51
0.8	0.2	16	109	80	63	162	0.3	0.1	11	27	0.08	0	0.05	0.2	0.1	0.05	2	0.51
0.8	0.1	9	92	72	56	139	0.3	0.1	10	31	0	1	0.04	0.18	0.1	0.04	4	0.44
0.7	0.1	11	138	106	62	194	0.5	0.1	12	26	0	1	0.05	0.17	0.1	0.04	5	0.44
0	0	0	4	2	42	6	0	0.3	2	0	0	2	0	0	0	0	0	0
—	—	0	1	0	3	13	0	0.1	1	0	0	0	0	0	0.1	0	0	0
0	0	0	4	2	42	6	0	0.3	2	0	0	2	0	0	0	0	0	0
0	0.1	0	12	24	42	12	0.1	6.2	2	0	0	0	0.02	0.02	0.3	0.01	6	0
0	0	36	4869	1390	1253	3478	41.9	62.7	1112	7311	70	376	4.19	1.88	69.7	5.56	1390	8.35
0.9	0.1	14	406	393	266	731	4.1	4.9	118	698	5.36	31	0.41	0.48	5.5	0.53	118	1.53
1.5	0.2	23	401	390	264	726	4.1	4.9	118	693	5.41	31	0.41	0.48	5.5	0.53	118	1.52
0.3	0	9	407	406	268	755	4.1	4.8	112	703	5.3	31	0.4	0.42	5.5	0.52	118	1.56
2.5	0.3	38	396	385	262	719	4.1	4.9	117	630	5.51	31	0.41	0.47	5.5	0.52	118	1.5
4.8	2.4	185	200	—	890	220	—	2.7	—	80	—	9	0.47	0.41	3	—	—	—
13	8	65	100	—	700	450	—	4.5	—	40	—	6	0.36	0.29	1.8	—	—	—
15	9	80	200	—	780	460	—	5.4	—	60	—	6	0.36	0.44	1.6	—	—	—
15.7	8.7	110	250	—	1240	540	—	5.4	—	80	—	9	0.24	0.48	8.8	0.39	—	—
—	—	55	250	—	1050	490	—	2.7	—	80	—	2	—	—	—	—	—	—
—	—	45	150	—	1290	180	—	1.8	—	40	—	0	—	—	—	—	—	—
—	—	20	20	—	200	170	—	5.4	—	0	—	0	—	—	—	—	—	—
3.6	1.4	35	250	—	700	430	—	2.7	—	100	—	6	0.75	0.17	6	—	—	—
—	—	35	60	—	890	270	—	2.7	—	20	—	5	—	—	—	—	—	—
17.8	7.9	110	200	—	1140	510	—	4.5	—	150	—	6	0.65	0.48	8	0.33	—	—
—	—	75	300	—	1270	500	—	3.6	—	80	—	5	—	—	—	—	—	—
—	—	235	250	—	1120	260	—	3.6	—	150	—	9	—	—	—	—	—	—
—	—	455	250	—	1800	450	—	4.5	—	150	—	9	—	—	—	—	—	—
0	0.1	0	39	41	3	344	0.5	0.7	42	34	0.17	8	0.03	0.12	0.5	0.12	16	0
—	—	0	4	2	2	18	—	0.2	—	0	—	3	0	0.01	0	—	—	—
0	0	0	4	2	2	18	0	0.2	1	0	0.02	0	0	0.01	0	0	2	0
0	0	0	2	2	0	14	0	0.1	1	0	0.01	0	0	0	0	0	2	0
0	0	0	4	2	8	15	0	0.1	1	0	0	2	0	0	0	0	7	0
0	0.1	0	1	1	5	12	0	0.2	1	0	0.03	8	0	0.02	0.1	0.03	2	0
—	—	0	2	2	1	7	0	0	1	0	—	1	0	0	0	0	—	0
0	0	0	1	1	6	12	0	0	1	0	0	0	0	0	0	0	0	0
0	0	0	1	1	0	12	0	0	1	0	0.02	0	0	0	0	0.01	0	0
0	0	0	1	1	5	9	0	0	1	0	0	0	0	0	0	0	0	0
0	0	0	1	1	0	13	0	0	1	0	0	0	0	0	0	0.01	0	0
0	0	0	7	11	2	90	0.1	0.4	7	1	2.74	12	0.01	0.02	0.1	0.02	7	0
0	0	0	6	8	2	68	0.1	0.3	6	1	0.23	7	0.01	0.01	0.1	0.02	4	0
0	0	0	7	11	2	90	0.1	0.4	7	1	0.27	12	0.01	0.02	0.1	0.02	7	0
0	0	0	18	8	5	68	0.1	0.2	5	1	0	81	0.01	0.05	0.2	0.05	1	0
0	0	0	18	8	5	68	0.1	0.2	5	1	0	81	0.01	0.05	0.2	0.05	1	0
0	0	0	18	8	5	68	0.1	0.2	5	1	0	81	0.01	0.05	0.2	0.05	1	0
0	0	0	18	8	5	68	0.1	0.2	5	1	0	81	0.01	0.05	0.2	0.05	1	0
0	0	0	0	—	21	92	—	0	—	0	—	0	—	—	—	—	—	0
0.2	0.2	0	24	22	7	235	0.2	1.2	29	123	0.1	3872	0.05	0.14	1	0.01	34	0
0	0.1	0	14	17	17	301	0.1	0.6	12	0	0.02	60	0.01	0.04	0.1	0.08	1	0
0	0.1	0	17	17	7	295	0.1	0.9	7	0	0.02	103	0.05	0.04	0.2	0.07	0	0
0.1	0.2	0	21	24	6	308	0.1	0.9	12	13	0.12	3	0.05	0.06	0.5	0.08	4	0
0	0.1	0	19	21	7	303	0.1	0.8	14	1	0.02	1	0.06	0.06	0.4	0.11	3	0

Esha Code	Food Item	Qty	Meas	Wgt (g)	Wtr (g)	Cals	Prot (g)	Carb (g)	Fib (g)	Fat (g)	SatF (g)
3320	Juice, apple-raspberry	1	cup	239	212	108	0	26	0.2	0	0
20057	Juice, beef broth & tomato, canned	0.5	cup	122	110	45	1	10	0.1	0	0
20042	Juice, clam and tomato	1	cup	241	210	115	1	26	0.5	0	0.1
3165	Juice, grapefruit, canned, sweetened	0.5	cup	125	109	58	1	14	0.1	0	0
3092	Juice, orange, chilled	1	cup	249	220	110	2	25	0.5	1	0.1
3090	Juice, orange, fresh	1	cup	248	219	112	2	26	0.5	0	0.1
3091	Juice, orange, frozen concentrate, prepared	1	cup	249	219	112	2	27	0.5	0	0
3093	Juice, orange, unsweetened, canned	1	cup	249	222	105	1	24	0.5	0	0
3094	Juice, orange, unsweetened, frozen concentrate	0.5	cup	106	62	169	3	41	0.9	0	0
3200	Juice, passion fruit, purple, fresh	0.5	cup	124	106	63	0	17	0.2	0	0
3201	Juice, passion fruit, yellow	0.5	cup	124	104	74	1	18	0.2	0	0
3120	Juice, pineapple, canned, unsweetened	1	cup	250	214	140	1	34	0.5	0	0
3119	Juice, pineapple, frozen concentrate, prepared	1	cup	250	216	130	1	32	0.5	0	0
3323	Juice, pineapple, sweetened	1	cup	252	211	158	1	39	0.2	0	0
3128	Juice, prune, bottled	1	cup	256	208	182	2	45	2.6	0	0
3324	Juice, strawberry	1	cup	237	217	71	1	17	0.2	1	0
3140	Juice, tangerine, canned, sweetened	0.5	cup	124	108	62	1	15	0.2	0	0
3347	Juice, tangerine, fresh, unsweetened	1	cup	247	220	106	1	25	0.5	0	0.1
3141	Juice, tangerine, frozen, sweetened, prepared	1	cup	241	212	111	1	27	0.5	0	0
3345	Juice, tangerine, frozen, unswt, prepared	1	cup	247	220	106	1	25	0.5	0	0.1
3144	Juice, watermelon, fresh	1	cup	238	218	76	1	17	1.2	1	0.1
3250	Jujube fruit, raw	4	oz.	113	88	90	1	23	1.4	0	—
5420	Jute/potherb, cooked	0.5	cup	43	38	16	2	3	0.9	0	0
15165	KFC chicken leg, original	1	each	57	30	152	14	3	0.2	8	2.2
56450	KFC, Chicken Little sandwich	1	each	47	16	169	6	14	0.4	10	2
15163	KFC, Chicken breast, side, original	1	each	90	42	266	20	10	0.2	16	4.5
56599	KFC, Chicken sandwich, Colonel's	1	each	166	76	482	21	39	—	27	6
56683	KFC, Red beans & rice	1	each	111	84	113	4	18	3	3	1
15164	KFC, chicken breast, center, original	1	each	115	60	290	28	10	0.1	16	4.2
15169	KFC, chicken breast, crispy	1	each	135	65	378	30	16	0.1	22	5.5
15170	KFC, chicken leg, crispy	1	each	69	34	202	14	6	0.1	13	3.4
15188	KFC, chicken, dark quarter, no skin, Rotisserie Gol	1	each	117	77	217	27	0	0	12	3.5
15177	KFC, chicken, hot wings pieces (6)	1	each	119	45	415	24	16	—	29	—
15191	KFC, chicken, white quarter, no skin, rotisserie go	1	each	117	73	199	37	0	0	6	1.7
15187	KFC, chicken, wing, whole, Hot and Spicy	1	each	61	23	220	14	5	—	16	4
5208	Kale, fresh, chopped	0.5	cup	34	28	17	1	3	0.7	0	0
5075	Kale, fresh, cooked, drained, no added salt	0.5	cup	65	59	18	1	4	1.3	0	0
5076	Kale, frozen, cooked, drained, no added salt	0.5	cup	65	59	20	2	3	1.3	0	0
3065	Kiwi fruit, freshly harvested	1	each	76	63	46	1	11	2.6	0	0
3357	Kiwi fruit, raw slices	10	piece	70	58	43	1	10	2.4	0	0
3356	Kiwi fruit, raw, stored	1	each	76	63	46	1	11	2.6	0	0
5078	Kohlrabi slices, raw	0.5	cup	70	64	19	1	4	2.5	0	0
5079	Kohlrabi, cooked, drained, no added salt	0.5	cup	82	74	24	1	6	0.9	0	0
20298	Kool-aid, mix, unsweetened, grape, prepared	1	cup	246	221	100	0	25	0	0	0
23065	Kudos nutty fudge snack bar	1	each	37	1	200	3	20	—	12	—
3252	Kumquat, raw	1	each	19	16	12	0	3	1.2	0	0
15199	LJS, chicken plank, 2 piece	1	each	112	62	240	16	22	—	12	3.2
56459	LJS, clam dinner	1	each	361	168	990	24	114	—	52	10.9
56467	LJS, fish & fryes, batter fried, 2 piece	1	each	261	142	610	27	52	—	37	7.9
56462	LJS, fish & more, 2 piece w/fries & slaw	1	each	407	233	890	31	92	—	48	10.1
69030	LJS, fish sandwich, batter dipped	1	each	159	86	340	18	40	—	13	3.1
57009	LJS, fish shrimp chicken dinner	1	each	513	—	1160	45	113	—	65	14.2
57003	LJS, fish w/lemon dinner, 3 piece	1	each	493	352	610	39	86	—	13	2.2
56461	LJS, fish, batter fried, svg	1	each	88	52	180	12	12	—	11	2.7
57004	LJS, fish, light portion dinner	1	each	334	257	330	24	46	—	5	0.9
57010	LJS, fish-shrimp-clams dinner	1	each	512	—	1240	44	123	—	70	15.2
15198	LJS, herb chicken a la carte	1	each	100	74	120	22	—	—	4	1.2
27110	LJS, malt vinegar, serving	1	each	8	—	1	0	0	0	—	—
19118	LJS, seafood gumbo w/cod	1	each	198	175	120	9	4	—	8	2.1
13900	Lamb curry	0.5	cup	118	93	141	14	1	0.3	9	2.2
13522	Lamb kabob meat, broiled, lean	4	oz.	113	72	211	32	0	0	8	3
13523	Lamb stew meat, braised, lean	4	oz.	113	64	253	38	0	0	10	3.6
13519	Lamb, arm chop, broiled, lean	1	each	74	46	148	20	0	0	7	2.5
13519	Lamb, arm chop, broiled, lean	3	oz.	85	53	170	24	0	0	8	2.9
13513	Lamb, chop, loin, broiled, lean	1	each	46	28	99	14	0	0	4	1.6

MonoF	PolyF	Choles	Calc	Phos	Sod	Pot	Zn	Iron	Magn	VitA	VitE	VitC	Thia	Ribo	Nia	B6	Fola	B12
(g)	(g)	(mg)	(mg)	(mg)	(mg)	(mg)	(mg)	(mg)	(mg)	(µg RE)	(mg α-TE)	(mg)	(mg)	(mg)	(mg)	(mg)	(µg)	(µg)
0	0.2	0	19	19	6	309	0.1	1.1	16	7	0.09	6	0.05	0.05	0.3	0.08	5	0
0	0	0	13	16	160	117	0	0.7	4	16	0.49	1	0	0.04	0.2	0.03	5	0.06
0	0	0	29	188	871	217	2.6	1.4	53	53	1.2	10	0.1	0.07	0.5	0.2	38	73.6
0	0	0	10	14	2	203	0.1	0.4	12	0	0.06	34	0.05	0.03	0.4	0.02	13	0
0.1	0.2	0	25	27	2	473	0.1	0.4	27	20	0.47	82	0.28	0.05	0.7	0.13	45	0
0.1	0.1	0	27	42	2	496	0.1	0.5	27	50	0.22	124	0.22	0.07	1	0.1	75	0
0	0	0	22	40	2	473	0.1	0.2	25	20	0.47	97	0.2	0.04	0.5	0.11	109	0
0.1	0.1	0	20	35	5	436	0.2	1.1	27	45	0.22	86	0.15	0.07	0.8	0.22	45	0
0	0	0	34	61	3	718	0.2	0.4	36	30	0.34	147	0.3	0.07	0.8	0.17	165	0
0	0	0	5	16	7	343	0.1	0.3	21	89	0.06	37	0	0.16	1.8	0.06	9	0
0	0.1	0	5	31	7	343	0.1	0.4	21	298	0.06	22	0	0.12	2.8	0.07	10	0
0	0.1	0	42	20	2	335	0.3	0.6	32	1	0.05	27	0.14	0.06	0.6	0.24	58	0
0	0	0	28	20	2	340	0.3	0.8	22	2	0.02	30	0.18	0.05	0.5	0.18	26	0
0	0.1	0	42	20	3	331	0.3	0.6	32	1	0.05	26	0.14	0.06	0.6	0.24	57	0
0.1	0	0	31	64	10	707	0.5	3	36	1	0.03	10	0.04	0.18	2	0.56	1	0
0.1	0.4	0	33	45	2	393	0.3	0.9	24	5	0.33	67	0.05	0.14	0.5	0.12	21	0
0	0	0	22	17	1	222	0	0.2	10	52	0.11	27	0.08	0.02	0.1	0.04	6	0
0.1	0.1	0	44	35	2	440	0.1	0.5	20	104	0.22	77	0.15	0.05	0.2	0.1	11	0
0	0	0	19	19	2	272	0.1	0.2	19	137	0.1	58	0.12	0.05	0.2	0.1	11	0
0.1	0.1	0	44	35	2	440	0.1	0.5	20	104	0.22	77	0.15	0.05	0.2	0.1	11	0
0.3	0.3	0	19	21	5	276	0.2	0.4	26	88	0.36	23	0.19	0.05	0.5	0.34	5	0
—	—	0	24	26	3	284	0.1	0.5	11	5	—	78	0.02	0.04	1	0.09	—	0
0	0	0	91	31	5	237	0.3	1.4	27	223	0.3	14	0.04	0.08	0.4	0.24	45	0
4.1	1.3	75	21	—	269	—	—	1.1	—	15	—	—	0.05	0.12	3.2	—	—	—
4.7	3.4	18	23	—	331	—	—	1.7	—	5	—	—	0.16	0.12	2.2	—	—	—
9.4	2.4	85	74	—	655	—	—	1.3	—	16	—	—	0.06	0.14	7.5	—	—	—
—	—	47	50	—	1060	—	—	1.3	—	15	—	6	—	—	—	—	—	—
—	—	4	10	—	312	—	—	0.7	—	—	—	—	—	—	—	—	—	—
8.7	2.2	103	34	—	680	—	—	0.8	—	17	—	—	0.1	0.19	12.8	—	—	—
12.4	2.4	86	38	—	847	—	—	0.9	—	17	—	—	0.13	0.15	15	—	—	—
7.7	1.7	69	21	—	329	—	—	0.4	—	32	—	—	0.06	0.13	3.9	—	—	—
—	—	128	10	—	772	—	—	0.2	—	15	—	1	—	—	—	—	—	—
—	—	132	35	—	1084	—	—	2.9	—	13	—	5	—	—	—	—	—	—
—	—	97	10	—	667	—	—	0.2	—	15	—	1	—	—	—	—	—	—
—	—	65	20	—	440	—	—	0.7	—	30	—	—	—	—	—	—	—	—
0	0.1	0	45	19	14	150	0.1	0.6	11	298	0.27	40	0.04	0.04	0.3	0.09	10	0
0	0.1	0	47	18	15	148	0.2	0.6	12	481	0.55	27	0.03	0.05	0.3	0.09	9	0
0	0.2	0	90	18	10	209	0.1	0.6	12	413	0.12	16	0.03	0.07	0.4	0.06	9	0
0	0.2	0	20	30	4	252	0.1	0.3	23	14	0.85	74	0.02	0.04	0.4	0.07	29	0
0	0.2	0	18	28	4	232	0.1	0.3	21	13	0.78	52	0.01	0.04	0.4	0.04	7	0
0	0.2	0	20	30	4	252	0.1	0.3	23	14	0.85	57	0.02	0.04	0.4	0.04	8	0
0	0	0	17	32	14	245	0	0.3	13	3	0.34	43	0.04	0.01	0.3	0.1	11	0
0	0	0	21	37	17	281	0.3	0.3	16	3	1.38	45	0.03	0.02	0.3	0.13	10	0
0	0	0	0	—	15	0	—	0	—	0	—	6	—	—	—	—	—	0
—	—	—	40	—	55	—	—	0.4	—	—	—	—	—	0.1	—	—	—	—
0	0	0	8	4	1	37	0	0.1	2	6	0.05	7	0.02	0.02	0.1	0.01	3	0
8.4	0.2	30	—	—	790	320	0.6	1.1	—	—	—	—	0.15	0.26	7	—	—	—
31.3	9.9	75	200	—	1830	910	3	4.5	—	40	—	12	0.75	0.42	12	—	—	—
23.5	5.3	60	40	—	1480	900	1.2	1.8	—	—	—	9	0.38	0.34	8	—	—	—
28.5	9.5	75	200	—	1790	1230	2.2	3.6	—	40	—	9	0.52	0.51	12	—	—	—
8.9	1	30	80	—	890	370	1.5	3.6	—	—	—	1	0.38	0.34	6	—	—	—
40.3	9.6	135	200	—	2590	1450	3.8	4.5	—	40	—	9	0.75	0.68	16	—	—	—
3.9	5.3	125	200	—	1420	990	2.2	5.4	—	700	—	6	0.75	0.6	24	—	—	—
8.1	0.2	30	—	—	490	260	0.3	0.4	—	—	—	—	0.15	0.17	3	—	—	—
1.6	1.2	75	80	—	640	440	0.9	1.8	—	1000	—	18	0.3	0.26	14	—	—	—
44.2	9.9	140	200	—	2630	1390	3.8	5.4	—	40	—	9	0.9	0.68	16	—	—	—
1.7	1.1	60	—	—	570	270	0.6	0.7	—	—	—	—	0.09	0.26	—	—	—	—
—	—	—	—	—	15	10	—	—	—	—	—	—	—	—	—	—	—	—
3.2	2.6	25	100	—	740	310	1.5	1.8	—	200	—	—	0.15	0.17	3	—	—	—
2.9	2.8	44	15	137	237	235	3.2	1.3	18	0	1	1	0.04	0.14	3.9	0.09	13	1.41
3.4	0.8	102	15	254	86	380	6.5	2.6	35	0	0.23	0	0.12	0.34	7.5	0.16	26	3.44
4	0.9	122	17	232	79	295	7.5	3.2	32	0	0.23	0	0.08	0.27	6.8	0.14	24	3.1
2.7	0.6	68	13	162	61	252	4.2	1.7	22	0	0.15	0	0.07	0.22	5	0.1	17	2.22
3.1	0.7	78	14	186	70	289	4.9	2	26	0	0.17	0	0.08	0.25	5.8	0.12	20	2.55
2	0.3	44	9	104	39	173	1.9	0.9	13	0	0.07	0	0.05	0.13	3.2	0.07	11	1.16

A

Esha Code	Food Item	Qty	Meas	Wgt (g)	Wtr (g)	Cals	Prot (g)	Carb (g)	Fib (g)	Fat (g)	SatF (g)
13513	Lamb, chop, loin, broiled, lean	3	oz.	85	52	184	26	0	0	8	3
13512	Lamb, chop, loin, broiled, lean & fat	1	each	64	33	202	16	0	0	15	6.3
13512	Lamb, chop, loin, broiled, lean & fat	3	oz.	85	44	269	21	0	0	20	8.4
13524	Lamb, ground, broiled	4	oz.	113	62	321	28	0	0	22	9.2
13501	Lamb, leg, roasted, lean	3	oz.	85	54	162	24	0	0	7	2.4
13518	Lamb, leg, sirloin, roasted, lean	4	oz.	113	71	231	32	0	0	10	3.7
13517	Lamb, leg, sirloin, roasted, lean & fat	4	oz.	113	61	331	28	0	0	24	9.9
13511	Lamb, rib, roast, cooked, lean	4	oz.	113	68	263	30	0	0	15	5.4
13510	Lamb, rib, roast, cooked, lean & fat	4	oz.	113	54	407	24	0	0	34	14.5
13503	Lamb, shoulder, roasted, lean	4	oz.	113	72	231	28	0	0	12	4.6
13502	Lamb, shoulder, roasted, lean & fat	4	oz.	113	64	313	26	0	0	23	9.6
5353	Lambsquarter, raw, chopped	0.5	cup	28	24	12	1	2	1.1	0	0
5354	Lambsquarters, cooked, drained	0.5	cup	90	80	29	3	4	1.9	1	0
8006	Lard, pork fat	1	Tbs	13	0	116	0	0	0	13	5.1
56108	Lasagna, w/meat, recipe	1	piece	245	165	382	22	39	3.3	15	7.8
81079	Lasagna, zucchini, Healthy Choice	1	each	397	330	290	14	49	5.2	4	2.6
5204	Leek, whole, drained	1	each	124	113	38	1	9	1.2	0	0
5206	Leek, whole, raw	1	each	124	103	76	2	18	2.2	0	0
5203	Leeks, chopped, cooked, drained	0.5	cup	52	47	16	0	4	0.5	0	0
5205	Leeks, chopped, raw	0.5	cup	52	43	32	1	7	0.9	0	0
6130	Lemon grass, leaves	1	oz.	28	20	19	0	4	—	0	—
3069	Lemon juice, bottled	1	cup	244	226	51	1	16	1	1	0.1
3068	Lemon juice, fresh	1	cup	244	221	61	1	21	1	0	0
3070	Lemon juice, frozen, unsweetened	1	cup	244	225	54	1	16	1	1	0.1
3463	Lemon peel, candied	1.5	oz.	43	7	134	0	34	—	0	0
3067	Lemon peel, fresh	1	Tbs	6	5	3	0	1	0.6	0	0
26099	Lemon pepper	0.25	tsp	1	0	2	0	0	0	0	—
45553	Lemon turnover	1	each	78	33	238	3	29	0.6	12	3.1
3066	Lemon, fresh, peeled	1	each	58	52	17	1	5	1.6	0	0
20104	Lemonade drink, powder	1	Tbs	15	0	56	0	14	0	0	0
20045	Lemonade flavor drink, dry, prepared	1	cup	266	237	112	0	29	0	0	0
20083	Lemonade, low calorie	1	cup	240	228	43	0	11	0.2	0	0
20083	Lemonade, low calorie	1	cup	240	228	43	0	11	0.2	0	0
20047	Lemonade, low calorie, dry, prepared (Country Time)	1	cup	238	236	5	0	1	0	0	0
20117	Lemonade, pink, frozen, prepared	1	cup	248	221	99	0	26	0	0	0
20102	Lemonade, powder	1	Tbs	14	0	51	0	14	0	0	0
20046	Lemonade, powder, prepared, Country Time	1	cup	264	237	103	0	27	0	0	0
20000	Lemonade, white, frozen, prepared	1	cup	248	221	99	0	26	0.2	0	0
7086	Lentil loaf	1	piece	47	30	82	4	9	3.1	3	0.4
5389	Lentil sprouts, raw	0.5	cup	38	26	41	3	9	1.6	0	0
1956	Lentil, sprouted, stir fried	4	oz.	113	78	115	10	24	4.4	1	0.1
7005	Lentils, dry	0.25	cup	48	5	162	14	27	14.6	0	0.1
7006	Lentils, dry, cooked	0.5	cup	99	69	115	9	20	7.8	0	0.1
5080	Lettuce, butterhead, chopped	0.5	cup	28	27	4	0	1	0.3	0	0
5081	Lettuce, butterhead, leaves	2	piece	15	14	2	0	0	0.2	0	0
5082	Lettuce, butterhead, whole head	1	each	163	156	21	2	4	1.6	0	0
5084	Lettuce, iceberg/crisphead leaves	1	piece	20	19	2	0	0	0.3	0	0
5083	Lettuce, iceberg/crisphead, chopped	0.5	cup	28	27	3	0	1	0.4	0	0
5085	Lettuce, iceberg/crisphead, whole head	1	each	539	517	65	5	11	7.6	1	0.1
5086	Lettuce, looseleaf, chopped	0.5	cup	28	26	5	0	1	0.5	0	0
5087	Lettuce, looseleaf, leaves	1	piece	10	9	2	0	0	0.2	0	0
5088	Lettuce, romaine, chopped	0.5	cup	28	27	4	0	1	0.5	0	0
5089	Lettuce, romaine, inner leaf	1	piece	10	9	1	0	0	0.2	0	0
3073	Lime juice, bottled	1	cup	246	228	52	1	16	1	1	0.1
3072	Lime juice, fresh	1	cup	246	222	66	1	22	1	0	0
3071	Lime, fresh, peeled	0.5	each	67	59	20	0	7	1.9	0	0
20003	Limeade, concentrate, frozen	0.5	cup	145	73	272	0	72	0.6	0	0
20002	Limeade, from frozen	1	cup	247	220	101	0	27	0.2	0	0
22519	Liqueur, coffee, 53 proof	1	oz.	28	9	95	0	13	0	0	0
22544	Liqueur, coffee, 63 proof	1	oz.	28	12	87	0	9	0	0	0
22521	Liqueur, de menthe, 72 proof	1	oz.	28	8	105	0	12	0	0	0
22551	Liqueur, kahlua, 1 shot	1	each	30	9	106	0	13	0	0	0
56258	Liver, chopped, w/egg & onion	0.5	cup	104	66	230	13	3	0.4	18	5.5
13019	Liverwurst	1	oz.	28	15	92	4	1	0	8	3
13019	Liverwurst	1	piece	18	9	59	3	0	0	5	1.9

MonoF (g)	PolyF (g)	Choles (mg)	Calc (mg)	Phos (mg)	Sod (mg)	Pot (mg)	Zn (mg)	Iron (mg)	Magn (mg)	VitA (μg RE)	VitE (mg α-TE)	VitC (mg)	Thia (mg)	Ribo (mg)	Nia (mg)	B6 (mg)	Fola (μg)	B12 (μg)
3.6	0.5	81	16	192	71	320	3.5	1.7	24	0	0.14	0	0.09	0.24	5.8	0.14	20	2.14
6.2	1.1	64	13	125	49	209	2.2	1.2	15	0	0.08	0	0.06	0.16	4.5	0.08	12	1.58
8.2	1.4	85	17	167	66	278	3	1.5	20	0	0.11	0	0.08	0.21	6	0.11	15	2.1
9.4	1.6	110	25	228	92	384	5.3	2	27	0	0.28	0	0.11	0.28	7.6	0.16	22	2.96
2.9	0.4	76	7	175	58	287	4.2	1.8	22	0	0.15	0	0.09	0.25	5.4	0.14	20	2.24
4.6	0.7	104	9	230	80	378	5.5	2.5	28	0	0.19	0	0.14	0.35	7.1	0.19	24	2.93
9.9	1.7	110	12	208	77	341	4.7	2.3	25	0	0.15	0	0.12	0.32	7.5	0.16	19	2.87
6.6	1	100	24	221	92	357	5.1	2	26	0	0.17	0	0.1	0.26	7	0.17	25	2.45
14.2	2.5	110	25	188	83	307	4	1.8	23	0	0.11	0	0.1	0.24	7.6	0.12	17	2.53
4.9	1.1	99	22	227	77	301	6.8	2.4	28	0	0.2	0	0.1	0.3	6.5	0.17	28	3.06
9.3	1.8	104	23	209	75	285	5.9	2.2	26	0	0.16	0	0.1	0.27	7	0.15	24	2.99
0	0.1	0	86	20	12	127	0.1	0.3	10	325	0.43	22	0.04	0.12	0.3	0.08	8	0
0.1	0.3	0	232	40	26	259	0.3	0.6	21	873	1.21	33	0.09	0.23	0.8	0.16	12	0
5.4	1.8	12	0	0	0	0	0	0	0	0	0.15	0	0	0	0	0	0	0
5	0.9	56	258	289	745	461	3.2	3.2	50	158	1.15	16	0.23	0.33	4	0.21	19	0.78
—	—	10	207	—	321	—	—	1.9	—	259	—	0	—	—	—	—	—	—
0	0.1	0	37	21	12	108	0.1	1.4	17	6	0.76	5	0.03	0.02	0.2	0.14	30	0
0	0.2	0	73	43	25	223	0.1	2.6	35	12	1.14	15	0.07	0.04	0.5	0.29	80	0
0	0.1	0	16	9	5	45	0	0.6	7	3	0.32	2	0.01	0.01	0.1	0.06	13	0
0	0.1	0	31	18	10	94	0.1	1.1	15	5	0.48	6	0.03	0.02	0.2	0.12	33	0
—	—	—	46	12	—	—	—	1.5	—	1143	—	7	0.01	0.03	0.1	—	—	0
0	0.2	0	27	22	51	249	0.1	0.3	20	5	0.22	60	0.1	0.02	0.5	0.1	25	0
0	0	0	17	15	2	303	0.1	0.1	15	5	0.22	112	0.07	0.02	0.2	0.12	32	0
0	0.2	0	20	20	2	217	0.1	0.3	20	2	0.22	77	0.14	0.03	0.3	0.15	23	0
—	—	0	0	0	0	0	—	0	—	0	—	0	0	0	0	—	—	0
0	0	0	8	1	0	10	0	0	1	0	0.01	8	0	0	0	0.01	1	0
—	—	—	—	—	98	3	—	—	—	—	—	—	—	—	—	—	—	0
5.4	3.2	47	10	41	228	31	0.3	1.1	5	32	1.16	1	0.13	0.12	1.1	0.02	8	0.09
0	0.1	0	15	9	1	80	0	0.3	5	2	0.14	31	0.02	0.01	0.1	0.05	6	0
0	0	0	12	1	6	0	0	0	0	0	0	17	0	0	0	0	0	0
0	0	0	29	3	19	3	0.1	0.1	3	0	0	34	0	0	0	0	0	0
0	0	0	7	2	7	38	0.1	0.4	5	2	0	16	0.02	0.02	0	0	7	0
0	0	0	7	2	7	38	0.1	0.4	5	2	0	16	0.02	0.02	0	0	7	0
0	0	0	50	24	7	0	0.1	0.1	2	0	0	6	0	0	0	0	0	0
0	0	0	7	5	7	37	0.1	0.4	5	0	0	10	0.02	0.05	0	0.02	5	0
0	0	0	33	17	3	16	0	0.1	0	0	0	4	0	0	0	0	2	0
0	0	0	71	34	13	34	0.1	0.2	3	0	0	8	0	0	0	0.01	3	0
0	0	0	7	5	7	37	0.1	0.4	5	5	0	10	0.02	0.05	0	0.02	5	0
0.7	2.1	0	15	88	40	155	0.6	1.4	26	0	2.01	1	0.13	0.04	0.6	0.09	62	0
0	0.1	0	10	67	4	124	0.6	1.2	14	2	0.04	6	0.09	0.05	0.4	0.07	38	0
0.1	0.2	0	16	174	11	322	1.8	3.5	40	5	0.1	14	0.25	0.1	1.4	0.19	76	0
0.1	0.2	0	24	218	5	434	1.7	4.3	51	2	0.16	3	0.23	0.12	1.3	0.26	208	0
0.1	0.2	0	19	178	2	365	1.3	3.3	36	1	0.11	1	0.17	0.07	1	0.18	179	0
0	0	0	9	6	1	72	0	0.1	4	27	0.12	2	0.02	0.02	0.1	0.01	20	0
0	0	0	5	3	1	39	0	0	2	15	0.07	1	0.01	0.01	0	0.01	11	0
0	0.2	0	52	38	8	419	0.3	0.5	21	158	0.72	13	0.1	0.1	0.5	0.08	119	0
0	0	0	4	4	2	32	0	0.1	2	7	0.06	1	0.01	0.01	0	0.01	11	0
0	0	0	5	6	3	44	0.1	0.1	3	9	0.08	1	0.01	0.01	0.1	0.01	16	0
0	0.5	0	102	108	48	852	1.2	2.7	48	178	1.51	21	0.25	0.16	1	0.22	302	0
0	0	0	19	7	3	74	0.1	0.4	3	53	0.12	5	0.01	0.02	0.1	0.02	14	0
0	0	0	7	2	1	26	0	0.1	1	19	0.04	2	0	0.01	0	0.01	5	0
0	0	0	10	13	2	81	0.1	0.3	2	73	0.12	7	0.03	0.03	0.1	0.01	38	0
0	0	0	4	4	1	29	0	0.1	1	26	0.04	2	0.01	0.01	0	0	14	0
0.1	0.2	0	30	25	39	185	0.1	0.6	17	5	0.17	16	0.08	0.01	0.4	0.07	19	0
0	0.1	0	22	17	2	268	0.1	0.1	15	2	0.22	72	0.05	0.02	0.2	0.11	20	0
0	0	0	22	12	1	68	0.1	0.4	4	1	0.16	20	0.02	0.01	0.1	0.03	5	0
0	0	0	7	9	0	86	0.1	0.1	6	0	0	17	0.02	0.02	0.1	0	6	0
0	0	0	7	2	5	32	0	0.1	2	0	0	7	0	0	0.1	0	2	0
0	0	0	0	2	2	9	0	0	1	0	0	0	0	0	0	0	0	0
0	0	0	0	2	2	9	0	0	1	0	0	0	0	0	0	0	0	0
0	0	0	0	0	1	0	0	0	0	0	0	0	0	0	0	0	0	0
0	0	0	0	1	2	4	0	0	0	0	0	0	0	0	0	0	0	0
7.4	3.5	367	21	178	1078	125	2.2	4.1	14	2230	1.38	9	0.09	0.88	2	0.31	358	8.89
3.8	0.7	45	7	65	244	48	0.7	1.8	3	2353	0.08	0	0.08	0.29	1.2	0.05	9	3.83
2.4	0.5	28	5	41	155	31	0.4	1.2	2	1494	0.05	0	0.05	0.18	0.8	0.03	5	2.43

A

Esha Code	Food Item	Qty	Meas	Wgt (g)	Wtr (g)	Cals	Prot (g)	Carb (g)	Fib (g)	Fat (g)	SatF (g)
18800	Lobster newburg	0.5	cup	122	75	306	15	6	0.1	25	14.8
3033	Loganberries, canned w/heavy syrup	0.5	cup	128	98	113	1	28	3.3	0	0
3025	Loganberries, fresh	0.5	cup	75	64	39	1	10	4	0	0
3074	Loganberries, frozen	0.5	cup	74	62	40	1	10	3.6	0	0
3254	Longan, raw	1	each	3	3	2	0	0	0	0	—
3253	Loquat, raw	1	each	10	9	5	0	1	0.2	0	0
5392	Lotus root, cooked	10	each	89	72	59	1	14	2.8	0	0
5391	Lotus root, slices, raw	10	each	81	64	60	2	14	4	0	0
56938	Lunchables, bologna & American, regular	1	each	128	—	450	18	19	0	34	15
56935	Lunchables, ham & cheddar, regular	1	each	128	—	340	21	19	0	20	11
13105	Lunchmeat, Spam, canned	1	piece	28	14	95	4	1	0.1	9	—
13055	Lunchmeat, chicken/turkey sandwich spread	1	Tbs	13	9	26	2	1	0	2	0.4
13057	Lunchmeat, chopped ham, slices	2	piece	42	27	96	7	0	0	7	2.4
13051	Lunchmeat, pickle & pimento loaf	2	piece	57	32	149	7	3	0	12	4.5
3257	Lychee, raw	1	each	10	8	6	0	2	0.1	0	0
3166	Lychees, canned, sweetened	3.5	oz.	100	76	91	1	23	0.3	0	0.1
4516	Macadamia nut, dried	0.25	cup	34	1	235	3	5	3.1	25	3.7
4587	Macadamia nuts, oil roasted, salted	0.25	cup	34	1	241	2	4	3.1	26	3.8
4590	Macadamia nuts, oil roasted, unsalted	11	each	28	0	204	2	4	2.6	22	3.3
56084	Macaroni & cheese, canned	0.5	cup	120	96	114	5	13	0.7	5	2.1
56082	Macaroni & cheese, recipe, w/margarine	0.5	cup	100	58	215	8	20	0.6	11	4.4
26024	Mace, ground	0.25	tsp	0	0	2	0	0	0.1	0	0
3259	Mamey apple, raw	1	each	846	729	431	4	106	25.4	4	1.2
3303	Mango nectar	1	cup	250	210	147	1	38	2	0	0.1
3220	Mango, fresh slices	0.5	cup	82	67	54	0	14	1.5	0	0.1
3221	Mango, fresh, whole	1	each	207	169	135	1	35	3.7	1	0.1
8060	Margarine, Blue Bonnet, stick	1	Tbs	14	2	102	0	0	0	11	2.4
8061	Margarine, Fleischmann's corn oil, tub type	1	Tbs	14	2	102	0	0	0	11	2
8166	Margarine, Parkay Squeeze	1	Tbs	14	2	102	0	0	0	11	1.9
8169	Margarine, Parkay, soft, tub	1	Tbs	14	2	102	0	0	0	11	1.9
8159	Margarine, Saffola, stick	1	Tbs	14	2	102	0	0	0	11	1.9
8173	Margarine, Saffola, tub	1	Tbs	14	2	102	0	0	0	11	1.5
8002	Margarine, hard, pat	1	each	3	0	22	0	0	0	2	0.4
8179	Margarine, hard, stick	1	Tbs	14	2	102	0	0	0	11	1.9
8134	Margarine, hard, unsalted	1	Tbs	14	3	101	0	0	0	11	2.1
8165	Margarine, liquid	1	Tbs	14	2	102	0	0	0	11	1.9
8168	Margarine, soft, tub	1	Tbs	14	2	102	0	0	0	11	1.9
8154	Margarine, spread, Blue Bonnet, tub	1	Tbs	14	8	49	0	0	0	6	0.9
8155	Margarine, spread, Fleischmann's light, tub	1	Tbs	14	8	49	0	0	0	6	0.9
8176	Margarine, spread, Shedd's Spread, tub	1	Tbs	14	8	60	0	0	0	6	0.8
8175	Margarine, spread, Touch of Butter, stick	1	Tbs	14	4	90	0	0	0	10	2
8131	Margarine, spread, Weight Watcher's XLight, tub	1	Tbs	14	8	49	0	0	0	6	1.1
8549	Margarine, unsalted, Saffola	1	Tbs	14	3	101	0	0	0	11	2
26025	Marjoram, dried	0.25	tsp	0	0	0	0	0	0.1	0	0
23005	Marmalade, orange	1	Tbs	20	7	49	0	13	0	0	0
23006	Marmalade, orange, packet	1	each	14	5	34	0	9	0	0	0
23007	Marshmallow	4	each	28	5	90	1	23	0	0	0
23064	Marshmallow creme, Kraft	1	oz.	28	5	93	0	23	0	0	0
23008	Marshmallow, minature, not packed	0.5	cup	23	4	73	0	19	0	0	0
8069	Mayonnaise, fat free (Kraft Free)	1	Tbs	16	14	10	0	2	0	0	0
8032	Mayonnaise, imitation	1	Tbs	15	9	35	0	2	0	3	0.5
8033	Mayonnaise, low calorie	1	Tbs	16	10	36	0	2	0	3	0.5
8148	Mayonnaise, low calorie, low sodium	1	Tbs	14	9	32	0	2	0	3	0.5
8046	Mayonnaise, soybean, w/salt	1	Tbs	14	2	99	0	0	0	11	1.6
69005	McDonald's Egg McMuffin	1	each	137	78	289	17	27	1.5	13	0.7
69013	McDonald's Fillet-O-Fish sandwich	1	each	145	71	364	14	41	1.5	16	3.7
47147	McDonald's McDonaldland cookies	1	each	56	2	258	4	41	1	9	1.7
69001	McDonald's McLean Deluxe, w/cheese	1	each	228	143	397	26	38	2.2	16	6.8
69000	McDonald's McLean deluxe	1	each	214	137	345	24	37	2.2	12	4.4
69006	McDonald's Sausage McMuffin	1	each	112	48	361	13	26	1.5	23	8.3
69009	McDonald's cheeseburger	1	each	122	56	319	15	36	1.9	13	5.6
2166	McDonald's frozen yogurt cone, vanilla	1	each	90	61	118	4	24	0.4	1	0.5
2167	McDonald's frozen yogurt shake, small, choc	1	each	295	—	348	13	62	0.9	6	3.5
2168	McDonald's frozen yogurt shake, small, strawberry	1	each	294	—	343	12	63	0.3	5	3.4
2169	McDonald's frozen yogurt shake, small, vanilla	1	each	293	—	308	12	54	0.3	5	3.3

MonoF (g)	PolyF (g)	Choles (mg)	Calc (mg)	Phos (mg)	Sod (mg)	Pot (mg)	Zn (mg)	Iron (mg)	Magn (mg)	VitA (μg RE)	VitE (mg α-TE)	VitC (mg)	Thia (mg)	Ribo (mg)	Nia (mg)	B6 (mg)	Fola (μg)	B12 (μg)
7.3	1.1	184	120	199	323	304	2	0.6	28	261	1	0	0.05	0.21	0.8	0.08	16	2.01
0	0.1	0	23	13	4	115	0.2	0.6	14	5	0.91	8	0.03	0.04	0.3	0.05	44	0
0	0.2	0	24	16	0	146	0.2	0.4	15	12	0.53	16	0.02	0.03	0.3	0.04	25	0
0	0.1	0	19	19	1	107	0.2	0.5	15	3	1.62	11	0.04	0.02	0.6	0.05	19	0
—	—	0	0	1	0	9	0	0	0	0	—	3	0	0	0	—	—	0
0	0	0	2	3	0	26	0	0	1	15	0.09	0	0	0	0	0.01	1	0
0	0	0	23	69	40	323	0.3	0.8	20	0	0.01	24	0.11	0.01	0.3	0.19	7	0
0	0	0	36	81	32	450	0.3	0.9	19	0	0.01	36	0.13	0.18	0.3	0.21	10	0
—	—	85	300	—	1620	—	—	2.7	—	60	—	0	—	—	—	—	—	—
—	—	75	250	—	1830	—	—	1.8	—	60	—	—	—	—	—	—	—	—
—	—	16	2	—	445	54	0.7	0.4	3	5	—	—	0.03	0.05	0.9	—	—	—
0.4	0.8	4	1	4	49	24	0.1	0.1	1	5	0.29	0	0	0.01	0.2	0.01	1	0.05
3.4	0.9	21	3	65	576	134	0.8	0.3	7	0	0.11	0	0.26	0.09	1.6	0.15	0	0.39
5.5	1.5	21	54	80	792	194	0.8	0.6	10	4	0.14	0	0.17	0.14	1.2	0.11	3	0.67
0	0	0	0	3	0	16	0	0	1	0	0.07	7	0	0.01	0.1	0.01	1	0
0	0.1	0	4	20	1	100	0.1	0.2	7	0	0.45	32	0.01	0.04	0.4	0.06	5	0
19.5	0.4	0	24	46	2	123	0.6	0.8	39	0	0.14	0	0.12	0.04	0.7	0.07	5	0
20.2	0.4	0	15	67	87	110	0.4	0.6	39	0	0.14	0	0.07	0.04	0.7	0.07	5	0
17.1	0.4	0	13	57	2	93	0.3	0.5	33	0	0.12	0	0.06	0.03	0.6	0.06	5	0
1.5	0.7	12	100	91	365	70	0.6	0.5	16	37	0.07	0	0.06	0.12	0.5	0.01	4	0.1
4.4	1.8	21	181	161	543	120	0.6	0.9	18	117	0.06	0	0.1	0.2	0.9	0.02	5	0.15
0	0	0	1	0	0	2	0	0.1	1	0	0.01	0	0	0	0	0	0	0
1.7	0.7	0	93	93	127	398	0.8	5.9	135	195	4.99	118	0.17	0.34	3.4	0.85	118	0
0.1	0.1	0	12	11	6	141	0.1	0.2	10	292	1.12	19	0.05	0.06	0.5	0.12	7	0
0.1	0	0	8	9	2	129	0	0.1	7	321	0.92	23	0.05	0.05	0.5	0.11	12	0
0.2	0.1	0	21	23	4	323	0.1	0.3	19	805	2.32	57	0.12	0.12	1.2	0.28	29	0
5.6	3	0	4	3	134	6	0	0	0	113	1.48	0	0	0	0	0	0	0.01
4.5	4.4	0	4	3	153	5	0	0	0	113	2.13	0	0	0	0	0	0	0.01
4	5.1	0	9	7	111	13	0	0	1	113	0.74	0	0	0.01	0	0	0	0.03
5.2	3.8	0	4	3	153	5	0	0	0	113	1.85	0	0	0	0	0	0	0.01
3.3	5.8	0	4	3	134	6	0	0	0	113	2.7	0	0	0	0	0	0	0.01
4.4	5	0	4	3	153	5	0	0	0	113	2.41	0	0	0	0	0	0	0.01
1.1	0.8	0	1	1	28	1	0	0	0	24	0.49	0	0	0	0	0	0	0
5.3	3.7	0	4	3	134	6	—	0	0	113	1.82	0	0	0	0	0	0	0.01
5.2	3.6	0	2	2	0	4	0	0	0	113	1.82	0	0	0	0	0	0	0.01
4	5.1	0	9	7	111	13	0	0	1	113	0.74	0	0	0.01	0	0	0	0.03
5.2	3.8	0	4	3	153	5	0	0	0	113	1.85	0	0	0	0	0	0	0.01
2.4	2	0	3	2	136	4	0	0	0	113	1.21	0	0	0	0	0	0	0.01
2.1	2.3	0	3	2	136	4	0	0	0	113	1.56	0	0	0	0	0	0	0.01
2.4	2.4	0	3	2	110	4	0	0	0	144	0.48	0	0	0	0	0	0	0.01
—	—	0	0	—	110	0	—	0	—	122	—	0	—	—	—	—	—	—
2.2	2	0	3	2	136	4	0	0	0	154	0.33	0	0	0	0	0	0	0.01
3	4.6	—	0	—	0	—	—	0	—	52	—	0	—	—	—	—	—	—
0	0	0	3	0	0	2	0	0.1	0	1	0	0	0	0	0	0	0	0
0	0	0	8	1	11	7	0	0	0	1	0	1	0	0	0	0	7	0
0	0	0	5	1	8	5	0	0	0	1	0	1	0	0	0	0	5	0
0	0	0	1	2	13	1	0	0.1	1	0	0	0	0	0	0	0	0	0
0	0	0	0	—	23	0	—	0	—	0	0	0	—	—	—	—	—	—
0	0	0	1	2	11	1	0	0.1	0	0	0	0	0	0	0	0	0	0
0	0	0	0	—	105	5	—	0	—	0	—	0	—	—	—	—	—	—
0.7	1.6	4	0	0	75	2	0	0	0	0	0.96	0	0	0	0	0	0	0
0.7	1.6	4	0	0	78	2	0	0	0	0	1	0	0	0	0	0	0	0
0.6	1.4	3	0	0	15	1	0	0	0	1	0.53	0	0	0	0	0	0	0.01
3.1	5.7	8	2	4	78	5	0	0.1	0	12	1.63	0	0	0	0	0.08	1	0.04
4.5	1.6	234	151	270	730	199	1.6	2.4	24	100	0.85	2	0.49	0.45	3.3	0.15	33	0.67
3.8	5.6	37	124	183	708	266	0.7	1.8	32	21	1.52	0	0.32	0.23	2.6	0.07	30	0.58
6.3	0.8	0	10	70	267	62	0.4	1.7	11	0	0.99	0	0.24	0.16	2	0.03	—	—
4.6	1.3	72	139	291	1045	558	5.3	4.3	43	115	0.85	8	0.42	0.39	7.2	0.3	47	2.05
3.6	1.2	59	131	226	809	537	4.9	4.3	40	74	0.63	8	0.42	0.34	7.2	0.29	44	1.9
8.2	2.8	46	132	157	751	191	1.5	2.1	22	48	0.66	0	0.56	0.27	3.8	0.14	16	0.5
3.8	1.1	42	134	178	768	282	2.6	2.7	27	64	0.46	2	0.33	0.31	3.8	0.15	24	1.2
0.2	0	3	132	101	84	175	—	0.2	—	4	—	1	0	0.02	0.2	—	—	—
0.1	0.7	24	371	354	241	542	—	1	—	46	—	3	0.12	0.51	0.4	0.1	—	—
0.1	0.6	24	366	329	170	542	—	0.3	—	46	—	3	0.12	0.51	0.4	0.11	—	—
0.1	0.6	24	360	327	194	534	—	0.3	—	45	—	3	0.12	0.51	0.3	—	—	—

Esha Code	Food Item	Qty	Meas	Wgt (g)	Wtr (g)	Cals	Prot (g)	Carb (g)	Fib (g)	Fat (g)	SatF (g)
6155	McDonald's hashed browns	1	each	53	29	130	1	14	1.4	8	1.4
48022	McDonald's turnover, apple	1	each	85	40	225	2	32	1.2	11	2.6
69010	McDonald's, Big Mac sandwich	1	each	216	115	510	25	46	3.3	26	9.3
15174	McDonald's, Chicken McNuggets	4	piece	73	37	198	12	10	0	12	2.5
56676	McDonald's, Fajita, chicken	1	each	82	42	190	11	20	1	8	2
69041	McDonald's, McChicken sandwich	1	each	189	98	492	17	42	1.7	29	5.5
69011	McDonald's, Quarter-Pounder	1	each	171	89	415	23	36	1.7	20	7.8
69012	McDonald's, Quarter-Pounder, w/cheese	1	each	199	100	520	28	37	1.7	29	12.6
42332	McDonald's, biscuit w/spread	1	each	76	24	260	4	32	1.1	13	3.8
56675	McDonald's, burrito, breakfast	1	each	105	52	290	12	21	1	17	5
52070	McDonald's, chicken salad, chunky	1	each	296	259	164	23	8	3.2	5	1.3
69014	McDonald's, chicken sandwich, McGrilled	1	each	188	126	254	24	33	2	3	0.7
15184	McDonald's, chicken, drumstick, hot & spicy	1	each	63	29	180	14	6	—	12	3
42335	McDonald's, danish pastry, apple	1	each	105	—	360	5	51	1.5	17	5.2
42336	McDonald's, danish pastry, cinnamon raisin	1	each	105	20	435	5	56	1.4	22	7.4
42338	McDonald's, danish pastry, raspberry	1	each	105	24	396	5	58	1.4	16	5.2
6157	McDonald's, french fries, regular order	1	each	97	37	320	4	36	1.7	17	3.5
69008	McDonald's, hamburger	1	each	108	54	266	12	36	1.9	9	3.2
19579	McDonald's, scrambled eggs, serving	1	each	102	75	170	13	1	0	12	3.6
7994	Meatless hot dog, Tofu Pups, Lightlife	1	each	42	3	60	8	28	0	2	1
7504	Meatless patty, Garden Burger	2.5	oz.	71	41	130	8	18	5	3	1
7652	Meatless patty, Garden Burger, Veggie Medley	2.5	oz.	71	41	130	8	18	5	3	1
7782	Meatless patty, Garden Burger, vegan	2.5	oz.	71	36	140	11	23	4	0	0
3167	Melon balls, mixed, frozen	0.5	cup	86	78	28	1	7	0.6	0	0.1
3075	Melon, cantaloupe, cubes	0.5	cup	80	72	28	1	7	0.6	0	0.1
3076	Melon, cantaloupe, cubes	0.5	each	267	240	94	2	22	2.1	1	0.2
3079	Melon, casaba/crenshaw	1	each	1640	1508	426	15	102	13.1	2	0.4
3078	Melon, casaba/crenshaw cubes	0.5	cup	85	78	22	1	5	0.7	0	0
3081	Melon, honeydew, 1/10th melon=piece	1	piece	129	116	45	1	12	0.8	0	0
3080	Melon, honeydew, cubes	0.5	cup	85	76	30	0	8	0.5	0	0
38	Milk drink, malted, chocolate (Ovaltine)	1	cup	265	215	225	9	29	0.3	9	5.5
34	Milk drink, malted, chocolate, unfortified	1	cup	265	215	228	9	30	0.3	9	5.5
36	Milk drink, malted, natural (Ovaltine)	1	cup	265	215	231	10	28	0	9	5.4
54	Milk, 1% fat, low lactose	1	cup	246	222	103	9	12	0	3	1.6
55	Milk, 1% fat, low lactose	1	cup	247	222	103	9	12	0	3	1.6
4	Milk, 1% lowfat	1	cup	244	220	102	8	12	0	3	1.6
64	Milk, 1% lowfat, protein fortified	1	cup	246	218	119	10	14	0	3	1.8
2	Milk, 2% lowfat	1	cup	244	218	121	8	12	0	5	2.9
63	Milk, 2% lowfat, protein+vitamin A fortified	1	cup	246	216	137	10	14	0	5	3
23	Milk, Goat	1	cup	244	212	168	9	11	0	10	6.5
19	Milk, chocolate, 1% lowfat	1	cup	250	211	158	8	26	1.2	2	1.5
18	Milk, chocolate, 2% lowfat	1	cup	250	209	179	8	26	1.2	5	3.1
59	Milk, chocolate, nonfat	1	cup	250	211	144	9	27	1.5	1	0.7
70	Milk, chocolate, syrup w/milk	1	cup	263	220	197	8	24	0.3	8	5.2
20	Milk, chocolate, whole fat	1	cup	250	206	209	8	26	2	8	5.2
11	Milk, condensed, sweetened, canned	3	Tbs	57	16	184	5	31	0	5	3.2
8	Milk, dry, nonfat, instant, w/vitamin A added	1	Tbs	4	0	15	1	2	0	0	0
80	Milk, evaporated, 2% fat	2	Tbs	32	25	29	2	4	0	1	0.4
10	Milk, evaporated, skim, canned	0.5	cup	128	101	99	10	14	0	0	0.2
22	Milk, human breast, mature	1	cup	246	215	171	3	17	0	11	4.9
82	Milk, imitation, (Vitamite)	1	cup	244	220	112	4	13	0	5	1
81	Milk, imitation, fluid, soy based	1	cup	244	215	150	4	15	0	8	1.9
29	Milk, malted, natural, powder, unfortified	1	cup	265	5	1097	30	201	1.6	21	11.1
6	Milk, nonfat skim	1	cup	245	222	86	8	12	0	0	0.3
57	Milk, nonfat, dry, reconstituted,	1	cup	245	223	82	8	12	0	0	0.1
56	Milk, nonfat, low lactose	1	cup	245	222	86	9	12	0	0	0.3
38362	Milk, rice, Arroz con leche	1	cup	245	219	100	0	25	0.2	0	0
65	Milk, skim, protein fortified	1	cup	245	219	100	10	14	0	1	0.4
41	Milk, strawberry mix w/milk (Nestle's Quik)	1	cup	250	202	220	8	31	0	8	4.8
1	Milk, whole, 3.3% fat	1	cup	244	215	150	8	11	0	8	5.1
62	Milk, whole, extra rich, 3.7% fat	1	cup	244	214	157	8	11	0	9	5.6
52	Milk, whole, fluid, low sodium	1	cup	244	215	149	8	11	0	8	5.2
2020	Milkshake, chocolate	1	cup	226	162	288	8	46	1.8	8	5.2
2022	Milkshake, strawberry	1	cup	226	168	256	8	43	0.9	6	3.9
2024	Milkshake, vanilla	1	cup	226	169	251	8	40	0.9	7	4.2

MonoF (g)	PolyF (g)	Choles (mg)	Calc (mg)	Phos (mg)	Sod (mg)	Pot (mg)	Zn (mg)	Iron (mg)	Magn (mg)	VitA (μg RE)	VitE (mg α-TE)	VitC (mg)	Thia (mg)	Ribo (mg)	Nia (mg)	B6 (mg)	Fola (μg)	B12 (μg)
2.3	1.9	0	7	51	332	213	0.2	0.3	11	0	0.58	3	0.08	0.02	0.9	0.08	8	0
4.6	2.8	0	6	24	179	67	0.2	1	6	10	1.62	1	0.13	0.09	1	0.03	20	0
7.5	4.1	76	202	267	931	455	4.8	4.3	46	66	1.01	3	0.49	0.44	6.1	0.25	49	2.25
3.7	2.4	42	9	199	353	210	0.7	0.6	17	0	0.96	0	0.08	0.11	5.2	0.21	—	0.21
—	—	35	80	—	310	—	—	0.7	—	20	—	6	—	—	—	—	—	—
8.5	10.2	52	129	223	799	320	1.1	2.5	33	29	6.17	1	0.91	0.24	7.8	0.39	37	0.05
6.7	1.3	70	127	207	692	405	4.7	4.3	34	33	0.36	3	0.39	0.32	6.8	0.24	27	2.58
8.7	1.6	97	143	—	1160	—	—	4.5	—	115	0.81	3	0.39	0.43	6.8	0.26	33	2.89
3.7	0.8	0	68	353	836	105	0.3	1.8	9	2	0.81	0	0.29	0.23	2.2	0.03	5	—
—	—	135	100	—	580	—	—	1.4	—	100	—	6	—	—	—	—	—	—
1.6	1	76	54	277	318	673	1.5	1.6	44	1973	1.28	30	0.51	0.21	8.5	0.52	83	0.28
0.5	1.1	47	117	327	506	433	0.9	2.4	42	46	0.3	5	0.43	0.28	12.1	0.55	38	0.16
—	—	55	—	—	320	—	—	—	—	15	—	6	—	—	—	—	—	—
—	—	42	78	0	291	113	—	1	—	100	—	1	0.3	0.17	2	—	—	—
—	—	51	92	0	280	112	—	1.6	—	100	—	1	0.3	0.26	3	—	—	—
—	—	44	86	0	296	94	—	1	—	101	—	1	0.3	0.17	2	—	—	—
12	1.5	0	14	—	150	—	—	0.7	—	0	—	12	0.23	0	3	—	—	0
2.8	0.9	28	126	113	533	261	2.3	2.7	24	23	0.23	2	0.33	0.26	3.8	0.14	21	1.05
5.3	1.7	424	50	172	143	126	1.1	1.2	10	168	0.92	0	0.07	0.51	0.1	0.12	44	1.11
—	—	0	20	—	140	—	—	1.8	—	0	—	2	—	—	—	—	—	—
1.5	0.5	11	84	132	290	193	0.9	0	30	10	0.2	0	0.11	0.15	1.1	0.08	10	0.11
1.5	0.5	11	84	132	290	193	0.9	0	30	10	0.2	1	0.11	0.15	1.1	0.08	10	0.11
0	0	0	20	—	250	—	—	1.1	—	0	—	0	—	—	—	—	—	—
0	0.1	0	9	10	27	242	0.1	0.3	12	153	0.13	5	0.14	0.02	0.6	0.09	22	0
0	0.1	0	9	14	7	247	0.1	0.2	9	258	0.12	34	0.03	0.02	0.5	0.09	14	0
0	0.3	0	29	45	24	825	0.4	0.6	29	860	0.4	113	0.1	0.06	1.5	0.31	45	0
0	0.6	0	82	115	197	3444	2.6	6.6	131	49	2.46	262	0.98	0.33	6.6	1.97	279	0
0	0	0	4	6	10	179	0.1	0.3	7	3	0.13	14	0.05	0.02	0.3	0.1	14	0
0	0	0	8	13	13	350	0.1	0.1	9	5	0.19	32	0.1	0.02	0.8	0.08	8	0
0	0	0	5	8	8	230	0.1	0.1	6	3	0.13	21	0.06	0.02	0.5	0.05	5	0
2.6	0.4	34	384	313	244	620	1.2	3.8	53	901	0.32	34	0.73	1.26	10.9	1.02	32	0.88
2.6	0.4	34	305	265	172	498	1.1	0.6	48	80	0.26	3	0.13	0.44	0.6	0.14	16	0.93
2.5	0.4	34	371	307	204	572	1.1	3.6	48	742	0.32	29	0.71	1.14	10.4	0.87	22	1.03
0.8	0.1	10	303	237	124	384	1	0.1	34	145	0.1	2	0.1	0.41	0.2	0.11	12	0.9
0.8	0.1	10	550	237	125	385	1	0.1	34	146	0.1	2	0.1	0.41	0.2	0.11	13	0.91
0.7	0.1	10	300	235	123	381	1	0.1	34	144	0.1	2	0.1	0.41	0.2	0.1	12	0.9
0.8	0.1	10	349	273	143	443	1.1	0.1	39	145	0.1	3	0.11	0.47	0.2	0.12	14	1.05
1.4	0.2	18	298	232	122	376	1	0.1	33	139	0.17	2	0.1	0.4	0.2	0.1	12	0.89
1.4	0.2	19	352	276	145	448	1.1	0.1	40	140	0.17	3	0.11	0.48	0.2	0.12	15	1.05
2.7	0.4	28	327	271	122	498	0.7	0.1	34	137	0.22	3	0.12	0.34	0.7	0.11	1	0.16
0.8	0.1	7	288	258	152	425	1	0.6	33	148	0.06	2	0.1	0.42	0.3	0.1	12	0.86
1.5	0.2	17	285	255	151	423	1	0.6	33	143	0.13	2	0.09	0.41	0.3	0.1	12	0.85
0.4	0	4	292	265	121	486	1.2	0.7	46	142	0.11	2	0.09	0.34	0.3	0.1	14	0.88
2.4	0.3	34	292	229	147	460	0.9	2.7	32	321	0.21	2	0.1	0.55	6.5	0.1	12	0.87
2.5	0.3	30	280	253	149	418	1	0.6	32	72	0.23	2	0.09	0.4	0.3	0.1	12	0.84
1.4	0.2	20	163	145	73	213	0.5	0.1	15	46	0.12	1	0.05	0.24	0.1	0.03	6	0.26
0	0	1	52	42	23	72	0.2	0	5	30	0	0	0.02	0.07	0	0.02	2	0.17
0.2	0	3	90	60	36	103	0.3	0.1	8	41	0.02	0	0.01	0.1	0.1	0.02	3	0.07
0.1	0	5	370	249	147	423	1.2	0.4	34	149	0.01	2	0.06	0.39	0.2	0.07	11	0.3
4.1	1.2	34	79	34	42	126	0.4	0.1	8	157	2.21	12	0.03	0.09	0.4	0.03	13	0.11
2.7	0.9	0	200	244	134	366	0.2	0.2	2	149	0	0	0	0	0.2	0	0	0
4.9	1.2	0	79	181	191	278	2.9	1	16	0	2.56	0	0.03	0.22	0	0	0	0
5.4	3.2	53	790	949	1306	2008	2.6	1.9	246	233	1.06	8	1.34	2.44	13.9	1.09	122	2.07
0.1	0	4	301	247	126	407	1	0.1	28	149	0.1	2	0.09	0.34	0.2	0.1	13	0.93
0.1	0	4	284	224	131	388	1.1	0.1	29	162	0	1	0.09	0.4	0.2	0.08	11	0.91
0.1	0	4	302	247	126	406	1	0.1	28	149	0.1	2	0.09	0.34	0.2	0.1	13	0.93
0	0	0	12	5	7	6	0.1	0.3	4	0	0	0	0.02	0.01	0.1	0.01	0	0
0.2	0	5	350	274	144	446	1.1	0.1	39	149	0.1	3	0.11	0.48	0.2	0.12	15	1.05
2.2	0.3	30	275	215	120	348	0.9	0.2	30	70	0.25	2	0.09	0.4	0.2	0.1	12	0.82
2.4	0.3	33	290	228	120	371	0.9	0.1	33	76	0.24	2	0.09	0.4	0.2	0.1	12	0.87
2.6	0.3	35	290	227	119	368	0.9	0.1	33	83	0.24	4	0.09	0.39	0.2	0.1	12	0.87
2.4	0.3	33	246	209	6	617	0.9	0.1	12	78	0.24	2	0.05	0.26	0.1	0.08	12	0.88
2.4	0.3	29	256	231	220	453	0.9	0.7	38	52	0.15	1	0.13	0.56	0.4	0.11	8	0.77
1.8	0.3	25	256	226	188	412	0.8	0.2	29	66	0.29	2	0.1	0.44	0.4	0.1	7	0.7
2	0.3	25	276	231	186	394	0.8	0.2	27	72	0.13	2	0.1	0.41	0.4	0.12	7	0.82

Esha Code	Food Item	Qty	Meas	Wgt (g)	Wtr (g)	Cals	Prot (g)	Carb (g)	Fib (g)	Fat (g)	SatF (g)
38052	Millet, cooked	0.5	cup	120	86	143	4	28	1.6	1	0.2
7503	Miso (soybean)	1	Tbs	17	7	36	2	5	0.9	1	0.2
7563	Miso sauce	0.25	cup	62	36	96	3	18	1.5	2	0.2
3344	Mixed fruit canned in heavy syrup	0.5	cup	128	103	92	0	24	1.3	0	0
3168	Mixed fruit, dried	0.5	cup	68	21	165	2	44	5.3	0	0
3169	Mixed fruit, frozen-sweetened-thawed	0.5	cup	125	92	123	2	30	2.4	0	0
4595	Mixed nuts, no peanuts, oil roasted, salted	0.25	cup	36	1	221	6	8	2	20	3.3
4594	Mixed nuts, no peanuts, oil roasted, unsalted	0.25	cup	36	1	221	6	8	2	20	3.3
4592	Mixed nuts, w/peanuts, dry roasted, salted	0.25	cup	34	1	203	6	9	3.1	18	2.4
4591	Mixed nuts, w/peanuts, dry roasted, unsalted	0.25	cup	34	1	203	6	9	3.1	18	2.4
4593	Mixed nuts, w/peanuts, oil roasted, salted	0.25	cup	36	1	219	6	8	3.2	20	3.1
4533	Mixed nuts, w/peanuts, oil roasted, unsalted	0.5	cup	71	1	438	12	15	7	40	6.2
6462	Mixed vegetables, Chinese, LaChoy	4	oz.	113	108	14	1	3	1.7	0	0
5305	Mixed vegetables, canned, drained	0.5	cup	82	71	38	2	8	2.4	0	0
5516	Mixed vegetables, canned, low sodium	0.5	cup	91	82	33	1	6	2.8	0	0
5548	Mixed vegetables, canned, w/liquid	0.5	cup	122	110	44	2	9	4.7	0	0.1
5521	Mixed vegetables, dried-Salad Crunchies	1	Tbs	6	0	22	1	3	0.8	1	0.1
5549	Mixed vegetables, frozen	4	oz.	113	93	73	4	15	4.5	1	0.1
5187	Mixed vegetables, frozen, cooked	0.5	cup	91	76	54	3	12	4	0	0
70230	Mocha mix, vanilla	1	Tbs	8	5	17	0	2	—	1	0.2
56323	Mock chicken leg, cooked	4	oz.	113	66	262	23	6	0.2	16	4.9
25004	Molasses, blackstrap cane	1	Tbs	20	6	48	0	12	0	0	0
25003	Molasses, light cane	1	Tbs	20	5	54	0	14	0	0	0
56250	Moo goo gai pan	0.5	cup	108	84	140	8	6	1.4	10	2.4
7090	Mothbean, cooked, no salt	0.5	cup	88	61	103	7	18	3.3	0	0.1
56080	Moussaka, lamb & eggplant	1	cup	250	205	237	16	13	3.6	13	4.6
2667	Mousse, chocolate, recipe	0.5	cup	202	125	446	9	33	1.2	33	18.5
44569	Muffin, blueberry, Weight Watchers	1	each	71	14	250	4	46	4	5	1
44516	Muffin, blueberry, commercial	1	each	57	22	158	3	27	1.5	4	0.8
44505	Muffin, blueberry, mix, prepared	1	each	45	16	135	2	22	0.5	4	0.7
44520	Muffin, blueberry, recipe, w/2% milk	1	each	57	22	162	4	23	1.1	6	1.2
44501	Muffin, blueberry, recipe, w/whole milk	1	each	45	18	131	3	18	0.8	5	1.1
44532	Muffin, buckwheat	1	each	47	16	144	4	20	1.4	6	1.7
44537	Muffin, carrot w/raisins & nuts	1	each	58	20	177	4	26	1	7	1.1
44534	Muffin, cheese	1	each	58	21	184	5	23	0.7	8	3
44530	Muffin, chocolate chip	1	each	58	18	190	4	27	1	8	2.8
44521	Muffin, cornmeal, commercial	1	each	57	19	174	3	29	1.9	5	0.8
44504	Muffin, cornmeal, mix, prepared	1	each	45	14	144	3	22	1.1	5	1.3
44524	Muffin, cornmeal, recipe w/2% milk	1	each	57	19	180	4	25	1.9	7	1.3
44503	Muffin, cornmeal, recipe, w/whole milk	1	each	45	15	144	3	20	1.5	6	1.2
44529	Muffin, cranberry nut	1	each	58	22	164	4	25	0.8	5	1.5
70762	Muffin, egg-bacon-cheese, Great Starts	1	each	116	59	290	14	25	2	15	6
44514	Muffin, oat bran	1	each	57	20	154	4	28	2.6	4	0.6
44533	Muffin, oatmeal	1	each	47	22	112	3	17	0.7	3	1
44515	Muffin, plain, recipe, w/2% milk	1	each	57	22	169	4	24	1.5	6	1.2
44500	Muffin, plain, recipe, w/whole milk	1	each	45	17	135	3	19	1.2	5	1.2
44535	Muffin, pumpkin, w/raisins	1	each	58	16	181	3	34	1.1	4	0.8
44518	Muffin, toaster type, blueberry	1	each	33	10	103	2	18	0.6	3	0.5
44519	Muffin, toaster type, blueberry, toasted	1	each	31	8	103	2	18	0.6	3	0.5
44522	Muffin, toaster type, corn	1	each	33	8	114	2	19	0.5	4	0.6
44523	Muffin, toaster type, cornmeal, toasted	1	each	31	6	114	2	19	0.5	4	0.6
44526	Muffin, toaster type, wheat bran-raisin	1	each	36	11	106	2	19	2.8	3	0.5
44527	Muffin, toaster type, wheat bran-raisin, toasted	1	each	34	9	106	2	19	2.8	3	0.5
44506	Muffin, wheat bran, mix, prepared	1	each	45	16	124	3	21	1.9	4	1.1
44528	Muffin, wheat bran, recipe, w/2% milk	1	each	57	20	161	4	24	2.2	7	1.3
44502	Muffin, wheat bran, recipe, w/whole milk	1	each	45	16	130	3	19	3.2	6	1.2
44531	Muffin, whole wheat	1	each	47	16	142	4	20	2.5	6	1.7
44536	Muffin, zucchini	1	each	58	17	210	3	26	0.8	10	1.7
3309	Mulberries, raw	0.5	cup	70	61	30	1	7	1.2	0	0
5092	Mushroom pieces, cooked, drained	0.5	cup	78	71	21	2	4	1.7	0	0
5090	Mushroom pieces, raw	0.5	cup	35	32	9	1	2	0.4	0	0
5657	Mushroom pieces, steamed	0.5	cup	78	72	20	2	4	0.9	0	0
5658	Mushroom pieces, stir fried, no oil	0.5	cup	78	72	20	2	4	0.9	0	0
5514	Mushroom, batter-dipped, fried	5	each	70	46	148	2	8	0.7	12	2.1
6113	Mushroom, chanterelle, dried	0.5	cup	72	9	246	13	38	14.2	5	0.5

MonoF (g)	PolyF (g)	Choles (mg)	Calc (mg)	Phos (mg)	Sod (mg)	Pot (mg)	Zn (mg)	Iron (mg)	Magn (mg)	VitA (μg RE)	VitE (mg α-TE)	VitC (mg)	Thia (mg)	Ribo (mg)	Nia (mg)	B6 (mg)	Fola (μg)	B12 (μg)
0.2	0.6	0	4	120	2	74	1.1	0.8	53	0	0.22	0	0.13	0.1	1.6	0.13	23	0
0.2	0.6	0	11	26	629	28	0.6	0.5	7	2	0	0	0.02	0.04	0.1	0.04	6	0
0.4	0.9	0	19	43	1003	52	0.9	0.8	13	2	0	0	0.03	0.07	0.2	0.06	9	0
0	0.1	0	1	13	5	107	0.1	0.5	6	24	0.51	88	0.02	0.05	0.8	0.05	4	0
0.2	0.1	0	26	52	12	541	0.3	1.8	26	166	0.43	3	0.03	0.11	1.3	0.11	3	0
0	0.1	0	9	15	4	164	0.1	0.4	8	40	0.75	94	0.02	0.04	0.5	0.03	10	0
11.9	4.1	0	38	162	252	196	1.7	0.9	90	1	2.16	0	0.18	0.18	0.7	0.06	20	0
11.9	4.1	0	38	162	4	196	1.7	0.9	90	1	2.16	0	0.18	0.18	0.7	0.06	20	0
10.8	3.7	0	24	149	229	204	1.3	1.3	77	0	2.06	0	0.07	0.07	1.6	0.1	17	0
10.8	3.7	0	24	149	4	204	1.3	1.3	77	0	2.06	0	0.07	0.07	1.6	0.1	17	0
11.3	4.7	0	38	165	231	206	1.8	1.1	83	1	2.13	0	0.18	0.08	1.8	0.08	30	0
22.5	9.4	0	77	329	8	413	3.6	2.3	167	1	4.26	0	0.35	0.16	3.6	0.17	59	0
—	—	0	14	—	59	—	—	0.2	—	1	—	8	—	—	—	—	—	0
0	0.1	0	22	34	121	237	0.3	0.9	13	949	0.49	4	0.04	0.04	0.5	0.06	19	0
0	0.1	0	19	34	24	126	0.5	0.6	14	462	0.19	3	0.03	0.04	0.4	0.07	16	0
0	0.1	0	26	45	274	169	0.6	0.8	18	622	0.55	5	0.04	0.05	0.6	0.09	22	0
0.1	0.4	0	17	23	28	106	0.2	0.8	10	194	0.47	13	0.05	0.03	0.4	0.06	13	0.01
0	0.3	0	28	67	53	240	0.5	1.1	27	576	0.34	12	0.14	0.1	1.4	0.11	33	0
0	0.1	0	23	46	32	154	0.4	0.7	20	389	0.33	3	0.06	0.11	0.8	0.07	17	0
0.3	0.4	0	3	5	10	12	—	0.1	0	0	—	0	0	0	0	—	—	—
6.5	2.6	98	24	211	648	320	3.8	1.3	24	4	0.78	0	0.31	0.34	5.6	0.31	11	1.25
0	0	0	176	8	11	511	0.2	3.6	44	0	0	0	0.01	0.01	0.2	0.14	0	0
0	0	0	42	6	8	300	0.1	1	50	0	0	0	0.01	0	0.2	0.14	0	0
3.2	3.7	19	65	98	163	238	0.8	0.8	16	101	1.03	17	0.07	0.16	2.2	0.16	22	0.18
0	0.2	0	3	132	9	268	0.5	2.8	92	1	0.09	1	0.11	0.02	0.6	0.08	126	0
5.4	1.9	97	68	179	432	557	2.6	1.8	40	105	0.81	6	0.15	0.31	4.1	0.23	45	1.41
10.3	1.7	299	202	259	87	297	1.4	1.3	44	323	0.98	1	0.08	0.41	0.3	0.13	32	0.93
3	1	45	480	—	384	92	—	0.1	—	540	—	0	—	—	—	—	—	—
1.1	1.4	17	32	112	255	70	0.3	0.9	9	5	0.6	1	0.08	0.07	0.6	0.01	26	0.33
1.6	1.4	21	11	85	197	35	0.2	0.5	5	10	0.63	0	0.07	0.14	1	0.03	5	0.04
1.5	3.1	21	108	83	251	70	0.3	1.3	9	22	0.97	1	0.16	0.16	1.3	0.02	27	0.08
1.2	2.4	18	85	65	198	55	0.2	1	7	13	0.81	1	0.12	0.13	1	0.02	5	0.06
2.4	1.3	21	88	85	284	106	0.5	1	31	14	0.6	0	0.1	0.12	1.1	0.07	8	0.07
1.6	3.6	18	82	69	251	112	0.3	1.2	10	263	0.61	1	0.15	0.15	1.2	0.04	7	0.08
3	1.4	30	111	115	274	80	0.5	1.3	11	35	0.6	0	0.16	0.2	1.3	0.03	8	0.11
3	1.4	24	74	75	186	92	0.4	1.4	16	17	0.65	0	0.17	0.18	1.4	0.03	7	0.09
1.2	1.8	15	42	162	297	39	0.3	1.6	18	20	1.05	0	0.16	0.19	1.2	0.05	35	0.05
2.4	0.6	28	34	173	358	59	0.3	0.9	9	20	0.68	0	0.11	0.12	0.9	0.05	5	0.07
1.7	3.5	24	148	101	333	83	0.3	1.5	13	29	1.03	0	0.17	0.18	1.4	0.05	35	0.09
1.4	2.8	20	116	79	263	65	0.3	1.2	10	18	0.86	0	0.14	0.14	1.1	0.04	8	0.07
2	1.1	39	81	72	326	71	0.3	1.2	9	23	0.61	0	0.16	0.18	1.3	0.03	8	0.11
—	—	95	150	—	750	—	—	1.8	—	0	—	0	—	—	—	—	—	—
1	2.4	0	36	214	224	289	1	2.4	90	0	0.75	0	0.15	0.05	0.2	0.09	30	0.01
1.2	0.7	18	69	62	161	58	0.3	0.9	10	13	0.32	0	0.13	0.13	0.9	0.02	6	0.07
1.6	3.3	22	114	87	266	69	0.3	1.4	10	23	1.03	0	0.16	0.17	1.3	0.02	29	0.09
1.3	2.6	19	90	68	210	54	0.3	1.1	7	13	0.81	0	0.13	0.14	1	0.02	5	0.07
1	2.1	26	31	40	154	87	0.2	1.1	9	331	0.59	1	0.1	0.11	0.8	0.03	6	0.05
0.7	1.8	2	4	20	158	27	0.1	0.2	4	22	0.57	0	0.08	0.1	0.7	0.01	18	0.01
0.7	1.7	2	4	60	158	27	0.1	0.2	5	20	0.24	0	0.06	0.09	0.6	0.01	15	0
0.9	2.1	4	6	50	142	30	0.1	0.5	5	7	0.53	0	0.1	0.12	0.8	0.02	19	0.01
0.9	1.9	2	6	80	142	30	0.1	0.5	4	6	0.5	0	0.08	0.11	0.7	0.01	3	0.01
0.7	1.7	6	13	71	178	60	0.2	1	11	18	0.62	0	0.09	0.11	0.9	0.04	12	0.01
0.8	1.7	3	13	97	179	60	0.2	1	7	16	0.42	0	0.07	0.1	0.8	0.02	7	0.01
2.1	0.6	31	14	150	210	66	0.5	1.1	26	14	0.68	0	0.09	0.11	1.3	0.08	7	0.06
1.7	3.6	19	107	162	335	181	1.6	2.4	44	143	1.31	4	0.19	0.25	2.3	0.18	30	0.08
1.4	2.8	16	84	128	265	143	1.2	1.9	35	108	1.04	4	0.15	0.2	1.8	0.14	23	0.06
2.3	1.4	21	89	110	283	119	0.7	0.9	31	14	0.7	0	0.08	0.09	1.2	0.07	9	0.07
2.6	5.7	37	41	44	169	69	0.3	1.2	8	22	0.84	1	0.12	0.12	0.9	0.03	9	0.07
0	0.1	0	27	27	7	136	0.1	1.3	13	2	0.32	26	0.02	0.07	0.4	0.04	4	0
0	0.1	0	5	68	2	278	0.7	1.4	9	0	0.09	3	0.06	0.23	3.5	0.07	14	0
0	0.1	0	2	36	1	130	0.3	0.4	4	0	0.04	1	0.04	0.16	1.4	0.03	7	0
0	0.1	0	4	81	3	289	0.6	1	8	0	0.09	2	0.07	0.34	3.1	0.07	14	0
0	0.1	0	4	81	3	289	0.6	1	8	0	0.09	2	0.07	0.33	3.1	0.07	13	0
3	6.4	14	54	103	121	180	0.4	0.8	8	10	0.92	1	0.07	0.22	1.6	0.05	8	0.06
2.3	2	1	34	—	23	—	—	8.2	—	2	—	1	—	—	—	—	—	0

A

Esha Code	Food Item	Qty	Meas	Wgt (g)	Wtr (g)	Cals	Prot (g)	Carb (g)	Fib (g)	Fat (g)	SatF (g)
5440	Mushroom, enoki, raw	1	each	3	3	1	0	0	0.1	0	0
6110	Mushroom, oyster, dried	0.5	cup	72	5	262	20	39	7.5	3	0.3
6115	Mushroom, patty straw, dried	0.5	cup	72	9	228	17	35	5.2	2	0.4
6494	Mushroom, raw, sliced	0.5	cup	34	31	8	1	2	0.4	0	0
5385	Mushroom, shiitake, cooked pieces	0.5	cup	72	60	40	1	10	1.5	0	0
5384	Mushroom, shiitake, cooked, whole	4	each	72	60	40	1	10	1.5	0	0
5383	Mushroom, shiitake, dried	4	each	15	1	44	1	11	1.7	0	0
6114	Mushroom, shiitake, dried	0.5	cup	72	9	241	19	37	9.1	2	0.3
5615	Mushroom, whole, pickled	1	each	12	11	3	0	1	0.1	0	0
5094	Mushrooms, canned, drained	0.5	cup	78	71	19	1	4	1.9	0	0
5095	Mushrooms, canned, drained	10	each	120	109	29	2	6	2.9	0	0
5093	Mushrooms, whole, cooked, drained	10	each	120	109	32	3	6	2.6	1	0.1
5091	Mushrooms, whole, raw	5	each	90	83	22	2	4	1.1	0	0
5096	Mustard greens, cooked, drained, no added salt	0.5	cup	70	66	10	2	1	1.4	0	0
5097	Mustard greens, frozen, cooked, drained	0.5	cup	75	70	14	2	2	2.1	0	0
5207	Mustard greens, raw	0.5	cup	28	25	7	1	1	0.9	0	0
26110	Mustard seed, yellow	1	tsp	4	0	18	1	1	0.5	1	0.1
6313	Mustard, Chinese Gai Choy	1	tsp	5	5	1	0	0	—	0	—
27094	Mustard, brown, prepared	1	tsp	5	4	5	0	0	0.1	0	0
27005	Mustard, yellow, prepared	1	tsp	5	4	4	0	0	0.1	0	0
49041	Nacho chips, w/cinnamon & sugar	7	piece	109	1	592	7	63	3.3	36	18.2
56639	Nachos, w/cheese	7	piece	113	46	346	9	36	—	19	7.8
3215	Nectarine, fresh	1	each	136	117	67	1	16	2.2	1	0.1
38150	Noodle roni, prepared	0.5	cup	82	55	123	4	20	1.8	3	0.6
38094	Noodles, Japanese soba, buckwheat, cooked	0.5	cup	57	42	56	3	12	0.6	0	0
38095	Noodles, Japanese somen, wheat, cooked	0.5	cup	88	60	115	4	24	1.4	0	0
38067	Noodles, Ramen, cooked	5	cup	114	93	78	3	15	1.4	1	0.2
38219	Noodles, buckwheat, dry, cooked	0.5	cup	70	50	81	2	17	0.1	0	—
38048	Noodles, chow mein, dry	0.25	cup	11	0	59	1	6	0.4	3	0.5
38047	Noodles, egg, enriched, cooked	0.5	cup	80	55	106	4	20	0.9	1	0.2
38149	Noodles, mug-o-lunch, prepared	1	each	198	132	295	9	48	4.2	7	1.5
38147	Noodles, rice, cooked	0.5	cup	80	65	62	0	15	0.1	0	0
38210	Noodles, rice, freshly made	0.5	cup	70	36	142	2	32	0.4	0	—
26026	Nutmeg, ground	0.25	tsp	1	0	3	0	0	0.1	0	0.2
38078	Oat bran, cooked	1	Tbs	14	12	5	0	2	0.4	0	0
38064	Oat bran, dry	2	Tbs	12	1	29	2	8	1.8	1	0.2
38043	Oats, rolled, baked value	1	cup	80	7	307	13	54	8.5	5	0.9
38008	Oats, rolled, dry	0.25	cup	20	2	78	3	14	2.2	1	0.2
38080	Oats, whole grain	0.5	cup	78	6	303	13	52	8.3	5	1
8078	Oil, almond	1	Tbs	14	0	120	0	0	0	14	1.1
8079	Oil, apricot kernel	1	Tbs	14	0	120	0	0	0	14	0.9
8031	Oil, butter	1	Tbs	13	0	112	0	0	0	13	7.9
8084	Oil, canola	1	Tbs	14	0	120	0	0	0	14	1
8080	Oil, cocoa butter	1	Tbs	14	0	120	0	0	0	14	8.1
8037	Oil, coconut	1	Tbs	14	0	117	0	0	0	14	11.8
8067	Oil, cod liver	1	Tbs	14	0	123	0	0	0	14	3.1
8009	Oil, corn	1	Tbs	14	0	120	0	0	0	14	1.7
8081	Oil, cottonseed	1	Tbs	14	0	120	0	0	0	14	3.5
8047	Oil, grapeseed	1	Tbs	14	0	120	0	0	0	14	1.3
8071	Oil, herring	1	Tbs	14	0	123	0	0	0	14	2.9
8072	Oil, menhaden, not fully hydrogenated	1	Tbs	14	0	123	0	0	0	14	4.1
8008	Oil, olive	1	Tbs	14	0	119	0	0	0	14	1.8
8082	Oil, palm	1	Tbs	14	0	120	0	0	0	14	6.7
8083	Oil, palm kernel	1	Tbs	14	0	117	0	0	0	14	11.1
8026	Oil, peanut	1	Tbs	14	0	119	0	0	0	14	2.3
8010	Oil, safflower	1	Tbs	14	0	120	0	0	0	14	1.2
8073	Oil, salmon	1	Tbs	14	0	123	0	0	0	14	2.7
8074	Oil, sardine	1	Tbs	14	0	123	0	0	0	14	4.1
8027	Oil, sesame	1	Tbs	14	0	120	0	0	0	14	1.9
8028	Oil, soybean & cottonseed	1	Tbs	14	0	120	0	0	0	14	2.4
8012	Oil, soybean (Crisco/Wesson)	1	Tbs	14	0	120	0	0	0	14	2
8011	Oil, sunflower (Wesson Sunlite)	1	Tbs	14	0	120	0	0	0	14	1.4
8085	Oil, walnut	1	Tbs	14	0	120	0	0	0	14	1.2
8038	Oil, wheat germ	1	Tbs	14	0	120	0	0	0	14	2.6
5100	Okra pods, frozen, cooked, drained	0.5	cup	92	84	26	2	5	2.6	0	0.1

MonoF (g)	PolyF (g)	Choles (mg)	Calc (mg)	Phos (mg)	Sod (mg)	Pot (mg)	Zn (mg)	Iron (mg)	Magn (mg)	VitA (μg RE)	VitE (mg α-TE)	VitC (mg)	Thia (mg)	Ribo (mg)	Nia (mg)	B6 (mg)	Fola (μg)	B12 (μg)
0	0	0	0	3	0	11	0	0	0	0	0	0	0	0	0.1	0	1	0
0.7	1.9	1	7	—	70	—	—	6.8	—	1	—	5	—	—	—	—	—	0
0.1	1.6	1	29	—	65	—	—	45.9	—	1	—	1	—	—	—	—	—	0
0	0.1	0	2	35	1	126	0.2	0.4	3	0	0.04	1	0.04	0.15	1.4	0.03	7	0
0	0	0	2	21	3	85	1	0.3	10	0	0.09	0	0.03	0.12	1.1	0.12	15	0
0	0	0	2	21	3	84	1	0.3	10	0	0.09	0	0.03	0.12	1.1	0.11	15	0
0	0	0	2	44	2	230	1.2	0.3	20	0	0.02	1	0.04	0.19	2.1	0.14	24	0
0.1	1.5	1	28	—	61	—	—	11.5	—	1	—	1	—	—	—	—	—	0
0	0	0	1	10	24	36	0.1	0.1	1	0	0.01	0	0.01	0.04	0.4	0.01	1	0
0	0.1	0	9	52	332	101	0.6	0.6	12	0	0.09	0	0.07	0.02	1.2	0.05	10	0
0	0.1	0	13	79	510	155	0.9	0.9	18	0	0.14	0	0.1	0.02	1.9	0.07	15	0
0	0.2	0	7	104	2	427	1	2.1	14	0	0.14	5	0.09	0.36	5.4	0.11	22	0
0	0.2	0	4	94	4	333	0.7	1.1	9	0	0.11	3	0.09	0.4	3.7	0.09	19	0
0.1	0	0	52	29	11	141	0.1	0.5	10	212	1.41	18	0.03	0.04	0.3	0.07	51	0
0.1	0	0	76	18	19	104	0.2	0.8	10	335	1.31	10	0.03	0.04	0.2	0.08	52	0
0	0	0	29	12	7	99	0.1	0.4	9	148	0.56	20	0.02	0.03	0.2	0.05	52	0
0.7	0.2	0	19	31	0	25	0.2	0.4	11	0	0.09	0	0.02	0.01	0.3	0.01	3	0
—	—	—	—	—	—	—	—	—	—	—	—	—	—	—	—	—	—	0
0	0.2	0	6	7	65	6	—	0.1	—	0	—	0	0	0	0	—	—	—
0.2	0	0	4	4	65	7	0	0.1	2	0	0.09	0	0	0	0	0	0	0
11.9	4.1	39	85	33	439	78	0.6	2.9	20	11	—	8	0.18	0.45	3.9	0.17	8	1.72
8	2.2	18	272	276	816	172	1.8	1.3	55	92	—	1	0.19	0.37	1.5	0.2	10	0.82
0.2	0.3	0	7	22	0	288	0.1	0.2	11	101	1.21	7	0.02	0.06	1.4	0.03	5	0
1.2	0.9	26	10	56	163	23	0.5	1.3	15	30	0.34	0	0.15	0.07	1.2	0.03	6	0.07
0	0	0	2	14	34	20	0.1	0.3	5	0	—	0	0.05	0.02	0.3	0.02	4	0
0	0.1	0	7	24	142	26	0.2	0.5	2	0	0.01	0	0.02	0.03	0.1	0.01	2	0
0.2	0.2	19	10	41	675	25	0.4	0.9	12	102	0.04	0	0.11	0.05	0.9	0.03	5	0.05
—	—	—	7	56	—	—	—	0.7	—	—	—	0	0.04	0.02	0.3	—	—	—
0.9	2	0	2	18	49	14	0.2	0.5	6	1	0.02	0	0.06	0.05	0.7	0.01	10	0
0.3	0.3	26	10	55	6	22	0.5	1.3	15	5	0.04	0	0.15	0.07	1.2	0.03	51	0.07
2.8	2.2	63	25	133	391	56	1.2	3	37	72	0.82	0	0.36	0.16	2.8	0.07	14	0.18
0	0	0	5	5	3	1	0.1	0.3	1	0	0.02	0	0.02	0	0	0.01	0	0
—	—	—	7	26	—	—	—	1.7	—	—	—	0	0.03	0.01	0.9	—	—	—
0	0	0	1	1	0	2	0	0	1	0	0.02	0	0	0	0	0	0	0
0	0	0	1	16	0	13	0.1	0.1	5	0	0.03	0	0.02	0	0	0	1	0
0.3	0.3	0	7	86	0	66	0.4	0.6	28	0	0.2	0	0.14	0.03	0.1	0.02	6	0
1.6	1.8	0	42	379	3	280	2.5	3.4	118	8	0.91	0	0.47	0.1	0.6	0.09	18	0
0.4	0.5	0	10	96	1	71	0.6	0.9	30	2	0.14	0	0.15	0.03	0.2	0.02	6	0
1.7	2	0	42	408	2	335	3.1	3.7	138	0	0.55	0	0.6	0.11	0.8	0.09	44	0
9.5	2.4	0	0	0	0	0	0	0	0	0	5.36	0	0	0	0	0	0	0
8.2	4	0	0	0	0	0	0	0	0	0	1.18	0	0	0	0	0	0	0
3.7	0.5	33	0	0	0	1	0	0	0	118	0.36	0	0	0	0	0	0	0
8	4	0	0	0	0	0	0	0	0	0	2.86	0	0	0	0	0	0	0
4.5	0.4	0	0	0	0	0	0	0	0	0	0.24	0	0	0	0	0	0	0
0.8	0.2	0	0	0	0	0	0	0	0	0	0.04	0	0	0	0	0	0	0
6.4	3.1	78	0	0	0	0	0	0	0	4080	2.99	0	0	0	0	0	0	0
3.3	8	0	0	0	0	0	0	0	0	0	2.88	0	0	0	0	0	0	0
2.4	7.1	0	0	0	0	0	0	0	0	0	5.22	0	0	0	0	0	0	0
2.2	9.5	0	0	0	0	0	0	0	0	0	4.36	0	0	0	0	0	0	0
7.7	2.1	104	0	0	0	0	0	0	0	0	1.25	0	0	0	0	0	0	0
3.6	4.6	71	0	0	0	0	0	0	0	0	1.77	0	0	0	0	0	0	0
10	1.1	0	0	0	0	0	0	0.1	0	0	1.67	0	0	0	0	0	0	0
5	1.3	0	0	0	0	0	0	0	0	0	2.97	0	0	0	0	0	0	0
1.6	0.2	0	0	0	0	0	0	0	0	0	0.52	0	0	0	0	0	0	0
6.2	4.3	0	0	0	0	0	0	0	0	0	1.74	0	0	0	0	0	0	0
1.6	10.2	0	0	0	0	0	0	0	0	0	5.87	0	0	0	0	0	0	0
3.9	5.5	66	0	0	0	0	0	0	0	0	2.6	0	0	0	0	0	0	0
4.6	4.3	97	0	0	0	0	0	0	0	0	1.63	0	0	0	0	0	0	0
5.4	5.7	0	0	0	0	0	0	0	0	0	0.56	0	0	0	0	0	0	0
4	6.6	0	0	0	0	0	0	0	0	0	3.84	0	0	0	0	0	0	0
3.2	7.9	0	0	0	0	0	0	0	0	0	2.48	0	0	0	0	0	0	0
2.7	9	0	0	0	0	0	0	0	0	0	6.9	0	0	0	0	0	0	0
3.1	8.6	0	0	0	0	0	0	0	0	0	0.44	0	0	0	0	0	0	0
2	8.4	0	0	0	0	0	0	0	0	0	26.1	0	0	0	0	0	0	0
0	0.1	0	88	42	3	215	0.6	0.6	47	47	0.64	11	0.09	0.11	0.7	0.04	134	0

Esha Code	Food Item	Qty	Meas	Wgt (g)	Wtr (g)	Cals	Prot (g)	Carb (g)	Fib (g)	Fat (g)	SatF (g)
5528	Okra, Chinese/luffa, cooked	0.5	cup	89	80	28	2	6	2.8	0	0
5644	Okra, batter-dipped, fried	0.5	cup	46	32	88	1	6	1	7	1.1
5098	Okra, fresh pods, cooked, drained	8	each	85	76	27	2	6	2.1	0	0
5099	Okra, fresh slices, cooked, drained	0.5	cup	80	72	26	2	6	2	0	0
27008	Olive, green, no pits	10	each	39	30	45	1	1	0.4	5	0.5
27042	Olive, green, stuffed	5	each	20	16	21	0	0	0.2	2	0.2
27022	Olive, ripe, jumbo/super colossal	1	each	15	13	12	0	1	0.4	1	0.1
27009	Olive, ripe, large, no pits	10	each	45	36	52	0	3	1.4	5	0.6
27010	Olive, ripe, large, no pits, slices	0.5	cup	68	54	78	1	4	2.2	7	1
6486	Olives, Calamata	1	oz.	28	16	80	0	3	0.2	7	0.9
5113	Onion flakes, dehydrated	0.25	cup	14	1	49	1	12	1.3	0	0
26008	Onion powder	0.25	tsp	1	0	2	0	0	0	0	0
6186	Onion rings, breaded, fried, serving	8.5	piece	83	31	276	4	31	—	16	7
6176	Onion rings, breaded, fried, svg	1	each	83	31	276	4	31	—	16	7
5190	Onion rings, heated from frozen	2	each	20	6	81	1	8	0.3	5	1.7
5111	Onion slices, cooked	2	piece	24	21	11	0	2	0.3	0	0
5106	Onion slices, raw	1	piece	14	13	5	0	1	0.3	0	0
5575	Onion, canned w/liquid	1	each	63	59	12	1	3	0.8	0	0
5300	Onion, chopped, frozen, cooked	0.5	cup	105	97	29	1	7	1.9	0	0
5649	Onion, chopped, steamed	0.5	cup	105	94	40	1	9	1.9	0	0
5650	Onion, chopped, stir fried	0.5	cup	105	94	40	1	9	1.9	0	0
5532	Onion, creamed	0.5	cup	114	94	100	3	11	1.3	5	1.7
5110	Onion, medium size, cooked	1	each	94	83	41	1	10	1.3	0	0
5529	Onion, pearl, cooked, whole	3	each	45	39	20	1	5	0.7	0	0
5101	Onion, raw, chopped	0.5	cup	80	72	30	1	7	1.4	0	0
6491	Onion, raw, red, chopped	0.5	cup	80	72	30	1	7	1.4	0	0
5104	Onion, raw, whole, medium size	1	each	110	99	42	1	9	2	0	0
5103	Onion, red, raw	0.5	cup	80	72	30	1	7	1.4	0	0
140	Onion, red, slices	2	piece	28	25	11	0	2	0.5	0	0
141	Onion, red, whole	1	each	110	99	42	1	9	2	0	0
5114	Onion, spring/green, chopped	0.5	cup	50	45	16	1	4	1.3	0	0
5210	Onion, spring/green, top only	0.5	cup	50	46	17	1	3	1.2	0	0.1
5209	Onion, spring/green, white part	0.5	cup	50	46	25	0	5	1.2	0	0
5576	Onion, welsh, raw	0.5	cup	80	72	27	2	5	1.1	0	0.1
5301	Onion, whole, frozen, cooked	1	each	63	58	18	0	4	0.9	0	0
5108	Onions, cooked, drained	0.5	cup	105	92	46	1	11	1.5	0	0
20058	Orange & apricot juice drink, canned	1	cup	250	217	128	1	32	0.2	0	0
20211	Orange Julius	1	cup	215	183	133	0	33	0.2	0	0.1
20111	Orange breakfast drink, frozen, prepared	1	cup	248	216	122	0	30	0.2	0	0.1
20107	Orange breakfast drink, powder	1	Tbs	12	0	44	0	11	0	0	0
20004	Orange breakfast drink, prepared w/water	1	cup	248	218	114	0	29	0	0	0
20070	Orange drink, Sunny Delight	1	cup	249	216	127	0	32	0.2	0	0
20029	Orange drink, carbonated	1	cup	248	217	119	0	30	0	0	0
20113	Orange drink, frozen, prepared	1	cup	248	218	112	0	28	0	0	0
20070	Orange drink/Sunny Delight	1	cup	248	216	126	0	32	0.2	0	0
23237	Orange peel, candied	1.5	oz.	43	7	134	0	34	—	0	0
3088	Orange peel, fresh, grated	1	Tbs	6	4	6	0	2	0.6	0	0
3083	Orange sections, fresh, cup measure	0.5	cup	90	78	42	1	11	2.2	0	0
3228	Orange, California Navel	1	each	140	122	64	1	16	3.4	0	0
3229	Orange, California Valencia	1	each	121	104	59	1	14	3	0	0
3230	Orange, Florida	1	each	151	132	70	1	17	3.6	0	0
3082	Orange, fresh	1	each	131	114	62	1	16	3.1	0	0
3089	Orange, mandarin, canned	0.5	cup	126	113	47	1	12	0.9	0	0
3170	Orange-grapefruit juice, canned	0.5	cup	124	109	53	1	13	0.1	0	0
26487	Oregano, Mexican	0.25	tsp	0	0	1	0	0	0.1	0	—
26310	Oregano, fresh	0.25	cup	18	15	12	0	2	—	0	—
26009	Oregano, ground	0.25	tsp	0	0	1	0	0	0.2	0	0
44036	Oriental snack mix	1	oz.	28	1	156	5	15	3.7	7	1.1
19403	Oysters rockefeller	0.5	cup	112	84	131	8	11	1.8	6	2.4
5522	Palm heart, cooked slices	0.5	cup	73	51	75	2	19	1.1	0	0.1
45000	Pancake mix, buckwheat, prepared	1	each	27	14	56	2	8	0.6	2	0.5
45044	Pancake, Chinese	1	each	28	14	58	1	13	0.2	0	0
45006	Pancake, French/crepe	1	each	102	57	239	9	22	0.6	12	4
45045	Pancake, Indian	1	each	29	16	52	2	10	0.7	0	0.2
45023	Pancake, blueberry, recipe	2	each	76	40	169	5	22	0.9	7	1.5

MonoF	PolyF	Choles	Calc	Phos	Sod	Pot	Zn	Iron	Magn	VitA	VitE	VitC	Thia	Ribo	Nia	B6	Fola	B12
(g)	(g)	(mg)	(mg)	(mg)	(mg)	(mg)	(mg)	(mg)	(mg)	(μg RE)	(mg α-TE)	(mg)	(mg)	(mg)	(mg)	(mg)	(μg)	(μg)
0	0	0	56	50	210	285	0.5	0.4	50	51	0.61	14	0.12	0.05	0.8	0.17	40	0
1.7	3.6	8	52	53	68	107	0.2	0.4	18	21	1.54	5	0.07	0.05	0.4	0.06	19	0.04
0	0	0	54	48	4	274	0.5	0.4	48	49	0.59	14	0.11	0.05	0.7	0.16	39	0
0	0	0	50	45	4	258	0.4	0.4	46	46	0.55	13	0.11	0.04	0.7	0.15	37	0
3.8	0.3	0	24	7	936	22	0	0.6	9	12	1.17	0	0	0	0	0.01	0	0
1.6	0.2	0	11	3	413	16	0	0.3	4	12	0.54	3	0	0	0	0.01	1	0
0.8	0.1	0	14	0	136	1	0	0.5	1	5	0.46	0	0	0	0	0	0	0
3.6	0.4	0	40	1	392	4	0.1	1.5	2	18	1.35	0	0	0	0	0	0	0
5.3	0.6	0	59	2	589	5	0.1	2.2	3	27	2.03	1	0	0	0	0.01	0	0
5.7	0.9	0	10	—	462	—	—	0.2	—	2	—	0	—	—	—	—	—	—
0	0	0	36	42	3	227	0.3	0.2	13	0	0.19	10	0.07	0.01	0.1	0.22	23	0
0	0	0	2	2	0	5	0	0	1	0	0	0	0	0	0	0.01	1	0
6.6	0.7	14	73	86	430	129	0.3	0.8	16	1	0.33	1	0.08	0.1	0.9	0.06	55	0.12
6.6	0.7	14	73	86	430	129	0.3	0.8	16	1	0.33	1	0.08	0.1	0.9	0.06	55	0.12
2.2	1	0	6	16	75	26	0.1	0.3	4	5	0.14	0	0.06	0.03	0.7	0.02	13	0
0	0	0	5	8	1	40	0	0.1	3	0	0.03	1	0.01	0.01	0	0.03	4	0
0	0	0	3	5	0	22	0	0	1	0	0.02	1	0.01	0	0	0.02	3	0
0	0	0	28	18	234	70	0.2	0.1	4	0	0.05	3	0.02	0	0	0.09	6	0
0	0	0	17	20	13	113	0.1	0.3	6	3	0.2	3	0.02	0.03	0.1	0.07	14	0
0	0.1	0	21	35	3	165	0.2	0.2	10	0	0.33	5	0.04	0.02	0.1	0.12	16	0
0	0.1	0	21	35	3	165	0.2	0.2	10	0	0.33	5	0.04	0.02	0.1	0.12	16	0
2.2	1.3	5	65	64	334	177	0.3	0.3	13	58	0.66	4	0.05	0.09	0.2	0.11	13	0.14
0	0.1	0	21	33	3	156	0.2	0.2	10	0	0.12	5	0.04	0.02	0.2	0.12	14	0
0	0	0	10	16	105	74	0.1	0.1	5	0	0.06	2	0.02	0.01	0.1	0.06	7	0
0	0	0	16	26	2	126	0.2	0.2	8	0	0.1	5	0.03	0.02	0.1	0.09	15	0
0	0	0	16	26	2	126	0.2	0.2	8	0	0.1	5	0.03	0.02	0.1	0.09	15	0
0	0.1	0	22	36	3	173	0.2	0.2	11	0	0.14	7	0.05	0.02	0.2	0.13	21	0
0	0	0	16	26	2	126	0.2	0.2	8	0	0.1	5	0.03	0.02	0.1	0.09	15	0
0	0	0	6	9	1	44	0.1	0.1	3	0	0.04	2	0.01	0.01	0	0.03	5	0
0	0.1	0	22	36	3	173	0.2	0.2	11	0	0.14	7	0.05	0.02	0.2	0.13	21	0
0	0	0	36	18	8	138	0.2	0.7	10	20	0.06	9	0.03	0.04	0.3	0.03	32	0
0	0.1	0	28	20	4	130	0.1	1.1	10	20	0.15	26	0.04	0.05	0.3	0	40	0
0	0	0	20	20	4	115	0.1	0.4	8	0	0.06	13	0.03	0.02	0.2	0.05	18	0
0	0.1	0	14	39	14	170	0.4	1	18	93	0.04	22	0.04	0.07	0.3	0.06	13	0
0	0	0	17	1	5	64	0.1	0.2	5	1	0.08	3	0.01	0.01	0.1	0.04	8	0
0	0.1	0	23	37	3	174	0.2	0.3	12	0	0.14	5	0.04	0.02	0.2	0.14	16	0
0.1	0.1	0	12	20	5	200	0.1	0.2	10	145	0	50	0.05	0.02	0.5	0.07	14	0
0	0	0	32	—	8	145	—	0.1	—	0	—	29	0.07	0.07	—	0.04	—	0
0.2	0.1	0	82	55	22	308	0.1	0.2	2	0	0.74	172	0.3	0.09	0	0	56	0
0	0	0	44	20	1	23	0	0	0	72	0.96	29	0	0.08	1	0.1	0	0
0	0	0	62	37	12	50	0.1	0.2	2	551	0	121	0	0.04	0	0	143	0
0	0	0	15	2	40	45	0.2	0.7	5	5	0	85	0.02	0.01	0.1	0.02	5	0
0	0	0	12	2	30	5	0.2	0.1	2	0	0	0	0	0	0	0	0	0
0	0	0	290	82	25	335	0.1	0.2	27	2	0.01	137	0.26	2.58	0.6	0.18	80	0
0	0	0	15	2	40	45	0.2	0.7	5	5	0	85	0.02	0.01	0.1	0.02	5	0
—	—	0	0	0	0	0	—	0	—	0	—	0	0	0	0	—	—	—
0	0	0	10	1	0	13	0	0	1	3	0.01	8	0.01	0	0.1	0.01	2	0
0	0	0	36	13	0	163	0.1	0.1	9	19	0.22	48	0.08	0.04	0.3	0.05	27	0
0	0	0	56	27	1	249	0.1	0.2	14	25	0.17	80	0.12	0.06	0.4	0.1	47	0
0.1	0.1	0	48	21	0	217	0.1	0.1	12	28	0.36	59	0.1	0.05	0.3	0.08	47	0
0.1	0.1	0	65	18	0	255	0.1	0.1	15	30	0.36	68	0.15	0.06	0.6	0.08	26	0
0	0	0	52	18	0	237	0.1	0.1	13	28	0.31	70	0.11	0.05	0.4	0.08	40	0
0	0	0	14	13	6	168	0.6	0.3	14	107	0.63	43	0.1	0.04	0.6	0.05	6	0
0	0	0	10	17	4	195	0.1	0.6	12	15	0.09	36	0.07	0.04	0.4	0.03	18	0
—	—	—	4	—	0	—	—	0.1	—	3	—	0	—	—	—	—	—	0
—	—	—	56	7	1	59	0.2	—	10	24	—	8	0.01	—	—	—	—	0
0	0	0	6	1	0	6	0	0.2	1	3	0.01	0	0	0	0	0	1	0
2.8	3	0	15	74	117	93	0.8	0.7	34	0	2.39	0	0.09	0.04	0.9	0.02	11	0
2.1	1	39	89	130	445	331	50.2	5.1	62	423	1.05	16	0.19	0.21	1.8	0.12	64	10.6
0	0	0	13	102	10	1318	2.7	1.2	7	5	0.36	5	0.03	0.12	0.6	0.53	15	0
0.5	0.8	18	69	110	144	63	0.3	0.5	15	18	0.56	0	0.05	0.07	0.4	0.04	5	0.09
0	0	0	5	18	1	18	0.2	0.1	4	0	0.02	0	0.01	0.01	0.3	0.03	1	0
4.9	2.4	163	93	145	274	159	0.8	1.6	17	88	1.43	0	0.17	0.37	1.3	0.08	19	0.48
0.1	0.1	1	29	40	59	84	0.3	0.2	10	2	0.06	0	0.04	0.04	0.3	0.04	9	0.08
1.8	3.2	43	157	115	313	105	0.4	1.3	12	39	0.76	2	0.15	0.21	1.2	0.04	27	0.15

Esha Code	Food Item	Qty	Meas	Wgt (g)	Wtr (g)	Cals	Prot (g)	Carb (g)	Fib (g)	Fat (g)	SatF (g)
45025	Pancake, buttermilk, recipe	2	each	76	40	173	5	22	0.6	7	1.4
45034	Pancake, cornmeal	1	each	21	12	43	1	7	0.3	1	0.3
45067	Pancake, frozen, ready to eat, 6 inch	2	each	146	66	334	8	64	2.6	5	1.1
45021	Pancake, mix, incomplete, prepared	2	each	76	40	166	6	22	1.4	6	1.6
45027	Pancake, mix, prepared, low calorie	2	each	44	22	88	2	19	0.7	0	0.1
45002	Pancake, plain, mix, prepared	1	each	27	14	52	1	10	0.4	1	0.1
45001	Pancake, plain, recipe	1	each	27	14	61	2	8	0.4	3	0.6
45036	Pancake, rye, 4 inch	1	each	21	7	63	1	9	0.6	2	0.6
45035	Pancake, sourdough, 4 inch	1	each	21	11	46	1	7	0.3	1	0.3
45008	Pancake, whole wheat, mix, prepared	1	each	52	28	108	4	15	1.5	3	0.9
45069	Pancakes w/butter & syrup, Fast Food	3	each	232	101	582	9	105	2	14	2.5
42190	Pannetone-Italian sweetbread	1	piece	27	8	86	2	15	0.7	2	1.2
3095	Papaya nectar, canned	1	cup	250	213	143	0	36	1.5	0	0.1
3172	Papaya, fresh slices	0.5	cup	70	62	27	0	7	1.3	0	0
3171	Papaya, whole, fresh	1	each	304	270	119	2	30	5.5	0	0.1
26010	Paprika	0.25	tsp	1	0	2	0	0	0.1	0	0
26035	Parsley, dried	0.25	tsp	0	0	0	0	0	0	0	0
26011	Parsley, freeze dried	0.25	tsp	0	0	0	0	0	0	0	0
26013	Parsley, fresh sprigs	10	each	10	9	4	0	1	0.3	0	0
26012	Parsley, fresh, chopped	0.5	cup	30	26	11	1	2	1	0	0
5212	Parsnip, cooked from raw, drained	0.5	cup	78	61	63	1	15	3.1	0	0
5211	Parsnip, sliced, raw	0.5	cup	66	53	50	1	12	3.3	0	0
3199	Passion fruit, purple, fresh	1	each	18	13	18	0	4	1.9	0	0
38060	Pasta, spaghetti, whole wheat, cooked	0.5	cup	70	47	87	4	19	3.2	0	0.1
38066	Pasta/Noodle, spaghetti, spinach, cooked	0.5	cup	70	48	91	3	18	2.4	0	0.1
38146	Pasta/Noodles, cellophane, cooked	0.5	cup	95	75	80	0	20	0.1	0	0
38152	Pasta/Noodles, corn-based, cooked	0.5	cup	60	41	75	2	17	2.9	0	0.1
38153	Pasta/Noodles, corn-based, spaghetti, cooked	0.5	cup	60	41	75	2	17	2.9	0	0.1
38310	Pasta/Noodles, egg, fried	0.5	cup	84	63	129	2	10	0.4	10	1.7
38160	Pasta/Noodles, egg, spinach, cooked	0.5	cup	80	55	106	4	19	1.8	1	0.3
38092	Pasta/Noodles, fresh, cooked	2	oz.	57	39	74	3	14	1	1	0.1
38159	Pasta/Noodles, homemade w/egg, cooked	0.5	cup	80	55	104	4	19	3.1	1	0.3
38093	Pasta/Noodles, homemade, no egg, cooked	2	oz.	57	39	70	2	14	0.9	1	0.1
38109	Pasta/Noodles, jumbo shells, enriched, cooked	2.5	oz.	70	46	99	3	20	0.9	0	0.1
38108	Pasta/Noodles, lasagna cuts, cooked	0.5	cup	70	46	99	3	20	0.9	0	0.1
38103	Pasta/Noodles, lasagna, enriched, cooked	2.5	oz.	70	46	99	3	20	0.9	0	0.1
38119	Pasta/Noodles, linguini, cooked	0.5	cup	70	46	99	3	20	1.2	0	0.1
38151	Pasta/Noodles, macaroni, corn-based, cooked	0.5	cup	60	41	75	2	17	2.9	0	0.1
38102	Pasta/Noodles, macaroni, enriched, cooked	1	cup	140	92	197	7	40	1.8	1	0.1
38117	Pasta/Noodles, macaroni, vegetable, cooked	0.5	cup	67	46	86	3	18	2.9	0	0
38104	Pasta/Noodles, rotini, enriched, cooked	0.5	cup	70	46	99	3	20	0.9	0	0.1
38105	Pasta/Noodles, small shells, enriched, cooked	0.5	cup	58	38	81	3	16	0.7	0	0.1
38118	Pasta/Noodles, spaghetti, cooked	0.5	cup	70	46	99	3	20	1.2	0	0.1
38121	Pasta/Noodles, spaghetti, cooked w/salt	0.5	cup	70	46	99	3	20	1.2	0	0.1
38069	Pasta/Noodles, spinach, fresh, cooked	2	oz.	57	39	74	3	14	1.3	1	0.1
38107	Pasta/Noodles, spirals, enriched, cooked	0.5	cup	67	44	94	3	19	0.9	0	0.1
38120	Pasta/Noodles, vermicelli, cooked	0.5	cup	70	46	99	3	20	1.2	0	0.1
38106	Pasta/Noodles, wagon wheels, enriched, cooked	0.5	cup	70	46	99	3	20	0.9	0	0.1
38116	Pasta/Noodles, whole wheat, lasagna cuts, cooked	0.5	cup	70	47	87	4	19	2	0	0.1
38111	Pasta/Noodles, whole wheat, lasagna, cooked	2.5	oz.	70	47	87	4	19	2	0	0.1
38110	Pasta/Noodles, whole wheat, macaroni, cooked	0.5	cup	70	47	87	4	19	2	0	0.1
38112	Pasta/Noodles, whole wheat, rotini, cooked	0.5	cup	70	47	87	4	19	2	0	0.1
38113	Pasta/Noodles, whole wheat, shells, cooked	0.5	cup	70	47	87	4	19	2	0	0.1
38115	Pasta/Noodles, whole wheat, spirals, cooked	0.5	cup	70	47	87	4	19	2	0	0.1
38114	Pasta/Noodles, whole wheat, wagon wheels, cooked	0.5	cup	70	47	87	4	19	2	0	0.1
13020	Pastrami, turkey	2	piece	57	40	80	10	1	0	4	1
47021	Pastry cookie, apple, dietetic	1	each	24	3	115	1	12	0.2	7	3.5
45557	Pastry, Chinese	1	oz.	28	13	67	1	13	0.1	1	0.2
45510	Patty tart shell, frozen, baked	1	each	71	5	396	5	32	1.1	27	3.9
45542	Patty tart shells, frozen	1	each	47	4	259	3	21	0.7	18	4.5
5666	Pea pod (snow pea), stir fried	0.5	cup	82	73	35	2	6	2.2	0	0
5299	Pea sprouts, cooked	4	oz.	113	84	134	8	25	4.9	1	0.1
5298	Pea sprouts, raw	0.5	cup	60	37	77	5	17	2.4	0	0.1
49009	Peach crisp, piece, 3x3 in	1	piece	139	104	155	2	27	2	5	0.9
3214	Peach halves, cooked from dry	0.5	cup	129	101	99	2	25	3.5	0	0

A

MonoF	PolyF	Choles	Calc	Phos	Sod	Pot	Zn	Iron	Magn	VitA	VitE	VitC	Thia	Ribo	Nia	B6	Fola	B12
(g)	(g)	(mg)	(mg)	(mg)	(mg)	(mg)	(mg)	(mg)	(mg)	(μg RE)	(mg α-TE)	(mg)	(mg)	(mg)	(mg)	(mg)	(μg)	(μg)
1.8	3.4	44	119	106	397	110	0.5	1.3	11	23	1.06	0	0.16	0.22	1.2	0.03	29	0.14
0.5	0.4	9	25	19	42	21	0.1	0.4	4	19	0.21	0	0.05	0.05	0.4	0.02	3	0.03
1.8	1.4	13	90	543	743	107	1	5.1	20	42	0.58	0	0.55	0.68	5.8	0.12	73	0.26
1.6	2.2	54	163	238	384	151	0.6	1	17	55	0.65	0	0.15	0.24	0.9	0.08	8	0.26
0.1	0.2	0	26	150	115	170	0.3	0.8	12	4	0.04	0	0.07	0.05	0.7	0.01	2	0
0.2	0.2	3	34	90	170	47	0.1	0.4	5	2	0.23	0	0.06	0.06	0.5	0.02	2	0.05
0.7	1.2	16	59	43	119	36	0.2	0.5	4	15	0.26	0	0.05	0.08	0.4	0.01	10	0.06
0.9	0.6	8	22	24	54	96	0.2	0.5	15	4	0.26	0	0.04	0.05	0.3	0.04	2	0.03
0.4	0.6	8	3	16	46	17	0.1	0.5	3	4	0.12	0	0.06	0.06	0.5	0.02	8	0.02
0.9	1.2	32	130	194	297	145	0.5	1.6	24	33	0.44	0	0.1	0.28	1.2	0.06	11	0.15
4.9	6.1	11	113	525	780	298	0.6	2.1	28	125	1.25	0	0.25	0.27	2	0.09	0	0.28
0.6	0.2	19	16	39	96	53	0.2	0.8	6	22	0.13	0	0.1	0.12	1	0.05	24	0.05
0.1	0.1	0	25	0	12	78	0.4	0.8	8	28	0.05	8	0.02	0.01	0.4	0.02	5	0
0	0	0	17	4	2	180	0	0.1	7	20	0.78	43	0.02	0.02	0.2	0.01	27	0
0.1	0.1	0	73	15	9	781	0.2	0.3	30	85	3.4	188	0.08	0.1	1	0.06	116	0
0	0	0	1	2	0	14	0	0.1	1	35	0	0	0	0.01	0.1	0.01	1	0
0	0	0	2	0	0	4	0	0.1	0	3	0	0	0	0	0	0	0	0
0	0	0	0	0	0	2	0	0	0	2	0	0	0	0	0	0	0	0
0	0	0	14	6	6	55	0.1	0.6	5	52	0.18	13	0.01	0.01	0.1	0.01	15	0
0.1	0	0	41	17	17	166	0.3	1.9	15	156	0.54	40	0.03	0.03	0.4	0.03	46	0
0.1	0	0	29	54	8	286	0.2	0.5	23	0	0.78	10	0.06	0.04	0.6	0.07	45	0
0.1	0	0	24	47	7	249	0.4	0.4	19	0	0.66	11	0.06	0.03	0.5	0.06	44	0
0	0.1	0	2	12	5	63	0	0.3	5	13	0.2	5	0	0.02	0.3	0.02	3	0
0.1	0.1	0	10	62	2	31	0.6	0.7	21	0	0.04	0	0.08	0.03	0.5	0.06	4	0
0	0.2	0	21	76	10	41	0.8	0.7	43	10	0.01	0	0.07	0.07	1.1	0.07	8	0
0	0	0	7	7	4	2	0.1	0.5	1	0	0.03	0	0.03	0	0	0.01	0	0
0.1	0.2	0	1	45	0	18	0.4	0.1	21	4	0.2	0	0.03	0.01	0.3	0.04	4	0
0.1	0.2	0	1	45	0	18	0.4	0.1	21	4	0.2	0	0.03	0.01	0.3	0.04	4	0
2	2.8	4	5	—	71	24	0.3	0.3	—	2	—	0	0.01	0.01	—	0.01	1	0
0.4	0.3	26	15	46	10	30	0.5	0.9	19	11	0.04	0	0.2	0.1	1.2	0.09	51	0.11
0.1	0.2	19	3	36	3	14	0.3	0.6	10	3	0.08	0	0.12	0.08	0.6	0.02	36	0.08
0.4	0.4	33	8	42	66	17	0.4	0.9	11	14	0.17	0	0.14	0.14	1	0.03	34	0.08
0.1	0.3	0	3	23	42	11	0.2	0.6	8	0	0.08	0	0.1	0.08	0.8	0.02	24	0
0.1	0.2	0	5	38	1	22	0.4	1	13	0	0.02	0	0.14	0.07	1.2	0.02	49	0
0.1	0.2	0	5	38	1	22	0.4	1	13	0	0.02	0	0.14	0.07	1.2	0.02	49	0
0.1	0.2	0	5	38	1	22	0.4	1	13	0	0.02	0	0.14	0.07	1.2	0.02	49	0
0.1	0.2	0	5	38	1	22	0.4	1	13	0	0.04	0	0.14	0.07	1.2	0.02	49	0
0.1	0.2	0	1	45	0	18	0.4	0.1	21	4	0.2	0	0.03	0.01	0.3	0.04	4	0
0.1	0.4	0	10	76	1	43	0.7	2	25	0	0.04	0	0.29	0.14	2.3	0.05	98	0
0	0	0	7	34	4	21	0.3	0.3	13	3	0.03	0	0.08	0.04	0.7	0.02	44	0
0.1	0.2	0	5	38	1	22	0.4	1	13	0	0.02	0	0.14	0.07	1.2	0.02	49	0
0	0.2	0	4	31	1	18	0.3	0.8	10	0	0.02	0	0.12	0.06	1	0.02	40	0
0.1	0.2	0	5	38	1	22	0.4	1	13	0	0.04	0	0.14	0.07	1.2	0.02	49	0
0.1	0.2	0	5	38	70	22	0.4	1	13	0	0.19	0	0.14	0.07	1.2	0.02	49	0
0.2	0.1	19	10	32	3	21	0.4	0.6	14	8	0.12	0	0.1	0.08	0.6	0.06	36	0.08
0.1	0.2	0	5	36	1	21	0.4	0.9	12	0	0.02	0	0.14	0.07	1.1	0.02	47	0
0.1	0.2	0	5	38	1	22	0.4	1	13	0	0.04	0	0.14	0.07	1.2	0.02	49	0
0.1	0.2	0	5	38	1	22	0.4	1	13	0	0.02	0	0.14	0.07	1.2	0.02	49	0
0.1	0.1	0	10	62	2	31	0.6	0.7	21	0	0.07	0	0.08	0.03	0.5	0.06	4	0
0.1	0.1	0	10	62	2	31	0.6	0.7	21	0	0.07	0	0.08	0.03	0.5	0.06	4	0
0.1	0.1	0	10	62	2	31	0.6	0.7	21	0	0.07	0	0.08	0.03	0.5	0.06	4	0
0.1	0.1	0	10	62	2	31	0.6	0.7	21	0	0.07	0	0.08	0.03	0.5	0.06	4	0
0.1	0.1	0	10	62	2	31	0.6	0.7	21	0	0.07	0	0.08	0.03	0.5	0.06	4	0
0.1	0.1	0	10	62	2	31	0.6	0.7	21	0	0.07	0	0.08	0.03	0.5	0.06	4	0
0.1	0.1	0	10	62	2	31	0.6	0.7	21	0	0.07	0	0.08	0.03	0.5	0.06	4	0
1.2	0.9	31	5	114	596	148	1.2	0.9	8	0	0.12	0	0.03	0.14	2	0.15	3	0.14
2.6	0.6	0	2	12	0	22	0.1	0.3	7	0	1.54	0	0.04	0.02	0.3	0.01	2	0.02
0.4	0.8	0	8	16	3	28	0.2	0.5	6	0	0.25	0	0.05	0	0.4	0.02	1	0
6.3	15.8	0	7	43	180	44	0.4	1.8	11	0	1.69	0	0.23	0.18	2.7	0.01	33	0
10.2	2.3	0	5	28	117	29	0.2	1.2	8	0	2.4	0	0.19	0.13	2	0.01	44	0
0	0.1	0	36	44	3	165	0.2	1.7	20	11	0.32	42	0.11	0.06	0.5	0.12	28	0
0.1	0.3	0	30	27	3	304	0.9	1.9	46	12	0.01	7	0.24	0.32	1.2	0.14	41	0
0	0.2	0	22	99	12	229	0.6	1.4	34	10	0.01	6	0.14	0.09	1.8	0.16	86	0
2.5	1.8	0	20	31	70	189	0.2	0.9	12	108	1.13	5	0.06	0.05	1.1	0.03	6	0.01
0.1	0.2	0	12	49	3	413	0.2	1.7	17	26	0	5	0.01	0.03	2	0.05	0	0

A

Esha Code	Food Item	Qty	Meas	Wgt (g)	Wtr (g)	Cals	Prot (g)	Carb (g)	Fib (g)	Fat (g)	SatF (g)
3100	Peach halves, dried	10	each	130	41	311	5	80	10.7	1	0.1
3101	Peach nectar, canned	1	cup	249	213	134	1	35	1.5	0	0
3102	Peach nectar, canned, sweetened	1	cup	249	213	134	1	35	1.5	0	0
3358	Peach nectar, canned, vit C added	1	cup	249	213	134	1	35	1.5	0	0
3234	Peach slices, frozen, sweetened	1	each	284	212	267	2	68	5.1	0	0
45554	Peach turnover	1	each	78	28	261	3	33	1.3	13	3.3
3096	Peach, fresh, whole (2.5in)	1	each	87	76	37	1	10	1.7	0	0
3097	Peach, peeled slices, fresh	0.5	cup	85	74	37	1	9	1.7	0	0
3098	Peaches, canned in heavy syrup	0.5	cup	128	102	95	1	26	1.7	0	0
3175	Peaches, canned in juice	0.5	cup	124	109	55	1	14	1.6	0	0
3173	Peaches, canned in light syrup	0.5	cup	126	106	68	1	18	1.6	0	0
4626	Peanut butter, chunky, salted	2	Tbs	32	0	188	8	7	2.1	16	3.1
4576	Peanut butter, chunky, unsalted	2	Tbs	32	0	188	8	7	2.1	16	3.1
4637	Peanut butter, natural, salted	2	Tbs	32	0	187	8	7	2.1	16	2.2
4668	Peanut butter, natural, unsalted	2	Tbs	32	0	187	8	7	2.1	16	2.2
4627	Peanut butter, smooth, salted	2	Tbs	32	0	190	8	6	1.9	16	3.3
4636	Peanut butter, smooth, unsalted	2	Tbs	32	0	190	8	6	1.9	16	3.3
4517	Peanut, Spanish, raw	0.5	cup	36	2	208	10	6	3.5	18	2.8
4665	Peanuts, Spanish, oil roasted, unsalted	0.25	cup	37	1	213	10	6	3.3	18	2.8
4666	Peanuts, Valencia, oil roasted, unsalted	0.25	cup	36	1	212	10	6	3.2	18	2.8
4667	Peanuts, Virginia, oil roasted, unsalted	0.25	cup	36	1	207	9	7	3.2	17	2.3
4541	Peanuts, dry roasted, unsalted	0.25	cup	36	1	214	9	8	2.9	18	2.5
4542	Peanuts, oil roasted, unsalted	0.25	cup	36	1	209	10	7	2.5	18	2.5
3349	Pear halves canned in water	1	each	77	71	22	0	6	1.2	0	0
3109	Pear halves, dried	10	each	175	47	459	3	122	13.1	1	0.1
3110	Pear nectar, canned	1	cup	250	210	150	0	40	1.5	0	0
3359	Pear nectar, canned, vit C added	1	cup	250	210	150	0	40	1.5	0	0
3272	Pear, Asian, raw	1	each	122	108	51	1	13	4.4	0	0
23238	Pear, candied	1.5	oz.	43	9	129	1	32	—	0	0
3107	Pear, canned in heavy syrup	0.5	cup	128	103	94	0	24	2	0	0
3104	Pear, fresh slices	0.5	cup	82	69	49	0	12	2	0	0
3103	Pear, fresh, Bartlett	1	each	166	139	98	1	25	4	1	0
3105	Pear, fresh, Bosc	1	each	139	116	82	1	21	3.3	1	0
3106	Pear, fresh, D'Anjou	1	each	209	175	123	1	32	5	1	0
3179	Pears, canned in juice	0.5	cup	124	107	62	0	16	2	0	0
3177	Pears, canned in light syrup	0.5	cup	126	106	72	0	19	2	0	0
5308	Peas & carrots, canned w/liquid, low sodium	0.5	cup	128	113	49	3	11	4.2	0	0.1
5281	Peas & carrots, canned, not drained	0.5	cup	128	113	49	3	11	2.6	0	0.1
5123	Peas & carrots, frozen, cooked	0.5	cup	80	69	38	2	8	2.5	0	0.1
5282	Peas & carrots, frozen, unheated	0.5	cup	70	59	37	2	8	2.4	0	0.1
5577	Peas & onions, canned w/liquid	0.5	cup	60	52	31	2	5	1.4	0	0
5122	Peas edible pod/snow pea, cooked	0.5	cup	80	71	34	3	6	2.2	0	0
7016	Peas, blackeyed/cowpea, canned w/liquid	0.5	cup	120	96	92	6	16	4	1	0.2
7017	Peas, blackeyed/cowpea, dry	0.5	cup	84	10	281	20	50	8.8	1	0.3
7018	Peas, blackeyed/cowpea, dry, cooked	0.5	cup	86	60	99	7	18	5.6	0	0.1
5296	Peas, edible pod/snow pea, frozen, cooked	0.5	cup	80	69	42	3	7	2.5	0	0.1
5120	Peas, edible pod/snow pea, raw	0.5	cup	72	64	30	2	5	1.9	0	0
5665	Peas, edible pods/snow peas, steamed	0.5	cup	82	73	35	2	6	2.2	0	0
5119	Peas, green, canned, drained	0.5	cup	85	69	59	4	11	3.5	0	0.1
5395	Peas, green, canned, low sodium	0.5	cup	85	69	59	4	11	3.5	0	0.1
5214	Peas, green, canned, not drained	0.5	cup	124	107	66	4	12	4	0	0.1
5267	Peas, green, canned, not drained, low sodium	0.5	cup	124	107	66	4	12	4	0	0.1
5118	Peas, green, frozen, cooked	0.5	cup	80	64	62	4	11	4.4	0	0
5280	Peas, green, frozen, unheated	0.5	cup	72	58	55	4	10	3.4	0	0
5116	Peas, green, raw	0.5	cup	72	57	59	4	10	3.7	0	0.1
5117	Peas, green, raw, cooked	0.5	cup	80	62	67	4	12	4.4	0	0
7062	Peas, pigeon/red gram, cooked	0.5	cup	84	58	102	6	20	5.6	0	0.1
5279	Peas, seasoned, canned, not drained	0.5	cup	114	99	57	4	10	2.3	0	0.1
7019	Peas, split, dry	0.5	cup	98	11	336	24	60	25.1	1	0.2
7020	Peas, split, dry, cooked	0.5	cup	98	68	116	8	21	8.1	0	0.1
4585	Pecan halves, oil roasted, unsalted	15	each	28	1	194	2	5	1.9	20	1.6
4583	Pecan, dry roasted, salted	0.25	cup	28	0	187	2	6	2.6	18	1.5
4578	Pecans, dried halves	0.25	cup	27	1	180	2	5	2	18	1.5
4577	Pecans, dried, chopped	0.25	cup	30	1	198	2	5	2.3	20	1.6
4579	Pecans, dried, ground	0.25	cup	24	1	158	2	4	1.8	16	1.3

MonoF	PolyF	Choles	Calc	Phos	Sod	Pot	Zn	Iron	Magn	VitA	VitE	VitC	Thia	Ribo	Nia	B6	Fola	B12
(g)	(g)	(mg)	(mg)	(mg)	(mg)	(mg)	(mg)	(mg)	(mg)	(µg RE)	(mg α-TE)	(mg)	(mg)	(mg)	(mg)	(mg)	(µg)	(µg)
0.4	0.5	0	36	155	9	1294	0.7	5.3	55	281	0	6	0	0.28	5.7	0.09	0	0
0	0	0	12	15	17	100	0.2	0.5	10	65	0.02	13	0.01	0.04	0.7	0.02	3	0
0	0	0	12	15	17	100	0.2	0.5	10	65	0.02	13	0.01	0.04	0.7	0.02	3	0
0	0	0	12	15	17	100	0.2	0.5	10	65	0.2	67	0.01	0.04	0.7	0.02	3	0
0.1	0.2	0	9	31	17	369	0.1	1	14	80	2.53	268	0.04	0.1	1.8	0.05	9	0
5.9	3.5	0	6	32	218	89	0.2	1.2	8	14	1.4	2	0.16	0.13	1.7	0.02	5	0
0	0	0	4	10	0	171	0.1	0.1	6	47	0.61	6	0.02	0.04	0.9	0.02	3	0
0	0	0	4	10	0	167	0.1	0.1	6	46	0.6	6	0.01	0.04	0.8	0.02	3	0
0	0.1	0	4	14	8	118	0.1	0.3	6	42	1.14	4	0.01	0.03	0.8	0.02	4	0
0	0	0	7	21	5	159	0.1	0.3	9	47	1.86	4	0.01	0.02	0.7	0.02	4	0
0	0	0	4	14	6	122	0.1	0.5	6	44	1.12	3	0.01	0.03	0.7	0.02	4	0
7.6	4.5	0	13	101	156	239	0.9	0.6	51	0	2.4	0	0.04	0.04	4.4	0.14	29	0
7.6	4.5	0	13	101	5	239	0.9	0.6	51	0	3.2	0	0.04	0.04	4.4	0.14	29	0
7.9	5	0	17	114	80	210	1.1	0.7	56	0	2.59	0	0.04	0.03	4.3	0.13	46	0
7.9	5	0	17	115	2	211	1.1	0.7	56	0	2.4	0	0.14	0.03	4.3	0.13	46	0
7.8	4.4	0	12	118	149	214	0.9	0.6	51	0	3.2	0	0.03	0.03	4.3	0.14	24	0
7.8	4.4	0	12	118	5	214	0.9	0.6	51	0	3.2	0	0.03	0.03	4.3	0.14	24	0
8.1	6.3	0	39	142	8	272	0.8	1.4	69	0	2.7	0	0.25	0.05	5.8	0.13	88	0
8.1	6.2	0	37	142	2	285	0.7	0.8	62	0	2.72	0	0.12	0.03	5.5	0.09	46	0
8.3	6.4	0	19	115	2	220	1.1	0.6	58	0	2.77	0	0.03	0.06	5.2	0.09	45	0
9	5.3	0	31	181	2	233	2.4	0.6	67	0	2.61	0	0.1	0.04	5.3	0.09	45	0
9	5.7	0	20	131	297	240	1.2	0.8	64	0	2.7	0	0.16	0.04	4.9	0.09	53	0
8.8	5.6	0	32	186	2	246	2.4	0.7	67	0	2.67	0	0.09	0.04	5.2	0.09	45	0
0	0	0	3	5	2	41	0.1	0.2	3	0	0.38	1	0.01	0.01	0	0.01	1	0
0.2	0.3	0	60	103	10	933	0.7	3.7	58	1	0	12	0.01	0.25	2.4	0.13	0	0
0	0	0	12	8	10	32	0.2	0.6	8	0	0.25	3	0	0.03	0.3	0.04	3	0
0	0	0	12	8	10	32	0.2	0.6	8	0	0.25	68	0	0.03	0.3	0.04	3	0
0.1	0.1	0	5	13	0	148	0	0	10	0	0.61	5	0.01	0.01	0.3	0.03	10	0
—	—	0	15	20	3	244	—	0.6	—	3	—	3	0	0.08	0.3	—	—	—
0	0	0	6	9	6	83	0.1	0.3	5	0	0.64	1	0.01	0.03	0.3	0.02	2	0
0.1	0.1	0	9	9	0	103	0.1	0.2	5	2	0.41	3	0.02	0.03	0.1	0.02	6	0
0.1	0.2	0	18	18	0	208	0.2	0.4	10	3	0.83	7	0.03	0.07	0.2	0.03	12	0
0.1	0.1	0	15	15	0	174	0.2	0.3	8	3	0.7	6	0.03	0.06	0.1	0.02	10	0
0.2	0.2	0	23	23	0	261	0.3	0.5	12	4	1.05	8	0.04	0.08	0.2	0.04	15	0
0	0	0	11	15	5	119	0.1	0.4	9	1	0.62	2	0.01	0.01	0.2	0.02	1	0
0	0	0	6	9	6	83	0.1	0.4	5	0	0.63	1	0.01	0.02	0.2	0.02	2	0
0	0.2	0	29	59	5	128	0.7	1	18	739	0.54	8	0.1	0.07	0.7	0.11	23	0
0	0.2	0	29	59	333	128	0.7	1	18	739	0.24	8	0.1	0.07	0.7	0.11	23	0
0	0.2	0	18	39	54	126	0.4	0.8	13	621	0.26	6	0.18	0.05	0.9	0.07	21	0
0	0.2	0	19	42	55	136	0.4	0.8	13	665	0.22	8	0.13	0.06	1	0.07	25	0
0	0.1	0	10	31	265	58	0.3	0.5	10	10	0.17	2	0.06	0.04	0.8	0.12	16	0
0	0.1	0	34	44	3	192	0.3	1.6	21	10	0.31	38	0.1	0.06	0.4	0.12	23	0
0.1	0.3	0	24	84	359	206	0.8	1.2	34	1	0.12	3	0.09	0.09	0.4	0.05	61	0
0.1	0.5	0	92	354	13	929	2.8	6.9	154	4	0.33	1	0.71	0.19	1.7	0.3	529	0
0	0.2	0	20	133	3	238	1.1	2.2	45	2	0.24	0	0.17	0.05	0.4	0.09	178	0
0	0.1	0	47	46	4	174	0.4	1.9	22	14	0.17	18	0.05	0.1	0.4	0.14	28	0
0	0.1	0	31	38	3	145	0.2	1.5	17	10	0.28	44	0.11	0.06	0.4	0.12	30	0
0	0.1	0	36	44	3	165	0.2	1.7	20	11	0.32	42	0.11	0.06	0.5	0.12	29	0
0	0.1	0	17	57	214	147	0.6	0.8	14	66	0.32	8	0.1	0.07	0.6	0.05	38	0
0	0.1	0	17	57	2	147	0.6	0.8	14	66	0.32	8	0.1	0.07	0.6	0.05	38	0
0	0.2	0	22	66	310	124	0.9	1.3	21	47	0.34	12	0.14	0.09	1	0.08	35	0
0	0.2	0	22	66	11	124	0.9	1.3	21	47	0.47	12	0.14	0.09	1	0.08	35	0
0	0.1	0	19	72	70	134	0.8	1.3	23	54	0.14	8	0.23	0.08	1.2	0.09	47	0
0	0.1	0	16	58	81	107	0.6	1.1	18	53	0.12	13	0.19	0.07	1.2	0.09	38	0
0	0.1	0	18	78	4	177	0.9	1.1	24	46	0.28	29	0.19	0.1	1.5	0.12	47	0
0	0.1	0	22	94	2	217	1	1.2	31	48	0.31	11	0.21	0.12	1.6	0.17	51	0
0	0.2	0	36	100	4	323	0.8	0.9	39	0	0.08	0	0.12	0.05	0.7	0.04	93	0
0	0.1	0	17	62	290	139	0.7	1.4	17	49	0.34	13	0.11	0.08	0.8	0.11	33	0
0.2	0.5	0	54	361	15	966	3	4.4	113	15	0.3	2	0.72	0.21	2.8	0.17	270	0
0.1	0.2	0	14	97	2	355	1	1.3	35	1	0.38	0	0.19	0.06	0.9	0.05	64	0
12.6	5	0	10	83	0	102	1.6	0.6	37	4	0.94	1	0.09	0.03	0.3	0.05	11	0
11.4	4.5	0	10	86	222	105	1.6	0.6	38	4	0.85	1	0.09	0.03	0.3	0.06	12	0
11.4	4.5	0	10	79	0	106	1.5	0.6	35	4	0.84	1	0.23	0.04	0.2	0.05	11	0
12.6	5	0	11	87	0	117	1.6	0.6	38	4	0.92	1	0.25	0.04	0.3	0.06	12	0
10	4	0	9	69	0	93	1.3	0.5	30	3	0.74	0	0.2	0.03	0.2	0.04	9	0

Esha Code	Food Item	Qty	Meas	Wgt (g)	Wtr (g)	Cals	Prot (g)	Carb (g)	Fib (g)	Fat (g)	SatF (g)
4582	Pecans, dry roasted, unsalted	0.24	cup	28	0	187	2	6	2.6	18	1.5
4586	Pecans, oil roasted, salted	0.25	cup	28	1	188	2	4	1.8	20	1.6
4584	Pecans, oil roasted, unsalted	0.25	cup	28	1	188	2	4	1.8	20	1.6
26016	Pepper, black	0.25	tsp	1	0	1	0	0	0.1	0	0
26027	Pepper, cayenne/red	0.25	tsp	0	0	1	0	0	0.1	0	0
5063	Pepper, hot green chili, canned, w/liquid, no seeds	0.5	cup	68	63	14	1	3	0.9	0	0
5400	Pepper, hot green chili, raw, whole	1	each	45	40	18	1	4	0.7	0	0
27043	Pepper, hot jalapeno, pickled	2	each	16	13	8	0	2	0.2	0	0
5291	Pepper, hot red chili, canned, not drained	1	Tbs	8	8	2	0	0	0.1	0	0
5289	Pepper, hot red chili, raw pod	1	each	45	40	18	1	4	0.7	0	0
5288	Pepper, hot red chili, raw, chopped	1	Tbs	9	8	4	0	1	0.1	0	0
6310	Pepper, hot red, dried pods	0.25	cup	2	0	5	0	1	—	0	0
5293	Pepper, jalapeno, chopped, canned	1	Tbs	8	8	2	0	0	0.2	0	0
6099	Pepper, jalapeno, raw	1	each	45	40	11	0	2	—	0	—
26604	Pepper, lemon	0.25	tsp	0	0	1	0	0	0	0	0
5617	Pepper, pickled	1	each	20	18	8	0	2	0.3	0	0
6100	Pepper, serrano, raw	1	each	45	40	20	—	—	—	—	—
5248	Pepper, sweet green bell, freeze dried	0.5	cup	3	0	10	1	2	0.7	0	0
5284	Pepper, sweet green bell, frozen, cooked	0.5	cup	68	64	12	1	3	0.6	0	0
5578	Pepper, sweet green, canned w/liquid	0.5	cup	70	64	13	1	3	0.8	0	0
5126	Pepper, sweet green, chopped, cooked	0.5	cup	68	62	19	1	5	0.8	0	0
5661	Pepper, sweet green, chopped, steamed	0.5	cup	68	63	18	1	4	1.2	0	0
5662	Pepper, sweet green, chopped, stir fried	0.5	cup	68	63	18	1	4	1.2	0	0
5124	Pepper, sweet green, raw, chopped	0.5	cup	50	46	14	0	3	0.9	0	0
5125	Pepper, sweet green, raw, whole	1	each	74	68	20	1	5	1.3	0	0
5127	Pepper, sweet green, whole, cooked	1	each	73	67	20	1	5	0.9	0	0
5568	Pepper, sweet red bell, canned, w/liquid	0.5	cup	70	64	13	1	3	0.8	0	0
5278	Pepper, sweet red bell, chopped, cooked	0.5	cup	68	62	19	1	5	0.8	0	0
5307	Pepper, sweet red bell, freeze dried	0.5	cup	3	0	10	1	2	0.7	0	0
5286	Pepper, sweet red bell, frozen, cooked	0.5	cup	68	64	12	1	3	1.1	0	0
5663	Pepper, sweet red bell, steamed	0.5	cup	68	63	18	1	4	1.2	0	0
5664	Pepper, sweet red bell, stir fried, no oil	0.5	cup	68	63	18	1	4	1.2	0	0
5128	Pepper, sweet red, raw, chopped	0.5	cup	50	46	14	0	3	1	0	0
5442	Pepper, sweet yellow, raw strips	10	piece	52	48	14	1	3	0.5	0	0
5441	Pepper, sweet yellow, raw, large	1	each	186	171	50	2	12	1.7	0	0.1
26037	Pepper, white	0.25	tsp	1	0	2	0	0	0.2	0	0
6485	Pepperoncini, Greek	1	oz.	28	26	8	0	1	0.4	0	0
6484	Pepperoncini, Italian	1	oz.	28	26	6	0	1	0.2	0	0
5399	Peppers, hot green chili, raw, chopped	1	Tbs	9	8	4	0	1	0.1	0	0
6482	Peppers, sweet cherry	1	oz.	28	24	16	1	2	0.5	0	0.1
3351	Persimmon, Japanese, dried	1	each	34	8	93	0	25	4.9	0	0.1
3193	Persimmon, Japanese, large, raw	1	each	168	135	118	1	31	6	0	0
3194	Persimmon, native, fresh	1	each	25	16	32	0	8	0.4	0	—
45582	Phyllo dough	1	each	19	6	57	1	10	0.4	1	0.3
27046	Pickle, chow chow	1	Tbs	15	10	18	0	4	0.2	0	0
27037	Pickle, cucumber, dill, low sodium, slices	4	each	30	28	3	0	1	0.4	0	0
27038	Pickle, cucumber, dill, low sodium, spears	1	each	30	28	3	0	1	0.4	0	0
27039	Pickle, cucumber, dill, low sodium, whole	1	each	65	61	7	0	1	0.8	0	0
27015	Pickle, cucumber, fresh slices	4	piece	30	24	22	0	5	0.4	0	0
27012	Pickle, dill	1	each	65	60	12	0	3	0.8	0	0
27013	Pickle, dill slices	10	piece	60	55	11	0	2	0.7	0	0
27028	Pickle, dill, low sodium	1	each	65	60	12	0	3	0.8	0	0
27029	Pickle, dill, low sodium, slices	10	piece	60	55	11	0	2	0.7	0	0
27047	Pickle, mustard	0.25	cup	61	42	71	1	16	0.9	1	0
27023	Pickle, sour	1	each	35	33	4	0	1	0.4	0	0
27024	Pickle, sour cucumber, slices	10	piece	70	66	8	0	2	0.8	0	0
27026	Pickle, sour, low sodium	1	each	35	33	4	0	1	0.4	0	0
27027	Pickle, sour, low sodium, slices	10	piece	70	66	8	0	2	0.8	0	0
27040	Pickle, sweet butter chips, low sodium	5	each	30	20	35	0	10	0.4	0	0
27041	Pickle, sweet cucumber, low sodium, slices	5	each	30	20	35	0	10	0.4	0	0
27062	Pickle, sweet relish	1	Tbs	15	10	21	0	5	0.3	0	0
27030	Pickle, sweet, low sodium	1	each	35	23	41	0	11	0.4	0	0
27031	Pickle, sweet, low sodium, slices	10	piece	60	39	70	0	19	0.7	0	0
27016	Pickle, sweet, medium size	1	each	35	23	41	0	11	0.4	0	0
27049	Pickles, Japanese, tsukemono	0.5	cup	68	62	14	1	3	1.8	0	0

MonoF	PolyF	Choles	Calc	Phos	Sod	Pot	Zn	Iron	Magn	VitA	VitE	VitC	Thia	Ribo	Nia	B6	Fola	B12
(g)	(g)	(mg)	(mg)	(mg)	(mg)	(mg)	(mg)	(mg)	(mg)	(μg RE)	(mg α-TE)	(mg)	(mg)	(mg)	(mg)	(mg)	(μg)	(μg)
11.4	4.5	0	10	86	0	105	1.6	0.6	38	4	0.88	1	0.09	0.03	0.3	0.06	12	0
12.2	4.8	0	9	81	208	99	1.5	0.6	36	4	0.91	1	0.08	0.03	0.2	0.05	11	0
12.2	4.8	0	9	81	0	99	1.5	0.6	36	4	0.91	1	0.08	0.03	0.2	0.05	11	0
0	0	0	2	1	0	7	0	0.2	1	0	0	0	0	0	0	0	0	0
0	0	0	1	1	0	9	0	0	1	18	0.02	0	0	0	0	0.01	0	0
0	0	0	5	12	798	127	0.1	0.3	10	42	0.47	46	0.01	0.03	0.5	0.1	7	0
0	0	0	8	21	3	153	0.1	0.5	11	35	0.31	109	0.04	0.04	0.4	0.12	10	0
0	0	0	3	6	121	43	0	0.1	3	124	0.08	28	0.01	0.01	0.1	0.03	3	0
0	0	0	1	1	100	16	0	0	1	101	0.06	6	0	0	0.1	0.01	1	0
0	0	0	8	21	3	153	0.1	0.5	11	484	0.31	109	0.04	0.04	0.4	0.12	10	0
0	0	0	2	4	1	32	0	0.1	2	101	0.06	23	0.01	0.01	0.1	0.03	2	0
—	—	0	2	4	6	19	—	0.1	—	123	—	0	0	0.02	0.2	—	—	0
0	0	0	2	2	142	16	0	0.2	1	14	0.06	1	0	0	0	0.02	1	0
—	—	—	—	—	2	2	—	—	—	30	0.37	53	—	—	—	—	—	0
0	0	0	1	0	115	1	0	0	0	0	0	0	0	0	0	0	0	0
0	0	0	2	4	26	31	0	0.1	2	46	0.1	21	0.01	0	0.1	0.04	4	0
—	—	—	—	—	2	2	—	—	—	63	—	37	—	—	—	—	—	0
0	0.1	0	4	10	6	101	0.1	0.3	6	20	0.13	61	0.04	0.04	0.2	0.07	7	0
0	0.1	0	5	9	3	49	0	0.4	5	20	0.42	28	0.04	0.02	0.7	0.07	7	0
0	0.1	0	29	14	958	102	0.1	0.6	8	11	0.42	33	0.02	0.02	0.4	0.12	11	0
0	0.1	0	6	12	1	113	0.1	0.3	7	40	0.47	51	0.04	0.02	0.3	0.16	11	0
0	0.1	0	6	13	1	120	0.1	0.3	7	41	0.47	52	0.04	0.02	0.3	0.15	13	0
0	0.1	0	6	13	1	120	0.1	0.3	7	39	0.47	52	0.04	0.02	0.3	0.15	12	0
0	0.1	0	4	10	1	88	0.1	0.2	5	32	0.34	45	0.03	0.02	0.3	0.12	11	0
0	0.1	0	7	14	1	131	0.1	0.3	7	47	0.51	66	0.05	0.02	0.4	0.18	16	0
0	0.1	0	7	13	1	121	0.1	0.3	7	43	0.5	54	0.04	0.02	0.3	0.17	12	0
0	0.1	0	29	14	958	102	0.1	0.6	8	36	0.48	33	0.02	0.02	0.4	0.12	11	0
0	0.1	0	6	12	1	113	0.1	0.3	7	256	0.47	116	0.04	0.02	0.3	0.16	11	0
0	0.1	0	4	10	6	101	0.1	0.3	6	247	0.14	61	0.04	0.04	0.2	0.07	7	0
0	0.1	0	5	9	3	49	0	0.4	5	227	0.42	28	0.04	0.02	0.7	0.07	7	0
0	0.1	0	6	13	1	120	0.1	0.3	7	368	0.47	110	0.04	0.02	0.3	0.15	13	0
0	0.1	0	6	13	1	120	0.1	0.3	7	349	0.47	110	0.04	0.02	0.3	0.15	12	0
0	0.1	0	4	10	1	88	0.1	0.2	5	285	0.34	95	0.03	0.02	0.3	0.12	11	0
0	0.1	0	6	12	1	110	0.1	0.2	6	12	0.36	96	0.02	0.01	0.5	0.09	14	0
0	0.2	0	20	45	4	394	0.3	0.9	22	45	1.28	342	0.05	0.05	1.7	0.31	48	0
0	0	0	2	1	0	0	0	0.1	1	0	0.02	0	0	0	0	0	0	0
0	0.1	0	11	—	369	—	—	0.2	—	7	—	2	—	—	—	—	—	—
0	0.1	0	14	—	598	—	—	0.4	—	12	—	0	—	—	—	—	—	—
0	0	0	2	4	1	32	0	0.1	2	7	0.06	23	0.01	0.01	0.1	0.03	2	0
0	0.3	0	4	—	323	—	—	0.5	—	52	—	12	—	—	—	—	—	—
0	0.1	0	8	28	1	273	0.1	0.3	10	19	0.34	0	—	0.01	0.1	0.04	3	0
0.1	0.1	0	13	29	2	270	0.2	0.3	15	365	0.99	13	0.05	0.03	0.2	0.17	13	0
—	—	0	7	6	0	78	—	0.6	—	0	0.25	16	—	—	—	—	2	0
0.6	0.2	0	2	14	92	14	0.1	0.6	3	0	0.19	0	0.1	0.06	0.8	0.01	14	0
0.1	0	0	4	3	81	31	0	0.2	3	1	0.02	1	0	0	0	0	1	0
0	0	0	0	4	5	7	0	0.1	1	4	0.02	0	0	0	0	0	0	0
0	0	0	0	4	5	7	0	0.1	1	4	0.02	0	0	0	0	0	0	0
0	0.1	0	0	9	12	15	0	0.3	3	10	0.03	1	0	0.01	0	0.01	0	0
0	0	0	10	8	202	60	0	0.5	2	4	0.05	3	0	0.01	0	0	0	0
0	0	0	6	14	833	75	0.1	0.3	7	22	0.1	1	0.01	0.02	0	0.01	1	0
0	0	0	5	13	769	70	0.1	0.3	7	20	0.1	1	0.01	0.02	0	0.01	1	0
0	0	0	6	14	12	75	0.1	0.3	7	22	0.1	1	0.01	0.02	0	0.01	1	0
0	0	0	5	13	11	70	0.1	0.3	7	20	0.09	1	0.01	0.02	0	0.01	1	0
0.3	0.1	0	14	14	323	123	0.1	0.9	13	6	0.1	4	0	0.01	0	0.01	3	0
0	0	0	0	5	423	8	0	0.1	1	5	0.06	0	0	0	0	0	0	0
0	0.1	0	0	10	846	16	0	0.3	3	10	0.11	1	0	0.01	0	0.01	0	0
0	0	0	0	5	6	8	0	0.1	1	5	0.02	0	0	0	0	0	0	0
0	0.1	0	0	10	13	16	0	0.3	3	10	0.04	1	0	0.01	0	0.01	0	0
0	0	0	1	4	5	10	0	0.2	1	4	0.05	0	0	0.01	0.1	0	0	0
0	0	0	1	4	5	10	0	0.2	1	4	0.05	0	0	0.01	0.1	0	0	0
0	0	0	3	2	109	31	0	0.1	1	2	0.02	1	0	0	0	0	0	0
0	0	0	1	4	6	11	0	0.2	1	5	0.06	0	0	0.01	0.1	0	0	0
0	0.1	0	2	7	11	19	0	0.4	2	8	0.1	1	0	0.02	0.1	0.01	1	0
0	0	0	1	4	329	11	0	0.2	1	5	0.06	0	0	0.01	0.1	0	0	0
0	0.1	0	26	25	360	400	0.1	0.2	7	6	0.04	0	0.01	0.02	0.2	0.07	17	0

Esha Code	Food Item	Qty	Meas	Wgt (g)	Wtr (g)	Cals	Prot (g)	Carb (g)	Fib (g)	Fat (g)	SatF (g)
45502	Pie crust, double, recipe, baked	1	each	320	31	1686	20	152	5.4	111	27.6
45536	Pie crust, frozen, baked	1	piece	21	2	108	1	10	0.2	7	2.2
45535	Pie crust, frozen, ready to bake	1	each	14	3	64	1	6	0.1	4	0.6
45538	Pie crust, homemade, not baked, double	1	each	194	38	910	11	82	6.6	60	14.9
45537	Pie crust, homemade, not baked, single	1	each	320	63	1500	18	135	10.9	99	24.5
45503	Pie crust, mix, prepared, baked	1	each	180	19	902	12	91	3.2	55	13.9
45501	Pie crust, single, recipe, baked	1	each	180	18	949	12	86	3	62	15.5
48002	Pie filling, apple	1	cup	255	187	258	0	67	2.6	0	0.1
48019	Pie filling, blueberry	1	cup	262	190	272	2	68	3.7	1	0.1
48016	Pie filling, cherry	1	cup	264	184	304	1	77	1.6	1	0.1
48018	Pie filling, cherry, low calorie	1	cup	264	208	211	2	51	1.6	2	0.4
48017	Pie filling, lemon	1	cup	266	49	927	13	185	1.2	18	4.4
48044	Pie filling, pumpkin, canned	0.5	cup	135	96	140	1	36	11.2	0	0.1
70557	Pie, Boston cream, thaw'n serve, Mrs. Smith	1	piece	106	51	240	3	48	0.8	4	1.5
48151	Pie, Plush Pippin, 9, apple	1	piece	126	—	350	2	41	2	21	4
48153	Pie, Plush Pippin, 9, cherry	1	piece	120	—	340	3	45	1	22	4
48154	Pie, Plush Pippin, chocolate creme	1	piece	124	—	280	4	36	1	14	4
48155	Pie, Plush Pippin, lemon meringue	1	piece	119	—	250	2	41	0.5	9	2
48156	Pie, Plush Pippin, pumpkin	1	piece	121	—	260	3	34	1	13	3
48023	Pie, banana cream, mix, no bake, prepared .	125	each	92	47	231	3	29	0.6	12	6.4
48023	Pie, banana cream, mix, no bake, prepared	1	each	737	375	1849	25	233	4.6	95	50.9
48143	Pie, blackberry, 1/5th pie, Banquet	1	piece	113	47	300	3	45	3	12	5
49004	Pie, cheesecake	1	piece	92	42	295	5	24	0.4	21	9.1
49017	Pie, cheesecake, chocolate	1	piece	128	37	501	8	48	1.9	32	15.5
49001	Pie, cheesecake, no bake mix, prepared	1	piece	103	46	282	6	37	2	13	6.9
49010	Pie, cheesecake, recipe	1	piece	128	52	457	9	32	0.5	33	18.4
46234	Pie, cheesecake, triple chocolate, svg, Weight Watc	1	each	89	46	200	7	32	1	5	2.5
49011	Pie, cheesecake, w/cherry topping, recipe	1	piece	142	70	408	7	38	0.6	26	14.5
48014	Pie, cherry, fried, turnover	1	each	85	32	269	3	36	2.2	14	2.1
48046	Pie, chocolate cream, individual	1	each	117	47	357	6	44	1.7	19	6.7
48034	Pie, chocolate mousse, mix, no bake, prepared .	125	each	95	47	247	3	28	—	15	7.8
48034	Pie, chocolate mousse, mix, no bake, prepared	1	each	760	378	1976	27	225	—	117	62.3
48036	Pie, coconut cream, mix, no bake, prepared .	125	each	94	47	260	3	27	0.5	17	8.4
48036	Pie, coconut cream, mix, no bake, prepared	1	each	754	375	2081	21	215	3.8	133	67.3
48013	Pie, fried, apple, turnover	1	each	85	34	266	2	33	1.5	14	6.5
48058	Pie, pecan, individual, Bama pie	1	each	85	14	366	4	45	1.4	20	3.4
5227	Pimento/pimiento, canned	1	Tbs	12	11	3	0	1	0.2	0	0
5228	Pimento/pimiento, canned slices	20	piece	20	19	5	0	1	0.4	0	0
4529	Pine nut, pignola, dried	1	oz.	28	2	160	7	4	1.3	14	2.2
4554	Pine nut, pinon, dried	1	oz.	28	2	178	3	5	3	17	2.7
3111	Pineapple chunks, fresh	0.5	cup	78	67	38	0	10	0.9	0	0
3118	Pineapple chunks, frozen, sweetened	0.5	cup	122	94	104	0	27	1.4	0	0
20059	Pineapple grapefruit juice drink, canned	1	cup	250	220	118	0	29	0.2	0	0
3360	Pineapple juice, canned, vit C, unsweetened	1	cup	250	214	140	1	34	0.5	0	0
20025	Pineapple orange drink, canned	1	cup	250	217	125	3	30	0.2	0	0
3114	Pineapple pieces in heavy syrup	0.5	cup	128	101	100	0	26	1	0	0
3115	Pineapple rings in heavy syrup	1	each	58	46	45	0	12	0.5	0	0
3113	Pineapple slices, fresh	1	piece	84	73	41	0	10	1	0	0
3183	Pineapple, canned in juice	0.5	cup	125	104	75	1	20	1	0	0
3181	Pineapple, canned in light syrup	0.5	cup	126	108	66	0	17	1	0	0
4520	Pistachio nut, dried, meat	0.25	cup	32	1	185	7	8	3.5	16	2
4540	Pistachio nut, dry roasted, salted	0.25	tsp	32	1	194	5	9	3.5	17	2.1
4654	Pistachio nuts, dry roasted, unsalted	0.25	cup	32	1	194	5	9	3.5	17	2.1
3261	Pitanga, raw	1	each	7	6	2	0	1	0.1	0	—
56481	Pizza Hut, Pizza, cheese, pan	2	piece	205	106	495	23	53	3.8	21	9.5
56482	Pizza Hut, Pizza, pepperoni, pan	2	piece	211	103	539	22	57	4.1	24	8.1
56483	Pizza Hut, Pizza, supreme, pan	2	piece	255	143	581	28	52	5.6	28	11.2
56490	Pizza Hut, pizza, pepperoni, hand-tossed	2	piece	197	100	452	23	55	3.8	15	7.6
56493	Pizza Hut, pizza, pepperoni, personal pan	1	each	256	128	639	27	69	5	28	10
56494	Pizza Hut, pizza, supreme, personal pan	1	each	264	152	582	27	56	4.8	27	9.7
56487	Pizza Hut, pizza, supreme, thin/crispy	2	piece	200	114	443	24	36	3.4	22	8.6
57166	Pizza, deluxe, Tombstone	2	piece	250	131	597	28	54	3.7	30	13.1
57215	Pizza, supreme, light, Tombstone	2	piece	276	—	540	50	60	4	18	7
44062	Plantain chips	32	piece	35	1	180	1	20	2.7	12	10
3196	Plantain slices, cooked	0.5	cup	77	52	89	1	24	1.8	0	0.1

MonoF	PolyF	Choles	Calc	Phos	Sod	Pot	Zn	Iron	Magn	VitA	VitE	VitC	Thia	Ribo	Nia	B6	Fola	B12
(g)	(g)	(mg)	(mg)	(mg)	(mg)	(mg)	(mg)	(mg)	(mg)	(µg RE)	(mg α-TE)	(mg)	(mg)	(mg)	(mg)	(mg)	(µg)	(µg)
48.6	29.2	0	32	214	1734	214	1.4	9.2	45	0	17.7	0	1.25	0.89	10.6	0.08	214	0
3.3	0.8	0	4	12	136	23	0.1	0.5	4	0	1.07	0	0.06	0.08	0.5	0.02	8	0
1.7	1.5	0	3	7	81	14	0	0.3	2	0	0.74	0	0.04	0.05	0.3	0.01	10	0
26.2	15.8	0	18	116	935	114	0.8	5	23	0	4.93	0	0.68	0.48	5.7	0.04	122	0
43.2	26	0	29	192	1542	189	1.2	8.2	38	0	8.13	0	1.11	0.79	9.4	0.07	202	0
31.1	6.9	0	108	151	1312	112	0.7	3.9	27	0	9.94	0	0.55	0.34	4.3	0.1	22	0
27.4	16.4	0	18	121	976	121	0.8	5.2	25	0	9.94	0	0.7	0.5	6	0.04	121	0
0	0.1	0	10	18	112	115	0.1	0.7	5	3	0	3	0.03	0.03	0.1	0.04	0	0
0.1	0.3	0	13	26	68	97	0.2	1	10	16	2.45	3	0.08	0.13	0.3	0.08	5	0
0.2	0.2	0	29	40	24	277	0.1	0.6	18	55	0.58	10	0.07	0.04	0.4	0.1	11	0
1	0.7	0	24	21	24	201	0.2	0.6	13	53	0.58	4	0.03	0.08	0.4	0.08	11	0
7.3	4.2	349	58	177	216	198	1.1	2.2	16	284	3.31	28	0.18	0.53	1.2	0.15	38	0.67
0	0	0	50	61	281	186	0.4	1.4	22	1120	1.08	5	0.02	0.16	0.5	0.22	47	0
1.7	0.8	4	43	—	240	105	—	0.5	—	7	—	1	0.02	0.12	0.3	0.05	—	—
6	0.5	0	—	—	220	75	—	1.1	—	—	—	1	—	—	—	—	—	—
7	0.5	0	—	—	220	90	—	1.4	—	—	—	1	—	—	—	—	—	—
4	0	45	80	—	300	130	—	1.1	—	20	—	—	—	—	—	—	—	—
3	0	35	—	—	180	25	—	0.7	—	—	—	—	—	—	—	—	—	—
4	0	55	60	—	210	180	—	1.4	—	200	—	2	—	—	—	—	—	—
4.2	0.7	27	67	154	267	104	0.3	0.4	11	92	1.47	0	0.09	0.14	0.7	0.03	19	0.19
33.6	5.6	214	538	1230	2137	833	2.4	3.4	88	737	11.8	4	0.75	1.08	5.2	0.26	155	1.55
—	—	5	80	—	430	—	—	1.1	—	0	—	4	0.02	0.03	0.3	—	—	—
7.9	1.5	51	47	86	190	83	0.5	0.6	10	134	1.45	0	0.03	0.18	0.2	0.05	17	0.16
11	3.9	118	72	144	403	188	0.9	2.2	37	347	2.31	0	0.16	0.29	1.3	0.05	14	0.23
4.7	0.8	30	177	241	391	217	0.5	0.5	20	102	1.13	1	0.12	0.27	0.5	0.05	31	0.32
10.4	2.6	155	74	123	362	131	0.7	1.6	10	411	2.94	1	0.04	0.27	0.5	0.06	15	0.32
—	—	10	80	—	200	170	—	1.1	—	0	—	0	—	—	—	—	—	—
8.3	2.2	121	61	101	288	132	0.6	1.8	10	342	2.27	1	0.04	0.23	0.5	0.06	14	0.24
6.3	4.6	0	19	37	318	55	0.2	1	8	14	0.37	1	0.12	0.09	1.2	0.03	15	0.07
7.5	3.6	58	81	126	277	169	0.8	1.8	34	41	1.31	0	0.18	0.24	1.5	0.05	12	0.21
4.8	0.8	33	73	219	437	271	0.6	1	30	96	1.43	0	0.05	0.14	0.6	0.03	25	0.2
38.6	6.2	266	585	1755	3496	2166	4.6	8.2	243	768	11.4	4	0.39	1.12	4.5	0.22	198	1.6
6.2	1.2	22	68	159	310	133	0.4	0.4	16	94	1.41	1	0.03	0.1	0.1	0.04	14	0.2
49.4	9.2	173	543	1274	2480	1063	2.9	3	128	754	11.3	5	0.21	0.78	1	0.34	113	1.58
5.8	1.2	13	13	37	325	51	0.2	0.9	8	33	0.37	1	0.1	0.08	1	0.03	4	0.08
10.7	5.1	38	19	83	210	104	1	1.4	27	19	1.47	0	0.23	0.15	1.1	0.05	11	0.07
0	0	0	1	2	2	19	0	0.2	1	32	0.08	10	0	0.01	0.1	0.03	1	0
0	0	0	1	3	3	32	0	0.3	1	53	0.14	17	0	0.01	0.1	0.04	1	0
5.4	6	0	7	144	1	170	1.2	2.6	66	1	0.99	1	0.23	0.05	1	0.03	16	0
6.5	7.3	0	2	10	20	178	1.2	0.9	66	1	0.99	1	0.35	0.06	1.2	0.03	16	0
0	0.1	0	5	5	1	88	0.1	0.3	11	2	0.08	12	0.07	0.03	0.3	0.07	8	0
0	0	0	11	5	2	123	0.1	0.5	12	4	0.12	10	0.12	0.04	0.4	0.09	13	0
0	0.1	0	18	15	35	153	0.2	0.8	15	10	0	115	0.08	0.04	0.7	0.1	26	0
0	0.1	0	42	20	2	335	0.3	0.6	32	1	0.05	60	0.14	0.06	0.6	0.24	58	0
0	0	0	12	10	8	115	0.2	0.7	15	133	0	56	0.08	0.05	0.5	0.12	27	0
0	0.1	0	18	9	1	133	0.2	0.5	20	1	0.13	9	0.12	0.03	0.4	0.09	6	0
0	0	0	8	4	1	60	0.1	0.2	9	1	0.06	4	0.05	0.02	0.2	0.04	3	0
0	0.1	0	6	6	1	95	0.1	0.3	12	2	0.08	13	0.08	0.03	0.4	0.07	9	0
0	0	0	18	8	1	153	0.1	0.4	18	5	0.12	12	0.12	0.02	0.4	0.09	6	0
0	0	0	18	9	1	132	0.2	0.5	20	1	0.13	9	0.12	0.03	0.4	0.09	6	0
10.5	2.3	0	43	161	2	350	0.4	2.2	51	7	1.67	2	0.26	0.06	0.3	0.08	19	0
11.4	2.6	0	22	152	250	310	0.4	1	42	8	2.06	2	0.14	0.08	0.5	0.08	19	0
11.4	2.6	0	22	152	2	310	0.4	1	42	8	1.67	2	0.14	0.08	0.5	0.08	19	0
—	—	0	1	1	0	7	—	0	1	10	—	2	0	0	0	—	—	0
6.4	3.2	48	273	—	951	320	4.1	2.8	60	200	—	7	0.57	0.61	5.2	0.17	—	—
10.1	3.8	49	209	—	1156	405	4.2	3.2	56	193	—	8	0.63	0.49	5.4	0.16	0	—
11.2	3.9	56	219	—	1428	580	5.6	4.3	76	182	—	10	0.8	0.78	6	0.31	—	—
—	—	46	192	—	1307	578	5.7	3	80	177	—	12	0.68	0.53	7.2	—	—	—
11.8	4.5	55	251	—	1344	408	3.8	4	60	234	—	10	0.56	0.66	8.2	0.2	—	—
11.9	4.5	53	223	—	1419	487	3.8	4.2	60	194	—	11	0.59	0.66	8	0.32	—	—
—	—	54	205	—	1371	544	4.7	3.1	68	170	—	10	0.6	0.49	5.4	—	—	—
—	—	56	466	—	1194	—	—	2.7	—	187	—	17	—	—	—	—	—	—
—	—	40	800	—	1420	—	—	3.6	—	400	—	12	—	—	—	—	—	—
0.7	0.2	0	6	19	2	185	0.3	0.4	26	3	1.87	2	0.03	0.01	0.2	0.09	5	0
0	0	0	2	22	4	358	0.1	0.4	25	70	0.11	8	0.04	0.04	0.6	0.18	20	0

Esha Code	Food Item	Qty	Meas	Wgt (g)	Wtr (g)	Cals	Prot (g)	Carb (g)	Fib (g)	Fat (g)	SatF (g)
3195	Plantain slices, raw	0.5	cup	74	48	90	1	24	1.7	0	0.1
5632	Plantain, ripe, fried	0.5	cup	84	40	216	1	30	2.2	12	1.8
3123	Plum slices, fresh	0.5	cup	82	70	45	1	11	1.2	1	0
3121	Plum, fresh	1	each	66	56	36	1	9	1	0	0
3187	Plum, purple, canned in light syrup	0.5	cup	126	105	79	0	20	1.3	0	0
3124	Plums, canned in heavy syrup	0.5	cup	129	98	115	0	30	1.3	0	0
3185	Plums, purple, canned in juice	0.5	cup	126	106	73	1	19	1.3	0	0
56285	Pochito, frank w/chili in tortilla	1	each	122	72	268	9	22	3.3	16	5.9
5580	Pokeberry shoots/poke greens, cooked	0.5	cup	78	72	16	2	2	1.2	0	0.1
5581	Pokeberry shoots/poke greens, cooked, drained	0.5	cup	82	77	16	2	3	1.2	0	0.1
5579	Pokeberry shoots/poke greens, raw	0.5	cup	80	73	18	2	3	1.4	0	0.1
38311	Polenta, dry	1	piece	57	7	190	5	39	1.6	1	—
3197	Pomegranate, raw (3.5 diameter)	1	each	154	125	105	1	26	0.9	0	0.1
45604	Pop Tarts, raspberry frosted	1	each	52	6	210	2	37	1	6	1
44022	Popcorn cake	1	each	10	0	38	1	8	0.3	0	0
44012	Popcorn, air popped, plain	1	cup	8	0	31	1	6	1.2	0	0
44014	Popcorn, caramel corn	1	cup	35	1	152	1	28	1.8	5	1.3
44037	Popcorn, caramel-coated, w/peanuts, Cracker Jacks	1	oz.	28	1	113	2	23	1.1	2	0.3
44038	Popcorn, cheese-flavored	1	cup	11	0	58	1	6	1.1	4	0.7
44013	Popcorn, cooked in oil, salted	1	cup	11	0	55	1	6	1.1	3	0.5
44066	Popcorn, microwave, lowfat, low sodium	1	cup	6	0	24	1	4	0.8	1	0.1
44065	Popcorn, microwave, pop & serve bag	1	each	87	2	435	8	50	8.7	24	4.2
44072	Popcorn, white, air-popped	1	cup	8	0	31	1	6	1.2	0	0
45540	Popover mix, prepared, 2 x 2	1	each	33	18	67	3	10	0.3	1	0.4
45541	Popover, homemade, w/2% milk	1	each	40	22	88	3	11	0.4	3	0.8
42017	Popover, homemade, w/whole milk	1	each	54	29	122	5	15	0.4	5	1.4
26015	Poppyseed	0.25	tsp	1	0	4	0	0	0.1	0	0
23050	Popsicle/ice pop, double stick	1	each	128	102	92	0	24	0	0	0
7023	Pork & beans, w/sweet sauce, canned	0.5	cup	126	89	140	7	27	6.6	2	0.7
7004	Pork & beans, w/tomato sauce, canned	0.5	cup	126	92	124	7	24	6.1	1	0.5
12065	Pork loin, top roast, prime, roasted, lean	1	piece	42	26	82	13	0	0	3	1.1
44039	Pork skins/rinds, BBQ flavor	1	cup	32	1	172	18	1	—	10	3.7
12021	Pork, blade chop, fried, lean & fat	1	each	89	44	304	19	0	0	25	9.1
12040	Pork, chop, blade, fried, lean	1	each	62	37	149	15	0	0	9	3.2
12082	Pork, chop, breaded, baked/broiled, lean	1	each	80	44	184	21	5	0.2	8	2.9
12026	Pork, chop, center loin, fried, lean	1	each	67	38	155	22	0	0	7	2.4
12044	Pork, chop, center loin, fried, lean & fat	1	each	89	47	247	27	0	0	15	5.4
12035	Pork, chop, loin, broiled, lean	1	each	66	40	139	19	0	0	6	2.4
12031	Pork, chop, loin, roasted, lean & fat	1	piece	42	24	104	11	0	0	6	2.3
12086	Pork, chop, smoked/cured, cooked, lean	1	each	67	43	114	17	0	0	5	1.6
12118	Pork, composite cuts, cooked, lean	4	oz.	113	68	240	33	0	0	11	3.9
12036	Pork, loin, slice, roasted, lean	1	piece	42	26	88	12	0	0	4	1.5
12098	Pork, loin, sparerib, braised, lean	4	oz.	113	67	265	30	0	0	15	5.6
12236	Pork, rib, country style, roasted, lean	4	oz.	113	66	280	30	0	0	17	6
13016	Pork, sausage link, cooked	1	each	13	6	48	3	0	0	4	1.4
13017	Pork, sausage patty, cooked	1	each	27	12	100	5	0	0	8	2.9
12004	Pork, shoulder, braised, lean	4	oz.	113	62	281	37	0	0	14	4.7
12108	Pork, sirloin steak, broiled, lean	4	oz.	113	69	242	32	0	0	12	4.1
12010	Pork, sparerib, braised, lean & fat	4	oz.	113	46	450	33	0	0	34	12.6
12087	Pork, steak/cutlet, breaded, fried	4	oz.	113	56	325	26	10	0.6	20	6.2
12238	Pork, tenderloin, roasted, lean & fat	4	oz.	113	74	196	32	0	0	7	2.4
12094	Pork, tenderloin, tipless, roasted, lean	4	oz.	113	75	186	32	0	0	5	1.9
44006	Potato chips	10	piece	20	0	107	1	11	0.9	7	2.2
44040	Potato chips, BBQ flavor	20	piece	26	0	128	2	14	1.1	8	2.1
44044	Potato chips, Pringles, can	1	each	198	3	1104	12	101	7.1	76	18.7
44042	Potato chips, cheese flavor	1	cup	20	0	99	2	12	1	5	1.7
44045	Potato chips, cheese, Pringles, can	1	each	191	4	1052	13	97	6.4	71	18.3
44008	Potato chips, crushed	0.25	cup	14	0	75	1	7	0.6	5	1.5
44007	Potato chips, grab bag	1	each	57	1	304	4	30	2.6	20	6.2
44043	Potato chips, light	20	piece	40	0	188	3	27	2.3	8	1.7
44024	Potato chips, light, Pringle, can	1	each	170	2	852	10	110	6.1	44	8.7
44024	Potato chips, light, Pringle, can	1	oz.	28	0	142	2	18	1	7	1.4
6023	Potato chips, no salt added	10	each	20	1	105	1	10	1	7	1.8
44076	Potato chips, plain, unsalted	1	oz.	28	1	152	2	15	1.4	10	3.1
44011	Potato chips, rippled	10	piece	30	1	161	2	16	1.4	10	3.3

MonoF	PolyF	Choles	Calc	Phos	Sod	Pot	Zn	Iron	Magn	VitA	VitE	VitC	Thia	Ribo	Nia	B6	Fola	B12
(g)	(g)	(mg)	(mg)	(mg)	(mg)	(mg)	(mg)	(mg)	(mg)	(μg RE)	(mg α-TE)	(mg)	(mg)	(mg)	(mg)	(mg)	(μg)	(μg)
0	0.1	0	2	25	3	369	0.1	0.4	27	84	0.2	14	0.04	0.04	0.5	0.22	16	0
2.7	6.6	0	3	32	4	427	0.1	0.6	35	81	0.96	12	0.04	0.05	0.6	0.26	10	0
0.3	0.1	0	3	8	0	142	0.1	0.1	6	26	0.5	8	0.04	0.08	0.4	0.07	2	0
0.3	0.1	0	3	7	0	114	0.1	0.1	5	21	0.4	6	0.03	0.06	0.3	0.05	1	0
0.1	0	0	11	16	25	117	0.1	1.1	6	33	0.88	1	0.02	0.05	0.4	0.03	3	0
0.1	0	0	12	17	24	117	0.1	1.1	6	34	0.9	1	0.02	0.05	0.4	0.04	3	0
0	0	0	13	19	1	194	0.1	0.4	10	127	0.88	4	0.03	0.07	0.6	0.03	3	0
7.3	1.8	30	86	211	728	279	2	2.4	46	20	0.54	10	0.13	0.12	1.7	0.18	16	0.5
0	0.1	0	41	26	14	143	0.1	0.9	11	674	0.66	64	0.05	0.19	0.9	0.09	7	0
0	0.1	0	44	27	15	152	0.2	1	12	718	0.7	68	0.06	0.21	0.9	0.09	7	0
0	0.1	0	42	35	18	194	0.2	1.4	14	696	0.68	109	0.06	0.26	1	0.12	13	0
—	—	0	2	—	1	86	0.3	0.4	24	12	—	0	0.35	0.01	0.3	—	—	—
0.1	0.1	0	5	12	5	399	0.2	0.5	5	0	0.85	9	0.05	0.05	0.5	0.16	9	0
—	—	0	0	40	210	—	0.6	1.8	8	150	—	0	0.15	0.17	2	0.2	40	—
0.1	0.1	0	1	28	29	33	0.4	0.2	16	1	0.01	0	0.01	0.02	0.6	0.02	2	0
0.1	0.2	0	1	24	0	24	0.3	0.2	10	2	0.01	0	0.02	0.02	0.2	0.02	2	0
1	1.6	2	15	29	72	38	0.2	0.6	12	4	0.42	0	0.02	0.02	0.8	0.01	1	0
0.8	0.9	0	19	36	84	101	0.4	1.1	23	2	0.42	0	0.01	0.04	0.6	0.05	5	0
1.1	1.7	1	12	40	98	29	0.2	0.2	10	5	0.01	0	0.01	0.03	0.2	0.03	1	0.06
0.9	1.5	0	1	28	97	25	0.3	0.3	12	2	0.01	0	0.02	0.02	0.2	0.02	2	0
0.2	0.3	0	1	15	28	14	0.2	0.1	9	1	0.06	0	0.02	0.01	0.1	0.01	1	0
7.1	11.7	0	9	218	769	196	2.3	2.4	94	13	0.1	0	0.12	0.12	1.4	0.18	15	0
0.1	0.2	0	1	24	0	24	0.3	0.2	10	0	0.01	0	0.02	0.02	0.2	0.02	2	0
0.6	0.2	37	9	30	143	25	0.2	0.6	5	16	0.36	0	0.05	0.06	0.4	0.02	6	0.08
0.9	1	46	38	56	82	65	0.3	0.8	7	34	0.43	0	0.09	0.15	0.7	0.03	7	0.13
1.3	1.4	64	50	75	110	87	0.4	1	10	37	0.2	0	0.12	0.2	1	0.04	10	0.18
0	0.2	0	11	6	0	5	0.1	0.1	2	0	0.02	0	0.01	0	0	0	0	0
0	0	0	0	0	15	5	0	0	1	0	0	0	0	0	0	0	0	0
0.8	0.2	9	77	133	425	336	1.9	2.1	43	14	0.68	4	0.06	0.08	0.4	0.11	47	0
0.6	0.2	9	71	148	557	380	7.4	4.2	44	15	0.68	4	0.07	0.06	0.6	0.09	28	0
1.4	0.2	33	2	93	19	149	1	0.4	10	1	0.15	0	0.27	0.13	2.2	0.17	4	0.23
4.8	1.1	37	14	70	853	58	0.2	0.3	0	58	—	0	0.03	0.14	1.1	0.05	10	0.04
10.4	2.8	76	27	183	60	295	2.8	0.8	19	3	0.23	1	0.55	0.26	3.5	0.3	4	0.75
3.9	1.2	51	14	137	48	226	2.4	0.7	16	1	0.16	0	0.45	0.22	2.8	0.25	2	0.6
3.7	0.9	57	17	197	333	331	1.8	0.8	22	1	0.36	1	0.68	0.25	4	0.36	5	0.52
3	0.9	62	15	182	58	301	1.6	0.7	21	1	0.17	1	0.83	0.22	4	0.34	4	0.51
6.3	1.7	82	24	231	71	378	2.1	0.8	26	2	0.23	1	1.01	0.27	5	0.42	5	0.65
2.9	0.5	52	11	167	42	289	1.6	0.6	19	1	0.17	0	0.61	0.22	3.5	0.32	4	0.48
2.7	0.5	34	8	102	25	171	1	0.4	11	1	0.11	0	0.42	0.13	2.3	0.22	3	0.3
2.2	0.5	32	7	163	825	196	2	0.7	11	0	0.17	0	0.49	0.15	3.2	0.25	3	0.74
4.9	0.9	98	24	269	67	425	3.4	1.2	30	2	0.3	0	0.96	0.39	5.9	0.49	7	0.85
1.8	0.3	34	8	105	24	179	1.1	0.5	12	1	0.11	0	0.43	0.14	2.5	0.23	3	0.31
6.7	1.2	98	28	191	71	391	4.5	1.6	20	2	0.5	1	0.62	0.32	4.6	0.41	3	0.84
7.3	1.2	105	33	251	33	396	4.3	1.5	27	2	0.55	0	0.65	0.39	5.3	0.5	6	0.91
2	0.4	11	4	24	168	47	0.3	0.2	2	0	0.03	0	0.1	0.03	0.6	0.04	0	0.23
4.2	0.8	22	9	50	349	98	0.7	0.3	5	0	0.07	0	0.2	0.07	1.2	0.09	1	0.47
6.6	1.3	129	9	256	116	459	5.6	2.2	25	2	0.3	0	0.68	0.41	6.7	0.46	6	0.8
5	1	96	15	291	82	455	3.1	1.2	35	2	0.3	1	1.17	0.42	5.4	0.68	6	0.9
15.3	3.1	137	53	296	105	363	5.2	2.1	27	3	0.3	0	0.46	0.43	6.2	0.4	5	1.22
7.7	3.7	109	44	233	458	343	3.3	1.7	28	15	0.71	1	0.77	0.4	4.4	0.38	11	0.86
2.8	0.6	90	7	291	62	491	3	1.6	31	2	0.3	0	1.05	0.44	5.3	0.47	7	0.62
2.2	0.5	90	7	294	64	496	3	1.7	32	2	0.3	0	1.07	0.44	5.3	0.48	7	0.62
2	2.4	0	5	33	119	255	0.2	0.3	13	0	0.98	6	0.03	0.04	0.8	0.13	9	0
1.7	4.3	0	13	48	195	328	0.2	0.5	20	6	1.3	9	0.06	0.06	1.2	0.16	22	0
14.4	39.6	0	48	311	1298	1995	1.2	3	115	0	9.66	16	0.41	0.24	6.2	0.29	14	0
1.5	1.9	1	14	60	159	306	0.2	0.4	15	2	0.98	11	0.03	0.03	1	0.07	0	0
13.6	35.7	8	210	311	1442	728	1.2	3.1	101	0	9.32	16	0.34	0.23	5	1	34	0
1.4	1.7	0	3	23	83	179	0.2	0.2	9	0	0.68	4	0.02	0.03	0.5	0.09	6	0
5.6	6.9	0	14	94	337	723	0.6	0.9	38	0	2.77	18	0.1	0.11	2.2	0.37	26	0
1.9	4.4	0	8	77	197	698	0	0.5	36	0	1.16	10	0.08	0.11	2.8	0.27	11	0
10.1	23	0	58	262	728	1708	1	2.6	107	0	8.5	20	0.32	0.1	7.1	1.33	39	0
1.7	3.8	0	10	44	121	285	0.2	0.4	18	0	1.42	3	0.05	0.02	1.2	0.22	7	0
1.2	3.6	0	5	31	2	260	0.2	0.2	12	0	0.86	8	0.03	0	0.8	0.1	9	0
2.8	3.5	0	7	47	2	361	0.3	0.5	19	0	1.38	9	0.05	0.06	1.1	0.19	13	0
3	3.7	0	7	50	178	383	0.3	0.5	20	0	1.46	9	0.05	0.06	1.2	0.2	14	0

Esha Code	Food Item	Qty	Meas	Wgt (g)	Wtr (g)	Cals	Prot (g)	Carb (g)	Fib (g)	Fat (g)	SatF (g)
5437	Potato chips, sour cream & onion	1	oz.	28	1	151	2	15	1.5	10	2.5
44046	Potato chips, sour cream & onion, Pringles, can	1	each	191	4	1044	13	98	2.3	71	18.1
5263	Potato pancake, large	1	each	76	36	207	5	22	1.5	12	2.3
5352	Potato pieces, canned, drained	0.5	cup	90	76	54	1	12	2.1	0	0
56005	Potato salad w/mayonnaise & eggs	0.5	cup	125	95	179	3	14	1.6	10	1.8
56319	Potato salad, German	0.5	cup	88	68	79	2	15	1.4	2	0.6
5368	Potato skin, cooked	1	each	34	26	26	1	6	1.1	0	0
5350	Potato skin, microwave cooked	1	each	58	37	77	3	17	3.2	0	0
5339	Potato skin, oven baked	1	each	58	27	115	2	27	4.6	0	0
44025	Potato skins, chips, Tato Skins	10	piece	20	0	112	1	10	0.7	7	1.9
5266	Potato, Tater Tots, frozen, oven heated	10	each	70	37	155	2	21	2.2	7	3.6
5276	Potato, au gratin, prep from dry mix	0.5	cup	122	97	114	3	16	1.1	5	3.2
5275	Potato, au gratin, recipe, w/margarine	0.5	cup	122	91	162	6	14	2.2	9	4.3
5130	Potato, baked, flesh only, medium size	1	each	122	92	113	2	26	1.8	0	0
5134	Potato, boiled in skin, peeled after, diced	0.5	cup	78	60	68	1	16	1.4	0	0
5133	Potato, boiled, peeled after	1	each	136	105	118	3	27	2.4	0	0
5351	Potato, canned, 1 in diam, drained	2	each	70	59	42	1	10	1.6	0	0
5332	Potato, cottage fries, frozen, oven heated	10	each	50	26	109	2	17	1.6	4	2
5582	Potato, flesh, raw, diced	0.5	cup	75	59	59	2	14	1.2	0	0
5460	Potato, french fried, veg oil, reg svg	1	each	76	31	232	3	29	2.7	11	2
5139	Potato, french fries, frozen, oven heated	10	piece	50	18	167	2	20	1.6	9	3
5329	Potato, french fries, frozen, restaurant fried	10	each	50	19	158	2	20	1.6	8	1.9
5331	Potato, french fries, frted in animal&veg oil	10	each	50	19	158	2	20	1.6	8	1.9
5463	Potato, hash browns-fast food serving	1	each	65	39	137	2	15	—	8	3.9
5141	Potato, hashed brown patty, frozen, fried	1	each	66	37	144	2	18	1.3	8	3
5591	Potato, hashed brown w/butter sce, frozen, cooked	0.5	cup	72	46	129	2	18	2.8	6	2.4
5140	Potato, hashed browns, frozen, cooked	0.5	cup	78	44	170	2	22	1.6	9	3.5
5272	Potato, mashed w/milk & margarine	0.5	cup	105	80	111	2	18	2.1	4	1.1
5137	Potato, mashed w/whole milk	0.5	cup	105	82	81	2	18	2.1	1	0.4
5569	Potato, mashed w/whole milk & butter	0.5	cup	105	80	111	2	18	2.1	4	2.9
5464	Potato, mashed, flakes prep w/milk & butter	0.5	cup	105	80	119	2	16	2.4	6	3.6
5138	Potato, mashed, flakes prep w/whole milk & margarin	0.5	cup	110	84	124	2	16	2.5	6	1.6
5585	Potato, mashed, granules w/whole milk & butter	0.5	cup	105	81	113	2	15	2.3	5	3.2
5347	Potato, microwaved w/skin, flesh only, medium size	1	each	92	68	92	2	21	1.5	0	0
5269	Potato, o'brien, frozen, cooked	0.5	cup	97	60	198	2	21	1.6	13	3.2
5268	Potato, o'brien, recipe	0.5	cup	97	77	79	2	15	1	1	0.8
5136	Potato, peeled, boiled, diced	0.5	cup	78	60	67	1	16	1.4	0	0
5135	Potato, peeled, boiled, whole	1	each	135	105	116	2	27	2.4	0	0
5540	Potato, prepared mix, Twice Baked	0.5	cup	118	54	324	8	33	2.7	18	9
5271	Potato, scalloped, prep from dry mix	0.5	cup	122	97	114	3	16	1.4	5	3.2
5270	Potato, scalloped, recipe w/margarine	0.5	cup	122	99	105	4	13	2.3	5	1.7
5328	Potato, small, whole, frozen, cooked	1	each	70	58	46	1	10	1	0	0
5337	Potato, w/skin, medium size, baked	1	each	122	87	133	3	31	2.9	0	0
5342	Potato, w/skin, medium size, microwaved	1	each	93	67	98	2	22	2.1	0	0
5512	Potato, white, roasted	1	each	93	58	132	3	30	2.7	0	0
5584	Potato, whole, canned w/liquid	0.5	cup	150	132	66	2	15	2.1	0	0
5583	Potato, whole, raw, flesh only	1	each	112	88	88	2	20	1.8	0	0
26028	Poultry seasoning	0.25	tsp	0	0	1	0	0	0	0	0
62206	Power bar	1	each	65	—	230	10	45	3	2	—
62280	Power bar, Mocha	1	each	65	7	230	10	45	3	2	1
62275	Power bar, apple cinnamon	1	each	65	7	230	10	45	3	2	0.5
44078	Pretzel, hard twist, unenriched, unsalted	10	each	60	2	229	5	48	1.7	2	0.4
44016	Pretzel, hard, twist	10	each	60	2	229	5	48	1.9	2	0.4
44048	Pretzel, hard, whole wheat	1	oz.	28	1	103	3	23	2.2	1	0.2
42093	Pretzel, soft	1	each	55	8	190	5	38	0.9	2	0.7
44017	Pretzel, sticks	10	each	5	0	19	0	4	0.2	0	0
44015	Pretzel, thick dutch twist	1	each	16	1	61	1	13	0.5	1	0.1
44067	Pretzel, yogurt-covered	6	each	25	1	115	2	17	0.2	5	3.6
44033	Pretzels, cheddar, Combos snack	10	piece	30	1	139	3	20	—	5	—
3198	Prickly pear fruit, raw	1	each	103	90	42	1	10	3.7	1	0.1
3352	Prunes, canned in heavy syrup	0.5	cup	117	83	123	1	32	4.4	0	0
3126	Prunes, dried	10	each	84	27	201	2	53	6	0	0
3127	Prunes, dry, stewed, no sugar added	0.5	cup	106	74	113	1	30	7	0	0
2026	Pudding pop, chocolate	1	each	47	30	72	2	12	0.2	2	2.1
2027	Pudding pop, vanilla	1	each	47	30	75	2	13	0	2	2.1

MonoF	PolyF	Choles	Calc	Phos	Sod	Pot	Zn	Iron	Magn	VitA	VitE	VitC	Thia	Ribo	Nia	B6	Fola	B12
(g)	(g)	(mg)	(mg)	(mg)	(mg)	(mg)	(mg)	(mg)	(mg)	(μg RE)	(mg α-TE)	(mg)	(mg)	(mg)	(mg)	(mg)	(μg)	(μg)
1.7	4.9	2	20	50	177	377	0.3	0.5	21	6	1.38	11	0.05	0.06	1.1	0.19	18	0.28
13.6	35.9	6	122	323	1375	947	1.4	2.7	105	187	9.32	18	0.34	0.19	4.8	0.91	44	0
3.5	5	73	18	84	386	597	0.6	1.2	25	11	1.52	17	0.1	0.13	1.6	0.29	12	0.14
0	0.1	0	4	25	197	206	0.3	1.1	13	0	0.04	5	0.06	0.01	0.8	0.17	6	0
3.1	4.7	85	24	65	661	318	0.4	0.8	19	41	2.33	12	0.1	0.08	1.1	0.18	8	0
0.7	0.2	3	7	42	201	277	0.3	0.3	18	1	0.07	10	0.09	0.02	1.1	0.21	9	0.05
0	0	0	15	18	5	138	0.2	2.1	10	0	0.01	2	0.01	0.01	0.4	0.08	3	0
0	0	0	27	48	9	377	0.3	3.4	22	0	0.02	9	0.04	0.04	1.3	0.28	10	0
0	0	0	20	59	12	332	0.3	4.1	25	0	0.02	8	0.07	0.06	1.8	0.36	12	0
1.2	3.9	0	5	31	131	202	0.1	0.3	12	0	0.98	2	0.04	0.02	0.6	0.03	1	0
3	0.6	0	21	34	522	266	0.2	1.1	13	1	0.04	5	0.14	0.05	1.5	0.16	12	0
1.4	0.2	18	102	116	538	268	0.3	0.4	18	38	1.47	4	0.02	0.1	1.2	0.05	8	0
3.2	1.3	18	146	138	530	485	0.8	0.8	24	47	0.65	12	0.08	0.14	1.2	0.21	14	0
0	0.1	0	6	61	6	477	0.4	0.4	30	0	0.05	16	0.13	0.03	1.7	0.37	11	0
0	0	0	4	34	3	296	0.2	0.2	17	0	0.04	10	0.08	0.02	1.1	0.23	8	0
0	0.1	0	7	60	5	515	0.4	0.4	30	0	0.07	18	0.14	0.03	2	0.41	14	0
0	0.1	0	4	20	153	160	0.2	0.9	10	0	0.04	4	0.05	0.01	0.6	0.13	4	0
1.7	0.3	0	5	32	22	240	0.2	0.7	11	0	0.1	5	0.06	0.02	1.2	0.12	8	0
0	0	0	5	34	4	407	0.3	0.6	16	0	0.04	15	0.07	0.03	1.1	0.2	10	0
5	2.8	0	11	98	150	524	0.4	0.6	30	0	0.93	9	0.06	0.03	2.2	0.27	29	0
5.6	0.7	0	6	48	307	270	0.2	0.8	12	0	0.25	3	0.04	0.02	1.3	0.11	11	0
4.7	0.7	0	10	46	108	366	0.2	0.4	17	0	0.25	5	0.09	0.01	1.6	0.12	14	0
4.7	0.7	6	10	46	108	366	0.2	0.4	17	0	0.25	5	0.09	0.01	1.6	0.12	14	0
3.5	0.4	8	6	62	262	241	0.2	0.4	14	3	0.11	5	0.07	0.01	1	0.15	7	0.01
3.4	0.9	0	10	48	22	288	0.2	1	11	0	0.12	4	0.07	0.01	1.6	0.08	4	0
2.3	1.3	17	24	28	73	237	0.2	0.7	11	12	0.1	3	0.04	0.02	1	0.19	10	0
4	1	0	12	56	26	340	0.2	1.2	13	0	0.15	5	0.09	0.02	1.9	0.1	5	0
1.9	1.3	2	27	48	310	303	0.3	0.3	19	21	0.32	6	0.09	0.04	1.1	0.24	8	0
0.2	0.1	2	27	50	318	314	0.3	0.3	19	6	0.05	7	0.09	0.04	1.2	0.24	9	0
1.2	0.2	13	27	48	310	303	0.3	0.3	19	21	0.32	6	0.09	0.04	1.1	0.24	8	0
1.7	0.3	15	52	59	349	245	0.2	0.2	19	22	0.73	10	0.12	0.05	0.7	0.01	8	0.08
2.5	1.7	4	54	62	365	256	0.2	0.2	20	23	0.77	11	0.12	0.06	0.7	0.01	8	0
1.5	0.2	15	37	63	270	151	0.3	0.2	20	20	0.03	6	0.08	0.08	0.8	0.01	8	0
0	0	0	5	100	6	378	0.3	0.4	23	0	0.04	14	0.12	0.02	1.5	0.29	11	0
5.6	3.4	0	19	90	42	459	0.5	0.9	33	18	0.18	10	0.05	0.13	1.4	0.37	12	0
0.3	0.1	4	35	48	210	258	0.3	0.5	18	55	0.12	16	0.07	0.05	1	0.21	8	0
0	0	0	6	31	4	256	0.2	0.2	16	0	0.04	6	0.08	0.02	1	0.21	7	0
0	0.1	0	11	54	7	443	0.4	0.4	27	0	0.07	10	0.13	0.03	1.8	0.36	12	0
6.5	1.3	155	83	153	936	515	0.7	0.8	34	155	1.38	25	0.34	0.26	2.2	0.32	23	0.36
1.5	0.2	14	44	69	418	249	0.3	0.5	17	26	0.18	4	0.02	0.07	1.3	0.05	12	0
1.6	0.9	7	70	77	410	463	0.5	0.7	23	23	0.4	13	0.08	0.11	1.3	0.22	14	0
0	0	0	5	18	14	201	0.2	0.6	8	0	0.04	7	0.07	0.02	0.9	0.14	6	0
0	0.1	0	12	70	10	510	0.4	1.7	33	0	0.06	16	0.13	0.04	2	0.42	13	0
0	0	0	10	98	7	416	0.3	1.2	25	0	0.05	14	0.11	0.03	1.6	0.32	11	0
0	0.1	0	12	77	10	905	0.6	1.3	35	0	0.1	26	0.12	0.06	2.4	0.41	19	0
0	0.1	0	58	33	326	308	0.6	1.1	21	0	0.06	11	0.05	0.03	1.3	0.21	7	0
0	0	0	8	52	7	608	0.4	0.9	24	0	0.07	22	0.1	0.04	1.7	0.29	14	0
0	0	0	3	1	0	2	0	0.1	1	1	0	0	0	0	0	0	0	0
—	—	0	300	350	110	150	5.2	5.4	140	—	—	60	1.5	1.7	20	2	400	6
1	0.5	0	300	350	90	145	5.2	6.3	140	0	20	60	1.5	1.7	20	2	400	6
1.5	0.5	0	300	350	90	110	5.2	6.3	140	0	20	60	1.5	1.7	20	2	400	6
0.8	0.7	0	22	68	173	88	0.5	1	21	0	0.13	0	0.11	0.06	1.2	0.07	50	0
0.8	0.7	0	22	68	1029	88	0.5	2.6	21	0	0.13	0	0.28	0.37	3.2	0.07	103	0
0.3	0.2	0	8	35	58	122	0.2	0.8	9	0	0.07	0	0.12	0.08	1.8	0.08	15	0
0.8	0.2	2	13	44	772	48	0.5	2.2	12	0	0.02	0	0.23	0.16	2.4	0.01	8	0
0.1	0.1	0	2	6	86	7	0	0.2	2	0	0.01	0	0.02	0.03	0.3	0.01	9	0
0.2	0.2	0	6	18	274	23	0.1	0.7	6	0	0.03	0	0.07	0.1	0.8	0.02	27	0
0.5	0.1	1	37	36	16	60	0.2	0.4	5	19	0.17	0	0.08	0.09	0.7	0.01	4	0.12
—	—	2	59	43	335	39	0.2	0.3	7	2	0.06	0	0.09	0.17	1	0.01	2	0.04
0.1	0.2	0	58	25	5	227	0.1	0.3	88	5	0.01	14	0.01	0.06	0.5	0.06	6	0
0.2	0	0	20	30	4	264	0.2	0.5	18	94	0.29	3	0.04	0.14	1	0.24	0	0
0.3	0.1	0	43	66	3	626	0.4	2.1	38	167	1.22	3	0.07	0.14	1.6	0.22	3	0
0.2	0.1	0	24	37	2	354	0.3	1.2	21	33	0	3	0.02	0.11	0.8	0.23	0	0
0	0	1	66	53	78	105	0.2	0.2	10	16	0.01	0	0.02	0.08	0.1	0.02	1	0.25
0	0	1	61	48	50	65	0.2	0	5	24	0.01	0	0.02	0.09	0	0.02	2	0.17

Esha Code	Food Item	Qty	Meas	Wgt (g)	Wtr (g)	Cals	Prot (g)	Carb (g)	Fib (g)	Fat (g)	SatF (g)
2628	Pudding, banana, instant w/2% milk	0.5	cup	147	110	153	4	29	0	2	1.5
2629	Pudding, banana, instant w/whole milk	0.5	cup	147	108	166	4	29	0	4	2.6
2620	Pudding, banana, mix w/whole milk	0.5	cup	140	104	157	4	25	0	4	2.6
2631	Pudding, banana, regular w/2% milk	0.5	cup	140	106	143	4	26	0	2	1.5
2617	Pudding, bread, w/raisins	0.5	cup	126	79	212	7	31	1.3	7	2.9
2634	Pudding, chocolate, instant w/2% milk	0.5	cup	147	110	150	5	28	0.6	3	1.6
2605	Pudding, chocolate, instant w/whole milk	0.5	cup	147	108	163	5	28	1.5	5	2.7
2637	Pudding, chocolate, recipe w/2% milk	0.5	cup	157	106	206	5	40	1.4	4	2
2604	Pudding, chocolate, reg mix w/whole milk	0.5	cup	142	106	158	5	26	1.4	5	3
2636	Pudding, chocolate, regular w/2% milk	0.5	cup	142	105	151	5	28	0.4	3	1.8
2601	Pudding, chocolate, w/whole milk, recipe	0.5	cup	157	105	221	5	40	1.3	6	3.1
2639	Pudding, coconut cream, instant w/2% milk	0.5	cup	147	109	157	4	28	0.1	3	2
2641	Pudding, coconut cream, reg w/2% milk	0.5	cup	140	106	146	4	25	0.3	4	2.5
2615	Pudding, coconut, instant w/whole milk	0.5	cup	147	108	172	4	28	0.1	5	3.1
2644	Pudding, lemon, instant w/2% milk	0.5	cup	147	109	154	4	30	0	2	1.5
2616	Pudding, lemon, instant w/whole milk	0.5	cup	147	108	169	4	30	0	4	2.6
2646	Pudding, lemon, mix+sugar+egg yolk+water	0.5	cup	146	106	164	1	36	0	2	0.6
2614	Pudding, low cal mix w/milk, D-Zerta	0.5	cup	130	110	88	4	12	0	2	1.5
2666	Pudding, low calorie mix w/milk, D-Zerta	0.5	cup	125	108	60	5	11	1	0	0
2650	Pudding, rice w/raisins, recipe	0.5	cup	152	101	217	5	40	0.8	4	2.6
2649	Pudding, rice, mix w/2% milk	0.5	cup	144	105	161	5	30	0.1	2	1.4
2606	Pudding, rice, mix w/whole milk, cooked	0.5	cup	144	104	176	5	30	0.1	4	2.5
2653	Pudding, tapioca, mix w/2% milk	0.5	cup	141	105	147	4	28	0	2	1.5
2607	Pudding, tapioca, reg mix w/whole milk	0.5	cup	141	104	161	4	28	0	4	2.5
2603	Pudding, tapioca, w/whole milk, recipe	0.5	cup	82	60	103	4	14	0	4	1.8
2764	Pudding, vanilla, fat free, snack size, Jell-o	1	each	113	87	100	2	23	0	0	0
2655	Pudding, vanilla, instant w/2% milk	0.5	cup	142	106	148	4	28	0	2	1.4
2608	Pudding, vanilla, instant w/whole milk	0.5	cup	142	104	162	4	28	0	4	2.5
2657	Pudding, vanilla, reg mix w/2% milk	0.5	cup	140	106	141	4	26	0	2	1.5
2609	Pudding, vanilla, reg mix w/whole milk	0.5	cup	140	104	155	4	26	0	4	2.6
2602	Pudding, vanilla, w/whole milk, recipe	0.5	cup	123	94	130	4	20	0	4	2.5
45543	Puff pastry, frozen	1	each	47	4	259	3	21	0.7	18	4.5
45583	Puff pastry, frozen, baked	1	each	40	3	223	3	18	0.6	15	2.2
3262	Pummelo, raw sections	0.5	cup	95	85	36	1	9	1	0	—
5422	Pumpkin leaves, cooked	0.5	cup	35	32	7	1	1	0.9	0	0
5421	Pumpkin leaves, raw	0.5	cup	20	19	4	1	0	0.2	0	0
26029	Pumpkin pie spice	0.25	tsp	0	0	2	0	0	0.1	0	0
4522	Pumpkin seed kernel, dry roasted, unsalted	0.25	cup	34	2	187	8	6	1.4	16	3
4625	Pumpkin seed kernels, roasted, salted	0.25	cup	57	4	296	19	8	2.2	24	4.5
4565	Pumpkin seed kernels, roasted, unsalted	0.25	cup	57	4	296	19	8	2.2	24	4.5
4564	Pumpkin seeds, roasted, salted	0.25	cup	16	1	71	3	9	0.8	3	0.6
45556	Pumpkin turnover	1	each	78	41	198	4	20	1.3	11	3.5
5142	Pumpkin, canned, low sodium	0.5	cup	123	111	42	1	10	3.6	0	0.2
5396	Pumpkin, fresh, cooked	0.5	cup	122	115	24	1	6	1.4	0	0
56122	Quesadilla	1	each	54	16	199	6	21	1.2	10	3.6
56098	Quiche Lorraine, 1/8th pie	1	piece	176	95	508	20	20	0.6	39	17.6
14004	Rabbit, domestic, roasted	4	oz.	113	69	223	33	0	0	9	2.7
5452	Radicchio leaf, raw	10	each	80	74	18	1	4	0.7	0	0
5451	Radicchio, raw, shredded	0.5	cup	20	19	5	0	1	0.2	0	0
5593	Radish, Daikon/Chinese, cooked slices	0.5	cup	74	70	12	0	3	1.2	0	0.1
5143	Radish, red	10	each	45	43	9	0	2	0.7	0	0
5144	Radish, red, slices	0.5	cup	58	55	12	0	2	0.9	0	0
5550	Radish, white icicle, raw slices	0.5	cup	50	48	7	1	1	0.7	0	0
5551	Radish, white icicle, raw, whole	3	each	51	49	7	1	1	0.7	0	0
5216	Radishes, Chinese/Daikon, slices, raw	0.5	cup	44	42	8	0	2	0.7	0	0
5217	Radishes, Daikon/Chinese, whole, raw	1	each	338	320	61	2	14	5.4	0	0.1
3129	Raisin, seedless, packed	0.5	cup	82	13	248	3	65	3.3	0	0.1
3130	Raisin, seedless, unpacked	0.5	cup	72	11	218	2	57	2.9	0	0.1
3202	Raisins, golden seedless, packed	0.5	cup	82	12	249	3	66	3.3	0	0.1
3132	Raspberries, canned in heavy syrup	0.5	cup	128	96	116	1	30	4.2	0	0
3131	Raspberries, fresh	0.5	cup	62	53	30	1	7	4.2	0	0
3235	Raspberries, frozen, sweetened	10	oz.	284	207	293	2	74	12.5	0	0
56128	Ravioli, cheese-filled, w/tomato sauce, serving	1	each	250	178	336	14	38	2.2	14	6.3
56303	Ravioli, meat filled	0.5	cup	125	85	194	10	18	1.3	9	3
56638	Refried beans/frijoles, w/cheese	8	oz.	167	115	225	11	29	—	8	4.1

MonoF	PolyF	Choles	Calc	Phos	Sod	Pot	Zn	Iron	Magn	VitA	VitE	VitC	Thia	Ribo	Nia	B6	Fola	B12
(g)	(g)	(mg)	(mg)	(mg)	(mg)	(mg)	(mg)	(mg)	(mg)	(μg RE)	(mg α-TE)	(mg)	(mg)	(mg)	(mg)	(mg)	(μg)	(μg)
0.7	0.2	9	150	318	435	193	0.5	0.1	18	66	0.07	1	0.05	0.2	0.1	0.05	6	0.44
1.2	0.2	16	147	315	434	188	0.5	0.1	18	37	0.07	1	0.05	0.2	0.1	0.05	6	0.44
1.2	0.2	17	151	116	231	189	0.5	0.1	18	38	0.07	1	0.04	0.2	0.1	0.05	6	0.35
0.7	0.1	10	154	118	232	193	0.5	0.1	18	70	0.07	1	0.04	0.2	0.1	0.05	6	0.36
2.7	1.2	83	144	137	291	282	0.7	1.4	24	82	0.63	1	0.12	0.28	0.8	0.09	16	0.33
0.9	0.2	9	153	353	417	247	0.6	0.4	26	56	0.15	1	0.05	0.21	0.1	0.06	6	0.46
1.4	0.3	16	150	351	417	244	0.6	0.4	26	31	0.09	1	0.05	0.21	0.1	0.06	6	0.44
1.3	0.4	9	155	149	138	256	0.8	0.7	39	78	0.11	1	0.05	0.22	0.2	0.05	6	0.36
1.4	0.2	17	158	132	146	231	0.6	0.5	21	37	0.08	1	0.04	0.25	0.1	0.05	6	0.36
0.8	0.1	10	160	138	149	240	0.7	0.5	30	68	0.08	1	0.04	0.21	0.2	0.05	6	0.36
1.8	0.5	17	152	148	137	253	0.8	0.7	38	49	0.14	1	0.05	0.22	0.2	0.05	6	0.34
0.9	0.3	9	150	295	362	194	0.5	0.2	21	69	0.06	1	0.05	0.2	0.1	0.06	6	0.44
0.7	0.1	10	158	125	228	223	0.5	0.3	22	70	0.1	1	0.04	0.2	0.1	0.2	6	0.36
1.4	0.4	16	147	294	362	190	0.5	0.2	21	37	0.09	1	0.05	0.2	0.1	0.05	6	0.44
0.7	0.1	9	148	304	394	190	0.5	0.1	16	69	0.07	1	0.05	0.2	0.1	0.05	6	0.44
1.2	0.2	16	146	301	392	187	0.5	0.1	16	38	0.07	1	0.05	0.2	0.1	0.05	6	0.44
0.7	0.2	77	12	31	93	7	0.2	0.3	3	35	0.07	0	0.01	0.05	0	0.02	9	0.19
0.7	0.1	9	151	211	303	191	0.5	0.1	18	70	0.09	1	0.05	0.2	0.1	0.05	6	0.45
0	0	0	150	210	65	290	0.5	0.4	27	40	0.09	1	0.05	0.2	0.1	0.05	6	0.42
1.2	0.2	17	155	143	85	269	0.7	1	24	38	0.08	1	0.12	0.21	0.8	0.08	6	0.24
0.6	0.1	9	151	127	158	190	0.6	0.5	19	52	0.06	1	0.11	0.2	0.6	0.05	6	0.36
1.2	0.2	16	148	124	157	186	0.5	0.5	19	29	0.09	1	0.11	0.2	0.6	0.05	6	0.35
0.7	0.1	8	149	117	172	189	0.5	0.1	17	69	0.07	1	0.04	0.2	0.1	0.06	6	0.35
1.2	0.2	17	147	116	171	186	0.5	0.1	17	38	0.11	1	0.04	0.2	0.1	0.05	6	0.35
1.2	0.3	68	86	87	157	117	0.4	0.3	11	47	0.07	0	0.03	0.18	0.1	0.04	7	0.3
0	0	0	80	—	240	125	—	0	—	20	—	0	—	—	—	—	—	—
0.7	0.1	9	146	283	406	185	0.5	0.1	17	64	0.07	1	0.05	0.2	0.1	0.05	6	0.43
1.2	0.2	16	143	280	406	182	0.5	0.1	17	36	0.08	1	0.05	0.19	0.1	0.05	6	0.43
0.7	0.1	10	153	118	224	193	0.5	0.1	18	70	0.07	1	0.04	0.2	0.1	0.05	6	0.36
1.2	0.2	17	150	115	224	190	0.5	0.1	18	38	0.08	1	0.04	0.2	0.1	0.05	6	0.35
1.2	0.2	16	145	114	113	185	0.5	0.1	16	37	0.1	1	0.03	0.2	0.1	0.04	5	0.23
10.2	2.3	0	5	28	117	29	0.2	1.2	8	0	2.4	0	0.19	0.13	2	0.01	44	0
3.5	8.9	0	4	24	101	25	0.2	1	6	0	0.95	0	0.13	0.1	1.5	0.01	19	0
—	—	0	4	16	1	205	0.1	0.1	6	0	0.09	58	0.03	0.03	0.2	0.03	25	0
0	0	0	15	28	3	153	0.1	1.1	13	86	0.34	0	0.02	0.05	0.3	0.07	9	0
0	0	0	8	21	2	87	0	0.4	8	39	0.35	2	0.02	0.03	0.2	0.04	7	0
0	0	0	3	1	0	3	0	0.1	1	0	0	0	0	0	0	0	0	0
4.9	7.2	0	15	405	6	278	2.6	5.2	185	13	0.34	1	0.07	0.11	0.6	0.08	20	0
7.4	10.9	0	24	665	326	457	4.2	8.5	303	22	0.57	1	0.12	0.18	1	0.05	33	0
7.4	10.9	0	24	665	10	457	4.2	8.5	303	22	0.57	1	0.12	0.18	1	0.05	33	0
1	1.4	0	9	15	92	147	1.6	0.5	42	1	0.08	0	0	0.01	0	0.01	1	0
4.7	2.5	34	72	84	103	153	0.4	1.3	16	635	1.26	1	0.12	0.19	1	0.04	10	0.07
0	0	0	32	43	6	253	0.2	1.7	28	2713	1.3	5	0.03	0.07	0.5	0.07	15	0
0	0	0	18	37	1	282	0.3	0.7	11	132	1.3	6	0.04	0.1	0.5	0.05	10	0
3.6	2.3	14	123	112	255	66	0.7	1.3	13	55	1.16	3	0.15	0.14	1.2	0.03	5	0.06
13.8	4.9	205	201	271	549	271	1.7	1.9	27	243	1.91	3	0.23	0.44	4.7	0.2	17	0.99
2.5	1.8	93	22	298	53	434	2.6	2.6	24	0	0.96	0	0.1	0.24	9.6	0.53	12	9.41
0	0.1	0	15	32	18	242	0.5	0.5	10	2	1.81	6	0.01	0.02	0.2	0.05	48	0
0	0	0	4	8	4	60	0.1	0.1	3	1	0.45	2	0	0.01	0.1	0.01	12	0
0	0.1	0	12	18	10	209	0.1	0.1	7	0	0	11	0	0.02	0.1	0.03	13	0
0	0	0	9	8	11	104	0.1	0.1	4	0	0	10	0	0.02	0.1	0.03	12	0
0	0	0	12	10	14	135	0.2	0.2	5	1	0	13	0	0.03	0.2	0.04	16	0
0	0	0	14	14	8	140	0.1	0.4	4	0	0	14	0.02	0.01	0.2	0.04	7	0
0	0	0	14	14	8	143	0.1	0.4	5	0	0	15	0.02	0.01	0.2	0.04	7	0
0	0	0	12	10	9	100	0.1	0.2	7	0	0	10	0.01	0.01	0.1	0.02	12	0
0.1	0.2	0	91	78	71	767	0.5	1.4	54	0	0	74	0.07	0.07	0.7	0.16	95	0
0	0.1	0	40	80	10	620	0.2	1.7	27	1	0.58	3	0.13	0.07	0.7	0.2	3	0
0	0.1	0	36	70	9	544	0.2	1.5	24	1	0.51	2	0.11	0.06	0.6	0.18	2	0
0	0.1	0	44	95	10	615	0.3	1.5	29	3	0.58	3	0.01	0.16	0.9	0.27	3	0
0	0.1	0	14	12	4	120	0.2	0.5	15	4	0.58	11	0.03	0.04	0.6	0.05	13	0
0	0.2	0	14	7	0	94	0.3	0.4	11	8	0.28	15	0.02	0.06	0.6	0.04	16	0
0	0.3	0	43	48	3	324	0.5	1.8	37	17	1.28	47	0.05	0.13	0.7	0.1	74	0
4.8	2	160	166	214	1541	400	1.4	3.1	32	245	2.36	9	0.31	0.42	2.9	0.19	30	0.38
3.6	1	84	32	109	619	259	1.7	2	20	94	1.52	11	0.15	0.22	3	0.14	14	0.81
2.6	0.7	37	189	175	882	605	1.7	2.2	85	70	—	2	0.13	0.33	1.5	0.2	112	0.68

A

Esha Code	Food Item	Qty	Meas	Wgt (g)	Wtr (g)	Cals	Prot (g)	Carb (g)	Fib (g)	Fat (g)	SatF (g)
27045	Relish, corn	1	Tbs	15	11	13	0	3	0.4	0	0
27019	Relish, cranberry orange	0.5	cup	138	73	245	0	64	0	0	0
27063	Relish, hotdog	1	Tbs	15	10	18	0	4	0.2	0	0
27017	Relish, pickle, sweet	1	Tbs	15	10	21	0	5	0.3	0	0
27018	Relish, sweet pickle, 2/3 Tbsp packet	1	each	10	6	14	0	3	0.2	0	0
27048	Relish, vegetable	1	Tbs	9	8	4	0	1	0.1	0	0
27035	Relish/preserves, tomato	1	Tbs	20	10	30	0	8	0.4	0	0
2659	Rennin dessert mix w/2% milk, chocolate	0.5	cup	136	109	110	4	18	0.7	3	1.7
2662	Rennin dessert mix w/2% milk, vanilla	0.5	cup	133	109	101	4	16	0	2	1.5
2660	Rennin dessert mix w/whole milk, chocolate	0.5	cup	136	108	125	4	18	0.7	4	2.8
2663	Rennin dessert mix w/whole milk, vanilla	0.5	cup	133	108	116	4	16	0	4	2.5
49024	Rhubarb crisp	1	cup	246	130	513	3	96	4.2	16	3.1
3133	Rhubarb, frozen, cooked w/sugar	0.5	cup	120	81	139	0	37	2.4	0	0
3209	Rhubarb, raw, diced	0.5	cup	61	57	13	1	3	1.1	0	0
38050	Rice bran, crude	0.25	cup	21	1	66	3	10	4.4	4	0.9
44049	Rice cake, brown, buckwheat	2	each	18	1	68	2	14	0.7	1	0.1
44050	Rice cake, brown, corn	2	each	18	1	69	2	15	0.5	1	0.1
44051	Rice cake, brown, multi-grain	2	each	18	1	70	2	14	0.5	1	0.1
44021	Rice cake, brown, plain	1	each	9	1	35	1	7	0.4	0	0.1
44052	Rice cake, brown, rye	2	each	18	1	70	1	14	0.7	1	0.1
44053	Rice cake, brown, sesame seed	2	each	18	1	71	1	15	1	1	0.1
44064	Rice cake, puffed, w/o salt	2	each	18	1	70	1	15	0.8	1	0.1
23171	Rice krispie bar	1	each	28	3	109	1	21	0.1	3	0.5
38148	Rice paste (mochi)	1	Tbs	17	7	40	1	9	0.3	0	0
56316	Rice pilaf	0.5	cup	103	73	134	2	23	0.6	3	0.7
38051	Rice polishings	1	Tbs	7	1	17	1	4	0.5	1	0.2
57356	Rice w/cheddar/broccoli sauce, Lipton	0.5	cup	63	5	250	6	48	1	3	1
56131	Rice, Spanish	0.5	cup	122	95	108	2	21	1.9	2	0.3
38344	Rice, basmati, brown, premium, dry	0.25	cup	49	5	173	4	38	2.3	2	0.4
38343	Rice, basmati, white, premium, dry	0.25	cup	51	6	183	4	41	0.3	1	0.2
38207	Rice, brown, glutinous	0.5	cup	92	11	333	7	71	0.7	2	—
38010	Rice, brown, long grain, cooked	0.5	cup	98	71	108	3	22	1.8	1	0.2
38011	Rice, brown, long grain, cooked, cold	0.5	cup	72	53	80	2	17	1.3	1	0.1
38009	Rice, brown, long grain, dry	0.25	cup	46	5	171	4	36	1.6	1	0.3
38082	Rice, brown, med grain, cooked	0.5	cup	98	72	110	2	23	1.8	1	0.2
38145	Rice, fried, meatless	0.5	cup	83	57	132	3	17	0.7	6	0.9
38342	Rice, organic, basmati CA white, dry	0.25	cup	51	7	179	4	39	1.1	1	—
38341	Rice, organic, basmati, CA brown, dry	0.25	cup	49	6	167	4	36	2.2	2	0.4
38013	Rice, white, enriched, long grain, cooked, hot	0.5	cup	102	70	133	3	29	0.4	0	0.1
38012	Rice, white, enriched, long grain, dry	0.25	cup	46	5	169	3	37	0.6	0	0.1
38083	Rice, white, glutinous/sticky, cooked	0.5	cup	120	92	117	2	25	1.2	0	0
38020	Rice, white, instant, long grain, cooked, cold	0.5	cup	65	50	64	1	14	0.4	0	0
38019	Rice, white, instant, long grain, cooked, hot	0.5	cup	82	63	81	2	18	0.5	0	0
38018	Rice, white, instant, long grain, dry	0.25	cup	24	2	90	2	20	0.4	0	0
38014	Rice, white, long grain, cooked, cold	0.5	cup	72	50	94	2	20	0.3	0	0.1
38017	Rice, white, long grain, parboiled, cooked, cold	0.5	cup	72	53	83	2	18	0.3	0	0.1
38016	Rice, white, long grain, parboiled, cooked, hot	0.5	cup	88	63	100	2	22	0.4	0	0.1
38015	Rice, white, long grain, parboiled, dry	0.25	cup	46	5	172	3	38	0.8	0	0.1
38097	Rice, white, med grain, unenriched, cooked	0.5	cup	102	70	133	2	29	0.3	0	0.1
38157	Rice, white, short grain, cooked	1	cup	205	140	267	5	59	2.1	0	0.1
38021	Rice, wild, cooked	0.5	cup	82	61	83	3	18	1.5	0	0
1707	Rockfish, Pacific, baked/broiled	1	each	149	109	180	36	0	0	3	0.7
42166	Roll dough, cinnamon, frosted, refrigerated, baked	1	each	30	7	109	2	17	0.6	4	1
42165	Roll dough, sweet, cinnamon, w/frosting, refrigerat	1	each	30	9	100	2	16	0.6	4	0.9
42161	Roll, French	1	each	38	13	105	3	19	1.2	2	0.4
42185	Roll, Mexican bolillo	1	each	117	46	295	10	58	2.2	2	0.4
42094	Roll, Mexican sweet (pan dulce), crumb topping	1	each	79	17	291	5	48	1.1	9	2
42187	Roll, butterhorn	1	each	55	17	174	5	27	0.7	5	1.3
42183	Roll, cheese bread	1	each	41	13	124	4	21	0.7	3	1
42167	Roll, cinnamon w/raisins & nuts, homemade	1	each	57	15	196	4	30	1.1	7	1.4
42157	Roll, dinner	1	each	28	9	85	2	14	0.9	2	0.5
42169	Roll, dinner, bran	1	each	28	10	76	3	14	1.2	2	0.2
42170	Roll, dinner, bran, toasted	1	each	25	8	73	2	12	1.2	1	0.2
42159	Roll, dinner, egg	1	each	35	11	107	3	18	1.3	2	0.6
42158	Roll, dinner, homemade, w/2% milk	1	each	35	10	111	3	19	0.7	3	0.6

MonoF (g)	PolyF (g)	Choles (mg)	Calc (mg)	Phos (mg)	Sod (mg)	Pot (mg)	Zn (mg)	Iron (mg)	Magn (mg)	VitA (μg RE)	VitE (mg α-TE)	VitC (mg)	Thia (mg)	Ribo (mg)	Nia (mg)	B6 (mg)	Fola (μg)	B12 (μg)
0	0	0	2	7	55	28	0	0.1	3	9	0.03	4	0.01	0.01	0.1	0.02	4	0
0	0.1	0	15	11	44	52	0.1	0.3	6	10	0.07	25	0.04	0.03	0.1	0.03	4	0
0.1	0	0	4	3	81	31	0	0.2	3	1	0.02	1	0	0	0	0	1	0
0	0	0	3	2	109	31	0	0.1	1	2	0.02	1	0	0	0	0	0	0
0	0	0	2	1	71	20	0	0.1	0	1	0.02	1	0	0	0	0	0	0
0	0	0	2	2	41	16	0	0	1	2	0.02	1	0	0	0	0	1	0
0	0	0	9	9	452	79	0	0.3	6	25	0.1	10	0.01	0.01	0.1	0.03	2	0
0.8	0.1	10	171	133	71	248	0.7	0.4	27	60	0.07	1	0.05	0.21	0.1	0.06	7	0.45
0.7	0.1	9	161	126	61	189	0.5	0.1	17	69	0.07	1	0.05	0.2	0.1	0.05	7	0.44
1.3	0.2	16	169	132	69	243	0.7	0.4	27	33	0.11	1	0.05	0.21	0.1	0.06	7	0.44
1.2	0.2	17	158	124	61	186	0.5	0.1	16	33	0.11	1	0.05	0.2	0.1	0.05	7	0.44
6.9	5	0	294	46	193	289	0.3	1.8	34	221	2.9	6	0.15	0.14	1.4	0.05	14	0.02
0	0	0	174	10	1	115	0.1	0.3	14	8	0.24	4	0.02	0.03	0.2	0.02	6	0
0	0.1	0	52	9	2	176	0.1	0.1	7	6	0.12	5	0.01	0.02	0.2	0.02	4	0
1.6	1.6	0	12	348	1	308	1.2	3.8	162	0	1.26	0	0.57	0.06	7.1	0.84	13	0
0.2	0.2	0	2	68	21	54	0.4	0.2	27	0	0.02	0	0.01	0.02	1.5	0.02	4	0
0.2	0.2	0	2	58	52	50	0.4	0.2	20	0	0	0	0.01	0.02	1.2	0.02	3	0
0.2	0.3	0	4	67	45	53	0.5	0.4	25	0	0	0	0.01	0.03	1.2	0.02	4	0
0.1	0.1	0	1	32	29	26	0.3	0.1	12	0	0.06	0	0	0.02	0.7	0.01	2	0
0.2	0.3	0	4	68	20	56	0.5	0.3	26	0	0	0	0.02	0.02	1.3	0.03	1	0
0.2	0.2	0	2	68	41	52	0.5	0.3	24	0	0.02	1	0.01	0.02	1.3	0.03	3	0
0.2	0.2	0	2	65	5	52	0.5	0.3	24	1	0.02	0	0.01	0.03	1.4	0.03	4	0
1.2	0.8	0	3	12	141	11	0.2	0.6	3	103	0.42	5	0.11	0.13	1.5	0.16	30	0
0	0	0	6	16	1	37	0.2	0.6	7	0	0.02	0	0.01	0	0.5	0.02	1	0
1.5	1.1	0	13	39	377	54	0.4	1.2	10	43	0.56	0	0.14	0.02	1.3	0.06	4	0
0.3	0.3	0	5	73	0	47	0.5	0.7	39	0	0.4	0	0.12	0.01	1.8	0.03	7	0
—	—	2	40	—	940	—	—	1.8	—	0	—	2	—	—	—	—	—	—
0.7	0.7	0	35	47	162	271	0.4	1.2	20	58	0.65	20	0.12	0.04	1.5	0.16	10	0
0.7	0.6	0	5	—	3	—	—	0.5	—	0	—	0	—	—	—	—	—	—
0.2	0.2	0	4	—	—	—	—	0.2	—	0	—	0	—	—	—	—	—	—
—	—	—	19	225	10	266	—	3.2	—	0	0.48	—	0.28	0.11	4.6	—	—	—
0.3	0.3	0	10	81	5	42	0.6	0.4	42	0	0.7	0	0.09	0.02	1.5	0.14	4	0
0.2	0.2	0	7	60	4	31	0.5	0.3	31	0	0.52	0	0.07	0.02	1.1	0.1	3	0
0.5	0.5	0	11	154	3	103	0.9	0.7	66	0	0.33	0	0.18	0.04	2.4	0.24	9	0
0.3	0.3	0	10	76	1	77	0.6	0.5	43	0	0.32	0	0.1	0.01	1.3	0.15	4	0
1.5	3.2	21	15	47	143	67	0.4	0.9	12	10	1.23	2	0.1	0.05	1.1	0.08	11	0.06
—	—	0	4	—	4	—	—	0.2	—	0	—	1	—	—	—	—	—	—
0.6	0.6	0	4	—	4	—	—	0.7	—	0	—	0	—	—	—	—	—	—
0.1	0.1	0	10	44	1	36	0.5	1.2	12	0	0.05	0	0.17	0.01	1.5	0.1	60	0
0.1	0.1	0	13	53	2	53	0.5	2	12	0	0.06	0	0.27	0.02	1.9	0.08	107	0
0.1	0.1	0	2	10	6	12	0.5	0.2	6	0	0.04	0	0.02	0.02	0.3	0.03	1	0
0	0	0	5	9	2	3	0.2	0.4	3	0	0.03	0	0.05	0.03	0.6	0.01	27	0
0	0	0	7	12	2	3	0.2	0.5	4	0	0.04	0	0.06	0.04	0.7	0.01	34	0
0	0	0	4	16	1	4	0.2	1	3	0	0.03	0	0.15	0.01	1.3	0.01	55	0
0.1	0.1	0	7	31	1	25	0.4	0.9	9	0	0.04	0	0.12	0.01	1.1	0.07	42	0
0.1	0.1	0	14	30	2	27	0.2	0.8	9	0	0.04	0	0.18	0.01	1	0.01	36	0
0.1	0.1	0	17	37	3	32	0.3	1	10	0	0.04	0	0.22	0.02	1.2	0.02	44	0
0.1	0.1	0	28	63	2	56	0.4	1.6	14	0	0.06	0	0.28	0.03	1.7	0.16	107	0
0.1	0.1	0	3	38	0	30	0.4	1.5	13	0	0.05	0	0.17	0.02	1.9	0.05	60	0
0.1	0.1	0	2	68	0	53	0.8	3	16	0	0.09	0	0.34	0.03	3	0.12	121	0
0	0.2	0	2	67	2	83	1.1	0.5	26	0	0.19	0	0.04	0.07	1.1	0.11	21	0
0.7	0.9	66	18	340	115	775	0.8	0.8	51	98	1.86	0	0.07	0.12	5.8	0.4	16	1.79
2.2	0.5	0	10	104	250	19	0.1	0.8	4	0	0.48	0	0.12	0.07	1.1	0.01	2	0.02
2	0.5	0	9	96	230	17	0.1	0.7	3	0	0.45	0	0.14	0.08	1.1	0.01	15	0.01
0.7	0.3	0	35	32	231	43	0.3	1	8	0	0.17	0	0.2	0.11	1.6	0.02	36	0
0.2	0.6	1	14	88	347	96	0.8	3.7	22	4	0.05	0	0.67	0.45	6.3	0.06	47	0
3.9	2.7	26	13	56	140	57	0.4	1.8	10	88	1.35	0	0.23	0.21	2	0.04	22	0.06
2.6	0.7	18	58	59	214	68	0.3	1.2	10	12	0.66	0	0.2	0.18	1.2	0.06	17	0
1.3	0.4	2	54	44	210	39	0.3	1.1	9	6	0.04	0	0.16	0.1	1.3	0.02	15	0.01
2.7	2.8	13	36	63	185	123	0.4	1.5	16	60	0.91	0	0.16	0.16	1.3	0.05	18	0.06
1	0.3	0	34	33	148	38	0.2	0.9	7	0	0.25	0	0.14	0.09	1.1	0.02	27	0.02
0.6	0.6	0	6	54	126	53	0.3	0.9	15	0	0.22	0	0.13	0.1	1.1	0.04	22	0
0.5	0.6	0	6	52	118	50	0.3	0.9	14	0	0.21	0	0.1	0.09	0.9	0.04	15	0
1	0.4	18	21	35	191	36	0.4	1.2	9	3	0.25	0	0.18	0.18	1.2	0.02	37	0.08
1	0.7	12	21	44	145	53	0.2	1	7	32	0.34	0	0.14	0.14	1.2	0.02	32	0.05

Esha Code	Food Item	Qty	Meas	Wgt (g)	Wtr (g)	Cals	Prot (g)	Carb (g)	Fib (g)	Fat (g)	SatF (g)
42019	Roll, dinner, recipe, w/whole milk	1	each	35	10	112	3	19	1	3	0.8
42160	Roll, dinner, wheat	1	each	28	10	77	2	13	1.1	2	0.4
42057	Roll, dinner, whole wheat	1	each	35	12	93	3	18	2.6	2	0.3
42184	Roll, garlic	1	each	35	11	104	3	18	0.7	2	0.5
42022	Roll, hard, white, enriched	1	each	50	16	147	5	26	1.2	2	0.3
42188	Roll, jelly filled	1	each	55	17	173	4	28	0.9	5	1.2
42070	Roll, oatmeal, toasted	1	each	33	14	78	3	13	1.4	2	0.2
42058	Roll, rye, light	1	each	28	9	81	3	15	1.4	1	0.2
42186	Roll, sourdough	1	each	45	14	131	4	25	1.2	1	0.3
42034	Roll, submarine/hoagie	1	each	135	41	392	12	75	3.6	4	0.9
42164	Roll, sweet, cheese	1	each	66	19	238	5	29	0.8	12	4
42033	Roll, sweet, cinnamon raisin, commercial	1	each	39	10	145	2	20	0.9	6	1.2
3264	Rose apple, raw	4	oz.	113	105	28	1	6	1.5	0	—
26030	Rosemary, dried	0.25	tsp	0	0	1	0	0	0.1	0	0
5219	Rutabaga, cooked cubes	0.5	cup	85	76	33	1	7	1.5	0	0
5220	Rutabaga, cooked, mashed	0.5	cup	120	107	47	2	10	2.2	0	0
5218	Rutabaga, raw, cubes/pieces	0.5	cup	70	63	25	1	6	1.8	0	0
38084	Rye, whole grain	0.5	cup	79	9	265	12	55	11.5	2	0.2
26111	Saffron	0.25	tsp	0	0	1	0	0	0	0	0
26306	Saffron safflower, flowers	1	oz.	28	4	68	5	—	—	1	—
26311	Sage, fresh	0.25	cup	8	5	10	0	1	—	0	—
26031	Sage, ground	0.25	tsp	0	0	1	0	0	0.1	0	0
8128	Salad dressing, Blue Cheese, low calorie	2	Tbs	31	24	30	2	1	0	2	0.3
8498	Salad dressing, Catalina, fat free, Kraft	2	Tbs	35	4	124	5	24	1.6	1	0.5
8017	Salad dressing, Dijon Vinegrarette Lite	2	Tbs	30	25	32	0	1	0	3	0.4
8491	Salad dressing, Italian, fat free, Kraft	2	Tbs	35	32	11	0	2	0	0	0
8641	Salad dressing, Italian, fat free, Lipton	2	Tbs	30	28	15	0	2	0	0	0
8020	Salad dressing, Seven Seas Viva	2	Tbs	30	12	140	0	3	0	14	2.1
8147	Salad dressing, bacon & tomato, low calorie	2	Tbs	32	24	65	1	1	0.1	7	1.1
8013	Salad dressing, blue cheese	2	Tbs	31	10	154	1	2	0	16	3
8140	Salad dressing, buttermilk, light	2	Tbs	29	21	58	1	2	—	5	—
8066	Salad dressing, caesar's	2	Tbs	23	8	107	3	1	0.1	10	1.9
8138	Salad dressing, caesar, low calorie	2	Tbs	30	22	33	0	6	0	1	0.2
8034	Salad dressing, cooked	2	Tbs	32	22	50	1	5	0	3	0.9
8126	Salad dressing, creamy Italian	2	Tbs	29	11	143	0	2	0	16	2.3
8125	Salad dressing, creamy bacon	2	Tbs	29	11	143	0	2	0	16	2.3
8127	Salad dressing, creamy cucumber	2	Tbs	29	11	143	0	2	0	16	2.3
8152	Salad dressing, creamy cucumber, low calorie	2	Tbs	30	22	48	0	2	0	4	0.6
8153	Salad dressing, creamy, oil free, low calorie	2	Tbs	30	22	48	0	2	0	4	0.6
8015	Salad dressing, french	2	Tbs	31	12	134	0	5	0	13	3
8499	Salad dressing, french, fat free, Kraft	2	Tbs	35	23	40	0	12	0.5	0	0
8146	Salad dressing, french, homemade	2	Tbs	28	7	177	0	1	0	20	3.5
8014	Salad dressing, french, low calorie	2	Tbs	32	23	44	0	7	0	2	0.3
8504	Salad dressing, honey dijon, fat free, Kraft	2	Tbs	35	23	50	0	11	1	0	0
8124	Salad dressing, honey mustard	2	Tbs	31	11	101	0	14	0.2	6	0.8
8018	Salad dressing, italian	2	Tbs	29	11	137	0	3	0	14	2.1
8016	Salad dressing, italian, low calorie	2	Tbs	30	25	32	0	1	0	3	0.4
8149	Salad dressing, light, cholesterol free	1	Tbs	15	9	48	0	2	0	4	1.1
8122	Salad dressing, low calorie, Miracle Whip Light	1	Tbs	14	8	36	0	3	0	3	0.4
8021	Salad dressing, mayonnaise type	1	Tbs	15	6	57	0	4	0	5	0.7
8141	Salad dressing, oil free, low calorie	2	Tbs	30	26	7	0	2	0	0	0
8030	Salad dressing, ranch	2	Tbs	30	16	109	1	1	0	11	1.7
8493	Salad dressing, ranch, fat free, Kraft	2	Tbs	35	23	50	0	11	0.5	0	0
8129	Salad dressing, roquefort, low calorie	2	Tbs	31	24	30	2	1	0	2	0.3
8022	Salad dressing, russian	2	Tbs	31	11	151	0	3	0	16	2.2
8139	Salad dressing, russian, low calorie	2	Tbs	33	21	46	0	9	0.1	1	0.2
8144	Salad dressing, sesame seed	2	Tbs	31	12	136	1	3	0.3	14	1.9
8024	Salad dressing, thousand island	2	Tbs	31	14	118	0	5	0	11	1.9
8023	Salad dressing, thousand island, low calorie	2	Tbs	31	21	49	0	5	0.4	3	0.5
8019	Salad dressing, vinaigrette	2	Tbs	29	11	137	0	3	0	14	2.1
8035	Salad dressing, vinegar & oil	2	Tbs	32	15	144	0	1	0	16	2.9
8150	Salad dressing, vinegar & sugar & water	2	Tbs	32	27	16	0	4	0	0	0
8123	Salad dressing, yogurt	2	Tbs	31	26	22	1	2	0	1	0.6
8151	Salad dressing/marinade, Korean	2	Tbs	30	27	10	0	2	0.2	0	0
27050	Salad topping, Bac-O-Bits	2	Tbs	12	1	50	5	3	—	2	—

MonoF (g)	PolyF (g)	Choles (mg)	Calc (mg)	Phos (mg)	Sod (mg)	Pot (mg)	Zn (mg)	Iron (mg)	Magn (mg)	VitA (μg RE)	VitE (mg α-TE)	VitC (mg)	Thia (mg)	Ribo (mg)	Nia (mg)	B6 (mg)	Fola (μg)	B12 (μg)
1.1	0.7	13	21	44	145	53	0.2	1	7	28	0.35	0	0.14	0.14	1.2	0.02	15	0.05
0.9	0.3	0	50	30	96	33	0.3	1	10	0	0.27	0	0.12	0.08	1.2	0.02	14	0
0.4	0.8	0	37	78	167	95	0.7	0.8	30	0	0.48	0	0.09	0.05	1.3	0.07	11	0
1	0.3	0	35	30	176	34	0.3	1	7	0	0.03	0	0.14	0.08	1.2	0.02	13	0
0.6	0.9	0	48	50	272	54	0.5	1.6	14	0	0.16	0	0.24	0.17	2.1	0.02	48	0
2.4	0.7	17	56	58	199	92	0.3	1.2	10	11	0.64	0	0.2	0.17	1.2	0.07	16	0
0.5	0.5	0	28	38	136	40	0.3	1.4	11	0	0.23	0	0.15	0.1	1.6	0.02	31	0
0.4	0.2	0	9	45	253	51	0.3	0.8	15	0	0.1	0	0.11	0.08	1.1	0.02	24	0
0.4	0.5	0	40	38	261	40	0.3	1.3	9	0	0.03	0	0.18	0.11	1.5	0.02	14	0
1.3	1.4	0	122	115	783	122	0.9	3.8	27	0	0.1	0	0.54	0.33	4.5	0.05	40	0
6	1.3	50	78	65	236	90	0.4	0.5	12	51	1.25	0	0.1	0.09	0.5	0.05	28	0.2
1.9	2.9	26	28	30	149	43	0.2	0.6	7	25	1.68	1	0.13	0.1	0.9	0.04	20	0.06
—	—	0	33	9	0	139	0.1	0.1	6	39	—	25	0.02	0.03	0.9	—	—	0
0	0	0	4	0	0	3	0	0.1	1	1	—	0	0	—	0	—	—	0
0	0.1	0	41	48	17	277	0.3	0.5	20	48	0.13	16	0.07	0.04	0.6	0.09	13	0
0	0.1	0	58	67	24	391	0.4	0.6	28	67	0.18	23	0.1	0.05	0.9	0.12	18	0
0	0.1	0	33	41	14	236	0.2	0.4	16	41	0.21	18	0.06	0.03	0.5	0.07	15	0
0.2	0.9	0	26	295	5	209	3	2.1	96	0	1.48	0	0.25	0.2	3.4	0.23	47	0
0	0	0	0	0	0	3	0	0	0	0	0	0	0	0	0	0	0	0
—	—	—	175	73	—	—	—	5.7	—	5	—	6	0.04	0.11	2.4	—	—	0
—	—	—	48	3	0	31	0.1	—	13	17	—	—	0.01	—	—	—	—	0
0	0	0	3	0	0	2	0	0	1	1	0	0	0	0	0	0	0	0
0.9	0.8	0	27	25	367	2	0.1	0.2	2	1	0.28	0	0.01	0.03	0	0.01	1	0.07
0.5	0.3	0	162	188	48	78	2.8	3.4	75	0	10.8	32	0.81	0.92	10.8	1.08	215	3.23
0.6	1.8	2	1	2	236	4	0	0.1	0	0	0.45	0	0	0	0	0	0	0
0	0	0	0	—	327	45	—	0	—	0	—	0	—	—	—	—	—	—
0	0	0	0	—	280	—	—	0	—	0	—	0	—	—	—	—	—	—
3.4	8.4	0	3	2	236	4	0	0.1	0	7	3.12	0	0	0.01	0	0	1	0.05
1.8	3.6	1	1	8	351	35	0.1	0.1	2	9	1.3	3	0.01	0.01	0.2	0.03	0	0.03
3.8	8.5	5	25	23	335	11	0.1	0.1	0	20	2.85	1	0	0.03	0	0.01	2	0.08
—	—	—	—	—	167	35	—	—	—	—	—	—	—	—	—	—	—	—
7.2	1	24	43	37	396	40	0.2	0.4	5	13	1.38	1	0.01	0.05	1	0.02	3	0.11
0.6	0.5	1	7	6	323	9	0	0.1	1	1	0.12	0	0	0	0	0	1	0.01
1.2	0.7	18	27	28	235	39	0.1	0.2	3	39	0.61	0	0.02	0.05	0.1	0.01	3	0.11
3.8	8.7	1	4	3	347	8	0	0	1	6	3.15	0	0	0	0	0	0	0.01
3.8	8.7	1	4	3	347	8	0	0	1	6	3.15	0	0	0	0	0	0	0.01
3.8	8.7	1	4	3	347	8	0	0	1	6	3.15	0	0	0	0	0	0	0.01
1.8	1.6	0	2	2	307	11	0	0	1	2	0.57	0	0	0	0	0.01	4	0.02
1.8	1.6	0	2	2	307	11	0	0	1	2	0.57	0	0	0	0	0.01	4	0.02
2.5	6.8	0	3	4	428	25	0	0.1	0	41	2.63	0	0	0	0	0	1	0.04
0	0	0	0	—	300	40	—	0	—	150	—	0	—	—	—	—	—	—
5.8	9.4	0	2	1	184	7	0	0.1	0	43	3.36	0	0	0.01	0	0	0	0
0.5	1.1	0	4	5	256	26	0.1	0.1	0	42	0.39	0	0	0	0	0	0	0
0	0	0	0	—	330	50	—	0.4	—	0	—	0	—	—	—	—	—	—
1.4	3.2	0	6	5	181	20	0.1	0.2	3	0	0.44	0	0	0.01	0.1	0.01	1	0
3.3	8.2	0	3	1	231	4	0	0.1	0	7	3.06	0	0	0.01	0	0	1	0.05
0.6	1.8	2	1	2	236	4	0	0.1	0	0	0.45	0	0	0	0	0	0	0
1.1	2.1	0	0	0	102	0	0	0	0	2	0.64	0	0	0	0	0	0	0
0.7	1.4	4	2	4	99	1	0	0	0	9	0.6	0	0	0	0	0	1	0.03
1.3	2.6	4	2	4	104	1	0	0	0	12	0.59	0	0	0	0	0	1	0.03
0	0	0	2	2	512	15	0	0.1	3	0	0	0	0	0	0	0	0	0
4.8	4.2	12	30	25	131	40	0.1	0.1	3	22	1.19	0	0.01	0.04	0	0.01	2	0.08
0	0	0	0	—	310	50	—	0	—	0	—	0	—	—	—	—	—	—
0.9	0.8	0	27	25	367	2	0.1	0.2	2	1	0.28	0	0.01	0.03	0	0.01	1	0.07
3.6	9	6	6	11	266	48	0.1	0.2	0	63	3.12	2	0.02	0.02	0.2	0.01	3	0.09
0.3	0.8	2	6	12	283	51	0	0.2	0	5	0.25	2	0	0	0	0	1	0.04
3.6	7.7	0	6	11	306	48	0	0.2	0	63	1.53	0	0	0	0	0	0	0
2.6	6.2	8	3	5	219	35	0	0.2	1	30	0.36	0	0	0.01	0	0	2	0.06
0.7	1.9	5	3	5	306	35	0	0.2	0	29	0.36	0	0	0.01	0	0	2	0.06
3.3	8.2	0	3	1	231	4	0	0.1	0	7	3.06	0	0	0.01	0	0	1	0.05
4.7	7.7	0	0	0	0	2	0	0	0	0	2.82	0	0	0	0	0	0	0
0	0	0	1	1	331	9	0	0.1	2	0	0	0	0	0	0	0	0	0
0.3	0.2	3	31	24	118	45	0.1	0.1	4	7	0.04	1	0.01	0.04	0	0.01	2	0.09
0	0	0	8	8	77	31	0	0.2	4	41	0.03	9	0.01	0.01	0.2	0.03	3	0
—	—	0	26	—	205	328	—	0.8	—	—	—	—	1.03	0.04	0.2	—	—	—

A

Esha Code	Food Item	Qty	Meas	Wgt (g)	Wtr (g)	Cals	Prot (g)	Carb (g)	Fib (g)	Fat (g)	SatF (g)
56109	Salad, carrot raisin	0.5	cup	88	50	202	1	21	2	14	2
56628	Salad, chef style w/turkey+ham+cheese	1.5	cup	326	269	267	26	5	—	16	8.2
19402	Salad, crab, w/imitation crab	0.5	cup	104	72	150	9	14	0.4	6	0.9
44023	Salad, fruit, canned, juice pack	0.5	cup	124	107	62	1	16	1.2	0	0
5637	Salad, mixed greens/lettuce	0.5	cup	28	26	5	0	1	0.5	0	0
5537	Salad, spinach, no dressing	0.5	cup	37	27	44	2	5	0.8	2	0.5
56643	Salad, taco	1.5	cup	198	143	279	13	24	—	15	6.8
56118	Salad, three bean	0.5	cup	75	61	70	2	7	1.5	4	0.6
5677	Salad, tossed green	0.5	cup	69	66	12	1	2	0.8	0	0
56006	Salad, waldorf	0.5	cup	68	40	204	2	6	1.2	20	2.1
13023	Salami, beef, cooked	1	piece	23	13	60	3	1	0	5	2.1
13026	Salami, dry, beef & pork	2	piece	20	7	84	5	1	0	7	2.4
13025	Salami, turkey, cooked	2	piece	57	38	112	9	0	0	8	2.3
11063	Salisbury steak, 4-compartment, Swanson	1	each	298	231	325	15	33	5.7	14	5.7
27020	Salsa cruda (uncooked salsa)	2	Tbs	30	28	6	0	1	0.3	0	0
5221	Salsify, cooked, drained	0.5	cup	68	55	46	2	10	2.1	0	0
26014	Salt	0.25	tsp	1	0	0	0	0	0	0	0
26101	Salt Free 17	0.25	tsp	2	0	5	0	1	0.2	0	—
26113	Salt blend, light, Papa Dash	0.25	tsp	2	0	1	0	0	—	0	0
26090	Salt substitute, Morton	0.25	tsp	1	0	0	0	0	—	0	0
26273	Salt, Sea	1	Tbs	16	0	0	0	0	0	0	0
26048	Salt, light, Morton	0.25	tsp	2	0	0	0	0	—	0	0
26089	Salt, light, Morton Lite	0.25	tsp	1	—	—	—	—	—	—	—
26091	Salt, seasoning, Morton	0.25	tsp	0	0	0	0	0	—	0	—
56008	Sandwich, BLT, on firm white	1	each	145	75	366	12	35	2	19	4.9
56022	Sandwich, avocado & cheese, on wheat	1	each	196	116	433	14	34	6.5	28	8.4
56281	Sandwich, bologna	1	each	83	34	257	7	26	1.2	14	4.2
13093	Sandwich, chicken frank on bun	1	each	85	38	235	9	24	0.8	11	3
56016	Sandwich, chicken salad, on firm white	1	each	114	45	381	11	34	1.6	22	3.5
56020	Sandwich, corned beef & swiss, on rye	1	each	147	73	396	26	20	0.1	24	8.9
56024	Sandwich, egg salad, on firm white	1	each	121	50	394	10	34	1.5	24	4.2
66011	Sandwich, fish w/tartar sauce & cheese	1	each	183	83	523	21	48	0.4	28	8.1
56268	Sandwich, french dip au jus	1	each	193	118	359	26	34	1.7	12	4.8
56012	Sandwich, grilled cheese, on firm white	1	each	127	46	426	19	34	1.5	24	13.1
69017	Sandwich, grilled chicken, Weight Watchers	1	each	113	65	210	18	24	2	5	2
56272	Sandwich, gyro	1	each	105	67	169	12	20	1.1	4	1.5
56033	Sandwich, ham & swiss, on rye	1	each	145	79	328	22	21	0.1	18	6.3
56066	Sandwich, ham salad, on wheat	1	each	126	60	343	10	34	3.3	19	4.4
56031	Sandwich, ham, on wheat	1	each	123	68	259	17	22	2.7	11	2.2
66004	Sandwich, hotdog, plain	1	each	98	53	242	10	18	—	14	5.1
56267	Sandwich, pastrami	1	each	134	71	334	14	27	1.7	18	6.3
56038	Sandwich, patty melt, on rye	1	each	177	81	546	36	21	2.9	36	12.9
56040	Sandwich, peanut butter & jam, on soft white	1	each	101	26	351	12	47	3	15	3.1
56266	Sandwich, reuben	1	each	181	91	496	23	31	4.1	31	10.6
56046	Sandwich, roast beef, on wheat	1	each	123	57	314	23	25	2.6	13	2.5
56671	Sandwich, submarine w/coldcuts	1	each	228	132	456	22	51	1.7	19	6.8
56047	Sandwich, tuna salad, on firm white	1	each	126	57	342	14	38	1.8	14	2.3
56059	Sandwich, turkey ham & cheese, on wheat	1	each	152	76	385	22	27	3.3	21	8
56103	Sandwich, turkey ham, on rye	1	each	116	70	217	16	16	0.1	10	1.9
56053	Sandwich, turkey, on whole wheat	1	each	136	72	294	21	26	3.5	12	1.8
3266	Sapodilla, raw	1	each	170	133	141	1	34	9	2	0.3
3267	Sapotes, raw	1	each	170	106	228	4	58	4.4	1	0.2
53388	Sauce, Alfredo, Di Girono	0.5	cup	124	—	460	8	4	0	44	20
53396	Sauce, Alfredo, low fat, Di Girono	0.5	cup	138	—	340	10	32	0	20	12
53085	Sauce, Tabasco brand pepper	1	tsp	5	5	1	0	0	0	0	0
57271	Sauce, alfredo, Progresso	0.5	cup	124	81	310	10	5	0	27	15
53133	Sauce, armanino pesto	0.25	cup	58	30	195	4	4	0.9	18	3
53000	Sauce, barbecue	2	Tbs	31	25	23	1	4	0.4	1	0.1
53018	Sauce, bechamel	0.25	cup	72	61	71	1	3	0.2	6	3.7
53100	Sauce, black bean	1	tsp	6	5	5	0	1	0.1	0	0
53019	Sauce, bordelaise	0.25	cup	116	100	104	1	5	0.3	6	3.9
53015	Sauce, cheese	0.25	cup	50	32	110	5	4	0.1	8	4.6
53029	Sauce, cheese, dry mix w/milk	0.25	cup	70	54	77	4	6	0.2	4	2.3
53097	Sauce, cheese, low fat	1	cup	243	177	338	23	16	0.3	20	8.2
53227	Sauce, chili, hot green	1	tsp	5	5	1	0	0	—	0	0

MonoF	PolyF	Choles	Calc	Phos	Sod	Pot	Zn	Iron	Magn	VitA	VitE	VitC	Thia	Ribo	Nia	B6	Fola	B12
(g)	(g)	(mg)	(mg)	(mg)	(mg)	(mg)	(mg)	(mg)	(mg)	(μg RE)	(mg α-TE)	(mg)	(mg)	(mg)	(mg)	(mg)	(μg)	(μg)
3.9	7.2	10	26	46	117	315	0.2	0.7	14	1444	5	5	0.08	0.05	0.6	0.22	9	0.05
5.2	1.4	140	235	401	743	401	3.1	2	49	137	—	16	0.39	0.39	6	0.42	101	0.85
1.6	3.4	37	37	110	892	211	0.3	0.4	33	22	0.86	1	0.03	0.1	1.5	0.14	7	1.41
0	0	0	14	17	6	144	0.2	0.3	10	74	0.74	4	0.01	0.02	0.4	0.03	3	0
0	0	0	15	9	7	87	0.1	0.4	7	75	0.18	4	0.02	0.03	0.1	0.02	32	0
0.7	0.4	30	26	37	78	138	0.3	0.8	17	120	0.5	5	0.06	0.13	0.7	0.05	38	0.08
5.2	1.8	44	192	143	762	416	2.7	2.3	52	77	—	4	0.1	0.36	2.5	0.22	83	0.63
1	2.4	0	18	32	257	112	0.3	0.7	13	11	0.98	2	0.04	0.05	0.2	0.02	26	0.01
0	0.1	0	10	16	7	134	0.1	0.3	7	139	0.26	7	0.04	0.03	0.3	0.04	24	0
3.7	13.5	10	21	42	118	135	0.3	0.4	20	20	4.34	3	0.05	0.02	0.2	0.18	14	0.04
2.2	0.2	15	2	26	270	52	0.5	0.5	3	0	0.04	0	0.02	0.04	0.7	0.04	0	0.7
3.4	0.6	16	2	28	372	76	0.6	0.3	3	0	0.06	0	0.12	0.06	1	0.1	0	0.38
2.6	2	47	11	60	572	139	1	0.9	9	0	0.32	0	0.04	0.1	2	0.14	2	0.12
—	—	29	76	—	879	—	—	2.6	—	955	—	6	—	—	—	—	—	—
0	0	0	3	6	117	48	0	0.1	3	44	0.08	11	0.01	0.01	0.1	0.02	4	0
0	0	0	32	38	11	191	0.2	0.4	12	0	0.13	3	0.04	0.12	0.3	0.15	10	0
0	0	0	0	0	535	0	0	0	0	0	0	0	0	0	0	0	0	0
—	—	—	—	—	1	18	—	—	—	—	—	—	—	—	—	—	—	0
0	0	0	—	—	694	0	—	—	—	0	0	0	0	0	0	0	0	0
0	0	—	8	6	0	694	—	—	—	—	—	—	—	—	—	—	—	0
0	0	0	6	0	6905	3	0	0	1	0	0	0	0	0	0	0	0	0
0	0	—	1	—	293	390	—	—	1	—	—	—	—	—	—	—	—	0
—	—	—	0	—	290	386	—	—	1	—	—	—	—	—	—	—	—	0
—	—	—	—	—	0	217	—	—	—	—	—	—	—	—	—	—	—	0
6.7	6.6	24	73	145	686	275	1.1	2.4	24	34	2.95	13	0.42	0.23	3.8	0.16	41	0.36
11.1	7.2	30	284	254	512	602	1.9	3	65	137	4.44	11	0.34	0.38	3.8	0.34	78	0.26
6.2	2.5	16	63	79	608	111	0.8	1.9	16	54	0.73	6	0.28	0.21	2.7	0.08	18	0.38
5	2.2	45	83	82	819	76	0.8	2	13	17	0.13	0	0.19	0.15	2.7	0.16	17	0.1
5.8	11.5	32	73	110	478	152	0.8	2.2	19	23	6.27	1	0.28	0.19	3.8	0.24	28	0.12
7	5.9	77	252	257	1311	212	3.4	2.9	26	77	2.44	1	0.18	0.31	2.6	0.16	18	1.63
6.5	11.5	152	84	129	545	128	0.8	2.3	17	73	4.74	0	0.28	0.32	2.2	0.19	40	0.42
8.9	9.4	68	185	311	939	353	1.2	3.5	37	97	1.83	3	0.46	0.42	4.2	0.11	92	1.08
5.2	0.9	58	66	212	608	355	5.3	3.7	31	0	0.15	0	0.3	0.31	5.4	0.24	26	2.11
7.4	2	56	412	488	1174	173	2.1	2.1	26	210	1.52	0	0.28	0.36	2.2	0.06	28	0.4
—	—	20	60	—	420	220	—	1.4	—	0	—	0	—	—	—	—	—	—
1.4	0.4	34	44	117	212	209	2.3	2.2	20	11	0.28	4	0.21	0.25	3.5	0.16	30	0.9
5	5.8	55	249	317	1548	333	2.5	2.2	28	76	2.43	15	0.7	0.35	3.9	0.34	15	1.13
6.6	7.2	28	66	160	901	207	1.3	2.3	32	8	3.55	4	0.5	0.23	3.6	0.2	25	0.48
3.5	4.7	36	56	218	1285	332	1.8	2.1	34	6	2.15	17	0.81	0.28	5.1	0.39	22	0.52
6.8	1.7	44	24	97	670	143	2	2.3	13	0	0.27	0	0.24	0.27	3.6	0.05	48	0.51
8.9	1.2	53	71	142	1341	242	2.7	2.6	24	3	0.21	4	0.29	0.27	4.8	0.13	21	0.99
11.4	8.2	110	215	319	682	380	6.9	4.1	35	119	3.4	0	0.24	0.45	6	0.34	24	2.36
6.7	3.9	2	60	141	293	245	1.1	2.2	56	0	0.12	0	0.27	0.17	5.3	0.13	40	0
9.9	7.6	89	319	321	1308	247	4.2	2.9	36	101	0.7	11	0.18	0.32	3.1	0.22	30	1.45
3.4	6.5	34	56	183	1267	382	3.2	3.4	34	9	2.91	10	0.24	0.25	5.4	0.33	27	1.76
8.2	2.3	36	189	287	1650	394	2.6	2.5	68	80	—	12	1	0.8	5.5	0.14	87	1.09
3.6	7.6	15	74	161	582	174	0.7	2.4	24	22	3	1	0.28	0.2	5.6	0.12	28	0.64
5.1	6.6	62	239	400	1350	345	3.1	3.6	43	88	3.11	0	0.26	0.39	4.2	0.26	29	0.35
2.2	5.4	42	40	166	917	264	2.3	3.1	19	6	2.16	0	0.17	0.26	3.3	0.22	13	0.21
2.8	6.8	35	47	289	1340	336	1.9	2.2	62	9	2.8	0	0.23	0.18	7.9	0.41	32	1.43
0.9	0	0	36	20	20	328	0.2	1.4	20	10	0.42	25	0	0.03	0.3	0.06	24	0
0.5	0	0	66	48	17	585	0.2	1.7	51	70	0.73	34	0.02	0.03	3.1	0.1	41	0
—	—	90	200	200	1100	150	—	0	0	160	—	0	0	0.2	0	—	—	—
—	—	60	300	200	1200	160	—	0	16	160	—	0	0	0.2	0	—	—	—
0	0	0	1	1	31	7	0	0.1	0	22	0.04	0	0	0	0	0.01	0	3.12
7	1	75	300	—	670	—	—	0	—	150	—	0	—	—	—	—	—	—
—	—	11	169	—	372	—	—	1.2	—	279	—	0	—	—	—	—	—	—
0.2	0.2	0	6	6	255	54	0.1	0.3	6	27	0.35	2	0.01	0.01	0.3	0.02	1	0
1.8	0.3	16	7	9	563	14	0	0.2	2	57	0.14	0	0.03	0.03	0.3	0	2	0.02
0.1	0.1	0	1	2	55	8	0	0	1	0	0.03	0	0	0	0	0	1	0
1.9	0.3	16	16	23	261	102	0.1	0.8	9	63	0.19	4	0.04	0.05	0.8	0.03	6	0.06
2.5	1.1	18	134	101	258	63	0.6	0.3	9	84	0.59	0	0.04	0.12	0.2	0.02	5	0.22
1.3	0.4	13	142	110	391	138	0.2	0.1	12	29	0.08	1	0.04	0.14	0.1	0.04	3	0.28
7.5	3.6	44	661	724	1549	397	2.9	1	40	231	2.18	2	0.14	0.56	0.6	0.12	16	1.08
—	—	0	0	1	1	29	—	0	—	3	—	3	0	0	0	—	—	—

Esha Code	Food Item	Qty	Meas	Wgt (g)	Wtr (g)	Cals	Prot (g)	Carb (g)	Fib (g)	Fat (g)	SatF (g)
27003	Sauce, chili, tomato base	1	tsp	6	4	6	0	1	0.1	0	0
53226	Sauce, chili, unsalted, bottled	0.25	cup	68	46	71	2	17	—	0	0
53016	Sauce, curry	0.25	cup	58	51	37	1	2	0.1	3	0.5
53103	Sauce, enchilada, green	0.5	cup	62	54	44	1	4	0.7	3	1.8
53102	Sauce, enchilada, red	0.25	cup	62	50	83	1	3	0.6	8	4.1
53104	Sauce, fish/bagoong	0.25	cup	68	44	71	14	0	0	1	0.2
53351	Sauce, hoisin	2	Tbs	34	16	70	1	14	0	2	0
53110	Sauce, hollandaise, dry mix w/water	2	Tbs	32	27	30	1	2	0.1	2	1.4
53098	Sauce, horseradish	1	tsp	5	3	10	0	0	0	1	0.6
53408	Sauce, horseradish, Kraft	1	tsp	5	5	0	0	0	0	0	0
27002	Sauce, hot chili/red pepper	1	tsp	5	5	1	0	0	0	0	0
50199	Sauce, lobster	0.25	cup	58	41	95	6	4	0.3	6	1.3
53120	Sauce, marinara tomato	0.5	cup	125	103	85	2	13	—	4	0.6
53125	Sauce, mole poblano	0.25	cup	66	47	109	2	9	2.8	7	2.2
53126	Sauce, mole verde	0.25	cup	66	57	39	2	4	1.1	2	0.4
53017	Sauce, mornay	0.25	cup	86	57	183	6	6	0.2	15	7
53106	Sauce, pesto	0.25	cup	58	12	311	10	4	0.9	29	7.3
53002	Sauce, soy (wheat & soy)	1	Tbs	18	13	10	1	2	0.1	0	0
53267	Sauce, soy, lite, LaChoy	1	Tbs	18	13	15	1	2	0	0	0
53063	Sauce, soy, tamari	1	Tbs	14	10	9	2	1	0.1	0	0
53010	Sauce, spaghetti w/meat, recipe	0.5	cup	124	94	144	8	11	2.1	8	2.3
53012	Sauce, spaghetti w/meatballs, canned	0.5	cup	125	94	128	6	14	0.9	5	1.3
53344	Sauce, spaghetti, Prego	0.5	cup	125	94	135	2	22	1.9	4	1.4
53009	Sauce, spaghetti, canned	0.5	cup	124	94	136	2	20	4.2	6	0.8
53011	Sauce, spaghetti, meat flavor, canned	0.5	cup	125	92	150	4	19	4	7	1.4
53014	Sauce, spaghetti, w/mushrooms, canned	0.5	cup	123	103	108	2	13	1.2	3	0.4
53008	Sauce, spaghetti/marinara	0.5	cup	125	102	94	2	13	2.5	5	0.7
53058	Sauce, stroganoff w/milk & water	0.25	cup	62	48	57	2	7	0.1	2	1.4
53001	Sauce, szechuan	1	Tbs	16	13	12	0	2	0.2	0	0
53003	Sauce, tartar	2	Tbs	28	10	149	0	1	0.1	16	3.1
53415	Sauce, tartar, nonfat, Kraft	2	Tbs	30	—	23	0	5	0.5	0	0
53004	Sauce, teriyaki	1	Tbs	18	12	15	1	3	0	0	0
53109	Sauce, teriyaki, dry w/water	1	Tbs	18	15	8	0	2	—	0	0
5180	Sauce, tomato, canned, no added salt	0.5	cup	122	109	37	2	9	1.7	0	0
53101	Sauce, white clam	0.25	cup	60	34	149	11	2	0	11	1.4
53025	Sauce, white, dry mix, prep w/milk	0.25	cup	66	54	60	3	5	0.1	3	1.6
53007	Sauce, white, recipe	0.25	cup	62	48	89	2	5	0.1	7	2
53099	Sauce, worcestershire	1	tsp	6	4	4	0	1	0	0	0
5531	Sauerkraut, canned, low sodium	0.5	cup	71	66	14	1	3	1.8	0	0
5145	Sauerkraut, canned, w/liquid	0.5	cup	118	109	22	1	5	3	0	0
13022	Sausage, Polish, pork	1	oz.	28	15	93	4	0	0	8	2.9
13066	Sausage, braunschweiger	2	piece	57	27	205	8	2	0	18	6.2
13070	Sausage, chorizo, link	1	each	60	19	273	14	1	0	23	8.6
13043	Sausage, kielbasa	1	piece	26	14	81	3	1	0	7	2.6
13021	Sausage, pepperoni, pork/beef	4	piece	22	6	109	5	1	0	10	3.5
13099	Sausage, pork, Chinese	4	oz.	113	44	403	24	7	0	33	—
13015	Sausage, pork, Italian link, cooked	1	each	67	34	216	13	1	0	17	6.1
13030	Sausage, summer, thuringer, beef & pork	1	piece	23	12	77	4	0	0	7	2.8
13052	Sausage, turkey, breakfast type	1	piece	28	17	65	6	0	0	5	1.6
13053	Sausage, turkey, smoked	1	oz.	28	19	55	4	0	0	4	1.3
26112	Savory, ground	0.25	tsp	0	0	1	0	0	0.2	0	0
42071	Scone	1	each	42	12	150	4	18	0.6	7	2.1
49095	Scone, apple kiwi, fat free, Health Valley	1	each	60	35	80	7	15	7	0	0
42072	Scone, whole wheat	1	each	42	11	145	5	18	2.8	7	2.1
56257	Seafood salad	0.5	cup	104	76	166	12	2	0.4	12	1.6
18816	Seafood souffle	0.5	cup	80	57	129	9	4	0.1	8	2.4
5255	Seaweed, Irishmoss, raw	0.5	cup	40	32	20	1	5	0.5	0	0
5254	Seaweed, agar, dried	0.5	cup	8	1	23	0	6	0.6	0	0
5253	Seaweed, agar, raw	0.5	cup	40	36	10	0	3	0.2	0	0
5256	Seaweed, kelp, raw	0.5	cup	40	33	17	1	4	0.5	0	0.1
5257	Seaweed, laver, raw	0.5	cup	40	34	14	2	2	0.1	0	0
5260	Seaweed, spirulina, dried	0.5	cup	8	0	22	4	2	0.3	1	0.2
7089	Seeds, lupin, cooked, no salt	0.5	cup	83	59	99	13	8	2.3	2	0.3
62000	Sego diet drink	1	cup	256	—	180	9	27	0	4	0.1
62001	Sego lite diet drink	1	cup	256	—	120	9	16	0	2	0.4

MonoF	PolyF	Choles	Calc	Phos	Sod	Pot	Zn	Iron	Magn	VitA	VitE	VitC	Thia	Ribo	Nia	B6	Fola	B12
(g)	(g)	(mg)	(mg)	(mg)	(mg)	(mg)	(mg)	(mg)	(mg)	(μg RE)	(mg α-TE)	(mg)	(mg)	(mg)	(mg)	(mg)	(μg)	(μg)
0	0	0	1	3	76	21	0	0	1	8	0.02	1	0	0	0.1	0.01	0	0
—	—	0	14	36	14	253	—	0.5	—	96	—	11	0.06	0.05	1.1	—	—	—
1.3	0.9	0	4	19	196	52	0.1	0.3	2	31	0.41	0	0.01	0.03	0.8	0.01	1	0.06
0.9	0.3	10	20	30	92	146	0.2	0.4	11	138	0.26	27	0.03	0.04	0.7	0.05	4	0.03
2.4	0.8	22	16	22	84	98	0.1	0.3	8	195	0.43	5	0.02	0.05	0.3	0.06	6	0.03
0.2	0.3	42	126	157	5440	442	1.4	2.2	7	29	2.63	0	0.02	0.15	4	0.09	12	5.24
—	—	0	0	—	500	—	—	0	—	0	—	0	—	—	—	—	—	—
0.7	0.1	6	16	16	196	16	0.1	0.1	1	28	0.08	0	0.01	0.02	0	0.06	3	0.1
0.3	0	2	5	4	14	7	0	0	1	9	0.03	0	0	0.01	0	0	0	0.01
0	0	0	0	—	47	9	—	0	—	0	—	1	—	—	—	—	—	—
0	0	0	0	1	1	29	0	0	1	50	0.04	2	0	0	0	0.01	1	0
1.8	2.5	42	11	67	484	114	0.6	0.5	8	12	0.43	1	0.1	0.1	1.2	0.09	13	0.2
2.1	1.2	0	22	44	786	530	0.3	1	30	120	2	16	0.06	0.07	2	0.31	17	0
3.2	1.9	1	16	54	89	216	0.3	1.2	21	254	0.96	0	0.02	0	1.1	0.17	19	0.03
0.6	0.8	0	11	67	235	191	0.4	0.9	25	41	0.22	12	0.03	0.04	1.3	0.06	9	0.04
5	2.6	79	158	127	402	108	0.6	0.4	12	163	1.14	1	0.06	0.16	0.3	0.05	10	0.39
18.1	2.1	18	417	207	422	206	1	2.4	33	86	2.9	5	0.02	0.1	0.4	0.09	16	0.32
0	0	0	3	20	1028	32	0.1	0.4	6	0	0	0	0.01	0.02	0.6	0.03	3	0
—	—	0	3	—	505	—	—	0.1	—	0	—	0	—	—	—	—	—	—
0	0	0	3	19	810	31	0.1	0.3	6	0	0	0	0.01	0.02	0.6	0.03	3	0
2.8	2.4	23	29	86	565	542	1.7	2	31	229	2.14	18	0.09	0.13	2.9	0.26	12	0.71
2.4	0.8	16	26	56	553	123	1.1	1.6	14	220	2	2	0.08	0.1	1.2	0.16	7	1.18
—	—	0	38	—	587	—	—	1.4	—	96	—	9	—	—	—	—	—	0
3	1.6	0	35	45	618	478	0.3	0.8	30	153	2.49	14	0.07	0.07	1.9	0.44	27	0
3.5	1.6	8	34	57	590	476	0.7	1	30	288	2.96	13	0.07	0.08	2.2	0.44	26	0.25
1.5	0.8	0	15	30	496	333	0.3	1	15	241	1.36	9	0.08	0.08	0.9	0.16	13	0
1.1	2.7	0	32	51	657	565	0.5	1.6	31	138	2.52	21	0.09	0.1	1.7	0.23	12	0
0.6	0.1	8	109	63	381	140	0.2	0.3	8	26	—	0	0.18	0.16	0.2	0.02	2	0.12
0.1	0.1	0	3	3	127	27	0	0.1	3	14	0.17	1	0	0	0.1	0.01	1	0
5.2	8.1	14	5	9	198	22	0	0.3	1	18	4.48	0	0	0.01	0	0.01	1	0
0	0	0	0	—	197	14	—	0	—	0	—	0	—	—	—	—	—	—
0	0	0	4	28	690	40	0	0.3	11	0	0	0	0	0.01	0.2	0.02	4	0
0	0	0	7	13	299	13	0	0.2	5	0	0	0	0	0	0.1	0.01	2	0
0	0.1	0	17	39	741	454	0.3	0.9	23	120	1.72	16	0.08	0.07	1.4	0.19	12	0
7.3	1.1	28	42	141	245	265	1.2	11.7	8	72	1.6	9	0.06	0.18	1.4	0.05	12	40.8
1.2	0.4	9	106	64	199	111	0.1	0.1	66	23	0.4	1	0.02	0.11	0.1	0.02	4	0.26
2.3	2.2	7	65	54	92	86	0.2	0.2	8	78	0.85	1	0.05	0.1	0.2	0.02	4	0.19
0	0	0	6	3	56	45	0	0.3	1	1	0	1	0	0.01	0	0	0	0
0	0	0	21	14	219	121	0.1	1	9	1	0.07	10	0.01	0.01	0.1	0.06	17	0
0	0.1	0	35	24	780	201	0.2	1.7	15	2	0.12	17	0.02	0.03	0.2	0.15	28	0
3.8	0.9	20	3	39	249	67	0.5	0.4	4	0	0.06	0	0.14	0.04	1	0.05	1	0.28
8.5	2.1	89	5	96	652	113	1.6	5.3	6	2405	0.2	0	0.14	0.87	4.8	0.19	25	11.5
11	2.1	53	5	90	741	239	2	1	11	0	0.13	0	0.38	0.18	3.1	0.32	1	1.2
3.4	0.8	17	11	38	280	70	0.5	0.4	4	0	0.06	0	0.06	0.06	0.7	0.05	1	0.42
4.6	1	17	2	26	449	76	0.6	0.3	4	0	0.05	0	0.07	0.06	1.1	0.06	1	0.55
—	—	—	27	245	998	—	—	3.4	—	0	—	0	0.52	0.31	5.3	—	—	—
8	2.2	52	16	114	618	204	1.6	1	12	0	0.17	1	0.42	0.16	2.8	0.22	3	0.87
3	0.3	17	3	26	286	62	0.6	0.6	3	0	0.05	0	0.04	0.08	1	0.06	0	1.27
1.8	1.2	23	5	52	191	76	1	0.5	6	0	0.14	0	0.03	0.08	1.4	0.08	1	0.5
1.6	1	19	5	37	219	59	0.7	0.4	5	0	0.14	0	0.02	0.06	1.2	0.06	1	0.56
—	—	0	8	1	0	4	0	0.1	1	2	—	0	0	—	0	—	—	0
2.5	1.4	51	62	61	246	50	0.3	1.2	7	85	0.9	0	0.14	0.16	1.2	0.03	8	0.1
0	0	0	20	—	160	—	—	0.1	—	200	—	12	—	—	—	—	—	—
2.5	1.5	50	55	153	174	189	0.8	1	32	84	1.07	0	0.09	0.11	1.3	0.08	11	0.1
8.3	1.2	64	45	137	274	249	1.6	1	27	27	2.29	7	0.04	0.05	1.2	0.09	16	0.89
3.3	2	112	65	116	303	136	0.8	0.8	14	117	1.49	1	0.05	0.19	1.3	0.08	13	0.53
0	0	0	29	63	27	25	0.8	3.6	58	5	0.35	1	0.01	0.19	0.2	0.03	73	0
0	0	0	47	4	8	84	0.4	1.6	58	0	0.38	0	0	0.02	0	0.02	44	0
0	0	0	22	2	4	90	0.2	0.7	27	0	0.35	0	0	0.01	0	0.01	34	0
0	0	0	67	17	93	36	0.5	1.1	48	5	0.35	1	0.02	0.06	0.2	0	72	0
0	0	0	28	23	19	142	0.4	0.7	1	208	0.4	16	0.04	0.18	0.6	0.06	58	0
0.1	0.2	0	9	9	79	102	0.2	2.1	15	4	0.38	1	0.18	0.28	1	0.03	7	0
1	0.6	0	42	106	3	203	1.2	1	45	1	0.08	1	0.11	0.04	0.4	0.01	49	0
1.7	1.5	3	200	200	289	481	3	3.6	80	300	—	12	0.3	0.34	4	0.4	80	1.2
0.4	0.9	3	200	200	289	481	3	3.6	80	300	—	12	0.3	0.34	4	0.4	80	1.2

Esha Code	Food Item	Qty	Meas	Wgt (g)	Wtr (g)	Cals	Prot (g)	Carb (g)	Fib (g)	Fat (g)	SatF (g)
4655	Sesame butter, tahini, f/roasted/toasted kernels	1	Tbs	15	0	89	3	3	1.4	8	1.1
4619	Sesame meal, partially defatted	1	oz.	28	1	161	5	7	1.1	14	1.9
4524	Sesame seed kernels, dried	0.25	cup	38	2	221	10	4	4.4	21	2.9
4523	Sesame seed, whole, dried	0.25	cup	36	2	206	6	8	4.2	18	2.5
5428	Shallot, freeze dried, chopped	0.25	cup	4	0	12	0	3	0.2	0	0
5427	Shallot, raw, chopped	1	Tbs	10	8	7	0	2	0.1	0	0
20186	Shasta Soda, cherry cola, diet	1	cup	240	239	0	0	0	0	0	0
20189	Shasta Soda, cream soda, diet	1	cup	240	239	0	0	0	0	0	0
20190	Shasta Soda, ginger ale, diet	1	cup	240	239	0	0	0	0	0	0
2011	Sherbet, orange	0.5	cup	96	64	132	1	29	0	2	1.1
22506	Sherry, medium	1	cup	240	206	336	1	19	0	0	0
8007	Shortening, vegetable (Crisco/Fluffo)	1	Tbs	13	0	113	0	0	0	13	3.2
56239	Shrimp jambalaya	0.5	cup	122	88	153	14	13	0.9	5	0.9
19426	Shrimp marinara dinner, Healthy Choice	1	each	298	243	250	10	44	5	4	2
19418	Shrimp patty burger	1	each	120	72	248	18	15	1.3	13	3.4
56256	Shrimp salad	0.5	cup	91	65	141	13	3	0.4	8	1.3
19410	Shrimp w/lobster sauce	0.25	cup	46	32	72	9	2	0.1	3	0.6
19408	Shrimp, curried	0.5	cup	118	88	157	14	7	0.2	8	2.5
20208	Soda, 7-Up, Gold	1	cup	240	215	104	0	25	—	0	0
20209	Soda, 7-Up, Gold, diet	1	cup	240	239	3	0	1	—	0	0
20207	Soda, 7-Up, diet	1	cup	240	240	2	0	0	0	0	0
20055	Soda, 7-Up, regular	1	cup	240	233	28	0	7	0	0	0
20147	Soda, Coca Cola, can/bottle	1	cup	240	215	100	0	26	0	0	0
20148	Soda, Coca Cola, classic, can/bottle	1	cup	240	218	94	0	26	0	0	0
20150	Soda, Coca Cola, diet, can/bottle	1	cup	240	240	1	0	0	0	0	0
20027	Soda, Dr. Pepper type	1	cup	245	219	101	0	26	0	0	0.2
20086	Soda, Dr. Pepper type, decaf, sugar free, 12 oz can	1	each	355	354	4	0	0	0	0	0
20167	Soda, Pepsi, diet	1	cup	240	239	0	0	0	0	0	0
20166	Soda, Pepsi, regular	1	cup	240	212	100	0	27	0	0	0
22508	Soda, Slice, apple, diet	1	cup	237	233	0	0	0	0	0	0
20125	Soda, Slice, mandarin orange, diet	1	cup	237	233	0	0	0	0	0	0
20125	Soda, Slice, mandarin orange, diet	1	cup	240	236	0	0	0	0	0	0
20163	Soda, Sprite, can/bottle	1	cup	240	213	93	0	25	0	0	0
20164	Soda, Sprite, diet, can/bottle	1	cup	240	240	3	0	0	0	0	0
20165	Soda, Tab, can/bottle	1	cup	240	239	1	0	0	0	0	0
20066	Soda, cherry cola, Slice	1	cup	248	217	119	0	30	0	0	0
20006	Soda, club	1	cup	237	236	0	0	0	0	0	0
20054	Soda, cola, caffeine-free, can/bottle	1	cup	240	212	107	0	27	0	0	0
20049	Soda, cola, diet, w/aspartame+saccharin	1	cup	237	236	2	0	0	0	0	0
20005	Soda, cola-type, regular	1	cup	247	221	101	0	26	0	0	0
20056	Soda, cola/coke, diet, caffeine-free	1	cup	240	239	0	0	0	0	0	0
20030	Soda, cola/coke, diet, w/aspartame, can/bottle	1	cup	237	236	2	0	0	0	0	0
20007	Soda, cola/pepper type, diet, w/saccharin	1	cup	237	236	0	0	0	0	0	0
20028	Soda, cream	1	cup	247	214	126	0	33	0	0	0
20085	Soda, cream, sugar-free, 12 fl oz can	1	each	355	354	0	0	0	0	0	0
20068	Soda, diet, lemon lime, Slice	1	cup	240	234	0	0	1	0	0	0
20008	Soda, ginger ale	1	cup	244	223	83	0	21	0	0	0
20084	Soda, ginger ale, sugar-free, 12 fl oz can	1	each	355	354	0	0	0	0	0	0
20031	Soda, grape, carbonated	1	cup	248	220	107	0	28	0	0	0
20032	Soda, lemon lime	1	cup	245	220	98	0	26	0	0	0
20271	Soda, mountain dew	1	cup	240	—	113	0	31	0	0	0
20160	Soda, orange, Minute Maid, can/bottle	1	cup	240	209	113	0	31	0	0	0
20269	Soda, pepsi, diet, caffeine free	1	cup	240	239	0	0	0	0	0	0
20009	Soda, root beer	1	cup	247	220	101	0	26	0	0	0
2066	Sorbet, fruit, citrus flavor	0.5	cup	100	76	92	0	23	0.1	0	0
2065	Sorbet, fruit, non-citrus flavor	0.5	cup	100	82	70	1	17	0	0	0
56075	Souffle, cheese	0.5	cup	56	40	98	6	3	0	7	2.8
56076	Souffle, spinach	0.5	cup	68	50	109	5	1	1.4	9	3.6
50575	Soup, Home Cookin', hearty lentil, RTS	0.5	cup	122	105	65	4	12	2.5	0	0.2
50624	Soup, Pasta Fagioli, fat free, Health Valley	0.5	cup	120	107	40	3	8	2	0	0
50124	Soup, Scotch broth, w/water	0.5	cup	120	111	40	2	5	0.6	1	0.6
50065	Soup, bean & ham, RTS, can	1	each	546	429	519	28	61	25.1	19	7.5
50064	Soup, bean & ham, chunky, RTS	0.5	cup	122	96	115	6	14	5.6	4	1.7
50063	Soup, bean and 'frank', w/water	0.5	cup	125	104	94	5	11	2.9	3	1.1
50063	Soup, bean and 'frank', w/water	1	cup	150	125	113	6	13	3.4	4	1.3

MonoF (g)	PolyF (g)	Choles (mg)	Calc (mg)	Phos (mg)	Sod (mg)	Pot (mg)	Zn (mg)	Iron (mg)	Magn (mg)	VitA (μg RE)	VitE (mg α-TE)	VitC (mg)	Thia (mg)	Ribo (mg)	Nia (mg)	B6 (mg)	Fola (μg)	B12 (μg)
3	3.5	0	64	110	17	62	0.7	1.3	14	1	0.34	0	0.18	0.07	0.8	0.02	15	0
5.1	6	0	43	219	11	115	2.9	4.1	98	2	0.64	0	0.73	0.08	3.6	0.04	8	0
7.8	9	0	49	291	15	153	3.9	2.9	130	3	0.85	0	0.27	0.03	1.8	0.06	36	0
6.8	7.8	0	351	226	4	168	2.8	5.3	126	0	0.82	0	0.28	0.09	1.6	0.28	35	0
0	0	0	7	11	2	59	0.1	0.2	4	202	0.01	1	0.01	0	0	0.06	4	0
0	0	0	4	6	1	33	0	0.1	2	12	0.01	1	0.01	0	0	0.04	3	0
0	0	0	—	49	37	0	—	—	—	—	—	—	—	—	—	—	—	0
0	0	0	—	0	37	0	—	—	—	—	—	—	—	—	—	—	—	0
0	0	0	—	—	37	0	—	—	—	—	—	—	—	—	—	—	—	0
0.5	0.1	6	52	38	44	92	0.5	0.1	8	13	0.08	3	0.02	0.08	0.1	0.02	5	0.18
0	0	0	19	16	18	200	0.2	0.6	19	0	0	0	0.02	0.06	0.3	0.02	0	0
5.7	3.3	0	0	0	0	0	0	0	0	0	1.06	0	0	0	0	0	0	0
1.8	1.6	93	51	158	327	227	0.9	2.7	31	82	2.12	9	0.09	0.05	2.3	0.12	5	0.6
—	—	55	60	—	260	—	—	1.8	—	60	—	1	—	—	—	—	—	—
5.4	3.5	143	58	197	299	328	1.1	2.3	39	29	2.7	5	0.1	0.1	2.7	0.22	9	0.78
2.2	4.2	103	43	140	195	183	0.8	1.7	26	21	2.56	3	0.02	0.03	1.6	0.14	8	0.65
0.8	1.3	64	21	91	248	105	0.6	0.9	15	10	0.86	1	0.05	0.05	1.2	0.07	6	0.39
2.9	2	91	113	181	316	218	0.9	1.5	30	94	2.04	2	0.06	0.15	1.6	0.08	6	0.67
0	0	—	—	45	47	—	—	—	—	0	—	—	—	—	—	—	—	0
0	0	—	—	45	47	—	—	—	—	0	—	—	—	—	—	—	—	0
0	0	0	5	—	7	18	—	0.1	—	0	—	0	0	0	—	0	—	0
0	0	0	1	—	2	5	—	0	—	0	0	0	0	0	—	0	—	0
0	0	0	7	35	5	2	0	0.1	2	0	0	0	0	0	0	0	0	0
0	0	0	9	40	9	0	0	0.1	3	0	0	0	0	0	0	0	0	0
0	0	0	10	18	4	12	0.2	0.1	2	0	0	0	0.02	0.05	0	0	0	0
0	0	0	7	27	24	2	0.1	0.1	0	0	0	0	0	0	0	0	0	0
0	0	0	14	32	21	0	0.3	0.1	4	0	0	0	0.02	0.08	0	0	0	0
0	0	0	0	27	23	5	—	0	—	0	—	0	—	—	—	—	—	0
0	0	0	0	35	23	—	—	0	—	0	—	0	—	—	—	—	—	0
0	0	0	0	0	33	—	—	0	—	0	—	0	—	—	—	—	—	0
0	0	0	0	0	33	—	—	0	—	0	—	0	—	—	—	—	—	0
0	0	0	0	0	33	—	—	0	—	0	—	0	—	—	—	—	—	0
0	0	0	5	0	22	0	0.1	0.2	2	0	0	0	0	0	0	0	0	0
0	0	0	10	0	0	67	0.1	0.1	—	0	0	0	0	0	0	0	0	0
0	0	0	8	30	4	12	—	0.1	—	0	0	0	0	0	—	0	0	0
0	0	0	12	2	30	5	0.2	0.1	2	0	0	0	0	0	0	0	0	0
0	0	0	12	0	50	5	0.2	0	2	0	0	0	0	0	0	0	0	0
0	0	0	—	33	30	0	—	—	—	—	—	—	—	—	—	—	—	0
0	0	0	9	21	21	0	0.2	0.1	2	0	0	0	0.01	0.05	0	0	0	0
0	0	0	7	30	10	2	0	0.1	2	0	0	0	0	0	0	0	0	0
0	0	0	—	33	37	36	—	—	—	—	—	—	—	—	—	—	—	0
0	0	0	9	21	14	0	0.2	0.1	2	0	0	0	0.01	0.05	0	0	0	0
0	0	0	9	26	38	5	0.1	0.1	2	0	0	0	0	0	0	0	0	0
0	0	0	12	0	30	2	0.2	0.1	2	0	0	0	0	0	0	0	0	0
0	0	0	14	39	57	7	0.2	0.1	4	0	0	0	0	0	0	0	0	0
0	0	0	0	0	23	—	—	0	—	0	—	0	—	—	—	—	—	0
0	0	0	7	0	17	2	0.1	0.4	2	0	0	0	0	0	0	0	0	0
0	0	0	14	39	57	7	0.2	0.1	4	0	0	0	0	0	0	0	0	0
0	0	0	7	0	37	2	0.2	0.2	2	0	0	0	0	0	0	0	0	0
0	0	0	5	0	27	2	0.1	0.2	2	0	0	0	0	0	0	0	0	0
0	0	—	0	0	47	—	—	0	—	0	—	0	—	—	—	—	—	0
0	0	0	5	0	0	13	0.1	0.2	2	0	0	0	0	0	0	0	0	0
0	0	—	0	27	23	—	—	0	—	0	—	0	—	—	—	—	—	0
0	0	0	12	0	32	2	0.2	0.1	2	0	0	0	0	0	0	0	0	0
0	0	0	9	13	8	100	0	0.5	8	27	0.05	26	0.01	0.03	0.2	0.02	22	0
0	0	0	2	0	46	2	0	0	1	0	0	0	0	0	0	0	0	0
2.4	1.4	97	105	100	149	73	0.5	0.4	8	84	0.64	0	0.04	0.18	0.1	0.04	12	0.39
3.4	1.5	92	115	116	381	101	0.6	0.7	19	337	0.61	2	0.05	0.15	0.2	0.06	40	0.68
0	0	0	20	—	430	—	—	1.8	—	200	—	0	—	—	—	—	—	—
0	0	0	20	—	125	—	—	0.1	—	200	—	8	—	—	—	—	—	—
0.4	0.3	2	7	28	506	80	0.8	0.4	2	108	0.04	0	0.01	0.02	0.6	0.04	5	0.13
8.6	2.1	49	175	322	2184	956	2.4	7.3	104	890	0.27	10	0.33	0.33	3.8	0.27	66	0.16
1.9	0.5	11	39	72	486	213	0.5	1.6	23	198	0.06	2	0.07	0.07	0.9	0.06	15	0.04
1.4	0.8	6	44	82	546	239	0.6	1.2	24	44	—	0	0.06	0.03	0.5	0.07	15	0.04
1.6	1	8	52	99	656	287	0.7	1.4	28	52	—	1	0.07	0.04	0.6	0.08	18	0.04

Esha Code	Food Item	Qty	Meas	Wgt (g)	Wtr (g)	Cals	Prot (g)	Carb (g)	Fib (g)	Fat (g)	SatF (g)
50151	Soup, bean w/bacon, dry, w/water	0.5	cup	132	119	53	3	8	4.5	1	0.5
50000	Soup, bean with bacon, prep w/water	0.5	cup	126	107	86	4	11	4.3	3	0.8
50198	Soup, beef and mushroom, w/water	0.5	cup	122	113	37	3	3	0.1	2	0.7
50001	Soup, beef broth/bouillon, condensed, prepared	0.5	cup	120	117	8	1	0	0	0	0.1
50002	Soup, beef broth/bouillon, ready to serve can	1	cup	236	230	16	3	0	0	1	0.3
50002	Soup, beef broth/bouillon, ready to serve can	1	each	397	387	28	5	0	0	1	0.4
50153	Soup, beef noodle, dry, w/water	0.5	cup	126	120	20	1	3	0.4	0	0.1
50003	Soup, beef noodle, prep w/water	0.5	cup	122	112	42	2	4	0.4	2	0.6
50206	Soup, beef stroganoff, chunky style	0.5	cup	120	96	118	6	11	0.7	6	2.5
50066	Soup, beef, chunky, RTS	0.5	cup	120	100	85	6	10	0.7	3	1.3
50066	Soup, beef, chunky, RTS	1	cup	240	200	170	12	20	1.4	5	2.5
50067	Soup, beef, chunky, RTS, can	1	each	539	449	383	26	44	3.2	12	5.7
50134	Soup, bisque, tomato, prepared, w/milk	0.5	cup	126	102	99	3	15	0.3	3	1.6
50135	Soup, bisque, tomato, w/water	0.5	cup	124	108	62	1	12	0.2	1	0.3
50060	Soup, black bean, w/water	0.5	cup	124	108	58	3	10	2.2	1	0.2
50204	Soup, bouillabaisse	0.5	cup	114	88	121	17	2	0.3	4	1
50035	Soup, broth, chicken, dry cube, prepared	0.5	cup	122	118	6	0	1	0	0	0
50183	Soup, broth/bouillon, beef, canned, low sodium	0.5	cup	120	115	19	2	0	0	1	0.2
50220	Soup, broth/bouillon, beef, condensed	1	each	298	286	36	7	2	0	0	0
50033	Soup, broth/bouillon, beef, dry cube, prepared	0.5	cup	120	118	4	0	0	0	0	0
50032	Soup, broth/bouillon, beef, dry, w/water	0.5	cup	122	118	10	1	1	0	0	0.2
50004	Soup, broth/bouillon, chicken, condensed, prepared	0.5	cup	122	117	20	2	0	0	1	0.2
50155	Soup, cauliflower, dry, w/water	0.5	cup	128	119	35	1	5	0.1	1	0.1
50651	Soup, cheese, condensed	1	cup	257	198	311	11	21	2.1	21	13.3
50070	Soup, cheese, condensed, can	1	each	312	241	378	13	26	2.5	25	16.2
50071	Soup, cheese, prepared w/milk	0.5	cup	126	103	115	5	8	0.5	7	4.6
50072	Soup, cheese, prepared w/water	0.5	cup	124	109	78	3	5	0.5	5	3.3
50089	Soup, chicken & vegetable chunky, RTS	1	each	539	450	372	28	42	0.5	11	3.2
50088	Soup, chicken & vegetable, chunky, RTS	1	cup	240	200	166	12	19	0.2	5	1.4
50074	Soup, chicken and dumpling, prep w/water	0.5	cup	120	111	48	3	3	0.2	3	0.7
50077	Soup, chicken gumbo, prep w/water	0.5	cup	122	114	28	1	4	1	1	0.2
50080	Soup, chicken mushroom, w/water	0.5	cup	122	110	66	2	5	0.1	5	1.2
50084	Soup, chicken noodle & meatballs, RTS	0.5	cup	124	112	50	4	4	0.3	2	0.5
50081	Soup, chicken noodle, chunky, RTS	0.5	cup	120	101	88	6	9	1.9	3	0.7
50081	Soup, chicken noodle, chunky, RTS	1	cup	240	202	175	13	17	3.8	6	1.4
50082	Soup, chicken noodle, chunky, RTS, can	1	each	539	453	393	29	38	8.6	14	3.1
50037	Soup, chicken noodle, dry, prep w/water	0.5	cup	126	119	26	1	4	0.4	1	0.1
50005	Soup, chicken noodle, prep w/water	0.5	cup	120	111	37	2	5	0.4	1	0.3
50085	Soup, chicken rice, chunky, RTS	0.5	cup	120	104	64	6	6	0.5	2	0.5
50086	Soup, chicken rice, chunky, RTS, can	1	each	539	468	286	28	29	2.2	7	2.2
50161	Soup, chicken rice, dry, w/water	0.5	cup	126	119	30	1	5	0.4	1	0.2
50020	Soup, chicken rice, w/water	0.5	cup	120	113	30	2	4	0.4	1	0.2
50038	Soup, chicken vegetable, dry, prep w/water	0.5	cup	126	119	25	1	4	0.3	0	0.1
50091	Soup, chicken vegetable, prep w/water	0.5	cup	120	112	37	2	4	0.5	1	0.4
50052	Soup, chicken, chunky, ready to serve	0.5	cup	126	106	89	6	9	0.8	3	1
50052	Soup, chicken, chunky, ready to serve	1	cup	251	211	178	13	17	1.5	7	2
50053	Soup, chicken, chunky, ready to serve, can	1	each	305	257	217	15	21	1.8	8	2.4
50007	Soup, chili beef, w/water	0.5	cup	125	106	85	3	11	4.8	3	1.7
50166	Soup, consomme, w/gelatin, prepared mix	0.5	cup	124	118	9	1	1	0	0	0
50213	Soup, crab bisque	0.5	cup	124	100	127	10	6	0.2	7	2.3
50099	Soup, crab, RTS	0.5	cup	122	112	38	3	5	0.4	1	0.2
50099	Soup, crab, RTS	1	cup	244	223	76	5	10	0.7	2	0.4
50100	Soup, crab, RTS, can	1	each	369	338	114	8	16	1.1	2	0.6
50645	Soup, cream of asparagus, condensed	1	cup	251	211	173	5	21	1	8	2.1
50056	Soup, cream of asparagus, condensed, can	1	each	305	257	210	6	26	1.2	10	2.5
50149	Soup, cream of asparagus, dry, w/water	0.5	cup	126	118	29	1	4	0.2	1	0
50057	Soup, cream of asparagus, w/milk	0.5	cup	124	107	81	3	8	0.4	4	1.7
50058	Soup, cream of asparagus, w/water	0.5	cup	122	112	43	1	5	0.2	2	0.5
50188	Soup, cream of bacon, prepared w/water	0.5	cup	122	111	59	2	5	0.1	4	1
50189	Soup, cream of broccoli	0.5	cup	118	96	117	4	8	0.9	8	3
50650	Soup, cream of celery, condensed	1	cup	251	213	181	3	18	1.5	11	2.8
50017	Soup, cream of celery, condensed, can	1	each	305	259	220	4	21	1.8	14	3.4
50157	Soup, cream of celery, dry, w/water	0.5	cup	127	119	32	1	5	0.2	1	0.1
50015	Soup, cream of celery, w/milk	0.5	cup	124	107	82	3	7	0.4	5	2
50016	Soup, cream of celery, w/water	0.5	cup	122	113	45	1	4	0.4	3	0.7

MonoF	PolyF	Choles	Calc	Phos	Sod	Pot	Zn	Iron	Magn	VitA	VitE	VitC	Thia	Ribo	Nia	B6	Fola	B12
(g)	(g)	(mg)	(mg)	(mg)	(mg)	(mg)	(mg)	(mg)	(mg)	(μg RE)	(mg α-TE)	(mg)	(mg)	(mg)	(mg)	(mg)	(μg)	(μg)
0.5	0.1	1	28	45	464	163	0.3	0.7	15	3	0.13	1	0.03	0.13	0.2	0.01	4	0.01
1.1	0.9	1	40	66	476	201	0.5	1	23	44	0.04	1	0.04	0.02	0.3	0.02	16	0.02
0.6	0.1	4	2	17	471	77	0.7	0.4	5	0	—	2	0.02	0.03	0.5	0.02	5	0.1
0.1	0	0	7	16	391	65	0	0.2	2	0	0	0	0	0.02	0.9	0.01	2	0.08
0.2	0	0	14	31	769	127	0	0.4	5	0	0	0	0	0.05	1.8	0.02	5	0.16
0.4	0	0	24	52	1294	214	0	0.7	8	0	0	0	0.01	0.08	3.1	0.04	8	0.28
0.2	0.1	1	3	20	521	40	0	0.2	5	1	0.01	0	0.06	0.03	0.3	0.02	8	0
0.6	0.2	2	7	23	476	50	0.8	0.5	2	32	0	0	0.03	0.03	0.5	0.02	10	0.1
2.1	1.2	25	24	60	522	168	1.3	1.1	2	98	0.76	0	0.05	0.11	0.1	0.07	7	0.31
1.1	0.1	7	16	60	433	168	1.3	1.2	2	131	0.08	3	0.03	0.08	1.4	0.07	7	0.31
2.1	0.2	14	31	120	866	336	2.6	2.3	5	262	0.17	7	0.06	0.15	2.7	0.13	13	0.62
4.8	0.5	32	70	270	1945	755	5.9	5.2	11	588	0.38	16	0.13	0.34	6.1	0.3	30	1.4
0.9	0.6	11	93	87	555	302	0.3	0.4	13	55	0.5	4	0.06	0.13	0.6	0.07	11	0.21
0.3	0.6	2	20	30	524	209	0.3	0.4	5	36	0.37	3	0.03	0.04	0.6	0.04	7	0
0.3	0.2	0	22	53	599	137	0.7	1.1	21	25	0.04	0	0.04	0.03	0.3	0.05	12	0.01
2	0.7	45	41	170	208	366	0.9	2	37	44	1.15	6	0.12	0.09	2.5	0.19	14	5.21
0.1	0	0	6	6	396	12	0	0.1	1	2	0.02	0	0.01	0.01	0.1	0	1	0.01
0.3	0.1	0	5	36	36	103	0.1	0.3	1	0	0.02	0	0	0.04	1.6	0.01	2	0.12
0	0	12	0	39	2162	161	0	0.9	6	0	0	0	0	0.05	2.3	0.02	6	0.22
0	0	0	1	6	578	10	0	0.1	1	0	0	0	0	0.01	0.1	0	1	0
0.1	0	0	5	12	681	18	0	0	4	1	0.01	0	0	0.01	0.2	0	0	0
0.3	0.1	0	5	37	388	105	0.1	0.3	1	0	0.02	0	0	0.04	1.7	0.01	2	0.12
0.4	0.3	0	5	26	421	52	0.1	0.3	1	0	—	1	0.04	0.04	0.3	0.01	1	0.09
5.9	0.6	59	285	272	1919	308	1.3	1.5	8	218	0.41	0	0.03	0.27	0.8	0.05	8	0
7.2	0.7	72	346	331	2330	374	1.6	1.8	9	265	0.5	0	0.04	0.33	1	0.06	9	0
2	0.2	24	144	126	510	171	0.3	0.4	10	74	0.13	1	0.03	0.17	0.3	0.04	5	0.21
1.5	0.1	15	70	68	479	77	0.3	0.4	2	54	—	0	0.01	0.07	0.2	0.01	2	0
4.8	2.3	38	59	237	2398	825	4.8	3.3	22	1347	0.16	12	0.09	0.37	7.4	0.22	27	0.54
2.2	1	17	26	106	1068	367	2.2	1.5	10	600	0.07	6	0.04	0.17	3.3	0.1	12	0.24
1.3	0.7	17	7	30	430	58	0.2	0.3	2	26	0.07	0	0.01	0.04	0.9	0.02	1	0.08
0.3	0.2	2	12	12	477	38	0.2	0.5	2	7	0.02	2	0.01	0.02	0.3	0.03	2	0.01
2	1.2	5	15	13	471	77	0.5	0.4	5	56	0.61	0	0.01	0.06	0.8	0.02	0	0.02
0.8	0.4	5	15	42	520	77	0.2	0.9	5	117	—	4	0.06	0.06	1.2	0.02	11	0.12
1.3	0.8	10	12	36	425	54	0.5	0.7	5	61	0.4	0	0.04	0.08	2.2	0.02	19	0.16
2.7	1.5	19	24	72	850	108	1	1.4	10	122	0.79	0	0.07	0.17	4.3	0.05	38	0.31
6	3.4	43	54	162	1908	243	2.2	3.2	22	275	1.78	0	0.16	0.38	9.7	0.11	86	0.7
0.3	0.2	1	16	16	641	15	0.1	0.3	4	3	0.01	0	0.04	0.03	0.4	0	9	0
0.6	0.3	4	8	18	553	28	0.2	0.4	2	36	0.04	0	0.03	0.03	0.7	0.01	11	0.07
0.7	0.3	6	17	36	444	54	0.5	0.9	5	293	0.04	2	0.01	0.05	2	0.02	2	0.16
3.2	1.5	27	76	162	1994	243	2.2	4.2	22	1315	0.19	9	0.05	0.22	9.2	0.11	9	0.7
0.3	0.2	1	4	5	491	5	0.1	0	0	0	0.02	0	0	0	0.2	0.01	0	0.04
0.5	0.2	4	8	11	407	51	0.1	0.4	0	32	0.03	0	0.01	0.01	0.6	0.01	0	0.07
0.2	0.1	1	8	16	404	34	0.1	0.3	11	1	—	1	0.04	0.02	0.3	0.04	1	0.05
0.6	0.3	5	8	20	472	77	0.2	0.4	4	133	0.04	0	0.02	0.03	0.6	0.02	2	0.06
1.5	0.7	15	13	56	444	88	0.5	0.9	4	65	0.09	1	0.04	0.09	2.2	0.02	2	0.13
3	1.4	30	25	113	889	176	1	1.7	8	131	0.18	1	0.08	0.17	4.4	0.05	5	0.25
3.6	1.7	37	30	137	1079	214	1.2	2.1	9	159	0.21	2	0.1	0.21	5.4	0.06	5	0.3
1.4	0.1	6	21	74	518	263	0.7	1.1	15	75	0.09	2	0.03	0.04	0.5	0.08	9	0.16
0	0	0	4	20	1649	29	0	0.1	4	0	0	0	0	0.01	0.3	0.01	2	0.06
2.5	1.5	46	125	149	290	242	1.9	0.5	23	74	1.06	2	0.08	0.15	1.5	0.1	23	2.9
0.3	0.2	5	33	44	617	163	0.7	0.6	7	26	0.12	0	0.1	0.04	0.7	0.06	7	0.1
0.7	0.4	10	66	88	1234	327	1.5	1.2	15	51	0.24	0	0.2	0.07	1.3	0.12	15	0.2
1	0.6	15	100	133	1867	494	2.2	1.8	22	78	0.37	0	0.3	0.11	2	0.18	22	0.3
1.9	3.7	10	58	78	1962	346	1.8	1.6	8	90	1.26	6	0.11	0.16	1.6	0.02	48	0.1
2.3	4.4	12	70	95	2385	421	2.1	2	9	110	1.53	7	0.13	0.19	1.9	0.03	58	0.12
0.4	0.3	0	11	15	400	66	0.3	0.3	1	14	—	0	0.02	0.02	0.3	0	4	0.01
1	1.1	11	87	77	521	180	0.5	0.4	10	42	0.42	2	0.05	0.14	0.4	0.03	15	0.25
0.5	0.9	2	15	20	490	87	0.4	0.4	2	22	0.33	1	0.03	0.04	0.4	0.01	11	0.02
1.6	0.7	5	17	18	493	44	0.3	0.3	1	28	0.1	0	0.02	0.03	0.4	0.01	1	0.05
3	1.7	12	123	104	394	214	0.4	0.3	18	104	0.74	22	0.05	0.19	0.3	0.08	19	0.31
2.6	5	28	80	75	1900	246	0.3	1.3	13	60	0.38	1	0.06	0.1	0.7	0.02	5	0.1
3.1	6.1	34	98	92	2308	299	0.4	1.5	15	73	0.46	1	0.07	0.12	0.8	0.03	6	0.12
0.4	0.3	0	18	16	419	55	0.1	0.3	3	14	0.13	0	0.01	0.02	0.2	0	1	0.02
1.2	1.3	16	93	76	505	155	0.1	0.3	11	34	0.48	1	0.04	0.12	0.2	0.03	4	0.25
0.6	1.3	7	20	18	475	61	0.1	0.3	4	16	0.45	0	0.02	0.02	0.2	0.01	1	0.12

Esha Code	Food Item	Qty	Meas	Wgt (g)	Wtr (g)	Cals	Prot (g)	Carb (g)	Fib (g)	Fat (g)	SatF (g)
50019	Soup, cream of chicken, condensed, can	1	each	305	249	284	8	22	0.6	18	5.1
50036	Soup, cream of chicken, dry, prep w/water	0.5	cup	130	119	54	1	7	0.1	3	1.7
50006	Soup, cream of chicken, w/milk	0.5	cup	124	105	96	4	7	0.1	6	2.3
50018	Soup, cream of chicken, w/water	0.5	cup	122	111	59	2	5	0.1	4	1
50666	Soup, cream of mushroom, condensed	1	cup	251	204	259	4	19	0.8	19	5.2
50010	Soup, cream of mushroom, condensed, can	1	each	305	248	314	5	23	0.9	23	6.2
50588	Soup, cream of mushroom, low sodium, RTS	1	each	298	262	200	3	18	3	14	4
50011	Soup, cream of mushroom, w/milk	0.5	cup	124	105	102	3	8	0.2	7	2.6
50049	Soup, cream of mushroom, w/water	0.5	cup	122	110	65	1	5	0.2	4	1.2
50184	Soup, cream of mushroom, w/water	0.5	cup	122	110	65	1	5	0.2	5	1.2
50191	Soup, cream of onion, condensed, can	1	each	305	247	268	7	32	1.2	13	3.6
50194	Soup, cream of onion, w/milk	0.5	cup	124	105	93	3	9	0.4	5	2
50196	Soup, cream of onion, w/water	0.5	cup	122	110	54	1	6	0.5	3	0.7
50026	Soup, cream of potato, w/milk	0.5	cup	124	108	74	3	9	0.2	3	1.9
50197	Soup, cream of potato, w/water	0.5	cup	122	113	37	1	6	0.2	1	0.6
50216	Soup, cream of salmon	0.5	cup	124	96	129	14	3	0.1	6	1.7
50127	Soup, cream of shrimp, w/milk	0.5	cup	124	107	82	3	7	0.1	5	2.9
50128	Soup, cream of shrimp, w/water	0.5	cup	122	112	45	1	4	0.1	3	1.6
50045	Soup, cream of vegetable, dry, prep w/water	0.5	cup	130	119	53	1	6	0.3	3	0.7
50190	Soup, egg drop	0.5	cup	122	114	36	4	1	0	2	0.6
50101	Soup, escarole, RTS	0.5	cup	124	120	14	1	1	—	1	0.3
50102	Soup, escarole, RTS, can	1	each	553	536	61	3	4	—	4	1.2
50103	Soup, gazpacho, RTS	0.5	cup	122	114	23	4	2	0.2	0	0
50104	Soup, gazpacho, RTS, can	1	each	369	346	70	11	7	0.7	0	0
50117	Soup, green pea, canned, w/milk	0.5	cup	127	99	119	6	16	1.4	4	2
50050	Soup, green pea, w/water	0.5	cup	125	104	82	4	13	1.4	1	0.7
50182	Soup, hot & sour/hot & spicy	0.5	cup	122	107	66	6	3	0.2	3	1
50168	Soup, leek, dry, w/water	0.5	cup	127	118	36	1	6	1.5	1	0.5
50105	Soup, lentil & ham, RTS	0.5	cup	124	106	69	5	10	1	1	0.6
50106	Soup, lentil & ham, RTS, can	1	each	567	486	318	21	46	4.3	6	2.6
50214	Soup, lobster bisque	0.5	cup	124	98	136	10	6	0.1	8	2.9
50215	Soup, lobster gumbo	0.5	cup	122	102	89	5	10	2	4	0.7
50295	Soup, minestrone, Real Italian, Health Valley	4	oz.	113	99	38	4	10	5.2	0	0
50107	Soup, minestrone, chunky, RTS	0.5	cup	120	104	64	3	10	2.9	1	0.7
50108	Soup, minestrone, chunky, RTS, can	1	each	539	467	286	12	47	12.9	6	3.3
50170	Soup, minestrone, dry, prepared	0.5	cup	127	116	39	2	6	0.7	1	0.4
50009	Soup, minestrone, w/water	0.5	cup	120	110	41	2	6	0.5	1	0.3
50113	Soup, mushroom & beef stock, w/water	0.5	cup	122	112	43	2	5	0.4	2	0.8
50111	Soup, mushroom barley, w/water	0.5	cup	122	113	37	1	6	0.4	1	0.2
50039	Soup, mushroom, dry, prep w/water	0.5	cup	126	116	48	1	6	0.4	2	0.4
50023	Soup, onion, canned, condensed, can	1	each	298	257	137	9	20	2.1	4	0.6
50054	Soup, onion, dry packet	1	each	7	0	21	1	4	0.7	0	0.1
50040	Soup, onion, dry, prep w/water	0.5	cup	123	118	14	1	3	0.5	0	0.1
50022	Soup, onion, w/water	0.5	cup	120	112	29	2	4	0.5	1	0.1
50173	Soup, oxtail, dry, w/water	0.5	cup	126	118	35	1	4	0.3	1	0.6
50185	Soup, pea, prepared w/water, low sodium	0.5	cup	125	104	82	4	13	0.4	2	0.7
50122	Soup, pepper pot, prep w/water	0.5	cup	120	109	52	3	5	0.2	2	1
50207	Soup, pork rice and vegetable	0.5	cup	122	109	61	6	4	0.5	2	0.7
50118	Soup, split pea & ham, chunky, RTS	0.5	cup	120	97	92	6	13	2	2	0.8
50119	Soup, split pea & ham, chunky, RTS, can	1	each	539	437	415	25	60	9.2	9	3.6
50300	Soup, split pea and carrot, Health Valley	4	oz.	113	101	52	4	8	1.9	0	0
50025	Soup, split pea and ham, w/water	0.5	cup	126	103	95	5	14	1.1	2	0.9
50590	Soup, split pea, low sodium, RTS	1	each	305	250	240	12	38	5	4	3
50041	Soup, split pea, prep w/watery	0.5	cup	128	111	62	4	11	1.4	1	0.2
50130	Soup, stock pot, w/water	0.5	cup	124	112	50	2	6	0.2	2	0.4
50209	Soup, sweet and sour	0.5	cup	122	110	37	2	8	0.9	0	0.1
50132	Soup, tomato beef noodle, w/water	0.5	cup	122	106	70	2	11	0.7	2	0.8
50137	Soup, tomato rice, w/water	0.5	cup	124	109	59	1	11	0.7	1	0.3
50043	Soup, tomato vegetable, dry, prep w/water	0.5	cup	126	118	28	1	5	0.3	0	0.2
50042	Soup, tomato, dry, prep w/water	0.5	cup	132	119	52	1	10	0.3	1	0.5
50591	Soup, tomato, low sodium, RTS	0.5	cup	122	105	70	2	12	0.8	2	1
50012	Soup, tomato, w/milk	0.5	cup	124	105	81	3	11	1.4	3	1.4
50028	Soup, tomato, w/water	0.5	cup	122	110	43	1	8	0.2	1	0.2
50141	Soup, turkey noodle, w/water	0.5	cup	122	113	34	2	4	0.4	1	0.3
50143	Soup, turkey vegetable, w/water	0.5	cup	120	112	36	2	4	0.2	2	0.4

MonoF (g)	PolyF (g)	Choles (mg)	Calc (mg)	Phos (mg)	Sod (mg)	Pot (mg)	Zn (mg)	Iron (mg)	Magn (mg)	VitA (μg RE)	VitE (mg α-TE)	VitC (mg)	Thia (mg)	Ribo (mg)	Nia (mg)	B6 (mg)	Fola (μg)	B12 (μg)
8	3.6	24	82	92	2397	214	1.5	1.5	6	137	0.4	0	0.07	0.15	2	0.04	4	0.21
0.6	0.2	1	38	48	592	107	0.8	0.1	3	61	0.07	0	0.05	0.1	1.3	0.03	3	0.13
2.2	0.8	14	90	76	523	136	0.3	0.3	9	47	0.12	1	0.04	0.13	0.5	0.03	4	0.27
1.6	0.7	5	17	18	493	44	0.3	0.3	1	28	0.1	0	0.02	0.03	0.4	0.01	1	0.05
3.6	8.9	3	65	85	1736	168	1.2	1	10	0	2.61	2	0.06	0.17	1.6	0.02	8	0.25
4.4	10.8	3	79	104	2110	204	1.4	1.3	12	0	3.17	3	0.07	0.2	2	0.03	9	0.3
—	—	20	60	—	65	—	—	1.1	—	0	—	0	—	—	—	—	—	—
1.5	2.3	10	89	78	459	135	0.3	0.3	10	19	0.67	1	0.04	0.14	0.5	0.03	5	0.25
0.9	2.1	1	23	24	440	50	0.3	0.3	2	0	0.62	0	0.02	0.04	0.4	0.01	2	0.02
0.9	0.9	1	23	24	24	50	0.3	0.3	2	0	0.62	0	0.02	0.05	0.4	0.01	2	0.02
5.1	3.5	37	82	92	2318	299	0.4	1.5	15	73	2.07	3	0.12	0.18	1.2	0.06	17	0.12
1.6	0.8	16	89	77	502	155	0.3	0.3	11	35	0.04	1	0.05	0.14	0.3	0.04	11	0.25
1	0.7	7	17	18	464	60	0.1	0.3	2	15	0.37	1	0.03	0.04	0.3	0.01	3	0.02
0.9	0.3	11	83	81	531	161	0.3	0.3	9	34	0.05	1	0.04	0.12	0.3	0.04	5	0.25
0.3	0.2	2	10	23	500	68	0.3	0.2	1	15	0.01	0	0.02	0.02	0.3	0.02	1	0.02
2.2	1.8	37	144	225	767	262	0.8	0.8	22	30	0.89	0	0.03	0.14	4.8	0.2	11	2.77
1.3	0.2	17	82	73	518	124	0.4	0.3	11	27	0.43	1	0.03	0.11	0.3	0.22	5	0.52
0.7	0.1	9	9	16	488	29	0.4	0.3	5	7	0.42	0	0.01	0.01	0.2	0.02	2	0.29
1.3	0.7	0	16	27	585	48	0.1	0.3	5	1	0.62	2	0.61	0.05	0.3	0.01	4	0.06
0.8	0.3	52	10	54	364	110	0.2	0.4	2	20	0.26	0	0.01	0.09	1.5	0.03	8	0.25
0.4	0.2	1	16	40	1931	133	1.1	0.4	2	109	—	2	0.04	0.02	1.2	0.11	17	0.25
1.8	0.8	6	72	177	8615	592	5	1.7	11	487	—	10	0.17	0.11	5.1	0.5	77	1.11
0	0	0	12	18	370	112	0.1	0.5	4	131	0.23	4	0.02	0.01	0.5	0.07	5	0
0	0.1	0	37	55	1118	339	0.4	1.5	11	395	0.7	11	0.07	0.04	1.4	0.22	15	0
1.1	0.3	9	86	119	485	188	0.9	1	28	29	0.09	1	0.08	0.13	0.7	0.05	4	0.22
0.5	0.2	0	14	62	459	95	0.9	1	20	10	0.05	1	0.05	0.03	0.6	0.03	1	0
1.2	0.5	11	15	80	781	176	0.6	0.9	14	1	0.06	0	0.1	0.11	2.3	0.07	6	0.17
0.4	0	1	15	15	483	44	0.1	0.3	5	0	0.08	1	0.02	0.01	0.1	0.01	4	0.01
0.6	0.2	4	21	92	660	179	0.4	1.3	11	17	0.12	2	0.09	0.06	0.7	0.11	25	0.15
3	0.7	17	96	420	3016	816	1.7	6.1	51	79	0.57	10	0.4	0.26	3.1	0.51	113	0.68
2.9	1.6	36	135	153	429	269	1.3	0.3	25	97	1.14	1	0.05	0.18	0.5	0.07	9	1.29
1.5	1.2	12	54	64	335	305	0.8	0.9	27	103	1.11	14	0.1	0.06	1.1	0.1	34	0.51
0	0	0	19	—	99	—	—	1.7	—	945	—	2	—	—	—	—	—	—
0.5	0.1	2	30	55	432	306	0.7	0.9	7	217	0.36	2	0.03	0.06	0.6	0.12	26	0
2	0.6	11	135	248	1940	1374	3.2	4	32	976	1.62	11	0.12	0.26	2.6	0.54	119	0
0.4	0.1	1	19	30	513	170	0.4	0.5	4	15	0.02	1	0.04	0.02	0.5	0.05	18	0
0.3	0.6	1	17	28	455	157	0.4	0.5	4	117	0.04	1	0.03	0.02	0.5	0.05	18	0
0.7	0.4	4	5	18	484	79	0.7	0.4	5	62	0.28	0	0.02	0.05	0.6	0.02	5	0
0.5	0.4	0	6	30	445	46	0.2	0.3	5	10	0.18	0	0.01	0.04	0.4	0.08	2	0
1.1	0.8	0	33	38	510	100	0	0.3	3	0	0.32	1	0.14	0.06	0.2	0.01	3	0.13
1.8	1.6	0	66	27	2562	167	1.5	1.6	6	0	0.68	3	0.08	0.06	1.5	0.12	37	0
0.2	0	0	10	23	636	47	0	0.1	5	0	0.08	0	0.02	0.04	0.4	0.01	1	0
0.2	0	0	6	15	424	32	0	0.1	2	0	0.05	0	0.01	0.03	0.2	0	1	0
0.4	0.3	0	13	6	527	34	0.3	0.3	1	0	0.14	1	0.02	0.01	0.3	0.02	8	0
0.5	0.1	1	5	30	605	42	0	0.1	5	2	0.04	0	0.01	0.01	0.4	0.01	3	0.13
0.5	0.2	0	14	62	12	95	0.8	1	20	10	0.05	1	0.05	0.04	0.6	0.02	1	0
1	0.2	5	12	20	486	76	0.6	0.4	2	43	0.04	1	0.03	0.02	0.6	0.03	5	0.08
1	0.2	19	9	48	301	110	1	0.5	8	247	0.11	1	0.12	0.07	1.2	0.11	4	0.12
0.8	0.3	4	17	89	482	152	1.6	1.1	19	244	0.07	3	0.06	0.05	1.3	0.11	2	0.12
3.7	1.3	16	76	399	2166	685	7	4.8	86	1094	0.32	16	0.26	0.21	5.7	0.48	10	0.54
0	0	0	19	—	109	208	—	2.6	—	945	—	4	0.05	0.08	2.7	0.21	—	—
0.9	0.3	4	11	106	503	200	0.7	1.1	24	23	0.08	1	0.07	0.04	0.7	0.03	1	0.13
—	—	5	40	—	50	—	—	1.8	—	250	—	0	—	—	—	—	—	—
0.3	0.1	1	10	62	574	112	0.3	0.5	22	3	0.06	0	0.1	0.07	0.6	0.02	20	0.13
0.5	0.9	2	11	27	526	119	0.6	0.4	2	200	—	1	0.02	0.03	0.6	0.04	5	0
0.1	0.1	2	14	24	661	139	0.2	0.3	9	15	0.26	9	0.04	0.03	0.5	0.06	9	0.02
0.9	0.3	2	9	28	459	110	0.4	0.6	4	27	0.39	0	0.04	0.04	0.9	0.04	10	0.1
0.3	0.7	1	11	17	408	165	0.3	0.4	2	38	0.4	7	0.03	0.02	0.5	0.04	7	0
0.2	0	0	4	15	573	52	0.1	0.3	10	10	0.4	3	0.03	0.02	0.4	0.02	5	0
0.5	0.1	0	26	33	472	147	0.1	0.2	7	41	0.42	2	0.03	0.02	0.4	0.05	3	0.04
—	—	4	16	—	25	—	—	0.6	—	51	—	15	—	—	—	—	—	—
0.8	0.6	9	79	74	372	224	0.1	0.9	11	55	1.3	34	0.07	0.12	0.8	0.08	10	0.22
0.2	0.5	0	6	17	348	132	0.1	0.9	4	34	1.24	33	0.04	0.03	0.7	0.06	7	0
0.4	0.2	2	6	24	407	38	0.3	0.5	2	15	0.03	0	0.04	0.03	0.7	0.02	10	0.07
0.7	0.3	1	8	20	453	88	0.3	0.4	2	122	0.07	0	0.01	0.02	0.5	0.02	2	0.08

Esha Code	Food Item	Qty	Meas	Wgt (g)	Wtr (g)	Cals	Prot (g)	Carb (g)	Fib (g)	Fat (g)	SatF (g)
50138	Soup, turkey, chunky, RTS	0.5	cup	118	102	67	5	7	0.5	2	0.6
50139	Soup, turkey, chunky, RTS, can	1	each	532	460	303	23	32	2.3	10	2.8
50212	Soup, turtle and vegetable	0.5	cup	122	110	59	6	2	0.3	2	0.4
50147	Soup, vegetable & beef broth, w/water	0.5	cup	120	110	41	1	7	0.2	1	0.2
50044	Soup, vegetable beef, dry, prep w/water	0.5	cup	126	119	27	1	4	0.3	1	0.3
50014	Soup, vegetable beef, w/water	0.5	cup	122	112	39	3	5	0.2	1	0.4
50219	Soup, vegetable chicken, low sodium, w/water	0.5	cup	120	100	83	6	10	0.5	2	0.7
50186	Soup, vegetable, canned, low sodium	0.5	cup	120	110	41	1	6	0.4	1	0.2
50144	Soup, vegetable, chunky, RTS	0.5	cup	120	105	61	2	10	0.6	2	0.3
50145	Soup, vegetable, chunky, RTS, can	1	each	539	472	275	8	43	2.7	8	1.2
50187	Soup, vegetable, from dry mix, low sodium	0.5	cup	126	118	28	1	5	0.3	0	0.2
50013	Soup, vegetable, vegetarian, w/water	0.5	cup	120	111	36	1	6	0.2	1	0.1
50027	Soup, vichyssoise	0.5	cup	124	108	74	3	9	0.2	3	1.9
50181	Soup, won ton	0.5	cup	120	101	94	7	8	0.5	3	1.1
8177	Sour cream, nonfat	2	Tbs	28	21	31	2	5	0	0	0
3268	Soursop, raw pulp	1	each	225	183	149	2	38	7.4	1	0.1
20145	Soy drink, So Good Lite	1	cup	260	229	114	9	17	2.1	2	0.3
20144	Soy drink, So Good	1	cup	255	222	158	8	13	2	8	0.8
7514	Soy flour, defatted, stirred	1	cup	88	6	290	41	34	15.4	1	0.1
20033	Soy milk	1	cup	240	224	79	7	4	3.1	5	0.5
7584	Soy milk, fat-free, Soy Moo, Health Valley	1	cup	54	48	25	1	5	0.2	0	0
5458	Soybean sprouts, raw	0.5	cup	35	24	43	5	3	0.4	2	0.3
5459	Soybean sprouts, steamed	0.5	cup	47	37	38	4	3	0.4	2	0.3
7508	Soybean, fermented/Natto	0.5	cup	88	48	186	16	13	4.7	10	1.4
7015	Soybeans, dry, cooked	0.5	cup	86	54	149	14	9	5.2	8	1.1
7063	Soybeans, dry, roasted	0.5	cup	86	1	387	34	28	7	19	2.7
5259	Soybeans, green, cooked	0.5	cup	90	62	127	11	10	3.8	6	0.7
56099	Spaghetti, w/meatballs, canned	1	cup	250	195	258	12	28	5.8	10	2.2
56096	Spaghetti, w/sauce & cheese, canned	1	cup	250	200	190	6	38	2.5	2	0
56306	Spaghetti, w/white clam sauce	0.5	cup	124	78	228	13	21	1.1	10	1.3
26490	Spearmint leaves	1	oz.	28	3	94	7	14	8.5	1	—
5595	Spinach, canned w/liquid	0.5	cup	117	109	22	2	3	1.9	0	0.1
5973	Spinach, canned w/liquid, low sodium	0.5	cup	117	109	22	2	3	2.6	0	0.1
5149	Spinach, canned, drained, no added salt	0.5	cup	107	98	25	3	4	2.6	1	0.1
5147	Spinach, cooked, drained, no added salt	0.5	cup	90	82	21	3	3	2.2	0	0
5148	Spinach, frozen, cooked, drained, no added salt	0.5	cup	95	86	27	3	5	2.8	0	0
5596	Spinach, frozen, unprepared	0.5	cup	78	71	19	2	3	2.3	0	0
5146	Spinach, raw, chopped	0.5	cup	28	26	6	1	1	0.8	0	0
5670	Spinach, steamed	0.5	cup	14	13	3	0	0	0.4	0	0
5669	Spinach, stir fried	0.5	cup	90	82	20	3	3	2.4	0	0
20423	Sport drink, orange, All Sport	1	cup	240	—	47	0	13	0	0	0
62205	Sports bar, Tiger	1	each	65	11	230	11	40	4	2	—
8132	Spread, Touch of Butter, tub	1	Tbs	14	5	77	0	0	0	9	2
56291	Spring roll w/meat	1	each	64	42	114	5	9	0.7	6	1.5
5314	Squash, acorn, baked cubes	0.5	cup	102	85	57	1	15	4.5	0	0
5315	Squash, acorn, baked, mashed	0.5	cup	122	102	69	1	18	5.4	0	0
5316	Squash, acorn, boiled, mashed	0.5	cup	122	110	42	1	11	3.2	0	0
5317	Squash, butternut, baked cubes	0.5	cup	102	90	41	1	11	2.9	0	0
5318	Squash, butternut, baked, mashed	0.5	cup	122	108	49	1	13	3.4	0	0
5274	Squash, butternut, frozen, cooked	0.5	cup	120	105	47	1	12	3.4	0	0
5597	Squash, crookneck, canned slices, drained	0.5	cup	108	104	14	1	3	1.5	0	0
5322	Squash, crookneck, cooked	0.5	cup	90	84	18	1	4	1.3	0	0.1
5453	Squash, hubbard, baked	0.5	cup	120	102	60	3	13	3.2	1	0.2
5325	Squash, scallop, cooked, mashed	0.5	cup	120	114	19	1	4	2.3	0	0
5324	Squash, scallop, slices, cooked	0.5	cup	90	86	14	1	3	1.7	0	0
5455	Squash, spaghetti, cooked	0.5	cup	78	72	21	1	5	1.1	0	0
5152	Squash, summer, cooked slices	0.5	cup	90	84	18	1	4	1.3	0	0.1
5151	Squash, summer, raw slices	0.5	cup	65	61	13	1	3	1.2	0	0
5303	Squash, winter, baked cubes	0.5	cup	102	91	40	1	9	2.9	1	0.1
5153	Squash, winter, cooked w/salt, no sugar, no fat	0.5	cup	120	106	46	1	10	3.3	1	0.2
5667	Squash, zucchini slices, steamed	0.5	cup	90	86	13	1	3	1.1	0	0
5598	Squash, zucchini w/peel, frozen, cooked	0.5	cup	112	106	19	1	4	1.4	0	0
5443	Squash, zucchini, baby, raw	1	each	16	15	3	0	0	0.2	0	0
5599	Squash, zucchini, canned, Italian style	0.5	cup	114	103	33	1	8	2.3	0	0
5327	Squash, zucchini, cooked	0.5	cup	90	85	14	1	4	1.3	0	0

MonoF (g)	PolyF (g)	Choles (mg)	Calc (mg)	Phos (mg)	Sod (mg)	Pot (mg)	Zn (mg)	Iron (mg)	Magn (mg)	VitA (μg RE)	VitE (mg α-TE)	VitC (mg)	Thia (mg)	Ribo (mg)	Nia (mg)	B6 (mg)	Fola (μg)	B12 (μg)
0.9	0.5	5	25	52	461	181	1.1	1	12	358	0.06	3	0.02	0.05	1.8	0.15	6	1.06
4	2.4	21	112	234	2080	814	4.8	4.3	53	1611	0.27	14	0.08	0.24	8.1	0.69	25	4.79
0.6	0.9	30	34	59	236	140	0.3	0.6	9	21	0.33	3	0.04	0.08	0.8	0.05	9	0.28
0.3	0.4	1	8	19	405	96	0.4	0.5	4	105	0.16	1	0.02	0.02	0.5	0.03	5	0
0.2	0	0	6	18	501	38	0.1	0.4	11	11	0.02	1	0.02	0.02	0.2	0.03	4	0.13
0.4	0.1	2	9	21	395	87	0.8	0.6	2	95	0.16	1	0.02	0.02	0.5	0.04	5	0.16
1.1	0.5	8	13	53	42	184	1.1	0.7	5	301	0.06	3	0.02	0.08	1.6	0.05	6	0.12
0.5	0.5	0	19	11	21	133	1.1	0.6	3	198	0.27	2	0.02	0.02	0.4	0.06	6	0
0.8	0.7	0	28	36	505	198	1.6	0.8	4	294	0.3	3	0.04	0.03	0.6	0.1	8	0
3.6	3.1	0	124	162	2269	889	7	3.7	16	1320	1.35	14	0.16	0.15	2.7	0.43	37	0
0.1	0	0	4	15	25	52	0.1	0.3	10	10	0.4	3	0.02	0.02	0.4	0.02	5	0
0.4	0.4	0	11	17	411	105	0.2	0.5	4	151	0.4	1	0.03	0.02	0.5	0.03	5	0
0.9	0.3	11	83	81	531	161	0.3	0.3	9	34	0.05	1	0.04	0.12	0.3	0.04	5	0.25
1.5	0.5	27	16	77	380	157	0.6	0.9	10	48	0.26	2	0.21	0.14	2.3	0.1	10	0.2
0	0	0	36	36	22	62	—	0	—	43	—	0	0	0.06	—	—	—	0.11
0.2	0.2	0	32	61	32	626	0.2	1.4	47	0	0.9	46	0.16	0.11	2	0.13	32	0
0.5	1	0	257	—	94	322	0.5	2.1	—	101	—	5	0.16	0.49	—	0.16	26	0.78
2	4.6	0	252	—	92	316	0.5	2	—	100	—	5	0.15	0.48	—	0.15	26	0.76
0.2	0.5	0	212	593	18	2097	2.2	8.1	255	4	0.17	0	0.61	0.22	2.3	0.5	268	0
0.8	2	0	10	118	29	338	0.6	1.4	46	7	0.02	0	0.39	0.17	0.4	0.1	4	0
0	0	0	90	—	14	4	—	0.3	—	0	—	0	0.02	0.02	0.7	—	—	0
0.5	1.3	0	24	57	5	169	0.4	0.7	25	0	0	5	0.12	0.04	0.4	0.06	60	0
0.5	1.2	0	28	64	5	167	0.5	0.6	28	0	0	4	0.1	0.02	0.5	0.05	38	0
2.1	5.4	0	190	152	6	638	2.6	7.5	101	0	0.01	11	0.14	0.17	0	0.11	7	0
1.7	4.4	0	88	211	1	443	1	4.4	74	1	1.68	1	0.13	0.24	0.3	0.2	46	0
4.1	10.5	0	120	558	2	1173	4.1	3.4	196	2	3.96	4	0.37	0.65	0.9	0.19	176	0
1.1	2.7	0	131	142	13	485	0.8	2.2	54	14	0.01	15	0.23	0.14	1.1	0.05	100	0
3.9	3.9	22	52	113	1220	245	2.4	3.2	20	100	1.5	5	0.15	0.18	2.2	0.12	5	0.82
0.4	0.5	8	40	88	955	303	1.1	2.8	21	120	2.13	10	0.35	0.28	4.5	0.13	6	0
6.6	1.1	24	42	162	218	256	1.4	11.3	20	64	1.46	8	0.19	0.22	2.4	0.07	16	36.2
—	—	—	471	—	99	—	—	54.4	—	184	—	0	—	—	—	—	—	0
0	0.2	0	97	37	373	269	0.5	1.8	66	752	1.25	16	0.02	0.12	0.3	0.09	68	0
0	0.2	0	97	37	88	269	0.5	1.8	66	752	1.13	16	0.02	0.12	0.3	0.09	68	0
0	0.2	0	136	47	29	370	0.5	2.5	81	939	1.39	15	0.02	0.15	0.4	0.11	105	0
0	0.1	0	122	50	63	419	0.7	3.2	78	737	0.86	9	0.09	0.21	0.4	0.22	131	0
0	0.1	0	139	46	82	283	0.7	1.4	66	739	0.91	12	0.06	0.16	0.4	0.14	103	0
0	0.1	0	87	32	58	252	0.3	1.6	45	605	0.74	19	0.07	0.12	0.3	0.11	94	0
0	0	0	28	14	22	156	0.1	0.8	22	188	0.53	8	0.02	0.05	0.2	0.06	54	0
0	0	0	13	6	11	73	0.1	0.4	11	89	0.26	2	0.01	0.02	0.1	0.02	18	0
0	0.1	0	89	44	71	502	0.5	2.4	71	545	1.7	22	0.06	0.16	0.6	0.17	149	0
0	0	—	0	23	37	37	—	0	—	0	—	0	—	—	—	—	—	0
—	—	—	350	400	100	280	—	4.5	140	50	20	60	1.5	1.7	20	2	400	6
4.4	1.9	1	3	2	140	4	0	0	0	152	0.43	0	0	0	0	0	0	0.01
2.7	1.6	37	13	58	304	124	0.5	0.8	10	14	0.78	2	0.16	0.13	1.3	0.1	9	0.12
0	0.1	0	45	46	4	448	0.2	1	44	44	0.12	11	0.17	0.01	0.9	0.2	19	0
0	0.1	0	54	55	5	535	0.2	1.1	53	53	0.15	13	0.2	0.02	1.1	0.24	23	0
0	0	0	32	33	4	322	0.1	0.7	32	32	0.15	8	0.12	0.01	0.6	0.14	14	0
0	0	0	42	28	4	291	0.1	0.6	30	718	0.17	16	0.07	0.02	1	0.13	20	0
0	0	0	50	33	5	348	0.2	0.7	36	858	0.21	18	0.09	0.02	1.2	0.15	24	0
0	0	0	23	17	2	160	0.1	0.7	11	401	0.16	4	0.06	0.05	0.6	0.08	20	0
0	0	0	13	23	5	104	0.3	0.8	14	13	0.13	3	0.02	0.03	0.5	0.04	11	0
0	0.1	0	24	35	1	173	0.4	0.3	22	26	0.11	5	0.04	0.04	0.5	0.08	18	0
0.1	0.3	0	20	28	10	430	0.2	0.6	26	725	0.14	11	0.09	0.06	0.7	0.21	19	0
0	0.1	0	18	34	1	168	0.3	0.4	23	11	0.14	13	0.06	0.03	0.6	0.1	25	0
0	0.1	0	14	25	1	126	0.2	0.3	17	8	0.11	10	0.05	0.02	0.4	0.08	19	0
0	0.1	0	16	11	14	91	0.2	0.3	9	9	0.09	3	0.03	0.02	0.6	0.08	6	0
0	0.1	0	24	35	1	173	0.4	0.3	22	26	0.11	5	0.04	0.04	0.5	0.06	18	0
0	0.1	0	13	23	1	127	0.2	0.3	15	13	0.08	10	0.04	0.02	0.4	0.07	17	0
0	0.3	0	14	20	1	448	0.3	0.3	8	365	0.12	10	0.09	0.02	0.7	0.07	29	0
0.1	0.3	0	17	24	279	521	0.3	0.4	10	425	0.14	12	0.1	0.03	0.8	0.09	33	0
0	0.1	0	14	29	3	223	0.2	0.4	20	29	0.11	7	0.06	0.03	0.3	0.07	17	0
0	0.1	0	19	28	2	216	0.2	0.5	14	48	0.34	4	0.05	0.04	0.4	0.05	9	0
0	0	0	3	15	0	73	0.1	0.1	5	8	0.04	5	0.01	0.01	0.1	0.02	3	0
0	0.1	0	19	33	424	311	0.3	0.8	16	61	0.11	3	0.05	0.04	0.6	0.17	34	0
0	0	0	12	36	3	228	0.2	0.3	20	22	0.11	4	0.04	0.04	0.4	0.07	15	0

Esha Code	Food Item	Qty	Meas	Wgt (g)	Wtr (g)	Cals	Prot (g)	Carb (g)	Fib (g)	Fat (g)	SatF (g)
5326	Squash, zucchini, raw	0.5	cup	65	62	9	1	2	0.8	0	0
5668	Squash, zucchini, stir fried, no oil	0.5	cup	90	86	13	1	3	1.1	0	0
50047	Stew, beef & vegetable, canned	1	cup	245	202	194	14	17	2.4	8	2.4
50048	Stew, brunswick	1	cup	250	208	174	16	21	3.2	4	1
50200	Stew, lamb, tomato base sauce	0.5	cup	126	96	136	9	14	2.9	5	2.2
50024	Stew, oyster, prep w/milk	1	cup	245	218	135	6	10	0	8	5
50115	Stew, oyster, prep w/water	0.5	cup	120	114	29	1	2	0	2	1.2
50205	Stew, seafood, tomato base sauce	0.5	cup	126	104	84	10	8	1.2	1	0.4
50201	Stew, veal, tomato base sauce	0.5	cup	126	105	95	8	8	1.3	3	1.4
50202	Stew, venison, tomato base sauce	0.5	cup	126	105	81	9	9	1.5	1	0.3
3316	Strawberries, cooked, unsweetened	0.5	cup	121	114	24	0	6	2.1	0	0
3135	Strawberries, fresh	0.5	cup	83	76	25	1	6	1.9	0	0
3136	Strawberries, fresh slices	1	each	32	29	10	0	2	0.7	0	0
3137	Strawberries, frozen, unsweetened	0.5	cup	74	67	26	0	7	1.6	0	0
3236	Strawberries, sliced, frozen, sweetened, thawed	0.5	cup	128	93	122	1	33	2.4	0	0
20212	Strawberry Julius	1	cup	215	183	170	0	41	0.4	0	0.1
49025	Strudel, berry	1	piece	64	28	159	2	29	1.4	4	0.8
49027	Strudel, cheese	1	piece	64	24	195	6	24	0.4	8	3.9
49026	Strudel, cherry	1	piece	64	25	179	3	29	1.1	6	0.9
49028	Strudel, peach	1	piece	64	36	123	2	23	1.2	3	0.6
42147	Stuffing mix, cornbread, prepared	0.5	cup	100	65	179	3	22	2.9	9	1.8
69117	Subway, Club sandwich on a 6 white roll	1	each	246	179	297	21	40	3	5	1
52120	Subway, Cold Cut Trio salad	1	each	330	294	191	13	11	1	11	3
69123	Subway, Spicy Italian sandwich on a 6 white roll	1	each	232	148	467	20	38	3	24	9
69109	Subway, Veggie Delite sandwich on a 6 white roll	1	each	175	124	222	9	38	3	3	0
52127	Subway, chicken taco salad	1	each	370	322	250	18	15	2	14	5
69129	Subway, meatball sandwich on a 6 white roll	1	each	260	181	404	18	44	3	16	6
52121	Subway, pizza salad	1	each	335	288	277	12	13	2	20	8
52116	Subway, seafood & crab salad w/light mayonnaise	1	each	331	298	161	13	11	2	8	1
52118	Subway, tuna salad w/light mayonnaise	1	each	331	294	205	12	11	1	13	2
69107	Subway, tuna sandwich w/light mayonnaise	1	each	178	119	279	11	38	2	9	2
5251	Succotash, cooked from fresh	0.5	cup	96	66	110	5	23	4.3	1	0.1
5154	Succotash, frozen, cooked	0.5	cup	85	63	79	4	17	3.5	1	0.1
5601	Succotash, whole corn & lima beans, canned	0.5	cup	128	105	80	3	18	3.3	1	0.1
3270	Sugar apple (sweetsop), raw	1	each	155	113	146	3	37	6.8	0	0.1
25118	Sugar cane juice	8	oz.	227	198	79	0	21	—	0	—
25040	Sugar, brown, Sugar Twin	1	tsp	0	0	1	0	0	0	0	0
25005	Sugar, brown, packed	1	tsp	3	0	11	0	3	0	0	0
25043	Sugar, maple, piece	1	each	28	2	100	0	26	0	0	0
25071	Sugar, raw	1	tsp	4	0	15	0	4	0	0	0
25006	Sugar, white, granulated	1	tsp	4	0	16	0	4	0	0	0
25008	Sugar, white, powdered, sifted	0.25	cup	25	0	97	0	25	0	0	0
25009	Sugar, white, powdered, unsifted	0.25	cup	30	0	117	0	30	0	0	0
56244	Sukiyaki	0.5	cup	81	63	88	10	3	0.6	4	1.5
4661	Sunflower seed butter, salted	1	Tbs	16	0	93	3	4	2	8	0.8
4550	Sunflower seed butter, unsalted	2	Tbs	32	0	185	6	9	2	15	1.6
4545	Sunflower seed kernels, dry	0.25	cup	36	2	205	8	7	3.8	18	1.9
4546	Sunflower seed kernels, oil roasted, unsalted	0.25	cup	34	1	208	7	5	2.3	19	2
4551	Sunflower seed, dry roasted	0.25	cup	32	0	186	6	8	3.6	16	1.7
4552	Sunflower seed, oil roasted, salted	0.25	cup	34	1	208	7	5	2.3	19	2
4597	Sunflower seeds, dry roasted, salted	0.25	cup	32	0	186	6	8	2.9	16	1.7
62150	Supplement, Osmolite, prepared, Ross Labs	1	cup	253	199	250	9	36	—	8	—
62214	Supplement, shake, vanilla, prepared, MenuMagic	1	cup	260	172	400	12	63	0	12	2
56315	Sushi, w/egg, rolled in seaweed	0.5	cup	83	62	102	5	12	0.2	4	1
56313	Sushi, w/vegetables & fish	0.5	cup	83	53	119	4	24	0.7	0	0.1
56314	Sushi, w/vegetables, rolled in seaweed	0.5	cup	83	59	97	2	22	0.5	0	0.1
5602	Swamp cabbage, chopped, cooked	0.5	cup	49	46	10	1	2	0.9	0	0
15921	Sweet & sour chicken breast	1	each	131	103	117	8	15	0.8	3	0.6
5429	Sweet potato leaves, raw	0.5	cup	18	15	6	1	1	0.4	0	0
5430	Sweet potato leaves, steamed	0.5	cup	32	28	11	1	2	0.6	0	0
5155	Sweet potato, baked, then peeled	1	each	114	83	117	2	28	3.4	0	0
5158	Sweet potato, baked, then peeled	0.5	cup	100	73	103	2	24	3	0	0
5166	Sweet potato, candied	1	piece	52	35	71	0	14	1.2	2	0.7
5167	Sweet potato, candied, cup measure	0.5	cup	98	66	134	1	27	2.4	3	1.3
5554	Sweet potato, canned, w/syrup	0.5	cup	114	88	101	1	24	2.8	0	0

MonoF (g)	PolyF (g)	Choles (mg)	Calc (mg)	Phos (mg)	Sod (mg)	Pot (mg)	Zn (mg)	Iron (mg)	Magn (mg)	VitA (μg RE)	VitE (mg α-TE)	VitC (mg)	Thia (mg)	Ribo (mg)	Nia (mg)	B6 (mg)	Fola (μg)	B12 (μg)
0	0	0	10	21	2	161	0.1	0.3	14	22	0.08	6	0.05	0.02	0.3	0.06	14	0
0	0.1	0	14	29	3	223	0.2	0.4	20	28	0.11	7	0.06	0.03	0.3	0.07	16	0
3.1	0.4	34	29	110	1006	426	4.2	2.2	39	262	0.34	7	0.07	0.12	2.4	0.2	31	1.59
1.3	1	34	37	168	451	538	1.4	1.7	46	51	0.57	18	0.12	0.16	5.8	0.37	44	0.18
1.9	0.4	26	18	100	512	361	1.6	1.1	27	157	0.54	7	0.12	0.14	2.7	0.2	17	0.74
2.1	0.3	32	167	162	1041	235	10.3	1	20	44	0.49	4	0.07	0.23	0.3	0.06	10	2.62
0.5	0.1	7	11	24	490	24	5.2	0.5	2	4	0.12	2	0.01	0.02	0.1	0.01	1	1.1
0.5	0.3	48	40	111	493	405	0.9	4.7	22	266	1.27	16	0.09	0.1	1.7	0.17	17	12.2
1.3	0.3	28	18	96	303	273	1	0.7	18	307	0.25	6	0.07	0.12	3.5	0.2	13	0.28
0.2	0.2	29	16	104	339	383	1	1.8	22	267	0.43	13	0.11	0.2	2.8	0.2	15	1.61
0	0.2	0	12	15	2	135	0.1	0.3	9	2	0.11	44	0.02	0.05	0.2	0.05	14	0
0	0.2	0	12	16	1	138	0.1	0.3	8	2	0.12	47	0.02	0.06	0.2	0.05	15	0
0	0.1	0	4	6	0	53	0	0.1	3	1	0.04	18	0.01	0.02	0.1	0.02	6	0
0	0	0	12	10	1	110	0.1	0.6	8	3	0.2	31	0.02	0.03	0.3	0.02	12	0
0	0.1	0	14	17	4	125	0.1	0.8	9	3	0.18	53	0.02	0.06	0.5	0.04	19	0
0.1	0.1	0	27	—	8	82	—	0.1	—	0	—	6	0.01	0.06	—	0.01	—	0
1.7	1.2	11	15	26	103	55	0.2	0.8	6	53	1.04	5	0.09	0.09	0.8	0.02	6	0.03
2.8	1.1	42	90	87	116	64	0.6	0.8	8	95	0.69	0	0.08	0.16	0.7	0.03	8	0.12
2	2.9	9	19	40	88	100	0.3	0.8	15	79	0.7	3	0.09	0.08	0.8	0.05	8	0.02
1.2	0.9	8	12	22	75	102	0.2	0.6	7	59	0.82	3	0.06	0.07	1	0.02	4	0.02
3.9	2.7	0	26	34	455	62	0.2	0.9	13	85	1.39	1	0.12	0.09	1.2	0.04	97	0.01
—	—	26	29	—	1341	—	—	4	—	120	—	15	—	—	—	—	—	—
—	—	64	46	—	1127	—	—	2	—	282	—	33	—	—	—	—	—	—
—	—	57	40	—	1592	—	—	4	—	169	—	15	—	—	—	—	—	—
—	—	0	25	—	582	—	—	3	—	120	—	15	—	—	—	—	—	—
—	—	52	115	—	990	—	—	3	—	361	—	35	—	—	—	—	—	—
—	—	33	32	—	1035	—	—	4	—	142	—	16	—	—	—	—	—	—
—	—	50	100	—	1336	—	—	2	—	390	—	33	—	—	—	—	—	—
—	—	32	25	—	599	—	—	2	—	284	—	32	—	—	—	—	—	—
—	—	32	29	—	654	—	—	2	—	298	—	32	—	—	—	—	—	—
—	—	16	26	—	583	—	—	3	—	126	—	14	—	—	—	—	—	—
0.1	0.4	0	16	112	16	394	0.6	1.5	51	28	0.32	8	0.16	0.09	1.3	0.11	32	0
0.1	0.4	0	13	60	38	225	0.4	0.8	20	20	0.31	5	0.06	0.06	1.1	0.08	28	0
0.1	0.3	0	14	70	282	208	0.6	0.7	24	19	0.26	6	0.04	0.07	0.8	0.06	40	0
0.2	0.1	0	37	50	14	383	0.2	0.9	33	2	0.92	56	0.17	0.18	1.4	0.31	22	0
—	—	—	30	20	—	—	—	0.2	—	—	—	—	0.02	0.02	0.2	—	—	—
0	0	0	4	0	2	0	0	0	0	0	0	0	0	0	0	0	0	0
0	0	0	3	1	1	10	0	0.1	1	0	0	0	0	0	0	0	0	0
0	0	0	26	1	3	78	1.7	0.5	5	1	0	0	0	0	0	0	0	0
0	0	0	3	1	2	14	0	0.1	1	0	0	0	0	0	0	0	0	0
0	0	0	0	0	0	0	0	0	0	0	0	0	0	0	0	0	0	0
0	0	0	0	0	0	0	0	0	0	0	0	0	0	0	0	0	0	0
0	0	0	0	1	0	1	0	0	0	0	0	0	0	0	0	0	0	0
1.6	0.4	77	31	105	381	234	1.8	1.7	24	132	0.55	2	0.06	0.21	1.6	0.18	31	0.78
1.5	5	0	20	118	83	12	0.8	0.8	59	1	7.68	0	0.05	0.04	0.9	0.13	38	0
2.9	10.1	0	39	236	1	23	1.7	1.5	118	2	15.4	1	0.1	0.09	1.7	0.26	76	0
3.4	11.8	0	42	254	1	248	1.8	2.4	127	2	18.1	1	0.82	0.09	1.6	0.28	82	0
3.7	12.8	0	19	384	1	163	1.8	2.3	43	2	17	0	0.11	0.1	1.4	0.27	79	0
3	10.5	0	22	370	1	272	1.7	1.2	41	0	16.1	0	0.03	0.08	2.2	0.26	76	0
3.7	12.8	0	19	384	204	163	1.8	2.3	43	2	13.5	0	0.11	0.1	1.4	0.27	79	0
3	10.5	0	22	370	250	272	1.7	1.2	41	0	16.1	0	0.03	0.08	2.2	0.26	76	0
—	—	—	125	125	150	240	2.8	2.2	50	125	3.78	38	0.38	0.43	5	0.5	100	1.5
—	—	5	400	267	267	467	4	4.8	160	267	5.33	16	0.4	0.45	5.3	0.53	107	1.6
1.6	0.9	98	22	72	274	70	0.6	0.9	12	66	0.8	1	0.07	0.14	0.8	0.07	14	0.21
0.1	0.1	6	13	55	172	108	0.4	1.2	14	86	0.3	2	0.14	0.04	1.5	0.08	8	0.17
0.1	0.1	0	12	34	76	56	0.4	0.8	11	33	0.07	1	0.11	0.02	1	0.07	5	0
0	0	0	26	21	60	139	0.1	0.6	15	255	0.01	8	0.02	0.04	0.2	0.04	17	0
0.8	1.5	23	16	75	732	187	0.7	0.8	21	20	0.39	12	0.06	0.08	3.1	0.18	6	0.08
0	0	0	6	16	2	91	0.1	0.2	11	18	0.17	2	0.03	0.06	0.2	0.03	14	0
0	0	0	8	19	4	153	0.1	0.2	20	29	0.31	0	0.04	0.08	0.3	0.05	16	0
0	0.1	0	32	63	11	397	0.3	0.5	23	2487	0.32	28	0.08	0.14	0.7	0.28	26	0
0	0	0	28	55	10	348	0.3	0.4	20	2182	0.28	25	0.07	0.13	0.6	0.24	23	0
0.3	0.1	4	14	14	36	98	0.1	0.6	6	218	1.98	3	0.01	0.02	0.2	0.02	6	0
0.6	0.1	8	26	26	69	185	0.1	1.1	11	411	3.72	7	0.02	0.04	0.4	0.04	11	0
0	0.1	0	17	31	50	211	0.2	0.9	15	652	0.26	12	0.03	0.05	0.5	0.06	7	0

Esha Code	Food Item	Qty	Meas	Wgt (g)	Wtr (g)	Cals	Prot (g)	Carb (g)	Fib (g)	Fat (g)	SatF (g)
5555	Sweet potato, canned, w/syrup, drained	0.5	cup	98	71	106	1	25	2.9	0	0.1
90067	Sweet potato, flakes prep w/water	0.5	cup	128	96	121	1	29	—	0	0
5161	Sweet potato, peeled, boiled, mashed	0.5	cup	100	73	105	2	24	1.8	0	0.1
5159	Sweet potato, peeled, boiled, medium size	1	each	156	114	164	3	38	2.8	0	0.1
25036	Sweetener, NutraSweet, low calorie	5	grams	5	0	19	5	0	0	0	0
25041	Sweetener, saccharin, tablet	1	each	0	0	0	0	0	0	0	0
25070	Sweetener, sugar substitute, saccharin-based, liqui	1	tsp	5	5	0	0	0	0	0	0
5057	Swiss chard, chopped, raw	0.5	cup	18	17	3	0	1	0.3	0	0
5059	Swiss chard, cooked, no added salt	0.5	cup	88	81	18	2	4	1.8	0	0
5058	Swiss chard, raw leaf	1	each	48	44	9	1	2	0.8	0	0
23013	Syrup, chocolate, thin	2	Tbs	38	14	82	1	22	0.7	0	0.2
23056	Syrup, chocolate, thin	2	Tbs	38	11	92	1	25	0.7	0	0.3
25010	Syrup, corn, dark	1	Tbs	20	5	58	0	16	0	0	0
25000	Syrup, corn, light	2	Tbs	41	9	116	0	31	0	0	0
25002	Syrup, maple	2	Tbs	40	13	105	0	27	0	0	0
23042	Syrup, pancake	2	Tbs	39	9	113	0	30	0	0	0
23177	Syrup, pancake, Pillsbury Lite	2	Tbs	39	25	55	0	14	0.5	0	0
23176	Syrup, pancake, Pillsbury regular	2	Tbs	39	14	103	0	26	0.1	0	0
23090	Syrup, pancake, buttery, Mrs. Butterworth's	2	Tbs	39	9	117	0	29	0	1	0.4
23091	Syrup, pancake, buttery, low cal, Butterworth's	2	Tbs	36	20	58	0	15	0	0	0
23172	Syrup, pancake, reduced-calorie	2	Tbs	36	20	59	0	16	0	0	0
23161	Syrup, pancake, w/2% maple	2	Tbs	39	12	104	0	27	0	0	0
56916	Tabbouleh/tabbuli	0.5	cup	80	62	93	2	8	2.3	7	0.9
56536	Taco Bell, Pintos & cheese	1	each	128	87	203	10	19	10.7	10	4.3
56690	Taco Bell, burrito, big beef supreme	1	each	298	192	520	24	54	11	23	10
56688	Taco Bell, burrito, chicken	1	each	171	99	345	17	41	—	13	5
56691	Taco Bell, burrito, seven layer	1	each	234	143	438	13	55	10.7	19	5.8
45585	Taco Bell, cinnamon twist	1	each	35	2	175	1	24	0	8	0
56531	Taco Bell, mexican pizza	1	each	223	119	578	21	43	8.1	36	10.1
56534	Taco Bell, nachos, bellgrande, svg	1	each	287	148	708	19	77	15.6	36	10.1
56684	Taco Bell, nachos, supreme, serving	1	each	145	81	330	10	33	6.6	18	5.9
56524	Taco Bell, taco	1	each	78	46	180	9	12	3	10	4
56689	Taco Bell, taco, soft, chicken	1	each	128	81	212	15	22	2.1	7	2.6
56693	Taco Bell, taco, soft, steak	1	each	100	63	180	12	16	1.6	8	2
56526	Taco Bell, taco, soft, supreme	1	each	124	79	227	10	20	2.6	12	6.1
56692	Taco Bell, taco, supreme	1	each	106	68	206	9	13	2.8	13	6.6
56553	Taco Time, Mexi-fries, svg	1	each	130	75	330	3	31	1	20	7
56540	Taco Time, burrito, bean, crispy	1	each	149	82	354	11	34	4	21	4
56541	Taco Time, burrito, beef, crispy	1	each	149	65	466	22	32	1	28	10
56544	Taco Time, burrito, combo, soft	1	each	255	153	520	27	48	4	25	10
56555	Taco Time, chicken fajita salad	1	each	297	198	541	28	39	2	31	7
56546	Taco Time, taco, natural super	1	each	283	173	575	28	49	4	31	13
42359	Taco shell, Ortega	2	each	30	0	140	2	20	2	7	1
42168	Taco shell, baked	2	each	26	2	122	2	16	2	6	0.8
56061	Taco, chicken	1	each	78	44	174	16	9	1.2	8	3.2
4532	Tahini (sesame butter)	1	Tbs	15	0	91	3	3	1.4	8	1.2
56113	Tamale, w/meat	1	each	70	36	183	7	16	2.9	10	3.7
82035	Tamales, Old El Paso	1	each	69	49	110	2	10	1.7	6	2.3
3269	Tamarind, raw	5	each	10	3	24	0	6	0.5	0	0
3087	Tangelo, fresh	1	each	95	82	45	1	11	2.3	0	0
3237	Tangerine, canned in light syrup	0.5	cup	126	105	77	1	20	0.9	0	0
3138	Tangerine, fresh	1	each	84	74	37	1	9	1.9	0	0
44020	Taro chips	10	each	23	0	115	1	16	1.7	6	1.5
5543	Taro shoots, cooked slices	0.5	cup	70	67	10	1	2	0.4	0	0
5302	Taro slices, cooked	0.5	cup	66	42	94	0	23	3.4	0	0
5369	Taro, raw slices	0.5	cup	52	37	58	1	14	2.1	0	0
5544	Taro, tahitian, cooked slices	0.5	cup	68	59	30	3	5	0.7	0	0.1
26032	Tarragon, ground	0.25	tsp	0	0	1	0	0	0	0	0
48057	Tart, lemon meringue	1	each	117	53	329	4	43	0.6	16	4
20014	Tea, brewed	1	cup	240	239	2	0	1	0	0	0
20118	Tea, camomile	1	cup	240	239	2	0	0	0	0	0
20079	Tea, decaff, low calorie, frozen, prepared	1	cup	245	243	7	0	2	0	0	0
20022	Tea, from instant, sweetened, w/lemon	1	cup	262	239	89	0	22	0	0	0
20020	Tea, from instant, unsweetened	1	cup	237	236	2	0	0	0	0	0
20036	Tea, herbal, brewed	1	cup	237	237	2	0	0	0	0	0

MonoF (g)	PolyF (g)	Choles (mg)	Calc (mg)	Phos (mg)	Sod (mg)	Pot (mg)	Zn (mg)	Iron (mg)	Magn (mg)	VitA (μg RE)	VitE (mg α-TE)	VitC (mg)	Thia (mg)	Ribo (mg)	Nia (mg)	B6 (mg)	Fola (μg)	B12 (μg)
0	0.1	0	17	24	38	189	0.2	0.9	12	702	0.27	11	0.02	0.04	0.3	0.06	8	0
0	0.1	0	19	26	57	179	—	0.8	—	1530	—	14	0.03	0.04	0.4	—	—	0
0	0.1	0	21	27	13	184	0.3	0.6	10	1705	0.28	17	0.05	0.14	0.6	0.24	11	0
0	0.2	0	33	42	20	287	0.4	0.9	16	2659	0.44	27	0.08	0.22	1	0.38	17	0
0	0	0	0	0	2	0	—	0.1	—	0	—	0	0	0	0	—	—	0
0	0	0	0	0	0	1	0	0	0	0	0	0	0	0	0	0	0	0
0	0	0	0	0	1	5	0	0	0	0	0	0	0	0	0	0	0	0
0	0	0	9	8	38	68	0.1	0.3	15	59	0.34	5	0.01	0.02	0.1	0.02	2	0
0	0	0	51	29	157	480	0.3	2	75	275	1.65	16	0.03	0.08	0.3	0.07	8	0
0	0	0	24	22	102	182	0.2	0.9	39	158	0.91	14	0.02	0.04	0.2	0.05	7	0
0.1	0	0	5	48	36	84	0.3	0.8	24	1	0.01	0	0	0.02	0.1	0	2	0
0.2	0	0	5	48	57	180	0.3	5.1	24	488	0.01	0	0	0.31	12.6	0.01	2	0
0	0	0	4	2	32	9	0	0.1	2	0	0	0	0	0	0	0	0	0
0	0	0	1	1	50	2	0	0	1	0	0	0	0	0	0	0	0	0
0	0	0	27	1	4	82	1.7	0.5	6	0	0	0	0	0	0	0	0	0
0	0	0	0	4	33	1	0	0	1	0	0	0	0	0	0	0	0	0
0	0	0	2	—	104	—	—	0	—	0	—	0	—	—	—	—	—	—
0	0	0	1	—	45	—	—	0.2	—	0	—	0	—	—	—	—	—	—
0.2	0	2	1	4	39	1	0	0	1	6	0.01	0	0	0	0	0	0	0
0	0	0	3	2	74	12	0	0.6	2	0	0	0	0.02	0.01	0	0	0	0
0	0	0	0	16	72	1	0	0	0	0	0	0	0	0	0	0	0	0
0	0	0	2	4	24	2	0.1	0	1	0	0	0	0	0.01	0	0	0	0
4.7	0.6	0	27	37	321	168	0.3	1.2	23	83	1.08	26	0.04	0.03	0.7	0.06	29	0
—	—	16	160	—	693	384	2.2	1.9	110	267	—	0	0.05	0.15	0.4	0.21	68	0
—	—	55	150	—	1520	—	—	2.7	—	600	—	5	—	—	—	—	—	—
—	—	57	140	—	854	—	—	2.5	—	440	—	1	—	—	—	—	—	—
—	—	21	165	—	1058	—	—	3	—	248	—	5	—	—	—	—	—	—
—	—	0	0	—	238	28	—	0.4	—	50	—	0	0.1	0.04	0.7	0.04	—	—
—	—	46	253	—	1054	408	5.4	3.6	80	405	—	5	0.32	0.34	3	1.12	60	—
—	—	32	184	—	1205	674	—	3.3	—	138	—	3	0.1	0.34	2.2	—	—	—
—	—	22	110	—	593	—	—	2	—	73	—	3	—	—	—	—	—	—
—	—	25	80	—	330	159	—	1.1	—	100	—	0	0.05	0.14	1.2	0.12	—	—
—	—	37	85	—	571	—	—	0.8	—	64	—	1	—	—	—	—	—	—
—	—	20	62	—	797	—	—	1.1	—	31	—	0	—	—	—	—	—	—
—	—	31	87	—	515	—	—	1.6	—	131	—	3	—	—	—	—	—	—
—	—	33	94	—	328	—	—	1	—	141	—	0	—	—	—	—	—	—
9	4	—	13	46	360	315	—	1	—	0	—	4	0.06	0.01	1	—	—	0
11	6	11	143	216	302	347	2	4	—	12	—	—	0.33	0.2	2	0.35	13	—
12	6	52	180	253	571	463	4	4	—	28	—	2	0.24	0.37	5	0.33	68	—
14	1	54	271	392	826	713	5	7	—	90	—	5	0.45	0.44	5	0.6	70	—
10	11	73	177	267	490	442	2	3	—	127	—	20	0.26	0.36	9	0.44	66	—
17	1	66	300	414	763	749	5	7	—	107	—	5	0.46	0.48	5	0.58	74	—
3	1	0	60	—	200	70	—	0.7	—	20	—	—	—	—	—	—	—	—
2.3	2.2	0	42	64	95	46	0.4	0.6	27	0	0.95	0	0.06	0.01	0.4	0.08	27	0
3.2	1.4	46	95	154	106	167	1.3	1	28	39	0.85	1	0.08	0.13	4.2	0.25	16	0.2
3.2	3.7	0	21	119	0	69	1.6	1	53	1	0.34	0	0.24	0.02	0.8	0.02	15	0
4.3	1.4	24	32	80	229	154	1.1	1.9	29	18	0.43	4	0.24	0.18	2.9	0.12	5	0.18
2.7	0.5	10	13	—	197	—	—	0.6	—	—	—	—	—	—	—	—	—	—
0	0	0	7	11	3	63	0	0.3	9	0	0.07	0	0.04	0.02	0.2	0.01	1	0
0	0	0	38	13	0	172	0.1	0.1	10	20	0.23	50	0.08	0.04	0.3	0.06	29	0
0	0	0	9	13	8	98	0.3	0.5	10	106	0.43	25	0.07	0.06	0.6	0.05	6	0
0	0	0	12	8	1	132	0.2	0.1	10	77	0.2	26	0.09	0.02	0.1	0.06	17	0
1	3	0	14	30	79	174	0.1	0.3	19	0	1.13	1	0.04	0.01	0.1	0.1	5	0
0	0	0	10	18	1	241	0.4	0.3	6	4	0.7	13	0.03	0.04	0.6	0.08	2	0
0	0	0	12	50	10	319	0.2	0.5	20	0	0.29	3	0.07	0.02	0.3	0.22	13	0
0	0	0	22	44	6	307	0.1	0.3	17	0	1.24	2	0.05	0.01	0.3	0.15	12	0
0	0.2	0	102	46	37	427	0.1	1.1	35	121	1.85	26	0.03	0.14	0.3	0.08	5	0
0	0	0	5	1	0	12	0	0.1	1	2	0.01	0	0	0	0	0	1	0
6.8	3.9	74	14	56	272	54	0.4	1.3	8	34	1.56	3	0.15	0.19	1.2	0.04	11	0.14
0	0	0	0	2	7	89	0	0	7	0	0	0	0	0.03	0	0	12	0
0	0	0	5	0	2	22	0.1	0.2	2	5	0.19	0	0.02	0.01	0	0	1	0
0	0	0	0	2	7	90	0	0	7	0	0	0	0	0.03	0	0	13	0
0	0	0	5	3	8	50	0.1	0.1	5	0	0	0	0	0.05	0.1	0	10	0
0	0	0	5	2	7	47	0.1	0	5	0	0	0	0	0	0.1	0	1	0
0	0	0	5	0	2	21	0.1	0.2	2	0	0	0	0.02	0.01	0	0	1	0

Esha Code	Food Item	Qty	Meas	Wgt (g)	Wtr (g)	Cals	Prot (g)	Carb (g)	Fib (g)	Fat (g)	SatF (g)
20040	Tea, instant, w/lemon, diet, dry, prepared	1	cup	238	236	5	0	1	0	0	0
20038	Tea, instant, w/lemon, prepared	1	cup	238	237	5	0	1	0	0	0
20078	Tea, presweetened, w/low calorie sweetener	1	cup	245	243	5	0	1	0	0	0
7564	Tempeh	0.5	cup	83	46	165	16	14	4.5	6	0.9
26312	Thyme, fresh	0.25	cup	17	12	16	1	3	—	0	—
26033	Thyme, ground	0.25	tsp	0	0	1	0	0	0.1	0	0
45544	Toaster pastry, Pop Tarts, brown sugar cinnamon	1	each	50	5	220	3	32	1	9	1
45504	Toaster pastry, fruit filled, Poptart	1	each	52	6	204	2	37	1.1	5	0.8
7500	Tofu (soybean curd, reg)	0.5	cup	124	108	76	8	2	0.2	5	0.7
7546	Tofu yogurt	1	cup	262	203	254	9	43	0.5	5	0.7
7520	Tofu, fried, w/Nigari	1	oz.	28	14	77	5	3	1.1	6	0.8
7520	Tofu, fried, w/Nigari	1	piece	13	7	35	2	1	0.5	3	0.4
7521	Tofu, okara, w/Nigari	0.5	cup	61	50	47	2	8	2.5	1	0.1
7518	Tofu, raw, firm, prepared, w/Nigari	0.5	cup	126	105	97	10	4	0.5	6	0.8
7522	Tofu, salted, fermented (fuyu), w/Nigari, block	1	each	11	8	13	1	1	0	1	0.1
5444	Tomatillo, raw, chopped	0.5	cup	66	60	21	1	4	1.2	1	0.1
5445	Tomatillo, raw, whole	1	each	34	31	11	0	2	0.6	0	0
5397	Tomato juice, canned, low sodium	1	cup	244	229	42	2	10	2	0	0
5188	Tomato juice, canned, w/salt	1	cup	244	229	42	2	10	1	0	0
5473	Tomato paste, canned	0.25	cup	66	48	54	2	13	2.7	0	0.1
5181	Tomato paste, canned, no added salt	0.5	cup	66	48	54	2	13	2.7	0	0.1
5225	Tomato puree, canned, low sodium	0.5	cup	125	109	50	2	12	2.5	0	0
5476	Tomato puree, canned, w/salt	0.5	cup	125	109	50	2	12	2.5	0	0
53113	Tomato sauce w/mushrooms, canned	0.5	cup	122	108	43	2	10	1.8	0	0
5173	Tomato slices, raw	2	piece	40	38	8	0	2	0.4	0	0
5545	Tomato wedge w/tomato juice, canned	0.5	cup	130	120	34	1	8	1.3	0	0
5172	Tomato, Italian/plum, raw, whole	1	each	62	58	13	1	3	0.7	0	0
6492	Tomato, Roma, raw	1	each	62	58	13	1	3	0.7	0	0
5171	Tomato, cherry	10	each	170	159	36	1	8	1.9	1	0.1
5468	Tomato, fresh, stewed w/bread crumbs	0.5	cup	50	41	40	1	7	0.9	1	0.3
5536	Tomato, green, fried	1	each	144	104	237	4	16	2	18	4.7
5518	Tomato, green, raw slices	1	piece	44	41	11	1	2	0.5	0	0
5519	Tomato, green, raw, chopped	0.5	cup	90	84	22	1	5	1	0	0
5520	Tomato, green, raw, whole	1	each	123	114	30	1	6	1.4	0	0
5170	Tomato, raw, chopped	0.5	cup	90	84	19	1	4	1	0	0
5174	Tomato, raw, wedge	1	piece	31	29	7	0	1	0.3	0	0
5169	Tomato, raw, whole, medium size	1	each	123	115	26	1	6	1.4	0	0.1
5628	Tomato, red, fried	1	each	101	74	164	3	11	1.2	13	3.3
5467	Tomato, ripe (June-Oct)	1	each	123	115	26	1	6	1.4	0	0.1
5466	Tomato, ripe (Nov-May)	1	each	123	115	26	1	6	1.4	0	0.1
5474	Tomato, stewed, canned, low sodium	0.5	cup	128	116	36	1	9	1.3	0	0
5447	Tomato, sun dried pieces	10	piece	20	3	52	3	11	2.5	1	0.1
5448	Tomato, sun dried, oil pack, drained	10	each	30	16	64	2	7	1.7	4	0.6
6116	Tomato, yellow, sun dried	0.5	cup	27	6	79	3	15	3.2	1	0.2
5546	Tomatoes w/green chilies, canned	0.5	cup	120	114	18	1	4	1.2	0	0
5179	Tomatoes, canned, no salt added	0.5	cup	120	112	23	1	5	1.2	0	0
5178	Tomatoes, raw, diced, cooked	0.5	cup	120	111	32	1	7	1.2	0	0.1
5446	Tomatoes, sun dried, whole	0.5	cup	27	4	70	4	15	3.3	1	0.1
23071	Topping, Marshmallow creme	2	Tbs	38	8	122	0	30	0	0	0
23069	Topping, butterscotch	2	Tbs	41	13	103	1	27	0.4	0	0
23070	Topping, caramel	2	Tbs	41	13	103	1	27	0.4	0	0
23014	Topping, chocolate hot fudge	2	Tbs	42	9	149	2	27	1.2	4	1.7
23162	Topping, nuts in syrup	2	Tbs	41	8	167	2	22	0.7	9	0.8
23163	Topping, pineapple	2	Tbs	42	14	108	0	28	0.4	0	0
23164	Topping, strawberry	2	Tbs	42	14	108	0	28	0.4	0	0
56129	Tortellini, spinach	0.5	cup	61	37	116	6	13	0.5	4	1.6
44018	Tortilla chips, Doritos	20	piece	36	1	180	3	23	2.3	9	1.8
44019	Tortilla chips, Doritos, grab bag	1	each	64	1	319	4	40	4.1	17	3.2
44266	Tortilla chips, baked, low fat, Tostitos	1	oz.	28	—	111	3	24	2	1	0
44267	Tortilla chips, baked, low fat, unsalted, Tostitos	1	oz.	28	—	111	3	24	2	1	0
44004	Tortilla chips, nacho flavor (Doritos)	1	cup	26	0	129	2	16	1.4	7	1.3
44005	Tortilla chips, nacho flavor (Doritos), grab bag	1	each	64	1	317	5	40	3.4	16	3.1
44054	Tortilla chips, nacho flavor, light	10	each	16	0	71	1	12	0.8	2	0.5
44055	Tortilla chips, ranch flavor, Doritos	10	piece	18	0	88	1	12	0.7	4	0.8
44056	Tortilla chips, taco flavor, Doritos	1	oz.	28	0	136	2	18	1.5	7	1.3

MonoF	PolyF	Choles	Calc	Phos	Sod	Pot	Zn	Iron	Magn	VitA	VitE	VitC	Thia	Ribo	Nia	B6	Fola	B12
(g)	(g)	(mg)	(mg)	(mg)	(mg)	(mg)	(mg)	(mg)	(mg)	(μg RE)	(mg α-TE)	(mg)	(mg)	(mg)	(mg)	(mg)	(μg)	(μg)
0	0	0	5	2	24	40	0.1	0.1	5	0	0	0	0	0.01	0.1	0	5	0
0	0	0	5	2	14	50	0.1	0	5	0	0	0	0	0.02	0.1	0	1	0
0	0	0	5	2	24	42	0.1	0.1	5	0	0	0	0	0.01	0.1	0	5	0
1.4	3.6	0	77	171	5	305	1.5	1.9	58	57	0.02	0	0.11	0.09	3.8	0.25	43	0.83
—	—	—	108	12	3	46	0.4	—	13	22	—	—	0.03	—	—	—	—	0
0	0	0	7	1	0	3	0	0.4	1	1	0.01	0	0	0	0	0	1	0
—	—	0	0	40	210	—	0.6	1.8	—	150	—	0	0.15	0.17	2	0.2	40	—
2.2	2	0	14	58	218	58	0.3	1.8	9	150	1.19	0	0.15	0.19	2	0.2	34	0
1	2.6	0	138	114	10	149	0.8	1.4	34	1	0.01	0	0.06	0.05	0.7	0.06	55	0
1.1	2.7	0	309	100	92	123	0.8	2.8	105	8	0.81	7	0.16	0.05	0.6	0.05	16	0
1.3	3.2	0	105	81	5	41	0.6	1.4	17	0	0.01	0	0.05	0.01	0	0.03	8	0
0.6	1.5	0	48	37	2	19	0.3	0.6	8	0	0	0	0.02	0.01	0	0.01	3	0
0.2	0.5	0	49	37	5	130	0.3	0.8	16	0	0	0	0.01	0.01	0.1	0.07	16	0
1.2	3.2	0	204	185	10	222	1.3	1.8	58	1	0.02	0	0.12	0.13	0	0.08	42	0
0.2	0.5	0	5	8	316	8	0.2	0.2	6	2	0	0	0.02	0.01	0	0.01	3	0
0.1	0.3	0	5	26	1	177	0.1	0.4	13	7	0.25	8	0.03	0.02	1.2	0.04	5	0
0.1	0.1	0	2	13	0	91	0.1	0.2	7	4	0.13	4	0.02	0.01	0.6	0.02	2	0
0	0.1	0	22	46	24	537	0.3	1.4	27	137	2.22	45	0.12	0.08	1.6	0.27	49	0
0	0.1	0	22	46	881	537	0.3	1.4	27	137	2.22	45	0.12	0.08	1.6	0.27	49	0
0.1	0.1	0	23	52	517	614	0.5	1.3	33	160	2.82	28	0.1	0.12	2.1	0.25	15	0
0.1	0.1	0	23	52	58	614	0.5	1.3	33	160	2.82	28	0.1	0.12	2.1	0.25	15	0
0	0.1	0	21	50	42	533	0.3	1.6	30	160	3.15	13	0.09	0.07	2.2	0.19	14	0
0	0.1	0	21	50	499	533	0.3	1.6	30	160	3.15	13	0.09	0.07	2.2	0.19	14	0
0	0.1	0	16	39	554	466	0.3	1.1	23	116	1.72	15	0.09	0.13	1.6	0.16	12	0
0	0.1	0	2	10	4	89	0	0.2	4	25	0.15	8	0.02	0.02	0.3	0.03	6	0
0	0.1	0	34	30	283	328	0.2	0.6	14	76	0.5	19	0.07	0.04	0.9	0.15	13	0
0	0.1	0	3	15	6	138	0.1	0.3	7	38	0.24	12	0.04	0.03	0.4	0.05	9	0
0	0.1	0	3	15	6	138	0.1	0.3	7	38	0.24	12	0.04	0.03	0.4	0.05	9	0
0.1	0.2	0	8	41	15	377	0.2	0.8	19	105	0.65	32	0.1	0.08	1.1	0.14	26	0
0.5	0.4	0	13	19	230	125	0.1	0.5	8	34	0.64	9	0.06	0.04	0.6	0.04	6	0
7.7	4.5	32	85	84	242	269	0.3	1.3	17	81	1.93	24	0.15	0.16	1.2	0.1	12	0.11
0	0	0	6	12	6	90	0	0.2	4	28	0.17	10	0.03	0.02	0.2	0.04	4	0
0	0.1	0	12	25	12	184	0.1	0.5	9	58	0.34	21	0.05	0.04	0.4	0.07	8	0
0	0.1	0	16	34	16	251	0.1	0.6	12	79	0.47	29	0.07	0.05	0.6	0.1	11	0
0	0.1	0	4	22	8	200	0.1	0.4	10	56	0.34	17	0.05	0.04	0.6	0.07	14	0
0	0	0	2	7	3	69	0	0.1	3	19	0.12	6	0.02	0.02	0.2	0.02	5	0
0.1	0.2	0	6	30	11	273	0.1	0.6	14	76	0.47	24	0.07	0.06	0.8	0.1	18	0
5.4	3.2	23	54	56	167	202	0.2	0.8	12	58	1.35	14	0.1	0.12	0.9	0.07	12	0.08
0.1	0.2	0	6	30	11	273	0.1	0.6	14	76	0.47	32	0.07	0.06	0.8	0.1	18	0
0.1	0.2	0	6	30	11	273	0.1	0.6	14	76	0.47	12	0.07	0.06	0.8	0.1	18	0
0	0.1	0	42	26	282	303	0.2	0.9	15	69	0.48	14	0.06	0.04	0.9	0.02	7	0
0.1	0.2	0	22	71	419	685	0.4	1.8	39	17	0	8	0.11	0.1	1.8	0.07	14	0
2.6	0.6	0	14	42	80	470	0.2	0.8	24	39	0.16	31	0.06	0.12	1.1	0.1	7	0
0.4	0	0	32	—	23	—	—	2.3	—	49	—	5	—	—	—	—	—	0
0	0	0	24	17	483	129	0.2	0.3	13	47	0.46	7	0.04	0.02	0.8	0.12	11	0
0	0.1	0	36	23	178	265	0.2	0.7	14	72	0.38	17	0.05	0.04	0.9	0.11	9	0
0.1	0.2	0	7	37	13	335	0.1	0.7	17	89	0.46	27	0.08	0.07	0.9	0.11	16	0
0.1	0.3	0	30	96	566	925	0.5	2.4	52	24	0	11	0.14	0.13	2.4	0.09	18	0
0	0	0	1	3	19	2	0	0.1	1	0	0	0	0	0	0	0	0	0
0	0	0	22	19	143	34	0.1	0.1	3	11	0	0	0	0.04	0	0.01	1	0.04
0	0	0	22	19	143	34	0.1	0.1	3	11	0	0	0	0.04	0	0.01	1	0.04
1.6	0.1	1	34	57	147	154	0.3	0.6	22	2	1.24	0	0.02	0.09	0.1	0.03	2	0.09
2	5.6	0	16	46	17	86	0.4	0.4	26	2	0.36	0	0.07	0.05	0.2	0.08	9	0
0	0	0	9	3	27	135	0.2	0.2	1	1	0	25	0.01	0	0	0.01	1	0
0	0	0	10	6	9	31	0.2	0.4	2	1	0.06	11	0	0.01	0.1	0.01	1	0
1.6	0.7	79	72	84	126	69	0.5	1.2	12	95	0.66	1	0.12	0.19	0.9	0.05	17	0.24
5.6	1.3	0	55	74	190	71	0.6	0.5	32	7	0.49	0	0.03	0.07	0.5	0.1	4	0
9.9	2.3	0	98	131	336	125	1	1	56	13	0.87	0	0.05	0.12	0.8	0.18	6	0
—	—	0	—	—	142	—	—	—	—	—	—	—	—	—	—	—	—	—
—	—	0	—	—	0	—	—	—	—	—	—	—	—	—	—	—	—	—
3.9	0.9	1	38	63	184	56	0.3	0.4	21	11	0.35	0	0.03	0.05	0.4	0.07	4	0.01
9.6	2.2	2	94	155	451	138	0.8	0.9	52	26	0.87	1	0.08	0.12	0.9	0.18	9	0.03
1.4	0.3	0	25	51	160	44	—	0.3	16	7	0.13	0	0.04	0.04	0.1	0.04	4	0
2.5	0.6	0	25	43	110	44	0.2	0.3	16	5	0.24	0	0.02	0.04	0.3	0.04	3	0
4.1	1	1	44	68	224	62	0.4	0.6	25	26	0.39	0	0.07	0.06	0.6	0.08	6	0

Esha Code	Food Item	Qty	Meas	Wgt (g)	Wtr (g)	Cals	Prot (g)	Carb (g)	Fib (g)	Fat (g)	SatF (g)
42023	Tortilla, corn, 6 inch	1	each	30	13	67	2	14	1.6	1	0.1
42024	Tortilla, corn, thin	1	each	17	8	38	1	8	0.9	0	0.1
42027	Tortilla, corn/taco shell	1	each	14	1	62	1	9	1.1	3	0.4
42026	Tortilla, flour, 10.5 inch	1	each	57	15	185	5	32	1.9	4	1
42025	Tortilla, flour, 8 inch	1	each	35	9	115	3	20	1.2	3	0.6
42079	Tortilla, whole wheat	1	each	35	11	73	3	20	1.9	0	0.1
56062	Tostada, bean & chicken	1	each	157	106	250	20	18	3.4	11	5.4
56645	Tostada, beef & cheese	1	each	163	101	315	19	23	—	16	10.4
56646	Tostada, w/guacamole	2	each	261	189	360	12	32	—	23	9.9
44058	Trail mix, regular	0.5	cup	75	7	347	10	34	3.8	22	4.2
44085	Trail mix, regular, unsalted	0.5	cup	75	7	347	10	34	3.8	22	4.2
44059	Trail mix, regular, w/chocolate chips, salted	0.5	cup	73	5	353	10	33	4	23	4.4
44086	Trail mix, regular, w/chocolate chips, unsalted	0.5	cup	73	5	353	10	33	4	23	4.4
44060	Trail mix, tropical	0.5	cup	70	6	285	4	46	4.5	12	5.9
56089	Tuna noodle casserole, recipe	1	cup	202	151	237	17	25	1.4	7	1.9
56007	Tuna salad	0.5	cup	102	65	192	16	10	0	9	1.6
17029	Tuna, bass, freshwater, baked/broiled fillet	1	each	62	43	90	15	0	0	3	0.6
17027	Tuna, light, canned in water, drained	1	cup	154	115	179	39	0	0	1	0.4
13223	Turkey breast, roasted, Healthy Favorites	1	oz.	28	—	22	4	1	0	0	0
16011	Turkey patty, breaded, fried	1	each	64	32	181	9	10	0.3	12	3
16011	Turkey patty, breaded, fried	3	oz.	85	42	241	12	13	0.4	15	4
16928	Turkey pot pie, Banquet	1	each	198	129	370	10	38	3	20	8
16009	Turkey roll, light & dark meat	2	piece	57	40	84	10	1	0	4	1.2
16008	Turkey roll, light meat	2	piece	57	41	83	11	0	0	4	1.2
16276	Turkey, canned in water, Swanson	0.5	cup	124	78	180	32	8	2	4	1
16000	Turkey, dark & light meat, skinless, roasted	4	oz.	113	74	193	33	0	0	6	1.9
16028	Turkey, dark meat, roasted	4	oz.	113	68	251	31	0	0	13	4
16002	Turkey, dark meat, skinless, roasted	4	oz.	113	72	212	32	0	0	8	2.7
16038	Turkey, fryer, breast meat, roasted	1	each	612	419	826	184	0	0	5	1.5
16038	Turkey, fryer, breast meat, roasted	3	oz.	85	58	115	26	0	0	1	0.2
16003	Turkey, ground, cooked patty	1	each	82	49	194	23	0	0	11	2.8
13112	Turkey, hickory smoked, fat free, Louis Rich	1	piece	28	22	23	4	1	0	0	0.1
16027	Turkey, light meat, roasted	4	oz.	113	71	223	32	0	0	9	2.6
16012	Turkey, roast, seasoned, frozen, roasted	4	oz.	113	77	176	24	3	0	7	2.2
16026	Turkey, roasted	4	oz.	113	70	236	32	0	0	11	3.2
16045	Turkey, tom, breast, roasted	4	oz.	113	72	214	32	0	0	8	2.4
16046	Turkey, tom, leg, roasted	4	oz.	113	69	234	32	0	0	11	3.4
16039	Turkey, tom, roasted	4	oz.	113	70	229	32	0	0	10	3
16040	Turkey, tom, skinless, roasted	4	oz.	113	74	191	33	0	0	5	1.8
16010	Turkey, w/gravy, frozen, heated	1	cup	240	204	161	14	11	0	6	2
16001	Turkey, white meat, skinless, roasted	4	oz.	113	78	159	34	0	0	1	0.4
26034	Turmeric, ground	0.25	tsp	1	0	2	0	0	0.1	0	0
5186	Turnip greens, frozen, cooked	0.5	cup	82	74	25	3	4	2.8	0	0.1
5547	Turnip greens, raw, chopped	0.5	cup	28	25	7	0	2	0.9	0	0
5185	Turnip greens, raw, cooked	0.5	cup	72	67	14	1	3	2.5	0	0
5182	Turnip, raw cubes	0.5	cup	65	60	18	1	4	1.2	0	0
5183	Turnip, raw cubes, cooked, no added salt	0.5	cup	78	73	16	1	4	1.6	0	0
14030	Turtle meat, cooked	4	oz.	113	80	152	27	0	0	4	0.9
45533	Vanilla cookie crust, recipe, baked	1	each	173	12	936	6	89	2.4	64	13.1
45532	Vanilla cookie crust, recipe, chilled	1	piece	29	2	156	1	15	0	11	2.2
26087	Vanilla extract, Single Fold	1	tsp	5	3	9	0	0	0	0	0
26290	Vanillan (no alcohol)	1	tsp	5	0	22	—	5	—	—	—
11900	Veal patty, breaded, cooked	1	each	79	42	209	16	6	0.4	13	4.4
11900	Veal patty, breaded, cooked	3	oz.	85	45	225	18	7	0.4	14	4.8
11902	Veal scallopini	1	piece	96	55	257	18	1	0.2	19	5.6
11530	Veal, ground, broiled	4	oz.	113	76	195	28	0	0	9	3.4
11514	Veal, leg, pan fried, lean	1	each	85	52	156	28	0	0	4	1.1
11514	Veal, leg, pan fried, lean	3	oz.	85	52	156	28	0	0	4	1.1
11516	Veal, leg, roasted, lean	4	oz.	113	76	170	32	0	0	4	1.4
11509	Veal, leg, roasted, lean & fat	4	oz.	113	75	181	31	0	0	5	2.1
11518	Veal, loin chop, braised, lean	1	each	69	39	156	23	0	0	6	1.8
11517	Veal, loin, cutlet/chop, braised, lean & fat	1	each	80	42	227	24	0	0	14	5.4
11520	Veal, rib, roasted, lean	4	oz.	113	73	201	29	0	0	8	2.4
11519	Veal, rib, roasted, lean & fat	4	oz.	113	68	259	27	0	0	16	6.1
11522	Veal, shoulder, whole, braised, lean	4	oz.	113	67	226	38	0	0	7	1.9

MonoF	PolyF	Choles	Calc	Phos	Sod	Pot	Zn	Iron	Magn	VitA	VitE	VitC	Thia	Ribo	Nia	B6	Fola	B12
(g)	(g)	(mg)	(mg)	(mg)	(mg)	(mg)	(mg)	(mg)	(mg)	(μg RE)	(mg α-TE)	(mg)	(mg)	(mg)	(mg)	(mg)	(μg)	(μg)
0.2	0.3	0	52	94	48	46	0.3	0.4	20	0	0.05	0	0.03	0.02	0.4	0.07	34	0
0.1	0.2	0	30	54	28	27	0.2	0.2	11	0	0.03	0	0.02	0.01	0.3	0.04	20	0
1.5	0.6	0	34	31	24	33	0.2	0.4	14	6	0.57	0	0.04	0.02	0.2	0.04	4	0
2.1	0.6	0	71	70	272	74	0.4	1.9	15	0	0.52	0	0.3	0.17	2	0.03	70	0
1.3	0.4	0	44	44	169	46	0.3	1.2	9	0	0.32	0	0.19	0.1	1.3	0.02	44	0
0.1	0.2	0	10	82	171	82	0.5	0.7	26	0	0.43	0	0.1	0.02	0.9	0.07	8	0
4	1.6	54	169	239	436	367	2.3	1.8	48	87	1.88	4	0.11	0.2	4.6	0.32	54	0.26
3.3	1	41	217	179	897	572	3.7	2.9	64	96	—	3	0.1	0.55	3.2	0.23	75	1.17
8.5	3	39	423	232	799	650	4.1	1.6	73	217	—	4	0.13	0.57	2	0.26	115	0.99
9.4	7.2	0	58	259	172	514	2.4	2.3	119	2	2.66	1	0.35	0.15	3.5	0.22	53	0
9.4	7.2	0	58	259	8	514	2.4	2.3	119	2	2.66	1	0.35	0.15	3.5	0.22	53	0
9.9	8.2	3	80	283	88	473	2.3	2.5	118	4	7.81	1	0.3	0.16	3.2	0.19	48	0
9.9	8.2	3	80	283	20	473	2.3	2.5	118	4	7.81	1	0.3	0.16	3.2	0.19	48	0
1.7	3.6	0	40	130	7	496	0.8	1.8	67	4	1.55	5	0.32	0.08	1	0.23	29	0
1.5	3.2	41	34	155	772	182	1.2	2.3	30	13	1.18	1	0.18	0.15	7.8	0.2	10	1.52
3	4.2	13	17	182	412	182	0.6	1	20	28	0.97	2	0.03	0.07	6.9	0.08	8	1.23
1.1	0.8	54	64	159	56	283	0.5	1.2	24	22	0.46	1	0.05	0.06	0.9	0.09	10	1.43
0.2	0.5	46	17	251	521	365	1.2	2.4	42	26	0.82	0	0.05	0.11	20.5	0.54	6	4.6
0	0	8	—	—	333	—	—	0.4	—	—	—	—	—	—	—	—	—	—
4.8	3	40	9	173	512	176	0.9	1.4	10	7	1.53	0	0.06	0.12	1.5	0.13	18	0.14
6.4	4	53	12	230	680	234	1.2	1.9	13	9	2.03	0	0.08	0.16	2	0.17	24	0.19
—	—	45	40	—	850	—	—	1.1	—	150	—	0	—	—	—	—	—	—
1.3	1	31	18	95	332	153	1.1	0.8	10	0	0.19	0	0.05	0.16	2.7	0.15	3	0.13
1.4	1	24	23	104	277	142	0.9	0.7	9	0	0.08	0	0.05	0.13	4	0.18	2	0.14
—	—	70	0	—	440	—	—	0	—	0	—	0	—	—	—	—	—	—
1.2	1.6	86	28	242	79	338	3.5	2	30	0	0.37	0	0.07	0.21	6.2	0.52	8	0.42
4.1	3.5	101	37	222	86	311	4.7	2.6	26	0	0.69	0	0.07	0.27	4	0.36	10	0.41
1.9	2.4	96	36	231	90	329	5.1	2.6	27	0	0.73	0	0.07	0.28	4.1	0.41	10	0.42
0.8	1.2	508	73	1370	318	1787	10.6	9.4	177	0	0.55	0	0.26	0.8	45.8	3.43	37	2.39
0.1	0.2	71	10	190	44	248	1.5	1.3	25	0	0.08	0	0.04	0.11	6.4	0.48	5	0.33
4	2.7	84	21	162	88	222	2.4	1.6	20	0	0.28	0	0.04	0.14	4	0.32	6	0.27
0.1	0	10	3	70	304	62	0.3	0.3	8	0	—	0	—	—	—	—	—	—
3.2	2.3	86	24	236	71	323	2.3	1.6	30	0	0.15	0	0.06	0.15	7.1	0.53	7	0.4
1.4	1.9	60	6	277	771	338	2.9	1.8	25	0	0.43	0	0.05	0.18	7.1	0.31	6	1.72
3.6	2.8	93	30	230	77	318	3.4	2	28	0	0.38	0	0.06	0.2	5.8	0.46	8	0.4
2.8	2	85	24	238	76	328	2.4	1.6	31	0	0.2	0	0.07	0.15	6.9	0.56	7	0.41
3.2	3	102	40	227	91	319	4.9	2.6	26	0	0.92	0	0.07	0.29	3.9	0.39	10	0.42
3.4	2.6	93	31	230	82	320	3.4	2	28	0	0.47	0	0.07	0.21	5.6	0.48	8	0.41
1.1	1.5	87	28	243	84	341	3.6	2	30	0	0.48	0	0.08	0.21	6	0.53	9	0.43
2.3	1.1	43	34	194	1329	146	1.7	2.2	19	31	0.84	0	0.06	0.3	4.3	0.24	10	0.58
0.2	0.4	98	17	245	64	314	2.4	1.8	32	0	0.12	0	0.05	0.15	7.9	0.65	7	0.44
0	0	0	1	2	0	14	0	0.2	1	0	0	0	0	0	0	0.01	0	0
0	0.1	0	125	28	12	184	0.3	1.6	21	654	2.39	18	0.04	0.06	0.4	0.06	32	0
0	0	0	52	12	11	81	0.1	0.3	9	209	0.8	16	0.02	0.03	0.2	0.07	53	0
0	0.1	0	99	21	21	146	0.1	0.6	16	396	1.24	20	0.03	0.05	0.3	0.13	85	0
0	0	0	20	18	44	124	0.2	0.2	7	0	0.02	14	0.03	0.02	0.3	0.06	9	0
0	0	0	17	15	39	105	0.2	0.2	6	0	0.02	9	0.02	0.02	0.2	0.05	7	0
1.6	1.3	68	163	247	454	316	1.4	1.9	28	83	1.23	0	0.15	0.21	1.4	0.15	18	1.23
27.7	18.9	69	74	137	910	140	0.4	2.9	19	503	9	0	0.33	0.4	3.7	0.09	12	0.16
4.6	3.1	11	12	23	151	23	0.1	0.5	3	84	1.48	0	0.06	0.07	0.6	0.02	14	0.03
0	0	0	0	0	0	0	0	0	0	0	0	0	0	0	0	0	0	0
—	—	—	0	0	0	0	—	0	0	—	—	—	—	—	—	—	—	0
5.1	1.9	80	25	152	309	221	1.9	0.9	19	8	0.74	0	0.06	0.22	5.7	0.28	12	0.73
5.5	2	86	27	164	333	237	2.1	1	20	9	0.8	0	0.06	0.23	6.1	0.3	13	0.79
8.3	4.2	62	45	170	381	228	1.9	0.7	19	165	2.2	0	0.05	0.19	3.6	0.22	10	0.95
3.2	0.6	117	19	246	94	382	4.4	1.1	27	0	0.17	0	0.08	0.31	9.1	0.44	12	1.44
1.4	0.3	91	6	247	66	376	2.9	0.7	27	0	0.36	0	0.06	0.32	10.7	0.43	14	1.28
1.4	0.3	91	6	247	66	376	2.9	0.7	27	0	0.36	0	0.06	0.32	10.7	0.43	14	1.28
1.4	0.3	117	7	268	77	446	3.5	1	32	0	0.62	0	0.07	0.37	11.5	0.35	18	1.34
2	0.4	117	7	265	77	441	3.4	1	32	0	0.56	0	0.07	0.36	11.3	0.35	18	1.33
2.3	0.6	86	22	164	58	205	2.8	0.8	19	0	0.29	0	0.04	0.24	7	0.19	10	0.91
5.4	0.9	94	22	176	64	224	2.9	0.9	19	0	0.32	0	0.03	0.24	7.2	0.21	11	0.97
3	0.8	130	14	235	110	353	5.1	1.1	27	0	0.41	0	0.07	0.33	8.5	0.31	16	1.79
6.2	1.1	125	12	223	104	335	4.6	1.1	25	0	0.4	0	0.06	0.31	7.9	0.28	15	1.66
2.5	0.6	147	42	295	110	362	7.9	1.6	32	0	0.51	0	0.07	0.4	7.6	0.3	18	2.2

Esha Code	Food Item	Qty	Meas	Wgt (g)	Wtr (g)	Cals	Prot (g)	Carb (g)	Fib (g)	Fat (g)	SatF (g)
11579	Veal, sirloin, braised, lean	4	oz.	113	66	231	39	0	0	7	2.1
11528	Veal, sirloin, roasted, lean	4	oz.	113	74	191	30	0	0	7	2.7
11527	Veal, sirloin, roasted, lean & fat	4	oz.	113	71	229	28	0	0	12	5.1
20080	Vegetable juice cocktail (V8), low sodium	1	cup	242	226	46	2	11	1.9	0	0
5629	Vegetable tempura	0.5	cup	32	22	50	1	4	0.4	3	0.6
6208	Vegetables, Japanese stir fry, Bird's Eye	0.5	cup	58	53	18	1	4	1.1	0	0
5622	Vegetables, pickled, giardiniera	0.5	cup	82	74	22	1	5	1.7	0	0
7653	Vegetarian, Garden dog, hotdog	1	each	57	30	120	19	4	1	2	—
7652	Vegetarian, Garden veggie	1	each	96	56	176	11	24	6.8	4	1.3
7504	Vegetarian, Garden(R) burger, meat only	2.5	oz.	71	41	130	8	18	5	3	1
7505	Vegetarian, Garden(R) sausage patty, meat only	1	each	35	21	65	4	9	2	2	1
7506	Vegetarian, Garden(R) steak, meat only, large	1	each	142	115	369	23	51	14.2	8	2.8
7507	Vegetarian, Garden(R) taco/Veg Mexi 1	0.25	oz.	35	9	107	6	18	4.8	1	0.6
27044	Vegetarian, bacon bits	4	each	57	5	253	18	16	5.8	15	2.3
7509	Vegetarian, bacon strips	3	each	24	12	74	3	2	0.6	7	1.1
7511	Vegetarian, breakfast links	1	each	25	13	64	5	2	0.7	5	0.7
7512	Vegetarian, breakfast sausage patty	1	each	38	19	97	7	4	1.1	7	1.1
7548	Vegetarian, chicken, breaded, fried	1	oz.	28	20	48	3	1	1.2	3	0.5
7548	Vegetarian, chicken, breaded, fried	1	piece	57	40	97	6	3	2.5	7	1
7557	Vegetarian, chili	0.5	cup	107	69	141	19	15	3.9	2	0.3
7549	Vegetarian, fish sticks	2	each	57	26	165	13	5	3.5	10	1.6
7550	Vegetarian, frankfurter	1	each	51	30	102	10	4	2.4	5	0.8
7551	Vegetarian, luncheon slice	1	piece	67	31	188	17	6	3.4	11	1.7
7561	Vegetarian, meat loaf/patties	1	each	71	41	142	15	6	3.3	6	1
7552	Vegetarian, meatballs	7	each	70	41	140	15	6	3.2	6	1
7553	Vegetarian, scallops, breaded, fried	0.5	cup	85	36	257	20	8	5.4	16	2.5
7554	Vegetarian, soyburger	1	each	71	41	142	15	6	3.3	6	1
7554	Vegetarian, soyburger	1	oz.	28	16	57	6	2	1.3	3	0.4
7562	Vegetarian, soyburger, w/cheese, serving	1	each	135	67	316	21	30	4.1	13	4.2
7562	Vegetarian, soyburger, w/cheese, serving	1	oz.	28	14	66	4	6	0.9	3	0.9
22510	Vermouth, dry	0.5	cup	120	92	144	0	7	0	0	0
27129	Vinegar, balsamic	1	Tbs	15	13	10	0	2	0	0	—
27007	Vinegar, cider	1	Tbs	15	14	2	0	1	0	0	0
27067	Vinegar, palm	1	oz.	28	28	2	0	1	—	—	—
27095	Vinegar, rice, natural, Nakano	1	Tbs	15	14	0	0	0	0	0	0
45101	Waffle, Special K, Eggo	1	each	30	11	72	3	15	0	0	0
45038	Waffle, blueberry, 7 inch round	1	each	75	32	186	6	30	1.3	5	1.8
45039	Waffle, blueberry, 9 inch square	1	each	200	85	496	15	81	3.4	13	4.8
45093	Waffle, buttermilk, Eggo	1	each	39	16	110	2	15	0	4	0.8
45030	Waffle, buttermilk, recipe	1	each	75	32	217	6	25	1.1	10	1.9
45041	Waffle, cornmeal, 7 inch round	1	each	75	31	209	6	28	1.3	8	2
45042	Waffle, cornmeal, 9 inch square	1	each	200	83	557	17	75	3.4	21	5.2
45043	Waffle, cornmeal, frozen, 4 inch	1	each	38	16	106	3	14	0.6	4	1
45005	Waffle, frozen toasted	1	each	35	15	92	2	14	0.8	3	0.5
45004	Waffle, mix prepared w/water	1	each	75	32	218	5	26	1	10	1.7
45037	Waffle, mixed grain, frozen, 4 inch	1	each	38	12	116	3	17	2.1	5	1.2
45095	Waffle, oat bran, Common Sense	1	each	39	18	100	3	14	1.5	4	0.8
45018	Waffle, oat bran, Eggo	1	each	38	16	107	3	15	2.1	4	0.6
45003	Waffle, plain, recipe	1	each	75	32	218	6	25	1.1	11	2.2
45016	Waffle, whole grain, 4 inch round	1	each	39	17	107	4	13	1	5	1.6
45017	Waffle, whole grain, frozen	1	each	39	17	107	4	13	1	5	1.6
4556	Walnut, English/Persian, dried, chopped	0.25	cup	30	1	193	4	5	1.4	19	1.7
4557	Walnut, English/Persian, dried, cup measure	0.25	cup	25	1	161	4	5	1.2	16	1.4
4526	Walnut, black, dried, ground	0.25	cup	20	1	121	5	2	1	11	0.7
4525	Walnuts, black, dried	0.25	cup	31	1	190	8	4	1.6	18	1.1
20041	Water	1	cup	237	237	0	0	0	0	0	0
20050	Water, Perrier, 6.5floz bottle	1	each	192	192	0	0	0	0	0	0
20051	Water, bottled, Poland Springs	1	cup	237	237	0	0	0	0	0	0
20011	Water, sparkling mineral, sweet, bottled	1	each	488	445	166	0	43	0	0	0
20121	Water, tonic, sugar-free, 12 fl oz can	1	each	355	354	0	0	0	0	0	0
20010	Water, tonic/quinine/carbonated	1	cup	244	222	83	0	22	0	0	0
5386	Waterchestnut, Chinese, raw slices	0.5	cup	62	46	60	1	15	1.9	0	0
5387	Waterchestnut, Chinese, slices, canned w/liquid	0.5	cup	70	60	35	1	9	1.8	0	0
5388	Waterchestnut, Chinese, whole, canned w/liquid	4	each	28	24	14	0	4	0.7	0	0
5222	Watercress, fresh	0.5	cup	17	16	2	0	0	0.3	0	0

MonoF	PolyF	Choles	Calc	Phos	Sod	Pot	Zn	Iron	Magn	VitA	VitE	VitC	Thia	Ribo	Nia	B6	Fola	B12
(g)	(g)	(mg)	(mg)	(mg)	(mg)	(mg)	(mg)	(mg)	(mg)	(μg RE)	(mg α-TE)	(mg)	(mg)	(mg)	(mg)	(mg)	(μg)	(μg)
2.6	0.7	128	22	294	92	384	5.4	1.4	33	0	0.5	0	0.07	0.43	8	0.43	18	1.8
2.6	0.5	118	16	262	96	414	4	1	31	0	0.52	0	0.07	0.42	10.6	0.39	18	1.69
4.6	0.8	116	15	253	94	398	3.8	1	30	0	0.48	0	0.07	0.4	10.1	0.36	17	1.61
0	0.1	0	27	41	653	467	0.5	1	27	283	0.77	67	0.1	0.07	1.8	0.34	51	0
0.9	1.3	20	8	22	10	56	0.1	0.4	4	73	0.32	1	0.04	0.06	0.4	0.02	7	0.04
—	—	0	16	21	219	96	—	0.4	8	37	—	16	0.03	0.06	0.5	0.05	18	0
0	0.1	0	18	23	562	186	0.1	0.3	10	624	0.23	26	0.04	0.03	0.4	0.11	14	0
—	—	0	20	—	310	500	—	1.4	—	0	—	4	—	—	—	—	—	—
2	0.7	15	114	179	394	262	1.2	0	41	14	0.27	1	0.14	0.2	1.5	0.11	14	0.15
1.5	0.5	11	84	132	289	193	0.9	0	30	10	0.2	0	0.11	0.15	1.1	0.08	10	0.11
0.4	0.1	5	40	68	150	71	0.4	0.2	14	12	0.1	0	0.05	0.07	0.5	0.04	5	0.06
4.2	1.2	31	239	375	822	548	2.5	0	86	28	0.61	0	0.3	0.42	3	0.21	29	0.31
0.4	0.2	0	118	—	80	152	—	0.4	—	18	—	1	—	—	—	—	—	0
3.6	7.7	0	58	124	1008	83	1.1	0.4	54	0	3.93	1	0.34	0.04	0.9	0.05	72	0.68
1.7	3.7	0	6	17	352	41	0.1	0.6	5	2	1.66	0	1.06	0.12	1.8	0.12	10	0
1.1	2.3	0	16	56	222	58	0.4	0.9	9	16	0.52	0	0.58	0.1	2.8	0.21	6	0
1.7	3.5	0	24	86	337	88	0.6	1.4	14	24	0.8	0	0.89	0.15	4.3	0.32	10	0
1.5	1.3	0	7	70	113	85	0.2	0.5	3	0	0.55	0	0.2	0.14	1.3	0.14	16	0.6
2.9	2.5	0	13	140	228	171	0.4	1	7	0	1.11	0	0.4	0.27	2.7	0.28	32	1.2
0.6	0.9	0	53	216	526	362	1.3	4.2	36	78	1.24	16	0.12	0.07	1.2	0.15	82	0
2.5	5.4	0	54	257	279	342	0.8	1.1	13	0	2.25	0	0.63	0.51	6.8	0.86	58	2.39
1.2	2.7	0	17	175	219	76	0.6	0.9	9	0	0.98	0	0.56	0.61	8.2	0.5	40	1.22
2.6	5.6	0	28	296	576	188	1.1	1.5	15	0	2.01	0	0.64	0.37	7.4	0.74	67	1.74
1.5	3.3	0	21	244	391	128	1.3	1.5	13	0	1.23	0	0.64	0.43	7.1	0.85	55	1.7
1.5	3.3	0	20	241	385	126	1.3	1.5	13	0	1.21	0	0.63	0.42	7	0.84	55	1.68
3.8	8.3	0	84	398	434	531	1.2	1.8	20	0	3.5	0	0.97	0.8	10.6	1.33	90	3.72
1.5	3.3	0	21	244	391	128	1.3	1.5	13	0	1.23	0	0.64	0.43	7.1	0.85	55	1.7
0.6	1.3	0	8	98	156	51	0.5	0.6	5	0	0.49	0	0.26	0.17	2.8	0.34	22	0.68
4	3.7	13	146	372	931	211	2	2.7	26	45	1.43	1	0.77	0.55	8.1	0.86	70	1.71
0.8	0.8	3	31	78	196	44	0.4	0.6	6	9	0.3	0	0.16	0.12	1.7	0.18	15	0.36
0	0	0	8	8	20	48	0	0.4	6	0	0	0	0.02	0.02	0	0.01	0	0
—	—	0	5	—	4	12	—	0.1	—	0	—	0	—	—	—	—	—	—
0	0	0	1	1	0	15	0	0.1	3	0	0	0	0	0	0	0	0	0
—	—	—	3	2	—	—	—	0.9	—	—	—	—	0	0	0.1	—	—	—
0	0	0	—	—	1	—	—	—	—	—	—	—	—	—	—	—	—	—
0	0	0	21	—	129	16	—	1.9	—	155	—	0	0.16	0.18	2.1	0.21	41	0.62
1.6	0.9	34	219	262	523	154	0.5	1.2	16	29	0.89	2	0.15	0.23	1	0.06	7	0.2
4.2	2.4	90	584	699	1394	411	1.4	3.2	43	78	2.38	6	0.39	0.6	2.6	0.16	20	0.54
—	—	12	20	—	240	32	—	1.8	—	150	—	0	0.15	0.17	2	0.2	40	0.6
2.5	5.1	50	137	124	451	128	0.6	1.6	14	26	1.5	0	0.2	0.27	1.6	0.04	11	0.16
2.2	3	75	110	108	312	124	0.6	1.6	17	50	1.41	0	0.21	0.27	1.6	0.08	16	0.27
5.7	8.1	199	294	289	832	330	1.5	4.3	45	133	3.77	1	0.55	0.71	4.2	0.22	43	0.73
1.1	1.5	38	56	55	158	63	0.3	0.8	9	25	0.72	0	0.1	0.14	0.8	0.04	8	0.14
1.1	1	8	81	147	275	45	0.2	1.6	8	127	0.29	0	0.14	0.17	1.6	0.31	16	0.88
2.7	5.2	38	93	252	458	134	0.4	1.2	15	20	1.5	0	0.16	0.19	1.2	0.08	9	0.2
1.2	2	28	83	104	146	123	0.9	1.4	25	60	0.93	3	0.14	0.19	1.4	0.11	23	0.12
2.2	0.5	0	20	—	175	18	—	1.8	—	150	—	0	0.15	0.17	2	0.2	40	0.6
1.1	2	0	8	131	214	189	0.7	0.7	38	57	0.57	0	0.06	0.06	0.8	0.03	15	0.23
2.6	5.1	52	191	143	383	119	0.5	1.7	14	49	1.73	0	0.2	0.26	1.6	0.04	34	0.19
1.9	1	39	84	83	150	91	0.4	0.7	16	25	0.53	0	0.08	0.13	0.7	0.04	7	0.15
1.9	1	39	84	83	150	91	0.4	0.7	16	25	0.53	0	0.08	0.13	0.7	0.04	7	0.15
4.3	11.7	0	28	95	3	151	0.8	0.7	51	4	0.79	1	0.12	0.04	0.3	0.17	20	0
3.6	9.8	0	24	79	2	126	0.7	0.6	42	3	0.66	1	0.1	0.04	0.3	0.14	16	0
2.5	7.5	0	12	93	0	105	0.7	0.6	40	6	0.52	1	0.04	0.02	0.1	0.11	13	0
4	11.7	0	18	145	0	164	1.1	1	63	9	0.82	1	0.07	0.03	0.2	0.17	20	0
0	0	0	5	0	7	0	0.1	0	2	0	0	0	0	0	0	0	0	0
0	0	0	27	0	2	0	0	0	0	0	0	0	0	0	0	0	0	0
0	0	0	2	0	2	0	0	0	2	0	0	0	0	0	0	0	0	0
0	0	0	5	0	20	0	0.5	0	0	0	0	0	0	0	0	0	0	0
0	0	0	14	39	57	7	0.2	0.1	4	0	0	0	0	0	0	0	0	0
0	0	0	2	0	10	0	0.2	0	0	0	0	0	0	0	0	0	0	0
0	0	0	7	39	9	362	0.3	0	14	0	0.74	2	0.09	0.12	0.6	0.2	10	0
0	0	0	3	13	6	83	0.3	0.6	4	0	0.35	1	0.01	0.02	0.3	0.11	4	0
0	0	0	1	5	2	34	0.1	0.2	1	0	0.14	0	0	0.01	0.1	0.04	2	0
0	0	0	20	10	7	56	0	0	4	80	0.17	7	0.02	0.02	0	0.02	2	0

Esha Code	Food Item	Qty	Meas	Wgt (g)	Wtr (g)	Cals	Prot (g)	Carb (g)	Fib (g)	Fat (g)	SatF (g)
5223	Watercress, fresh sprigs	10	each	25	24	3	1	0	0.4	0	0
3142	Watermelon, fresh pieces	0.5	cup	80	73	26	0	6	0.4	0	0
5432	Waxgourd, cooked cubes	0.5	cup	87	84	11	0	3	0.9	0	0
5431	Waxgourd, raw, cubes	0.5	cup	66	63	9	0	2	1.9	0	0
56283	Weiner wraps, franks in dough	1	each	85	39	278	7	15	0.4	21	6.8
2177	Wendy's, Frosty dairy dessert, medium	1	each	324	219	478	12	79	0	12	7.6
69058	Wendy's, Jr cheeseburger, deluxe	1	each	179	104	358	18	36	3	17	6
56571	Wendy's, bacon cheeseburger, w/bun	1	each	170	94	389	20	35	2	20	7.2
69059	Wendy's, chicken sandwich, grilled	1	each	177	109	290	25	33	1.9	7	1.4
56574	Wendy's, hamburger, big classic, w/cheese	1	each	287	170	590	35	47	3	30	12.2
56566	Wendy's, hamburger, single, deluxe	1	each	219	136	420	25	37	3	20	7
69057	Wendy's, junior hamburger	1	each	117	56	268	15	34	2	10	3.5
38057	Wheat berries, whole, cooked	0.5	cup	75	65	42	2	10	1.7	0	0
38045	Wheat bran, baked value	0.5	cup	18	2	39	3	12	7.7	1	0.1
38024	Wheat bran, crude	0.25	cup	15	1	32	2	10	6.4	1	0.1
38025	Wheat germ, crude, raw	2	Tbs	12	1	45	3	6	1.6	1	0.2
38333	Wheat germ, defatted, Viobin	0.5	oz.	15	1	45	4	9	3	0	0
38026	Wheat germ, toasted	2	Tbs	14	1	54	4	7	1.8	2	0.3
38055	Wheat germ, w/brown sugar/honey	1	cup	113	4	420	30	66	11.5	9	1.5
38316	Wheat grain, cracked, dry	4	oz.	113	12	384	16	82	13.1	2	0.4
38068	Wheat sprouts	0.5	cup	54	26	107	4	23	0.6	1	0.1
22540	Whiskey sour mix, packet	1	each	17	0	64	0	16	0	0	0
22541	Whiskey sour, canned	2	Tbs	31	24	37	0	4	0	0	0
22518	Wine, dessert, dry	1	cup	236	189	297	0	10	0	0	0
22507	Wine, dessert, sweet	0.5	cup	118	86	181	0	14	0	0	0
20076	Wine, non-alcoholic	1	cup	232	228	14	1	3	0	0	0
20077	Wine, non-alcoholic, light	1	cup	251	246	15	1	3	0	0	0
22501	Wine, red	1	cup	236	209	170	0	4	0	0	0
22600	Wine, rice	4	oz.	113	89	152	1	6	0	0	0
22502	Wine, rose'	1	cup	236	210	168	0	3	0	0	0
22601	Wine, sangria	4	oz.	113	94	93	0	13	0	0	0
22509	Wine, sherry, dry	0.5	cup	117	104	82	0	2	0	0	0
22511	Wine, sweet vermouth	0.5	cup	120	87	184	0	14	0	0	0
22503	Wine, white, dry	1	cup	238	213	158	0	1	0	0	0
22504	Wine, white, medium	1	cup	236	211	160	0	2	0	0	0
5433	Winged bean/goabean leaves, raw	0.5	cup	50	38	37	3	7	1.2	1	0.1
5434	Winged bean/goabean tuber, raw	0.5	cup	50	29	74	6	14	2.8	0	0.1
56111	Wonton, fried, meat filled	3	piece	57	25	183	8	12	0.6	11	2.2
49016	Wonton/eggroll wrapper	3	each	24	7	70	2	14	0.4	0	0.1
5370	Yam, Hawaii Mountain, steamed	0.5	cup	72	56	60	1	14	2.2	0	0
5553	Yam, orange, canned in syrup	0.5	cup	114	88	101	1	24	2.8	0	0
5168	Yam, white, cooked	0.5	cup	68	48	79	1	19	2.6	0	0
5156	Yams, orange, baked, then peeled, mashed	0.5	cup	100	73	103	2	24	3	0	0
5163	Yams, orange, canned, mashed	0.5	cup	128	95	129	3	30	2.2	0	0.1
5160	Yams, orange, peeled, boiled, mashed	0.5	cup	100	73	105	2	24	1.8	0	0.1
28007	Yeast, baker's, compressed cake	1	each	17	12	18	1	3	1.4	0	0
28000	Yeast, baker's, dry active	1	Tbs	8	1	22	3	3	1.6	0	0
28002	Yeast, brewer's	1	Tbs	8	0	23	3	3	2.5	0	0
44068	Yogurt chips	1	oz.	28	1	146	3	16	0.5	8	2.1
2002	Yogurt, custard fruit, lowfat	1	cup	245	183	250	11	47	0	3	1.7
70637	Yogurt, frozen, banana-strawberry, HaagenDaz	0.5	cup	98	—	170	6	27	—	4	2
70633	Yogurt, frozen, peach, HaagenDaz	0.5	cup	98	—	170	6	26	—	4	2
2001	Yogurt, fruit, lowfat	1	cup	245	183	250	11	47	0	3	1.7
2034	Yogurt, fruit, nonfat, low cal sweetener	1	cup	241	208	122	12	19	1.3	0	0.2
2101	Yogurt, lowfat, fruit & nuts	1	cup	245	178	290	11	47	0.5	7	2
2015	Yogurt, lowfat, maple	1	cup	245	194	209	12	34	0	3	2
2014	Yogurt, lowfat, vanilla/lemon	1	cup	245	194	209	12	34	0	3	2
2282	Yogurt, mixed berry, nonfat, Knudsen	6	oz.	170	—	170	8	33	0	0	0
2096	Yogurt, nonfat, lemon	1	cup	245	187	223	12	43	0	0	0.3
2099	Yogurt, nonfat, lemon	1	cup	245	187	223	12	43	0	0	0.3
2098	Yogurt, nonfat, vanilla	1	each	227	173	207	12	40	0	0	0.2
2283	Yogurt, peach, nonfat, Knudsen	6	oz.	170	—	170	8	33	0	0	0
2000	Yogurt, plain, lowfat	1	cup	245	208	155	13	17	0	4	2.4
2012	Yogurt, plain, nonfat	1	cup	245	209	137	14	19	0	0	0.3
2013	Yogurt, plain, whole milk	1	cup	245	215	150	8	11	0	8	5.2

A

MonoF (g)	PolyF (g)	Choles (mg)	Calc (mg)	Phos (mg)	Sod (mg)	Pot (mg)	Zn (mg)	Iron (mg)	Magn (mg)	VitA (μg RE)	VitE (mg α-TE)	VitC (mg)	Thia (mg)	Ribo (mg)	Nia (mg)	B6 (mg)	Fola (μg)	B12 (μg)
0	0	0	30	15	10	82	0	0	5	118	0.25	11	0.02	0.03	0	0.03	2	0
0.1	0.1	0	6	7	2	93	0.1	0.1	9	30	0.12	8	0.06	0.02	0.2	0.12	2	0
0	0.1	0	16	15	93	4	0.5	0.3	9	0	0.34	9	0.03	0	0.3	0.03	3	0
0	0.1	0	12	12	73	4	0.4	0.3	7	0	0.26	9	0.03	0.07	0.3	0.02	3	0
9.6	3.4	22	137	103	818	131	1	1.2	10	14	0.82	10	0.19	0.16	2	0.06	5	0.59
—	—	54	446	356	260	776	1.4	1.6	65	217	—	0	0.15	0.67	0.5	0.17	25	1.2
—	—	50	179	—	885	—	—	3.4	—	99	—	6	—	—	—	—	—	—
10.5	1.4	61	174	342	870	384	6	3.5	39	82	—	6	0.31	0.32	6.6	0.27	29	2.04
—	—	61	94	—	740	—	—	2.5	—	38	—	6	—	—	—	—	—	—
—	—	102	254	—	1485	588	—	5.5	—	153	—	15	0.46	1.55	6.1	—	—	—
—	—	70	130	—	920	468	—	4.7	—	60	—	6	0.43	0.33	5.8	—	—	—
—	—	30	109	—	605	—	—	3	—	20	—	1	—	—	—	—	—	—
0	0.1	0	4	39	0	50	0.4	0.4	17	0	0.15	0	0.06	0.02	0.8	0.04	6	0
0.1	0.4	0	13	182	0	213	1.3	1.9	110	0	0.47	0	0.08	0.09	2.2	0.21	10	0
0.1	0.3	0	11	152	0	177	1.1	1.6	92	0	0.35	0	0.08	0.09	2	0.2	12	0
0.2	0.8	0	5	105	2	112	1.5	0.8	30	0	2.25	0	0.24	0.06	0.9	0.16	35	0
0	0.1	0	10	179	1	174	2.1	1.5	52	250	0.01	—	0.15	0.08	1.2	0.22	63	0.08
0.2	0.9	0	6	162	1	134	2.4	1.3	45	0	2.56	1	0.24	0.12	0.8	0.14	50	0
1.2	5.5	0	56	1142	12	1089	15.7	9.1	307	11	24.9	0	1.51	0.78	5.3	0.56	376	0
0.3	0.9	0	39	392	6	459	3.3	4.4	156	0	0.48	0	0.51	0.24	7.2	0.39	50	0
0.1	0.3	0	15	108	9	91	0.9	1.2	44	0	0.03	1	0.12	0.08	1.7	0.14	20	0
0	0	0	45	2	46	3	0	0.1	3	1	0	0	0	0	0	0	0	0
0	0	0	0	2	14	3	0	0	0	0	0	0	0	0	0	0	0	0
0	0	0	19	21	21	217	0.2	0.6	21	0	0	0	0.04	0.04	0.5	0	1	0
0	0	0	9	11	11	109	0.1	0.3	11	0	0	0	0.02	0.02	0.3	0	0	0
0	0	0	21	35	16	204	0.2	0.9	23	0	0	0	0	0.02	0.2	0.05	2	0
0	0	0	23	38	18	221	0.2	1	25	0	0	0	0	0.02	0.3	0.05	3	0
0	0	0	19	33	12	264	0.2	1	31	0	0	0	0.01	0.07	0.2	0.08	5	0.02
0	0	0	6	7	2	28	0	0.1	7	0	0	0	0	0	0	0	0	0
0	0	0	19	35	12	234	0.1	0.9	24	0	0	0	0.01	0.04	0.2	0.06	3	0.02
0	0	0	5	6	8	40	0.1	0.1	4	1	0.01	4	0.01	0.01	0	0.01	2	0
0	0	0	9	16	9	104	0.1	0.5	12	0	0	0	0	0.02	0.1	0.03	1	0.01
0	0	0	10	11	11	110	0.1	0.3	11	0	0	0	0.02	0.02	0.3	0	0	0
0	0	0	22	14	10	146	0.2	0.8	22	0	0	0	0	0.01	0.2	0.05	0	0
0	0	0	21	33	12	189	0.2	0.8	24	0	0	0	0.01	0.01	0.2	0.03	0	0
0.1	0.1	0	112	32	4	88	0.6	2	4	405	—	22	0.42	0.3	1.7	0.12	8	0
0.1	0.1	0	15	22	18	293	0.7	1	12	0	—	0	0.19	0.08	0.8	0.04	10	0
4.9	3.6	39	17	72	250	114	0.7	1.2	13	65	1.71	1	0.24	0.17	1.8	0.1	10	0.17
0	0.1	2	11	19	137	20	0.2	0.8	5	1	0.02	0	0.12	0.09	1.3	0.01	21	0
0	0	0	6	29	9	359	0.2	0.3	7	0	—	0	0.06	0.01	0.1	0.15	9	0
0	0.1	0	17	31	50	211	0.2	0.9	15	652	0.26	12	0.03	0.05	0.5	0.06	7	0
0	0	0	10	33	5	456	0.1	0.4	12	0	0.11	8	0.06	0.02	0.4	0.16	11	0
0	0	0	28	55	10	348	0.3	0.4	20	2182	0.28	25	0.07	0.13	0.6	0.24	23	0
0	0.1	0	38	67	96	269	0.3	1.7	31	1936	0.35	7	0.04	0.12	1.2	0.3	14	0
0	0.1	0	21	27	13	184	0.3	0.6	10	1705	0.28	17	0.05	0.14	0.6	0.24	11	0
0.2	0	0	3	57	5	102	1.7	0.6	7	0	0.01	0	0.32	0.19	2.1	0.07	133	0
0.2	0	0	5	97	4	150	0.5	1.2	7	0	0.01	0	0.18	0.41	3	0.12	176	0
0	0	0	17	140	10	151	0.6	1.4	18	0	—	0	1.25	0.34	3	0.4	313	0
3.5	2.1	1	37	47	13	63	0.3	0.9	7	3	0.69	0	0.12	0.12	1	0.02	5	0.08
0.7	0.1	10	372	292	143	478	1.8	0.2	36	27	0.07	2	0.09	0.44	0.2	0.1	23	1.14
2	0	60	146	195	50	170	—	0.4	—	—	—	4	—	0.17	—	—	—	—
2	0	40	146	146	45	160	—	0.4	—	—	—	—	—	0.17	—	—	—	—
0.7	0.1	10	372	292	143	478	1.8	0.2	36	27	0.07	2	0.09	0.44	0.2	0.1	23	1.14
0.1	0	3	369	291	139	550	1.8	0.6	41	6	0.17	26	0.1	0.45	0.5	0.11	32	1.11
3.7	1.3	10	364	305	139	490	2.2	0.3	44	27	0.29	2	0.15	0.43	0.3	0.11	25	1.11
0.8	0.1	12	419	331	161	537	2	0.2	40	32	0.08	2	0.1	0.49	0.3	0.11	26	1.29
0.8	0.1	12	419	331	161	537	2	0.2	40	32	0.08	2	0.1	0.49	0.3	0.11	26	1.29
0	0	5	250	200	105	370	—	0	—	0	—	0	0.03	0.26	—	—	—	0.9
0.1	0	4	436	343	168	559	2.1	0.2	42	4	0.01	2	0.1	0.52	0.3	0.12	27	1.34
0.1	0	4	436	343	168	559	2.1	0.2	42	4	0.01	2	0.1	0.52	0.3	0.12	27	1.34
0.1	0	4	404	318	155	518	2	0.2	39	4	0.01	2	0.1	0.48	0.3	0.11	25	1.24
0	0	5	250	200	105	370	—	—	—	0	—	0	0.03	0.26	—	—	—	0.9
1	0.1	15	448	353	172	573	2.2	0.2	43	39	0.1	2	0.11	0.52	0.3	0.12	27	1.38
0.1	0	4	488	385	187	625	2.4	0.2	47	5	0.01	2	0.12	0.57	0.3	0.13	30	1.5
2.2	0.2	31	296	233	114	380	1.4	0.1	28	74	0.22	1	0.07	0.35	0.2	0.08	18	0.91

A

Esha Code	Food Item	Qty	Meas	Wgt (g)	Wtr (g)	Cals	Prot (g)	Carb (g)	Fib (g)	Fat (g)	SatF (g)
2284	Yogurt, red raspberry, nonfat, Knudsen	6	oz.	170	—	160	8	31	0	0	0
2285	Yogurt, strawberry, nonfat, Knudsen	6	oz.	170	—	160	8	32	0	0	0

MonoF	PolyF	Choles	Calc	Phos	Sod	Pot	Zn	Iron	Magn	VitA	VitE	VitC	Thia	Ribo	Nia	B6	Fola	B12
(g)	(g)	(mg)	(mg)	(mg)	(mg)	(mg)	(mg)	(mg)	(mg)	(μg RE)	(mg α-TE)	(mg)	(mg)	(mg)	(mg)	(mg)	(μg)	(μg)
0	0	5	250	200	105	360	—	0	—	0	—	0	0.03	0.26	—	—	—	0.9
0	0	5	250	200	105	380	—	0	—	0	—	0	0.03	0.26	—	—	—	0.9

Appendix B

B Anthropometric Standards of Body Weight and Composition

1983 Metropolitan Life Insurance Co. Height and Weight Tables

Height	Small Frame	Medium Frame	Large Frame
	←	lb	→
Men°			
5′2″	128–134	131–141	138–150
5′3″	130–136	133–143	140–153
5′4″	132–138	135–145	142–156
5′5″	134–140	137–148	144–160
5′6″	136–142	139–151	146–164
5′7″	138–145	142–154	149–168
5′8″	140–148	145–157	152–172
5′9″	142–151	148–160	155–176
5′10″	144–154	151–163	158–180
5′11″	146–157	154–166	161–184
6′0″	149–160	157–170	164–188
6′1″	152–164	160–174	168–192
6′2″	155–168	164–178	172–197
6′3″	158–172	167–182	176–202
6′4″	162–176	171–187	181–207
Women†			
4′10″	102–111	109–121	118–131
4′11″	103–113	111–123	120–134
5′0″	104–115	113–126	122–137
5′1″	106–118	115–129	125–140
5′2″	108–121	118–132	128–143
5′3″	111–124	121–135	131–147
5′4″	114–127	124–138	134–151
5′5″	117–130	127–141	137–155
5′6″	120–133	130–144	140–159
5′7″	123–136	133–147	143–163
5′8″	126–139	136–150	146–167
5′9″	129–142	139–153	149–170
5′10″	132–145	142–156	152–173
5′11″	135–148	145–159	155–176
6′0″	138–151	148–162	158–179

°Weights at ages 25 to 59 based on lowest mortality. Weight in pounds according to frame (in indoor clothing weighing 5 lb, shoes with 1″ heels).

†Weights at ages 25 to 59 based on lowest mortality. Weight in pounds according to frame (in indoor clothing weighing 3 lb, shoes with 1″ heels).

Courtesy of Metropolitan Life Insurance Company.

Weight-for-Height Tables for Adults—Gerontology Center Recommendations

Height (ft and in)	Gerontology Research Center* (Age-Specific Weight Range in Pounds for Men and Women)				
	20–29 yr	30–39 yr	40–49 yr	50–59 yr	60–69 yr
4′10″	84–111	92–119	99–127	107–135	115–142
4′11″	87–115	95–123	103–131	111–139	119–147
5′0″	90–119	98–127	106–135	114–143	123–152
5′1″	93–123	101–131	110–140	118–148	127–157
5′2″	96–127	105–136	113–144	122–153	131–163
5′3″	99–131	108–140	117–149	126–158	135–168
5′4″	102–135	112–145	121–154	130–163	140–173
5′5″	106–140	115–149	125–159	134–168	144–179
5′6″	109–144	119–154	129–164	138–174	148–184
5′7″	112–148	122–159	133–169	143–179	153–190
5′8″	116–153	126–163	137–174	147–184	158–196
5′9″	119–157	130–168	141–179	151–190	162–201
5′10″	122–162	134–173	145–184	156–195	167–207
5′11″	126–167	137–178	149–190	160–201	172–213
6′0″	129–171	141–183	153–195	165–207	177–219
6′1″	133–176	145–188	157–200	169–213	182–225
6′2″	137–181	149–194	162–206	174–219	187–232
6′3″	141–186	153–199	166–212	179–225	192–238
6′4″	144–191	157–205	171–218	184–231	197–244

*Values in this table are for height without shoes and weight without clothes.

Healthy Weight Ranges for Men and Women

Height*	Weight (in pounds)†
4′10″	91–119
4′11″	94–124
5′0″	97–128
5′1″	101–132
5′2″	104–137
5′3″	107–141
5′4″	111–146
5′5″	114–150
5′6″	118–155
5′7″	121–160
5′8″	125–164
5′9″	129–169
5′10″	132–174
5′11″	136–179
6′0″	140–184
6′1″	144–189
6′2″	148–195
6′3″	152–200
6′4″	156–205
6′5″	160–211
6′6″	164–216

*Without shoes.
†Without clothes.

Source: Dietary Guidelines for Americans, USDA, DHS, 1995. Derived from National Research Council, 1989, for adults, p. 564.

B

B

BOYS: BIRTH TO 36 MONTHS
PHYSICAL GROWTH
NCHS PERCENTILES*

NAME ______________________ RECORD # ________

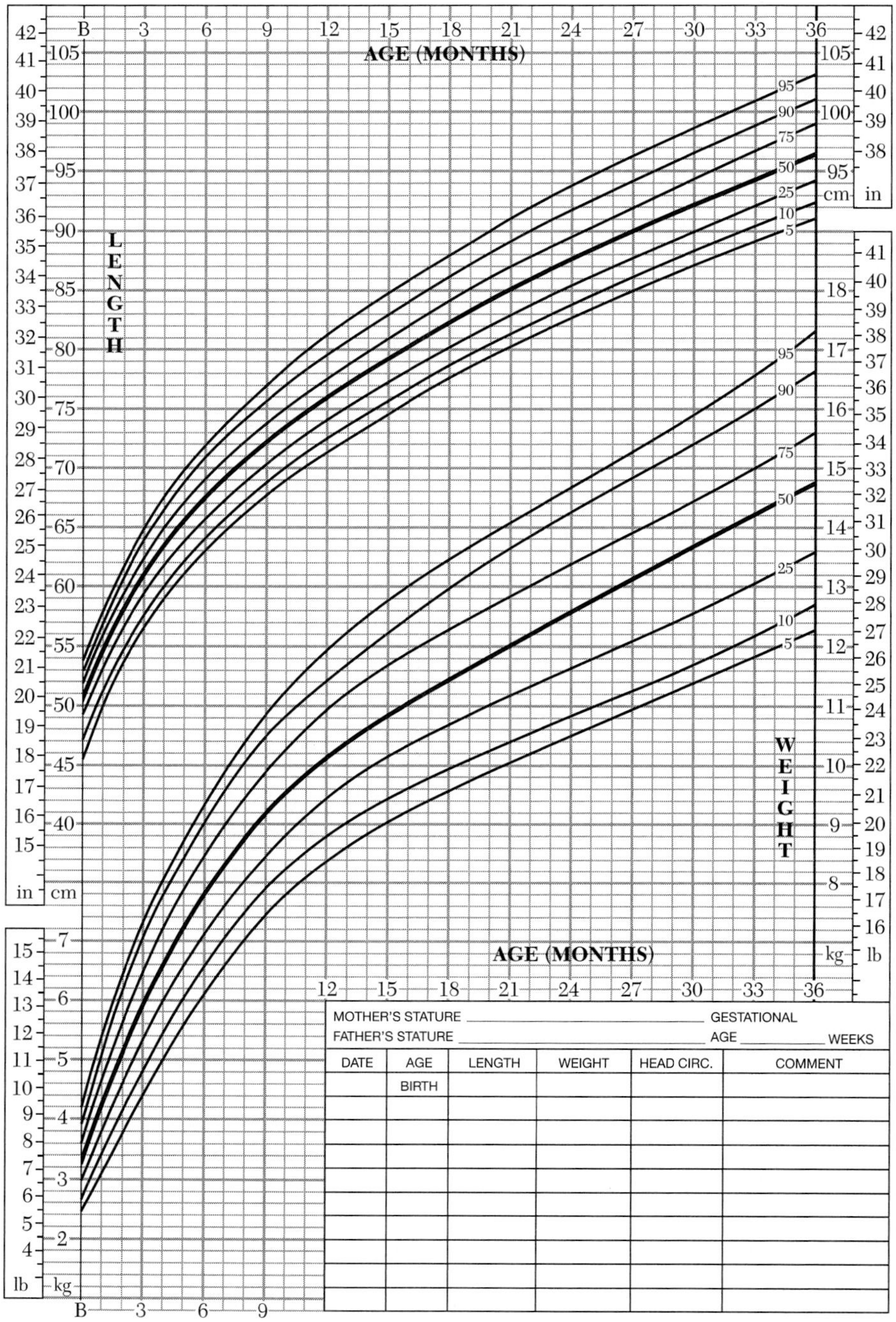

*Adapted from: Hamill PVV, Drizd TA, Johnson CL, Reed RB, Roche AF, Moore WM: Physical growth: National Center for Health Statistics percentiles. AM J CLIN NUTR 32: 607-629, 1979. Data from the Fels Research Institute, Wright State University School of Medicine, Yellow Springs, Ohio.

GIRLS: BIRTH TO 36 MONTHS
PHYSICAL GROWTH
NCHS PERCENTILES*

NAME ______________________ RECORD # ________

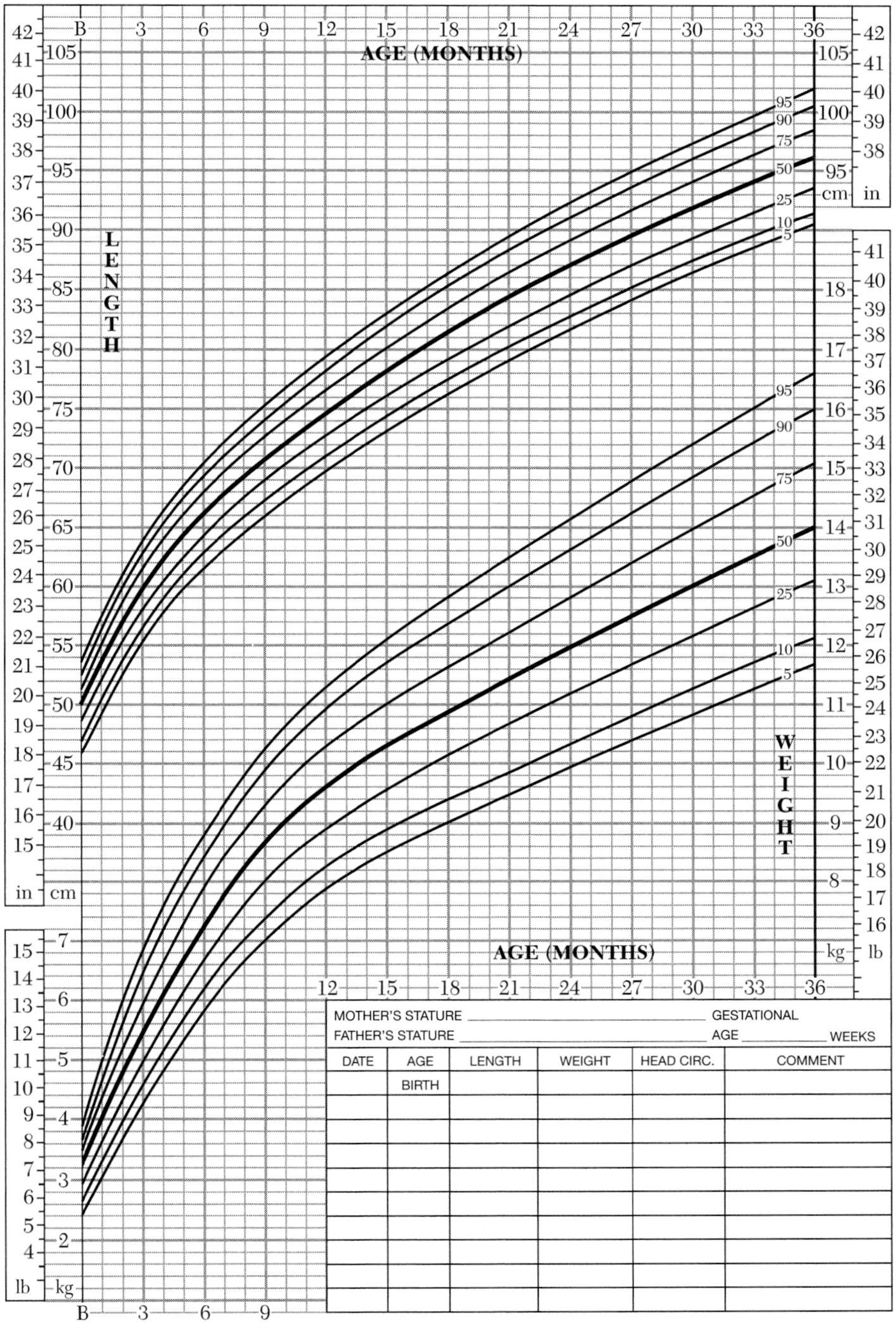

MOTHER'S STATURE ______________ GESTATIONAL
FATHER'S STATURE ______________ AGE ________ WEEKS

DATE	AGE	LENGTH	WEIGHT	HEAD CIRC.	COMMENT
	BIRTH				

*Adapted from: Hamill PVV, Drizd TA, Johnson CL, Reed RB, Roche AF, Moore WM: Physical growth: National Center for Health Statistics percentiles. AM J CLIN NUTR 32: 607-629, 1979. Data from the Fels Research Institute, Wright State University School of Medicine, Yellow Springs, Ohio.

BOYS: 2 TO 18 YEARS
PHYSICAL GROWTH
NCHS PERCENTILES*

NAME ______________________ RECORD # __________

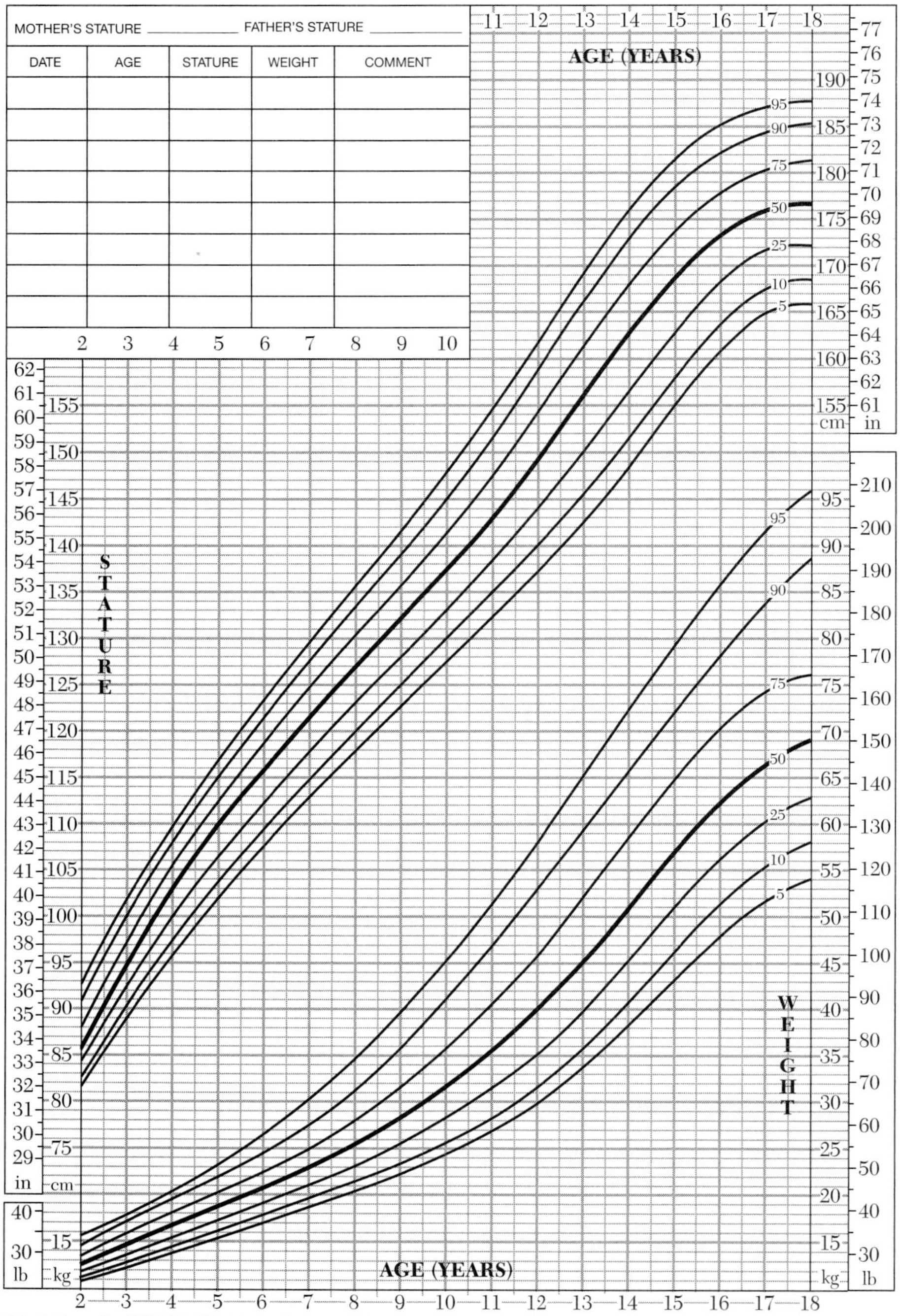

*Adapted from: Hamill PVV, Drizd TA, Johnson CL, Reed RB, Roche AF, Moore WM: Physical growth: National Center for Health Statistics percentiles. AM J CLIN NUTR 32: 607-629, 1979. Data from the Fels Research Institute, Wright State University School of Medicine, Yellow Springs, Ohio.

GIRLS: 2 TO 18 YEARS
PHYSICAL GROWTH
NCHS PERCENTILES*

NAME ____________ RECORD # ______

MOTHER'S STATURE ______	FATHER'S STATURE ______			
DATE	AGE	STATURE	WEIGHT	COMMENT

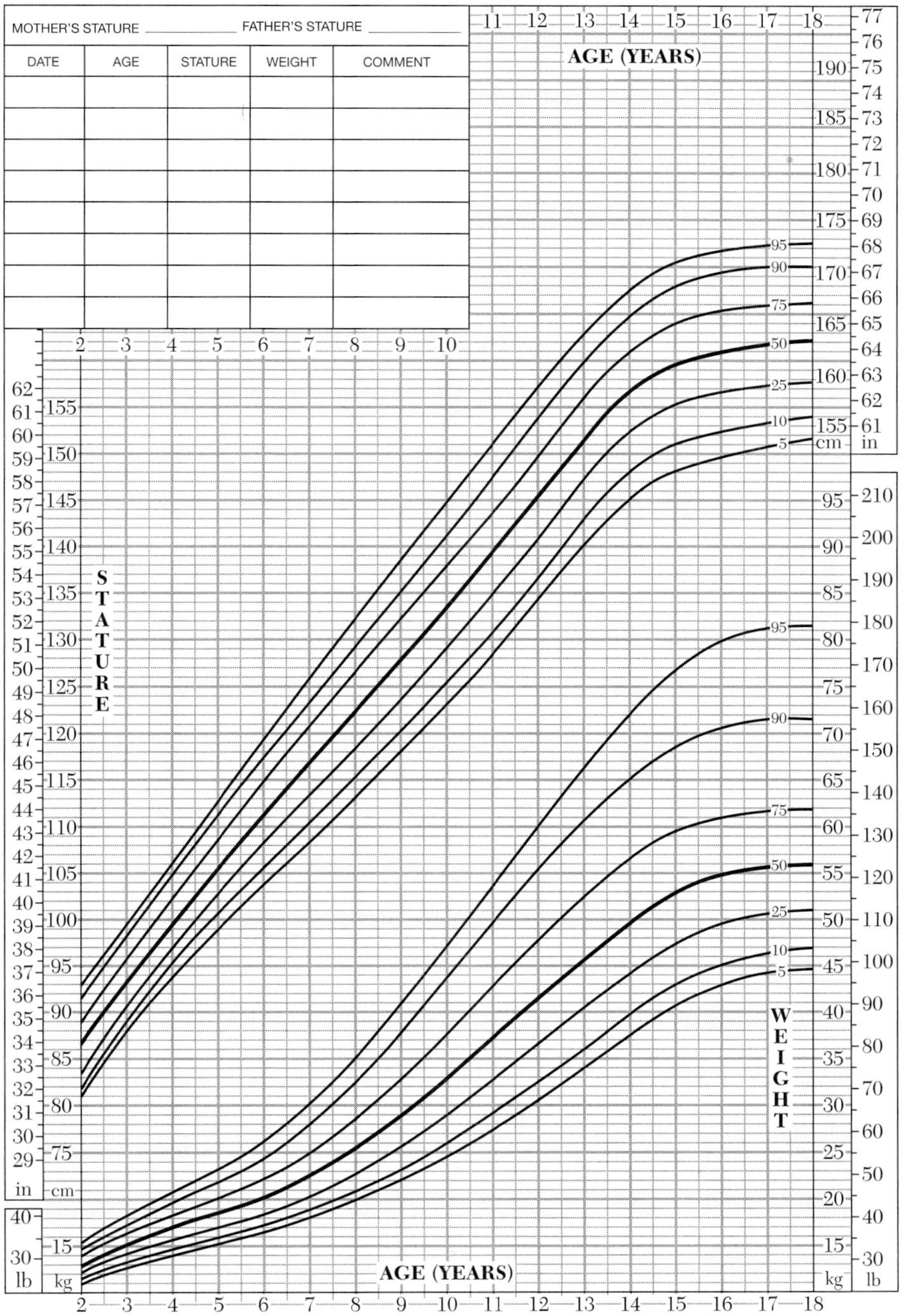

*Adapted from: Hamill PVV, Drizd TA, Johnson CL, Reed RB, Roche AF, Moore WM: Physical growth: National Center for Health Statistics percentiles. AM J CLIN NUTR 32: 607-629, 1979. Data from the National Center for Health Statistics (NCHS) Hyattsville, Maryland.

B

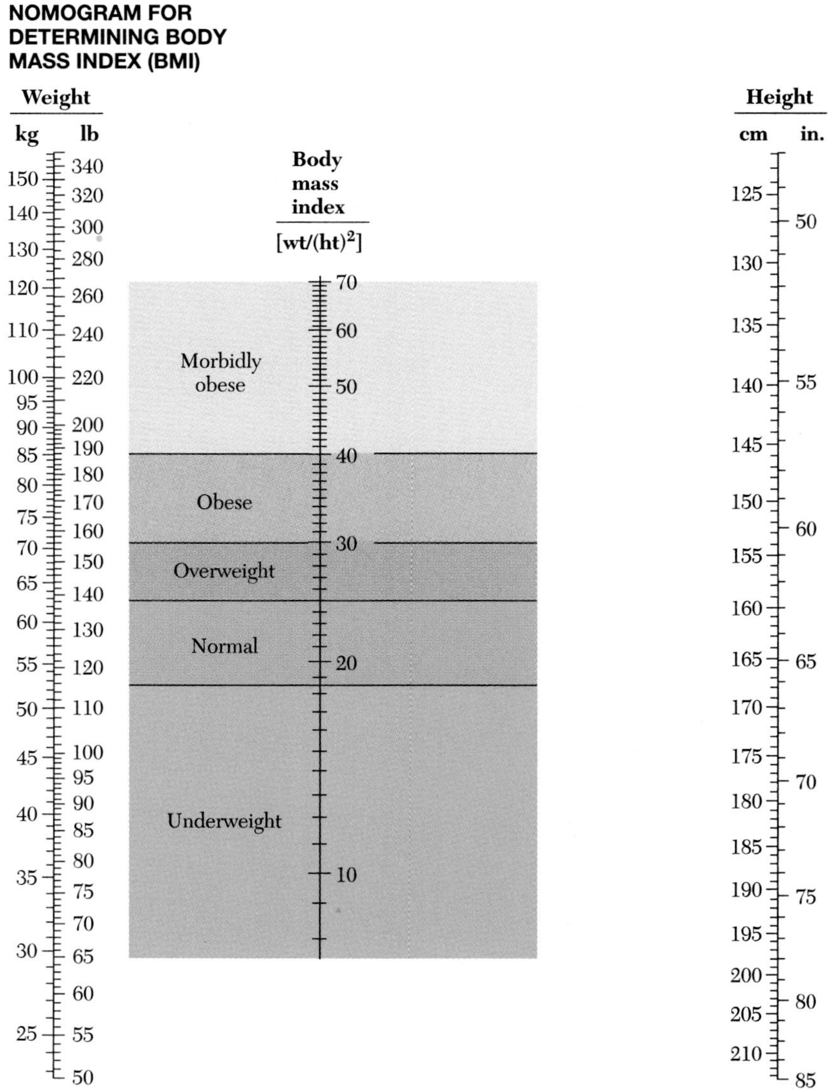

*Estimation of Frame Size Using Elbow Breadth**

MEN Height in 1-Inch Heels	Elbow Breadth	WOMEN Height in 1-Inch Heels	Elbow Breadth
5 ft 2 in. to 5 ft 3 in.	2½ to 2⅞ in.	4 ft 10 in. to 4 ft 11 in.	2¼ to 2½ in.
5 ft 4 in. to 5 ft 7 in.	2⅝ to 2⅞ in.	5 ft 0 in. to 5 ft 3 in.	2¼ to 2½ in.
5 ft 8 in. to 5 ft 11 in.	2¾ to 3 in.	5 ft 4 in. to 5 ft 7 in.	2⅜ to 2⅝ in.
6 ft 0 in. to 6 ft 3 in.	2¾ to 3⅛ in.	5 ft 8 in. to 5 ft 11 in.	2⅜ to 2⅝ in.
6 ft 4 in. and over	2⅞ to 3¼ in.	6 ft 0 in. and over	2½ to 2¾ in.

*If your measurement is within the range indicated, you have a medium frame. Measurements smaller than those listed indicate a small frame, and those larger indicate a large frame. Elbow breadth is measured as the distance between the bony protrusions of the elbow. For this measurement the right arm is raised to the horizontal, and the elbow flexed to 90 degrees, with the back of the hand facing the measurer.

Source: Metropolitan Life Insurance Company.

*Equation for Predicting Resting Metabolic Rate From Body Weight**

Sex and Age Range (years)	Equation to Derive RMR in kcal/day
Males	
0–3	$(60.9 \times wt^{\dagger}) - 54$
3–10	$(22.7 \times wt) + 495$
10–18	$(17.5 \times wt) + 651$
18–30	$(15.3 \times wt) + 679$
30–60	$(11.6 \times wt) + 879$
>60	$(13.5 \times wt) + 487$
Females	
0–3	$(61.0 \times wt) - 51$
3–10	$(22.5 \times wt) + 499$
10–18	$(12.2 \times wt) + 746$
18–30	$(14.7 \times wt) + 496$
30–60	$(8.7 \times wt) + 829$
>60	$(10.5 \times wt) + 596$

* From WHO (1985). These equations were derived from BMR data.
† Weight of person in kilograms.

Source: From National Research Council, *Recommended Dietary Allowances*, 10th ed. (Washington, D.C.: National Academy of Sciences, 1989).

Appendix C

Normal Blood Values of Nutritional Relevance

C

Red blood cells	
Men	4.6–6.2 million/mm^3
Women	4.2–5.2 million/mm^3
White blood cells	5,000–10,000/mm^3
Hematocrit	
Men	40–54 ml/100 ml
Women	36–47 ml/100 ml
Children	35–49 ml/100 ml
Hemoglobin	
Men	14–18 g/100 ml
Women	12–16 g/100 ml
Children	11.2–16.5 g/100 ml
Ferritin	
Men	20–300 ng/ml
Women	20–120 ng/ml
Calcium	9–11 mg/100 ml
Iodine	3.8–8 μg/100 ml
Iron	
Men	75–175 μg/100 ml
Women	65–165 μg/100 ml
Zinc	0.75–1.4 μg/ml
Magnesium	1.8–3.0 mg/100 ml
Potassium	3.5–5.0 mEq/liter
Sodium	136–145 mEq/liter
Chloride	100–108 mEq/liter
Vitamin A	20–80 μg/100 ml
Vitamin B_{12}	200–800 pg/100 ml
Vitamin C	0.6–2.0 mg/100 ml
Carotene	48–200 μg/liter
Folate	2–20 ng/ml
pH	7.35–7.45
Total protein	6.6–8.0 g/100 ml
Albumen	3.0–4.0 g/100 ml
Cholesterol	<200 mg/100 ml
LDL Cholesterol	<160 mg/100 ml
HDL Cholesterol	>35 mg/100 ml
Triglycerides	<150 mg/100 ml
Glucose	60–100 mg/100 ml blood, 70–120 mg/100 ml serum

Source: Handbook of Clinical Dietetics, American Dietetic Association, © 1981 by Yale University Press (New Haven, Conn.); and Committee on Dietetics of the Mayo Clinic, *Mayo Clinic Diet Manual* (Philadelphia: W. B. Saunders Company, 1981), pp. 275–277.

Blood Pressure Levels

Blood pressure is measured in millimeters of mercury (mm Hg). The classifications in the following table are for persons who are not taking antihypertensive drugs and are not acutely ill. When systolic and diastolic pressures fall into different categories, the physician will select the higher category to classify the person's blood pressure status. Diagnosis of high blood pressure is based on the average of two or more readings taken at each of two or more visits after an initial screening.

Classification of Blood Pressure for Adults Age 18 Years and Older, With Recommended Follow-Up

Category	Systolic (mm Hg)		Diastolic (mm Hg)	Follow-Up Recommended
Optimal*	<120	and	<80	Recheck in 2 years
Normal	<130	and	<85	Recheck in 2 years
High normal	130–139	or	85–89	Recheck in 1 year
Hypertension				
STAGE 1 (Mild)	140–159	or	90–99	Confirm within 2 months
STAGE 2 (Moderate)	160–179	or	100–109	Evaluate within 1 month
STAGE 3 (Severe)	≥180	or	≥110	Evaluate immediately or within 1 week depending on clinical situation

* Unusually low readings should be evaluated for clinical significance.

Source: Sixth Report of the Joint National Committee on Detection, Evaluation, and Treatment of High Blood Pressure, NIH, 1997.

Appendix D

Sources of Information on Nutrition

Many publications are available at little or no cost from the government. For individual publications or catalogs, write to:

Superintendent of Documents
U.S. Government Printing Office
Washington, DC 20402

National Technical Information Service
5285 Port Royal Road
Springfield, VA 22162

National Research Council
National Academy of Sciences
2102 Constitution Ave. N.W.
Washington, DC 20418

Consumer Information Service
Department 609K
Pueblo, CO 81009

Food Safety and Inspection Administration
USDA
Washington, DC 20250

Food and Nutrition Service
500 12th St. S.W.
Washington, DC 20250

Food and Drug Administration
5600 Fishers Lane
Rockville, MD 20852

The Food and Nutrition Information Center
National Agriculture Library
Room 304
10301 Baltimore Blvd.
Beltsville, MD 20705

Data Dissemination Branch
Division of Data Services
National Center for Health Statistics
6265 Belcrest Road
Hyattsville, MD 20782

Health Nutrition Information Service
Federal Center Building
Hyattsville, MD 20782

National Cancer Institute
Office of Cancer Communications
Building 31, Room 10A18
Bethesda, MD 20205

Agriculture Research Service
USDA
3700 East West Hwy.
Hyattsville, MD 20782

National Institute on Aging
Information Office
Building 31, Room 5C35
Bethesda, MD 20205

National Heart, Lung, and Blood Institute
Information Office
Building 31, Room 4A21
Bethesda, MD 20205

National Institute of Dental Research
Information Office
Building 31, Room 2C34
Bethesda, MD 20205

Health and Welfare Canada
Canadian Government Publishing Center
Minister of Supply and Services
Ottawa, Ontario K1A 0S9

Many private and international organizations also publish reputable food and nutrition information. Some of these include:

American Dietetic Association
216 W. Jackson Blvd.
Suite 800
Chicago, IL 60606-6995

National Dairy Council
6300 North River Road
Rosemont, IL 60018-4233

American Heart Association
7320 Grenville Ave.
Dallas, TX 75231

American Diabetes Association
Diabetes Information Service Center
1660 Duke St.
Alexandria, VA 22314

American Cancer Society
90 Park Ave.
New York, NY 10016

Canadian Dietetic Association
480 University Ave.
Suite 601
Toronto, Ontario M5G 1V2

The World Health Organization
1211 Geneva 27
Switzerland

The Food and Agriculture Organization
North American Regional Office
1325 C St. S.W.
Washington, DC 20025

These and many other sources of nutrition information are available online. For easy access to these, use the *Nutrition: Science and Applications* Web site at ***www.Wiley.com/college/Smolin*** and click on **Student Companion Site** for chapter-by-chapter links.

Appendix E

Canadian Nutritional Recommendations and Guidelines

Recommended Nutrient Intakes (RNI): Summary of Examples of Recommended Nutrient Intake Based on Energy Expressed as Daily Rates

Age	Sex	Energy (kcal)	Thiamin (mg)	Riboflavin (mg)	Niacin (NE[b])	N-3 PUFA[a] (g)	n-6 PUFA (g)
Months							
0–4	Both	600	0.3	0.3	4	0.5	3
5–12	Both	900	0.4	0.5	7	0.5	3
Years							
1	Both	1100	0.5	0.6	8	0.6	4
2–3	Both	1300	0.6	0.7	9	0.7	4
4–6	Both	1800	0.7	0.9	13	1.0	6
7–9	M	2200	0.9	1.1	16	1.2	7
	F	1900	0.8	1.0	14	1.0	6
10–12	M	2500	1.0	1.3	18	1.4	8
	F	2200	0.9	1.1	16	1.2	7
13–15	M	2800	1.1	1.4	20	1.5	9
	F	2200	0.9	1.1	16	1.2	7
16–18	M	3200	1.3	1.6	23	1.8	11
	F	2100	0.8	1.1	15	1.2	7
19–24	M	3000	1.2	1.5	22	1.6	10
	F	2100	0.8	1.1	15	1.2	7
25–49	M	2700	1.1	1.4	19	1.5	9
	F	1900	0.8[c]	1.0[c]	14[c]	1.1[c]	7[c]
50–74	M	2300	0.9	1.2	16	1.3	8
	F	1800	0.8[c]	1.0[c]	14[c]	1.1[c]	7[c]
75+	M	2000	0.8	1.0	14	1.1	7
	F[d]	1700	0.8[c]	1.0[c]	14[c]	1.1[c]	7[c]
Pregnancy (additional)							
1st trimester		100	0.1	0.1	1	0.05	0.3
2nd trimester		300	0.1	0.3	2	0.16	0.9
3rd trimester		300	0.1	0.3	2	0.16	0.9
Lactation (additional)		450	0.2	0.4	3	0.25	1.5

[a]PUFA: polyunsaturated fatty acids.
[b]Niacin equivalents.
[c]Level below which intake should not fall.
[d]Assumes moderate (more than average) physical activity.

Source: Reprinted from Health and Welfare Canada, *Nutrition Recommendations: The Report of the Scientific Review Committee* (Ottawa: Supply and Services Canada, 1990). Copyright, Health and Welfare Canada, with corrections.

Recommended Nutrient Intakes (RNI): Summary Examples of Recommended Nutrient Intake Based on Age and Body Weight Expressed as Daily Rates

Age	Sex	Weight (kg)	Protein (g)	Vit. A (RE[a])	Vit. D (μg)	Vit. E (mg)	Vit. C (mg)	Folate (μg)	Vit. B_{12} (μg)	Calcium (mg)	Phosphorus (mg)	Magnesium (mg)	Iron (mg)	Iodine (μg)	Zinc (mg)
Months															
0–4	Both	6.0	12[b]	400	10	3	20	25	0.3	250[c]	150	20	0.3[d]	30	2[d]
5–12	Both	9.0	12	400	10	3	20	40	0.4	400	200	32	7	40	3
Years															
1	Both	11	13	400	10	3	20	40	0.5	500	300	40	6	55	4
2–3	Both	14	16	400	5	4	20	50	0.6	550	350	50	6	65	4
4–6	Both	18	19	500	5	5	25	70	0.8	600	400	65	8	85	5
7–9	M	25	26	700	2.5	7	25	90	1.0	700	500	100	8	110	7
	F	25	26	700	2.5	6	25	90	1.0	700	500	100	8	95	7
10–12	M	34	34	800	2.5	8	25	120	1.0	900	700	130	8	125	9
	F	36	36	800	2.5	7	25	130	1.0	1100	800	135	8	110	9
13–15	M	50	49	900	2.5	9	30[e]	175	1.0	1100	900	185	10	160	12
	F	48	46	800	2.5	7	30[e]	170	1.0	1000	850	180	13	160	9
16–18	M	62	58	1000	2.5	10	40[e]	220	1.0	900	1000	230	10	160	12
	F	53	47	800	2.5	7	30[e]	190	1.0	700	850	200	12	160	9
19–24	M	71	61	1000	2.5	10	40[e]	220	1.0	800	1000	240	9	160	12
	F	58	50	800	2.5	7	30[e]	180	1.0	700	850	200	13	160	9
25–49	M	74	64	1000	2.5	9	40[e]	230	1.0	800	1000	250	9	160	12
	F	59	51	800	2.5	6	30[e]	185	1.0	700	850	200	13	160	9
50–74	M	73	63	1000	5	7	40[e]	230	1.0	800	1000	250	9	160	12
	F	63	54	800	5	6	30[e]	195	1.0	800	850	210	8	160	9
75+	M	69	59	1000	5	6	40[e]	215	1.0	800	1000	230	9	160	12
	F	64	55	800	5	5	30[e]	200	1.0	800	850	210	8	160	9
Pregnancy (additional)															
1st trimester			5	0	2.5	2	0	200	0.2	500	200	15	0	25	6
2nd trimester			20	0	2.5	2	10	200	0.2	500	200	45	5	25	6
3rd trimester			24	0	2.5	2	10	200	0.2	500	200	45	10	25	6
Lactation (additional)			20	400	2.5	3	25	100	0.2	500	200	65	0	50	6

[a] Retinol equivalents.
[b] Protein is assumed to be from breast milk and must be adjusted for infant formula.
[c] Infant formula with high phosphorus should contain 375 mg calcium.
[d] Breast milk is assumed to be the source of the mineral.
[e] Smokers should increase vitamin C by 50%.

Source: Reprinted from Health and Welfare Canada, *Nutrition Recommendations: The Report of the Scientific Review Committee* (Ottawa: Supply and Services Canada, 1990). Copyright, Health and Welfare Canada, with corrections.

Nutrition Recommendations for Canadians

- The Canadian diet should provide energy consistent with the maintenance of *body weight* within the recommended range.
- The Canadian diet should include *essential nutrients* in amounts recommended.
- The Canadian diet should include no more than 30 percent of energy as *fat* (33 grams/1000 kcalories or 39 grams/5000 kilojoules) and no more than 10 percent as saturated fat (11 grams/1000 kcalories or 13 grams/5000 kilojoules).
- The Canadian diet should provide 55 percent of energy as *carbohydrate* (138 grams/1000 kcalories or 165 grams/5000 kilojoules) from a variety of sources.
- The *sodium* content of the Canadian diet should be reduced.
- The Canadian diet should include no more than 5 percent of total energy as *alcohol*, or two drinks daily, whichever is less.
- The Canadian diet should contain no more *caffeine* than the equivalent of four regular cups of coffee per day.
- Community water supplies containing less than 1 milligram per liter should be *fluoridated* to that level.

Note: Italics added to highlight areas of concern.

Source: Health and Welfare Canada, *Nutrition Recommendations: The Report of the Scientific Review Committee* (Ottawa: Canadian Government Publishing Centre, 1990).

Canada's Guidelines for Healthy Eating

1. Enjoy a VARIETY of foods.
2. Emphasize cereals, breads, other grain products, vegetables, and fruit.
3. Choose lower-fat dairy products, leaner meats, and foods prepared with little or no fat.
4. Achieve and maintain a healthy body weight by enjoying regular physical activity and healthy eating.
5. Limit salt, alcohol, and caffeine.

Source: Minister of Supply and Services, Canada, 1992. Cat. No. 1139-252/1992E.

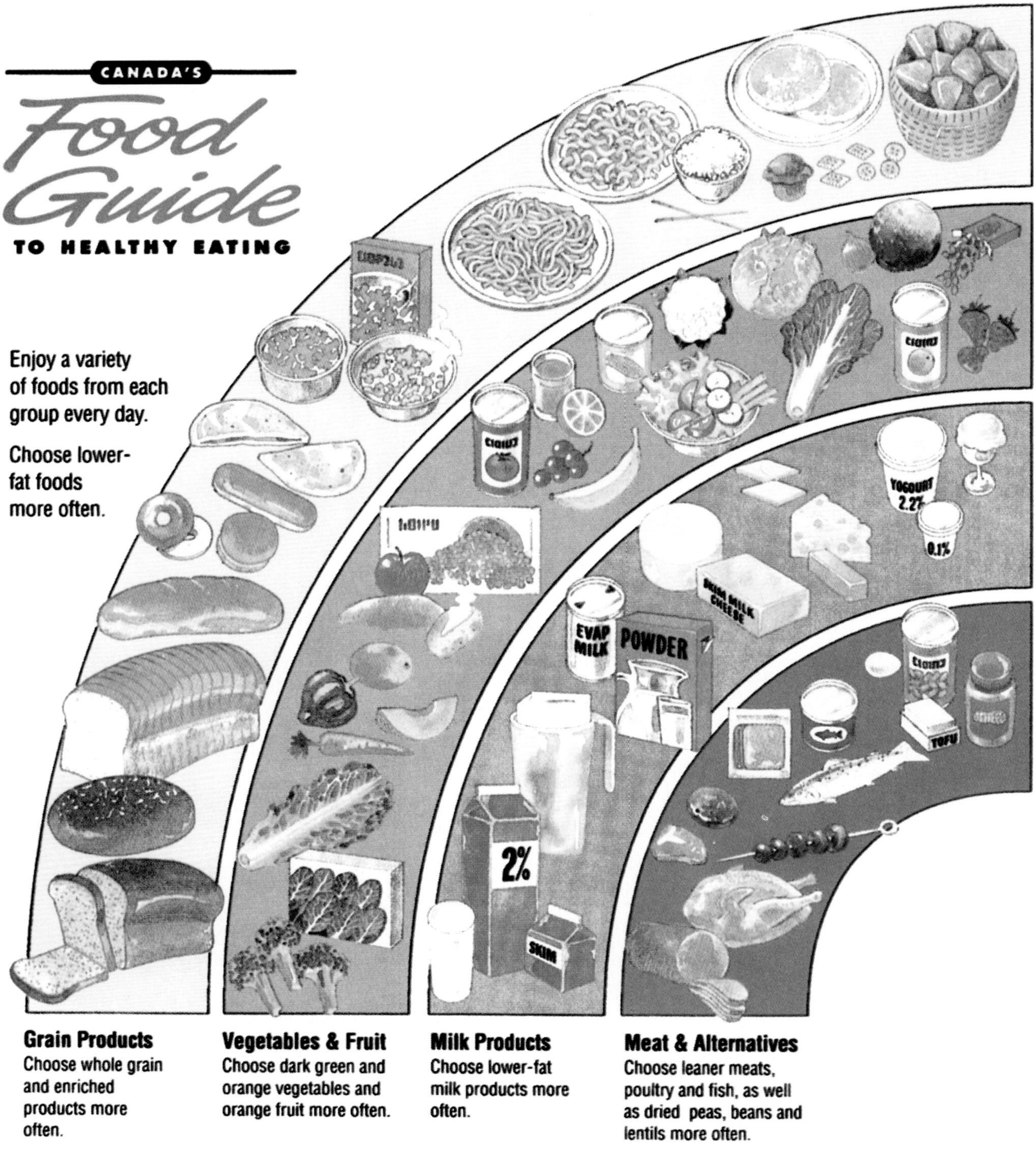
CANADA'S
Food Guide
TO HEALTHY EATING
Enjoy a variety of foods from each group every day.
Choose lower-fat foods more often.
YOGOURT 2.2%
0.1%
SKIM MILK CHEESE
EVAP MILK
POWDER
2%
SKIM
TOFU
Grain Products
Choose whole grain and enriched products more often.
Vegetables & Fruit
Choose dark green and orange vegetables and orange fruit more often.
Milk Products
Choose lower-fat milk products more often.
Meat & Alternatives
Choose leaner meats, poultry and fish, as well as dried peas, beans and lentils more often.

CANADA'S

Food Guide

TO HEALTHY EATING

FOR PEOPLE FOUR YEARS AND OVER

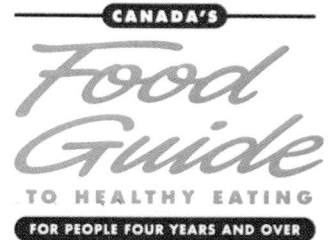

Different People Need Different Amounts of Food

The amount of food you need every day from the 4 food groups and other foods depends on your age, body size, activity level, whether you are male or female and if you are pregnant or breast-feeding. That's why the Food Guide gives a lower and higher number of servings for each food group. For example, young children can choose the lower number of servings, while male teenagers can go to the higher number. Most other people can choose servings somewhere in between.

Grain Products

5–12

SERVINGS PER DAY

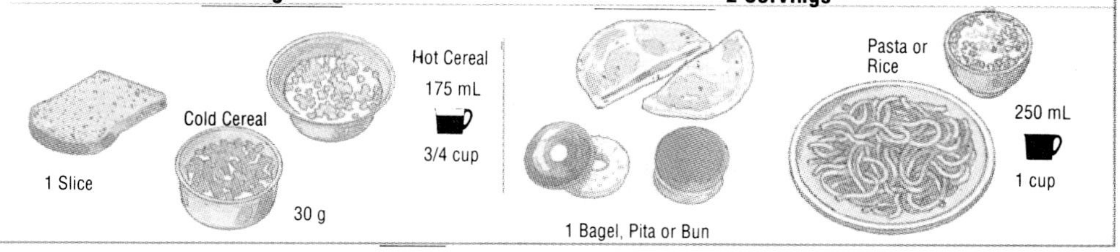

Vegetables & Fruit

5–10

SERVINGS PER DAY

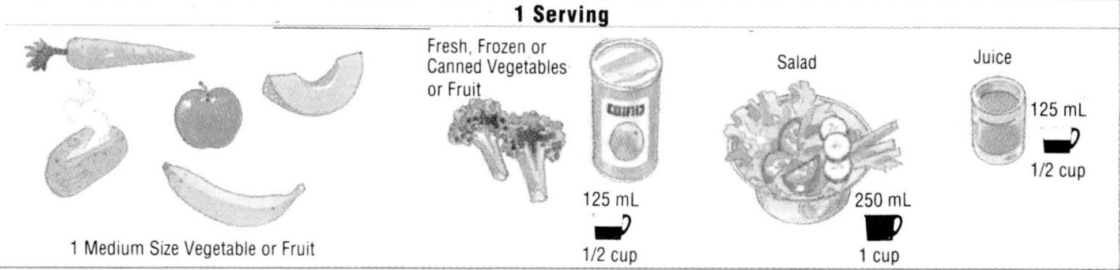

Milk Products

SERVINGS PER DAY

Children 4–9 years: 2–3
Youth 10–16 years: 3–4
Adults: 2–4
Pregnant & Breast-feeding Women: 3–4

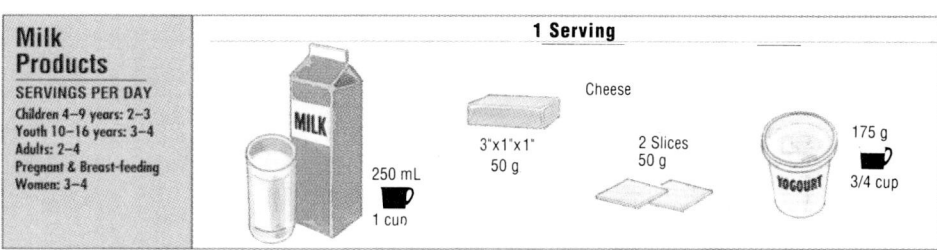

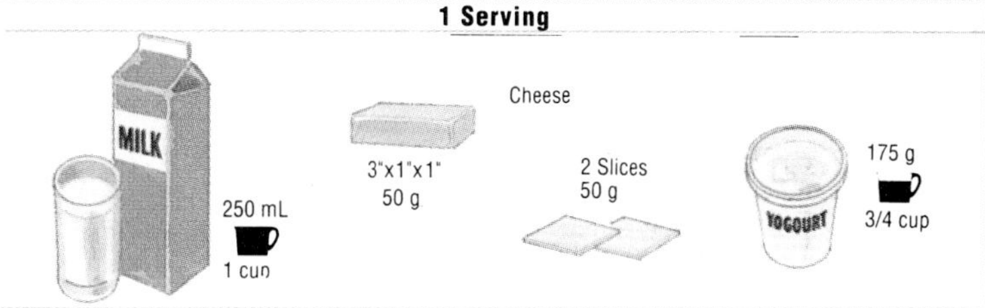

Meat & Alternatives

2–3

SERVINGS PER DAY

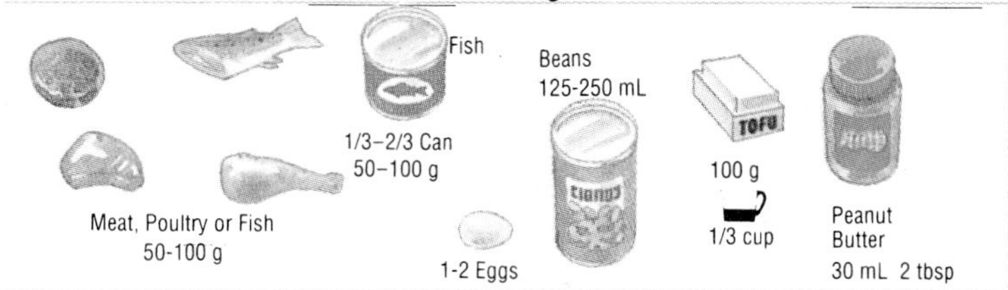

Other Foods

Taste and enjoyment can also come from other foods and beverages that are not part of the 4 food groups. Some of these foods are higher in fat or Calories, so use these foods in moderation.

Key Nutrients in Canada's Food Guide to Healthy Eating

Each food group is essential. That's because it provides its own set of nutrients.

Grain Products +	Vegetables & Fruits +	Milk Products +	Meat & Alternatives =	The Food Guide
protein		protein	protein	protein
		fat	fat	fat
carbohydrate	carbohydrate			carbohydrate
fibre	fibre			fibre
thiamin	thiamin		thiamin	thiamin
riboflavin		riboflavin	riboflavin	riboflavin
niacin			niacin	niacin
folacin	folacin		folacin	folacin
		vitamin B_{12}	vitamin B_{12}	vitamin B_{12}
	vitamin C			vitamin C
	vitamin A	vitamin A		vitamin A
		vitamin D		vitamin D
		calcium		calcium
iron	iron		iron	iron
zinc		zinc	zinc	zinc
magnesium	magnesium	magnesium	magnesium	magnesium

E

What Is Nutrition Labelling?

- It is a **standardized presentation** of the nutrient content of a food.
- It is designed to provide useful information that is **not misleading or deceptive.**
- It is **voluntary,** but if applied should comply with the Guidelines on Nutrition Labelling* and with the *Food and Drug Regulations*, which regulate the format, nutrient content information, nomenclature, units of measurement, per-serving basis and declaration of serving size.
- It consists of the **heading,** a statement of the **serving size,** the **"core list"** (energy, protein, fat, and carbohydrate) plus optional nutrient declarations given equal prominence, in a standardized order.

**Guidelines on Nutrition Labelling*, Guideline No. 2 (Ottawa: Health Canada, Health Protection Branch, May 2, 1996).

Nomenclature, Order of Listing, and Units

1. **Heading**
2. **Serving size:** metric units as sold (household measure should be declared in brackets).
3. **Energy** (expressed in both Calories and kilojoules), **protein, fat** and **carbohydrate** constitute the "core list" and must be included when the nutrition labelling format is used. All must be expressed in grams.
4. If one of these **fat components,** excluding linoleic acid, is listed, all four (in addition to fat) must be listed. Linoleic acid may be listed provided the four fat components and fat are also listed.
5. Declaration of one **carbohydrate** component does not require the declaration of any others. All sugar alcohols must be declared by name when used.
6. If either **sodium or potassium** is listed, both must be listed. Both must be expressed in milligrams.
7. **Vitamins and mineral nutrients** must be stated as % of Recommended Daily Intake. If less than 5% of Recommended Daily Intake, they may be listed provided no claims relate to them. Only the names shown may be used in nutrition labelling.

Source: Online at http://www.cfia-acia.agr.ca/english/ppc/label/5-0-0.html

Nutrition Information Nutritionnelle

per × g or mL per serving (× cups, item, etc.)
par portion de × g ou mL (× tasses, unités, etc.)

Energy/Énergie	× Cal × kJ
Protein/Protéines	× g
Fat/Matières grasses	× g
polyunsaturates/polyinsaturés	× g
linoleic acid/acide linoléique	× g
monounsaturates/monoinsaturés	× g
saturates/saturés	× g
cholesterol/cholestérol	× mg
Carbohydrate/Glucides	× g
sugars/sucres	× g
sugar alcohols (named)	× g
polydextrose	× g
starch/amidon	× g
dietary fibre/fibres alimentaires	× g
Sucralose	× mg
Aspartame	× mg
Acesulfame-potassium/acésulfame-potassium	× mg
Sodium	× mg
Potassium	× mg

Percentage of Recommended Daily Intake
Pourcentage de l'Apport Quotidien Recommandé

Vitamin A/Vitamine A	× %
Vitamin D/Vitamine D	× %
Vitamin E/Vitamine E	× %
Vitamin C/Vitamine C	× %
Thiamine or/ou Vitamin B1/Vitamine B1	× %
Riboflavin/Riboflavine or/ou Vitamin B2/Vitamine B2	× %
Niacin/Niacine	× %
Vitamin B6/Vitamine B6	× %
Folacin/Folacine	× %
Vitamin B12/Vitamine B12	× %
Pantothenic Acid or Pantothenate/ Acide Pantothénique ou Pantothénate	× %
Calcium	× %
Phosphorus/Phosphore	× %
Magnesium/Magnésium	× %
Iron/Fer	× %
Zinc	× %
Iodine/Iode	× %

THE CANADIAN DIABETES ASSOCIATION FOOD CHOICE SYSTEM

The Canadian Diabetes Association (CDA) Food Choice System is a method of meal planning that is based on *Canada's Food Guide to Healthy Eating*. Foods are divided into choices according to carbohydrate, fat, and protein content. An energy value is given for each choice group and foods are interchangeable within a group. Most foods are eaten in measured amounts. The Canadian Food Choice System tables are adapted from the Good Health Eating Guide Resource, copyright 1994, with permission of the Canadian Diabetes Association.

Canadian Food Choice System: Starch Foods

1 Starch Choice = 15 g carbohydrate (starch), 2 g protein, 290 kJ (68 kcal)

Food	Measure	Mass (weight)
Breads		
Bagels	½	30 g
Bread crumbs	50 mL (¼ c)	30 g
Bread cubes	250 mL (1 c)	30 g
Bread sticks	2	20 g
Brewis, cooked	50 mL (¼ c)	45 g
Chapati	1	20 g
Cookies, plain	2	20 g
English muffins, crumpets	½	30 g
Flour	40 mL (2½ tbs)	20 g
Hamburger buns	½	30 g
Hot dog buns	½	30 g
Kaiser rolls	½	30 g
Matzo, 15 cm	1	20 g
Melba toast, rectangular	4	15 g
Melba toast, rounds	7	15 g
Pita, 20-cm (8″) diameter	¼	30 g
Pita, 15-cm (6″) diameter	½	30 g
Plain rolls	1 small	30 g
Pretzels	7	20 g
Raisin bread	1 slice	30 g
Rice cakes	2	30 g
Roti	1	20 g
Rusks	2	20 g
Rye, coarse or pumpernickel	½ slice	30 g
Soda crackers	6	20 g
Tortillas, corn (taco shell)	1	30 g
Tortilla, flour	1	30 g
White (French and Italian)	1 slice	25 g
Whole-wheat, cracked-wheat, rye, white enriched	1 slice	30 g
Cereals		
Bran flakes, 100% bran	125 mL (½ c)	30 g
Cooked cereals, cooked	125 mL (½ c)	125 g
Dry	30 mL (2 tbs)	20 g
Cornmeal, cooked	125 mL (½ c)	125 g
Dry	30 mL (2 tbs)	20 g
Ready-to-eat unsweetened cereals	125 mL (½ c)	20 g
Shredded wheat biscuits, rectangular or round	1	20 g
Shredded wheat, bite size	125 mL (½ c)	20 g
Wheat germ	75 mL (⅓ c)	30 g
Cornflakes	175 mL (⅔ c)	20 g
Rice Krispies	175 mL (⅔ c)	20 g
Cheerios	200 mL (¾ c)	20 g

1 Starch Choice = 15 g carbohydrate (starch), 2 g protein, 290 kJ (68 kcal)

Food	Measure	Mass (weight)
Cereals *(continued)*		
Muffets	1	20 g
Puffed rice	300 mL (1¼ c)	15 g
Puffed wheat	425 mL (1⅔ c)	20 g
Grains		
Barley, cooked	125 mL (½ c)	120 g
Dry	30 mL (2 tbs)	20 g
Bulgur, kasha, cooked, moist	125 mL (½ c)	70 g
Cooked, crumbly	75 mL (⅓ c)	40 g
Dry	30 mL (2 tbs)	20 g
Rice, cooked, brown & white (short & long grain)	125 mL (½ c)	70 g
Rice, cooked, wild	75 mL (⅓ c)	70 g
Tapioca, pearl and granulated, quick cooking, dry	30 mL (2 tbs)	15 g
Couscous, cooked moist	125 mL (½ c)	70 g
Dry	30 mL (2 tbs)	20 g
Quinoa, cooked moist	125 mL (½ c)	70 g
Dry	30 mL (2 tbs)	20 g
Pastas		
Macaroni, cooked	125 mL (½ c)	70 g
Noodles, cooked	125 mL (½ c)	80 g
Spaghetti, cooked	125 mL (½ c)	70 g
Starchy Vegetables		
Beans and peas, dried, cooked	125 mL (½ c)	80 g
Breadfruit	1 slice	75 g
Corn, canned, whole kernel	125 mL (½ c)	85 g
Corn on the cob	½ medium cob	140 g
Cornstarch	30 mL (2 tbs)	15 g
Plantains	⅓ small	50 g
Popcorn, air-popped, unbuttered	750 mL (3 c)	20 g
Potatoes, whole (with or without skin)	½ medium	95 g
Yams, sweet potatoes (with or without skin)	½	75 g

Food	Exchanges per Serving	Measure	Mass (weight)
Note: Food items found in this category provide more than 1 starch exchange:			
Bran flakes	1 starch + ½ sugar	150 mL (⅔ c)	24 g
Croissant, small	1 starch + 1½ fats	1 small	35 g
Large	1 starch + 1½ fats	½ large	30 g
Corn, canned creamed	1 starch + ½ fruits and vegetables	12 mL (½ c)	113 g
Potato chips	1 starch + 2 fats	15 chips	30 g
Tortilla chips (nachos)	1 starch + 1½ fats	13 chips	20 g
Corn chips	1 starch + 2 fats	30 chips	30 g
Cheese twists	1 starch + 1½ fats	30 chips	30 g
Cheese puffs	1 starch + 2 fats	27 chips	30 g
Tea biscuit	1 starch + 2 fats	1	30 g
Pancakes, homemade using 50 mL (¼ c) batter (6″ diameter)	1½ starches + 1 fat	1 medium	50 g
Potatoes, french fried (homemade or frozen)	1 starch + 1 fat	10 regular size	35 g
Soup, canned° (prepared with equal volume of water)	1 starch	250 mL (1 c)	260 g
Waffles, packaged	1 starch + 1 fat	1	35 g

°Soup can vary according to brand and type. Check the label for Food Choice Values and Symbols or the core nutrient listing.

Canadian Food Choice System: Fruits and Vegetables

1 Fruits and Vegetables Choice = 10 g carbohydrate, 1 g protein, 190 kJ (44 kcal)

Food	Measure	Mass (weight)
Fruits (fresh, frozen, without sugar, canned in water)		
Apples, raw (with or without skin)	½ medium	75 g
Sauce unsweetened	125 mL (½ c)	120 g
Sweetened	see *Combined Food Choices*	
Apple butter	20 mL (4 tsp)	20 g
Apricots, raw	2 medium	115 g
Canned, in water	4 halves, plus 30 mL (2 tbs) liquid	110 g
Bake-apples (cloudberries), raw	125 mL (½ c)	120 g
Bananas, with peel	½ small	75 g
Peeled	½ small	50 g
Berries (blackberries, blueberries, boysenberries, huckleberries, loganberries, raspberries)		
Raw	125 mL (½ c)	70 g
Canned, in water	125 mL (½ c), plus 30 mL (2 tbs) liquid	100 g
Cantaloupe, wedge with rind	¼	240 g
Cubed or diced	250 mL (1 c)	160 g
Cherries, raw, with pits	10	75 g
Raw, without pits	10	70 g
Canned, in water, with pits	75 mL (⅓ c), plus 30 mL (2 tbs) liquid	90 g
Canned, in water, without pits	75 mL (⅓ c), plus 30 mL (2 tbs) liquid	85 g
Crabapples, raw	1 small	55 g
Cranberries, raw	250 mL (1 c)	100 g
Figs, raw	1 medium	50 g
Canned, in water	3 medium, plus 30 mL (2 tbs) liquid	100 g
Foxberries, raw	250 mL (1 c)	100 g
Fruit cocktail, canned, in water	125 mL (½ c), plus 30 mL (2 tbs) liquid	120 g
Fruit, mixed, cut-up	125 mL (½ c)	120 g
Gooseberries, raw	250 mL (1 c)	150 g
Canned, in water	250 mL (1 c), plus 30 mL (2 tbs) liquid	230 g
Grapefruit, raw, with rind	½ small	185 g
Raw, sectioned	125 mL (½ c)	100 g
Canned, in water	125 mL (½ c), plus 30 mL (2 tbs) liquid	120 g
Grapes, raw, slip skin	125 mL (½ c)	75 g
Raw, seedless	125 mL (½ c)	75 g
Canned, in water	75 mL (⅓ c), plus 30 mL (2 tbs) liquid	115 g
Guavas, raw	½	50 g
Honeydew melon, raw, with rind	½	225 g
Cubed or diced	250 mL (1 c)	170 g
Kiwis, raw, with skin	2	155 g
Kumquats, raw	3	60 g
Loquats, raw	8	130 g
Lychee fruit, raw	8	120 g
Mandarin oranges, raw, with rind	1	135 g
Raw, sectioned	125 mL (½ c)	100 g
Canned, in water	125 mL (½ c), plus 30 mL (2 tbs) liquid	100 g
Mangoes, raw, without skin and seed	⅓	65 g
Diced	75 mL (⅓ c)	65 g
Nectarines	½ medium	75 g

Canadian Food Choice System: Fruits and Vegetables (continued)

1 Fruits and Vegetables Choice = 10 g carbohydrate, 1 g protein, 190 kJ (44 kcal)

Food	Measure	Mass (weight)
Fruits *(continued)*		
Oranges, raw, with rind	1 small	130 g
Raw, sectioned	125 mL (½ c)	95 g
Papayas, raw, with skin and seeds	¼ medium	150 g
Raw, without skin and seeds	¼ medium	100 g
Cubed or diced	125 mL (½ c)	100 g
Peaches, raw, with seed and skin	1 large	100 g
Raw, sliced or diced	125 mL (½ c)	100 g
Canned in water, halves or slices	125 mL (½ c), plus 30 mL (2 tbs) liquid	120 g
Pears, raw, with skin and core	½	90 g
Raw, without skin and core	½	85 g
Canned, in water, halves	1 half plus 30 mL (2 tbs) liquid	90 g
Persimmons, raw, native	1	30 g
Raw, Japanese	¼	50 g
Pineapple, raw	1 slice	75 g
Raw, diced	125 mL (½ c)	75 g
Canned, in juice, diced	75 mL (⅓ c), plus 15 mL (1 tbs) liquid	55 g
Canned, in juice, sliced	1 slice, plus 15 mL (1 tbs) liquid	55 g
Canned, in water, diced	125 mL (½ c), plus 30 mL (2 tbs) liquid	100 g
Canned, in water, sliced	2 slices, plus 15 mL (1 tbs) liquid	100 g
Plums, raw	2 small	60 g
Damson	6	65 g
Japanese	1	70 g
Canned, in apple juice	2, plus 30 mL (2 tbs) liquid	70 g
Canned, in water	3, plus 30 mL (2 tbs) liquid	100 g
Pomegranates, raw	½	140 g
Strawberries, raw	250 mL (1 c)	150 g
Frozen/canned, in water	250 mL (1 c), plus 30 mL (2 tbs) liquid	240 g
Rhubarb	250 mL (1 c)	150 g
Tangelos, raw	1	205 g
Tangerines, raw	1 medium	115 g
Raw, sectioned	125 mL (½ c)	100 g
Watermelon, raw, with rind	1 wedge	310 g
Cubed or diced	250 mL (1 c)	160 g
Dried Fruit		
Apples	5 pieces	15 g
Apricots	4 halves	15 g
Banana flakes	30 mL (2 tbs)	15 g
Currants	30 mL (2 tbs)	15 g
Dates, without pits	2	15 g
Peaches	½	15 g
Pears	½	15 g
Prunes, raw, with pits	2	15 g
Raw, without pits	2	10 g
Stewed, no liquid	2	20 g
Stewed, with liquid	2, plus 15 mL (1 tbs) liquid	35 g
Raisins	30 mL (2 tbs)	15 g

Canadian Food Choice System: Fruits and Vegetables (continued)

1 Fruits and Vegetables Choice = 10 g carbohydrate, 1 g protein, 190 kJ (44 kcal)

Food	Measure	Mass (weight)
Juices (no sugar added or unsweetened)		
Apricot, grape, guava, mango, prune	50 mL (½ c)	55 g
Apple, carrot, papaya, pear, pineapple, pomegranate	75 mL (⅓ c)	80 g
Cranberry (see Sugars Section)		
Clamato (see Sugars Section)		
Grapefruit, loganberry, orange, raspberry, tangelo, tangerine	125 mL (½ c)	130 g
Tomato, tomato-based mixed vegetables	250 mL (1 c)	255 g
Vegetables (fresh, frozen, or canned)		
Artichokes, French, globe	2 small	50 g
Beets, diced or sliced	125 mL (½ c)	85 g
Carrots, diced, cooked or uncooked	125 mL (½ c)	75 g
Chestnuts, fresh	5	20 g
Parsnips, mashed	125 mL (½ c)	80 g
Peas, fresh or frozen	125 mL (½ c)	80 g
Canned	75 mL (⅓ c)	55 g
Pumpkin, mashed	125 mL (½ c)	45 g
Rutabagas, mashed	125 mL (½ c)	85 g
Sauerkraut	250 mL (1 c)	235 g
Snow peas	250 mL (1 c)	135 g
Squash, yellow or winter, mashed	125 mL (½ c)	115 g
Succotash	75 mL (⅓ c)	55 g
Tomatoes, canned	250 mL (1 c)	240 g
Tomato paste	50 mL (¼ c)	55 g
Tomato sauce*	75 mL (⅓ c)	100 g
Turnips, mashed	125 mL (½ c)	115 g
Vegetables, mixed	125 mL (½ c)	90 g
Water chestnuts	8 medium	50 g

*Tomato sauce varies according to brand name. Check the label or discuss with your dietitian.

Canadian Food Choice System: Sugars

1 Sugar Choice = 10 g carbohydrate (sugar), 167 kJ (40 kcal)

Food	Measure	Mass (weight)
Beverages		
Condensed milk	15 mL (1 tbs)	
Flavoured fruit crystals*	75 mL (⅓ c)	
Iced tea mixes*	74 mL (⅓ c)	
Regular soft drinks	125 mL (½ c)	
Sweet drink mixes*	75 mL (⅓ c)	
Tonic water	125 mL (½ c)	
Miscellaneous		
Bubble gum (large square)	1 piece	5 g
Cranberry cocktail	75 mL (⅓ c)	80 g
Cranberry cocktail, light	350 mL (1⅓ c)	260 g
Cranberry sauce	30 mL (2 tbs)	
Hard candy mints	2	5 g
Honey, molasses, corn & cane syrup	10 mL (2 tsp)	15 g
Jelly bean	4	10 g
Licorice	1 short stick	10 g
Marshmallows	2 large	15 g
Popsicle	1 stick (½ popsicle)	
Powdered gelatin mix		
Jello® (reconstituted)	50 mL (¼ c)	
Regular jam, jelly, marmalade	15 mL (1 tbs)	
Sugar, white, brown, icing, maple	10 mL (2 tsp)	10 g
Sweet pickles	2 small	100 g
Sweet relish	30 mL (2 tbs)	

Food	Exchanges per Serving	Measure	Mass (weight)
The following food items provide more than 1 sugar exchange:			
Brownie	1 sugar + 1 fat	1	20 g
Clamato juice	1½ sugars	175 mL (⅔ c)	
Fruit salad, light syrup	1 sugar + 1 fruits & vegetables	125 mL (½ c)	130 g
Aero® bar	2½ sugars + 2½ fats	1 bar	43 g
Smarties®	4½ sugars + 2 fats	1 box	60 g
Sherbet	3 sugars + ½ fat	125 mL (½ c)	95 g

*These beverages have been made with water.

Canadian Food Choice System: Protein Foods

1 Protein Choice = 7 g protein, 3 g fat, 230 kJ (55 kcal)

Food	Measure	Mass (weight)
Cheese		
Low-fat cheese, about 7% milkfat	1 slice	30 g
Cottage cheese, 2% milkfat or less	50 mL (¼ c)	55 g
Ricotta, about 7% milkfat	50 mL (¼ c)	60 g
Fish		
Anchovies (see *Extras*)		
Canned, drained (e.g., mackerel, salmon, tuna packed in water)	(⅓ of 6.5 oz can)	30 g
Cod tongues, cheeks	75 mL (⅓ c)	50 g
Fillet or steak (e.g., Boston blue, cod, flounder, haddock, halibut, mackerel, orange roughy, perch, pickerel, pike, salmon, shad, snapper, sole, swordfish, trout, tuna, whitefish)	1 piece	30 g
Herring	⅓ fish	30 g
Sardines, smelts	2 medium or 3 small	30 g
Squid, octopus	50 mL (¼ c)	40 g
Shellfish		
Clams, mussels, oysters, scallops, snails	3 medium	30 g
Crab, lobster, flaked	50 mL (¼ c)	30 g
Shrimp, fresh	5 large	30 g
Frozen	10 medium	30 g
Canned	18 small	30 g
Dry pack	50 mL (¼ c)	30 g
Meat and Poultry (e.g., beef, chicken, goat, ham, lamb, pork, turkey, veal, wild game)		
Back, peameal bacon	3 slices, thin	30 g
Chop	½ chop, with bone	40 g
Minced or ground, lean or extra-lean	30 mL (2 tbs)	30 g
Sliced, lean	1 slice	30 g
Steak, lean	1 piece	30 g
Organ Meats		
Hearts, liver	1 slice	30 g
Kidneys, sweetbreads, chopped	50 mL (¼ c)	30 g
Tongue	1 slice	30 g
Tripe	5 pieces	60 g
Soyabean		
Bean curd or tofu	½ block	70 g
Eggs		
In shell, raw or cooked	1 medium	50 g
Without shell, cooked or poached in water	1 medium	45 g
Scrambled	50 mL (¼ c)	55 g

Canadian Food Choice System: Protein Foods (continued)

1 Protein Choice = 7 g protein, 3 g fat, 230 kJ (55 kcal)

Food	Exchanges per Serving	Measures	Mass (weight)
Note: The following choices provide more than 1 protein exchange:			
Cheese			
Cheeses	1 protein + 1 fat	1 piece	25 g
Cheese, coarsely grated (e.g., cheddar)	1 protein + 1 fat	50 mL (¼ c)	25 g
Cheese, dry, finely grated (e.g., parmesan)	1 protein + 1 fat	45 mL	15 g
Cheese, ricotta, high fat	1 protein + 1 fat	50 mL (¼ c)	55 g
Fish			
Eel	1 protein + 1 fat	1 slice	50 g
Meat			
Bologna	1 protein + 1 fat	1 slice	20 g
Canned lunch meats	1 protein + 1 fat	1 slice	20 g
Corned beef, canned	1 protein + 1 fat	1 slice	25 g
Corned beef, fresh	1 protein + 1 fat	1 slice	25 g
Ground beef, medium-fat	1 protein + 1 fat	30 mL (2 tbs)	25 g
Meat spreads, canned	1 protein + 1 fat	45 mL	35 g
Mutton chop	1 protein + 1 fat	½ chop, with bone	35 g
Paté (see *Fats and Oils* group)			
Sausages, garlic, Polish or knockwurst	1 protein + 1 fat	1 slice	50 g
Sausages, pork, links	1 protein + 1 fat	1 link	25 g
Spareribs or shortribs, with bone	1 protein + 1 fat	1 large	65 g
Stewing beef	1 protein + 1 fat	1 cube	25 g
Summer sausage or salami	1 protein + 1 fat	1 slice	40 g
Wiener, hot dog	1 protein + 1 fat	½ medium	25 g
Miscellaneous			
Blood pudding	1 protein + 1 fat	1 slice	25 g
Peanut butter	1 protein + 1 fat	15 mL (1 tbs)	15 g

Canadian Food Choice System: Milk Foods

Type of Milk	Carbohydrate (g)	Protein (g)	Fat (g)	Energy
Nonfat (0%)	6	4	0	170 kJ (40 kcal)
1%	6	4	1	206 kJ (49 kcal)
2%	6	4	2	244 kJ (58 kcal)
Whole (4%)	6	4	4	319 kJ (76 kcal)

Food	Measure	Mass (weight)
Buttermilk (higher in salt)	125 mL (½ c)	125 g
Evaporated milk	50 mL (¼ c)	50 g
Milk	125 mL (½ c)	125 g
Powdered milk, regular	30 mL (2 tbs)	15 g
Instant	50 mL (¼ c)	15 g
Plain yogurt	125 mL (½ c)	125 g

Food	Exchanges per Serving	Measure	Mass (weight)
Note: Food items found in this category provide more than 1 milk exchange:			
Milkshake	1 milk + 3 sugars + ½ protein	250 mL (1 c)	300 g
Chocolate milk, 2%	2 milks 2% + 1 sugar	250 mL (1 c)	300 g
Frozen yogurt	1 milk + 1 sugar	125 mL (½ c)	125 g

Canadian Food Choice System: Fats and Oils

1 Fat Choice = 5 g fat, 190 kJ (45 kcal)

Food	Measure	Mass (weight)
Avocado°	⅛	30 g
Bacon, side, crisp°	1 slice	5 g
Butter°	5 mL (1 tsp)	5 g
Cheese spread	15 mL (1 tbs)	15 g
Coconut, fresh°	45 mL (3 tbs)	15 g
Coconut, dried°	15 mL (1 tbs)	10 g
Cream, half and half (cereal), 10%°	30 mL (2 tbs)	30 g
Light (coffee), 20%°	15 mL (1 tbs)	15 g
Whipping, 32% to 37%°	15 mL (1 tbs)	15 g
Cream cheese°	15 mL (1 tbs)	15 g
Gravy°	30 mL (2 tbs)	30 g
Lard°	5 mL (1 tsp)	5 g
Margarine	5 mL (1 tsp)	5 g
Nuts, shelled:		
Almonds	8	5 g
Brazil nuts	2	10 g
Cashews	5	10 g
Filberts, hazelnuts	5	10 g
Macadamia	3	5 g
Peanuts	10	10 g
Pecans	5 halves	5 g
Pignolias, pine nuts	25 mL (5 tsp)	10 g
Pistachios, shelled	20	10 g
Pistachios, in shell	20	20 g
Pumpkin and squash seeds	20 mL (4 tsp)	10 g
Nuts (*continued*):		
Sesame seeds	15 mL (1 tbs)	10 g
Sunflower seeds		
Shelled	15 mL (1 tbs)	10 g
In shell	45 mL (3 tbs)	15 g
Walnuts	4 halves	10 g
Oil, cooking and salad	5 mL (1 tsp)	5 g
Olives, green	10	45 g
Ripe black	7	57 g
Pâté, liverwurst, meat spread	15 mL (1 tbs)	15 g
Salad dressing: blue cheese, French, Italian, mayonnaise,	10 mL (2 tsp)	10 g
Thousand Island	5 mL (1 tsp)	5 g
Salad dressing, low-calorie	30 mL (2 tbs)	30 g
Salt pork, raw or cooked°	5 mL (1 tsp)	5 g
Sesame oil	5 mL (1 tsp)	5 g
Sour cream		
12% milkfat	30 mL (2 tbs)	30 g
7% milkfat	60 mL (4 tbs)	60 g
Shortening°	5 mL (1 tsp)	

°These items contain higher amounts of saturated fat.

Canadian Food Choice System: Extras

Extras have no more than 2.5 g carbohydrate, 60 kJ (14 kcal)

Vegetables 125 mL (½ c)

Artichokes
Asparagus
Bamboo shoots
Bean sprouts, mung or soya
Beans, string, green, or yellow
Bitter melon (balsam pear)
Bok choy
Broccoli
Brussels sprouts
Cabbage
Cauliflower
Celery
Chard
Cucumbers
Eggplant
Endive
Fiddleheads
Greens: beet, collard, dandelion, mustard, turnip, etc.
Kale
Kohlrabi
Leeks
Lettuce
Mushrooms
Okra
Onions, green or mature
Parsley
Peppers, green, yellow or red
Radishes
Rapini
Rhubarb
Sauerkraut
Shallots
Spinach
Sprouts: alfalfa, radish, etc.
Tomato wedges
Watercress
Zucchini

Free Foods (may be used without measuring)

Artificial sweetener, such as cyclamate or aspartame
Baking powder, baking soda
Bouillon from cube, powder, or liquid
Bouillon or clear broth
Chowchow, unsweetened
Coffee, clear
Consommé
Dulse
Flavorings and extracts
Garlic
Gelatin, unsweetened
Ginger root
Herbal teas, unsweetened
Horseradish, uncreamed
Lemon juice or lemon wedges
Lime juice or lime wedges
Marjoram, cinnamon, etc.
Mineral water
Mustard
Parsley
Pimentos
Salt, pepper, thyme
Soda water, club soda
Soya sauce
Sugar-free Crystal Drink
Sugar-free Jelly Powder
Sugar-free soft drinks
Tea, clear
Vinegar
Water
Worcestershire sauce

Condiments

Food	Measure
Anchovies	2 fillets
Barbecue sauce	15 mL (1 tbs)
Bran, natural	30 mL (2 tbs)
Brewer's yeast	5 mL (1 tsp)
Carob powder	5 mL (1 tsp)
Catsup	5 mL (1 tsp)
Chili sauce	5 mL (1 tsp)
Cocoa powder	5 mL (1 tsp)
Cranberry sauce, unsweetened	15 mL (1 tbs)
Dietetic fruit spreads	5 mL (1 tsp)
Maraschino cherries	1
Nondairy coffee whitener	5 mL (1 tsp)
Nuts, chopped pieces	5 mL (1 tsp)
Pickles	
Unsweetened dill	2
Sour mixed	11
Sugar substitutes, granular	5 mL (1 tsp)
Whipped toppings	15 mL (1 tbs)

Canadian Food Choice System: Combined Food Choices

Food	Exchanges per Serving	Measures	Mass (weight)
Angel food cake	½ starch + 2½ sugars	1⁄12 cake	50 g
Apple crisp	½ starch + 1½ fruits & vegetables + 1 sugar + 1–2 fats	125 mL (½ c)	
Applesauce, sweetened	1 fruits & vegetables + 1 sugar	125 mL (½ c)	
Beans and pork in tomato sauce	1 starch + ½ fruits & vegetables + ½ sugar + 1 protein	125 mL (½ c)	135 g
Beef burrito	2 starches + 3 proteins + 3 fats		110 g
Brownie	1 sugar + 1 fat	1	20 g
Cabbage rolls*	1 starch + 2 proteins	3	310 g
Caesar salad	2–4 fats	20 mL dressing (4 tsp)	
Cheesecake	½ starch + 2 sugars + ½ protein + 5 fats	1 piece	80 g
Chicken fingers	1 starch + 2 proteins + 2 fats	6 small	100 g
Chicken and snow pea Oriental	2 starches + ½ fruits & vegetables + 3 proteins + 1 fat	500 mL (2 c)	
Chili	1½ starches + ½ fruits & vegetables + 3½ protein	300 mL (1¼ c)	325 g
Chips			
Potato chips	1 starch + 2 fats	15 chips	30 g
Corn chips	1 starch + 2 fats	30 chips	30 g
Tortilla chips	1 starch + 1½ fats	13 chips	
Cheese twist	1 starch + 1½ fats	30 chips	30 g
Chocolate bar			
Aero®	2½ sugars + 2½ fats	bar	43 g
Smarties®	4½ sugars + 2 fats	package	60 g
Chocolate cake (without icing)	1 starch + 2 sugars + 3 fats	1⁄10 of a 8″ pan	
Chocolate devil's food cake (without icing)	2 starches + 2 sugars + 3 fats	9″ pan	
Chocolate milk	2 milks 2% + 1 sugar	250 mL (1 c)	300 g
Clubhouse (triple-decker) sandwich	3 starches + 3 proteins + 4 fats		
Cookies			
Chocolate chip	½ starch + ½ sugar + 1½ fats	2	22 g
Oatmeal	1 starch + 1 sugar + 1 fat	2	40 g
Donut (chocolate glazed)	1 starch + 1½ sugars + 2 fats	1	65 g
Egg roll	1 starch + ½ protein + 1 fat	1	75 g
Four bean salad	1 starch + ½ protein + 1 fat	125 mL (½ c)	
French toast	1 starch + ½ protein + 2 fats	1 slice	65 g
Fruit in heavy syrup	1 fruits & vegetables + 1½ sugars	125 mL (½ c)	
Granola bar	½ starch + 1 sugar + 1–2 fats	1	30 g
Granola cereal	1 starch + 1 sugar + 2 fats	125 mL (½ c)	45 g
Hamburger	2 starches + 3 proteins + 2 fats	junior size	
Ice cream and cone, plain flavour			
Ice cream	½ milk + 2–3 sugars + 1–2 fats		100 g
Cone	½ sugar		4 g
Lasagna			
Regular cheese	1 starch + 1 fruits & vegetables + 3 proteins + 2 fats	3″ × 4″ piece	
Low-fat cheese	1 starch + 1 fruits & vegetables + 3 proteins	3″ × 4″ piece	
Legumes			
Dried beans (kidney, navy, pinto, fava, chick peas)	2 starches + 1 protein	250 mL (1 c)	180 g

Canadian Food Choice System: Combined Food Choices (continued)

Food	Exchanges per Serving	Measures	Mass (weight)
Dried peas	2 starches + 1 protein	250 mL (1 c)	210 g
Lentils	2 starches + 1 protein	250 mL (1 c)	210 g
Macaroni and cheese	2 starches + 2 proteins + 2 fats	250 mL (1 c)	210 g
Minestrone soup	1½ starches + ½ fruits & vegetables + ½ fat	250 mL (1 c)	
Muffin	1 starch + ½ sugar + 1 fat	1 small	45 g
Nuts (dry or roasted without any oil added)			
Almonds, dried sliced	½ protein + 2 fats	50 mL (¼ c)	22 g
Brazil nuts, dried unblanched	½ protein + 2½ fats	5 large	23 g
Cashew nuts, dry roasted	½ starch + ½ protein + 2 fats	50 mL (¼ c)	28 g
Filbert hazelnuts, dry	½ protein + 3½ fats	50 mL (¼ c)	30 g
Macadamia nuts, dried	½ protein + 4 fats	50 mL (¼ c)	28 g
Peanuts, raw	1 protein + 2 fats	50 mL (¼ c)	30 g
Pecans, dry roasted	½ fruits & vegetables + 3 fats	50 mL (¼ c)	22 g
Pine nuts (pignolia) dried	1 protein + 3 fats	50 mL (¼ c)	34 g
Pistachio nuts, dried	½ fruits & vegetables + ½ protein + 2½ fats	50 mL (¼ c)	27 g
Pumpkin seeds, roasted	2 proteins + 2½ fats	50 mL (¼ c)	47 g
Sesame seeds, whole dried	½ fruits & vegetables + ½ protein + 2½ fats	50 mL (¼ c)	30 g
Sunflower kernel, dried	½ protein + 1½ fats	50 mL (¼ c)	17 g
Walnuts, dried chopped	½ protein + 3 fats	50 mL (¼ c)	26 g
Perogies	2 starches + 1 protein + 1 fat	3	
Pie, fruit	1 starch + 1 fruits & vegetables + 2 sugars + 3 fats	1 piece	120 g
Pizza, cheese	1 starch + 1 protein + 1 fat	1 slice (⅛ of a 12″)	50 g
Pork stir fry	½–1 fruits & vegetables + 3 proteins	200 mL (¾ c)	
Potato salad	1 starch + 1 fat	125 mL (½ c)	130 g
Potatoes, scalloped	2 starches + 1 milk + 1–2 fats	200 mL (¾ c)	210 g
Pudding, bread or rice	1 starch + 1 sugar + 1 fat	125 mL (½ c)	
Pudding, vanilla	1 milk + 2 sugars	125 mL (½ c)	
Raisin bran cereal	1 starch + ½ fruits & vegetables + ½ sugar	175 mL (⅔ c)	40 g
Rice Krispie squares	½ starch + 1½ sugars + ½ fat	1 square	30 g
Shepherd's pie	2 starches + 1 fruits & vegetables + 3 proteins	325 mL (1⅓ c)	
Sherbet, orange	3 sugars + ½ fat	125 mL (½ c)	
Spaghetti and meat sauce	2 starches + 1 fruits & vegetables + 2 proteins + 3 fats	250 mL (1 c)	
Stew	2 starches + 2 fruit & vegetables + 3 proteins + ½ fat	200 mL (¾ c)	
Sundae	4 sugars + 3 fats	125 mL (½ c)	
Tuna casserole	1 starch + 2 proteins + ½ fat	125 mL (½ c)	
Yogurt, fruit bottom	1 fruits & vegetables + 1 milk + 1 sugar	125 mL (½ c)	125 g
Yogurt, frozen	1 milk + 1 sugar	125 mL (½ c)	125 g

° If eaten with sauce, add ½ fruits & vegetables exchange.

E

Appendix F

Nutrient Intake Recommendations by the World Health Organization

Recommended Intakes of Nutrients—WHO—1974

Age	Body Weight (kg)	Energy[1] (kcal)	Energy[1] (mJ)	Protein[1,2] (gm)	Vitamin A[3,4] (μg)	Vitamin D[5,6] (μg)
Children						
<1	7.3	820	3.4	14	300	10.00
1–3	13.4	1360	5.7	16	250	10.0
4–6	20.2	1830	7.6	20	300	10.0
7–9	28.1	2190	9.2	25	400	2.5
Male adolescents						
10–12	36.9	2600	10.9	30	575	2.5
13–15	51.3	2900	12.1	37	725	2.5
16–19	62.9	3070	12.8	38	750	2.5
Female adolescents						
10–12	38.0	2350	9.8	29	575	2.5
13–15	49.9	2490	10.4	31	725	2.5
16–19	54.4	2310	9.7	30	750	2.5
Adult man (moderately active)	65.0	3000	12.6	37	750	2.5
Adult woman (moderately active)	55.0	2200	9.2	29	750	2.5
Pregnancy (later half)		+350	+1.5	38	750	10.0
Lactation (first 6 months)		+550	+2.3	46	1200	10.0

[1]Energy and Protein Requirements. Report of a Joint FAO/WHO Expert Group, FAO, Rome, 1972. [2]As egg or milk protein. [3]Requirements of vitamin A, thiamin, riboflavin and niacin. Report of a Joint FAO/WHO Expert Group, FAO, Rome, 1965. [4]As retinol. [5]Requirements of ascorbic acid, vitamin D, vitamin B_{12}, folate and iron. Report of a Joint Applied FAO/WHO Expert Group, FAO, Rome, 1970. [6]As cholecalciferol. [7]Calcium requirements. Report of a FAO/WHO Expert Group, FAO, Rome, 1961. [8]On each line the lower value applies when over 25 percent of calories in the diet come from animal foods, and the higher value when animal foods represent less than 10 percent of calories. [9]For women whose iron intake throughout life has been at the level recommended in this table, the daily intake of iron during pregnancy and lactation should be the

Thiamin[3] (mg)	Riboflavin[3] (mg)	Niacin[3] (mg)	Folic Acid[5] (μg)	Vitamin B_{12}[5] (μg)	Ascorbic Acid[5] (mg)	Calcium[7] (gm)	Iron[5,8] (mg)
0.3	0.5	5.4	60	0.3	20	0.5–0.6	5–10
0.5	0.8	9.0	100	0.9	20	0.4–0.5	5–10
0.7	1.1	12.1	100	1.5	20	0.4–0.5	5–10
0.9	1.3	14.5	100	1.5	20	0.4–0.5	5–10
1.0	1.6	17.2	100	2.0	20	0.6–0.7	5–10
1.2	1.7	19.1	200	2.0	30	0.6–0.7	9–18
1.2	1.8	20.3	200	2.0	30	0.5–0.6	5–9
0.9	1.4	15.5	100	2.0	20	0.6–0.7	5–10
1.0	1.5	16.4	200	2.0	30	0.6–0.7	12–24
0.9	1.4	15.2	200	2.0	30	0.5–0.6	14–28
1.2	1.8	19.8	200	2.0	30	0.4–0.5	5–9
0.9	1.3	14.5	200	2.0	30	0.4–0.5	14–28
+0.1	+0.2	+2.3	400	3.0	50	1.0–1.2	(9)
+0.2	+0.4	+3.7	300	2.5	50	1.0–1.2	(9)

same as that recommended for nonpregnant, nonlactating women of childbearing age. For women whose iron status is not satisfactory at the beginning of pregnancy, the requirement is increased, and in the extreme situation of women with no iron stores, the requirement can probably not be met without supplementation.

Source: Passmore, Nicol and Rao. *Handbook on Human Nutritional Requirements*. Geneva, WHO Monogr. Ser. No. 61, 1974, Table 1.

ADDENDUM: Dietary allowances, official or unofficial for many European countries, as of 1976 or earlier, appear in the Proceedings of the Second European Nutrition Conference, Munich, 1976. (Nutr. Metab. 21:210, 1977.)

The Population Nutrient Goals From WHO

	Limits for Population Average Intakes	
	Lower Limit	Upper Limit
Total fat	15% of energy	30% of energy[a]
Saturated fatty acids	0% energy	10% of energy
Polyunsaturated fatty acids	3% of energy	7% of energy
Dietary cholesterol	0 mg/day	300 mg/day
Total carbohydrate	55% of energy	75% of energy
Complex carbohydrates[b]	50% of energy	75% of energy
Dietary fibre[c]		
As non-starch polysaccharides (NSP)	16 g/day	24 g/day
As total dietary fibre	27 g/day	40 g/day
Free sugars[d]	0% of energy	10% of energy
Protein	10% of energy	15% of energy[e]
Salt	—[e]	6 g/day

Total energy
Energy intake needs to be sufficient to allow for normal childhood growth, for the needs of pregnancy and lactation, and for work and desirable physical activities, and to maintain appropriate body reserves of energy in children and adults. Adult populations on average should have a body-mass index (BMI) of 20–22.
(BMI = body mass in kg/[height in metres]^2).

The lower limit defines the minimum intake needed to prevent deficiency diseases, while the upper limit expressed the maximum intake compatible with the prevention of chronic diseases.

[a] An interim goal for nations with high fat intakes; further benefits would be expected by reducing fat intake towards 15% of total energy.
[b] A daily minimum intake of 400 g vegetables and fruits, including at least 30 g of pulses, nuts, and seeds, should contribute to this component.
[c] Dietary fibre includes the non-starch polysaccharides (NSP), the goals for which are based on NSP obtained from mixed food sources. Since the definition and measurement of dietary fibre remain uncertain, the goals for total dietary fibre have been estimated from the NSP values.
[d] These sugars include monosaccharides, disaccharides, and other short-chain sugars extracted from carbohydrates by refining. These refined, or purified, sugars do not include the natural sugars consumed when eating fruits and vegetables or drinking milk.
[e] Not defined.

Source: Diet, nutrition and the prevention of chronic diseases. A report of the WHO Study Group on Diet, Nutrition and Prevention of Noncommunicable Diseases. Nutr. Rev. 49:291–301, 1991.

F

Appendix G

Dietary Recommendations From Various Groups

*American Heart Association Eating Plan for Healthy Americans**

Total fat intake should be no more than 30% of total kcalories.

Saturated fatty acid intake should be 8 to 10% of total kcalories.

Polyunsaturated fatty acid intake should be up to 10% of total kcalories.

Monounsaturated fatty acids should make up the rest of the total fat intake, about 10 to 15% of total kcalories.

Cholesterol intake should be less than 300 milligrams per day.

Sodium intake should be less than 2400 milligrams per day, which is about 1¼ teaspoons of sodium chloride (salt).

Carbohydrate intake should make up 55 to 60% or more of kcalories, with emphasis on increasing sources of complex carbohydrates.

Total kcalories should be adjusted to achieve and maintain a healthy body weight.

* Recommendations available online at http://amhrt.org/Heart_and_Stroke_A_Z_Guide/dietg.html

G

*National Cholesterol Education Program Step I and Step II Diets**

	Recommended Intake as Percent of Total Kcalories	
Nutrient	**Step I**	**Step II**
Total Fat	30% or less	30% or less
Saturated fatty acids	8–10%	Less than 7%
Polyunsaturated fatty acids	Up to 10%	Up to 10%
Monounsaturated fatty acids	Up to 15%	Up to 15%
Carbohydrate	55% or more	55% or more
Protein	Approximately 15%	Approximately 15%
Cholesterol	Less than 300 mg/day	Less than 300 mg/day
Total kcalories	To achieve and maintain desired weight	To achieve and maintain desired weight

* Recommendations available online at http://amhrt.org/Heart_and_Stroke_A_Z_Guide/dietg.html

American Institute of Cancer Research Dietary Guidelines

Choose predominantly plant-based diets rich in a variety of vegetables and fruits, pulses (legumes), and minimally processed starchy staple foods.

Avoid being underweight or overweight and limit weight gain during adulthood to less than 5 kg (11 pounds).

If occupational activity is low or moderate, take an hour's brisk walk or similar exercise daily, and also exercise vigorously for a total of at least one hour in a week.

Eat 400–800 grams (15–30 ounces) or five or more portions (servings) a day of a variety of vegetables and fruits, all year round.

Eat 600–800 grams (20–30 ounces), or more than seven portions (servings), a day of a variety of cereals (grains), pulses (legumes), roots, tubers, and plantains. Prefer minimally processed foods. Limit consumption of refined sugar.

Alcohol consumption is not recommended. If consumed, limit alcoholic drinks to less than two drinks a day for men and one for women.

If eaten at all, limit intake of red meat to less than 80 grams (3 ounces) daily. It is preferable to choose fish, poultry, and meat from nondomesticated animals in place of red meat.

Limit consumption of fatty foods, particularly those of animal origin.

Choose modest amounts of appropriate vegetable oils.

Limit consumption of salted foods and use of cooking and table salt. Use herbs and spices to season foods.

Do not eat food which, as a result of prolonged storage at ambient temperatures, is liable to contamination with mycotoxins.

Use refrigeration and other appropriate methods to preserve perishable foods as purchased and at home.

When levels of additives, contaminants, and other residues are properly regulated, their presence in food and drink is not known to be harmful. However, unregulated or improper use can be a health hazard, and this applies particularly in economically developing countries.

Do not eat charred food. For meat and fish eaters, avoid burning of meat juices. Consume the following only occasionally: meat and fish grilled (broiled) in direct flame; cured and smoked meats.

For those who follow the recommendations presented here, dietary supplements are probably unnecessary, and possibly unhelpful, for reducing cancer risk.

Source: American Institute of Cancer Research. Online at http://www.aicr.org/aicrhst2.htm

G

*National Cancer Institute Dietary Guidelines**

Reduce fat intake to 30% of kcalories or less.

Increase fiber to 20–30 grams/day, with an upper limit of 35 grams.

Include a variety of fruits and vegetables in the daily diet.

Avoid obesity.

Consume alcoholic beverages in moderation, if at all.

Minimize consumption of salt-cured, salt-pickled, and smoked foods.

* Available online at http://rex.nci.nih.gov/NCI_Pub_Interface/ActionGd_Web/guidelns.html

American Cancer Society*

Choose most foods you eat from plant sources.

Limit your intake of high-fat foods, particularly from animal sources.

Be physically active: Achieve and maintain a healthy weight.

Limit consumption of alcoholic beverages, if you drink at all.

* Available online at http://www.cancer.org/statistics/cff98/nutrition.html

Dietary Approaches to Stop Hypertension: DASH Diet

When making changes, start small.

Center your meal around carbohydrates such as pasta, rice, beans, or vegetables.

Treat meat as one part of the whole meal, instead of the focus.

Use fruit and lowfat low-energy foods such as sugar-free gelatin for desserts and snacks.

A 2000-kcalorie diet should include
- 7–8 servings of grains and grain products
- 4–5 servings of vegetables
- 4–5 servings of fruit
- 2–3 servings of lowfat and nonfat dairy foods
- 2 or fewer servings of meat, poultry, and fish
- one-half serving of nuts, seeds, or legumes

Source: Dietary Approaches to Stop Hypertension. Online at http://dash.bwh.harvard.edu

Nutrition and Your Health: Dietary Guidelines for Americans

Eat a variety of foods.

Balance the food you eat with physical activity to maintain or improve your weight.

Choose a diet with plenty of grain products, vegetables, and fruits.

Choose a diet low in fat, saturated fat, and cholesterol.

Choose a diet moderate in sugars.

Choose a diet moderate in salt and sodium.

If you drink alcoholic beverages, do so in moderation.

Source: USDA, USDHHS. *Nutrition and Your Health: Dietary Guidelines for Americans*, 4th ed., 1995.

G

Appendix H

Healthy People 2010

Goals of Healthy People 2010

Increase quality and years of healthy life

Eliminate health disparities

Objectives of Healthy People 2010

- Promote healthy behaviors
  - Physical activity and fitness
  - Nutrition
  - Tobacoo use
- Promote healthy and safe communities
  - Educational and community-based programs
  - Environmental health
  - Food safety
  - Injury/violence prevention
  - Occupational safety and health
  - Oral health
- Improve systems for personal and public health
  - Access to quality health services
    - a. Preventive care
    - b. Primary care
    - c. Emergency services
    - d. Long-term care and rehabilitative services
  - Family planning
  - Maternal, infant, and child health
  - Medical product safety
  - Public health infrastructure
  - Health communication
- Prevent and reduce diseases and disorders
  - Arthritis, osteoporosis, and chronic back conditions
  - Cancer
  - Diabetes
  - Disability and secondary conditions
  - Heart disease and stroke
  - HIV
  - Immunization and infectious diseases
  - Mental health and mental disorders
  - Respiratory diseases
  - Sexually transmitted diseases

Specific Nutrition Objectives of Healthy People 2010

These Objectives Target the Following Areas:

- Healthy weight
- Obesity in adults
- Overweight and obesity in children
- Growth retardation
- Fat intake
- Saturated fat intake
- Vegetable and fruit intake
- Grain product intake
- Sodium intake
- Iron deficiency
- Anemia in pregnant women
- Meals and snacks at school
- Nutrition education, elementary schools
- Nutrition education, middle/junior high schools
- Nutrition education, senior high schools
- Worksite nutrition education and weight management programs
- Nutrition assessment and planning
- Food security

Source: Healthy People 2010 Objectives: Draft for public comment. Available online at http://web.health.gov/healthypeople/2010draft

Appendix I

Exchange Lists

Foods are listed with their serving sizes, which are usually measured after cooking. When you begin, you should measure the size of each serving. This may help you learn to "eyeball" correct serving sizes.

The following chart shows the amount of nutrients in one serving from each list.

The exchange lists provide you with a lot of food choices (foods from the basic food groups, foods with added sugars, free foods, combination foods, and fast foods). This gives you variety in your meals. Several foods, such as dried beans and peas, bacon, and peanut butter, are on two lists. This gives you flexibility in putting your meals together. Whenever you choose new foods or vary your meal plan, monitor your blood glucose to see how these different foods affect your blood glucose level.

Groups/Lists	Carbohydrate (grams)	Protein (grams)	Fat (grams)	Calories
Carbohydrate Group				
Starch	15	3	1 or less	80
Fruit	15	—	—	60
Milk				
Skim	12	8	0–3	90
Low-fat	12	8	5	120
Whole	12	8	8	150
Other carbohydrates	15	Varies	Varies	Varies
Vegetables	5	2	—	25
Meat and Meat Substitute Group				
Very lean	—	7	0–1	35
Lean	—	7	3	55
Medium-fat	—	7	5	75
High-fat	—	7	8	100
Fat Group	—	—	5	45

• Starch List

One starch exchange equals 15 grams carbohydrate, 3 grams protein, 0–1 grams fat, and 80 calories.

Bread

Bagel .... ½ (1 oz)
Bread, reduced-calorie .... 2 slices (1½ oz)
Bread, white, whole-wheat, pumpernickel, rye .... 1 slice (1 oz)
Bread sticks, crisp, 4 in. long × ½ in. .... 2 (⅔ oz)
English muffin .... ½
Hot dog or hamburger bun .... ½ (1 oz)
Pita, 6 in. across .... ½
Roll, plain, small .... 1 (1 oz)
Raisin bread, unfrosted .... 1 slice (1 oz)
Tortilla, corn, 6 in. across 1
Tortilla, flour, 7–8 in. across 1
Waffle, 4½ in. square, reduced-fat 1

Cereals and Grains

Bran cereals .... ½ cup
Bulgur .... ½ cup
Cereals .... ½ cup
Cereals, unsweetened, ready-to-eat .... ¾ cup
Cornmeal (dry) .... 3 Tbsp
Couscous .... ⅓ cup
Flour (dry) .... 3 Tbsp
Granola, low-fat .... ¼ cup
Grape-Nuts .... ¼ cup
Grits .... ½ cup
Kasha .... ½ cup
Millet .... ¼ cup
Muesli .... ¼ cup
Oats .... ½ cup
Pasta .... ½ cup
Puffed cereal .... 1½ cups
Rice milk .... ½ cup
Rice, white or brown .... ⅓ cup
Shredded Wheat .... ½ cup
Sugar-frosted cereal .... ½ cup
Wheat germ .... 3 Tbsp

Dried Beans, Peas, and Lentils

(Count as 1 starch exchange, plus 1 very lean meat exchange.)

Beans and peas (garbanzo, pinto, kidney, white, split, black-eyed) .... ½ cup
Lima beans .... ⅔ cup
Lentils .... ½ cup
Miso [salt shaker icon] .... 3 Tbsp

[salt shaker icon] = 400 mg or more of sodium per serving.

Starchy Vegetables

Baked beans .... ⅓ cup
Corn .... ½ cup
Corn on cob, medium .... 1 (5 oz)
Mixed vegetables with corn, peas, or pasta .... 1 cup
Peas, green .... ½ cup
Plantain .... ½ cup
Potato, baked or boiled .... 1 small (3 oz)
Potato, mashed .... ½ cup
Squash, winter (acorn, butternut) .... 1 cup
Yam, sweet potato, plain .... ½ cup

Crackers and Snacks

Animal crackers 8
Graham crackers, 2½ in. square 3
Matzoh .... ¾ oz

(continued)

Melba toast .... 4 slices
Oyster crackers 24
Popcorn (popped, no fat added or low-fat microwave) .... 3 cups
Pretzels .... ¾ oz
Rice cakes, 4 in. across 2
Saltine-type crackers 6
Snack chips, fat-free (tortilla, potato) .... 15–20 (¾ oz)
Whole-wheat crackers, no fat added .... 2–5 (¾ oz)

Starchy Foods Prepared With Fat
(Count as 1 starch exchange, plus 1 fat exchange.)

Biscuit, 2½ in. across 1
Chow mein noodles .... ½ cup
Corn bread, 2 in. cube .... 1 (2 oz)
Crackers, round butter type 6
Croutons .... 1 cup
French-fried potatoes .... 16–25 (3 oz)
Granola .... ¼ cup
Muffin, small .... 1 (1½ oz)
Pancake, 4 in. across 2
Popcorn, microwave .... 3 cups
Sandwich crackers, cheese or peanut butter filling 3
Stuffing, bread (prepared) .... ⅓ cup
Taco shell, 6 in. across 2
Waffle, 4½ in. square 1
Whole-wheat crackers, fat added .... 4–6 (1 oz)

Fruit List

One fruit exchange equals 15 grams carbohydrate and 60 calories. The weight includes skin, core, seeds, and rind.

Fruit

Apple, unpeeled, small .... 1 (4 oz)
Applesauce, unsweetened .... ½ cup
Applies, dried .... 4 rings
Apricots, fresh .... 4 whole (5½ oz)
Apricots, dried .... 8 halves
Apricots, canned .... ½ cup
Banana, small .... 1 (4 oz)
Blackberries .... ¾ cup
Blueberries .... ¾ cup
Cantaloupe, small .... ⅓ melon (11 oz) or 1 cup cubes
Cherries, sweet, fresh .... 12 (3 oz)
Cherries, sweet, canned .... ½ cup
Dates 3
Figs, fresh .... 1½ large or 2 medium (3½ oz)
Figs, dried 1½
Fruit cocktail .... ½ cup
Grapefruit, large .... ½ (11 oz)
Grapefruit sections, canned .... ¾ cup
Grapes, small .... 17 (3 oz)
Honeydew melon .... 1 slice (10 oz) or 1 cup cubes
Kiwi .... 1 (3½ oz)
Mandarin oranges, canned .... ¾ cup
Mango, small .... ½ fruit (5½ oz) or ½ cup
Nectarine, small .... 1 (5 oz)
Orange, small .... 1 (6½ oz)
Papaya .... ½ fruit (8 oz) or 1 cup cubes
Peach, medium, fresh .... 1 (6 oz)
Peaches, canned .... ½ cup
Pear, large, fresh .... ½ (4 oz)
Pears, canned .... ½ cup
Pineapple, fresh .... ¼ cup
Pineapple, canned .... ½ cup
Plums, small .... 2 (5 oz)
Plums, canned .... ½ cup
Prunes, dried 3
Raisins .... 2 Tbsp
Raspberries .... 1 cup
Strawberries .... 1¼ cup whole berries
Tangerines, small .... 2 (8 oz)
Watermelon .... 1 slice (13½ oz) or 1¼ cup cubes

Fruit Juice

Apple juice/cider .... ½ cup
Cranberry juice cocktail .... ⅓ cup
Cranberry juice cocktail, reduced-calorie .... 1 cup
Fruit juice blends, 100% juice .... ⅓ cup
Grape juice .... ⅓ cup
Grapefruit juice .... ½ cup
Orange juice .... ½ cup
Pineapple juice .... ½ cup
Prune juice .... ⅓ cup

Milk List

One milk exchange equals 12 grams carbohydrate and 8 grams protein.

Skim and Very Low-Fat Milk
(0–3 grams fat per serving)

Skim milk .... 1 cup
½% milk .... 1 cup
1% milk .... 1 cup
Nonfat or low-fat buttermilk .... 1 cup
Evaporated skim milk .... ½ cup
Nonfat dry milk .... ⅓ cup dry
Plain nonfat yogurt .... ¾ cup
Nonfat or low-fat fruit-flavored yogurt sweetened with aspartame or with a non-nutritive sweetener .... 1 cup

Low-Fat
(5 Grams Fat per Serving)

2% milk .... 1 cup
Plain low-fat yogurt .... ¾ cup
Sweet acidophilus milk .... 1 cup

Whole Milk
(8 grams fat per serving)

Whole milk .... 1 cup
Evaporated whole milk .... ½ cup
Goat's milk .... 1 cup
Kefir .... 1 cup

Other Carbohydrates List

One exchange equals 15 grams carbohydrate, or 1 starch, or 1 fruit, or 1 milk.

Food	Serving Size	Exchanges per Serving
Angel food cake, unfrosted	1/12 cake	2 carbohydrates
Brownie, small, unfrosted	2 in. square	1 carbohydrate, 1 fat
Cake, unfrosted	2 in. square	1 carbohydrate, 1 fat
Cake, frosted	2 in. square	2 carbohydrates, 1 fat
Cookie, fat-free	2 small	1 carbohydrate
Cookie or sandwich cookie with creme filling	2 small	1 carbohydrate, 1 fat
Cupcake, frosted	1 small	2 carbohydrates, 1 fat
Cranberry sauce, jellied	1/4 cup	2 carbohydrates
Doughnut, plain cake	1 medium (1½ oz)	1½ carbohydrates, 2 fats
Doughnut, glazed	3¾ in. across (2 oz)	2 carbohydrates, 2 fats
Fruit juice bars, frozen, 100% juice	1 bar (3 oz)	1 carbohydrate
Fruit snacks, chewy (pureed fruit concentrate)	1 roll (¾ oz)	1 carbohydrate
Fruit spread, 100% fruit	1 Tbsp	1 carbohydrate
Gelatin, regular	½ cup	1 carbohydrate
Gingersnaps	3	1 carbohydrate
Granola bar	1 bar	1 carbohydrate, 1 fat
Granola bar, fat-free	1 bar	2 carbohydrates
Hummus	1/3 cup	1 carbohydrate, 1 fat
Ice cream	½ cup	1 carbohydrate, 2 fats
Ice cream, light	½ cup	1 carbohydrate, 1 fat
Ice cream, fat-free, no sugar added	½ cup	1 carbohydrate
Jam or jelly, regular	1 Tbsp	1 carbohydrate
Milk, chocolate, whole	1 cup	2 carbohydrates, 1 fat
Pie, fruit, 2 crusts	1/6 pie	3 carbohydrates, 2 fats
Pie, pumpkin or custard	1/8 pie	1 carbohydrate, 2 fats
Potato chips	12–18 (1 oz)	1 carbohydrate, 2 fats
Pudding, regular (made with low-fat milk)	½ cup	2 carbohydrates
Pudding, sugar-free (made with low-fat milk)	½ cup	1 carbohydrate
Salad dressing, fat-free	¼ cup	1 carbohydrate
Sherbet, sorbet	½ cup	2 carbohydrates
Spaghetti or pasta sauce, canned	½ cup	1 carbohydrate, 1 fat
Sweet roll or Danish	1 (2½ oz)	2½ carbohydrates, 2 fats
Syrup, light	2 Tbsp	1 carbohydrate
Syrup, regular	1 Tbsp	1 carbohydrate
Syrup, regular	¼ cup	4 carbohydrates
Tortilla chips	6–12 (1 oz)	1 carbohydrate, 2 fats
Yogurt, frozen, low-fat, fat-free	1/3 cup	1 carbohydrate, 0–1 fat
Yogurt, frozen, fat-free, no sugar added	½ cup	1 carbohydrate
Yogurt, low-fat with fruit	1 cup	3 carbohydrates, 0–1 fat
Vanilla wafers	5	1 carbohydrate, 1 fat

= 400 mg or more of sodium per serving.

Vegetable List

Vegetables that contain small amounts of carbohydrates and calories are on this list. Vegetables contain important nutrients. Try to eat at least 2 or 3 vegetable choices each day. In general, one vegetable exchange is:

½ cup of cooked vegetable or vegetable juice, or
1 cup of raw vegetables

If you eat 1 to 2 vegetable choices at a meal or snack, you do not have to count the calories or carbohydrates because they contain small amounts of these nutrients.

One vegetable exchange equals 5 grams carbohydrate, 2 grams protein, 0 grams fat, and 25 calories.

Artichoke
Artichoke hearts
Asparagus
Beans (green, wax, Italian)
Bean sprouts
Beets
Broccoli
Brussels sprouts
Cabbage
Carrots
Cauliflower
Celery
Cucumber
Eggplant
Green onions or scallions
Greens(collard, kale, mustard, turnip)
Kohlrabi
Leeks
Mixed vegetables (without corn, peas, or pasta)
Mushrooms
Okra
Onions
Pea pods
Peppers (all varieties)
Radishes
Salad greens (endive, escarole, lettuce, romaine, spinach)
Sauerkraut
Spinach
Summer squash
Tomato
Tomatoes, canned
Tomato sauce
Tomato/vegetable juice
Turnips
Water chestnuts
Watercress
Zucchini

= 400 mg or more sodium per exchange.

Very Lean Meat and Substitutes List

One exchange equals 0 grams carbohydrate, 7 grams protein, 0–1 grams fat, and 35 calories.

One very lean meat exchange is equal to any one of the following items.

Poultry: Chicken or turkey (white meat, no skin), Cornish hen (no skin) ... 1 oz
Fish: Fresh or frozen cod, flounder, haddock, halibut, trout; tuna, fresh or canned in water ... 1 oz
Shellfish: Clams, crab, lobster, scallops, shrimp, imitation shellfish ... 1 oz
Game: Duck or pheasant (no skin), venison, buffalo, ostrich ... 1 oz
Cheese with 1 gram or less fat per ounce:
Nonfat or low-fat cottage cheese ... ¼ cup
Fat-free cheese ... 1 oz
Other: Processed sandwich meats with 1 gram or less fat per ounce, such as deli thin, shaved meats, chipped beef, turkey ham ... 1 oz
Egg whites ... 2
Egg substitutes, plain ... ¼ cup
Hot dogs with 1 gram or less fat per ounce ... 1 oz
Kidney (high in cholesterol) ... 1 oz
Sausage with 1 gram or less fat per ounce ... 1 oz

Count as one very lean meat and one starch exchange.

Dried beans, peas, lentils (cooked) ... ½ cup
= 400 mg or more sodium per exchange.

Lean Meat and Substitutes List

One exchange equals 0 grams carbohydrate, 7 grams protein, 3 grams fat, and 55 calories.

One lean meat exchange is equal to any one of the following items.

Beef: USDA Select or Choice grades of lean beef trimmed of fat, such as round, sirloin, and flank steak; tenderloin; roast (rib, chuck, rump); steak (T-bone, porterhouse, cubed), ground round ... 1 oz
Pork: Lean pork, such as fresh ham; canned, cured, or boiled ham; Canadian bacon; tenderloin, center loin chop ... 1 oz
Lamb: Roast, chop, leg ... 1 oz
Veal: Lean chop, roast ... 1 oz
Poultry: Chicken, turkey (dark meat, no skin), chicken white meat (with skin), domestic duck or goose (well-drained of fat, no skin) ... 1 oz
Fish:
Herring (uncreamed or smoked) ... 1 oz
Oysters ... 6 medium
Salmon (fresh or canned), catfish ... 1 oz
Sardines (canned) ... 2 medium
Tuna (canned in oil, drained) ... 1 oz
Game: Goose (no skin), rabbit ... 1 oz
Cheese:
4.5%-fat cottage cheese ... ¼ cup
Grated Parmesan ... 2 Tbsp
Cheeses with 3 grams or less fat per ounce ... 1 oz
Other:
Hot dogs with 3 grams or less fat per ounce ... 1½ oz
Processed sandwich meat with 3 grams or less fat per ounce, such as turkey pastrami or kielbasa ... 1 oz
Liver, heart (high in cholesterol) ... 1 oz
= 400 mg or more sodium per exchange.

Medium-Fat Meat and Substitutes List

One exchange equals 0 grams carbohydrate, 7 grams protein, 5 grams fat, and 75 calories.

One medium-fat meat exchange is equal to any one of the following items.

Beef: Most beef products fall into this category (ground beef, meatloaf, corned beef, short ribs, Prime grades of meat trimmed of fat, such as prime rib) ... 1 oz
Pork: Top loin, chop, Boston butt, cutlet ... 1 oz
Lamb: Rib roast, ground ... 1 oz
Veal: Cutlet (ground or cubed, unbreaded) ... 1 oz
Poultry: Chicken dark meat (with skin), ground turkey or ground chicken, fried chicken (with skin) ... 1 oz
Fish: Any fried fish product ... 1 oz
Cheese: With 5 grams or less fat per ounce
Feta ... 1 oz
Mozzarella ... 1 oz
Ricotta ... ¼ cup (2 oz)
Other:
Egg (high in cholesterol, limit to 3 per week) ... 1
Sausage with 5 grams or less fat per ounce ... 1 oz
Soy milk ... 1 cup
Tempeh ... ¼ cup
Tofu ... 4 oz or ½ cup

High-Fat Meat and Substitutes List

One exchange equals 0 grams carbohydrate, 7 grams protein, 8 grams fat, and 100 calories.

Remember, these items are high in saturated fat, cholesterol, and calories and may raise blood cholesterol levels if eaten on a regular basis. One high-fat meat exchange is equal to any one of the following items.

Pork: Spareribs, ground pork, pork sausage ... 1 oz
Cheese: All regular cheeses, such as American, cheddar, Monterey Jack, Swiss ... 1 oz
Other: Processed sandwich meats with 8 grams or less fat per ounce, such as bologna, pimento loaf, salami ... 1 oz
Sausage, such as bratwurst, Italian, knockwurst, Polish, smoked ... 1 oz
Hot dog (turkey or chicken) ... 1 (10/lb)
Bacon ... 2 slices (20 slices/lb)

Count as one high-fat meat plus one fat exchange.

Hot dog (beef, pork, or combination) ... 1 (10/lb)
Peanut butter (contains unsaturated fat) ... 2 Tbsp
= 400 mg or more sodium per exchange.

Fats List

Monounsaturated Fats

One fat exchange equals 5 grams fat and 45 calories.

Avocado, medium ... ⅛ (1 oz)
Oil (canola, olive, peanut) ... 1 tsp

(continued)

Olives: ripe (black) .... 8 large
Green, stuffed .... 10 large
Nuts
Almonds, cashews .... 6 nuts
Mixed (50% peanuts) .... 6 nuts
Peanuts .... 10 nuts
Pecans .... 4 halves
Peanut butter, smooth or crunchy .... 2 tsp
Sesame seeds .... 1 Tbsp
Tahini paste .... 2 tsp
= 400 mg or more sodium per exchange.

Polyunsaturated Fats

One fat exchange equals 5 grams fat and 45 calories.

Margarine: stick, tub, or squeeze .... 1 tsp
Lower-fat (30% to 50% vegetable oil) .... 1 Tbsp
Mayonnaise: regular .... 1 tsp
Reduced-fat .... 1 Tbsp
Nuts, walnuts, English .... 4 halves
Oil (corn, safflower, soybean) .... 1 tsp
Salad dressing: regular .... 1 Tbsp
Reduced-fat .... 2 Tbsp
Miracle Whip Salad Dressing®: regular .... 2 tsp
Reduced-fat .... 1 Tbsp
Seeds: pumpkin, sunflower .... 1 Tbsp
= 400 mg or more sodium per exchange.

Saturated Fats*

One fat exchange equals 5 grams of fat and 45 calories.

Bacon, cooked .... 1 slice (20 slices/lb)
Bacon, grease .... 1 tsp
Butter: stick .... 1 tsp
Whipped .... 2 tsp
Reduced-fat .... 1 Tbsp
Chitterlings, boiled .... 2 Tbsp (½ oz)
Coconut, sweetened, shredded .... 2 Tbsp
Cream, half and half .... 2 Tbsp
Cream cheese: regular .... 1 Tbsp (½ oz)
Reduced-fat .... 2 Tbsp (1 oz)
Fatback or salt pork, see below†
Shortening or lard .... 1 tsp
Sour cream: regular .... 2 Tbsp
Reduced-fat .... 3 Tbsp

* Saturated fats can raise blood cholesterol levels.
† Use a piece 1 in. × 1 in. × ¼ in. if you plan to eat the fatback cooked with vegetables. Use a piece 2 in. × 1 in. × ½ in. when eating only the vegetables with the fatback removed.

Free Foods List

A *free food* is any food or drink that contains less than 20 calories or less than 5 grams of carbohydrate per serving. Foods with a serving size listed should be limited to three servings per day. Be sure to spread them out throughout the day. If you eat all three servings at one time, it could affect your blood glucose level. Foods listed without a serving size can be eaten as often as you like.

Fat-Free or Reduced-Fat Foods

Cream cheese, fat-free .... 1 Tbsp
Creamers, nondairy, liquid .... 1 Tbsp
Creamers, nondairy, powdered .... 2 tsp
Mayonnaise, fat-free .... 1 Tbsp
Mayonnaise, reduced-fat .... 1 tsp
Margarine, fat-free .... 4 Tbsp
Margarine, reduced-fat .... 1 tsp
Miracle Whip®, nonfat .... 1 Tbsp
Miracle Whip®, reduced-fat .... 1 tsp
Nonstick cooking spray
Salad dressing, fat-free .... 1 Tbsp
Salad dressing, fat-free, Italian .... 2 Tbsp
Salsa .... ¼ cup
Sour cream, fat-free, reduced-fat 1Tbsp
Whipped topping, regular or light .... 2 Tbsp

Sugar-Free or Low-Sugar Foods

Candy, hard, sugar-free .... 1 candy
Gelatin dessert, sugar-free
Gelatin, unflavored
Gum, sugar-free
Jam or jelly, low-sugar or light .... 2 tsp
Sugar substitutes*
Syrup, sugar-free .... 2 Tbsp

* Sugar substitutes, alternatives, or replacements that are approved by the Food and Drug Administration (FDA) are safe to use. Common brand names include: Equal® (aspartame), Sprinkle Sweet® (saccharin), Sweet One® (acesulfame K), Sweet-10® (saccharin), Sugar Twin® (saccharin), Sweet 'n Low® (saccharin).

Drinks

Bouillon, broth, consommé
Bouillon or broth, low-sodium
Carbonated or mineral water
Cocoa powder, unsweetened .... 1 Tbsp
Coffee
Club soda
Diet soft drinks, sugar-free
Drink mixes, sugar-free
Tea
Tonic water, sugar-free

Condiments

Catsup .... 1 Tbsp
Horseradish
Lemon juice
Lime juice
Mustard
Pickles, dill .... 1½ large
Soy sauce, regular or light
Taco sauce .... 1 Tbsp
Vinegar

Seasonings

Be careful with seasonings that contain sodium or are salts, such as garlic or celery salt, and lemon pepper.

Flavoring extracts
Garlic
Herbs, fresh or dried
Pimento
Spices
Tabasco® or hot pepper sauce
Wine, used in cooking
Worcestershire sauce
= 400 mg or more of sodium per choice.

Combination Food List

Many of the foods we eat are mixed together in various combinations. These combination foods do not fit into any one exchange list. Often it is hard to tell what is in a casserole dish or prepared food item. This is a list of exchanges for some typical combination foods. This list will help you fit these foods into your meal plan. Ask your dietitian for information about any other combination foods you would like to eat.

Food	Serving Size	Exchanges per Serving
Entrees		
Tuna noodle casserole, lasagna, spaghetti with meatballs, chile with beans, macaroni and cheese	1 cup (8 oz)	2 carbohydrates, 2 medium-fat meats
Chow mein (without noodles or rice)	2 cups (16 oz)	1 carbohydrate, 2 lean meats
Pizza, cheese, thin crust	¼ of 10 in. (5 oz)	2 carbohydrates, 2 medium-fat meats, 1 fat
Pizza, meat topping, thin crust	¼ of 10 in. (5 oz)	2 carbohydrates, 2 medium-fat meats, 2 fats
Pot pie	1 (7 oz)	2 carbohydrates, 1 medium-fat meat, 4 fats
Frozen entrees		
Salisbury steak with gravy, mashed potato	1 (11 oz)	2 carbohydrates, 3 medium-fat meats, 3–4 fats
Turkey with gravy, mashed potato, dressing	1 (11 oz)	2 carbohydrates, 3 lean meats
Entree with less than 300 calories	1 (8 oz)	2 carbohydrates, 3 lean meats
Soups		
Bean	1 cup	1 carbohydrate, 1 very lean meat
Cream (made with water)	1 cup (8 oz)	1 carbohydrate, 1 fat
Split pea (made with water)	½ cup (4 oz)	1 carbohydrate
Tomato (made with water)	1 cup (8 oz)	1 carbohydrate
Vegetable beef, chicken noodle, or other broth-type	1 cup (8 oz)	1 carbohydrate

= 400 mg or more sodium per exchange.

Fast Foods List*

Food	Serving Size	Exchanges per Serving
Burritos with beef	2	4 carbohydrates, 2 medium-fat meats, 2 fats
Chicken nuggets	6	1 carbohydrate, 2 medium-fat meats, 1 fat
Chicken breast and wing, breaded and fried	1 each	1 carbohydrate, 4 medium-fat meats, 2 fats
Fish sandwich/tartar sauce	1	3 carbohydrates, 1 medium-fat meat, 3 fats
French fries, thin	20–25	2 carbohydrates, 2 fats
Hamburger, regular	1	2 carbohydrates, 2 medium-fat meats
Hamburger, large	1	2 carbohydrates, 3 medium-fat meats, 1 fat
Hot dog with bun	1	1 carbohydrate, 1 high-fat meat, 1 fat
Individual pan pizza	1	5 carbohydrates, 3 medium-fat meats, 3 fats
Soft-serve cone	1 medium	2 carbohydrates, 1 fat
Submarine sandwich	1 sub (6 in.)	3 carbohydrates, 1 vegetable, 2 medium-fat meats, 1 fat
Taco, hard shell	1 (6 oz)	2 carbohydrates, 2 medium-fat meats, 2 fats
Taco, soft shell	1 (3 oz)	1 carbohydrate, 1 medium-fat meat, 1 fat

= 400 mg or more of sodium per serving.

* Ask at your fast-food restaurant for nutrition information about your favorite fast foods.

I

Appendix J

Diet Planning Tools for Ethnic Diets and the Food Guide Pyramid for Young Children

The Mediterranean Diet Pyramid

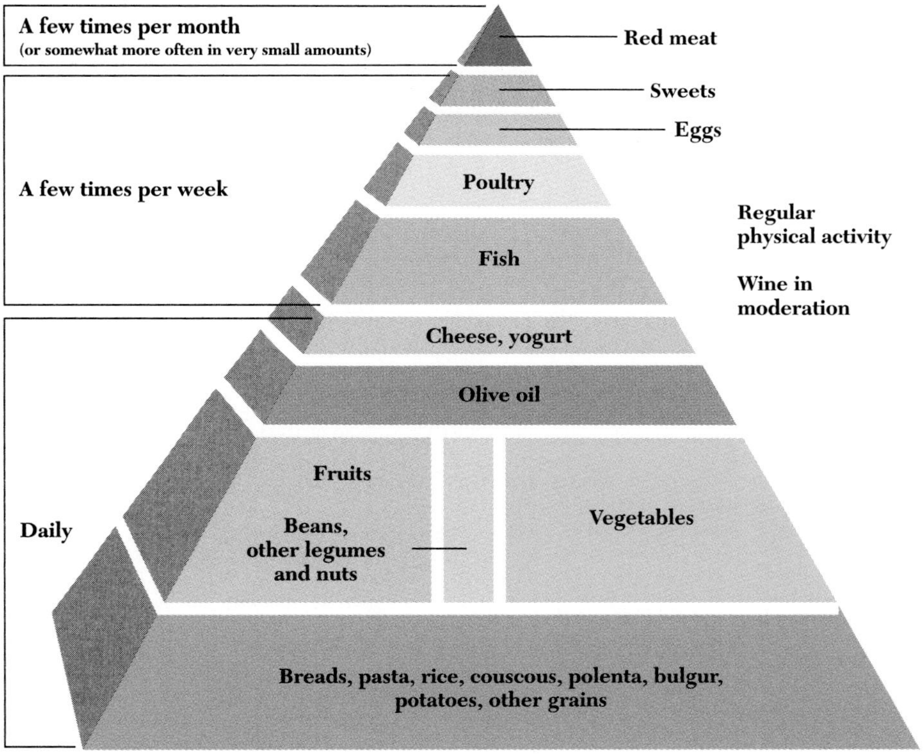

HEALTH HINTS FROM THE MEDITERRANEAN DIET PYRAMID

- Eat most food from plant sources, including fruits, vegetables, potatoes, breads, beans, nuts, and seeds.
- Use seasonally fresh, locally grown food with a minimum of processing.
- Let olive oil be your principal fat, replacing other fats, oils, butter, and margarine.
- Eat red meat only a few times per month and favor the lean cuts.
- If you drink wine, enjoy only 1 or 2 glasses a day, preferably with meals.
- Engage in regular exercise to promote a healthy weight, fitness, and well-being.

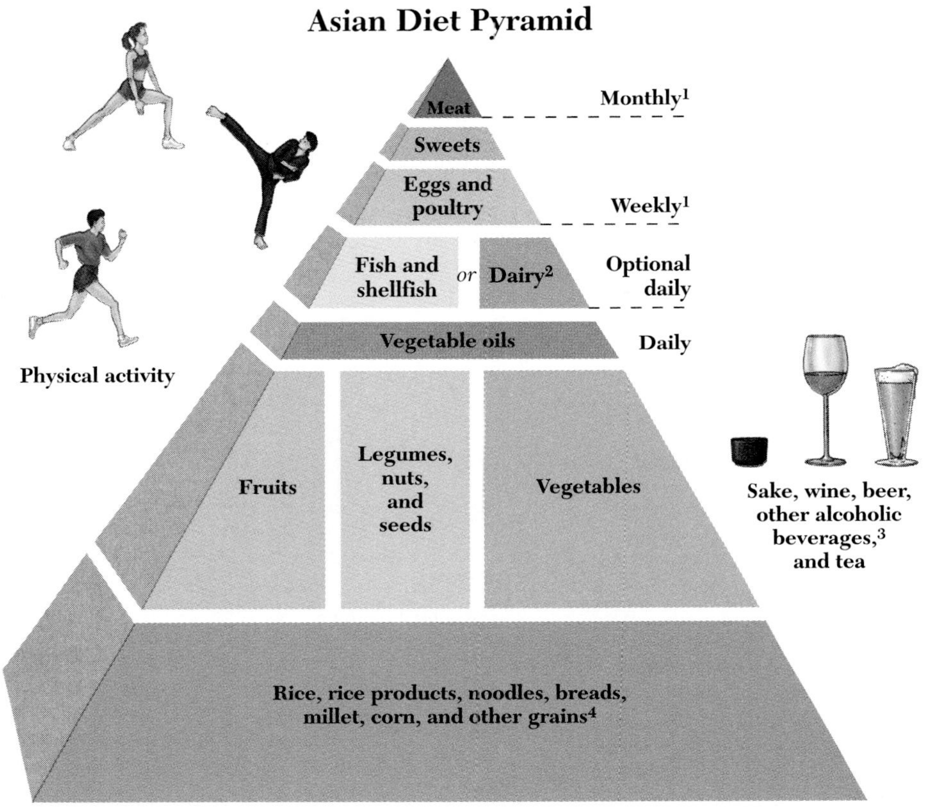

[1]Or more often in very small amounts.

[2]Dairy foods are generally not part of the healthy, traditional diets of Asia, with the notable exception of India. In light of current nutrition research, if dairy foods are consumed on a daily basis, they should be used in low to moderate amounts, and preferably be low in fat.

[3]Wine, beer, and other alcoholic beverages should be consumed in moderation and primarily with meals, and avoided whenever consumption would put an individual or others at risk.

[4]Minimally refined whenever possible.

Mexican American Foods and the Food Guide Pyramid

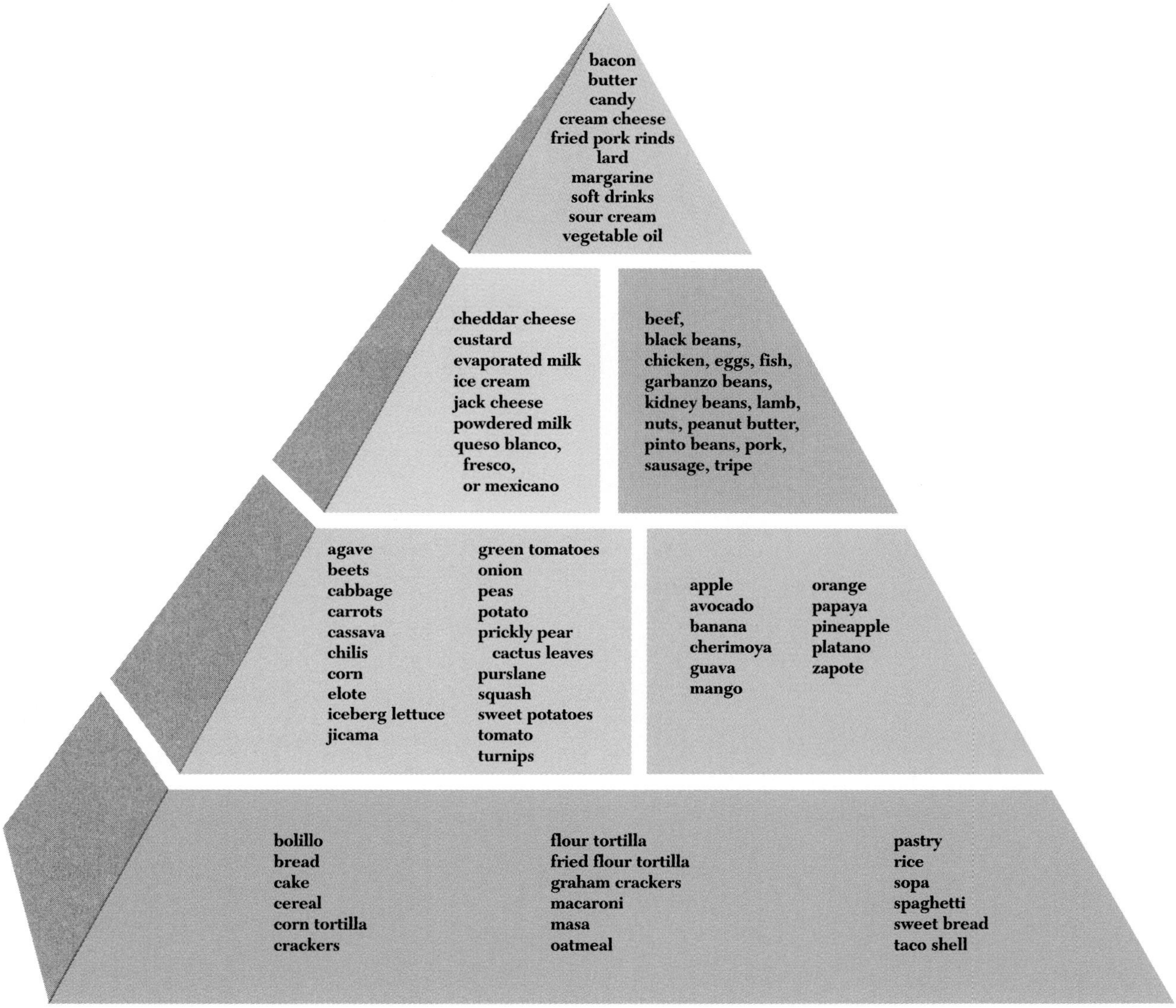

Sources: Algert, Susan J., and Teri Hall Ellison, Contributors. *Ethnic and Regional Food Practices—A Series: Mexican American Food Practices, Customs, and Holidays*; Diabetes Care and Education Practice Group of the American Dietetic Association, 1989; *Comidas Hispana en Dietas Diabetica (Spanish Foods in Diabetic Diets)*. Visiting Nurse Association of Milwaukee, 1975.

J

African American Foods and the Food Guide Pyramid

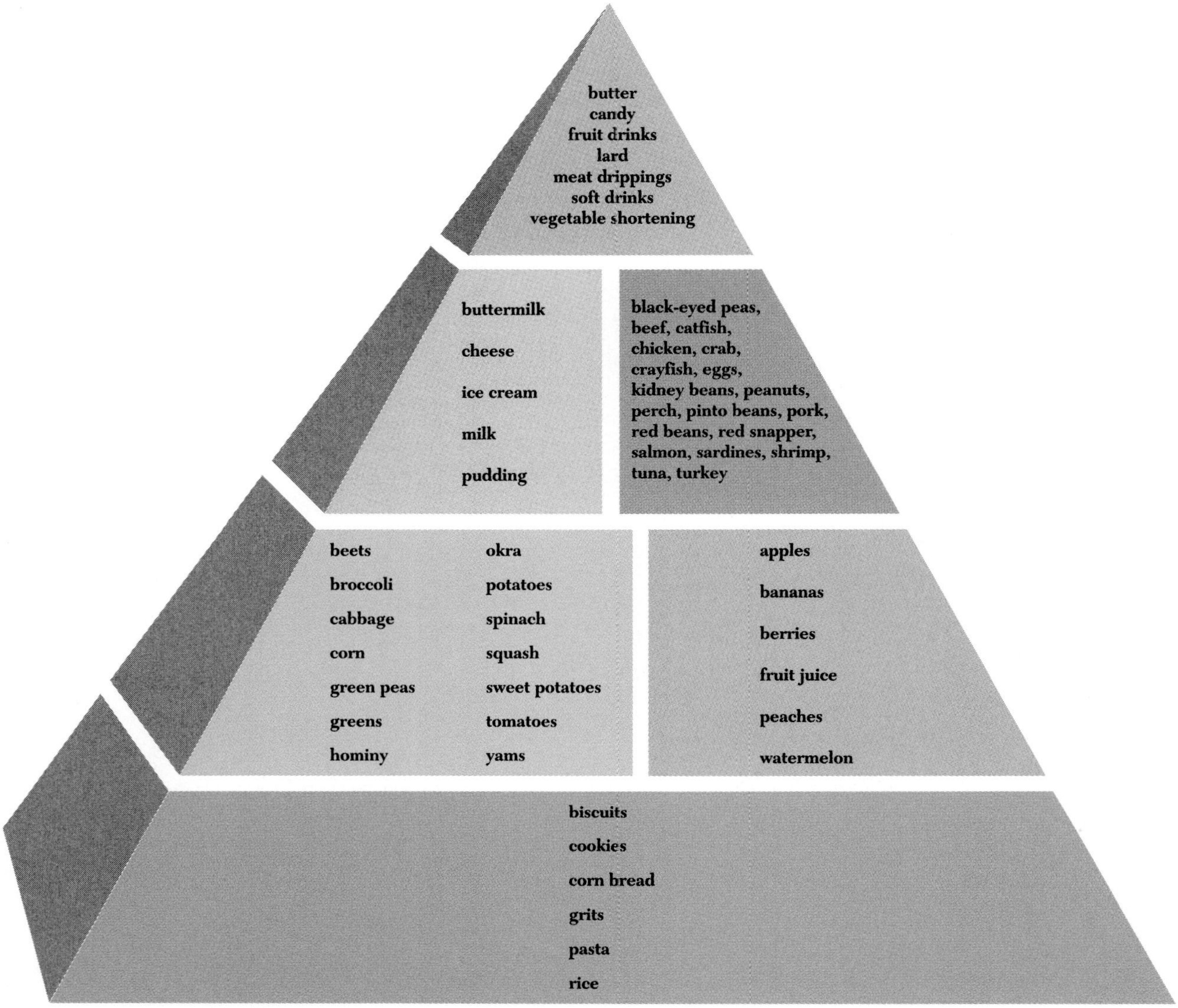

Source: Kittler, Pamela Goyan, and Kathryn Sucher. *Food and Culture in America* (New York: Van Nostrand Reinhold, 1989).

J

Chinese American Foods and the Food Guide Pyramid

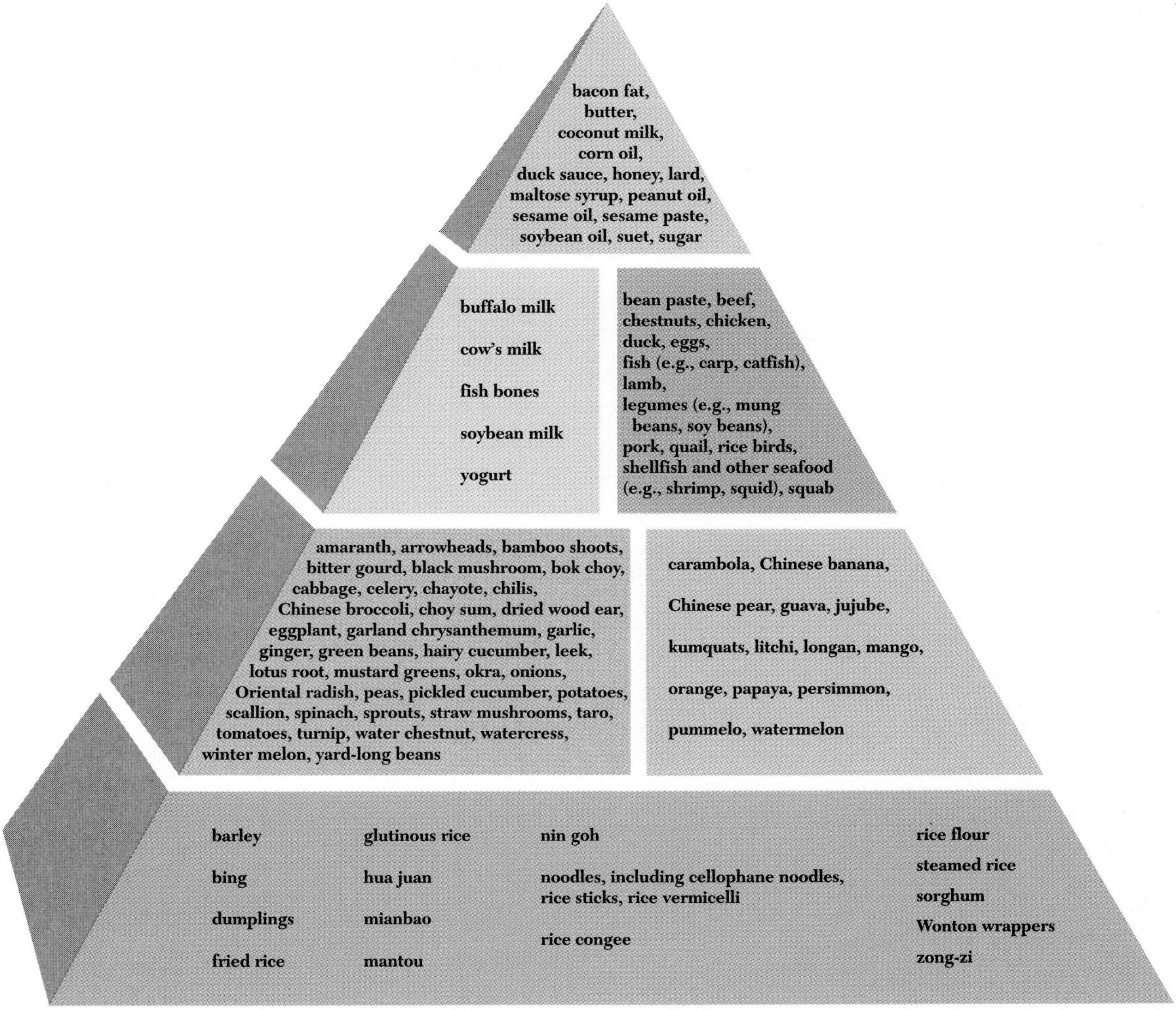

Sources: Kee Maggie Ma. *Ethnic and Regional Food Practices—A Series: Chinese American Food Practices, Customs and Holidays*. Diabetes Care and Education Practice Group of the American Dietetic Association, 1990; Kittler, Pamela Goyan, and Kathryn Sucher. *Food and Culture in America* (New York; Van Nostrand Reinhold, 1989).

Indian Foods and the Food Guide Pyramid

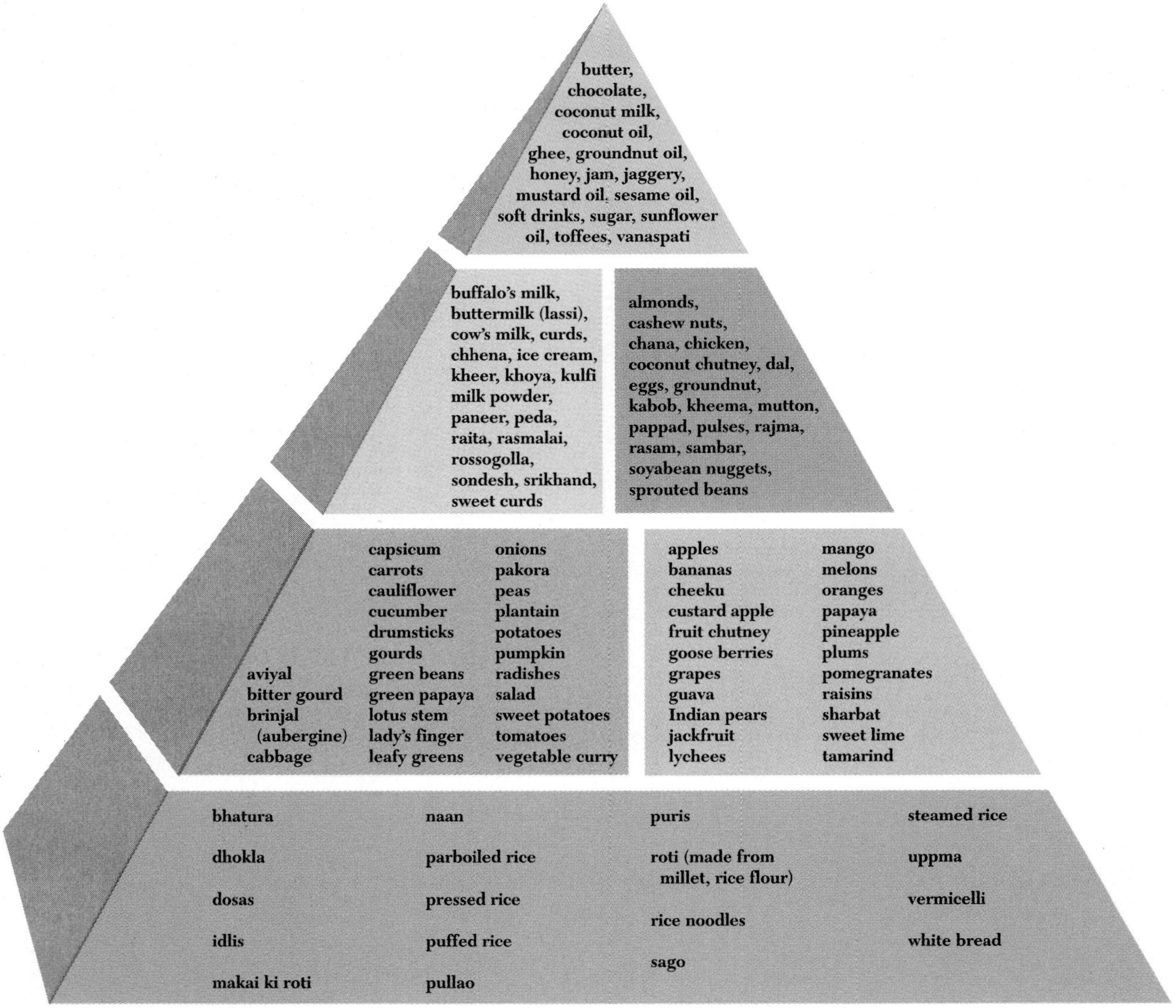

Sources: Barer-Stein, Thelma. *You Eat What You Are—A Study of Ethnic Food Traditions* (Toronto: McClelland and Stewart, Ltd., 1979); Dalal, *Tarla Dalal's New Indian Vegatarian Cooking* (Bombay: India Book Distributors, 1986); Kittler, Pamela Goyan, and Kathryn Sucher. *Food and Culture in America* (New York: Van Nostrand Reinhold, 1989); Madhur, Jaffrey. *A Taste of India* (London: Pan Books, Ltd., 1985); Sahni, Julie. *Classic Indian Cooking* (New York: William Morrow and Company, Inc. 1980); Santha, Rama Rau. *The Cooking of India* (New York: Time-Life Books [Foods of the World], 1969). Pyramid prepared by Uma Srinath.

Jewish Foods and the Food Guide Pyramid

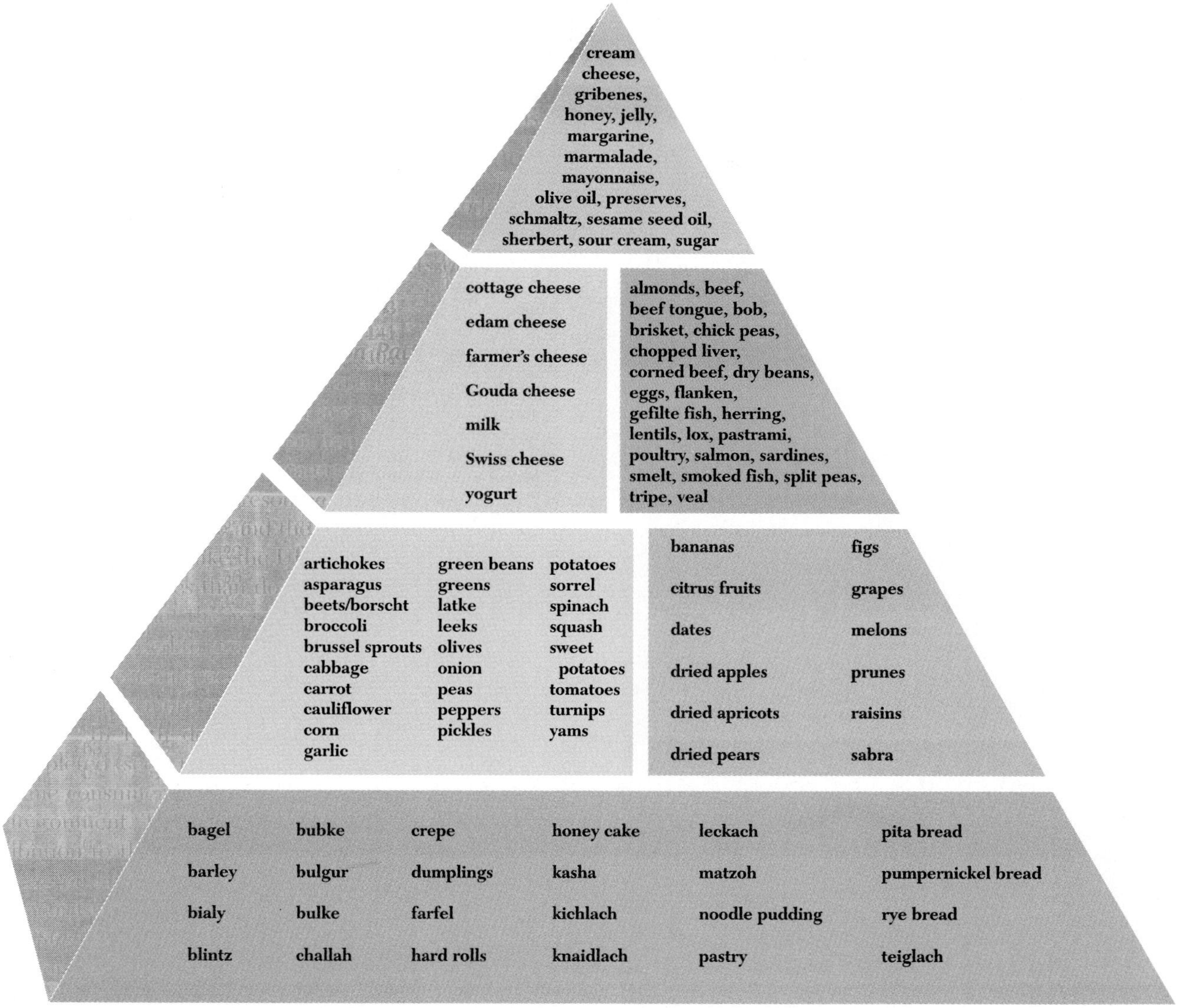

Sources: Higgins, Catherine, and Hope S. Warshaw, contributors. *Ethnic and Regional Food Practices—A Series: Jewish Food Practices, Customs, and Holidays.* Diabetes Care and Education Practice Group of the American Dietetic Association, 1989; Barer-Stein, Thelma. *You Eat What You Are—A Study of Ethnic Food Traditions* (Toronto: McClelland and Stewart Ltd., 1979).

J

Current Navajo Foods and the Food Guide Pyramid

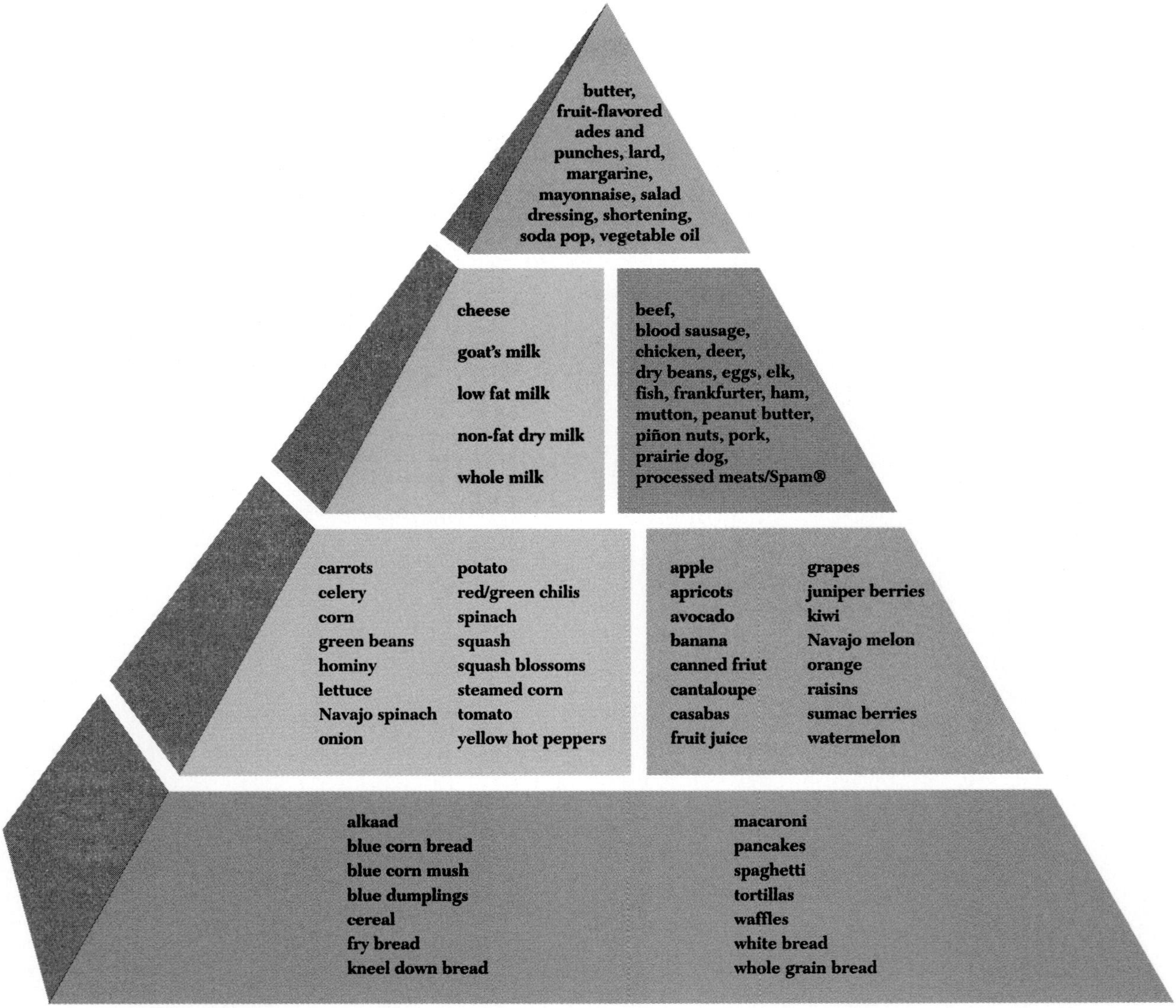

Sources: Pelican, Suzanne, and Karen Bachman-Carter. *Ethnic and Regional Food Practices—A Series: Navajo Food Practices, Customs, and Holidays.* Diabetes Care and Education Practice Group of the American Dietetic Association, 1991; Navajo Health and Nutrition Survey (unpublished). Navajo Area Indian Health Service.

Puerto Rican Foods and the Food Guide Pyramid*

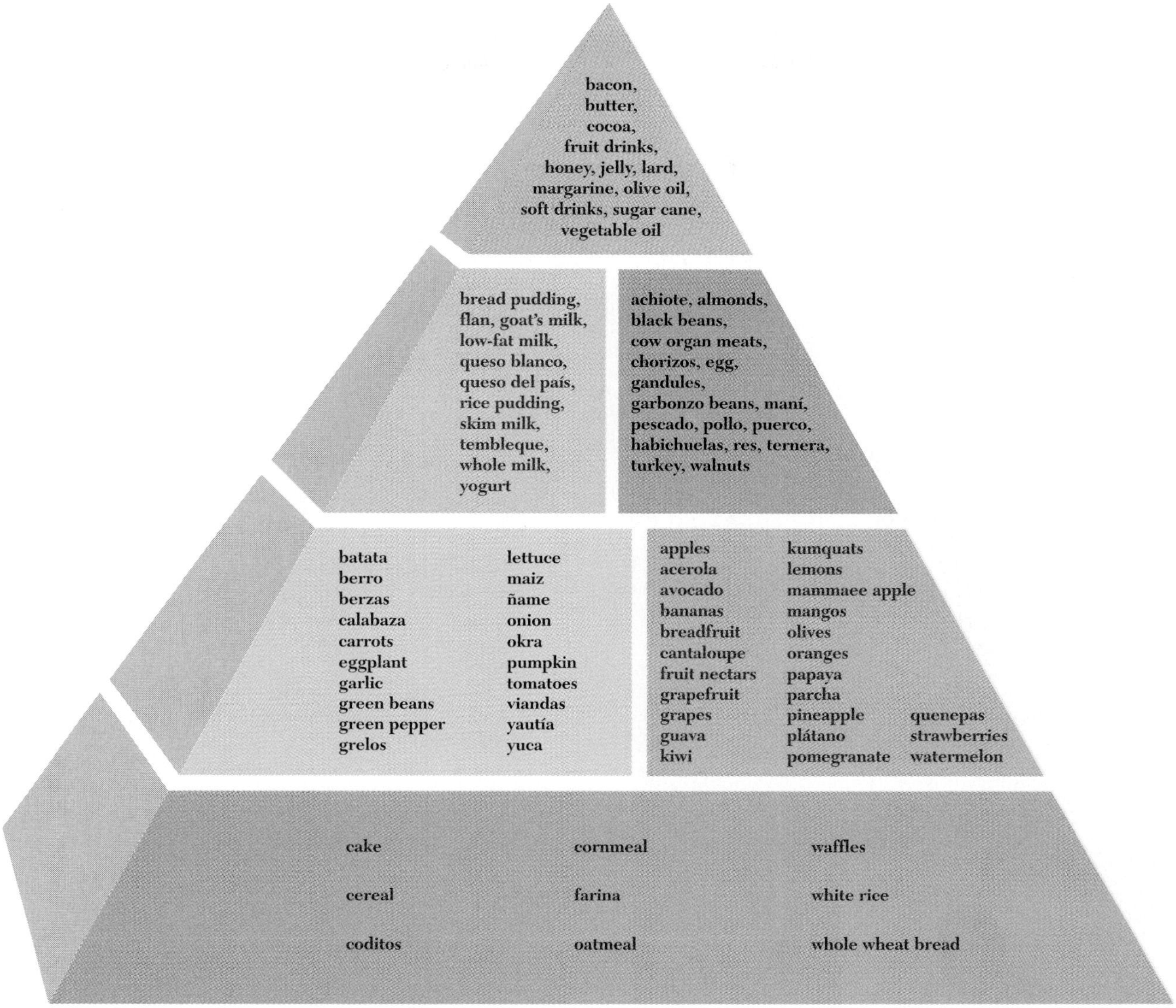

* May be used with Cuban and Dominican populations.

Sources: Dooley, Eliza B.K. *Puerto Rican Cookbook* (Virginia: Dietz, 1948); Internet: http://www.cu-online.com/~maggy/pr.html; Internet: http://pubweb.acns.nwu.edu/%7Ecotto/pr.html; Rivera, Jeanie. Personal interview, 1 April 1996; Ruíz, Leondro. Personal interview, 26 May 1996; "Buen Provecho..." *Bienvenidos* 1994; Vasquez, Susana. Personal Interview, 10 April 1996.

Vietnamese American Foods and the Food Guide Pyramid

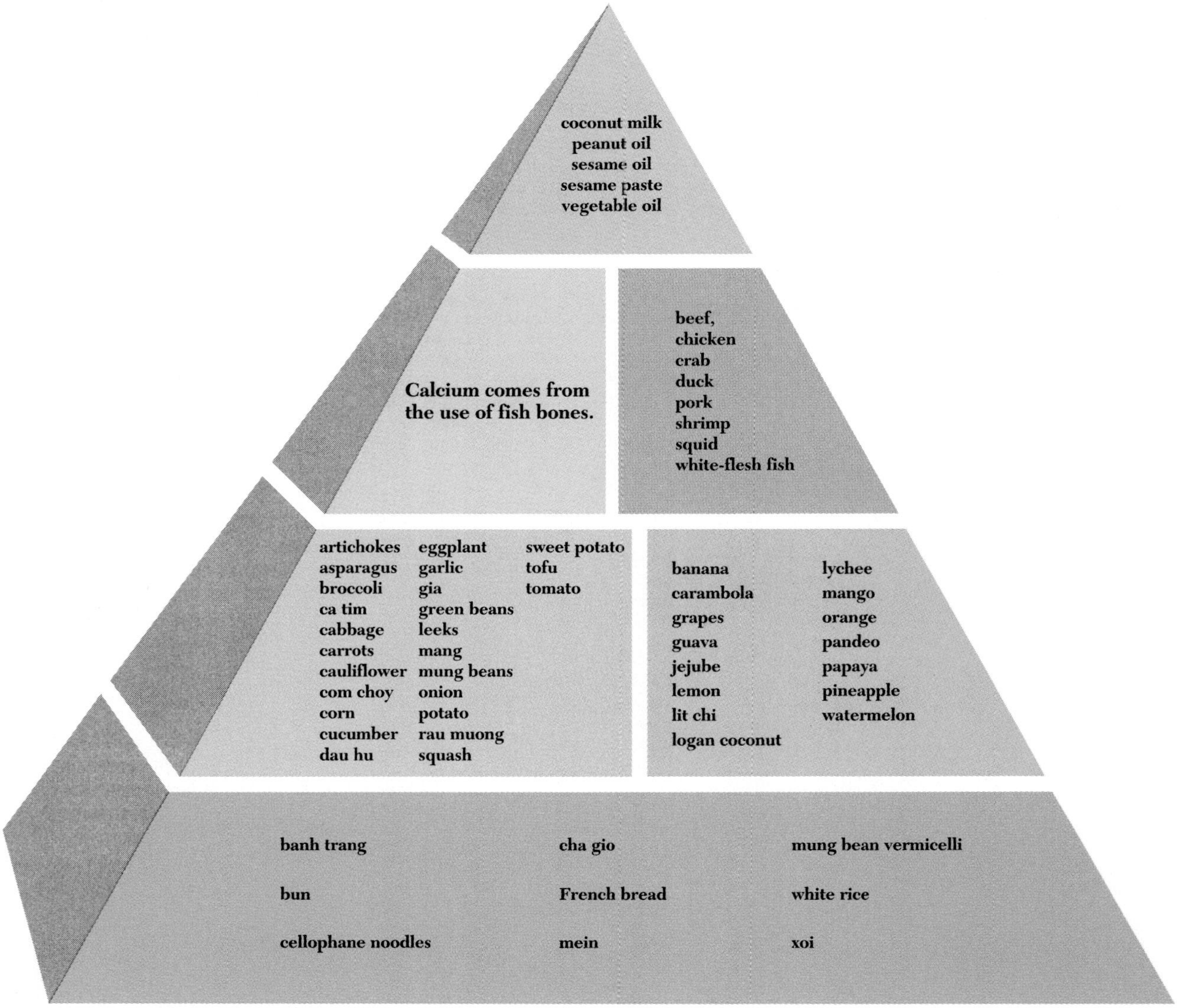

Sources: Passimore, Jackie. *Asia, the Beautiful Cookbook* (San Francisco: Collins Publishers, 1990); Routhier, Nicole. *The Foods of Vietnam* (New York: Stewart, Taborr and Chang, 1989); Solomon, Charmaine. *Complete Asian Cookbook* (New York: McGraw-Hill Book Co., 1982); Le, Laura, personal interview, April 1996; Le, Tuan, personal interview, April 1996; Waiter at The Pho Express Restaurant. personal interview, April 1996.

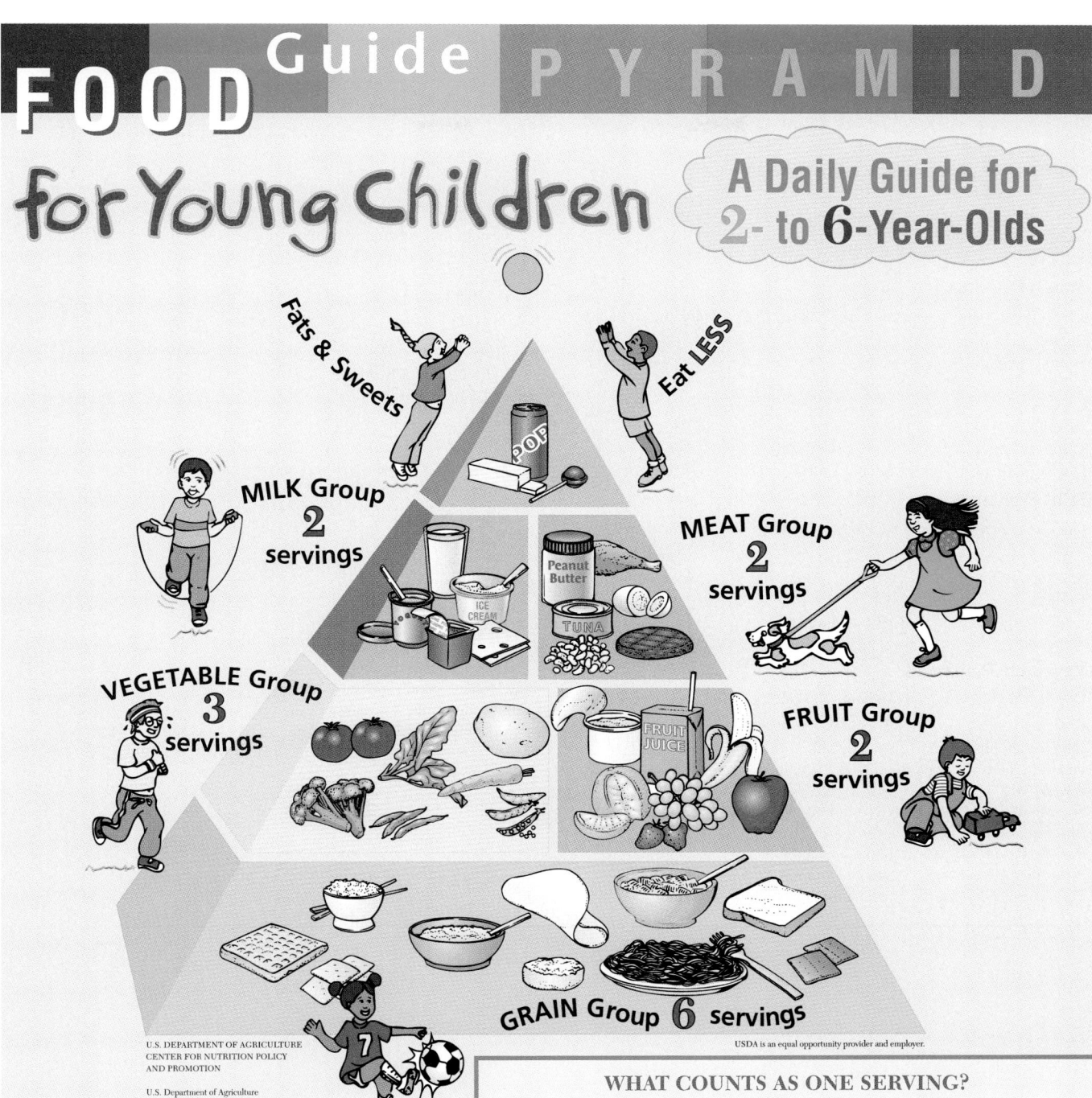

FOOD Guide PYRAMID

for Young Children

A Daily Guide for 2- to 6-Year-Olds

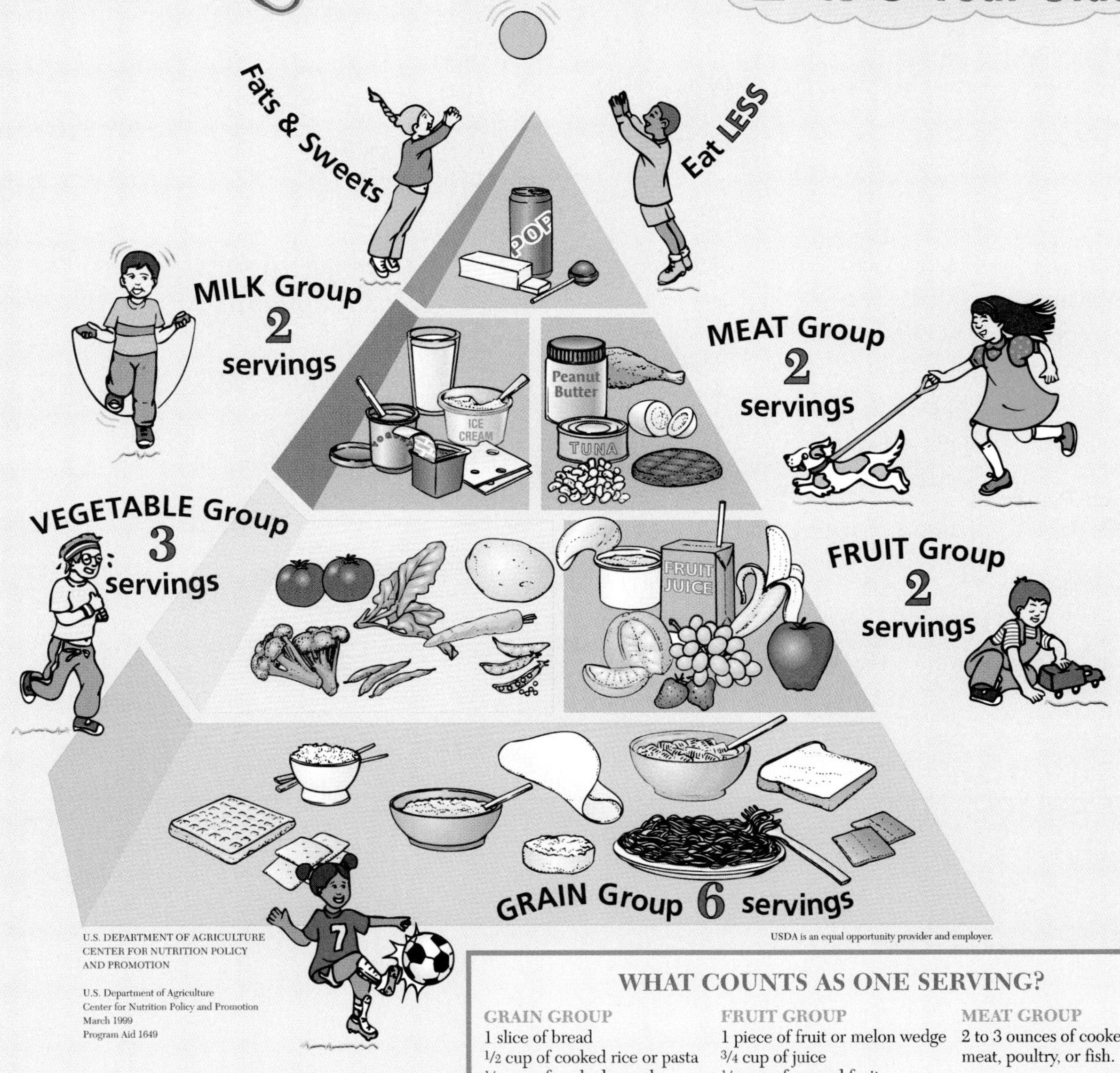
Fats & Sweets
Eat LESS
POP
MILK Group 2 servings
MEAT Group 2 servings
Peanut Butter
ICE CREAM
TUNA
VEGETABLE Group 3 servings
FRUIT Group 2 servings
FRUIT JUICE
GRAIN Group 6 servings

U.S. DEPARTMENT OF AGRICULTURE
CENTER FOR NUTRITION POLICY
AND PROMOTION

U.S. Department of Agriculture
Center for Nutrition Policy and Promotion
March 1999
Program Aid 1649

USDA is an equal opportunity provider and employer.

FOOD IS FUN and learning about food is fun, too. Eating foods from the Food Guide Pyramid and being physically active will help you grow healthy and strong.

WHAT COUNTS AS ONE SERVING?

GRAIN GROUP
1 slice of bread
1/2 cup of cooked rice or pasta
1/2 cup of cooked cereal
1 ounce of ready-to-eat cereal

VEGETABLE GROUP
1/2 cup of chopped raw or cooked vegetables
1 cup of raw leafy vegetables

FRUIT GROUP
1 piece of fruit or melon wedge
3/4 cup of juice
1/2 cup of canned fruit
1/4 cup of dried fruit

MILK GROUP
1 cup of milk or yogurt
2 onces of cheese

MEAT GROUP
2 to 3 ounces of cooked lean meat, poultry, or fish.

1/2 cup of cooked dry beans, or 1 egg counts as 1 ounce of lean meat. 2 tablespoons of peanut butter count as 1 ounce of meat.

FATS AND SWEETS
Limit calories from these.

Four- to 6-year-olds can eat these serving sizes. Offer 2- to 3-year-olds less, except for milk. Two- to 6-year-old children need a total of 2 servings from the milk group each day.

EAT a variety of FOODS AND ENJOY!

J

Samoan Foods in the Exchange Lists

Calcium/Milk Exchanges

One serving contains approximately 90 kcal, 12 g carbohydrate, 8 g protein, and a trace of fat.

Dark, green, leafy vegetables (calcium may not be readily absorbed)	3 c
Tofu, prepared with calcium (omit 1 fat group)	½ c
Fish, sardines, mackerel	3 oz
Salmon, canned with bones (omit 1 fat group)	3 oz

Starch Exchanges

One serving contains approximately 80 kcal, 15 g carbohydrate, and 3 g protein.

Banana, plantain (cooking banana)	1 medium (2″ × 1⅞″)
Cassava	⅓ c
Breadfruit	¼ c
Taro	½ c
O'o (sprouting coconut meat; omit 1 fat)	1¾ c

Fruit Exchanges

One serving contains approximately 60 kcal and 15 g carbohydrate.

Guava (good source of vitamin C)	1 medium
Soursop, pulp	⅓ c
Lychees	10 fruits
Passion fruit juice (good source of vitamin C)	½ c
Star fruit	1½ c, cubed

Vegetable Exchanges

One serving contains approximately 25 kcal, 5 g carbohydrate, and 2 g protein.

Bamboo shoot	½ c
Papaya, green	½ c
Banana bud	½ c
Squash, leaf tips (good source of vitamin A)	½ c
Bittermelon, fruit	½ c
Sweet potato leaves (good source of vitamin A)	½ c
Bittermelon, leaves (good source of vitamin A)	½ c
Taro leaves (good source of vitamin A)	½ c

Meat Exchanges

Meat exchanges are divided into three groups (A, B, and C) on the basis of fat content.

Meat Group A—one serving contains approximately 55 kcal, 7 g protein, and 3 g fat.

Clams, crab, lobster, prawns	1 oz
Fish (e.g., aku, opakapaka, mahimahi, tuna)	1 oz or 1 slice (3″ × 1″ × ¾″)
Cuttlefish, squid, octopus	1 oz
Sea slug	1 c

Meat Group B—one serving contains approximately 75 kcal, 7 g protein, and 5 g fat.

Chicken wing	1 wing
Tofu	⅓ c
Corned beef	1 oz

Meat Group C—one serving contains approximately 100 kcal, 7 g protein, and 8 g fat.

Canned luncheon meat	1 oz
Turkey tails	½ oz
Mutton flaps (flank of mature sheep)	1 oz
Turkey wings	½ wing

Fat Exchanges

One serving contains approximately 45 kcal and 5 g fat.

Coconut, mature meat	1 piece (1″ × 1″ × ⅜″)
Coconut, cream (no water added)	1 tbsp
Coconut, milk (1 c water, 1 c cream)	2 tbsp
Coconut, grated	2 tbsp

Mexican American Exchange Lists

Carbohydrate Group

Starch List

Bread	1 slice
Tortilla	1
Corn meal	2½ Tbsp
Rice	½ cup
Frijoles	½ cup

Milk List

Milk, yogurt	1 cup
Evaporated milk	½ cup

Fruit List

Fresh or canned, without sugar	½ cup
Guava	1
Papaya	½

Vegetable List

Pumpkin	½ cup
Beets	½ cup
Squash	½ cup
Jicama	½ cup
Chayote	½ cup

Meat Group

Meat, fish, or poultry	1 oz
Tripe	5 × 2 in.
Pork chop	1
Meatballs	2
Cheese	1 oz

Fat Group

Lard	1 tsp
Avocado	⅛
Nuts	6
Olives	5

Free Foods

Raw vegetables
Clear broth
Unsweetened gelatin
Sour pickles
Coffee
Tea
Seasoning and salts

Appendix K

Food Labeling Information

Sample Label for a Granola Bar

Nutrition Facts
Serving Size 1 bar (24g)
Servings Per Container 12

Amount Per Serving	
Calories 120	Calories from Fat 45
	% Daily Value*
Total Fat 5g	8%
Saturated Fat 1g	5%
Cholesterol 0mg	0%
Sodium 65mg	3%
Total Carbohydrate 17g	6%
Dietary Fiber 1g	4%
Sugars 6g	
Protein 2g	

Vitamin A 0% • Vitamin C 0%
Calcium 0% • Iron 4%

* Percent Daily Values are based on a 2,000 calorie diet. Your daily values may be higher or lower depending on your calorie needs:

	Calories:	2,000	2,500
Total Fat	Less than	65g	80g
Sat Fat	Less than	20g	25g
Cholesterol	Less than	300mg	300mg
Sodium	Less than	2,400mg	2,400mg
Total Carbohydrate		300g	375g
Dietary Fiber		25g	30g

Calories per gram:
Fat 9 • Carbohydrate 4 • Protein 4

Ingredients: Rolled oats, sugar, sunflower oil, brown sugar syrup, honey, salt, soy lecithin

Daily Reference Values

Food Component	Daily Reference Value (2000 kcal)
Total fat	Less than 65 g (30% of energy)
Saturated fat	Less than 20 g (10% of energy)
Cholesterol	Less than 300 mg
Total carbohydrate	300 g (60% of energy)
Dietary fiber	25 g (11.5 g/1000 kcal)
Sodium	Less than 2400 mg
Potassium	3500 mg
Protein	50 g (10% of energy)

K

Recommended Dietary Intakes (RDIs)*

Vitamins and Minerals	Units of Measurement	Adults and Children 4 or More Years of Age	Infants	Children Under 4 Years of Age	Pregnant or Lactating Women
Vitamin A	International Units (micrograms)†	5000 (1000 μg)	1500	2500	8000
Vitamin D	International Units (micrograms)†	400 (10 μg)	400	400	400
Vitamin E	International Units (micrograms)†	30 (10 μg)	5	10	30
Vitamin C	Milligrams	60	35	40	60
Folic acid	Micrograms	400	0.1	0.2	0.8
Thiamin	Milligrams	1.5	0.5	0.7	1.7
Riboflavin	Milligrams	1.7	0.6	0.8	2.0
Niacin	Milligrams	20	8	9	20
Vitamin B_6	Milligrams	2.0	0.4	0.7	2.5
Vitamin B_{12}	Micrograms	6.0	2	3	8
Biotin	Micrograms	300	0.05	0.15	0.30
Pantothenic acid	Milligrams	10	3	5	10
Calcium	Milligrams	1000	0.6	0.8	1.3
Phosphorus	Milligrams	1000	0.5	0.8	1.3
Iodine	Micrograms	150	45	70	150
Iron	Milligrams	18	15	10	18
Magnesium	Milligrams	400	70	200	450
Copper	Milligrams	20	0.6	1.0	2.0
Zinc	Milligrams	15	5	8	15
Vitamin K	Micrograms	80	—‡	—‡	—‡
Chromium	Micrograms	120	—	—	—
Selenium	Micrograms	70	—	—	—
Molybdenum	Micrograms	75	—	—	—
Manganese	Milligrams	2	—	—	—
Chloride	Milligrams	3400	—	—	—

* Based on National Academy of Sciences' 1968 Recommended Dietary Allowances.

†The RDIs for fat-soluble vitamins are expressed in International Units (IU). The current RDAs use a newer system of measurement. Values that are approximately equivalent are given in parentheses.

‡ No values yet established for vitamin K, chromium, selenium, molybdenum, manganese, or chloride for this population.

K

Nutrient Content Descriptors Commonly Used on Food Labels

Free	Means that a product contains no amount of, or a trivial amount of, fat, saturated fat, cholesterol, sodium, sugars, or kcalories. For example, "sugar free" and "fat free" both mean less than 0.5 g per serving. Synonyms for "free" include "without," "no," and "zero."
Low	Used for foods that can be eaten frequently without exceeding the Daily Value for fat, saturated fat, cholesterol, sodium, or kcalories. Specific definitions have been established for each of these nutrients. For example, "lowfat" means that the food contains 3 g or less per serving, and "low cholesterol" means that the food contains less than 20 mg of cholesterol per serving. Synonyms for "low" include "little," "few," and "low source of."
Lean and extra lean	Used to describe the fat content of meat, poultry, seafood, and game meats. "Lean" means that the food contains less than 10 g fat, less than 4.5 g saturated fat, and less than 95 mg of cholesterol per serving and per 100 g. "Extra lean" means that the food contains less than 5 g fat, less than 2 g saturated fat, and less than 95 mg of cholesterol per serving and per 100 g.
High	Can be used if a food contains 20% or more of the Daily Value for a particular nutrient. Synonyms for "high" include "rich in" and "excellent source of."
Good source	Means that a food contains 10 to 19% of the Daily Value for a particular nutrient per serving.
Reduced	Means that a nutritionally altered product contains 25% less of a nutrient or of energy than the regular or reference product.
Less	Means that a food, whether altered or not, contains 25% less of a nutrient or of energy than the reference food. For example, pretzels may claim to have "less fat" than potato chips. "Fewer" may be used as a synonym for "less."
Light	May be used in different ways. First, it can be used on a nutritionally altered product that contains one-third fewer kcalories or half the fat of a reference food. Second, it can be used when the sodium content of a low-calorie, lowfat food has been reduced by 50%. The term "light" can be used to describe properties such as texture and color as long as the label explains the intent—for example, "light and fluffy."
More	Means that a serving of food, whether altered or not, contains a nutrient that is at least 10% of the Daily Value more than the reference food. This definition also applies to foods using the terms "fortified," "enriched," or "added."
Healthy	May be used to describe foods that are low in fat and saturated fat and contain no more than 360 mg of sodium and no more than 60 mg of cholesterol per serving and provide at least 10% of the Daily Value for vitamins A or C, or iron, calcium, protein, or fiber.
Fresh	May be used on foods that are raw and have never been frozen or heated and contain no preservatives.

Source: Federal Register 58. Washington, D.C.: U.S. Government Printing Office, Superintendent of Documents, Jan. 6, 1993.

*Health Claims Allowed on Food Labels**

Calcium and osteoporosis	Adequate calcium intake throughout life helps maintain bone health and reduce the risk of osteoporosis.
Sodium and hypertension (high blood pressure)	Diets high in sodium may increase the risk of high blood pressure in some people.
Dietary fat and cancer	Diets high in fat increase the risk of some types of cancer.
Saturated fat and cholesterol and risk of coronary heart disease	Diets high in saturated fat and cholesterol increase blood cholesterol and, thus, the risk of heart disease.
Foods high in fiber and cancer	Diets low in fat and rich in fiber-containing grain products, fruits, and vegetables may reduce the risk of some types of cancer.
Foods high in fiber and risk of coronary heart disease	Diets low in saturated fat and cholesterol and rich in fruits, vegetables, and grain products that contain fiber, particularly soluble fiber, may reduce the risk of coronary heart disease.
Fruits and vegetables and cancer	Diets low in fat and rich in fruits and vegetables may reduce the risk of some types of cancer.
Folic acid and neural tube defect–affected pregnancy	Adequate folic acid intake by the mother reduces the risk of birth defects of the brain or spinal cord in her baby.
Foods high in soluble fiber from whole oats or psyllium husk and heart disease	Diets low in saturated fat and cholesterol that include soluble fiber from whole oats or psyllium husks may reduce the risk of heart disease.
Dietary sugar alcohol and dental caries	Sugar-free foods that are sweetened with sugar alcohols do not promote tooth decay and may reduce the risk of dental caries.

*A food carrying a health claim must be a naturally good source (10% or more of the Daily Value) for 1 of 6 nutrients (vitamin A, vitamin C, protein, calcium, iron, or fiber) and must not contain more than 20% of the Daily Value for fat, saturated fat, cholesterol, or sodium.

K

Appendix L

Energy Expenditure for Various Activities

Type of Activity	Kcalories per Hour (by body weight)				
	100 lb	120 lb	150 lb	180 lb	200 lb
Aerobics (heavy)	363	435	544	653	726
Aerobics (medium)	227	272	340	408	454
Aerobics (light)	136	163	204	245	272
Archery	159	190	238	286	317
Backpacking	408	490	612	735	816
Badminton (doubles)	181	218	272	327	363
Badminton (singles)	231	278	347	416	463
Basketball (nonvigorous)	431	517	646	776	862
Basketball (vigorous)	499	599	748	898	998
Bicycling (6 mph)	159	190	238	286	317
Bicycling (10 mph)	249	299	374	449	499
Bicycling (11 mph)	295	354	442	531	590
Bicycling (12 mph)	340	408	510	612	680
Bicycling (13 mph)	385	463	578	694	771
Billiards	91	109	136	163	181
Bowling	177	212	265	318	354
Boxing—competition	603	724	905	1086	1206
Boxing—sparring	376	452	565	678	753
Calisthenics (heavy)	363	435	544	653	726
Calisthenics (light)	181	218	272	327	363
Canoeing (2.5 mph)	150	180	224	269	299
Canoeing (5 mph)	340	408	510	612	680
Carpentry	227	272	340	408	454
Climbing (mountain)	454	544	680	816	907
Disco dancing	272	327	408	490	544
Ditch digging (hand)	263	316	395	473	526
Fencing	340	408	510	612	680
Fishing (bank/boat)	159	190	238	286	317
Fishing (in waders)	249	299	374	449	499
Football (touch)	340	408	510	612	680
Gardening	145	174	218	261	290
Golf (carry clubs)	227	272	340	408	454
Golf (pull cart)	163	196	245	294	327
Golf (ride in cart)	113	136	170	204	227
Handball (vigorous)	454	544	680	816	907
Hiking (X-country)	249	299	374	449	499
Hiking (mountain)	340	408	510	612	680
Horseback trotting	231	278	347	416	463
Housework	181	218	272	327	363

(continued)

Type of Activity	Kcalories per Hour (by body weight) 100 lb	120 lb	150 lb	180 lb	200 lb
Hunting (carry load)	272	327	408	490	544
Ice hockey (vigorous)	454	544	680	816	907
Ice skating (10 mph)	263	316	395	473	526
Jazzercize (heavy)	363	435	544	653	726
Jazzercise (medium)	227	272	340	408	454
Jazzercise (light)	136	163	204	245	272
Jog (9 min/mile)	499	599	748	898	998
Jog (10 min/mile)	454	544	680	816	907
Jog (12 min/mile)	385	463	578	694	771
Jog (13 min/mile)	317	381	476	571	635
Jog (14 min/mile)	272	327	408	490	544
Jog (15 min/mile)	227	272	340	408	454
Jog (17 min/mile)	181	218	272	327	363
Lawn mowing (hand)	295	354	442	531	590
Lawn mowing (power)	163	196	245	294	327
Musical instrument playing	113	136	170	204	227
Racquetball (social)	385	463	578	694	771
Racquetball (vigorous)	454	544	680	816	907
Roller skating	231	278	347	416	463
Rowboating (2.5 mph)	200	239	299	359	399
Rowing (11 mph)	590	707	884	1061	1179
Run (5 min/mile)	816	980	1224	1469	1633
Run (6 min/mile)	703	844	1054	1265	1406
Run (7 min/mile)	612	735	918	1102	1224
Run (8 min/mile)	544	653	816	980	1088
Sailing	159	190	238	286	317
Shuffleboard/skeet	136	163	204	245	272
Skiing (X-country)	454	544	680	816	907
Skiing (downhill)	363	435	544	653	726
Square dancing	272	327	407	490	544
Swimming (competitive)	680	816	1020	1224	1361
Swimming (fast)	426	512	639	767	853
Swimming (slow)	349	419	524	629	698
Table tennis	236	283	354	424	472
Tennis (doubles)	227	272	340	408	454
Tennis (singles)	295	354	442	531	590
Tennis (vigorous)	385	463	578	694	771
Volleyball	231	278	347	416	463
Walking (20 min/mile)	159	190	238	286	317
Walking (26 min/mile)	136	163	204	245	272
Water skiing	317	381	476	571	635
Weight lifting (heavy)	408	490	612	735	816
Weight lifting (light)	181	218	272	327	363
Wood chopping (sawing)	295	354	442	531	590

Data reprinted with permission from N-Squared Computing, First Databank Division of the Hearst Corporation.

L

Appendix M

Answers to Critical Thinking Exercises

Chapter 1: What Is Wrong With This Experiment?

Was the study well controlled? No. Although muscle strength was tested both before and after the supplement was given to establish any strength differences between groups that were not due to the supplement, other controls were missing. There was no placebo used to make the control group indistinguishable from the experimental group. The diet was not well controlled. No information was obtained about what the subjects were consuming before or during the study. Subjects were asked not to change their diets, but the study provided no way to assess whether some subjects changed their diets during the experiment. There was also no control of activity. If subjects in the experimental group began weight lifting during the study, the differences in muscle strength may have been due to this rather than to the supplement.

Was the proper number of subjects used? There is no mention of the statistical methods used to determine the correct number of subjects, but 25 in each group is probably enough to establish reliable results.

Were the experimental data objective? Yes. Muscle strength is an objective measure that can be tested repeatedly.

Is the conclusion valid? No. Since the diets and exercise regimens of the two groups were not evaluated and controlled, these variables could have caused the observed differences in muscle strength. In addition, because no statistics are presented, the 5-pound increase in leg strength may not have represented a true statistical difference between the two groups.

Chapter 2: Using the Food Guide Pyramid

Does Naomi's diet meet the minimum serving recommendations of the Food Guide Pyramid?

Grains:	6–11 are recommended; she had 7.
Vegetables:	3–5 are recommended; she had 1¾.
Fruits:	2–4 are recommended; she had 1.
Milk:	2–3 are recommended; she had 2½.
Meat:	2–3 are recommended; she had 2.

How many foods did she have during the day that contributed primarily sugar and/or fat? It is recommended that fats and sweets be consumed sparingly. She had 5.

What snacks could she substitute for doughnuts and french fries that would contribute less fat and sugar? She could have a bagel or a banana in the morning; baked tortilla chips and salsa, carrot sticks, or an apple in the afternoon.

Chapter 2: Nutritional Assessment

Should she be concerned about the nutrients she is consuming in excess of her goals? Use the DRI tables to determine if her 1300 mg of calcium is likely to pose a risk. Her vitamin C intake is 183% of goal; this amount has not been shown to produce side effects. Her vitamin A intake is 128% of goal. Too much vitamin A can be toxic, but only if it is consumed as preformed vitamin A (retinoids), which is found in animal products. Plant sources of vitamin A provide carotenoids, which are not toxic (see Chapter 9). The UL for calcium is 2.5 grams per day—her intake is well below this in a safe range of intake.

Chapter 3: Gastrointestinal Problems Can Affect Digestion and Absorption

What type of food should be avoided? Fatty foods should be avoided because fat in the GI tract causes the gallbladder to contract. This contraction results in pain when there are gallstones in the gallbladder.

Chapter 4: What Happens If You Consume Too Little Carbohydrate?

Why can type 1 diabetics develop ketosis even when consuming plenty of carbohydrate? Type 1 diabetics do not produce enough insulin. Without insulin, glucose cannot enter cells. Without adequate carbohydrate, fat cannot be completely broken down and ketones are formed.

Chapter 4: Carbohydrates in the Total Diet

Does Mercedes's original diet meet the recommendations of 2–4 servings of fruits, 3–5 servings of vegetables, and 6–11 servings of grains? No. She consumes only 1⅓ servings of fruit as orange juice and only 2 servings of vegetables (potatoes). Her intake of 6 servings of grains does meet the recommendation.

Are the carbohydrate sources in her modified diet from whole or refined sources? The white bread, tortillas, cookies, pretzels, canned pears, graham crackers, and frozen yogurt are primarily refined sources. The beans, potatoes, green beans, milk, and berries are primarily whole food sources.

How many grams of fiber are in Mercedes's modified diet? Does this meet the recommendations? Her modified diet provides approximately 21.5 grams of fiber, which meets her recommended intake of 20 to 26 grams.

Chapter 5: Dietary Fat and Heart Disease Risk

What risk factors does Rafael have for developing cardiovascular disease? He is a 35-year-old male. His mother died of a heart attack before the age of 65. His stress level is moderate. His total blood cholesterol is over 200 mg/dl, and his HDL cholesterol is less than 35 mg/dl. His diet exceeds the recommendations for fat, saturated fat, and cholesterol intake and contains fewer servings of fruits and vegetables and more meat than is recommended by the Food Guide Pyramid.

What dietary and lifestyle changes would you recommend to reduce his risks? He could increase the number of servings of fruits and vegetables he eats each day, use lowfat dairy products, and reduce his intake of meat to decrease his intake of fat, saturated fat, and cholesterol. He could increase his exercise level and reduce his stress level.

If Rafael were to replace all of the added fat in his diet with olive oil, would he reduce his risk of cardiovascular disease to the level found in Mediterranean countries? No. Olive oil is only one component of a total dietary pattern and lifestyle that is associated with a lower risk of cardiovascular disease. He would also need to change other aspects of his diet and lifestyle.

Chapter 5: Fats in the Total Diet

Does Stella's diet meet the serving recommendations of the Food Guide Pyramid for grains, vegetables, and fruits? Do her choices from these groups follow the selection tips of the Food Guide Pyramid? No. Stella's diet includes 4 servings of grains but should have at least 6. It contains 3 servings of vegetables, which meets recommendations, but only 1 serving of fruit, which is below the suggested 2 to 4 servings. Her choices do not follow the selection tips. All 3 vegetables are potatoes, so there is little variety; they are also fried, which increases fat and kcalories in the diet. Many of her other choices are also high in fat and low in nutrient density.

What is the percent kcalories from fat in her original diet?

$$81.6 \text{ g} \times 9 \text{ kcal/g} = 734 \text{ kcal}/2100 \text{ kcal} \times 100 = 35\%$$

What is the percent kcalories from fat in the modified diet, assuming it also contains 2100 kcalories? Does this diet meet the serving selection recommendations of the Food Guide Pyramid for grains, vegetables, and fruits?

$$34.8 \text{ g} \times 9 \text{ kcal/g} = 313 \text{ kcal}/2100 \text{ kcal} \times 100 = 15\%$$

Yes. Her modified diet does meet the Food Guide Pyramid recommendations. It includes about 8 servings of grains, 5 servings of vegetables, and 4 servings of fruit.

Chapter 6: What Does Nitrogen Balance Tell Us?

What is his nitrogen balance? His balance is 0. Intake is equal to output, so he is in nitrogen balance.

What is her nitrogen balance? She is in positive nitrogen balance by 2.4 grams.

Does this make sense metabolically? Yes. Subject C is pregnant, so she is retaining nitrogen that is being used to synthesize new tissue.

Chapter 6: Choosing a Vegetarian Diet

How much protein would his diet provide if he decided to eliminate dairy products? It would provide 46.7 grams.

Does his diet meet the serving recommendations of the vegetarian Food Guide Pyramid? Yes, with the exception of vegetables, whose amount he could increase slightly:

	Recommended	Ajay's Diet
Grains	6–11	9
Vegetable	3–5	2
Fruit	2–4	3
Milk	0–3	2½
Meat Substitutes	2–3	2

Chapter 7: Is She Destined to Be Obese?

What is her energy expenditure? According to Table 7.2, at age 23 and 140 pounds, April uses 1437 kcal/24 hours, or 59.9 kcal/hr, for basal metabolism. Using the equations in Table 7.3, this can be used to calculate the energy needed for activities throughout the day:

8 hours of sleep × 1 × 59.9 kcal/hr = 479 kcal

14 hours of very light activity = 14 × 1.5 × 59.9 kcal/hr
= 1258 kcal

2 hours of light activity = 2 × 2.5 × 59.9 kcal/hr = 300 kcal

RMR + activity = 2037 kcal

TEF = 10% × 2650 kcal = 265 kcal

Total = RMR + activity + TEF = 2302 kcal

If she replaces two hours of her very light activity with two hours of tennis (a moderate activity), how much additional energy will this burn? Two hours of very light activity uses 180 kcal. Replacing it with 2 hours of light activity, which uses 300 kcal, will cause her to expend an additional 120 kcals.

What other substitutions could she make to decrease her intake? She could have grilled chicken instead of chicken nuggets and pasta with tomato sauce instead of macaroni and cheese to further reduce her kcaloric intake.

Is she destined to be obese? What other recommendations would you give her about weight management? She is not destined to be obese, but to maintain her weight she probably has to monitor her kcaloric intake more carefully and exercise more than an individual with no genetic tendency to carry excess body fat. If she makes small changes in diet and exercise that she can stick with she is more likely to succeed.

Chapter 7: Do You Think This Diet Will Work?

Does the program promote changes in eating habits and lifestyle that will encourage achieving and maintaining a healthy weight? No. It tries for a quick fix rather than suggesting small changes that will last a lifetime.

Chapter 8: Four Hundred of Fortified Folate

List some substitutions that would increase Marcia's intake of naturally occuring folate and of folic acid from fortified foods? She could increase her intake of naturally occurring folate by replacing the french fries at lunch with a leafy green vegetable such as a salad. To increase her intake from fortified foods she must increase her intake of fortified grain products. She could replace the cake, a grain product that is high in energy, with more servings of more nutrient-dense choices.

Would you recommend Marcia take a folate supplement? Yes. Unless Marcia's diet is always carefully planned and well-balanced, she should take a folic acid supplement.

Chapter 9: Evaluating Vitamin Supplements

Will any of these prevent Miguel from getting sick or help boost his energy level? Vitamin C has been shown to reduce the duration and severity of cold symptoms but not to prevent colds. Some of the B vitamins and antioxidants such as vitamin E and beta-carotene are important for proper immune function; however, unless the diet was deficient in these nutrients to begin with, supplements are unlikely to enhance immune function and prevent Miguel from getting sick. The B vitamins and choline are necessary to produce energy from carbohydrate, fat, and protein but do not provide energy themselves.

Would you suggest Miguel stop taking any of these supplements? He should stop taking all supplements that exceed the UL. He is consuming 120 mg of vitamin B_6 daily (2 B50 tablets); the UL is 100 mg. He is consuming 200 mg of niacin daily (two B50s and two Brain Boosters); the UL is 35 mg.

Chapter 10: A Diet for Health

How does the modified diet compare to the Food Guide Pyramid? To Rashamel's current diet?

	FGP	Current	Modified
Grains	6–11	8	10
Vegetable	3–5	1	5
Fruit	2–4	3	5
Milk	2–3	1	4
Meat	2–3	2	2

How could this diet be changed to reduce energy content without reducing the calcium? Uka could use nonfat milk instead of lowfat milk and reduce the number of servings from other groups as shown in Table 10.3. Someone who needs only 1800 kcal should consume fewer servings of grains, vegetables, and fruits.

M

Chapter 11: Increasing Iron Intake

What dietary factors could contribute to Odelia's poor iron status?

1. Her iron intake is marginal at 12.0 mg per day compared with the 1989 RDA of 15 mg.
2. The iron in her diet comes from plant sources that contain only nonheme iron, which is less well absorbed than heme iron found in animal foods.
3. The diet is low in vitamin C–rich foods. Vitamin C enhances the absorption of nonheme iron in foods.
4. The switch to stainless steel cookware reduced the iron content of her diet because iron leaches into food from the cast iron cookware she used to use.

What modifications could Odelia make to increase the iron content of her dinner? She could cook the meal in an iron pot. She could add tomatoes or lime juice to the meal; the acid would increase the amount of iron leached from the cookware into the food. She could have orange juice instead of apple juice with dinner, which would also enhance iron absorption from foods in that meal. She could add beans (a good vegetarian source of iron) to the rice. Tea, which contains tannins that inhibit iron absorption, could be consumed later in the evening.

Does Odelia's diet meet the recommendations of the Food Guide Pyramid? She needs to add a serving of dairy products and of legumes or nuts to her diet to meet the recommendations. Also, the only fruit she consumes is apples and apple juice; she should add more variety from this group.

Are there other nutrient deficiencies for which she may be at risk? Because she consumes dairy products, she is unlikely to be at risk for calcium, vitamin D, or vitamin B_{12} deficiency, but the lack of meat in her diet puts her at risk of zinc deficiency.

Chapter 12: Incorporating Exercise Sensibly

If Nicole's food intake does not increase, how long will it take for her to lose 5 pounds? Each pound requires a deficit of 3500 kcal (for 5 pounds, 5×3500 kcal = 17,500 kcal). She is expending an additional 653 kcal/week, so it will take 17,500/653 = 26.8 weeks, or 6 to 7 months, to lose 5 pounds. If she also decreases her food intake, she can lose the weight more quickly.

Chapter 12: Evaluating Ergogenic Aids

What would you recommend Hector do? If Hector participates in a sport that requires short, rapid bursts of speed, bicarbonate may improve his performance. However, if he experiences the side effects of nausea and diarrhea, his performance will suffer. Hector should try the supplement during his practice schedule and evaluate his performance and any side effects before using it for a track meet.

Chapter 13: Nutrient Needs for a Successful Pregnancy

Chevon is overweight. Should she still add these foods to her diet? Yes. All pregnant women should gain weight during pregnancy to allow for the healthy growth of the fetus. Even though she is overweight, Chevon needs to slowly gain weight during the last two trimesters of her pregnancy.

How could her original diet be improved to increase its nutrient density? Chevon could reduce the number of french fries she has at lunch or replace them with a lower kcalorie vegetable such as carrots or celery. She could have juice instead of the orange soft drink, and she could skip the cookies or have them later in the day for a snack with a glass of lowfat milk. She could use reduced-fat mayonnaise and salad dressings and use milk rather than cream in her coffee.

Does this diet meet the iron needs of pregnancy without supplements? Her current diet provides 10.5 mg of iron—significantly less than the RDA of 30 mg for pregnant women.

Chapter 13: How to Nourish a New Baby

Why should Grandma wait until Henry is four to six months old before feeding him solid food? Infants' GI tracts are not ready to handle solid or semisolid food until this age. Introducing foods too early can increase the risk of developing food allergies.

Chapter 14: At Risk for Malnutrition

Suggest some dietary changes that would increase Bobby's iron intake and absorption. To increase the amount of iron in his diet, foods could be cooked in iron cookware. An extra serving of red meat might be included by adding it to spaghetti sauce or as a pizza topping. Dried fruit could be used for snacks. To increase iron absorption Bobby should consume high-iron foods with foods that are acidic to increase absorption. For instance, a snack of dry breakfast cereal and a glass of orange juice would provide iron and enhance its absorption.

Suggest some activities you enjoyed as a child that would help Bobby increase his activity level. He could try a family walk or a game of catch after dinner, a bike ride, a stroll to the park to play on the swings, or a weekend hike in the woods.

Chapter 14: Meeting Teen Needs

How could she modify her original diet to reduce her energy intake, provide the essential nutrients she needs, and still fit her busy schedule? Jenny's original breakfast is fast and easy. For lunch, she could have a turkey sandwich, apple, and glass of milk but skip the chips. For a snack, she could have either the burger, the shake, or the fries but not all three. If she has the ham sandwich from her original dinner and a glass of milk, she will be consuming fewer kcalories and more nutrients than she is with the candy bar and chips.

Chapter 15: Can Your Diet Keep You Young?

Why would fish oil supplements be dangerous for Marilyn? Marilyn is taking blood-thinning medication. Because fish oil may also thin the blood, the combination of her medications and these supplements could be dangerous.

Is it safe for them to reduce their meat intake to 3 ounces a week? As long as their diet provides other sources of iron and protein, it would be safe.

Chapter 15: Dietary Modifications to Meet the Needs of the Elderly

How would Shirley benefit from participating in a congregate meal program at the local senior center? Shirley would be guaranteed one hot meal a day from a varied menu. This provides nutrients and reduces the amount of cooking and shopping she needs to do for herself. In addition, the social interaction would probably cause her to eat more food and enjoy her meal more.

Chapter 16: Are These Choices Safe?

How might raw vegetables and fruit salad become contaminated? Because they are not cooked, bacteria that come in contact with them either directly or via cross-contamination will not be destroyed by cooking. Both fruits and vegetables can become contaminated with pathogens in the field or during transport. Produce may also become contaminated if cutting boards, knives, or other utensils used to prepare raw meats are used to cut the fruits and vegetables without washing.

After the party is over, what foods would you consider safe to keep as leftovers and what would you throw out? The fruit salad, raw vegetables, chips, crackers and cheese, and cookies would be the safest to keep. The cooked items that were left at room temperature for hours (lasagna, cheesecake, stuffed mushrooms, and tamales) should be discarded, as should the chicken salad and onion dip.

Chapter 16: Individual Risk-Benefit Analysis

What other changes can he make to minimize the risks associated with his family's typical diet while including foods that are beneficial? To decrease the risks associated with using raw eggs, he can advise his son that he does not need the protein shakes but that if he wants to drink them, he should use nonfat dry milk rather than raw eggs. He can have his daughter wait for the cookies to bake before tasting them. To decrease the risks associated with eating fish, he can try a wider variety of fresh and saltwater fish to avoid an excess of any one type. Because the risks of eating raw fish are greater, he can limit sushi to a rare treat purchased only from a restaurant that he knows buys the fish fresh daily. The pesticide risks from consuming produce are small compared with the benefits of a diet high in fruits and vegetables. To reduce the amounts of pesticides ingested, fruits and vegetables can be washed thoroughly or consumed without the skins. He can also reduce pesticide consumption by purchasing organic produce, but he must consider that it is more expensive. He can also buy locally grown produce and keep up his summer vegetable garden.

Chapter 17: What Can You Do?

What impact will the following changes Keesha makes have on the environment? By bringing her juice in a thermos, Keesha can reduce the amount of garbage (packaging, disposable cups and cans, etc.) she produces from her meals; composting reduces the amount of garbage sent to the dump; buying organically grown produce supports agricultural techniques that reduce the amount of chemical fertilizers and pesticides used; buying locally grown foods reduces the energy cost of transporting and storing produce grown at distant locations.

Suggest some other changes Keesha could make to decrease her impact on the environment. She could reduce energy usage in her home by buying a timer for her household thermostat and water heater to automatically turn both down during the hours when no one is home. Modifying her diet to consume smaller portions of animal products would save energy because animal products take more energy to produce than plant products. She could both buy foods in larger containers to reduce the amount of packaging and select products with less packaging. She could take her lunch to work in reusable plastic containers rather than in disposable lunch bags.

Chapter 17: Cutting Food Costs

Does her modified diet meet the recommendations of the Food Guide Pyramid? She meets the serving recommendations for grains, fruit, and milk. She may need to add an additional serving of vegetables, depending on the amount of salad and spaghetti sauce she consumes. She may also need to add a serving of dry beans (maybe some chick peas on her salad) because the meat in the spaghetti sauce plus the peanut butter in her sandwich may still fall short of the 2 to 3 servings recommended from this group.

What other changes could Cecelia make to reduce food costs without purchasing bulk items? She can make homemade salad dressing, use bread instead of rolls, buy store brands rather than brand-name products, and shop for items on sale.

Glossary

Absorption The process of taking substances from the gastrointestinal tract into the interior of the body.

Accidental contaminants Substances not regulated by the FDA that unexpectedly enter the food supply.

Accutane A drug that is used orally to treat severe acne. It is a derivative of vitamin A.

Acesulfame K (Acesulfame potassium) An artificial sweetener that contains no energy and is 200 times as sweet as sugar.

Acetylcholine A neurotransmitter that functions in the brain and other parts of the nervous system.

Acetyl-CoA A common intermediate consisting of a 2-carbon compound attached to a molecule of CoA that is produced from the metabolism of carbohydrate, fat, and protein.

Acid A substance that releases hydrogen ions (H^+) in solution.

Active transport The transport of substances across a cell membrane with the aid of a carrier molecule and the expenditure of energy. This may occur against a concentration gradient.

Acute Effects that develop rapidly.

Adaptive thermogenesis Adjustments in energy expenditure induced by factors such as changes in ambient temperature and food intake.

Adequate Intake (AI) A goal for intake that should be used when no RDA can be determined. These values are an approximation of the average nutrient intake that appears to sustain a desired indicator of health.

ADI (Acceptable Daily Intake) The amount of a sweetener that can be safely consumed over a lifetime without adverse effects.

Adipocytes Fat-storing cells.

Adipose tissue Tissue found under the skin and around body organs that is composed of fat-storing cells.

Adolescent growth spurt An 18- to 24-month period of peak growth velocity that begins at about ages 10 to 13 in girls and 12 to 15 in boys.

Adrenaline A hormone secreted by the adrenal gland in response to stress that causes changes, such as an increase in heart rate, in preparation for "fight or flight"; also called epinephrine.

Aerobic exercise Exercise such as jogging, swimming, or cycling that increases heart rate and requires oxygen in metabolism. This type of exercise improves cardiovascular fitness.

Aerobic metabolism Metabolism requiring oxygen. In aerobic metabolism, glycolysis, the citric acid cycle, and the electron transport chain break down carbohydrates, fatty acids, and amino acids to carbon dioxide and water and produce ATP.

Aflatoxin An extremely potent carcinogen that is produced by a mold that grows on peanuts, corn, and grains.

Agar A polysaccharide extract of seaweed that is used in foods as an emulsifier, stabilizer, and gel.

Age-related osteoporosis *See* Type II osteoporosis.

AIDS (acquired immune deficiency syndrome) The syndrome caused by HIV infection that causes the immune system to fail, resulting in frequent recurrent infections that ultimately result in death.

Alcohol An energy-containing molecule that contains 7 kcalories per gram and is made by the fermentation of carbohydrates from plant products; the type of alcohol that is consumed in the diet is called ethanol.

Alcohol dehydrogenase An enzyme with activity in the stomach and liver that converts ethanol to acetaldehyde.

Alcoholic hepatitis Inflammation of the liver caused by alcohol consumption.

Alcohol-related birth defects *See* Fetal alcohol effects.

Aldosterone A hormone secreted by the adrenal glands that increases sodium reabsorption and therefore enhances water reabsorption by the kidney.

Alginate A polysaccharide extract of brown algae used in the processing of food, primarily dairy products.

Alimentary canal *See* Gastrointestinal tract.

Allergen A foreign substance, usually a protein, that stimulates an immune response.

Allergy An adverse reaction involving the immune system that results from exposure to a specific allergen.

Alpha-carotene A carotenoid, some of which can be converted into vitamin A, that is found in leafy green vegetables, carrots, and squash.

Alpha-linolenic acid An 18-carbon omega-3 polyunsaturated fatty acid known to be essential in humans.

Alpha-tocopherol (α-tocopherol) The form of tocopherol (vitamin E) that is most common and has the greatest biological activity.

Alpha-tocopherol equivalent (α-TE) A unit of measure for vitamin E, equal to the amount of any form of tocopherol that provides the function of 1 mg of alpha-tocopherol.

Alzheimer's disease A disease that results in the relentless and irreversible loss of mental function.

Amenorrhea Delayed onset of menstruation or the absence of three or more consecutive menstrual cycles.

Amino acid pool All of the amino acids in body tissues and fluids that are available for protein synthesis.

Amino acids The building blocks of proteins. Each contains a carbon atom bound to a hydrogen atom, an amino group, an acid group, and a side chain.

Amniotic fluid The liquid in the amniotic sac that surrounds and protects the fetus during development.

Amniotic sac A membrane surrounding the fetus that contains the amniotic fluid.

Amylopectin A plant starch that is composed of long branched chains of glucose molecules.

Amylose A plant starch that is composed of long unbranched chains of glucose molecules.

Anabolic Energy-requiring processes in which simpler molecules are combined to form more complex substances.

Anabolic steroids Synthetic fat-soluble hormones that mimic testosterone and are used by some athletes to increase muscle strength and mass.

Anaerobic metabolism or **anaerobic glycolysis** Metabolism in the absence of oxygen. In glycolysis, two molecules of ATP are produced from each molecule of glucose. Glucose is metabolized in this way when the blood cannot deliver oxygen to the tissues quickly enough.

Androstenedione A compound (known as Andro) that can be converted into testosterone and estrogen inside the body. It is a dietary supplement used by athletes to increase muscle mass and strength.

Anecdotal Information based on a story of personal experience.

Anemia A condition in which there is a reduced number of red blood cells or a reduced amount of hemoglobin, which reduces the oxygen-carrying capacity of the blood.

Angiotensin II A compound that causes blood vessel walls to constrict and stimulates the release of the hormone aldosterone.

Anisakis disease A disease caused by infection of the gastrointestinal tract with an Anisakis roundworm that contaminates raw fish.

Anorexia nervosa An eating disorder characterized by self-starvation, a distorted body image, and low body weight.

Antacid A drug used to neutralize acidity in the gastrointestinal tract.

Anthropometric measurements External measurements of the body, such as height, weight, limb circumference, and skinfold thickness.

Antibiotic A substance that inhibits the growth of or destroys microorganisms; used to treat or prevent infection.

Antibodies Proteins produced by cells of the immune system that destroy or inactivate foreign substances in the body.

Anticaking agent A substance added to food to prevent clumping of dry products.

Anticarcinogen A compound that can counteract the effect of cancer-causing substances.

Anticoagulant A substance that delays or prevents blood coagulation.

Antidiuretic hormone (ADH) A hormone secreted by the pituitary gland that increases the amount of water reabsorbed by the kidney and therefore retained in the body.

Antioxidant A substance that is able to neutralize reactive oxygen molecules and protect the body from oxidative damage.

Antithiamin factors Substances in food that destroy the vitamin thiamin. Some are enzymes and are destroyed by cooking; others are not inactivated by cooking.

Anus The lower opening of the digestive tract through which the feces leave the body.

Apolipoprotein B A protein embedded in the outer shell of low-density lipoprotein (LDL) particles that binds to LDL receptor proteins on body cells.

Appetite The desire to consume specific foods that is independent of hunger.

Arachidonic acid A 20-carbon omega-6 polyunsaturated fatty acid that can be synthesized from linoleic acid.

Arginine A nonessential amino acid found in protein.

Ariboflavinosis The condition resulting from a deficiency of riboflavin.

Arteriole A small artery that carries blood to capillaries.

Artery A blood vessel that carries blood away from the heart.

Arthritis A disease characterized by inflammation of the joints, pain, and sometimes changes in structure.

Artificial sweetener A chemically manufactured sweetener that differs from simple sugars in chemical structure and often provides little or no energy when ingested.

Ascorbic acid The chemical term for vitamin C.

Aseptic processing A method that places sterilized food in a sterilized package using a sterile process.

Asparagine A nonessential amino acid found in protein.

Aspartame An artificial sweetener that is 200 times as sweet as sugar and is composed of the amino acids phenylalanine and aspartic acid.

Aspartic acid A nonessential amino acid found in protein.

Asthma A respiratory disorder characterized by wheezing and difficulty in breathing.

Atherosclerosis A type of cardiovascular disease that involves the buildup of fatty material in the artery walls.

Atoms The smallest units of an element that still retain the properties of that element.

ATP (adenosine triphosphate) The high-energy molecule used by the body to perform energy-requiring activities.

Atrophic gastritis An inflammation of the stomach lining that causes a reduction in stomach acid and allows bacterial overgrowth.

Attention deficit hyperactive disorder A condition that is characterized by a short attention span, a high level of activity, excitability, and distractibility.

Autoimmune disease A disease that results from immune reactions that destroy normal body cells.

Avidin A protein found in raw egg whites that binds biotin, preventing its absorption.

Bacteria (singular, **bacterium**) Tiny single-celled organisms found throughout the environment. Most are harmless or beneficial, but a few types can cause disease in humans.

Balance study A study that compares the total amount of a nutrient that enters the body with the total amount that leaves the body.

Basal metabolic rate (BMR) The minimum amount of energy that an awake, fasted (12 hours without food), resting body needs to maintain itself.

Base A substance that accepts hydrogen ions in solution.

Bee pollen A mixture of pollen, bee saliva, and plant nectar that collects on the legs of bees; sold as an ergogenic aid.

Behavior modification A process used to gradually and permanently change habitual behaviors.

Benzocaine A local anesthetic used in some weight-loss products.

Beriberi A thiamin deficiency disease that is characterized by muscle weakness, loss of appetite, and nerve degeneration.

Beta-carotene (β-carotene) A pigment found in many yellow and red-orange fruits and vegetables that acts as an antioxidant in the body and is a precursor of vitamin A.

Beta-cryptoxanthin A carotenoid found in corn, green peppers, and lemons that can provide some vitamin A activity.

Bile A substance made in the liver and stored in the gallbladder. It is released into the small intestine to aid in fat digestion and absorption.

Bile acids Emulsifiers present in bile that are synthesized by the liver from cholesterol.

Binge The consumption of a large amount of food in a discrete period of time associated with a feeling that eating is out of control.

Binge-eating disorder An eating disorder characterized by recurrent episodes of binge-eating in the absence of purging behavior.

Bioavailability A general term that refers to how well a nutrient can be absorbed and used by the body.

Bioelectric impedance analysis A technique for estimating body composition that measures body water by directing electric current through the body and calculating resistance to flow.

Biological value A measure of protein quality determined by comparing the amount of nitrogen retained in the body with the amount absorbed from the diet.

Biotechnology A set of techniques used to manipulate DNA for the purpose of changing the characteristics of an organism or creating a new product; also called genetic engineering.

Blood pressure The amount of force exerted by the blood against the artery walls.

Body mass index (BMI) An index of weight in relation to height that is used to compare body size with a standard; it is equal to body weight (in kilograms) divided by height (in meters squared).

Bolus A ball of chewed food mixed with saliva.

Bomb calorimeter An instrument used to determine the energy content of food. It measures the heat energy released when a food is combusted.

Bone remodeling The process whereby bone is continuously broken down and reformed to allow for growth and maintenance.

Bovine somatotropin (bST) A hormone naturally produced by cows that stimulates the production of milk. A synthetic version of this hormone is now being produced by genetic engineering.

Bran The protective outer layers of whole grains. It is a concentrated source of dietary fiber.

Brewer's yeast The type of yeast used in brewing beer; a good source of B vitamins and often used as a nutritional supplement.

Brown adipose tissue A type of fat tissue that has a greater number of mitochondria than the more common white adipose tissue. It can waste energy by producing heat and is believed to be responsible for some of the change in energy expenditure in adaptive thermogenesis in rodents.

Brush border Refers to the microvilli surface of the intestinal mucosa, which contains some digestive enzymes.

Buffer A substance that reacts with an acid or base by picking up or releasing hydrogen ions to prevent changes in pH.

Bulimia nervosa An eating disorder characterized by the consumption of large amounts of food at one time (bingeing), followed by purging behavior such as vomiting and the use of laxatives to eliminate food from the body.

Caffeine A bitter white substance found in coffee, tea, chocolate, and other foods; a stimulant and a diuretic.

Calcitonin A hormone produced by the thyroid gland that stimulates bone mineralization and inhibits bone breakdown, thus lowering blood calcium levels.

Calorie The amount of heat required to raise the temperature of 1 g of water 1 degree Celsius; equal to 4.18 joules.

Calorimetry A technique for measuring energy expenditure.

Campylobacter jejuni A bacterium common in raw milk and undercooked meat that causes food-borne illness.

Cancer A disease characterized by cells that grow and divide without restraint and have the ability to grow in different locations in the body.

Capillaries Small, thin-walled blood vessels where the exchange of gases and nutrients between blood and cells occurs.

Caprenin An artificial fat made from a triglyceride containing poorly absorbed fatty acids; provides 5 kcal per gram.

Carbohydrate A compound containing carbon, hydrogen, and oxygen in the same proportions as in water; includes sugars, starches, and most fibers.

Carbohydrate loading *See* Glycogen supercompensation.

Carbon dioxide A waste product produced by cellular respiration that is eliminated from the body by the lungs.

Carcinogen A substance that causes cells to multiply out of control, eventually resulting in cancer.

Cardiorespiratory system The circulatory and respiratory systems which together deliver oxygen and nutrients to cells.

Cardiovascular Refers to the heart and blood vessels.

Cardiovascular disease Any disease affecting the heart and blood vessels.

Caries or **dental caries** Cavities, or decay of the tooth enamel caused by acid produced when bacteria growing on the teeth metabolize carbohydrate.

Carnitine A molecule that is needed to transport fatty acids and some amino acids into the mitochondria for met abolism. Supplements of carnitine are marketed to athletes to enhance performance.

Carotenoids Natural pigments synthesized by plants and many microorganisms. They give yellow and red-orange fruits and vegetables their color.

Carpal tunnel syndrome Numbness, tingling, weakness, and pain in the hand caused by pressure on the nerves.

Carrageenan A seaweed polysaccharide extracted from the algae Irish moss and used as a thickener mainly in dairy products.

Casein The predominant protein in cow's milk.

Cash crops Crops grown to be sold for monetary return rather than to be used for food locally.

Cassava A starchy root that is the staple of the diet in many parts of Africa.

Catabolic Refers to the processes by which substances are broken down into simpler molecules releasing energy.

Catalase An iron-containing enzyme that destroys peroxides.

Cataracts A disease of the eye that results in cloudy spots on the lens (and sometimes the cornea) which obscure vision.

Cell differentiation Structural and functional changes that cause cells to mature into specialized cells.

Cell membrane The membrane that encloses the cell contents.

Cells The basic structural and functional units of plant and animal life.

Cellular respiration The reactions that break down carbohydrates, fats, and proteins in the presence of oxygen to produce carbon dioxide, water, and energy in the form of ATP.

Cellulite Subcutaneous fat that has a lumpy appearance because strands of connective tissue connect it to underlying structures.

Cellulose An insoluble fiber that is the most prevalent structural material of plant cell walls.

Cephalic phase The phase of gastric secretion that is stimulated by the sight, smell, and taste of food.

Certified food color A food color that has been tested and certified for safety, quality, consistency, and strength of color.

Ceruloplasmin A copper-containing protein that converts iron to the ferric form, which can bind to iron storage and iron transport proteins.

Cesarean section The surgical removal of the fetus from the uterus.

Chemical bonds Forces that hold atoms together.

Chemical score A measure of protein quality determined by comparing the amount of the limiting amino acid in a food with that in a reference protein.

Chinese restaurant syndrome *See* MSG symptom complex.

Choice grade A USDA-regulated grade of beef with a modest amount of marbled fat.

Cholecalciferol The chemical name for vitamin D_3. It can be formed in the skin of animals by the action of sunlight on a form of cholesterol called 7-dehydrocholesterol.

Cholecystokinin (CCK) A hormone released by the duodenum that signals the pancreas to secrete digestive enzymes and causes the gallbladder to contract and release bile into the duodenum.

Cholesterol A lipid made only by animal cells that consists of multiple chemical rings.

Cholic acid A bile acid.

Choline A compound needed for the synthesis of the phospholipid phosphatidylcholine and the neurotransmitter acetylcholine. It is important for a number of biochemical reactions and there is evidence that it is essential in the diet during certain stages of life.

Chromium picolinate A form of chromium sold as a supplement promoted to change body composition. Chromium is involved in insulin action, and supplements claim to increase lean body mass, decrease body fat, and delay fatigue. There is little evidence of their effectiveness as an ergogenic aid.

Chronic Effects that develop slowly over a long period.

Chylomicron A lipoprotein that transports lipids from the mucosal cells of the intestine and delivers triglycerides to other body cells.

Chyme A mixture of partially digested food and stomach secretions.

Chymotrypsin A protein-digesting enzyme produced in an inactive form in the pancreas and activated in the small intestine, where it aids digestion.

Circulatory system The organ system consisting of the heart, blood, and blood vessels, which transports material to and from cells.

Cirrhosis Chronic liver disease characterized by the loss of functioning liver cells and the accumulation of fibrous connective tissue.

Citric acid cycle Also known as the Krebs cycle or the tricarboxylic acid cycle, this is the stage of respiration in which 2 carbons of acetyl-CoA are broken down, producing carbon dioxide.

Clones Copies that are identical to the original.

Clostridium botulinum A bacterium that produces a deadly toxin and grows in a low-acid, low-oxygen environment, such as inside certain canned goods.

Clostridium perfringens A bacterium found in meat and poultry that can cause food-borne illness.

Coagulation The process of blood clotting.

Cobalamin The chemical term for vitamin B_{12}.

Coenzymes Small nonprotein organic molecules that act as carriers of electrons or atoms in metabolic reactions and are necessary for the proper functioning of many enzymes.

Cofactor An inorganic ion or coenzyme required for enzyme activity.

Colic A condition in young infants characterized by inconsolable crying. It is believed to be due to pain from gas buildup in the gastrointestinal tract or immaturity of the central nervous system.

Collagen The major protein in connective tissue.

Colon The largest portion of the large intestine.

Colostrum The first milk, which is secreted in late pregnancy and up to a week after birth. It is rich in protein and immune factors.

Complete dietary protein Dietary protein that provides essential amino acids in the proportions needed to support cellular protein synthesis.

Complex carbohydrates Carbohydrates composed of sugar molecules linked together in straight or branching chains. They include oligosaccharides, starches, and fibers.

Compression of morbidity The postponement of the onset of chronic disease so that disability occupies a smaller and smaller proportion of the life span.

Concentration gradient A condition that exists when the amount of a dissolved substance is greater in one area than it is in another.

Conception The union of sperm and egg (ovum) that results in pregnancy.

Condensation reaction A type of chemical reaction in which two molecules are joined to form a larger molecule and water is released.

Conditionally essential amino acid An amino acid that is essential in the diet only under certain conditions or at certain times of life; also called semiessential amino acids.

Connective tissue One of the four human tissue types; includes cartilage, bone, blood, adipose tissue, and the coverings of some organs.

Constipation Infrequent or difficult defecation.

Continuing Survey of Food Intakes by Individuals (CSFII) A survey conducted by the U.S. Department of Agriculture that collects data on the food intake of individuals within households for the purpose of monitoring the nutritional health of the population.

Control group The group of participants in an experiment receiving no experimental treatment; otherwise, members of the control group are identical to the experimental group. A control group is used as a basis of comparison.

Cornea The clear, transparent fibrous outer coat of the eye.

Coronary heart disease A disease of the heart and blood vessels that supply blood to the heart.

Correlation Two or more factors occurring together.

Cortical bone Dense compact bone that forms the sturdy outer surface layer of bone.

Covalent bond A type of chemical bond formed when two atoms share a pair of electrons.

Creatine A compound that can be converted into creatine-phosphate which replenishes ATP during short bursts of activity. Creatine is a dietary supplement used by athletes to increase muscle mass and delay fatigue during short intense exercise.

Creatine phosphate A high-energy compound found in muscle that can be broken down to make ATP.

Cretinism A condition resulting from deficient maternal iodine intake during pregnancy that causes stunted growth and poor mental development in offspring.

Criterion of adequacy A measure or outcome that can be examined to determine the biological effect of a particular level of nutrient intake; established for each nutrient and gender and life-stage group when developing Dietary Reference Intakes.

Critical control points Possible points in food production, manufacturing, and transportation where contamination could occur or be prevented or eliminated.

Critical periods Times in growth and development when an organism is more susceptible to harm from poor nutrition or other environmental factors.

Cross-contamination The transfer of contaminants from one food to another.

Cross-sectional data Information obtained by a single broad sampling of many different individuals in a population.

Crude fiber Fiber that remains after a food has been treated in the laboratory with acid and base. It consists primarily of cellulose and lignin.

Cyclamate An artificial sweetener that was common in the United States in the 1960s; banned after it was found to cause cancer in laboratory animals.

Cycle of malnutrition A cycle in which malnutrition is perpetuated by an inability to meet nutrient needs at all life stages.

Cysteine A conditionally essential sulfur-containing amino acid; when methionine is available in sufficient quantities, cysteine is not essential in the diet.

Cystic acne A chronic inflammatory disease of the skin in which cysts and nodules are common and scarring may occur.

Cytoplasm The cellular material outside the nucleus that is contained by the cell membrane.

Daily Reference Values (DRVs) Reference values established for protein and seven nutrients for which no RDA has been established. The values are based on dietary recommendations for reducing the risk of chronic disease.

Daily Values Nutrient reference values used on food labels to help consumers see how foods fit into their overall diets.

DASH diet A dietary pattern that is plentiful in fruits and vegetables and lowfat dairy products and therefore high in potassium, magnesium, calcium, and fiber, and low in saturated fat and cholesterol.

Deamination The removal of the amino group from an amino acid.

Dehydration A condition that results when the output of water exceeds water input, due to either low water intake or excessive loss.

Delaney Clause A clause added to the 1958 Food Additives Amendment of the Pure Food and Drug Act that prohibits the intentional addition to foods of any compound that has been shown to induce cancer in animals or humans at any dose.

Dementia A deterioration of mental state resulting in impaired memory, thinking, and/or judgment.

Denaturation The alteration of a protein's three-dimensional structure.

Dental caries *See* Caries.

Deoxyribose The 5-carbon sugar that is part of DNA.

Depletion-repletion study A study that feeds subjects a diet devoid of a nutrient until signs of deficiency appear, and then adds the nutrient back to the diet to a level at which symptoms disappear.

Dermatitis An inflammation of the skin.

DHEA (dehydroepiandosterone) A precursor of the sex hormones testosterone, estrogen, and progesterone; sold as a dietary supplement to slow aging and to increase muscle mass.

Diabetes mellitus A disease of carbohydrate metabolism caused by either insufficient insulin production or decreased sensitivity of cells to insulin. It results in elevated blood glucose levels.

Diacylglycerol or **diglyceride** A molecule of glycerol with two fatty acids attached.

Diaphragm A muscular wall separating the abdomen from the thoracic cavity containing the heart and lungs.

Diarrhea An intestinal disorder characterized by frequent or watery stools.

Dicumarol An anticoagulant that was isolated from moldy clover.

Dietary fiber *See* Fiber.

Dietary folate equivalent (DFE) The amount of folate equivalent to 1 μg of folate naturally occurring in food, 0.6 μg of synthetic folic acid from fortified food or supplements consumed with food, or 0.5 μg synthetic folic acid consumed on an empty stomach.

Dietary Guidelines for Americans A set of nutrition recommendations designed to promote population-wide dietary changes to reduce the incidence of nutrition-related chronic disease.

Dietary Reference Intakes (DRIs) A set of four reference values for the intake of nutrients and food components that can be used for planning and assessing the diets of healthy people in the United States and Canada.

Dietary supplement A product intended for ingestion in the diet that contains one or more of the following ingredients: vitamins, minerals, herbs, botanicals, or other plant-derived substance; amino acids; concentrates or extracts.

Diet history A dietary intake assessment method that collects information about dietary habits and patterns and combines methods such as 24-hour recall, food frequency, and a food diary in order to determine an individual's typical food intake.

Diet-induced thermogenesis *See* Thermic effect of food (TEF).

Diffusion The movement of molecules from an area of higher concentration to an area of lower concentration without the expenditure of energy.

Digestion The process of breaking food into components small enough to be absorbed into the body.

Digestive system The organ system responsible for the ingestion, digestion, and absorption of food and the elimination of food residues; includes the gastrointestinal tract as well as a number of accessory organs.

Digestive tract *See* Gastrointestinal tract.

Diglyceride *See* Diacylglycerol.

Dipeptide Two amino acids linked by a peptide bond.

Direct calorimetry A method of calculating energy use that measures the amount of energy released as heat.

Direct food additives Substances intentionally added to foods. They are regulated by the FDA.

Disaccharide A sugar formed by linking two monosaccharides.

Dissociate To separate two charged ions.

Diuretic A drug that promotes fluid excretion.

Diverticula Sacs or pouches that protrude from the wall of the large intestine.

Diverticulitis A condition in which diverticula in the large intestine become inflamed.

Diverticulosis A condition in which outpouchings (or sacs) form in the wall of the large intestine.

DNA (deoxyribonucleic acid) The genetic material found in the nucleus that codes for the synthesis of proteins.

Docosahexaenoic acid (DHA) A 22-carbon omega-3 polyunsaturated fatty acid found in fish that may be needed in the diet of newborns. It can be synthesized from alpha-linolenic acid.

Dolomite A calcium supplement composed of ground-up limestone.

Double-blind study An experiment in which neither the study participants nor the researchers know who is in a control or an experimental group.

Down syndrome A disorder caused by extra genetic material that results in distinctive facial characteristics, mental retardation, and other health problems.

Duodenum The upper segment of the small intestine that connects to the stomach.

Eating disorder A psychological disorder affecting eating behavior and the regulation of food intake or energy balance.

Eclampsia A life-threatening condition that may occur during pregnancy. It is characterized by high blood pressure, protein in the urine, convulsions, and coma.

Edema Swelling of body tissue due to the buildup of fluid in the intestitial space.

Eicosanoids Regulatory molecules that can be synthesized from omega-3 and omega-6 fatty acids.

Eicosapentaenoic acid (EPA) A 20-carbon omega-3 polyunsaturated fatty acid found in fish that can be synthesized from alpha-linolenic acid but may be essential in humans under some conditions.

Electrolytes Substances that separate in water to form positively and negatively charged ions. In nutrition this term refers to sodium, potassium, and chloride.

Electrons High-energy particles carrying a negative charge that orbit the nucleus of an atom.

Electron transport chain The final stage of cellular respiration in which electrons are passed down a chain of molecules to oxygen, forming water and producing ATP.

Elements Substances that cannot be broken down into products with different properties.

Elimination diet A diet that eliminates potential allergy-causing foods from an individual's diet and then systematically adds them back to identify any foods that cause an allergic reaction.

Embryo The developing human from two to eight weeks after fertilization. All organ systems are formed during this time.

Empty kcalories A term that refers to foods that contribute energy but few other nutrients.

Emulsifier A substance with both water-soluble and fat-soluble portions that can break fat into tiny droplets and suspend it in a watery fluid.

Endocrine system Organ system composed of cells, tissues, and organs that secrete hormones to help control body functions.

Endoplasmic reticulum A cellular organelle involved in the synthesis of proteins and lipids and composed of a system of membranous tubules, channels, and sacs in the cytoplasm; rough endoplasmic reticulum has ribosomes on its outside surface.

Endorphin A chemical released by the brain during exercise that acts as a natural tranquilizer; may be the cause of the euphoria known as runner's high.

Endosperm The largest portion of a kernel of grain. It is primarily starch and serves as a food supply for the sprouting seed.

Endurance The length of time one can perform a task.

Energy The capacity to do work.

Energy balance A state in which body weight remains stable because the amount of energy consumed in the diet equals the amount expended.

Enrichment The addition of nutrients to a food to restore those lost in processing to a level equal to or higher than originally present.

Environmental Protection Agency (EPA) U.S. government agency responsible for determining acceptable levels of environmental contaminants in the food supply and for establishing water quality standards.

Enzymes Protein molecules that accelerate the rate of specific chemical reactions without being changed themselves.

Epidemiology The study of the interrelationships between health and disease and other factors in the environment or lifestyle of different populations.

Epiglottis A flap of cartilage that serves as a valve during swallowing to prevent food from passing into the lung passage.

Epinephrine A hormone secreted by the adrenal gland in response to stress that causes changes, such as an increase in heart rate, in preparation for "fight or flight"; also called adrenaline.

Epithelial tissue One of the four human tissue types; includes the cells that cover external body surfaces and line internal cavities and tubes.

Ergogenic aids Anything designed to increase work or improve performance.

Ergot A toxin produced by a mold that grows on grains, particularly rye.

Esophagus A portion of the gastrointestinal tract that extends from the pharynx to the stomach.

Essential amino acid An amino acid that cannot be synthesized by the human body in sufficient amounts to meet needs and therefore must be included in the diet.

Essential fatty acid A fatty acid that must be consumed in the diet because it cannot be made by the body or cannot be made in sufficient quantities to meet needs.

Essential fatty acid deficiency The condition that results when the diet does not supply sufficient amounts of the essential fatty acids.

Essential hypertension High blood pressure that has no obvious external cause.

Essential nutrients Nutrients that must be provided in the diet because the body either cannot make them or cannot make them in sufficient quantities to satisfy its needs.

Essential or **indispensable amino acids** Amino acids that cannot be synthesized by the human body in sufficient amounts to meet needs and therefore must be included in the diet.

Estimated Average Requirements (EARs) Intakes that meet the estimated nutrient needs (as defined by a specific indicator of adequacy) of 50% of individuals in a gender and life-stage group.

Estimated safe and adequate daily dietary intakes (ESADDIs) Recommended intakes of essential nutrients established when data were sufficient to estimate a range of requirements but insufficient to develop a 1989 RDA.

Estrogen A steroid hormone secreted by the ovaries and by the placenta that is involved in the maintenance of pregnancy and the maintenance and development of female sex organs and secondary sex characteristics.

Exchange Lists A system of grouping foods based on their carbohydrate, protein, fat, and energy content.

Excretory system Organ system involved in the elimination of metabolic waste products; includes the lungs, skin, and kidneys.

Experimental controls Factors included in an experimental design that limit the number of variables, allowing an investigator to examine the effect of only the parameters of interest.

Experimental groups Groups of participants in an experiment who are subjected to an experimental treatment.

Extracellular fluid The fluid located outside cells. It includes fluid found in the blood, lymph, gastrointestinal tract, spinal column, eyes, and joints, and that found between cells and tissues.

Facilitated diffusion The movement of substances across a cell membrane from an area of greater concentration to an area of lower concentration with the aid of a carrier molecule. No energy is required.

Fad bulimia A type of bulimia that is more a trend than a psychological disorder; binge episodes are typically less dramatic and emotional than those of a true bulimic and are common among teenagers and young adults who are concerned about a few extra pounds of body weight.

Failure to thrive The inability of a child's growth to keep up with normal growth curves.

Fallopian tubes (oviducts) Narrow ducts leading from the ovaries to the uterus.

Famine A widespread lack of access to food due to a disaster that causes a collapse in the food production and marketing systems.

Fasting hypoglycemia Low blood sugar that is not related to food intake; often caused by an insulin-secreting tumor.

Fat A lipid that is solid at room temperature; commonly used to refer to all lipids or specifically to triglycerides.

Fat-free mass Body mass composed of all tissue except adipose tissue.

Fatigue The inability to continue an activity at an optimal level.

Fat-soluble vitamin A vitamin that does not dissolve in water; includes vitamins A, D, E, and K.

Fatty acid A lipid made up of a chain of carbons linked to hydrogens with an acid group at one end.

Fatty liver The accumulation of fat in the liver.

Fatty streak A cholesterol deposit in the artery wall.

FDA *See* Food and Drug Administration.

Feces Body waste, including unabsorbed food residue, bacteria, mucus, and dead cells, which is excreted from the gastrointestinal tract by way of the anus.

Fermentation A process in which microorganisms metabolize components of a food and therefore change the composition, taste, and storage properties of the food.

Ferritin The major iron storage protein.

Fertilization The union of sperm and egg (ovum).

Fetal alcohol effects (FAE) Also called alcohol-related birth defects (ARBD) and refers to mild symptoms such as learning disabilities, behavioral abnormalities, and motor impairments seen in an infant whose mother consumed alcohol during pregnancy.

Fetal alcohol syndrome (FAS) A characteristic group of severe physical and mental abnormalities in an infant resulting from alcohol consumed by the mother during pregnancy.

Fetus The developing human from the ninth week after conception to birth. Growth and refinement of structures occur during this time.

Fiber Substances in food that are not broken down by the digestive processes in the human stomach and small intestine.

Fitness The ability to perform routine physical activity without undue fatigue.

Flexibility Range of motion.

Fluorhydroxyapatite A fluoride-containing mineral deposit in the tooth enamel that is resistant to acid.

Foam cell A cholesterol-filled white blood cell.

Food additives Substances that can reasonably be expected to become a component of a food during processing. The foods that may contain them and the amounts that may be present are regulated by the FDA.

Food and Drug Administration (FDA) U.S. government agency responsible for the safety and wholesomeness of all food except red meat, poultry, and eggs; also sets standards and enforces regulations for food labeling and for food and color additives.

Food-borne illness An illness that can be transmitted to humans through food or water.

Food-borne infection Illness produced by the ingestion of food containing microorganisms that can multiply inside the body and produce effects that are injurious.

Food-borne intoxication Illness caused by consuming a food containing a toxin or organisms that produce a toxin inside the body.

Food Code A set of recommendations published by the FDA for the handling and service of food sold in restaurants and other establishments that serve food.

Food diary Dietary intake assessment method in which the individual is asked to keep a record of all food and beverage consumed for a defined period.

Food disappearance study A method of determining the food use by a population in which the amount of food that leaves the marketplace provides an estimate of the amount of food used by the population.

Food frequency A dietary intake assessment method which obtains information about an individual's typical food consumption patterns.

Food Guide Pyramid A system of food groups developed by the USDA as a guide to the number of servings of different types of foods needed to provide an adequate diet and comply with current nutrition recommendations.

Food insecurity An inability to acquire appropriate foods in a socially acceptable way.

Food intolerance An adverse reaction to a food that does not involve the immune system.

Food jag A temporary food fixation during which a child will eat only certain foods.

Food processing Any alteration of food from the way it is found in nature.

Food self-sufficiency The ability of an area to produce enough food to feed its population.

Food shortage Insufficient food to feed a population.

Fortification A term used generally to describe the addition of nutrients to foods, such as the addition of vitamin D to milk.

Frame size An estimation of the proportion of body weight due to bone.

Free radical One type of highly reactive molecule that causes oxidative damage to cells.

Fructose A monosaccharide found in fruits and honey that is composed of six carbon atoms arranged in a ring structure; commonly called fruit sugar.

Functional foods Foods that provide health benefits.

Galactose A monosaccharide composed of six carbon atoms arranged in a ring structure; when combined with glucose, it forms the disaccharide lactose.

Gallbladder An organ of the digestive system that stores bile, which is produced by the liver.

Gastric juice A substance produced by the gastric glands of the stomach that contains pepsinogen and hydrochloric acid.

Gastric phase The phase of gastric secretion triggered by the entry of food into the stomach; involves the release of gastrin and the secretion of mucus, acid, and enzymes from the gastric glands.

Gastrin A hormone secreted by the mucosa of the stomach that stimulates the secretion of enzymes and acid in the stomach.

Gastrointestinal tract A hollow tube consisting of the mouth, pharynx, esophagus, stomach, small intestine, large intestine, rectum, and anus in which digestion and absorption of nutrients occur; also called the alimentary canal and digestive tract.

Gastroplasty A surgical procedure that staples the lower part of the stomach, decreasing the storage capacity and consequently the amount of food that can be consumed at one time; also called stomach stapling.

Gel A jelly-like suspension of a liquid in a solid system that is semisolid in consistency.

Gelatin A protein derived from collagen that is deficient in the amino acid tryptophan.

Gene A length of DNA that contains the instructions for making a protein.

Gene expression Refers to the events of protein synthesis in which the information coded in a gene is used to synthesize a protein.

Generally recognized as safe (GRAS) A group of chemical additives that are generally recognized as safe based on their long-standing presence in the food supply without obvious harmful effects.

Genetic engineering *See* Biotechnology.

Germ The embryo or sprouting portion of a kernel of grain. It contains vegetable oil, vitamins, and minerals.

Gestation The time between conception and birth, which lasts about nine months (or about 40 weeks) in humans.

Gestational diabetes A consistently elevated blood glucose level that develops during pregnancy and returns to normal after delivery.

Ginseng An herb used in traditional Chinese medicine; claims are made that it improves athletic performance and increases sexual potency.

Glucagon A hormone secreted by the pancreas that stimulates the breakdown of liver glycogen and the synthesis of glucose to increase blood sugar

Gluconeogenesis The synthesis of glucose from simple noncarbohydrate molecules. Amino acids from protein are the primary source of carbons for glucose synthesis.

Glucose A monosaccharide that is the primary form of carbohydrate used to produce energy in the body. It is the sugar referred to as blood sugar.

Glutamic acid A nonessential amino acid that is found in protein and in monosodium glutamate (MSG).

Glutathione peroxidase A selenium-containing enzyme that protects the cell from oxidative damage by degrading reactive chemical species called peroxides.

Glycemic response or **glycemic index** A measure of how quickly blood glucose levels increase after a food or a meal is consumed.

Glyceride The most common type of lipid; consists of one, two, or three fatty acids attached to a molecule of glycerol.

Glycerol A 3-carbon molecule that forms the backbone of triglycerides and phosphoglycerides; also used as a humectant in food.

Glycogen A carbohydrate made of many glucose molecules linked together in a highly branched structure. It is the storage form of carbohydrate in animals.

Glycogen supercompensation or **carbohydrate loading** A regimen of diet and exercise training, followed in preparation for endurance activities, that is designed to maximize muscle glycogen stores.

Glycolysis A metabolic pathway in the cytoplasm of the cell that splits glucose into two 3-carbon pyruvate molecules. The energy released is used to make two ATP molecules.

Goiter An enlargement of the thyroid gland that is caused by a deficiency of iodine.

Goitrogens Substances that interfere with the utilization of iodine or the function of the thyroid gland.

GRAS *See* Generally recognized as safe.

Growth hormone A hormone secreted by the pituitary gland that stimulates growth.

Guar gum A branched polysaccharide from guar plants used as an additive to increase the viscosity of food.

Gum A plant polysaccharide and its derivatives that can dissolve in water and swell to form viscous solutions.

Gum arabic A branched polysaccharide from acacia trees; it is colorless, odorless, and tasteless, and is used as an additive to increase the viscosity of food.

Gum karaya A branched polysaccharide from trees; used as an additive to increase the viscosity of food.

Gum tragacanth A branched polysaccharide from thorny shrubs that grow in the semidesert of the Near East; used as an additive to thicken foods and to stabilize emulsions.

Hazard Analysis Critical Control Point (HACCP) A food safety system that focuses on identifying and preventing hazards that could cause food-borne illness.

Health claim A statement made about the relationship between a nutrient or food and a disease or health condition.

Healthy People A set of national health promotion and disease prevention objectives for the U.S. population.

Heart attack A condition in which an artery supplying blood to the heart becomes blocked, cutting off blood flow and hence oxygen and nutrients to a segment of the heart muscle, resulting in tissue death.

Heartburn A burning sensation in the chest caused when acidic stomach contents leak into the esophagus through the gastroesophageal sphincter.

Heat cramp A muscle cramp caused by an imbalance of sodium and potassium as a result of excessive exercise without adequate fluid and electrolyte replacement.

Heat exhaustion Low blood pressure, rapid pulse, fainting, and sweating caused when dehydration decreases blood volume so much that blood can no longer both cool the body and provide oxygen to the muscles.

Heat stroke Elevated body temperature as a result of fluid loss and the failure of the temperature regulatory center of the brain.

Heimlich maneuver A procedure used to dislodge an object blocking an air passage; involves the application of sharp, firm pressure to the abdomen just below the rib cage.

Heme iron A readily absorbed form of iron found in animal products that is chemically associated with proteins such as hemoglobin and myoglobin.

Hemicellulose An insoluble fiber that is a structural component of plant cell walls.

Hemochromatosis An inherited condition that results in increased iron absorption and leads to iron deposits throughout the body and tissue damage.

Hemoglobin An iron-containing protein in red blood cells that binds and transports oxygen through the bloodstream to cells.

Hemolytic anemia A condition in which there is an insufficient number of red blood cells because many have burst open.

Hemorrhoids Swollen veins in the anal or rectal area.

Hemosiderin An insoluble iron-protein compound formed in the liver when the iron storage capacity of ferritin is exceeded.

Hepatic portal circulation The system of blood vessels that collects nutrient-laden blood from the digestive organs and delivers it to the liver.

Hepatic portal vein The vein that transports blood from the gastrointestinal tract to the liver.

Hepatitis Inflammation of the liver.

Herb The leaves, flowers, stems, roots, seeds, or any other part of a nonwoody seed-bearing plant that dies down to the ground after flowering.

Herbicide An agent that kills weeds.

Heterocyclic amines (HAs) A class of mutagenic substances produced when there is incomplete combustion of amino acids during the cooking of meats—for example, when meat is charred.

High-density lipoprotein (HDL) A lipoprotein that picks up cholesterol from cells so that it can be eliminated from the body. A low level of HDL increases the risk of cardiovascular disease.

High-fructose corn syrup A sweetener made from corn syrup that is composed of approximately half fructose and half glucose.

Histamine A substance produced by cells of the immune system as part of a nonspecific response that leads to inflammation.

HIV (human immunodeficiency virus) A virus that infects cells of the immune system and eventually leads to AIDS.

Homeostasis A physiological state in which a stable internal body environment is maintained.

Homocysteine A sulfur-containing amino acid that is produced from the metabolism of methionine. Elevated blood levels increase the risk of cardiovascular disease.

Hormone A chemical messenger that is produced in one location, released into the blood, and elicits responses at other locations in the body.

Hormone sensitive lipase An enzyme present in adipose cells that responds to chemical signals by breaking down triglycerides into fatty acids and glycerol for release into the bloodstream.

Humectant A substance added to foods to retain moisture.

Hunger Internal signals that stimulate one to acquire and consume food.

Hydrochloric acid An acid secreted by the gastric glands of the stomach to aid in digestion.

Hydrogenation The process whereby hydrogens are added to the carbon-carbon double bonds of unsaturated fatty acids, making them more saturated.

Hydrogen peroxide A reactive oxygen-containing compound that can form free radicals and cause oxidative damage. It can be eliminated by the selenium-containing enzyme glutathione peroxidase.

Hydrolysis A type of reaction in which a large molecule is broken into two smaller molecules by the addition of water.

Hydrolyzed protein *See* Protein hydrolysate.

Hydroxyapatite A compound composed of calcium and phosphorus that is deposited in the protein matrix of bone to give it strength and rigidity.

Hyperactivity Overactive, excitable, distractible behavior that is characteristic of attention deficit hyperactive disorder.

Hypercarotenemia A condition caused by an accumulation of carotenoids in the adipose tissue, causing the skin to appear yellow-orange.

Hypertension Blood pressure that is consistently elevated to 140/90 mm of mercury or greater.

Hypoglycemia A symptomatic low blood glucose level, usually below 40 to 50 mg of glucose per 100 ml of blood.

Hypothalamus The region of the brain that monitors and regulates conditions and activities in the body, including food intake and energy expenditure.

Hypothermia A condition in which body temperature drops below normal. Hypothermia depresses the central nervous system, resulting in the inability to shiver, sleepiness, and eventually coma.

Hypothesis An educated guess made to explain an observation or to answer a question.

Ileocecal valve The structure that separates the ileum of the small intestine from the large intestine.

Ileum The 11-foot segment of the small intestine that connects the jejunum with the large intestine.

Immunization An injection of a killed or inactivated organism into the body to stimulate the immune system to develop antibodies against the active disease-causing organism.

Implantation The process that begins about a week after fertilization by which the developing ball of cells embeds in the uterine lining.

Incomplete protein A protein that is deficient in one or more of the amino acids required for protein synthesis in humans.

Indirect calorimetry A method of estimating energy use that compares the amount of oxygen consumed with the carbon dioxide expired.

Indirect food additives Substances that are expected to unintentionally enter foods during manufacturing or from packaging. They are regulated by the FDA.

Infant mortality rate The number of deaths during the first year of life per 1000 live births.

Inorganic Substances that contain no carbon atoms.

Inositol A compound that is often included in B vitamin supplements; functions as part of a phospholipid in the human brain but is not a dietary essential; also called myo-inositol.

Insensible losses Fluid losses that are not perceived by the senses, such as evaporation of water through the skin and lungs.

Insoluble fiber Fiber that, for the most part, does not dissolve in water. It includes cellulose, hemicelluloses, and lignin.

Insulin A hormone made in the pancreas that allows the uptake of glucose by body cells and has other metabolic effects such as stimulating the synthesis of glycogen in liver and muscle.

Insulin-dependent diabetes *See* Type 1 diabetes.

Integrated pest management (IPM) A method of agricultural pest control that reduces pesticide usage by integrating nonchemical and chemical techniques.

Intermediate-density lipoprotein (IDL) A lipoprotein produced by the removal of triglycerides from VLDLs, most of which are then transformed to LDLs.

International unit (IU) A unit of measure used to express requirements of some vitamins.

Interstitial fluid The portion of the extracellular fluid located in the spaces between cells.

Interstitial space The fluid-filled spaces between cells.

Intervention study A study of a population in which there is an experimental manipulation of some members of the population and observations and measurements are made to determine the effects of this manipulation.

Intestinal microflora Microorganisms that inhabit the large intestine.

Intestinal phase The phase of gastric secretion that is begun by the entry of food into the small intestine.

Intracellular fluid The fluid located inside cells.

Intrinsic factor A protein produced in the stomach that is needed for the absorption of adequate amounts of vitamin B_{12}.

Ion An atom or group of atoms that carries a negative or a positive electrical charge.

Iron deficiency anemia A condition that occurs when the oxygen-carrying capacity of the blood is decreased because there is insufficient iron to make hemoglobin. It is diagnosed clinically when red blood cells are small and pale and hemoglobin is less than normal.

Irradiation A process of exposing foods to high-energy waves to kill contaminating organisms and retard ripening and spoilage of fruits and vegetables.

Isoleucine An essential amino acid found in protein.

Isotope An alternative form of an element that has a different atomic mass, which may or may not be radioactive.

Jejunum The 8-foot-long section of the small intestine lying between the duodenum and the ileum.

Juvenile-onset diabetes *See* Type 1 diabetes.

Keratin A hard protein that makes up hair and nails.

Keratomalacia Advanced xerophthalmia, characterized by softening of the cornea and irreversible blindness.

Keshan disease A heart disease that occurs in an area of China where the soil is very low in selenium.

Ketones or **ketone bodies** Molecules formed when there is not sufficient carbohydrate to completely metabolize the acetyl-CoA produced from fat breakdown.

Ketosis High levels of ketones in the blood.

Kilocalorie (kcal) A unit of heat that is used to express the amount of energy provided by foods. It is the amount of heat required to raise the temperature of 1 kilogram of water 1 degree Celsius (1 kcalorie = 4.18 kjoules).

Kilojoule (kjoule or kJ) A measure of work that can be used to express energy intake and energy output. It is the amount of work required to move an object weighing 1 kilogram a distance of 1 meter under the force of gravity (4.18 kjoules = 1 kcalorie).

Kwashiorkor A form of protein-energy malnutrition in which only protein is deficient. It is most common in young children who are unable to meet their high protein needs with the available diet.

Lactase An enzyme located in the brush border of the small intestine that breaks the disaccharide lactose into glucose and galactose.

Lactation The production and secretion of milk by the mammary gland.

Lacteal A lymph vessel in the intestine that can accept large particles such as the products of fat digestion.

Lactic acid An end product of anaerobic metabolism and an additive used in food to maintain acidity or form curds.

Lactitol The sugar alcohol formed from lactose.

Lacto-ovo vegetarian One who eats no animal flesh but eats eggs and dairy products such as milk and cheese.

Lactose A disaccharide made of glucose linked to galactose that is found in milk.

Lactose intolerance The inability to digest lactose because of a deficiency of the enzyme lactase. It causes symptoms such as intestinal gas and bloating after dairy products are consumed.

Lacto-vegetarian One who eats no animal flesh or eggs but eats dairy products.

Large-for-gestational-age An infant weighing greater than 4 kg (8.8 lb) at birth.

Large intestine The portion of the gastrointestinal tract that includes the colon and rectum; some water and vitamins are absorbed and bacteria act on food residues here.

Laxative A substance that eases the excretion of feces.

LDL receptor *See* Low-density lipoprotein receptor.

Lean body mass Body mass attributed to nonfat body components such as bone, muscle, and internal organs. It is also called fat-free mass.

Leavening agent A substance added to food that causes the production of gas, resulting in an increase in volume.

Lecithin A phosphoglyceride composed of a glycerol backbone, two fatty acids, a phosphate group, and a molecule of choline; often used as an emulsifier in foods.

Legume The starchy seed of plants that produce bean pods; includes peas, peanuts, beans, soybeans, and lentils.

Leptin A protein hormone produced by adipocytes that signals information about the amount of body fat.

Leptin receptors Proteins that bind the hormone leptin. In response to this binding they trigger events that cause changes in food intake and energy expenditure.

Let-down A hormonal reflex triggered by the infant's suckling that causes milk to be released from the milk ducts and flow to the nipple.

Leucine An essential amino acid found in protein.

Life expectancy The average length of life for a population of individuals.

Life span The maximum age to which a member of a species can live.

Lignin An insoluble fiber responsible for the hard woody nature of plant stems.

Limiting amino acid The essential amino acid that is available in the lowest concentration in relation to the body's needs.

Linoleic acid An omega-6 essential fatty acid with 18 carbons and 2 double bonds.

Lipases Fat-digesting enzymes.

Lipid bilayer Two layers of phosphoglyceride molecules oriented so that the fat-soluble fatty acid tails are sandwiched between the water-soluble phosphate-containing heads.

Lipids Organic molecules, most of which do not dissolve in water, that provide energy and insulation and serve as precursors in the synthesis of certain hormones; include fatty acids, glycerides, phospholipids, and sterols.

Lipoic acid A coenzyme needed in the reaction that forms acetyl-CoA; not a dietary essential.

Lipoprotein lipase An enzyme that breaks down triglycerides into free fatty acids and glycerol; attached to the outside of the cells that line the blood vessels.

Lipoproteins Particles containing a core of lipids surrounded by a shell of protein and phospholipid.

Liposuction A procedure that suctions out adipose tissue from under the skin; used to decrease the size of local fat deposits such as on the abdomen or hips.

Locust bean gum A branched polysaccharide that is produced from the endosperm of the seed of the carob plant; used as an additive to increase viscosity in cheese products and sausages.

Longevity The duration of an individual's life.

Longitudinal data Information obtained by repeatedly sampling the same individuals in a population over time.

Low birth weight infant An infant born weighing less than 2.5 kg (5.5 lb).

Low-density lipoprotein (LDL) A lipoprotein that transports cholesterol to cells. Elevated LDL cholesterol increases the risk of cardiovascular disease.

Low-density lipoprotein receptor A protein on the surface of cells that binds to LDL particles and allows their contents to be taken up for use by the cell.

Low-input agriculture or **sustainable agriculture** Methods of producing food that leave the environment able to restore itself and continue to produce food for future generations.

Lumen The inside cavity of a tube, such as the gastrointestinal tract.

Lutein A carotenoid found in corn and green peppers that provides some protection against macular degeneration.

Lycopene A carotenoid that gives the red color to tomatoes. It cannot be converted to vitamin A.

Lymphatic system The system of lymph vessels and other lymph organs and tissues that drains excess fluid from the space between cells and provides immune function.

Lymph vessel or **lacteal** A tubular component of the lymphatic system that carries fluid away from body tissues. Lymph vessels in the intestine are known as lacteals and can transport large particles such as the products of fat digestion.

Lysosome A cellular organelle containing degradative enzymes.

Macrocytes Larger-than-normal mature red blood cells that have a shortened life span.

Macronutrients Nutrients needed by the body in large amounts. These include water and the energy-yielding nutrients carbohydrates, lipids, and proteins.

Macular degeneration Degeneration of a portion of the retina that results in a loss of visual detail and blindness.

Major minerals Minerals needed in the diet in amounts greater than 100 mg per day or present in the body in amounts greater than 0.01% of body weight.

Malnutrition Poor nutritional status resulting from a dietary intake either above or below that which is optimal.

Maltase An enzyme found in the brush border of the small intestine that breaks maltose into two molecules of glucose.

Maltose A disaccharide made of two glucose molecules linked together.

Mannitol The sugar alcohol formed from the sugar mannose.

Marasmus A form of protein-energy malnutrition in which a deficiency of energy in the diet causes severe body wasting.

Maturity-onset diabetes *See* Type 2 diabetes.

Maximal oxygen consumption or **VO_2 max** The maximum amount of oxygen that can be consumed by the tissues during exercise.

Maximum heart rate The maximum number of beats per minute that the heart can attain. It declines with age and can be estimated by subtracting age in years from 220.

Megaloblastic or **macrocytic anemia** A condition in which there are abnormally large immature and mature red blood cells and a reduction in the total number of red blood cells.

Megaloblasts Large immature red blood cells that are formed when developing red blood cells are unable to divide normally.

Melatonin A hormone involved in regulating the body's cycles of sleep and wakefulness. Levels decline with age. Supplements are claimed to boost antioxidant defenses, improve immune function, and slow aging.

Menaquinones The forms of vitamin K synthesized by bacteria and found in animals.

Menarche The onset of menstruation. It occurs normally in girls between the ages of 10 and 15.

Menopause Physiological changes that mark the end of a woman's capacity to bear children.

Menstruation The cyclic discharge of the uterine lining that, in the absence of pregnancy, occurs about every four weeks during the reproductive years of female humans.

Metabolism The sum of all the chemical reactions that take place in a living organism.

Metallothionein A protein that binds zinc and copper in intestinal cells and limits their absorption.

Methionine An essential sulfur-containing amino acid found in protein.

Methyl group A chemical group consisting of a carbon atom bound to three hydrogen atoms.

Micelles Particles formed in the small intestine when droplets of lipid are emulsified by bile acids.

Microbe An organism too small to be seen without a microscope; also called microorganism.

Microflora *See* Intestinal microflora.

Micronutrients Nutrients needed by the body in small amounts. These include vitamins and minerals.

Microorganism An organism such as a bacterium, too small to be seen without a microscope.

Microvilli Minute projections on the mucosal cell membrane that increase the absorptive surface area in the small intestine.

Mineral An element needed by the body in small amounts for structure and to regulate chemical reactions and body processes.

Miscarriage or **spontaneous abortion** Interruption of pregnancy prior to the seventh month.

Mitochondrion (mitochondria) The cellular organelle that is responsible for generating energy in the form of ATP via aerobic metabolism; the citric acid cycle and electron transport chain are located here.

Modified atmosphere packaging (MAP) A type of food packaging in which the gases inside the package are changed to control or retard chemical, physical, and microbiological changes.

Modified starch or **modified food starch** Starch that has been treated to enhance its ability to thicken or form a gel.

Molds Multicellular fungi that form a filamentous branching growth.

Molecular biology The study of cellular function at the molecular level.

Molecules Units of two or more atoms of the same or different elements bonded together.

Monoacylglycerol or **monoglyceride** A molecule of glycerol with one fatty acid attached.

Monosaccharide A single sugar molecule, such as glucose.

Monosodium glutamate (MSG) An additive used as a flavor enhancer, commonly used in Chinese food; made up of the amino acid glutamate bound to sodium.

Monounsaturated fatty acid A fatty acid containing one carbon-carbon double bond.

Morbidity The incidence or state of disease or disability.

Morbid obesity A condition in which an individual's body weight is 100 pounds (45.5 kg) above desirable body weight, or the body mass index is greater than 40.

Morning sickness Nausea and vomiting that affects many women during the first few months of pregnancy and that in some women can continue throughout the pregnancy.

mRNA (messenger RNA) A molecule that carries the information in a gene to ribosomes in the cytoplasm so proteins can be synthesized.

MSG symptom complex Symptoms of headache, flushing, tingling, burning sensations, and chest pain reported by some individuals after consuming monosodium glutamate (MSG); commonly referred to as Chinese restaurant syndrome.

Mucosa The layer of tissue lining the gastrointestinal tract and other body cavities.

Mucus A viscous fluid secreted by glands in the gastrointestinal tract and other parts of the body. It acts to lubricate, moisten, and protect cells from harsh environments.

Mutagen Any agent that causes a change in a cell's genetic material.

Mutations Changes in DNA caused by chemical or physical agents.

Myelin A soft, white fatty substance that covers nerve fibers and aids in nerve transmission.

Myocardial infarction Heart attack.

Myoglobin An iron-containing protein in muscle cells that binds oxygen.

Myo-inositol *See* Inositol.

National Health and Nutrition Examination Survey (NHANES) An ongoing set of surveys designed to monitor the overall nutritional status of the U.S. population; combines food consumption information with medical histories, physical examinations, and laboratory measurements.

Nervous system A system of nerve cells organized in message sending, message receiving, and information processing pathways.

Net protein utilization A measure of protein quality determined by comparing the amount of nitrogen retained in the body with the amount eaten in the diet.

Neural tube A portion of the embryo that develops into the brain and spinal cord.

Neural tube closure A developmental event in which neural tissue forms a groove and the sides fold together to form a tube; is completed about 28 days after fertilization.

Neural tube defect A defect in the formation of the neural tube that occurs early in development and results in defects of the brain and spinal cord such as anencephaly and spina bifida.

Neurotransmitter A chemical substance produced by a nerve cell that can stimulate or inhibit another cell.

Niacin equivalent (NEs) A unit used to express the amount of niacin present in food including that which can be made from its precursor, tryptophan. One NE is equal to 1 mg of niacin or 60 mg of tryptophan.

Nicotinamide A form of niacin.

Nicotinamide adenine dinucleotide (NAD) A coenzyme made from niacin that transports electrons.

Nicotinamide adenine dinucleotide phosphate (NADP) A coenzyme made from niacin that is needed as an electron carrier in synthetic reactions.

Nicotinic acid A form of niacin.

Nitrogen balance A state in which nitrogen intake is equal to nitrogen excretion.

Nitrosamines Carcinogenic compounds produced by reactions between nitrites and other molecules.

Nonessential or **dispensable amino acids** Amino acids that can be synthesized by the human body in sufficient amounts to meet needs.

Nonheme iron A poorly absorbed form of iron found in both plant and animal products that is not part of the iron complex found in hemoglobin and myoglobin.

Noninsulin-dependent diabetes *See* Type 2 diabetes.

Nucleus The central core of an atom, consisting of positively charged protons and electrically neutral neutrons. In cells, it is an organelle containing DNA.

Nursing bottle syndrome Extreme tooth decay in the upper teeth resulting from putting a child to bed with a bottle containing milk or other sweetened liquid.

Nutrient density A measure of the nutrients provided by a food relative to the energy it contains.

Nutrients Chemical substances in foods that provide energy, structure, and regulation of body processes.

Nutrification The process of adding one or more nutrients to commonly consumed foods with the goal of adding to the nutrient intake of a group of people.

Nutrition A science that studies the interactions that occur between living organisms and food.

Nutritional assessment The process of determining the nutritional status of individuals or groups for the purpose of identifying nutritional needs and planning personal health care or community programs to meet these needs.

Nutritional status State of health as it is influenced by the intake and utilization of nutrients.

Nutrition support claims Claims often included on the labels of dietary supplements that describe the relationship between a nutrient and a deficiency disease that could result if the nutrient were lacking in the diet.

Nutrition transition The shift in dietary pattern from a diet high in complex carbohydrates and fiber to a more varied diet higher in fats, saturated fat, and sugar that occurs as incomes increase.

Obese A condition characterized by excess body fat. It is defined as a body mass index of 30 kg/m^2 or greater, or a body weight that is 20% or more above the desirable body weight standard.

Obesity genes Genes that code for proteins involved in the regulation of body fat. When they are abnormal the result is abnormal amounts of body fat.

Oil A lipid that is liquid at room temperature.

Oleic acid A monounsaturated fatty acid with 18 carbons.

Olestra (sucrose polyester) An artificial fat made of sucrose with fatty acids linked to it that cannot be digested or absorbed. It has been approved by the FDA for use in certain snack foods.

Oligosaccharides Short chain carbohydrates containing 3 to 10 sugar units.

Omega-3 (ω-3) fatty acid A fatty acid containing a carbon-carbon double bond between the third and fourth carbons from the omega end; includes alpha-linolenic acid found in vegetable oils and eicosapentaenoic acid (EPA) and docosahexaenoic acid found in fish oils.

Omega-6 (ω-6) fatty acid A fatty acid containing a carbon-carbon double bond between the sixth and seventh carbons from the omega end; includes linoleic and arachidonic acid.

Opsin A protein in the retina of the eye involved in the visual cycle.

Organ A discrete structure composed of more than one tissue that performs a specialized function.

Organelles Cellular organs that carry out specific metabolic functions.

Organic food A food that contains no additives and that is produced without the use of chemical fertilizers, pesticides, or herbicides.

Organic molecules Substances that contain carbon atoms.

Osmosis The passive movement of water across a membrane to equalize the concentration of dissolved solutes on both sides.

Osteoarthritis The form of arthritis common in the elderly that is characterized by a wearing down of the joint surfaces and pain when the joint is moved.

Osteoblasts Cells responsible for the deposition of bone.

Osteoclasts Large cells responsible for bone breakdown.

Osteomalacia A vitamin D deficiency disease in adults that causes weak bones and an increase in bone fractures.

Osteoporosis A bone disorder characterized by a reduction in bone mass, an increase in bone fragility, and an increased risk of fractures.

Overnutrition Poor nutritional status resulting from a dietary intake in excess of that which is optimal for health.

Overweight A body mass index of 25 to 29.9 kg/m^2, or a body weight 10% to 19% above the desirable body weight standard.

Oviduct *See* Fallopian tube.

Ovum The female reproductive cell.

Oxalates Organic acids found in spinach, rhubarb, and other leafy green vegetables that can bind certain minerals and decrease their absorption.

Oxaloacetate A 4-carbon compound derived from carbohydrate that combines with acetyl-CoA in the first step of the citric acid cycle.

Oxidation The loss of electrons.

Oxidative damage Damage caused by highly reactive oxygen molecules that steal electrons from other compounds, causing changes in structure and function.

Oxidative stress A condition that occurs when there are more reactive oxygen molecules than can be neutralized by available antioxidant defenses. It occurs either because excessive amounts of reactive oxygen molecules are generated or because antioxidant defenses are deficient.

Oxidized LDL cholesterol A substance formed when the cholesterol in LDL particles is oxidized by reactive oxygen molecules. It is key in the development of atherosclerosis because it is taken up by scavenger receptors on white blood cells.

Oxytocin A hormone released by the posterior pituitary that stimulates the ejection or let-down of milk during lactation.

Palmitic acid A saturated fatty acid containing 16 carbons.

Pancreas An organ that secretes digestive enzymes and bicarbonate ions into the small intestine during digestion. It also secretes the hormones insulin and glucagon into the blood.

Pancreatic amylase A starch-digesting enzyme found in pancreatic juice.

Pancreatic juice The secretion of the pancreas containing bicarbonate to neutralize acid and enzymes for the digestion of carbohydrates, fats, and proteins.

Papain A protein-digesting enzyme found in papaya.

Para-aminobenzoic acid (PABA) A chemical that is part of the folic acid molecule but that alone has no vitamin activity and cannot be used by the body to synthesize folic acid; effective at blocking ultraviolet (UV) light and thus is used in topical sunscreens.

Parasites Organisms that live at the expense of others without contributing to the survival of the host.

Parathyroid hormone (PTH) A hormone secreted by the parathyroid gland that acts to increase blood calcium levels.

Parietal cells Large cells in the stomach lining that produce and secrete intrinsic factor and hydrochloric acid.

Partially hydrogenated vegetable oil Vegetable oil that has been modified by hydrogenation to decrease the number of unsaturated bonds, therefore raising the melting point and improving the storage characteristics.

Pasteurization The process of heating food products to kill disease-causing organisms.

Pathogen An organism capable of causing disease.

Peak bone mass The maximum bone density attained at any time in life, usually occurring in young adulthood.

Pectin A soluble fiber found in plant cell walls that forms a gel when mixed with acid and sugar.

Peer review Review of the design and validity of a research experiment by experts in the field of study who did not participate in the research.

Pellagra A niacin deficiency disease that is characterized by dermatitis, dementia, diarrhea, and, ultimately, death.

Pepsin A protein-digesting enzyme produced by the stomach. It is secreted in the gastric juice in an inactive form (pepsinogen) and activated by acid in the stomach.

Pepsinogen An inactive protein-digesting enzyme produced by gastric glands and activated to pepsin by acid in the stomach.

Peptic ulcer An open sore in the lining of the stomach, esophagus, or small intestine.

Peptide Two or more amino acids joined by peptide bonds.

Peptide bond A chemical linkage between the amino group of one amino acid and the acid group of another.

Periodontal disease A degeneration of the area surrounding the teeth, specifically the gum and supporting bone.

Peristalsis Coordinated muscular contractions that move food through the gastrointestinal tract.

Pernicious anemia An anemia resulting from vitamin B_{12} deficiency that occurs because dietary vitamin B_{12} cannot be absorbed due to a lack of intrinsic factor. If not treated with vitamin B_{12} injections, nerve damage will result.

Peroxide A reactive chemical that can form free radicals and cause cellular damage.

Pesticide A substance used to prevent or decrease damage to plants from insects and microorganisms.

pH A measure of the level of acidity or alkalinity of a solution compared to neutrality.

Pharynx A funnel-shaped opening that connects the nasal passages and mouth to the respiratory passages and esophagus. It is a common passageway for food and air and is responsible for swallowing.

Phenylalanine An essential amino acid found in protein that cannot be metabolized by individuals with phenylketonuria (PKU).

Phenylketone The product of phenylalanine breakdown produced when phenylalanine cannot be converted to tyrosine; when blood levels get too high, brain damage results.

Phenylketonuria (PKU) An inherited disease in which the body cannot metabolize the amino acid phenylalanine. If the disease is untreated, toxic byproducts accumulate in the blood and cause mental retardation.

Phenylpropanolamine A stimulant used in some weight-loss aids to blunt appetite.

Phosphoglyceride A phospholipid composed of a glycerol backbone with two fatty acids and a phosphate group attached; mixes well with both watery and oily substances and is an important component of cell membranes.

Phospholipid A lipid containing a phosphate group.

Photosynthesis The metabolic process by which plants trap energy from the sun and use it to make sugars from carbon dioxide and water.

Phylloquinones The forms of vitamin K found in plants.

Phytic acid or **phytate** An inorganic phosphorus-containing compound found in seeds and grains that can bind minerals and decrease their absorption.

Phytochemical A substance found in plant foods that is not an essential nutrient but has health-promoting properties.

Phytoestrogen An estrogen-like molecule produced by plants.

Phytosterol Compound produced by plants that has a structure similar to cholesterol.

Pica An abnormal craving for and ingestion of unusual food and nonfood substances such as clay, laundry starch, and paint chips.

Placebo A fake medicine or supplement that is indistinguishable in appearance from the real thing. It is used to disguise the control and experimental groups in an experiment.

Placenta An organ produced from both maternal and embryonic tissues. It secretes hormones, transfers nutrients and oxygen from the mother's blood to the fetus, and removes wastes.

Plaque The cholesterol-rich material that is deposited in the blood vessels of individuals with atherosclerosis. It consists of cholesterol, smooth muscle cells, fibrous tissue and, eventually, calcium.

Platelet A cell fragment found in blood that is involved in blood clotting.

Polar A term used to describe a molecule that has a positive charge at one end and a negative charge at the other.

Polychlorinated biphenyls (PCBs) Carcinogenic industrial compounds that have found their way into the environment and, subsequently, the food supply. Repeated exposure causes them to accumulate in biological tissues over time.

Polycyclic aromatic hydrocarbons (PAHs) A class of mutagenic substances produced during cooking when there is incomplete combustion of organic materials—for example, when fat drips on a grill.

Polypeptide A chain of three or more amino acids joined together by peptide bonds.

Polysaccharides Complex carbohydrates containing many sugar units linked together.

Polyunsaturated fatty acid A fatty acid that contains two or more double bonds.

Postmenopausal bone loss The accelerated bone loss that occurs in women for about five years after estrogen production decreases.

Postmenopausal osteoporosis *See* Type I osteoporosis.

Precursor Inactive form of a substance that can be converted into the active form.

Preeclampsia A form of pregnancy-induced hypertension that causes an increase in blood pressure, edema, and protein in the urine.

Pregnancy-induced hypertension A spectrum of conditions involving a rise in blood pressure during pregnancy.

Premature or **preterm infant** An infant born before 37 weeks of gestation.

Premenstrual syndrome (PMS) A syndrome of mood swings, food cravings, bloating, tension and depression, headaches, acne, and anxiety, among other symptoms, that results from the hormonal changes during the days prior to menstruation.

Preservative A compound that prevents spoilage and extends the shelf life of a product by retarding chemical, physical, or microbiological changes.

Preterm infant *See* Premature infant.

Prime grade A USDA-regulated grade of beef with the largest amount of marbled fat.

Progesterone A female sex hormone needed for development and function of the uterus and mammary glands.

Programmed cell death The death of cells at specific predictable times.

Prolactin A hormone released from the anterior pituitary that stimulates the breasts to produce milk.

Pro-oxidant A substance that promotes oxidative damage.

Protein An organic molecule made up of one or more intertwining chains of amino acids.

Protein complementation The process of combining proteins from different sources so that they collectively provide the proportions of amino acids required to meet needs.

Protein efficiency ratio A measure of protein quality determined by comparing the weight gain of a laboratory animal fed a test protein with the weight gain of an animal fed a reference protein.

Protein-energy malnutrition (PEM) A condition characterized by wasting and an increased susceptibility to infection that results from the long-term consumption of insufficient energy and protein to meet needs.

Protein hydrolysate or **hydrolyzed protein** A mixture of amino acids or amino acids and polypeptides that results when a protein is completely or partially broken down by treatment with acid or enzymes.

Protein quality A measure of how efficiently a protein in the diet can be used to make body proteins.

Protein-sparing modified fast A very-low-kcalorie diet of high protein content designed to maximize the loss of fat and minimize the loss of protein from the body.

Prothrombin A blood protein required for blood clotting.

Provitamin or **vitamin precursor** A compound that can be converted into the active form of a vitamin in the body.

Psyllium A plant product high in soluble fiber that is used in over-the-counter bulk-forming laxatives.

Puberty A period in life characterized by rapid growth and physical changes that ends in the attainment of sexual maturity.

Purging Behaviors such as self-induced vomiting and misuse of laxatives and diuretics used to rid the body of energy.

Pyloric sphincter A muscular valve that helps regulate the rate at which food leaves the stomach and enters the small intestine.

Pyridoxal phosphate The active coenzyme form of vitamin B_6.

Pyridoxamine A form of vitamin B_6.

Pyridoxine A form of vitamin B_6; a general name used to refer to vitamin B_6, including pyridoxal, pyridoxine, and pyridoxamine.

Pyruvate A 3-carbon molecule produced when glucose is broken down by glycolysis.

Raffinose An oligosaccharide found in beans and other legumes that cannot be digested by human enzymes in the stomach and small intestine.

Reactive hypoglycemia Low blood sugar that occurs an hour or so after the consumption of high-carbohydrate foods; results from an overproduction of insulin.

Recommended Dietary Allowances (RDAs) Intakes that are sufficient to meet the nutrient needs of almost all healthy people in a specific life-stage and gender group.

Recommended Nutrient Intakes (RNIs) Recommended intakes of nutrients established for Canadians by the Canadian government (Health Canada).

Rectum The portion of the large intestine that connects the colon and anus.

Reference Daily Intakes (RDIs) Reference values established for vitamins and minerals that are based on the highest amount of each nutrient recommended for any adult age group by the 1968 RDAs.

Refined Refers to the process whereby the coarse parts of foods are removed, leaving behind a product of more uniform composition.

Renewable resources Resources that are restored and replaced by natural processes and can therefore be used forever.

Renin An enzyme produced by the kidney that aids in the conversion of angiotensin to its active form, angiotensin II.

Rennin An enzyme produced by the stomach of infants and young children that acts on the milk protein casein to convert it to a curdy substance.

Reserve capacity The amount of functional capacity that an organ has above and beyond what is needed to sustain life.

Respiratory system Organ system that includes the lungs and air passageways involved in the exchange of oxygen from the environment with carbon dioxide waste from cells by way of the bloodstream.

Resting energy expenditure (REE) *See* Resting metabolic rate (RMR).

Resting heart rate The number of times that the heart beats per minute while a person is at rest.

Resting metabolic rate (RMR) or **resting energy expenditure (REE)** An estimate of basal metabolic rate that is determined by measuring energy utilization after 5 to 6 hours without food or exercise.

Retin-A A drug that is a vitamin A derivative used topically to treat acne.

Retinal The aldehyde form of vitamin A, which is needed for the visual cycle.

Retinoic acid The acid form of vitamin A, which is needed for cell differentiation, growth, and reproduction.

Retinoids The chemical forms of preformed vitamin A: retinol, retinal, and retinoic acid.

Retinol The alcohol form of vitamin A, which can be interconverted with retinal.

Retinol-binding protein A protein that is necessary to transport vitamin A in the blood.

Retinol equivalent (RE) A unit of measure for vitamin A equal to the amount of any form of vitamin A that provides the function of 1 μg of retinol.

Rhodopsin A light-sensitive compound found in the retina of the eye that is composed of the protein opsin loosely bound to retinal.

Ribose The 5-carbon sugar that is part of RNA.

Ribosome The cell organelle where protein synthesis occurs.

Rickets A vitamin D deficiency disease in children that is characterized by poor bone development due to inadequate calcium deposition.

Risk-benefit analysis The process of weighing the risk of ingesting a substance against the benefits it provides; if the risk is small and the benefits great, small amounts of this substance may be acceptable.

Risk factor A characteristic or circumstance that is associated with the occurrence of a particular disease.

RNA (ribonucleic acid) The single-stranded nucleic acid that carries information in DNA from the nucleus to the cytoplasm where it is translated into a sequence of amino acids to make a protein.

Royal jelly The substance that is produced by worker bees to feed the queen; marketed as an ergogenic aid.

Saccharin An artificial sweetener used in diet products that contains no energy and is about 300 times sweeter than sugar.

Saliva A watery fluid produced and secreted into the mouth by the salivary glands. It contains lubricants, enzymes, and other substances.

Salivary amylase An enzyme secreted by the salivary glands that breaks down starch into smaller units.

Salivary glands The internal structures that secrete saliva at the sides of and below the face and in front of the ears.

Salmonella A bacterium that commonly causes food-borne illness.

Satiety The feeling of fullness and satisfaction caused by food consumption that eliminates the desire to eat.

Saturated fatty acid A fatty acid in which the carbon atoms are bound to as many hydrogens as possible and which therefore contains no carbon-carbon double bonds.

Scavenger receptor A protein on white blood cells that binds to oxidized LDL cholesterol, allowing it to enter the cell.

Scientific method The general approach of science that is used to explain observations about the world around us.

Scurvy A vitamin C deficiency disease.

Seasonal affective disorder A disorder characterized by depression and carbohydrate cravings during the fall and winter months.

Secondary lactase deficiency Lactase deficiency that occurs as a result of disease and may resolve after the disease has ended.

Secretin A hormone released by the duodenum that signals the pancreas to secrete bicarbonate ions and stimulates the liver to secrete bile into the gallbladder.

Select grade A USDA-regulated grade of beef with a medium amount of marbled fat.

Selectively permeable Describes a membrane or barrier that will allow some substances to pass freely but will restrict the passage of others.

Semiessential amino acids *See* Conditionally essential amino acids.

Semivegetarian One who avoids only certain types of meat, fish, or poultry; e.g., an individual who avoids all red meat but continues to consume poultry and fish.

Serotonin A neurotransmitter that functions in the sleep center of the brain.

Set point A level at which body fat or body weight seems to resist change despite changes in energy intake or output.

Sickle cell anemia An inherited disease in which hemoglobin structure is altered. Red blood cells containing the altered hemoglobin are sickle-shaped; rupture easily, causing anemia; and block small blood vessels, causing inflammation and pain.

Simple carbohydrates Carbohydrates known as sugars that include monosaccharides and disaccharides.

Simple diffusion The movement of substances from an area of greater concentration to an area of lower concentration. No energy is required.

Simplesse An artificial fat made from egg and milk proteins that contains about 1.3 kcalories per gram.

Simple sugar *See* Simple carbohydrate.

Single-blind study An experiment in which either the study participants or the researchers (but not both) are unaware of who is in a control or an experimental group.

Skinfold thickness A measurement of subcutaneous fat used to estimate total body fat.

Small-for-gestational-age An infant born at term weighing less than 2.5 kg (5.5 lb).

Small intestine A tube-shaped organ of the digestive tract where digestion of ingested food is completed and most of the absorption occurs.

Smooth muscle Involuntary muscles that cause constriction of the gastrointestinal tract, blood vessels, and glands.

Sodium bicarbonate A compound that is part of an important buffer system in pancreatic juice and in the bloodstream.

Sodium caseinate A form of the milk protein casein that is frequently used as a food additive.

Sodium-potassium ATPase An energy-requiring protein pump in the cell membrane that pumps sodium out of the cell and potassium into the cell.

Solanine A toxic substance naturally occurring in potatoes; inhibits the action of neurotransmitters.

Soluble fiber Fiber that either dissolves when placed in water or absorbs water. It includes pectins, gums, and some hemicelluloses.

Solutes Dissolved substances.

Solution A solvent containing a dissolved substance.

Solvent A fluid in which one or more substances dissolve.

Sorbitol A sugar alcohol formed from the sugar sorbose; used as a sweetener or humectant in food.

Sperm The male reproductive cell.

Sphincter A muscular valve that helps control the flow of materials in the gastrointestinal tract.

Spina bifida A neural tube defect in which part of the spinal cord is exposed through a gap in the backbone, causing varying degrees of disability.

Spontaneous abortion *See* Miscarriage.

Spores A dormant state of some bacteria that is resistant to heat but can germinate and produce a new organism when environmental conditions are favorable.

Sports anemia A temporary decrease in hemoglobin concentration that occurs during exercise training. It occurs as an adaptation to training and does not impair delivery of oxygen to tissues.

Stabilizer A substance added to food to stabilize its consistency.

Standards of identity Regulations that define the allowable ingredients, composition, and other characteristics of foods.

Staphylococcus A bacterium, commonly found in the nasal passages, that can contaminate food and cause food-borne illness.

Starch A carbohydrate made of many glucose molecules linked in straight or branching chains. The bonds that hold the glucose molecules together can be broken by the human digestive enzymes.

Starchyose An oligosaccharide found in beans and other legumes that cannot be digested by human enzymes in the stomach and small intestine.

Starvation The condition that occurs when insufficient food is ingested to maintain health.

Stearic acid An 18-carbon saturated fatty acid that, unlike other saturated fats, does not raise blood cholesterol levels.

Steroid hormone A hormone that is made from cholesterol; includes the male and female sex hormones.

Sterol A lipid that contains multiple ring structures.

Stomach A muscular pouchlike organ of the digestive tract that mixes food and secretes gastric juice into the lumen and the hormone gastrin into the blood.

Stroke A blood clot or bleeding in the brain that causes brain tissue death.

Stroke volume The volume of blood pumped by each beat of the heart.

Stunting A decrease in linear growth rate which is an indicator of the nutritional well-being in populations of children.

Subcutaneous fat Adipose tissue located under the skin which is not associated with a great increase in the risk of chronic diseases.

Subscapular The region just below the shoulder blade that is a common location for measuring skinfold thickness.

Subsistence crops Crops grown as food for the local population.

Sucralose An artificial sweetener that is about 600 times sweeter than sucrose; trichlorogalactosucrose. It is heat stable, and so can be used in baked products.

Sucrase An enzyme in the brush border of the small intestine that breaks sucrose into glucose and fructose.

Sucrose A disaccharide commonly known as table sugar that is made of glucose linked to fructose.

Sudden infant death syndrome (SIDS or **crib death)** The unexplained death of infants, usually during sleep.

Sugar alcohol A sweetener that is structurally related to sugars but provides less energy than monosaccharides and disaccharides because it is not as well absorbed.

Sulfites Sulfur-containing compounds used as preservatives to prevent oxidation in dried fruits and vegetables and to prevent bacterial growth in wine.

Superoxide dismutase (SOD) An enzyme that protects the cell from oxidative damage by neutralizing superoxide radicals. One form of the enzyme requires zinc and copper for activity and another form requires manganese.

Superoxide radical A type of reactive oxygen molecule that can form free radicals leading to oxidative damage. They can be neutralized by the enzyme superoxide dismutase.

Sustainable Refers to methods of using resources that prevents overuse of natural systems and allows the environment to be maintained indefinitely without a decline.

Sustainable agriculture *See* Low-input agriculture.

Tannins Substances found in tea and some grains that can bind certain minerals and decrease their absorption.

Taurine An amino acid found only in animal foods that is not used in protein synthesis but is necessary for nerve function and vision and the synthesis of bile acids; made in the adult human in sufficient quantities but may be essential in premature infants.

Teratogen A chemical, biological, or physical agent that causes birth defects.

Testosterone A steroid hormone secreted by the testes that is involved in the maintenance and development of male sex organs and secondary sex characteristics.

Texturizer A substance added to food to change its texture.

Theory An explanation based on scientific study and reasoning.

Thermal distress A condition resulting from the inability of the body to dissipate heat as fast as it is produced.

Thermic effect of food (TEF) or **diet-induced thermogenesis** The energy required for the digestion, absorption, metabolism, and storage of food. It is equal to approximately 10% of daily energy intake.

Thiamin pyrophosphate The active coenzyme form of thiamin.

Threshold effect A reaction that occurs at a certain level of ingestion and increases as the dose increases. Below that level there is no reaction.

Thyroid gland A gland located in the neck that produces thyroid hormones and calcitonin.

Thyroid hormones Hormones produced by the thyroid gland that regulate metabolic rate.

Thyroid-stimulating hormone A hormone that stimulates the synthesis and secretion of thyroid hormones from the thyroid gland.

Tocopherol The chemical name for vitamin E.

Tolerable Upper Intake Level (UL) The maximum daily intake by an individual that is unlikely to pose risks of adverse health effects to almost all individuals in the specified life-stage and gender group.

Tolerances Allowable levels of pesticide residues in foods, set by the EPA.

Total parenteral nutrition (TPN) A method of providing complete nutrition without use of the gastrointestinal tract by infusing a nutrient-rich solution directly into the bloodstream.

Toxic The capacity to produce injury at some level of intake.

Toxin A substance with the ability to cause harm at some level of exposure; also called toxicant.

Trabecular bone The spongy bone that forms the inner bone lattice that supports the cortical shell.

Trace elements or **trace minerals** Minerals required in the diet in amounts less than 100 mg per day or present in the body in amounts less than 0.01% of body weight.

Transamination The process by which an amino group from one amino acid is transferred to a carbon compound to form a new amino acid.

Transcription The process of copying the information in DNA to a molecule of mRNA.

Trans fatty acid An unsaturated fatty acid in which the hydrogens are on opposite sides of the double bond.

Transferrin An iron transport protein in the blood.

Transit time The time between the ingestion of food and the elimination of the solid waste from that food.

Translation The process of translating the mRNA code into the amino acid sequence of a protein.

Treatment groups *See* Experimental groups.

Triacylglycerol or **triglyceride** The major form of lipid in food and the major storage form of lipid in the body. It consists of three fatty acids attached to a glycerol molecule.

Triceps Region at the back of the upper arm that is a common site for measuring skin-fold thickness.

Trichinosis The disease caused by infection with the roundworm *Trichinella spiralis* after eating undercooked contaminated pork or game meats; the juvenile form of this roundworm migrates to the muscles and causes flu-like symptoms and muscle pain and weakness.

Triglyceride *See* Triacylglycerol.

Trimester A term used to describe each third or three-month period of a pregnancy.

Tripeptide Three amino acids linked together by peptide bonds.

Tropical oils A term used in the popular press to refer to the saturated oils—coconut, palm, and palm kernel oil—that are derived from plants grown in tropical regions.

Trypsin A protein-digesting enzyme that is secreted from the pancreas in inactive form and activated in the small intestine.

Tuber The starchy underground storage organ of plants.

Tumor A growth of tissue that forms an abnormal mass that serves no physiological function.

Tumor initiator A substance that causes mutations and therefore may predispose a cell to becoming cancerous.

Tumor promoter A substance that stimulates a mutated cell to begin dividing.

Twenty-four-hour recall A dietary intake assessment method in which an interviewer asks an individual to recall all food and drink consumed for the past 24 hours.

Type 1 diabetes A disease that most commonly develops during childhood and is characterized by elevated blood glucose that results when insufficient insulin is produced by the pancreas; also called insulin-dependent diabetes and juvenile-onset diabetes.

Type 2 diabetes A disease that most commonly occurs in overweight adults and is characterized by elevated blood glucose resulting from an insensitivity of the cells to the action of insulin; also called noninsulin-dependent and maturity-onset diabetes.

Type I osteoporosis or **postmenopausal osteoporosis** A loss of bone serious enough to cause fractures; a disproportionate loss of trabecular bone related to the drop in estrogen that occurs with menopause.

Type II osteoporosis or **age-related osteoporosis** The loss of bone mass serious enough to cause fractures; occurs in both cortical and trabecular bone and is related to advanced age.

Tyrosine A conditionally essential amino acid; when phenylalanine is available in sufficient quantities, tyrosine is not essential in the diet.

Ubiquinone A compound that transports electrons in the electron transport chain but that is not essential in the diet; also called coenzyme Q.

UL *See* Tolerable Upper Intake Level (UL).

Ulcer An open sore.

Undernutrition Poor nutritional status resulting from a dietary intake below that which meets nutritional needs.

Underwater weighing A method that calculates body composition by comparing an individual's body weight while on land with his or her weight while submerged in water.

Underweight A body mass index of less than 18.5 kg/m^2, or a body weight 10% or more below the desirable body weight standard.

Unsaturated fatty acid A fatty acid that contains one or more carbon-carbon double bonds.

Urea A nitrogen-containing waste product from the breakdown of proteins that is excreted in the urine.

Urine A fluid produced by the kidneys consisting of metabolic wastes, excess water, and dissolved substances.

U.S. Department of Agriculture (USDA) U.S. government agency responsible for monitoring the safety and wholesomeness of meat, poultry, and eggs.

U.S. Recommended Daily Allowances (U.S. RDAs) Standard reference values for nutrients designed to be used on food labels; generally equal to the highest nutrient recommendations in any age or sex category from the published 1968 RDAs. Replaced by the RDIs.

Uterus A female organ for containing and nourishing the embryo and fetus from the time of implantation to the time of birth.

Variable A factor or condition that is changed in an experimental setting.

Vegan A pattern of food intake that eliminates all animal products.

Vegetarian One who eats either no animal products or limited categories of animal products.

Vegetarianism A pattern of food intake that eliminates some or all animal products.

Veins Vessels that carry blood toward the heart.

Venule A small vein that drains blood from capillaries and passes it to larger veins for return to the heart.

Very low birth weight infant An infant born weighing less than 1.5 kg (3.3 lb).

Very-low-density lipoproteins (VLDLs) A lipoprotein assembled by the liver that carries lipid from the liver and delivers triglycerides to body cells.

Very-low-kcalorie diet A weight-loss diet that provides fewer than 800 kcalories per day.

Villi (villus) Fingerlike protrusions of the lining of the small intestine that participate in the digestion and absorption of foodstuffs.

Viruses Minute particles not visible under an ordinary microscope that depend on body cells for their metabolic and reproductive needs.

Visceral fat Adipose tissue deposited in the abdominal cavity around the internal organs. High levels are associated with an increased risk of heart disease, high blood pressure, stroke, diabetes, and breast cancer.

Vitamins Organic compounds needed in the diet in small amounts to promote and regulate the chemical reactions and processes needed for growth, reproduction, and the maintenance of health.

Warfarin An anticoagulant drug that acts by inhibiting the action of vitamin K. It is a derivative of dicumarol; also used as rat poison.

Water A molecule composed of two hydrogen atoms and one oxygen atom; essential nutrient needed by the human body in large amounts.

Water-soluble vitamin A vitamin that dissolves in water; includes the B vitamins and vitamin C.

Wear and tear hypothesis A hypothesis that proposes that the changes that occur with age result from the accumulation of cellular damage over time.

Weight cycling or **yo-yo dieting** The cycle of repeatedly losing and regaining weight.

Wheat germ oil An oil pressed from the germ of wheat that is sold as an ergogenic aid.

Whole wheat flour A flour that contains all components of the wheat kernel: the bran, the germ, and the endosperm.

Xanthan gum A plant extract used as a stabilizer in processed foods.

Xerophthalmia A spectrum of eye conditions resulting from vitamin A deficiency. It is characterized by a lack of mucus, which leaves the eye dry and vulnerable to cracking and infection; may lead to blindness.

Xylitol The sugar alcohol formed from the sugar xylose; used in sugarless gum.

Yo-yo diet syndrome *See* Weight cycling.

Zeaxanthin A carotenoid found in corn and green peppers that provides some protection against macular degeneration.

Zygote The cell produced by the union of sperm and ovum during fertilization.

Index

Boldface numbers indicate the page where the term is defined. The letter "t" after a page number indicates a table.

C

D

G

H

M

O

P

T